Psychiatry in the Elderly

Edited by

ROBIN JACOBY
University of Oxford, The Warneford Hospital, Oxford, UK

CATHERINE OPPENHEIMER
The Warneford Hospital, Oxford, UK

THIRD EDITION

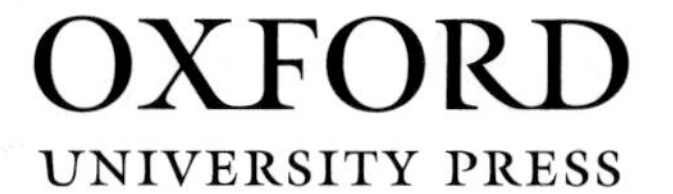

UNIVERSITY PRESS

OXFORD
UNIVERSITY PRESS

Great Clarendon Street, Oxford OX2 6DP

Oxford University Press is a department of the University of Oxford.
It furthers the University's objective of excellence in research, scholarship, and education by publishing worldwide in

Oxford New York

Auckland Bangkok Buenos Aires Cape Town Chennai Dar es Salaam Delhi Hong Kong Istanbul Karachi Kolkata Kuala Lumpur Madrid Melbourne Mexico City Mumbai Nairobi São Paulo Shanghai Singapore Taipei Tokyo Toronto

and an associated company in Berlin

Oxford is a registered trade mark of Oxford University Press in the UK and in certain other countries

Published in the United States
by Oxford University Press Inc., New York

First edition published 1991
Second edition published 1997
Third edition published 2002

A catalogue record for this title is available from the British Library

Library of Congress Cataloging in Publication Data

Psychiatry in the elderly/edited by Robin Jacoby and Catherine Oppenheimer. – 3rd ed.
1. Geriatric psychiatry. I. Jacoby, Robin. II. Oppenheimer, Catherine.
RC451.4.A5 P773 2001 618.97′689 – dc21 2001046498

ISBN 0 19 263151 9 (Hbk)
0 19 851563 4 (Pbk)

10 9 8 7 6 5 4 3 2 1

Typeset by EXPO Holdings, Malaysia
Printed in Great Britain
on acid-free paper by
The Bath Press, Avon

For our families
with love and gratitude
RJ & CO

Preface to the Third Edition

In the Preface to the second edition of this book we observed that in other books which have run into several editions, reproduction of preceding prefaces constitutes a kind of brief history of their development and the field they portray. With this one our own history continues.

The micro-development level we chronicle is the development of the book itself. We have been keen to introduce new elements and new authors, and to bear the changing needs of our readers in mind, while still preserving the sectional structure (Basic science, Clinical practice, Psychiatric services, and Specific disorders) which lends coherence, we hope, to the range of topics covered in the book. We have dispensed with certain chapters, such as those on nursing and occupational therapy, because these disciplines have developed to such an extent that they now merit their own specialized textbooks. For those subjects that have been retained from edition to edition we have engaged many new authors. This was a policy decision on our part; it is no reflection on our previous authors whose expertise and knowledge were crucial in establishing the book for what it is. Our intention, rather, is to maintain a fresh slant on the various topics, and always to afford opportunities to younger workers in the field. For this reason, we have also curtailed our own roles as contributors. All the chapters by authors who contributed to the second edition have been extensively revised and updated.

The macro-developmental level is the progress of old age psychiatry itself. We hope that this book reflects the development of the specialty over the last 5 years (1997–2001). As the number of old age psychiatrists increases in many countries, including the United Kingdom, the intellectual curiosity of its practitioners and their desire to seek a better deal for their patients also grows; so also does the range of professions involved in the field. This is manifest in the improvement in services and advances in research. Nothing is perfect, but opportunities for patients to be assessed, treated, and supported at home have increased, and more modern and home-like acute units and long-stay facilities have been opened. Better ways of monitoring and teaching improved standards of care of people in such facilities are emerging, and low standards of accommodation and care for sufferers are decreasingly acceptable to professionals, relatives, or the public in general. It is clear that the demand for better care is now louder in the halls of Western governments who, mindful that the increasing numbers of older people are also electors, have begun to pay attention to their voices, to assess unmet need, and to respond with more resources. Since resources go with power, the specialty is gradually finding its legitimate place among other branches of medicine. Old age psychiatry is being permitted to come in from the cold.

On the research front the exciting advances in molecular biology have continued, and much more is known now about the pathogenesis of the dementias, especially, but by no means exclusively, Alzheimer's disease (AD). This area of research has become one in which young scientists are eager to work, for the ultimate prizes are great. Over the past 5 years or so the search for a cure for AD has become passionate, comparable to the search for a cure for cancer. We have also seen the introduction of the central cholinesterase inhibitors, the first specific treatments for AD. As we write, we might have just learnt of one of the greatest advances in treatment for this condition ever made: immunization against Aβ protein. If this proves to be effective, the shadow of AD may really begin to lift. It may of course be a false dawn. What is sure, however, is that neuroscientists will be trying hard to prove wrong those who asserted that the cure for AD will come by serendipity rather than from systematic research. Whoever turns out to be correct, we remain optimistic that something approaching a cure will come within the foreseeable future, and what could be more exciting for our field than that?

Oxford
November 2001

R.J.
C.O.

Preface to the Second Edition

As good a reason as any for updating this book is to document the many advances in the scientific basis of old age psychiatry since the first edition was published. The most striking must surely be those in the molecular biology of dementia, especially Alzheimer's disease. Research in this area is moving at such a pace, it is likely that the time taken to prepare, print and publish this book will see developments too recent to be included. Nevertheless, it is important for *Psychiatry in the elderly* to give the practising old age psychiatrist a review of scientific progress which is as current as publishing technology allows.

One of our first steps in planning this second edition was to conduct a modest readership survey by asking for comments from consultants and senior trainees working in the UK. While it was not possible to implement all their suggestions, we hope that the respondents will recognize their contribution to the finished work. As to specific changes, these fall into four main categories. First, there are the chapters by the same authors on the same subjects as in the first edition. Each of these has been revised and updated; none remains unchanged.

Second, there are reviews of new topics by new authors. Our editorial choice here reflects the advances in the field, such as the molecular biology and molecular genetics of dementia (Chapter 7), or the changed context in which old age psychiatry is practised, for example the economics of long-term care provision (Chapter 23) and the links between medical and social services (Chapter 12). In 1988 when *Psychiatry in the elderly* was first mooted it was still possible for old age psychiatrists in this country to devote most of their energies to clinical work and to ignore the economic and managerial context in which they practised. In the mid- to late-1990s changes in the structure of the National Health Service, competition for resources, budgetary limitations, and legislation such as the Community Care Act 1992, have made it essential for old age psychiatrists to understand and participate in the economic as well as clinical management of services. Clearly, a textbook of old age psychiatry needs to reflect this change.

Third, there are new authors writing on subjects that were covered by others in the first edition. Old age psychiatry has been proud from the outset to encompass clinicians who practise in a wide variety of personal styles, while all are rooted firmly in the same philosophy and basic science. The second edition gave us the opportunity to ask new authors to write on 'old' topics, and so to introduce changes of perspective which reflect this diversity in clinical practice.

The fourth and final category of change is the exclusion of some themes which were dealt with in the first edition. These were descriptions of specific services, teaching, and research. Our first instinct was to have much more on services than in the first edition, in order to include accounts from the many developed and developing countries in which this book has been read. In the end, it became too difficult to draw the line between what should and should not be included. We have therefore narrowed the choice down to a description of the general principles of service provision which can be applied across local and national boundaries. Teaching and research are similarly large areas which are now comprehensively covered in specialist texts. Old age psychiatry has come of age, and research and teaching are part of the culture, as in other branches of medicine or psychiatry, so they need no special mention here.

We have chosen to reprint the preface to the first edition. In other books (on any subject), which have run into several editions, reproduction of preceding prefaces constitutes a kind of brief history of their development and of the field they portray. Without making immodest assumptions about the future we hope that the two prefaces will help our readers to see how *Psychiatry in the elderly* and psychiatry in old age are developing, whilst the underlying aims and design of the book remain the same. To choose a minor example, in the earlier preface (in the heyday of political correctness) we mentioned that our editorial ruling on gender references was non-restrictive to reflect the 'variety that corresponds to life' . We have applied a similar ruling to the second edition, but now, where authors are describing personal interactions (the heart of old age psychiatry), we have sought to avoid the awkward 'they/their' in favour of a *non-exclusive* he, or she, or him, or her.

The final paragraph of the first preface would serve just as well for this one. We hope to remain true to the spirit that informs, stimulates debate, and encourages enquiry. Old age psychiatry has indeed matured since the first edition, but science and practice continue to make such great advances that much remains to be learnt in what is still one of the most rewarding and enjoyable activities which medicine has to offer.

Oxford
February 1996

R.J.
C.O.

Preface to the First Edition

Old age psychiatry has become established as a specialty within its own right. Although many countries now recognize and practise it, Britain was one of the first. Here, the evolution and development were determined by demographic changes, academic advances, and service innovations. Academically there were the landmark studies of Roth, Post, and others. Service provision came in different forms, such as hospital joint assessment units, or domiciliary based services. The particular type of service was often dictated by the geographical nature of the district (urban or rural), and by the resources available, but above all by the drive and enthusiasm of individual practitioners. In 1973 the Royal College of Psychiatrists set up a special interest group, which in 1978 became the Section for the Psychiatry of Old Age. This has acted as a forum for debate and the exchange of ideas, as a channel of communication to the Government and to colleagues in other specialties and disciplines, and as a means of influencing opinion and setting standards. It was the Section of the College which in 1988 facilitated and organized recognition in Britain of old age psychiatry as a specialty, although unofficial recognition had come several years before. It was also prominent members of the Section who helped to ensure the representation of old age psychiatry at international conferences and in the World Psychiatric Association. The formative influence of consumer interests such as the Alzheimer's Disease Association and Age Concern, and of those interested in ethics, health economics, and gerontology should also be acknowledged in the drive to improve standards and focus attention on resource and research priorities.

In the USA interest in old age psychiatry followed that in Britain. The same demographic changes - 'the greying of America' - were a powerful motivating force but scientifically the origins were different and emerged more from the basic sciences of gerontology. In the United States, too, old age psychiatry has now become a specialty in its own right. Wherever it is practised, old age psychiatry has overlapping frontiers and works in the closest partnership with other medical specialties and other disciplines, such as social work.

Pari passu with the emergence of specialty status and increased service provision there came interesting and important findings from basic scientific research, clinical psychiatry, and therapeutics. The care of the elderly mentally ill ceased to focus exclusively on custodial management, and began to concentrate much more on active intervention in all types of cases, with consequent improvement in prognosis and quality of life. Such has been the importance of discoveries in neuropathology and neurochemistry that there is an increasing need for a good clinical base from which further advances can be made; a need which has been translated into a demand for more resources and more well trained specialists. Clinical training in old age psychiatry is now an integral part of basic postgraduate psychiatric education, and also forms part of the undergraduate curriculum. General practitioners are expected to acquire knowledge and experience in this field. There are also schemes and courses in many countries for higher professional training and for updating practising specialists. It is in the context of a relatively new, but now firmly established, specialty with increasing academic, service, and training needs that this book should find a useful place.

The book can be seen as a two-storey building on prepared foundations. Section I - Basic science, the first of the three main sections, provides the foundations: a broad underpinning from neurochemistry through to sociology. The ground floor, Section II - Clinical practice, deals with the three principal clinical activities : assessment, treatment, and the provision of services. These are covered in detail, and from the different professional viewpoints which make up psychiatry for elderly people. The top floor, Section III - Specific disorders and medico-legal issues, describes the specific disorders with which psychogeriatricians and their colleagues deal every working day: dementia, the functional psychoses, and other less common but no less important conditions.

The book has been written by 43 authors drawn from all the relevant specialties and disciplines. The choice of a large number of contributors was deliberate: reviewers often praise single-author books for their unity of style, but we believe that there is much to be gained from a rich variety of style and perspective. The conjunction of disparate viewpoints is a great strength of old age psychiatry rather than a weakness. One small way in which this is reflected is the editorial ruling on the use of pronouns to refer to women and men (he/she, him/her), or ways of avoiding gender reference (their, person, and so on). We chose not to impose an editorial rule for the simple reason that variety corresponds to life, where staff and patients are of either sex.

We should mention here that there are some points of this book which overlap with each other. This is not a matter of editorial oversight, but a considered decision to permit the reader to view topics from more than one side. Where such overlap occurs, however, we hope the reader will find it complementary rather than repetitive. An example of this would be the quotation of two different definitions of dementia in Chapter 17. In Section A (Epidemiology of dementia) Cooper quotes the WHO definition, whilst in Section B (Alzheimer's disease) Wilcock and Jacoby cite a Royal College of Physicians' report, each definition serving the points the authors wish to make and neither excluding the other.

Another reason for allowing this sort of overlap is to ensure that each contribution not only fits into the overall plan, but is also self-contained, We have no wish to force the reader into frequent cross-referencing moves a hundred pages forwards or backwards. Of course, appropriate cross-references are still made in the text, but we hope readers will be able to use the book in different ways. Some will follow it systematically from start to finish, whilst others should he able to dip into it to refresh themselves on a particular topic, or to turn to it by way of reference to a specific subject.

Where there are contradictory views, it is for the reader to decide which speaks with greater force. Our view of the reader is of a participant whose needs we have kept in mind at every stage in the composition of the book. We encouraged some contributors to write from personal experience because the body of knowledge in their field is still sparse. Moreover, there are some relatively uncharted areas that are mentioned only in passing and not given the prominence their clinical importance deserves, such as the quality of life in extended care or bereavement in old age. We hope that younger colleagues will feel stimulated in future to explore these areas and extend knowledge for all. Old age psychiatry is a young subject, many aspects of which are not established; some are well defined, but others are much less clear. We want the reader to be critical about what is known and inventive about what remains to be discovered.

We hope that this book will appeal to trainees in psychiatry. Because, however, the field is in its essence multidisciplinary, it should also be of value to a much wider readership. For instance, it may be useful to specialist teams in local area offices of social services departments, to nurses, general practitioners, general psychiatrists, managers, and care staff. We hope that these colleagues will be able to refer to the appropriate section of this book to supplement or refresh their knowledge.

Our authors have been chosen mostly but not exclusively from Britain. Because mental health legislation and the provision of services are essentially determined by national, social and political factors, we have been unable, nor have we wished, to avoid the British context. It simply has to be said that where required, for example with services, we have spelt out the principles on which specific provisions are based; principles which are generally and internationally recognized.

Much work has gone into the preparation of this book. Those who have contributed to it will be rewarded if it succeeds in its purpose of informing all those who read it, stimulating disagreement and enquiry, and enlightening and attracting many to what is a fascinating, worthwhile, and above all enjoyable field of endeavour.

London and Oxford R.J.
December 1990 C.O.

Acknowledgements

This edition

Once again it is a pleasure to thank all our contributors for the patient and forbearing way in which they have responded to our requests, entreaties, and still strict editorial discipline to submit their contributions to us in time to meet our deadline. They must take the major credit for this book. We are also grateful to our secretaries Carole Walton and Tracey Macready for assistance with editorial corrections. Our very longstanding friend, Anna Truelove, gave us invaluable editorial help which we acknowledge with affection and gratitude. As with the first two editions, the staff of Oxford University Press have been unfailingly helpful.

Russian edition

We are proud to inform our readers that a Russian translation of the second edition is almost complete, and will be published and distributed free of charge in Russian-speaking countries in 2001. We should like to express our gratitude for the efforts of our colleagues in Belarus, Professor R. Evsegneev and Dr V. Poznyak (currently seconded to WHO in Geneva), as well as to Dr Robert van Voren, Secretary General of the Geneva Initiative on Psychiatry, and most particularly to the Open Society Institute (Soros Foundation) whose generous funding has made the project possible. We are greatly encouraged by this clear evidence of international recognition of the importance of old age psychiatry, especially in countries of the former Soviet Union, where provision of psychiatric services for older people is very underdeveloped. We must also warmly thank Oxford University Press for their generosity in permitting us to have this translation made and distributed through a non-royalty bearing contract.

Contents

Contributors

Hema Ananth Specialist Registrar, Chase Farm Hospital, Enfield, Middlesex EN2 8JL, UK.

Mark Ardern Consultant in Old Age Psychiatry, St Charles Hospital, Exmoor Street, London W10 6DZ, UK.

Eia Asen Consultant Psychiatrist in Psychotherapy, The Maudsley Hospital, London SE5 8AZ, UK.

Janet Askham Professor of Gerontology, King's College London, Stamford Street, London SE1 9NN, UK.

Roland Atkinson Professor of Psychiatry, School of Medicine, Oregon Health and Science University, Portland, Oregon 97201, USA.

Robert Baldwin Consultant in Old Age Psychiatry and Honorary Professor, Manchester Mental Health Partnership, York House, Manchester Royal Infirmary, Manchester M13 9BX, UK.

Peter Bentham Consultant in Old Age Psychiatry, Queen Elizabeth Psychiatric Hospital, Birmingham B15 2QZ, UK.

Klaus Bergmann Emeritus Consultant Psychiatrist, The Bethlem Royal and Maudsley Hospitals, London SE5 8AZ, UK.

Alan Bittles Foundation Professor of Human Biology, Edith Cowan University, Perth, WA 6027, Australia.

Martin Bradshaw Service Manager, Yarnton House, Rutten Lane, Yarnton OX51LP, UK.

Alistair Burns Professor of Old Age Psychiatry, University of Manchester, Withington Hospital, Manchester M20 8LR, UK.

Patrick Campbell Formerly Consultant Psychiatrist, The Royal Free Hospital, Pond Street, London NW3 2QG, UK.

Harry Cayton Chief Executive, Alzheimer's Society, London SW1P 1PH, UK.

Georgina Charlesworth Alzheimer's Society Research Fellow, UCL Department of Psychiatry and Behavioural Sciences, Wolfson Building, London W1N 8AA.

Margaret Esiri Professor of Neuropathology, University of Oxford, Radcliffe Infirmary, Oxford OX2 6HE, UK.

Andrew Fairbairn Consultant in Old Age Psychiatry, Centre for the Health of the Elderly, Newcastle General Hospital, Newcastle-upon-Tyne NE4 6BE, UK.

Sebastian Fairweather Consultant Physician, Department of Clinical Geratology, The Radcliffe Infirmary, Oxford OX2 6HE, UK.

Seena Fazel Clinical Research Fellow, University of Oxford, The Warneford Hospital, Oxford OX3 7JX, UK.

Hans Förstl Professor of Psychiatry and Psychotherapy, Technical University of Munich, Klinikum rechts der Isar, Ismaninger Straße 22, D-81675 München, Germany.

Helen Graham Senior Lecturer in General Practice, Guys, Kings and St Thomas' School of Medicine, The Sherman Education Centre, Guy's Hospital, London SE1 9RT, UK.

Alastair Gray Reader in Health Economics, University of Oxford, Health Economics Research Centre, Institute of Health Sciences, Oxford OX3 7LF, UK.

Lars Gustafson Professor of Geriatric Psychiatry, Department of Psychogeriatrics, University Hospital of Lund, SE-221 85 Lund, Sweden.

Richard Harvey Director of Research, Alzheimer's Society, London SW1P 1PH; and Senior Research Fellow, University and Imperial Colleges London, Queen Square, London WC1N 3BG, UK.

Daniel Harwood Consultant Psychiatrist, Isle of Wight Healthcare NHS Trust, Isle Of Wight PO30 1YQ, UK.

Frank Hentschel Professor and Head of the Division of Neuroradiology, Zentralinstitut für Seelische Gesundheit, D-68072 Mannheim, Germany.

Nathan Herrmann Head, Division of Geriatric Psychiatry, University of Toronto, Sunnybrook and Women's College Health Sciences Centre, Toronto, Ontario M4N 3M5, Canada.

Rolf D. Hirsch Professor of Psychogerontology, University of Erlangen-Nürnberg, Rheinische Kliniken Bonn, D-5311 Bonn, Kaiser-Karl-Ring 20, Germany.

John Hodges Professor of Behavioural Neurology, MRC Cognition and Brain Sciences Unit, 15 Chaucer Rd, Cambridge CB1 2EF, UK.

Gareth Hoskins Principal, Gareth Hoskins Architects, Atlantic Chambers, 45 Hope Street, Glasgow G2 6AE, UK.

Robert Howard Reader in Old Age Psychiatry, Institute of Psychiatry, London SE5 8AF, UK.

Julian C. Hughes Research Fellow, ETHOX, University of Oxford and Consultant in Old Age Psychiatry, Newcastle General Hospital, Newcastle-upon-Tyne NE4 6BE, UK.

Susan Iversen Professor of Psychology, Department of Experimental Psychology, South Parks Road, Oxford OX1 3UD, UK.

Robin Jacoby Professor of Old Age Psychiatry, University of Oxford, The Warneford Hospital, Oxford OX3 7JX, UK.

Anthony Jorm Professor and Director, Centre for Mental Health Research, Australian National University, Canberra 0200, Australia.

James Lindesay Professor of Psychiatry for the Elderly, University of Leicester, Leicester General Hospital, Leicester LE5 4PW, UK.

Simon Lovestone Professor of Old Age Psychiatry, Institute of Psychiatry, London SE5 8AF, UK.

Denzil Lush Master of the Court of Protection, Stewart House, 24 Kingsway, London WC2B 6JX, UK.

Declan Lyons Specialist Registrar, The Maudsley Hospital, London SE5 8AZ, UK.

Rupert McShane Consultant Psychiatrist, The Fulbrook Centre, The Churchill Hospital, Oxford OX3 7JU, UK.

Mary Marshall Director of Dementia Services Development Centre, University of Stirling, Stirling FK9 4LA, UK.

Elizabeth Milwain Research Neuropsychologist, OPTIMA, The Radcliffe Infirmary, Oxford OX2 6HE, UK.

Zsuzsanna Nagy Queen Elizabeth The Queen Mother Fellow, University of Oxford, Departments of Pharmacology and Neuropathology, The Radcliffe Infirmary, Oxford OX2 6HE, UK.

John O'Brien Professor of Old Age Psychiatry, University of Newcastle-upon-Tyne, Wolfson Research Centre, Newcastle General Hospital, Newcastle-upon-Tyne NE4 6BE, UK.

Desmond O'Neill Senior Lecturer in Medical Gerontology, Trinity Centre for Health Sciences, Adelaide and Meath Hospital, Dublin 24, Ireland.

Catherine Oppenheimer Consultant Psychiatrist, The Warneford Hospital, Oxford OX3 7JX, UK.

Jane Pearce Consultant Psychiatrist, The Fulbrook Centre, The Churchill Hospital, Oxford OX3 7JU, UK.

Michael Philpot Consultant in Old Age Psychiatry, The Maudsley Hospital, London SE5 8AZ, UK.

Harvey Posener Solicitor, 31/32 Ely Place, London EC1 6TD, UK.

Martin Prince Senior Lecturer in Psychiatric Epidemiology, Institute of Psychiatry, De Crespigny Park, London SE5 8AF, UK.

Andrew Procter Consultant Psychiatrist, Manchester Royal Infirmary, Manchester M13 9WL, UK.

Tom Reynolds Consultant in Old Age Psychiatry, Clare Mental Health Services, Ennis, Co. Clare, Ireland.

Karen Ritchie Director Epidemiology of Pathologies of the Nervous System Research Group, French National Institute of Health and Medical Research (INSERM), Hôpital de la Colombière, Montpellier 34093, France.

Kenneth Shulman Professor of Psychiatry, University of Toronto, Sunnybrook and Women's College Health Sciences Centre, Toronto, Ontario M4N 3M5, Canada.

Neil Stewart Specialist Registrar, Department of Clinical Geratology, The Radcliffe Infirmary, Oxford OX2 6HE, UK.

Robert Stewart Wellcome Trust Research Training Fellow, Section of Epidemiology, Institute of Psychiatry, London SE5 8AF, UK.

Alan Thomas Lecturer in Old Age Psychiatry, University of Newcastle, Newcastle General Hospital, Newcastle-upon-Tyne NE4 6BE, UK.

Bodo R. Vollhardt Senior Psychiatrist, Department of Gerontopsychiatry, Rheinische Kliniken Bonn, D-5311 Bonn, Kaiser-Karl-Ring 20, Germany.

Gordon Wilcock Professor of Care of The Elderly, University of Bristol, Frenchay Hospital, Bristol, BS16 1LE, UK.

Simon Winner Consultant Physician, Department of Clinical Geratology, The Radcliffe Infirmary, Oxford OX2 6HE, UK.

Jane Wolstenholme Health Economist, Health Economics Research Centre, Institute of Health Sciences, University of Oxford, Oxford OX3 7LF, UK.

Philip Wood Senior Lecturer, Health Services for the Elderly, North Shore Hospital, Takapuna, New Zealand.

Robert Woods Professor of Clinical Psychology of Older People, Dementia Services Development Centre Wales, Neuadd Ardudwy, University of Wales, Bangor LL57 2PX, UK.

Abbreviations

5-HIAA	5-hydroxy-indoleacetic acid
5-HT	5-hydroxytryptamine (aka serotonin)
5mC	5-methyl cytosine
AA	Alcoholics Anonymous
AAMI	age-associated memory impairment
Aβ	amyloid protein fragment-β
ACE	Addenbrooke's Cognitive Examination; also angiotensin converting enzyme
AD	Alzheimer's disease; also autonomy–dependence
ADAS-Cog	Alzheimer's Disease Assessment Scale-cognitive subscale
ADL	activities of daily living
ADR	adverse drug reactions
ADRDA	Alzheimer's Disease and Related Disorders Association
AF	atrial fibrillation
AGE	advanced glycosylation endproducts
AIDS	acquired immunodeficiency syndrome
AIREN	Association Internationale pour la Recherche et l'Enseignement en Neurosciences
ALE	active life expectancy
AMT	Abbreviated Mental Test
APA	American Psychiatric Association (also American Psychological Association)
APA DCP	American Psychological Association Division of Clinical Psychology
APOE	apolipoprotein E gene
ApoE	apolipoprotein E protein
ApoE 2–4	apolipoprotein E protein isoforms
APOE ε*2–4*	apolipoprotein E gene alleles
APP	amyloid precursor protein
APP	Association for Psychoanalytic Psychotherapy
APS	Adult Protective Services
ASN	alpha-synuclein
ASP	aspartate
Astrid	A Social and Technological Response to meeting the needs of Individuals with Dementia and their carers
ASW	approved social workers
βA4	4-kDa β-amyloid protein
BACE	beta-site APP-cleaving enzyme (aka β-secretase)
BAS-DEP	Brief Assessment Scale for Depression
BASDEC	Brief Assessment Schedule Depression Cards
BBB	blood–brain barrier
BDI	Beck Depression Inventory
BFD	British familial dementia
BNF	*British national formulary*

BOD	burden of disease
bp	base pair
BPRS	Brief Psychiatric Rating Scale
BPSD	Behavioural and psychological symptoms of dementia
BSE	bovine spongiform encephalopathy
CADASIL	cerebral autosomal dominant arteriopathy with subcortical infarcts and leucoencephalopathy
CAMCOG	Cambridge Cognitive Capacity Scale
CAMDEX	Cambridge Mental Disorders of the Elderly Examination
cAMP	cyclic 3′,5′ adenosine monophosphate
CANE	Camberwell Assessment of Need for the Elderly
CAPE	Clifton Assessment Procedures for the Elderly
CARENAP-D	Care Needs Assessment Pack for Dementia
CAS	Caregiver Activity Survey
CAT	cognitive analytic therapy
CATS	Caregiver Activities Time Survey
CBA	cost–benefit analysis
CBD	corticobasal degeneration
CBS	Charles Bonnet syndrome
CBT	cognitive–behavioural therapy
Cdk	cyclin-dependent kinases
CDR	Clinical Dementia Rating (scale)
CEA	cost-effectiveness analyses
CEMH	Centre for the Economics of Mental Health
CER	Cost-effectiveness ratio
CES-D	Center for Epidemiological Studies of Depression
CGA	color graphics adapter
ChAT	choline acetyltransferase
ChEI	cholinesterase inhibitor
CJD	Creutzfeldt–Jakob disease
CMA	cost-minimization analysis
COI	cost-of-illness
COMT	catechol-O-methyl transferase
CPA	Care Programme Approach; also continuing powers of attorney
CPD	cell-population doublings
CPN	community psychiatric nurse
CPQ	Community Placement Questionnaire
CREB	cAMP responsive-element binding (protein)
CRH	corticotropin-releasing hormone
CRP	C-reactive protein
CSF	cerebrospinal fluid
CSP	caregiver support programme
CSRI	Client Service Receipt Interview
CT	computed tomography
CUA	cost-utility analyses
DA	dopamine
DALE	disability-adjusted life expectancy

DALY	disability-adjusted life year
DAT	dementia of the Alzheimer type
DCT	Digit Copying Test
DDPAC	disinhibition–dementia–parkinsonism–amyotrophy complex
DFT	dementia of frontal lobe type
DLB	dementia with Lewy bodies
DMVs	departments of motor vehicles
DRN	dorsal raphe nuclei
DRPLA	dentato-rubro-pallido-luysian atrophy
DSM	Diagnostic and statistical manual of mental disorders
DVLA	Driver and Vehicle Licensing Agency
e-PACT	electronic format of PACT
EATT	excitatory amino acid transporter
EBAS-DEP	Even Briefer Assessment Scale for Depression
ECA	Epidemiological Catchment Area
ECT	electroconvulsive therapy
EE	expressed emotion
EGA	enhanced graphics adapter
EMI	elderly mentally infirm
EOFAD	early-onset familial Alzheimer's disease
EPA	enduring power of attorney
ERP	event-related potentials
ESR	erythrocyte sedimentation rate
EURODEM	dementia in Europe
EURODEP	depression in Europe
FAD	familial Alzheimer's disease
FDA	(US) Food and Drug Administration
FDD	familial Danish dementia (aka heredopathia ophthalmo-oto-encephalica)
FFI	fatal familial insomnia
FLD	frontal lobe degeneration
fMRI	functional MRI
FTD	frontotemporal dementia
FTDP-17	frontotemporal dementia with Parkinson's
GABA	gamma-aminobutyric acid
GAD	generalized anxiety disorder; also glutamic acid decarboxylase, GLU decarboxylase
GAT	GABA transporter protein
GDP	gross domestic product
GDS	Geriatric Depression Scale
GFR	glomerular filtration rate
GHQ	General Health Questionnaire
GLU	glutamate
GP	general practitioner (aka primary-care physician)
GSK-3	glycogen synthase kinase-3
GSS	Gerstmann-Sträussler-Scheinker disease
HADS	Hospital Anxiety and Depression Scale
HCHWA-D	hereditary cerebral haemorrhage with amyloidosis—Dutch type
HD	Huntington's disease

HERNS	hereditary endotheliopathy with retinopathy, nephropathy, and stroke
HIV	human immunodeficiency virus
HLA	human leucocyte antigen
HMG CoA	3-hydroxy-3-methylglutaryl coenzyme A
HMPAO	hexamethyl propyleneamine oxime (
HPA	hypothalamic–pituitary–adrenal (axis)
HRT	hormone-replacement therapy
HUI	Health Utility Index
HVA	homovanilic acid
IADL	instrumental activities of daily living
ICD	International Classification of Diseases
ICER	incremental cost-effectiveness ratio
ICIDH	International Classification of Impairments, Disabilities, and Handicaps
INR	international normalized ratio
IPT	interpersonal psychotherapy
IQCODE	Informant Questionnaire on Cognitive Decline in the Elderly
IRT	item-response theory
kb	kilobase
kDa	kilodalton
KPI	Kunitz-type protease inhibitor
LB	Lewy body
LC	locus coeruleus
LOAD	late-onset Alzheimer's disease
MacCAT-T	MacArthur Competence Assessment Tool—Treatment
MADRS	Montgomery Asberg Depression Rating Scale
MAO-B	monoamino-oxidase B
MAOI	monoamine oxidase inhibitor
MAP	microtubule-associated protein
MAPK	mitogen-activated protein kinases
MAUS	multi-attribute utility scales
MCI	mild cognitive impairment
MEAMS	Middlesex Elderly Assessment of Mental State
MELAS	mitochondrial myopathy, encephalopathy, lactic acidosis, and stroke-like episodes
MHA	Mental Health Act 1983
MHPG	3-methoxy-4-hydroxyphenylglycol
MID	multi-infarct dementia
MMSE	Mini-Mental State Examination
MND	motor neuron disease
MRI	magnetic resonance imaging
MRS	magnetic resonance spectroscopy
MSA	multisystem atrophy
MSU	midstream urine
mtDNA	mitochondrial DNA
MTS	Mental Test Score
NA	noradrenaline
NAD	nicotinamide adenine dinucleotide
NATs	negative automatic thoughts

NB	nucleus basalis
nbM	nucleus basalis of Meynert
NCEA	National Council On Elder Abuse
nDNA	nuclear DNA
NE	norepinephrine
NEAIS	National Elder Abuse Incidence Study
NFT	neurofibrillary tangles
NGF	nerve growth factor
NHS	National Health Service
NIDDM	non-insulin-dependent diabetes mellitus
NIH	National Institutes of Health
NINCDS	National Institute of Neurological and Communicative Disorders and Stroke
NINDS	National Institute of Neurological Disorders and Stroke
NMDA	*N*-methyl-D-aspartate
NMS	neuroleptic malignant syndrome
NPC	negative–positive communication
NPH	normal-pressure hydrocephalus
NSAID	non-steroidal anti-inflammatory drug
OBRA-87	Omnibus Budget Reconciliation Act-1987
OCD	obsessive–compulsive disorder
OR	odds ratio
OT	occupational therapy
OTC	over-the-counter (medicines)
PACT	prescribing, analyses and costs
PAS	Periodic Acid Schiff
PCG	primary care group
PD	Parkinson's disease
PDE	personality disorder examination
PDI	peripheral decarboxylase inhibitor
PEG	percutaneous endoscopic gastrostomy
PEMA	palilalia, echolalia, mutism, and amimia
PEO	progressive external ophthalmoplegia
PET	positron emission tomography
PHF	paired helical filaments
PIP_2	phosphatidylinositol bisphosphate
PKB	protein kinase B
PKC	protein kinase C
PML	progressive multifocal leucoencephalopathy
PPA	Prescription Pricing Authority
PRODIGY	Prescribing RatiOnally with Decision support In General practice studY
PrP	prion protein
PrP^c	normal cellular prion protein
PrP^{sc}	disease-associated prion protein
PSP	progressive supranuclear palsy (also referred to as the Steele–Richardson–Olsiewski syndrome)
PSSRU	Personal Social Services Research Unit
PSVE	progressive subcortical vascular encephalopathy

PTO	person trade-off
PTSD	post-traumatic stress disorder
PVS	persistent vegetative state
QALY	quality-adjusted life years
QWB	Quality of Well-being Scale
R	raphe nuclei
RAID	Rating Anxiety in Dementia (scale)
rCBF	regional cerebral blood flow
RCT	randomized controlled trial
RO	reality orientation
RR	relative risk
RT	reaction time
RUD	Resource Utilization in Dementia
SAE	subcortical arteriosclerotic encephalopathy
SAILS	Structured Assessment of Independent Living Skills
SANS	Scale for Assessment of Negative Symptoms (SANS
SAST	Short Anxiety Screening Test
SCAN	Schedules for Assessment of Negative Symptoms
SD	submissiveness–dominance
SelfCARE-D	Self-admininistered depression scale
SG	standard gamble
SLIR	somatostatin-like immunoreactivity
SMAC	Standing Medical Advisory Committee
SMR	standardized mortality rate
SNRI	serotonin and norepinephrine reuptake inhibitor
SP	senile plaques
SPECT	single photon emission computed tomography (aka SPET)
SPET	single photon emission tomography (aka SPECT)
SSRI	selective serotonin-reuptake inhibitor
Syst-Eur	Systolic Hypertension in Europe (trial)
TAPS	Team for Assessment of Psychiatric Services
TAT	thrombin–antithrombin complex
Tc	technetium
TCA	tricarboxylic acid cycle; also tricyclic antidepressant
TIA	transient ischaemic attack
TNF-α	tumour necrosis factor-alpha
TOT	tip of the tongue
tPA	tissue plasminogen activator
TR	transcription factor
TRH	thyroid-releasing hormone
TSH	thyroid-stimulating hormone
TTO	time trade-off
VA	Veterans' Administration
VAS	visual analogue scale
VBR	ventricle-to-brain ratio
vCJD	variant CJD
VGA	visual graphics array

VLOSLP	very late-onset schizophrenia-like psychosis ()
WAIS	Wechsler Adult Intelligence Scale
WHIMS	Women's Health Initiative Memory Study
WMH	white matter hyperintensities
WML	white matter lesions
WTP	willingness to pay
YLD	years lost due to disability
YLL	years of life lost (due to premature mortality)

I | *Basic science*

1 Biological aspects of human ageing

Alan H. Bittles

Introduction

The overall goal of this chapter is to review our present knowledge of the biological processes that govern human ageing. The final product necessarily will reflect the underlying interests and assumptions of the investigators who are cited, the experimental techniques they have employed, and the specific foci of their fields of interest. At the outset, a key consideration that needs to be addressed is the nature of the relationship between ageing and evolution. Should ageing be considered as an adaptive or a non-adaptive trait? In other words, did senescence evolve as a direct result of natural selection in order to limit lifespan, or did increases in longevity follow random events which ordinarily would be expected to restrict that lifespan? At the species level, ageing has been claimed to be beneficial in permitting and/or promoting the turnover of generations. In the wild, however, few animals ever succeed in attaining old age and so it is difficult to perceive why genes coding for ageing, and in practice seldom expressed, should have been preserved through evolutionary time.

One explanation offered is that genes responsible for ageing may be pleiotropic in their action, exerting beneficial effects when the individual is young or in early, reproductive adulthood, but responsible for unfavourable consequences in the later, postreproductive years. Under these conditions a relatively small advantage acting early in life, when many individuals would potentially be placed at a selective advantage, could balance highly deleterious late-acting effects in the much smaller number of persons who survive to older ages. Although adaptive theories have their attractions, non-adaptive hypotheses, which primarily regard senescence as an evolutionary by-product, tend to be more strongly favoured (Johnson 1988; Kirkland 1989). In effect, it is the dichotomy between these two approaches which forms the basis of many of the divisions in rationale between the different theories of ageing that have been formulated.

A second underlying issue concerns the onset of ageing, and more specifically its timing. Is ageing in mammals and other genera part of an overall developmental process commencing at conception or birth, or can a specific switch be observed later in life? To some extent this question can be regarded as a re-statement of the adaptive/non-adaptive conundrum, and for a similar reason the idea of specific ageing genes and their activation in adulthood appears untenable. Despite this shortcoming, some early theories of ageing were based on the supposition of a chronological reduction of essential metabolites, with the concomitant development and expression of the ageing phenotype. The apparent correlation between the time taken to reach sexual maturity, reproductive lifespan, and species longevity has led to a variation of this concept being further employed to explain the human female menopause.

Ageing and the human lifespan

The nature of the relationship between ageing and lifespan is of potential importance in biological, clinical, and demographic terms. Although ageing cannot be adequately described merely in terms of lifespan, actuarial study of a population can provide valuable insights into the process of ageing, and it is widely accepted that lifespan is a constitutional feature of the phenotype of a species. Increases in maximum lifespan potential during the course of hominid evolution were estimated from allometric regressions on brain weight and body weight (Sacher 1959). According to this method, data derived from early hominid fossil remains suggest an approximate doubling of maximum lifespan potential over the past 3 million years, with the greatest increase occurring about 100 000 years ago (Cutler 1975; Brown 1988).

A formula to describe the exponential rise in death rate between sexual maturity and old age was derived by Gompertz in 1825 and, with the effective decline of extrinsic causes of mortality during the present century, evidence in support of an intrinsic mortality schedule has become more clearly apparent. Contrary to Gompertzian prediction, laboratory-based studies on *Drosophila* have shown a flattening in age-specific mortality rates at advanced ages (Carey *et al.* 1992), which has been interpreted as evidence that the lifespan of this species may not be rigidly defined (Curtsinger *et al.* 1992). However, further *Drosophila* work showed that in females, reproduction influenced both death rates and mortality, suggesting that ageing may have evolved primarily because of the damaging effects of reproduction earlier in life, rather than the action of late-acting detrimental mutations (Sgrò and Partridge 1999). This means that the deceleration in death rates reported in *Drosophila* at greater ages might, at least in part, reflect waning of the wave of mortality induced by reproduction (Reznick and Ghalambor 1999).

The maximum reported lifespan of humans is approximately 120 years (Jeune and Vaupel 1999), and there are conflicting opinions as to whether or not this apparent upper limit is likely to be extended within the foreseeable future (Olshansky and Carnes 1997; Manton and Yashin 2000). As discussed below, the direct genetic contribution to human longevity appears to be quite low. None the less, it was proposed by Alexander Graham Bell (1919) that in some families longevity was an inherited characteristic, and a study of centenarians has indicated that their siblings also had significantly increased life expectancies (Perls *et al.* 1998). A further example of this phenomenon is the family of Jeanne Calment who died in France in 1997 aged 122 years. Among her 55 immediate relatives whose life histories were studied, 24% lived to over 80 years of age compared to just 2% of a matched control group (Robine and Allard 1998). Of course, in families that exhibit above average longevity, their enhanced lifespan may be primarily associated with the absence of major life-threatening pathologies.

The differential in life expectancy between males and females provides an example of the influence of non-genetic factors. With the current exception of a very few less developed countries where maternal deaths in childbirth remains high, female life expectancy consistently exceeds that of males. In recent years the differential has, however, narrowed in countries such as the United States, Sweden, England and Wales, and Australia, due largely to declining rates of male mortality caused by heart disease, accidents, violence, and lung cancer, and with a concomitant increase in deaths due to breast cancer in women (Trovato and Lalu 1998).

The relationship between ageing and the human lifespan has important practical connotations. For example, in considering future geriatric medical and social support needs, Fries (1980) assumed a maximum human lifespan of approximately 85 years, and on this basis he predicted a future compression of mortality and morbidity in human populations. If this assumption was correct, no appreciable future increase in the numbers of very old individuals would be expected. In addition, the average period of reduced vigour in the elderly would decrease, a smaller proportion of the total lifespan would be occupied by chronic disease, and there would be an overall reduction in the requirement for health care by older persons.

In fact, although the rapid increases in mean life expectancy enjoyed by the populations of economically developed countries during the nineteenth and twentieth centuries may have peaked (Olshansky *et al.* 1990; Wilmoth and

Horiuchi 1999), there seems little doubt that in both developed and developing countries the numbers of the oldest old, i.e. persons who are over 80 years of age, will continue to increase to a significant degree. Indeed, changes of this nature have already been documented for a wide range of countries (Kannisto *et al.* 1994). Further, while an autopsy study on persons aged 85 years and over reported no diagnosable, fatal pathology in at least 30% of cases (Kohn 1982*a*), suggesting that in a sizeable proportion of individuals the ultimate causes of death were linked to normal, physiological decrements associated with ageing, it is generally accepted that any increase in the numbers of very old persons would be accompanied by disproportionately larger groups of individuals with major age-related pathologies (Schneider and Brody 1983; Brody 1985).

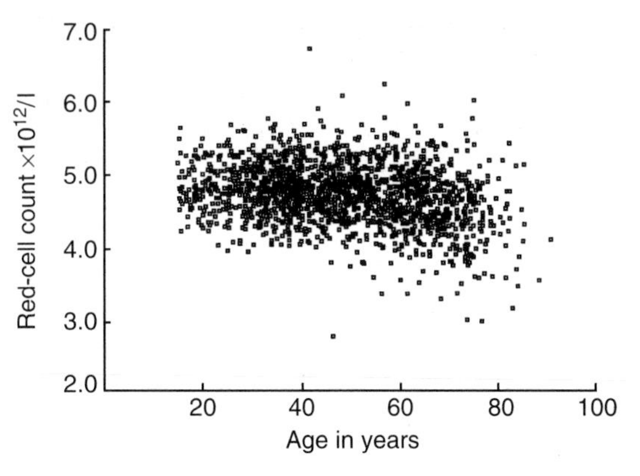

Fig. 1.1(a) Scatter plot of red cell counts for males by age.

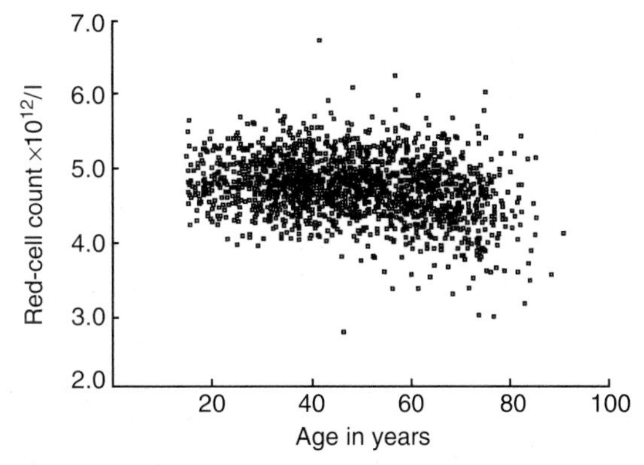

Fig. 1.1(b) Scatter plot of red cell counts for females by age.

Ageing and age-related pathologies

These studies raise a further problem in the assessment of ageing, namely differentiation between so-called normal ageing and pathological conditions which commonly are seen at greater frequency with advancing age. In many earlier texts it was the practice to refer collectively to atherosclerosis, cancers, type-2 diabetes mellitus, and degenerative arthritis as diseases of ageing. Although a positive correlation clearly exists between the incidence of these disorders and increasing age (Rogers 1995), it is difficult to identify specific causal mechanisms. With occult disease the task is even more problematic, especially among the elderly who frequently present with a wide spectrum of vague signs and symptoms. Yet for diagnostic and prognostic purposes it is highly desirable that the symptoms of ageing and disease be separated, which in turn necessitates the establishment of meaningful 'normal' ranges throughout the human lifespan.

This is illustrated in Figs 1.1(*a*) and (*b*), collated from data collected during 1994–95 as part of the Busselton Health Survey, an ongoing community-based study initiated in Western Australia in 1966 (Brightwell *et al.* 1998). The participants were ambulant volunteers, none of whom reported major disease symptoms. As illustrated in the scatter plots for red cell counts, at all ages there were a number of individuals whose red cell counts were beyond the commonly adopted normal ranges, $4.5–5.9 \times 10^{12}$/l for males and $4.1–5.1 \times 10^{12}$ for females. However, with advancing age the proportion of those outside the age-invariant normal ranges increased, especially among males. On this basis, sizeable numbers of males over 60 years and females over 70 years would be categorized as showing subnormal red cell counts. The question then arises whether or not these 'subnormal' values should be accepted as part of the ageing phenotype.

Methods utilized in the study of ageing

Three major approaches have been adopted for the study of ageing. The first involves direct measurements on human subjects, with either cross-sectional studies employed to compare anatomical, physiological, and biochemical parameters in young and old subjects, or longitudinal studies used with serial measurements conducted on given individuals over extended periods. A number of ethical and methodological problems are apparent with this approach. For example, at what age should the studies begin and, in cross-sectional studies, can any real knowledge of the ageing process be gained merely by comparing young and old subjects whose life experiences may have been very different? Particularly with elderly persons, to what extent is it permissible to impose the potentially stressful test protocols that may be needed to demonstrate age-dependent changes? How does one differentiate between age-dependent changes and age-related pathologies? Additional major factors to be considered in longitudinal studies include the costs and extended times involved, the required continuity in staff commitment and testing procedures, and the extent to which subjects initially recruited to the programme can be retained. For these reasons, and because of relatively large individual variations in the phenotype of elderly persons which may or may not be due to ageing *per se*, studies directly conducted on human subjects have marked limitations.

The second approach is to utilize non-human species for experimental procedures. The nature of the genetic code is near-universal in the living world and, since exposure to detrimental environmental agents has been shown adversely to affect lifespan to comparable extents across species, the use of mammalian, avian, and even invertebrate models is theoretically credible. The short lifespan of many of these species also permits studies on multiple generations, and non-human species have been used in experimental procedures which would not have received the requisite ethical permission in human subjects, an example being life-extension protocols utilizing food supplementation with synthetic antioxidants (Melov *et al.* 2000). There are, however, considerable problems in translating results obtained with non-human species, especially those of non-mammalian origin, to human ageing. This particular objection would be lessened if non-human primates were used, but information on ageing and longevity in primate species remains quite limited. Besides, costs would again be a problem and, given the present climate of opinion with respect to animal experimentation, stringent restrictions on the use of primates for ageing studies are predictable.

The third experimental approach to the study of human ageing is based on laboratory culture of normal human cells. The *in vitro* lifespan of human diploid cells was initially described in three stages: initiation of the culture, a period of rapid cell proliferation, and a gradual decline in growth potential (Hayflick and Moorhead 1961). The commencement of growth in primary culture from a tissue explant is most rapid with embryonic tissue, becoming slower and more difficult with advancing age of the donor. Once established, diploid cells grow exponentially until they form a confluent monolayer on the surface of the vessel; on subculture the cells undergo mitosis until the available growth area is again covered. Through time there is stochastic loss of replicative ability in a continuously increasing fraction of cells, so that after a specific number of subcultivations, which is characteristic of the cell strain, growth irreversibly ceases. This cessation of mitosis, which occurs independently of culture conditions, has been referred to as 'The Hayflick Limit' and it provides an important basis for theories of programmed ageing. By comparison, cells derived from tumour tissue, or cultures which have been transformed *in vitro*, do not display a finite growth pattern.

The triphasic cell lifespan *in vitro* was subsequently redefined into four phases, with differentiation between the period of declining growth potential (phase III), commencing after approximately two-thirds of the total lifespan *in vitro*, and phase IV during which cells are incapable of mitosis but may remain viable for an extended period (Macieira-Coelho 1988). In addition to human diploid fibroblasts, finite lifespan *in vitro* and specific age-dependent morphological changes have been reported for many cell types, including arterial smooth muscle, bronchial epithelium, epidermal keratinocytes, glial cells, lens cells, liver cells, and T lymphocytes. An inverse relationship between the age of the explant donor and the number of cell-population doublings (CPD) *in vitro* has been widely described, with both slower cell outgrowth from the explants of older donors and poorer recovery of cells after subcultivation, although the validity of this relationship has recently been questioned (Cristofalo *et al.* 1998).

Since their inception, human cell cultures have been of great importance in enabling the identification of progressive ageing changes at both the cellular and subcellular levels. Their human origin precludes problems of cross-specific comparisons and, given the rapid growth rate of cells *in vitro* combined with the option of long-term cryogenic storage, the method combines flexibility and cost-efficiency. Despite the close comparability observed between ageing changes *in vivo* and *in vitro*, it would however be inappropriate to consider cell-culture systems as complete models of ageing.

Theories of ageing

As noted earlier, theories of ageing often primarily reflect the view of a particular investigator in terms of the evolutionary significance of senescence, whether adaptive or non-adaptive. Superimposed on this bias are the particular mores of the scientific discipline in which the researcher has been trained and works. Thus geneticists espouse theories which emphasize age-dependent alterations in the genome, physiologists measure and assess the physiological decrements associated with ageing, immunologists describe changes in T- and B-cell populations in the elderly, and so on. Some of the very diverse approaches that have been utilized in the study of ageing are illustrated in Table 1.1, with a range of positive and negative associations with longevity listed.

It soon became apparent that belief in the existence of a single, 'magic bullet' cause of ageing was fallacious in complex biological species, and with this recognition earlier organ-

Table 1.1 Experimental studies on longevity in mammalian species

Test system	Test organism	Source
Positive association		
UV-induced DNA repair	Mammalian fibroblasts	Hart and Setlow (1974)
UV-induced DNA repair	Primate lymphocytes and fibroblasts	Hall *et al.* (1984)
Lifespan *in vivo* and *in vitro*	Mammalian erythrocytes and fibroblasts	Rohme (1981)
Superoxide dismutase activity	Primate liver, brain, heart	Tolmasoff *et al.* (1980)
Carotenoid level	Primate and other mammalian brain, sera	Cutler (1984)
Negative association		
Chromosomal abnormalities	Guinea pig liver cells	Curtis and Miller (1971)
DNA binding of activated 7.12 dimethyl benz(a) anthracene	Mammalian fibroblasts	Schwartz and Moore (1977)
Benzo(a)pyrene conversion to water-soluble metabolites	Mammalian fibroblasts	Moore and Schwartz (1978)
Cytochrome P-488 content	Mammalian fibroblasts	Pashko and Schwartz (1982)
Auto-oxidation	Mammalian brain and kidney	Cutler (1985)
Superoxide and hydrogen peroxide generation	Mammalian heart and kidney	Ku *et al.* (1993)

and system-based theories (reviewed in Bittles 1997) have gradually been discounted. Just as the ageing phenotype shows marked variation in different members of a species, so there are many influences, both genetic and non-genetic, which interact to produce that phenotype. For the purposes of discussion it is convenient to collate theories of ageing into groups with discrete topic headings, but it must be stressed that subdivisions of this nature have limited biological meaning, and the observations made and the conclusions drawn should be considered in that light.

Genome-based theories

As the name indicates, these theories are based on the postulate that ageing is primarily associated with changes in the genetic constitution of the organism, and originally they referred only to mutations in nuclear DNA. Much progress on ageing has recently been made in the area of genetics as a spin-off from the Human Genome Project. The major theories which have been advanced differ in relative emphasis as to whether ageing is encoded genetically, is the result of extrinsic damage to the genome, or represents an intrinsic failure in information flow.

Programmed ageing

The initial impetus for theories of programmed ageing was provided by lifespan studies which indicated remarkable constancy in the life expectation of various species, both mammalian and non-mammalian. Theories proposing a primarily genetic basis for ageing were greatly strengthened by the demonstration that human diploid cells exhibited a finite lifespan when cultured in the laboratory (Hayflick and Moorhead 1961; Hayflick 1965). Prior to these reports it was believed that explanted mammalian and avian tissue had the potential for infinite growth *in vitro*, an expectation subsequently discounted as stemming from flawed laboratory protocols and probable contamination of cultures by transformed, heteroploid cells which do not exhibit senescence. As detailed above in the discussion on cell-culture models of ageing, it seems appropriate to postulate a central monitoring system for ageing at the cellular level. By means of cell-fusion experiments on normal diploid fibroblasts with a defined lifespan and potentially immortal, transformed cells, it was shown that the phenotype of cellular senescence is dominant (Pereira-Smith and Smith 1983).

While there are strong evolutionary advantages for the species through genetic control of developmental changes from conception to reproductive adulthood, as noted in the introduction to this chapter, the case for 'ageing' genes is much less strong. The evolutionary compromise may be that, with the attainment of adulthood, the developmental programme gradually runs down, possibly as a result of increasing chromosomal instability.

Somatic mutation

Since DNA is responsible for specifying the production of peptides and proteins essential for the maintenance of life, it was reasoned that the characteristic, physiological decrements associated with ageing could have arisen from accumulated mutations in the nuclear DNA (nDNA) of somatic cells (Szilard 1959). Damage to nDNA induced, for example, by non-lethal doses of ionizing radiation, would be expected to reduce the longevity of experimental animals in a dose-dependent manner. But the relevance of this damage to normal ageing may be minimal as it is dividing cells, such as the bone marrow stem cells, which are most sensitive to radiation, whereas in old age non-dividing cells show the greatest functional declines.

As shown in Table 1.1, an inverse correlation was reported between the lifespan of a number of mammalian species and the incidence of chromosome abnormalities with increasing age (Curtis and Miller 1971). Rather than being indicative of a causal relationship, these findings could as readily be explained in terms of the ability of an animal to tolerate DNA damage via the repair of damaged molecules (Hart and Setlow 1974). While somatic mutation in nDNA can critically influence lifespan, whether 'spontaneous' or radiation-induced, its role in the ageing process would appear to be of limited direct significance.

Mitochondrial decline

A more feasible connection between nDNA and ageing may be via the critical role of the nucleus in the maintenance of mitochondrial structure and function. Mitochondria are the subcellular organelles primarily responsible for aerobic energy production in humans, and throughout animal and insect phyla. The mammalian mitochondrial genome is characterized by its extremely compact organization, with a virtual absence of introns. The 16 569 nucleotides that comprise the human mitochondrial genome encode 13 polypeptides, all of which are constituents of the respiratory chain: subunits I, II, and III of cytochrome *c* oxidase, subunits 6 and 8 of ATPase, cytochrome *b*, and 7 subunits of NAD dehydrogenase, along with 2 rRNAs and 22 tRNAs required for synthesis of the polypeptides (Anderson *et al.* 1981; Chomyn *et al.* 1986; Tzagoloff and Myers 1986).

Despite the obvious importance of mitochondrial DNA (mtDNA) in mitochondrial propagation and the maintenance of cellular respiration, the majority of proteins involved in the regulation of mtDNA transcription, translation, and replication are actually encoded in the nuclear genome, which also encodes 70 subunits of the mitochondrial respiratory chain. The nuclear-encoded precursors of mitochondrial proteins carry specific targeting sequences that are imported into the organelle via a specific, energy-dependent system located in the outer mitochondrial membrane (Voos *et al.* 1994). This implies the operation of a highly coordinated mechanism for the expression of the two genomes, with greatest vulnerability in those mitochondrial enzymes which include subunit polypeptides transcribed and translated from both nuclear and mitochondrial loci. For this reason it has been claimed that age-related mitochondrial dysfunction in humans is primarily associated with mutations in nDNA rather than mtDNA (Hayashi *et al.* 1994).

Across species, the mitochondria of old organisms show a decrease in number, an increase in size, and the occurrence of structural abnormalities. Given the central role occupied by mitochondria in energy production, these changes are of considerable metabolic significance. It is, however, the additional, proposed relationship between mitochondria and free-radical damage, discussed below under non-genetic theories, which has provoked most attention, with both the mitochondrial membrane and mtDNA proposed as targets (reviewed in Bittles 1992). Controlled experimental studies on the role of mitochondria in ageing have been somewhat equivocal, possibly reflecting differential rates of removal of damage or mutations in mtDNA by mitochondrial replication. None the less, there is a sufficiently large body of information to associate a decline in mitochondrial functional capacity with many of the features previously considered as central to the ageing process.

Information transfer

The ability of an organism to produce functional proteins is dependent on the fidelity of genetic information encoded in the DNA, on unimpaired transcription of this information from DNA to RNA, and on its subsequent translation into peptides and proteins. Transcription and translation are multi-step processes each of which must be considered as subject to error, and during the life-course of an organism the sequence of information transfer steps is continuously operational. The potential for mistakes is thus large and would be expected to grow exponentially with increasing chronological age. Further, since a number of the proteins produced may be involved as surveillance enzymes in maintaining the accuracy of the entire process, feedback mechanisms could lead to collapse of the system, resulting in a phenomenon initially termed error catastrophe (Orgel 1963, 1973). In support of this scenario, it was shown that the lifespan of mammalian species was inversely correlated with their rates of protein turnover (Spector 1974).

Although interest in the error theory gradually waned, it has received a major boost following the demonstration of an age-related, down-regulation of genes specifically involved in the G_2–M phase of the cell cycle (Ly *et al.* 2000). This finding has been interpreted as evidence of increasing mitotic errors in dividing cells during the postreproductive stage of life, which ultimately result in chromosomal abnormalities and the misregulation of genes centrally involved in the ageing process.

The codon-restriction theory, which takes into account the redundant nature of the genetic code with multiple, alternative triplets coding for specific amino acids, provided an additional hypothesis for age-related changes in the information processing ability of cells (Strehler *et al.* 1971). It was proposed that as organisms age there is altered availability of tRNA species and/or tRNA synthetases. Therefore, even though the DNA remains functionally intact, loss of translational ability effectively leaves certain codons stranded. Although some supportive experimental evidence was published (Sambuy and Bittles 1982), attention has gradually drifted from codon restriction to other research areas perceived to hold greater promise.

Epigenetic mechanisms

Rather than senescence involving defects in DNA or proteins, it was proposed that it is epigenetic errors, i.e. errors in the control of gene expression, which are the primary causal factors. The base 5-methyl cytosine (5mC) is the main candidate implicated in the control of gene activity in ageing, and it is predicted that loss of methylation by 5mC could lead to the expression of genes that otherwise are silent in somatic cells. If particular genes have a cluster of 5mC bases in adjacent promoter regions, their expression would require the sequential loss of several methyl groups. In this way, many silent epigenetic defects could be present in the genome that reveal their deleterious phenotype only after a given time or following a specific number of cell divisions (Holliday 1987).

The advantage of this model of ageing over other genetic theories is the lack of requirement for an evolutionary preservation of genes which, in former generations, would seldom have been expressed. Experimental evidence in support of the theory includes the reduced lifespan exhibited by cultured human diploid fibroblasts following treatment with 5-azacytidine, which inhibits methylation of cytosine in DNA (Holliday 1986), and the apparent relationship between 5mC loss and lifespan of diploid cells in culture (Catania and Fairweather 1991). However, the entire area of mammalian gene expression and its control is still poorly understood.

Telomere loss

Following the observation that diploid fibroblasts in culture exhibit a progressive loss of telomeres, (specialized structures located at the terminus of the DNA helix and critical to the maintenance of DNA stability and replication) it was proposed that telomere length could predict the potential number of divisions achievable by a cell strain (Harley *et al.* 1990). The hypothesis was then extended to suggest that loss of telomere sequences beyond a threshold limit would act as a signal for cells to undergo senescence (Harley 1991).

Human telomeres are arranged as a simple sequence (T_2AG_3) of tandem repeats that are approximately 10 kb in length in somatic tissues and 15 kb in sperm (Broccoli and Cooke 1993). They are synthesized by the enzyme telomerase, which is present in germline cells and in cells that have undergone immortalization, but not in somatic cells. To test whether the prevention of telomere loss would negate the limited replicative capacity of cells *in vitro*, vectors encoding the catalytic subunit of human telomerase were introduced into two telomerase-negative, normal, human cell strains (Bodnar *et al.* 1998). The resultant cell clones expressing telomerase activity continued to divide vigorously long after cessation of mitosis in the cells from which they were derived, and they also showed reduced staining for the enzyme β-galactosidase which is commonly used as a marker for senescence. Telomere shortening thus fulfilled the essential criteria for a candidate marker of cellular senescence, although, somewhat surprisingly, preliminary studies on peripheral blood leucocytes have indicated that telomerase loss occurred most rapidly in children under 5 years of age (Frenck *et al.* 1998).

Further twists in the telomere story that may have a direct bearing on human ageing emerged following the birth of cloned mammalian offspring. In the original set of experiments that resulted in the birth of the sheep Dolly, the telomeres of the cloned animal were shorter than normal, suggesting accelerated ageing (Shiels *et al.* 1999). By comparison, when bovine oocytes were reconstructed by nuclear transfer with senescent fibroblasts, they exhibited both a significant extension in replicative lifespan and increased telomere length (Lanza *et al.* 2000), which appears to indicate re-setting of the telomere clock. If this finding is confirmed across species, and if the loss of telomere sequences proves to be a causative process in mammalian ageing, then the possibility of 'rejuvenation' through cell and tissue replacement could arise.

Non-genetic/stochastic theories

Theories in this category are based on the assumption that cumulative minor, adverse random changes occur through time, which ultimately overwhelm the capacity of an organism to survive. Within this schema, ageing represents the preceding period of decline.

Rate-of-living theory

Initial evidence for the rate-of-living theory came from the observation that in a variety of poikilotherms, including *Drosophila* and rotifers, optimum lifespan was achieved when the organisms were maintained at suboptimal temperatures. As there is a general correlation between temperature and reaction rates, it was reasoned that the abbreviated lifespan observed at higher temperatures reflected the adverse effects of faster rates of living, presumably associated with energy expenditure. In mammals, a clear inverse relationship between basal metabolic rate and longevity has been shown (Sacher 1976), and taken as corroborative evidence of lifespan being governed by the rate of living of the particular species. Unfortunately, theories of this type tend to be notably imprecise in defining the nature of the salient factor(s) controlling ageing and lifespan, although it has been proposed that the rate-of-living theory could be convincingly reformulated as a stress theory of ageing (Parsons 1995). According to this modified theory, resistance to external stress is the primary inherited trait that determines lifespan, and so organisms which through time have evolved to a more stress-resistant genotype will exhibit the greatest longevity.

Accumulation theories

Ageing has been ascribed to the accumulation of waste products within cells, on the assumption that these products interfere with normal cellular metabolism and function in a mainly non-specific manner. Ultimately, this results in dysfunction and death at cellular and organ levels. The molecule that has been principally implicated in accumulation theories is lipofuscin, a highly insoluble, pigmented compound present with advancing age in the cells of many mammalian tissues, including neurons, cardiac muscle fibres, and the adrenal cortex. Lipofuscin is believed to be derived by auto-oxidation from incompletely degraded cellular materials, in particular the lipid component of cell mitochondrial membranes (Fleming *et al.* 1985). As such it appears probable that the build-up of lipofuscin, which has not been demonstrated to affect cell function critically, may be secondary to an age-related decline in the function of cellular catabolic processes.

Cross-linkage and postsynthetic modification theories

With increasing chronological age many macromolecules of biological importance gradually develop cross-links, either covalent in nature or via hydrogen bonding. The establishment of cross-linkage changes the chemical and physical properties of molecules; for example, cross-linkage of the extracellular protein collagen is held to be responsible for the loss of elasticity in mammalian blood vessels and skin with advancing age (Bjorksten 1968; Kohn 1982*b*). DNA and RNA are also believed to be potential intracellular targets for cross-linking agents, with serious implications for cellular information flow.

The existence of cross-linkage in older organisms is indisputable, and the resultant molecular aggregation and immobilization predictably could compromise cellular metabolism and function. Similar end-effects could result from postsynthetic modification of proteins, with non-enzymatic glycosylation (glycation) a potentially important example that has been associated with ageing. Glycation results from the initial reaction of glucose with the amino group of lysine residues, which then proceeds to form a Schiff base and progressively more complex compounds termed advanced glycosylation end (AGE) products (Martin *et al.* 1993).

In effect, cross-linkage or any modification of proteins that leads to decreased proteolysis could be considered a specific form of accumulation but, as with general accumulation theories, the extent to which abnormal proteins build up is uncertain. Progressive age-related increases in cross-linkage have been observed in collagen, which is subject to turnover throughout life (Schnider and Kohn 1981). By contrast, little change was reported in the level of glycation in lens crystallin proteins obtained from subjects aged between 10 and 80 years (Patrick *et al.* 1990). It has been claimed that the retardation of senescence effected by the dipeptide carnosine in human diploid fibroblast cultures may be due to its antiglycation effect (McFarland and Holliday 1994). However, in common with the majority of ageing theories, cross-linkage and postsynthetic mechanisms primarily appear to represent examples of the cause versus effect debate.

Free-radical theory

The role of free-radical damage as a significant factor in ageing was first advanced by Harman (1956). Free radicals are compounds with an unpaired electron in their outer orbital which renders them highly reactive, and they tend to attack neighbouring compounds autocatalytically. Free radicals can result from the exposure of cells and organelles to ionizing radiation, but the free-radical theory of ageing emphasizes the role of oxygen radical-initiated tissue damage. A number of reactive species are derived from molecular oxygen, including the superoxide and hydroperoxyl radicals, hydrogen peroxide, hydroxyl radical, and singlet oxygen. Polyunsaturated fatty-acid side chains of cell and organelle membranes serve as highly susceptible targets for the action of oxygen radicals, with the lipids undergoing a chain reaction, known as lipid peroxidation, that may result in severe damage and the eventual death of the cell (Gutteridge *et al.* 1986). It has also been proposed that DNA may be the critical target molecule for free-radical damage, with mtDNA especially susceptible because of its proximity to the site of free-radical production in the inner mitochondrial membrane.

In addition to the free radicals produced by enzymatic reactions of the respiratory chain, lesser concentrations of free radicals are formed during phagocytosis, in prostaglandin synthesis, and in the cytochrome P-450 system, and non-enzymatic reactions of oxygen with organic compounds provide a further minor source (Harman 1986). It has, however, been suggested that only terminally differentiated cells, such as those of the brain, heart, and muscle are severely affected, since in fast-replicating cells frequent turnover of macromolecules can take place during mitochondrial division at mitosis. Support for this idea is provided by marked age-dependent increases in oxidative damage to mtDNA, and to a lesser extent nDNA, in human brain (Mecocci *et al.* 1993), and there also is an age-associated decline in respiratory chain function in skeletal muscle (Trounce *et al.* 1989; Boffoli *et al.* 1994; Hsieh *et al.* 1994).

As noted in Table 1.1, an inverse correlation has been demonstrated between the longevity of mammalian species and rates of peroxidation, at least partially determined by the antioxidant defences utilized by each species (Cutler 1985). In humans, a wide variety of antioxidants have been identified including ascorbate, α-tocopherol,

β-carotene, glutathione, and the enzymes superoxide dismutase, peroxidase, and catalase. There has been little evidence that these antioxidants produce a significant extension in maximum lifespan, but a series of experiments in the nematode *Caenorhabditis elegans* using small, synthetic superoxide dismutase/catalase mimetics to augment their natural antioxidant systems succeeded in significantly extending both mean and maximum lifespan (Melov *et al.* 2000). Further work on the same model system has indicated that oxidative damage to neurons may act as a primary determinant of lifespan (Wolkow *et al.* 2000).

Considerable overlap is apparent between many of the theories that have been advanced to explain ageing. Earlier, non-genome theories such as wear and tear, rate of living, accumulation, and cross-linkage are to a large extent phenomenological, and the observations on which they were based can probably be more convincingly discussed in terms of free-radical damage. It is, however, difficult to conceive how the essentially stochastic free-radical theory can be evoked to explain all the characteristics of ageing. In particular, it would appear that free-radical damage should not critically intervene in the highly reproducible *in vitro* ageing of human diploid cells, since these mitotic cells must be presumed to have the capacity of mitochondrial macromolecular renewal. Indeed, various studies have confirmed that, even at the end of their *in vitro* lifespan, the mitochondria of human diploid fibroblasts remain potentially functional (Bittles *et al.* 1988; Flannery *et al.* 1989), and so the claim that ageing is due solely to free-radical damage appears exaggerated.

Apoptosis and ageing

Apoptosis, the activation of a gene-directed, self-destruct programme, is a rapidly emerging topic which may prove to be of both theoretical and practical significance in ageing at the cellular level. Experiments conducted on *Drosophila* have indicated that apoptosis is under epigenetic control (Steller 1995). In mammals this form of cell death appears to be initiated by cysteine proteases (caspases), with subsequent condensation and segregation of nuclei, condensation and fragmentation of the cytoplasm, and enzymatic degradation of chromosomal DNA to nucleosomes by endonucleases. To date, some 12 caspases have been identified in humans, of which two-thirds are believed to be apoptosis-related (Hengartner 2000). Since apoptosis can be induced in the absence of *de novo* protein synthesis, it has been assumed that the cellular components involved in the associated, characteristic morphological changes are continually present in the mammalian cell, although normally inhibited (Steller 1995).

From the specific perspective of ageing, the major interest in apoptosis lies in the association with diseases traditionally found in the elderly. For example, the increased cell accumulation found in cancers and autoimmune disorders has been ascribed to inhibition of apoptosis, whereas neurodegenerative disorders, including Alzheimer's disease, and ischaemic injury resulting in myocardial infarction and stroke are associated with an increase (Thompson 1995). In Alzheimer's disease the role of β-amyloid is of particular interest, since it has been proposed that its normal function is as an anti-apoptotic, extracellular antioxidant protecting neurons from trauma (Chan *et al.* 1999), thus complementing the action of the intracellular antioxidant superoxide dismutase (Dharmarajan *et al.* 1999). By comparison, at the higher concentrations found in the brains of persons with Alzheimer's disease, and especially in persons homozygous for the apolipoprotein ϵ4 allele, β-amyloid may actually promote apoptosis via oxidative stress (Cotman and Anderson 1995). However, as many degenerating neurons in Alzheimer's disease do not show evidence of apoptosis, other non-apoptotic, causative mechanisms may exist (Yuan and Yander 2000).

In addition, loss of mitochondrial function is observed during apoptosis and, since an outer mitochondrial protein Bcl-2 can block apoptosis induced by a wide range of stimuli (Halestrap 2000), it was suggested that mitochondria may play a significant role in its regulation.

Experimental support for this opinion has recently been produced with the demonstration that apoptosis is initiated following the translocation of a nuclear transcription factor, TR3, to the mitochondria (Li *et al.* 2000). The translocation of TR3 triggers mitochondrial membrane permeability and the consequent release of cytochrome *c*, whose normal cellular function is to act as an electron carrier in the respiratory chain.

The genetics of ageing and progeroid disorders

Genetic models of ageing and life expectancy

The main rationale behind the genetic study of ageing is the species-specific variation in maximum lifespan potential. This suggests there are underlying differences in the genetic constitution of species controlling the rate of ageing although, as noted earlier, the relationship between ageing and lifespan requires careful qualification. Attempts to specify the numbers of genes involved in the increment of maximum lifespan potential that accompanied the evolution of *Homo sapiens* were made using rates of amino acid substitution in proteins, an approach which yielded estimates of between 70 and 240 genes (Sacher 1975; Cutler 1975).

Subsequent studies on evolutionary changes in lifespan indicated the involvement of chromosomal rearrangements at a large number of gene loci, rather than the point mutations on which these estimates were based. By enumeration of the genetic variants associated with development of the senescent phenotype, it has been calculated that while approximately 1000 genes are implicated in regulating features of ageing, up to 6900 genes might be involved peripherally in the overall ageing phenotype (Martin 1985, 1989). As the human genome has been estimated to comprise 30 000 to 40 000 genes, it follows that if the suggested numbers of genes associated with ageing are even approximately correct, the potential degree of genetic heterogeneity involved in senescence is immense. To investigate this topic, DNA microarrays have been applied to the direct study of ageing in cultured human diploid fibroblasts. Of the approximately 6300 genes examined, the expression of 61 genes (~1% of those monitored) was found to change with ageing *in vitro*. As noted earlier, these included genes involved in control of the cell cycle, and a number of genes responsible for the formation and remodelling of collagen and other proteins of the extracellular matrix (Ly *et al.* 2000).

Further evidence against a simple genetic basis for longevity is provided by parent–offspring comparisons. Initially, a strong link was believed to exist between parental longevity and the lifespan of their children (Pearl and Pearl 1934), but in subsequent longitudinal studies on nonagenarians (Abbott *et al.* 1974) and in a French–Canadian isolate (Philippe 1978) the correlation was found to be very weak and as readily explicable in social and environmental terms as by inheritance (Murphy 1978). A long-term study of monozygotic and dizygotic twins did show greater similarity in the lifespan of identical twins than their non-identical counterparts (Jarvik *et al.* 1960). However, these findings are probably indicative only of the greater comparability in timing and causes of death among monozygotic twins. A more recent investigation in Denmark produced quite low heritability estimates for longevity of 0.26 for males and 0.23 for females (Herskind *et al.* 1996). All currently available data thus point to the inheritance of longevity as determined by variable numbers of interacting genes, whose expression is subject to major modification by environmental agents.

Support for this interpretation comes from data on the human leucocyte antigen (HLA) system which showed a significant excess of specific HLA antigens among nonagenarians, Cw7 in males and Cw1 in females, suggesting the association of certain haplotypes with increased survival (Proust *et al.* 1982). It was also reported that the apolipoprotein $\varepsilon 4$ allele, which promotes premature atherosclerosis and is a significant risk factor in the development of late-onset familial Alzheimer's disease, is less frequent in centenarians than in controls (Schächter *et al.* 1994). This has led to the intriguing hypothesis that the uniquely human apolipoprotein $\varepsilon 3$ allele evolved from the $\varepsilon 4$ of primate ancestors, concomitant with the rapid increase in human brain size and the emergence of grandmothering as an advantageous behavioural trait (Finch and Sapolsky 1999). While such studies can be taken as examples of genetic influences on differential survival, and possible pleiotropic age-dependent effects on longevity, at this time their precise biological significance and relevance is difficult to perceive.

Progeroid syndromes

Studies conducted on patients with Hutchinson–Gilford syndrome and Werner's syndrome provide a rather different perspective on the genetic contribution to ageing. In both disease states affected individuals exhibit a grossly premature spectrum of pathologies, usually regarded as typical only of the very old. Hutchinson–Gilford syndrome presents in childhood as severe growth retardation, with balding, loss of subcutaneous tissue, prominent veins, pigmented age spots, arthritis, and a very characteristic facial appearance. Severe atherosclerosis usually develops around 10 years of age and median lifespan is 13 years (Brown *et al.* 1985), although atypically a Japanese patient was described who lived to 45 years (Ogihara *et al.* 1986).

The onset of symptoms in individuals with Werner's syndrome occurs later in life and is typically observed as shortness in stature owing to absence of the adolescent growth spurt, accompanied by greying of the hair by 20 years. With increasing chronological age the disorder follows a fairly predictable course, which includes atrophy of the skin and connective tissue, hair loss, vocal changes, cataract formation, skin ulceration, and diabetes by the middle of the fourth decade of life. Osteoporosis and coronary artery disease are common, and affected females show early cessation of menstruation. The mean lifespan is 47 years (Epstein *et al.* 1966; Salk 1982). Cell cultures established from the skin of Werner's patients behave in a similar manner to those derived from very old persons. There is a long lag phase before fibroblasts begin to migrate from the explant, with the growth of the cells being both sparse and grossly restricted in duration, and associated with a variety of chromosomal rearrangements including deletions and multiple translocations (Salk 1982; Fukuchi *et al.* 1989; Scappaticci *et al.* 1990).

In both diseases, single gene mutations or small multigene deletions appear to be responsible for the early onset and very rapid development of the disease phenotype. Hutchinson–Gilford syndrome has been described both as a sporadic autosomal dominant (Brown *et al.* 1985) and an autosomal recessive disorder (Khalifa 1989), with the possibility that rare cases of affected siblings may result from germinal mosaicism. In Werner's syndrome the mode of inheritance is autosomal recessive (Epstein *et al.* 1966; Goto *et al.* 1981), and the disease gene has been mapped to chromosome 8p12–p11 (Goto *et al.* 1992). A range of mutations has been described in this gene, which has significant similarity to DNA helicases (Yu *et al.* 1996). In the yeast *Saccharomyces cerevisiae*, the gene *PIF1* encodes a 5'-to-3' DNA helicase believed to be associated with the inhibition of telomere lengthening, and it also affects mitochondrial DNA (Zhou *et al.* 2000). Therefore it seems possible that the basic defect in Werner's syndrome may be associated with overexpression of the enzymatically active gene product, Pif1p, which is known to cause telomere shortening.

It was argued that because of their apparent similarities to many aspects of normal ageing, both disorders should be regarded as segmental progeroid syndromes, i.e. diseases in which many, but not all, aspects of the senescent phenotype are present (Martin 1985). The contrary opinion was that, in view of the abnormalities which are specific to Hutchinson–Gilford and Werner's syndromes and their failure to meet the criteria used to define precocious or accelerated ageing, both syndromes could most appropriately be considered as caricatures of ageing (Epstein 1985). This debate appears to have been effectively settled in favour of the former viewpoint, by demonstration that the patterns of change in gene expression observed with ageing in cultured human diploid fibroblasts from normal individuals and from a person with Hutchinson–Gilford progeria overlapped to a large degree (Ly *et al.* 2000).

Experimental methods for the modification of rates of ageing

By definition, if ageing is mainly stochastic in nature then it should be possible to retard development of the ageing phenotype by altering the relative influence of contributory environmental variables. Although many theories have been proposed and experimentally tested, the only method so far proven to increase maximum lifespan in mammals is calorie restriction, the feeding of a diet low in calories but otherwise nutritionally adequate. This phenomenon was first reported in albino rats (McCay *et al.* 1935), and animals chronically underfed from birth remained prepubertal as a result of their retarded growth and development (McCay *et al.* 1939). In more recent food restriction experiments, rodents were typically fed a diet corresponding to approximately 60% of that ingested by *ad libitum* fed controls, commencing either soon after weaning or in young adulthood, with both regimens equally efficacious in increasing maximum lifespan (Yu *et al.* 1985). Dietary restriction in rodents has also been shown to retard the development of tumours and other chronic diseases of late adulthood (Weindruch and Walford 1982; Holehan and Merry 1986; Masoro 1988).

Food restriction has been associated with immune theories of ageing, since delayed maturation of the immune system is predicted to result from the general retardation in growth and development in treated animals. Although this may be beneficial to old animals in terms of reduced autoimmunity, it is difficult to comprehend how a delay in the development of full immune competence could be other than detrimental to young animals, especially when reared under natural conditions. This disadvantage may extend into adulthood, as preliminary human studies indicated that poor early growth resulted in lower adult levels of the hormone thymosin $\alpha 1$, produced by the thymus and essential both for T-cell function and in the overall regulation of the immune system (Clark *et al.* 1989).

A correlation between food restriction and diminished free-radical damage has also been claimed, secondary to lower metabolic activity and hence reduced oxygen consumption (Harman 1986). Dietary restriction has also been shown to attenuate age-related increases in rodent skeletal muscle enzyme activities (Luhtala *et al.* 1994). But long-term food restriction does not result in a sustained reduction in metabolic rate (McCarter *et al.* 1985), and the addition of antioxidants to the diet of rodents failed to increase maximum lifespan (Harman 1983). Nevertheless, it has been claimed that adoption of an appropriately nutritious diet supplemented by one or more free-radical reaction inhibitors would increase mean life expectancy at birth by five or more years (Harman 1992).

A general explanation for the central effect of caloric restriction in retarding mammalian ageing has recently been revealed by DNA microarray studies of over 6000 genes in the skeletal muscle of mice. In control animals, ageing resulted in differential gene-expression patterns indicative of a marked stress response and lower expression of metabolic and biosynthetic genes. By comparison, the transcriptional patterns of calorie-restricted animals indicated they had undergone a metabolic shift towards increased protein turnover and decreased macromolecular damage (Lee *et al.* 1999). Later, more specific work on *Saccharomyces cerevisiae* has suggested that the life extension role of caloric restriction may be mediated via the metabolic intermediate nicotinamide adenine dinucleotide (NAD), which acts to suppress DNA errors that arise during mitotic recombination (Lin *et al.* 2000).

Ageing as an energy crisis

The literature on ageing often appears as confusing and contradictory as it is vast. There has been an ongoing tendency to concentrate on theories that suppose a single cause of ageing. Given the widely variant nature of the ageing phenotype, it is difficult to perceive how such an extreme degree of pleiotropy could have been encoded or otherwise resulted from a unimodal origin. Much of the confusion inherent in theories of ageing also results from ambitious claims made on behalf of processes and systems that are only marginally testable, and so cannot readily be proved or disproved.

In evolutionary terms, senescence was suggested to be the end-result of an energy conservation strategy operating in somatic cells (Kirkwood 1977). During the course of an organism's lifespan, the total available energy has to be differentially allocated to a variety of functions, including macromolecular synthesis and degradation, cell and organ maintenance, and reproduction of the species. Since the energy supply is finite, and to ensure propagation of the species by the successful transmission of genes to future generations, a compromise has to be reached between the energy made available for each function. According to the disposable soma theory, the proposed accommodation in energy-saving is achieved by maintenance of absolute or near-absolute accuracy in germ-cell replication but less rigorous error correction in somatic cells (Kirkwood and Holliday 1986).

Minimally, this would provide an explanation for the puzzling inability of organisms to maintain their existing structure and function despite having completed morphogenesis (Williams 1957), and support for the theory is provided by the observation of a negative relationship between longevity and fecundity in mammals (Holliday 1996). Likewise, in a study of the British aristocracy, female longevity was negatively correlated with their number of progeny and positively correlated with age at first childbirth (Westendorp and Kirkwood 1998). Extending this line of reasoning, if maintenance of the energy supply is a critical factor in ageing, then in the event of a reduction in energy production or supply, all energy-dependent processes in somatic cells would suffer in proportion to their energy requirements. A simple check on the implications of this prediction can be made by reference to experimentally derived correlates of mammalian longevity, associated either with energy production or processes which appear to be energy-dependent.

For that reason, and given the integral role that appears to be played by the mitochondria in apoptosis, investigators have sought to link functional decline in mitochondria to free radical-induced damage, particularly to the inner mitochondrial membrane. As the inner membrane is the site of the electron transport chain, and enzymes of the tricarboxylic acid cycle (TCA) are located within the mitochondrial matrix, oxidative damage by free radicals generated as by-products of cell respiration could severely compromise the ability of an organism to produce ATP and so meet its energy requirements. Cross-sectional experimental studies on invertebrates and rodents have indicated major morphological and functional changes in mitochondria with ageing, and similar observations were reported in the mitochondria of individuals aged from 60 to 80 years of age (Tauchi and Sato 1985; Beregi 1986), and cultured human cells close to termination of their *in vitro* lifespan (Johnson 1979).

In humans, analysis of mtDNA after amplification revealed the age-dependent presence of a 4977 base pair (bp) deletion in mtDNA from a wide variety of tissues, including heart, brain, liver, kidney, spleen, and skeletal muscle (Cortopassi and Arnheim 1990; Ikebe *et al.* 1990; Linnane *et al.* 1990; Yen *et al.* 1991). This deletion was also detected in ovarian tissue, but only after onset of the menopause (Kitagawa *et al.* 1993). The mtDNA region deleted occurs between base pairs 8470 and 13 459 of the mitochondrial genome; genes encoded in this region include subunits 6 and 8 of ATP synthase, subunit *CO3* of the cytochrome oxidase complex, and subunits ND3, -4L, -4, and -5 of the NADH–coenzyme Q reductase complex (Linnane *et al.* 1990). Further age-dependent deletions have since been described, ranging in size from 6063 bp to 10 422 bp (Corral-Debrinski *et al.* 1992; Hsieh *et al.* 1994; Pang *et al.* 1994), and specific age-related point mutations in human mtDNA have also been detected (Münscher *et al.* 1993; Zhang *et al.* 1993).

This evidence provides valuable support for the hypothesis that the accumulation of somatic mtDNA deletions and other forms of mutation may be an important determinant of ageing (Linnane *et al.* 1989), and cytoplasmic segregation of the mutant genomes could lead to cells with variable bioenergetic capacities. Whether the appearance of mtDNA mutations is spontaneous and/or provoked by free-radical damage, it seems probable that once initiated the problem would be exacerbated by the organization of mtDNA, with its virtual absence of introns (Anderson *et al.* 1981), lack of histone protection (Richter *et al.* 1988), and no excision or recombinational repair (Clayton 1982). The subsequent segregation patterns of mutant mtDNA per cell via the process of heteroplasmy, and the effects on cellular bioenergetic capacities, would be largely dependent on the essentially stochastic process of mitochondrial replication in diluting out defective genomes (Hart and Turturro 1987). It has been claimed that non-availability of this option is a critical component in the age-dependent functional decline of fixed, postmitotic cells (Miquel 1991). Moreover, specific missense mutations in the *CO1* and *CO2* genes of cytochrome *c* oxidase, each of which is exclusively encoded in the mitochondria, have been shown to segregate at higher frequency with late-onset Alzheimer's disease (Davis *et al.* 1997). In other cell types, mitochondrial turnover may be a significant factor in reducing adverse age-related responses.

The number of mtDNA genomes per cell could equally be a critical factor in determining the extent to which respiration of the organism will be adversely affected. Human cells typically contain hundreds of mitochondria, all of which appear to be polyploid. The numbers of mitochondria and mitochondrial genomes are tissue-dependent, and their concentration is proportional to respiratory demand, being highest in tissues such as muscle (Holt and Jacobs 1994). Considered against the low observed frequency of mutant mtDNA molecules in humans, e.g. with an estimated 0.06% of muscle mtDNA showing the 4977 bp deletion in persons over 70 years (Lee *et al.* 1994), cells would appear to possess very considerable spare mtDNA capacity. Therefore, unless an extremely low functional threshold is operational, respiration should be adversely affected only to a limited extent.

As previously discussed, the role of the nuclear genome in mtDNA mutations may prove to be critical. An indication of the significance and complexity of this interactive role was demonstrated in progressive external ophthalmoplegia (PEO). Although this disease is characterized by multiple mtDNA deletions in tissues such as brain, muscle, and heart, and by a lack of respiratory chain proteins leading to defective energy production, the primary mutation in PEO actually occurs in the nuclear genome at chromosome 10q23.3–24.3. As a result, the disorder is inherited as an autosomal dominant (Suomalainen *et al.* 1995).

An alternative hypothesis to be considered is that the main driving force behind ageing is a gradual deficiency in available energy. As an organism ages, the demands being placed upon the free-energy pool alter and increase from a primarily anabolic role to meeting the requirements of ever-increasing repair and catabolic functions, including those imposed by specific disease-related insults. While damage to the mitochondrial inner membrane and/or mtDNA may well occur during the lifespan of an organism and contribute to development of the ageing phenotype, generally its role will only become critical late in life when the energy needs of the organism for repair and the catabolism of aberrant proteins can no longer be fully accommodated. Whether the energy crisis hypothesis is, or proves not to be, a major causative factor in age-related pathologies, the very low caloric intakes recorded by elderly persons in the USA, with 45% of those surveyed reporting mean caloric intakes that were less than two-thirds of the US Recommended Dietary Allowances (Ryan *et al.* 1989), may explain at least some of the behavioural correlates of old age.

Ageing and the concept of healthy life expectancy

Current progress in understanding the nature of the disorders that frequently accompany ageing is timely, given the projected global numbers of persons over 60 years of age, and more especially those aged over 80 years. Especially in the latter age group, a high rate of physical and psychiatric disability can be predicted, a prospect which is viewed with growing concern by many national governments. In fact, the scale of the potential problem may have been significantly underestimated, since it has been demonstrated that median forecasts of life expectancy in the G7 countries, which should have access to good data sources, are substantially larger than the official governmental statistics (Tuljapurkar *et al.* 2000).

Rather than concentrate only on life expectancy, there has been a major push by demographers, epidemiologists, and public health planners to develop ancillary measures that would be of greater practical value in assessing the adverse effects of ageing, and hence the potential capabilities or disabilities of older people. Active Life Expectancy (ALE) is defined as the period of life that is free of disabilities with respect to the basic Activities of Daily Living (ADL), e.g. eating, getting in and out of bed, bathing and toileting needs, dressing, and indoor mobility (Manton and Land 2000). This approach has been extended by weighting specific physical and cognitive dysfunctions to produce measures of Disability-Adjusted Life Years (DALY) and Quality-Adjusted Life Years (QALY).

In mid-2000 the World Health Organization published tables of healthy life expectancy for babies born in 1999, based on a comparable indicator, Disability-Adjusted Life Expectancy (DALE), which estimates the number of years that might be expected to be spent in 'full health'. Under this system the number of years of healthy life expectancy can be calculated after weighting the period of predicted ill health according to the perceived severity of the disorders(s). Applying the DALE measure across 191 countries, Japan ranked first with a healthy life expectancy of 74.5 years, by comparison with total mean life expectancies of 77 years for Japanese males and 84 years for females (PRB 1999). A common finding in the developed countries was that although females enjoyed higher DALE scores, they also could expect more years of disability than males, thus emphasizing the greater probability of disability at more advanced ages.

Measures such as DALE, DALY, and QALY have been criticized because of their dependence on subjective judgements regarding the level of health care required to maintain an individual in a given state of health, a criticism which can become even more significant in international, cross-cultural comparisons. Despite these limitations, the concept of healthy life expectancy should be useful in practical terms when applied to the general ageing population, and given access to better quality data the initial estimates can be readily adjusted and regularly updated. However, any attempted extension to specific population subgroups, such as people with intellectual disability, could prove difficult without major modifications in rationale.

Conclusions

It is important to note the remarkable, recent progress in elucidating the nature of the genomic changes which cause and/or accompany ageing. This is now proceeding at a pace which is exceeding even the most optimistic projections, to the extent where modification of the ageing phenotype at the cellular level no longer seems unrealistic. As a result, for the first time in human history the majority of those entering old age can look forward with some degree of confidence to an extended state of healthy life expectancy.

References

Abbott, M. H., Murphy, E. A., Bolling, D. R., and Abbey, H. (1974). The familial component in longevity. A study of offspring of nonagenarians. *Johns Hopkins Medical Journal*, **134**, 1–16.

Anderson, S., Bankier, A. T., Barrell, B. G., de Bruijn, M. H. L., Coulson, A. R., Drouin, J., *et al.* (1981). Sequence and organisation of the human mitochondrial genome. *Nature, London*, **290**, 457–65.

Bell, A. G. (1919). Who shall inherit long life? *The National Geographic Magazine*, **35**, 504–10.

Beregi, E. (1986). Relationship between ageing of the immune system and ageing of the whole organism. In *Dimensions in ageing* (ed. M. Bergener, M. Ermini, and H. B. Stahelin), pp. 35–50. Academic Press, London.

Bittles, A. H. (1992). Evidence for and against the causal involvement of mitochondrial DNA mutation in mammalian ageing. *Mutation Research*, **275**, 217–25.

Bittles, A. H. (1997). Biological aspects of human ageing. In *Psychiatry in the elderly* (2nd edn) (ed. R. Jacoby and C. Oppenheimer), pp. 3–23. Oxford University Press, Oxford.

Bittles, A. H., Monks, N., and Baum, H. (1988). Differential growth inhibition of human diploid fibroblasts by 2-deoxyglucose and antimycin A with ageing *in vitro*. *Gerontology*, **34**, 236–41.

Bjorksten, J. (1968). The crosslinkage theory of aging. *Journal of the American Geriatrics Society*, **16**, 408–27.

Bodnar, A. G., Ouellette, M., Frolkis, M., Holt, S. E., Chiu, C-P., Morin, G. B., *et al.* (1998). Extension of life-span by introduction of telomerase into normal human cells. *Science*, **279**, 349–52.

Boffoli, D., Scacco, S. C., Vergari, R., Solarino, G., Santacroce, G., and Papa, S. (1994). Decline with age of the respiratory chain activity in human skeletal muscle. *Biochimica et Biophysica Acta*, **1226**, 73–82.

Brightwell, R. F., Crawford, G. P. M., Cale, J. B., Pedler, P. J., and Bittles, A. H. (1998). Ageing, and the haematological profiles of an Australian community. *Annals of Human Biology*, **25**, 1–10.

Broccoli, D. and Cooke, H. (1993). Aging, healing, and the metabolism of telomeres. *American Journal of Human Genetics*, **52**, 657–60.

Brody, J. A. (1985). Prospects for an ageing population. *Nature, London*, **315**, 463–6.

Brown, W. T. (1979). Human genetic mutations affecting aging—a review. *Mechanisms of Development and Ageing*, **9**, 325–36.

Brown, W. T. (1988). Human genetic models for aging research. In *Human aging research, concepts, and techniques*, Aging series, Vol. 34 (ed. B. Kent and R. N. Butler), pp. 163–81. Plenum, New York.

Brown, W. T., Kieras, F. J., Houck, G. E., Dutkowski, R., and Jenkins, E. C. (1985). A comparison of adult, and childhood progerias: Werner Syndrome, and Hutchinson–Gilford Progeria. In *Werner's syndrome and human aging, advances in experimental medicine and biology*, Vol. 190 (ed. D. Salk, Y. Fujiwara, and G. M. Martin), pp. 229–44. Plenum, New York.

Carey, J. R., Liedo, P., Orozco, D., and Vaupel, J. W. (1992). Slowing of mortality rates at older ages in large Medfly cohorts. *Science*, **258**, 457–61.

Catania, J. and Fairweather, D. S. (1991). DNA methylation and cellular ageing. *Mutation Research*, **256**, 283–93.

Chan, C-W., Dharmarajan, A., Atwood, C. S., Huang, X., Tanzi, R. E., Bush, A. I., *et al.* (1999). Anti-apoptotic action of Alzheimer Aβ. *Alzheimer's Reports*, **2**, 113–19.

Chomyn, A., Cleeter, M. W. J., Ragan, C. I., Riley, M., Doolittle, R. F., and Attardi, G. (1986). URF6, last unidentified reading frame of human mtDNA, codes for an NADH dehydrogenase subunit. *Science*, **234**, 614–18.

Clark, G. A., Aldwin, C. M., Hall, N. R., Spiro, A., and Goldstein, A. (1989). Is poor early growth related to adult immune aging? *American Journal of Human Biology*, **1**, 331–7.

Clayton, D. A. (1982). Replication of animal mitochondrial DNA. *Cell*, **28**, 693–705.

Corral-Debrinski, M., Shoffner, J. M., Lott, M. T., and Wallace, D. C. (1992). Association of mitochondrial DNA damage with aging, and coronary atherosclerotic heart disease. *Mutation Research*, **275**, 169–80.

Cortopassi, G. A. and Arnheim, N. (1990). Detection of a specific mitochondrial DNA deletion in tissues of older humans. *Nucleic Acids Research*, **18**, 6927–33.

Cotman, C. W. and Anderson, A. J. (1995). A potential role for apoptosis in neurodegeneration and Alzheimer's disease. *Molecular Neurobiology*, **10**, 19–45.

Cristofalo, V. J., Allen, R. G., Pignolo, R. J., Martin, B. G., and Beck, J. (1998). Relationship between donor age, and the replicative lifespan of human cells in culture: a reevaluation. *Proceedings of the National Academy of Sciences, USA.*, **95**, 10614–19.

Curtis, J. H. and Miller, K. (1971). Chromosome aberrations in liver cells of guinea pigs. *Journal of Gerontology*, **26**, 292–4.

Curtsinger, J. W., Fukui, H. H., Townsend, D. R., and Vaupel, J. W. (1992). Demography of genotypes: failure of the limited life-span paradigm in *Drosophila melanogaster*. *Science*, **258**, 461–3.

Cutler, R. G. (1975). Evolution of human longevity, and the genetic complexity governing aging rate. *Proceedings of the National Academy of Sciences, USA.*, **72**, 4664–8.

Cutler, R. G. (1984). Carotenoids, and retinol: their possible importance in determining longevity of primate species. *Proceedings of the National Academy of Sciences, USA*, **81**, 7627–31.

Cutler, R. G. (1985). Peroxide-producing potential of tissues: inverse correlation with longevity of mammalian species. *Proceedings of the National Academy of Sciences, USA*, **82**, 4798–802.

Davis, R. E., Miller, S., Herrnstadt, C., Ghosh, S. S., Fahy, E., Shinobu, L. A., *et al.* (1997). Mutations in mitochondrial cytochrome *c* oxidase genes segregate with late-onset Alzheimer disease. *Proceedings of the National Academy of Sciences, USA*, **94**, 4526–31.

Dharmarajan, A. M., Hisheh, S., Singh, B., Parkinson, S., Tilly, K. I., and Tilly, J. L. (1999) Anti-oxidants mimic the ability of chorionic gonadotrophin to suppress apoptosis in the rabbit corpus luteum *in vitro*: a novel role for superoxide dismutase in regulating *bax* expression. *Endocrinology*, **140**, 2555–61.

Epstein, C. J. (1985). Werner's syndrome and aging: a reappraisal. In *Werner's syndrome and human aging, advances in experimental medicine and biology*, Vol. 190 (ed. D. Salk, Y. Fujiwara, and G. M. Martin), pp. 219–27. Plenum, New York.

Epstein, C. J., Martin, G. M., Schultz, A. L., and Motulsky, A. G. (1966). Werner's syndrome: a review of its symptomatology, natural history, pathologic features, genetics and relationship to the natural aging process. *Medicine*, **45**, 177–221.

Finch, C. E. and Sapolsky, R. M. (1999). The evolution of Alzheimer disease, the reproductive schedule, and apoE isoforms. *Neurobiology of Aging*, **20**, 407–28.

Flannery, G. R., Baum, H., and Bittles, A. H. (1989). Mitochondrial antigenic structure and enzyme activity in ageing human diploid fibroblasts. *Annals of Human Biology*, **16**, 259–64.

Fleming, J. E., Miquel, J., and Bensch, K. G. (1985). Age dependent changes in mitochondria. In *Molecular biology of aging* (ed. A. D. Woodhead, A. D. Blackett, and A. Hollaender), pp. 143–56. Plenum, New York.

Frenck, R. W., Blackburn, E. H., and Shannon, K. M. (1998). The rate of telomere sequence loss in human leukocytes varies with age. *Proceedings of the National Academy of Sciences, USA*, **95**, 5607–10.

Fries, J. F. (1980). Aging, natural death, and the compression of morbidity. *New England Journal of Medicine*, **303**, 130–5.

Fukuchi, K., Martin, G. M., and Monnat, R. J. (1989). Mutator phenotype of Werner syndrome is characterized by extensive deletions. *Proceedings of the National Academy of Sciences, USA*, **86**, 5893–7.

Goto, M., Tanimoto, K., Horiuchi, Y., and Sasazuki, T. (1981). Family analysis of Werner's syndrome: a survey of 42 Japanese families with a review of the literature. *Clinical Genetics*, **19**, 8–15.

Goto, M., Rubenstein, M., Weber, J., Woods, K., and Drayna, D. (1992). Genetic linkage of Werner's syndrome to five markers on chromosome 8. *Nature, London*, **355**, 735–8.

Gutteridge, J. M. C., Westermarck, T., and Halliwell, B. (1986). Oxygen radical damage in biological systems. In *Free radicals, aging and degenerative diseases*, Modern Aging Research Vol. 8 (ed. J. E. Johnson, R. Walford, D. Harman, and J. Miquel), pp. 99–139. Alan R. Liss, New York.

Halestrap, A. (2000). Mitochondria and cell death. *The Biochemist*, **22**, 19–24.

Hall, K. Y., Hart, R. W., Benirschke, A. K., and Walford, R. L. (1984). Correlation between ultraviolet-induced DNA repair in primate lymphocytes and fibroblasts and species maximum achievable life span. *Mechanisms of Ageing and Development*, **24**, 163–73.

Harley, C. B. (1991). Telomere loss: mitotic clock or genetic time bomb? *Mutation Research*, **256**, 271–82.

Harley, C. B., Futcher, A. B., and Greider, C. W. (1990). Telomeres shorten during ageing of human fibroblasts. *Nature, London*, **345**, 458–60.

Harman, D. (1956). Aging: a theory based on free radical and radiation chemistry. *Journal of Gerontology*, **11**, 298–300.

Harman, D. (1983). Free radical theory of aging: consequences of mitochondrial aging. *Age*, **6**, 86–94.

Harman, D. (1986). Free radical theory of aging: role of free radicals in the origination and evolution of life, aging, and disease processes. In *Free radicals, aging, and degenerative diseases*, Modern Aging Research Vol. 8 (ed. J. E. Johnston, R. Walford, D. Harman, and J. Miquel), pp. 3–49. Alan R. Liss, New York.

Harman, D. (1992). Free radical theory of aging. *Mutation Research*, **275**, 257–66.

Hart, R. W. and Setlow, R. B. (1974). Correlation between deoxyribonucleic acid excision repair and lifespan in a number of mammalian species. *Proceedings of the National Academy of Sciences, USA*, **71**, 2169–73.

Hart, R. W. and Turturro, A. (1987). Review of recent biological research in the theories of aging. In *Review of biological research in aging*, Vol. 3 (ed. M. Rothstein), pp. 15–21. Alan R. Liss, New York.

Hayashi, J. I., Ohta, S., Kagawa, Y., Kondo, H., Kaneda, H., Yonekawa, H., *et al.* (1994). Nuclear but not mitochondrial genome involvement in human age-related mitochondrial dysfunction. *Journal of Biological Chemistry*, **269**, 6878–83.

Hayflick, L. (1965). The limited *in vitro* lifetime of human diploid cell strains. *Experimental Cell Research*, **37**, 614–36.

Hayflick, L. and Moorhead, P. S. (1961). The serial cultivation of human diploid cell strains. *Experimental Cell Research*, **25**, 585–621.

Hengartner, M. O. (2000). The biochemistry of apoptosis. *Nature*, **407**, 770–6.

Herskind, A. M., McGue, M., Holm, N. V., Sørensen, T. I. A., Harvald, B., and Vaupel, J. W. (1996). The heritability of human longevity: a population-based study of 2872 Danish twin pairs born 1870–1900. *Human Genetics*, **97**, 319–23.

Holehan, A. M. and Merry, B. J. (1986) The experimental manipulation of ageing by diet. *Biological Reviews*, **61**, 329–68.

Holliday, R. (1986). Strong effects of 5-azacytidine on the *in vitro* life span of human diploid fibroblasts. *Experimental Cell Research*, **166**, 543–52.

Holliday, R. (1987). The inheritance of epigenetic defects. *Science*, **238**, 163–70.

Holliday, R. (1996). The evolution of human longevity. *Perspectives in Biology and Medicine*, **40**, 100–7.

Holt, I. J. and Jacobs, H. T. (1994). The structure and expression of normal and mutant mitochondrial genomes. In *Mitochondria: DNA, proteins and disease* (ed. V. Darley-Usmar and A. H. V. Schapira), pp. 27–54. Portland, London.

Hsieh, R-H., Hou, J-H., Hsu, H-S., and Wei, Y-H. (1994). Age-dependent respiratory function decline and DNA deletions in human muscle mitochondria. *Biochemistry and Molecular Biology International*, **32**, 1009–22.

Ikebe, S., Tanaka, M., Ohno, K., Sata, W., Hattori, K., Kondo, T., *et al.* (1990). Increase of deleted mitochondrial DNA in the striatum in Parkinson's disease and senescence. *Biochemistry and Biophysics Research Communications*, **170**, 1044–8.

Jarvik, L. F., Falek, A., Kallman, F. J., and Lorge, I. (1960). Survival trends in a senescent twin population. *American Journal of Human Genetics*, **12**, 170–9.

Jeune, B. and Vaupel, J. (ed.) (1999). *Validation of exceptional longevity.* Odense University Press, Odense.

Johnson, J. E. (1979). Fine structure of IMR-90 cells in culture as examined by scanning and transmission electron microscopy. *Mechanisms of Ageing and Development*, **10**, 405–43.

Johnson, T. E. (1988). Genetic specification of life span: processes, problems and potentials. *Journal of Gerontology: Biological Sciences*, **43**, B87–92.

Kannisto, V., Lauritsen, J., Thatcher, A. R., and Vaupel, J. W. (1994). Reductions in mortality at advanced ages. *Population and Development Review*, **20**, 793–810.

Khalifa, M. M. (1989). Hutchinson–Gilford progeria syndrome: report of a Libyan family and evidence of autosomal recessive inheritance. *Clinical Genetics*, **35**, 125–32.

Kirkland, J.L (1989). Evolution and ageing. *Genome*, **31**, 398–405.

Kirkwood, T. B. L. (1977). Evolution of ageing. *Nature, London*, **270**, 301–4.

Kirkwood, T. B. L. and Holliday, R. (1986). Ageing as a consequence of natural selection. In *The biology of human ageing* (ed. A. H. Bittles and K. J. Collins), pp. 1–16. Cambridge University Press, Cambridge.

Kitagawa, T., Suganuma, N., Nawa, A., Kikkawa, F., Tanaka, M., Ozawa, T., *et al.* (1993). Rapid accumulation of deleted mitochondrial deoxyribonucleic acid in postmenopausal ovaries. *Biology of Reproduction*, **49**, 730–6.

Kohn, R. R. (1982*a*). Causes of death in very old people. *Journal of the American Medical Association*, **247**, 2793–7.

Kohn, R. R. (1982*b*). *Principles of mammalian aging* (2nd edn). Prentice-Hall, Englewood Cliffs, NJ.

Ku, H-K., Brunk, U. T., and Sohal, R. S. (1993). Relationship between mitochondrial superoxide and hydrogen peroxide production and longevity of mammalian species. *Free Radicals in Biology and Medicine*, **15**, 621–7.

Lanza, R. P., Cibelli, J. B., Blackwell, C., Cristofalo, V. J., Francis, M. K., Baerlocher, G. M., *et al.* (2000). Extension of cell life-span and telomere length in animals cloned from senescent somatic cells. *Science*, **288**, 665–9.

Lee, C-K., Klopp, R. G., Weindruch, R., and Prolla, T. A. (1999). Gene expression profile of aging and its retardation by caloric restriction. *Science*, **285**, 1390–3.

Lee, H-C., Pang, C-Y., Hsu, H-S., and Wei, Y-H. (1994). Differential accumulations of 4,977 bp deletion in mitochondrial DNA of various tissues in human ageing. *Biochimica et Biophysica Acta*, **1226**, 37–43.

Li, H., Kolluri, S. K., Gu, J., Dawson, M. I., Cao, X., Hobbs, P. D., *et al.* (2000). Cytochrome *c* release and apoptosis induced by mitochondrial targeting of nuclear orphan receptor TR3. *Science*, **289**, 1159–64.

Lin, S-J., Defossez, P-A., and Guarente, L. (2000). Requirement of NAD and *SIR2* for life-extension by calorie restriction in *Saccharomyces cerevisiae*. *Science*, **289**, 2126–8.

Linnane, A. W., Marzuki, S., Ozawa, T., and Tanaka, M. (1989). Mitochondrial DNA mutations as an important contributor to ageing and degenerative diseases. *Lancet*, **1**, 642–5.

Linnane, A. W., Baumer, A., Maxwell, R. J., Preston, H., Zhang, C., and Marzuki, S. (1990). Mitochondrial gene mutation: the ageing process and degenerative diseases. *Biochemistry International*, **22**, 1067–76.

Luhtala, T. A., Roecker, E. B., Pugh, T., Feuers, R. J., and Weindruch, R. (1994). Dietary restriction attenuates age-related increases in rat skeletal muscle antioxidant enzyme activities. *Journal of Gerontology*, **49**, B231–8.

Ly, D. H., Lockhart, D. J., Lerner, R. A., and Schultz, P. G. (2000). Mitotic misregulation and human aging. *Science*, **287**, 2486–92.

McCarter, R., Masoro, E. J., and Yu, B. P. (1985). Does food restriction retard aging by reducing the metabolic rate? *American Journal of Physiology*, **248**, E488–90.

McCay, C. M., Crowell, M. F., and Maynard, L. A. (1935). The effect of retarded growth upon the length of lifespan and upon the ultimate body size. *Journal of Nutrition*, **10**, 63–79.

McCay, C. M., Ellis, G. H., Barnes, L. L., Smith, C. A. H., and Sperling, G. (1939). Clinical and pathological changes in aging and after retarded growth. *Journal of Nutrition*, **18**, 15–25.

McFarland, G. A. and Holliday, R. (1994). Retardation of the senescence of cultured human diploid fibroblasts by carnosine. *Experimental Cell Research*, **212**, 167–75.

Macieira-Coelho, A. (1988). *Biology of normal proliferating cells in vitro: relevance for in vivo aging*. Karger, Basel.

Manton, K. G. and Land, K. C. (2000). Active life expectancy estimates for the U. S. elderly population: a multidimensional continuous-mixture model of functional change applied to completed cohorts, 1982–1996. *Demography*, **37**, 253–65.

Manton, K. G. and Yashin, A. I. (2000) *Mechanisms of aging, and mortality: the search for new paradigms*. Odense University Press, Odense.

Martin, G. M. (1985). Genetics and aging: the Werner syndrome as a segmental progeroid syndrome. In *Werner's syndrome and human aging, advances in experimental medicine and biology*, Vol. 190 (ed. D. Salk, Y. Fujiwara, and G. M. Martin), pp. 161–70, Plenum, New York.

Martin, G. M. (1989). Genetic modulation of the senescent phenotype in *Homo sapiens*. *Genome*, **31**, 390–7.

Martin, G. R., Danner, D. B., and Holbrook, N. J. (1993). Aging—causes and defenses. *Annual Review of Medicine*, **44**, 419–29.

Masoro, E. J. (1988). Food restriction in rodents: an evaluation of its role in the study of aging. *Journal of Gerontology*, **43**, B59–64.

Mecocci, P., MacGarvey, U., Kaufman, A. E., Koontz, D., Shoffner, J. M., Wallace, D. C., *et al.* (1993). Oxidative damage to mitochondrial DNA shows marked age-dependent increases in human brain. *Annals of Neurology*, **34**, 609–6.

Melov, S., Ravenscroft, J., Malik, S., Gill, M. S., Walker, D. W., Clayton, P. E., *et al.* (2000). Extension of lifespan with superoxide dismutase/catalase mimetics. *Science*, **289**, 1567–9.

Miquel, J. (1991). An integrated theory of aging as the result of mitochondrial-DNA mutation in differentiated cells. *Archives of Gerontology and Geriatrics*, **12**, 99–117.

Moore, C. J. and Schwartz, A. G. (1978). Inverse correlation between species lifespan and capacity of cultured fibroblasts to convert benzo(a)pyrene to water-soluble metabolites. *Experimental Cell Research*, **116**, 359–64.

Münscher, C., Müller-Höcker, J., and Kadenbach, B. (1993). Human ageing is associated with various point mutations in tRNA genes of mitochondrial DNA. *Biological Chemistry Hoppe-Seyler*, **374**, 1099–104.

Murphy, E. A. (1978). Genetics of longevity in man. In *The genetics of ageing* (ed. E. L. Schneider), pp. 261–302. Plenum Press, New York.

Ogihara, T., Hata, T., Tanaka, K., Fukuchi, K., Tabuchi, Y., and Kumahara, Y. (1986). Hutchinson–Gilford progeria syndrome in a 45-year-old man. *American Journal of Medical Genetics*, **81**, 135–8.

Olshansky, S. J. and Carnes, B. A. (1997). Ever since Gompertz. *Demography*, **34**, 1–15.

Olshansky, S. J., Carnes, B. A., and Cassel, C. (1990). In search of Methusaleh: estimating the upper limits to human longevity. *Science*, **250**, 634–40.

Orgel, L. E. (1963). The maintenance of the accuracy of protein synthesis and its relevance to aging. *Proceedings of the National Academy of Sciences, USA*, **49**, 517–21.

Orgel, L. E. (1973). Ageing of clones of mammalian cells. *Nature, London*, **243**, 441–5.

Pang, C-Y., Lee, H-C., Yang, J-H., and Wei, Y-H. (1994). Human skin mitochondrial DNA deletions associated with light exposure. *Archives of Biochemistry and Biophysics*, **312**, 534–8.

Parsons, P. A. (1995). Inherited stress resistance and longevity: a stress theory of ageing. *Heredity*, **74**, 216–21.

Pashko, L. L. and Schwartz, A. G. (1982). Inverse correlation between species' lifespan and species' cytochrome P-488 content of cultured fibroblasts. *Journal of Gerontology*, **37**, 38–41.

Patrick, J. S., Thorpe, S. R., and Baynes, J. W. (1990). Nonenzymatic glycosylation of protein does not increase with age in normal lenses. *Journal of Gerontology*, **45**, B18–23.

Pearl, R. and Pearl, R. de W. (1934). Studies on human longevity. VI The distribution and correlation of variation in the total immediate ancestral longevity of nonagenarians and centenarians, in relation to the inheritance factor in duration of life. *Human Biology*, **6**, 98–222.

Pereira-Smith, O. M. and Smith, J. R. (1983). Evidence for the recessive nature of cellular immortality. *Science*, **221**, 964–6.

Perls, T. T., Bubrick, E., Wager, C. G., Vijg, J., and Kruglyak, L. (1998). Siblings of centenarians live longer. *Lancet*, **351**, 1560.

Philippe, P. (1978). Familial correlations of longevity: an isolate-based study. *American Journal of Medical Genetics*, **2**, 121–9.

PRB (1999). *World population data sheet, 1999*. Population Reference Bureau, Washington, DC.

Proust, J., Moulias, R., Fumeron, F., Bekkhoucha, F., Busson, M., Schmid, M., *et al.* (1982). HLA and longevity. *Tissue Antigens*, **19**, 168–73.

Reznick, D. N. and Ghalambor, C. (1999). Sex and death. *Science*, **286**, 2458–9.

Richter, C., Park, J. W., and Ames, B. N. (1988). Normal oxidative damage to mitochondrial and nuclear DNA is extensive. *Proceedings of the National Academy of Sciences, USA*, **85**, 6465–7.

Robine, J. M. and Allard, M. (1998). The oldest old. *Science*, **279**, 1834–5.

Rogers, R. G. (1995). Sociodemographic characteristics of long-lived and healthy individuals. *Population and Development Review*, **21**, 33–58.

Rohme, D. (1981). Evidence for a relationship between longevity of mammalian species and life spans of normal fibroblasts *in vitro* and erythrocytes *in vivo*. *Proceedings of the National Academy of Sciences, USA*, **78**, 5009–13.

Ryan, A. S., Martinez, G. A., Wysong, J. L., and Davis, M. A. (1989). Dietary patterns of older adults in the United States, NHANES II 1976–1980. *American Journal of Human Biology*, **1**, 321–30.

Sacher G. A. (1959). Relation of lifespan to brain weight and body weight in mammals. In *The lifespan of animals*, Ciba Foundation Colloquia on aging No. 5 (ed. G. E. W. Wolstenholme and M. O'Connor), pp. 114–41. Churchill, London.

Sacher, G. A. (1975). Maturation and longevity in relation to cranial capacity in hominid evolution. In *Antecedents of man and after*, Vol. 1 Primates: functional morphology and evolution (ed. R. Tuttle), pp. 417–41. Mouton, The Hague.

Sacher, G. A. (1976). Evaluation of the entropy and information terms governing mammalian longevity. In *Cellular ageing: concepts and mechanisms*, Interdisciplinary topics in gerontology, Vol. 9 (ed. R. G. Cutler), pp. 69–82. Karger, Basel.

Salk, D. (1982). Werner's syndrome: a review of recent research with an analysis of connective tissue metabolism, growth control of cultured cells and chromosomal aberrations. *Human Genetics*, **62**, 1–15.

Sambuy, Y. and Bittles, A. H. (1982). The effects of *in vitro* ageing on the composition of the intracellular free amino acid pool of human diploid fibroblasts. *Mechanisms of Ageing and Development*, **20**, 279–87.

Scappaticci, S., Forabosco, A., Borroni, G., Orecchia, G., and Fraccaro, M. (1990). Clonal structural chromosomal rearrangements in lymphocytes of four patients with Werner's syndrome. *Annals of Human Genetics*, **33**, 5–8.

Schächter, F., Faure-Delanef, L., Guénot, F., Rouger, H., Froguel, P., Lesueur-Ginot, L., *et al.* (1994). Genetic associations with human longevity at the APOE and ACE loci. *Nature Genetics*, **6**, 29–32.

Schneider, E. L. and Brody, J. A. (1983). Aging, natural death and the compression of morbidity: another view. *New England Journal of Medicine*, **309**, 854–5.

Schnider, S. L. and Kohn, R. R. (1981). Effects of age and diabetes mellitus on the solubility of collagen and nonenzymatic glycolysation of human skin collagen. *Journal of Clinical Investigation*, **67**, 1630–5.

Schwartz, A. G. and Moore, C. J. (1977). Inverse correlation between species life span and capacity of cultured fibroblasts to bind 7,12 dimethylbenz(a)anthracene to DNA. *Experimental Cell Research*, **109**, 448–50.

Sgrò, C. M. and Partridge, L. (1999). A delayed wave of death from reproduction in *Drosophila*. *Science*, **286**, 2521–4.

Shiels, P. G., Kind, A. J., Campbell, K. H. S., Waddington, D., Wilmut, I., Colman, A., *et al.* (1999). Analysis of telomere lengths in cloned sheep. *Nature, London*, **39**, 316–17.

Spector, I. M. (1974). Animal longevity and protein turnover rates. *Nature (New Biology)*, **249**, 66.

Steller, H. (1995). Mechanisms and genes of cellular suicide. *Science*, **267**, 1445–9.

Strehler, B., Birsch, G., Gussek, D., Johnson, R., and Bick, M. (1971). Codon-restriction theory of aging and development. *Journal of Theoretical Biology*, **33**, 429–74.

Suomalainen, A., Kaukonen, J., Amati, P., Timonen, R., Haltia, M., Weissenbach, J., *et al.* (1995). An autosomal locus predisposing to deletions of mitochondrial DNA. *Nature Genetics*, **9**, 146–51.

Szilard, L. (1959). On the nature of the ageing process. *Proceedings of the National Academy of Sciences, USA*, **45**, 30–45.

Tauchi, H. and Sato, T. (1985). Cellular changes in senescence: possible factors influencing the process of cellular ageing. In *Thresholds in ageing* (ed. M. Bergener, M. Ermini, and H. B. Stahelin), pp. 91–113. Academic Press, London.

Thompson, C. B. (1995). Apoptosis in the pathogenesis and treatment of disease. *Science*, **267**, 1456–62.

Tolmasoff, J. M., Ono, T., and Cutler, R. G. (1980). Superoxide dismutase: correlation with lifespan and specific metabolic rates in primate species. *Proceedings of the National Academy of Sciences, USA*, **77**, 2777–81.

Trounce, I., Bryne, E., and Marzuki, S. (1989). Decline in human skeletal muscle mitochondrial respiratory chain function: possible factor in ageing. *Lancet*, **1**, 637–9.

Trovato, F. and Lalu, N. M. (1998). Contributions of cause-specific mortality to changing sex differences in life expectancy: seven nations case study. *Social Biology*, **45**, 1–20.

Tuljapurkar, S., Li, N., and Boe, C. (2000). A universal pattern of mortality decline in the G7 countries. *Nature, London*, **405**, 789–92.

Tzagoloff, A. and Myers, A. M. (1986). Genetics of mitochondrial biogenesis. *Annual Review of Biochemistry*, **55**, 249–85.

Voos, W., Moczko, M., and Pfanner, N. (1994). Targeting, translocation and folding of mitochondrial preproteins. In *Mitochondria: DNA, proteins and disease* (ed. V. Darley-Usmar and A. H. V. Schapira), pp. 55–80. Portland, London.

Weindruch, R. and Walford, R. L. (1982). Life span and spontaneous cancer incidence in mice dietarily restricted beginning at one year of age. *Science*, **215**, 1415–8.

Westendorp, R. G. J. and Kirkwood, T. B. L. (1998). Human longevity at the cost of reproductive success. *Nature, London*, **396**, 743–6.

Williams, G. C. (1957). Pleiotropy, natural selection and the evolution of senescence. *Evolution*, **11**, 398–411.

Wilmoth, J. R. and Horiuchi, S. (1999). Rectangularization revisited: variability of age at death within human populations. *Demography*, **36**, 475–95.

Wolkow, C. A., Kimura, K. D., Lee, M-S., and Ruvkun, G. (2000). Regulation of *C. elegans* life-span by insulinlike signaling in the nervous system. *Science*, **290**, 147–50.

Yen, T. C., Su, J. H., King, K. L., and Wei, Y. H. (1991). Ageing-associated 5 kb deletion in human liver mitochondrial DNA. *Biochemistry and Biophysics Research Communications*, **178**, 124–31.

Yu, B. P., Masoro, E. J., and McMahan, C. A. (1985). Nutritional influences on aging of Fischer 344 rats: I. Physical, metabolic and longevity characteristics. *Journal of Gerontology*, **40**, 657–70.

Yu, C-E., Oshima, J., Fu, Y-H., Wijsman, E. M., Hisama, F., Alsich, R., *et al.* (1996). Positional cloning of the Werner's syndrome gene. *Science*, **272**, 258–62.

Yuan, J. and Yanker, B. A. (2000). Apoptosis in the nervous system. *Nature*, **407**, 802–9.

Zhang, C., Linnane, A. W., and Nagley, P. (1993). Occurrence of a particular base substitution (3243 A to G) in mitochondrial DNA of tissues of ageing humans. *Biochemical and Biophysical Research Communications*, **195**, 1104–10.

Zhou, J. Q., Monson, E. K., Teng, S-C., Schulz, V. P., and Zakian, V. A. (2000). Pif1p helicase, a catalytic inhibitor of telomerase in yeast. *Science*, **289**, 771–4.

2 The sociology of ageing

Janet Askham

...no science can ignore the fact that the explanation of real world phenomena requires interdisciplinary collaboration. Social relations never exist in isolation, even though they are the focus of sociological explanation. Sociologists can't ignore biology or economics, but the converse applies also.

(Albrow 1999)

Sociological investigation

Sociology is concerned with explaining and interpreting the impact of scientific, technological, environmental, and demographic changes on social life and with the way in which social relations respond to these changes. Ageing is a social as well as a biological phenomenon, and is constructed through social relationships. We know this—as we know about all other socially constructed phenomena—from the fact that the social standing and roles of older people have not always and everywhere been the same (Holmes and Holmes 1995; Minois 1989). Thus has developed a sociology of ageing. The topics such sociologists study have been influenced by what 'people' (either inside or outside their discipline) have considered problematic about older people or growing older. In addition, the problematic nature of the subject has tended to be led by social policy analysts or the health professions: why are some older people poor, living on their own, unable to manage in the community, liable to victimization, and so on. But there is more to social aspects of ageing than this. As well as studying the socially problematic, sociologists also investigate the intellectually problematic in a search for meaning, and they may indeed point out what is working to people's advantage and/or to the support of what they see as fundamental human values. The questions sociologists ask spring mainly from their theories about society, or from previous sociological research findings or current social trends or changes. Of course what we choose to study is a product of the kind of knowledge and the system of values prevailing in the society we inhabit. This is a very interesting time to be studying the sociology of ageing because the rapid social changes now occurring affect all aspects of social life including ageing and the social experiences of older people. The chapter begins therefore with a brief discussion of these broad social changes. It then—again briefly—reviews major theories affecting what is studied and how it is interpreted. Finally it examines some of the key areas of sociological research on ageing.

Although we shall present some statistical data in this chapter it should be remembered that 'statistical data by themselves do not make sociology...The enumerations are meaningful... only in terms of their much broader implications for an understanding of institutions and values in our society.' (Berger 1963)

The impact of social change/postmodernization

Western society has seen radical changes over the past 30 or 40 years, changes which have been gathering momentum in recent decades. These changes are often described as a move to a 'postmodern' society. Although it is impossible to be dogmatic or precise about them whilst we are in the midst of the process of transition, none the less there is a good deal of agreement about the key social trends.

'Postmodern' was preceded by 'modern' society, and by 'traditional' before that. 'Modernity' is distinguished by the key characteristics:

- rationality (based on knowledge derived from science) coupled with a belief in social progress;
- an impersonal bureaucratic style of management and administration, organized around capitalist industrialized economic production (leading crucially to major social divisions based on ownership and control of economic resources);
- and supported by a common culture through the institutions of religion (purveying, for example, the ethic of hard work and duty), family, education, and the nation state.

'Postmodern' society, seen to have been in growing ascendancy since around the 1960s (but of course with seeds inherent within 'modern' society), is characterized predominantly by a declining belief in the notion of social progress and a decreasing sense of societal direction (for example, with the development of science and technology merely for its own sake, and with many of its effects unknown or seen as detrimental to human well-being). The older overarching social structures and institutions are fragmenting and losing their control over individual experience. For example, the way in which we accord value to things is changing. Sociologists studying crime have shown that we are less likely to judge crimes by standards seen as inculcated by the church or educational institutions, but more according to our own standards of what is right and wrong. With this has come the vast proliferation of groups and subgroups within a more fragmented and increasingly dynamic society. Such societies have also been defined as risk societies because individuals are increasingly faced by choices which they must make in the absence of any certainty about outcomes (Beck 1992).

The old divisions of society organized around class are breaking up as industry, in Western societies, has moved away from the manufacture of goods towards service industry and as technological advances have changed the production process (with labour skills required to be flexible and responsive to the dynamism of technology and consumer choice). Consumption rather than production has become the prime organizing principle of the economy, with the need to create, inform, and satisfy a multitude of new and proliferating consumer markets. As a consequence, social differentiation is based not so much on its relation to the production process but on shared, shifting, and media-influenced lifestyles. Indeed in the postmodern world the culture of style and taste has achieved tremendous force through mass and global communication in the search for markets. Thomas and Walsh (1998), perhaps in an exaggeration of current social trends, express some of this change in the following way:

> So social differentiation in the postmodern world becomes a fluid mosaic of media-simulated and media-imagined multiple status identities which are based, not on location in society or work, but in consumption and access to codes which display themselves in mass participation and social movement politics. (p. 384)

The nation state is losing its prime position of authority and control as markets become more international and weapons of warfare can bring about global destructiveness. It is also losing control as welfare services become impossible to deliver: for whilst expectations rise, willingness to contribute through taxation declines along with the rising desire of citizens to control their own spending power, in the increasingly individualistic society of today.

The emphasis on individual identity is a key feature of postmodernization. It is becoming more possible to develop changing and flexible identities (again spearheaded by the search for ever new consumer markets). Difference has become acceptable, even encouraged, rather than repressed under the former domination of powerful institutions or particular groups, such as men or White ethnic communities. The body itself has become a prime site for these markets, partly because of the ageing of the population and consumer demands for treatment, body care, and the maintenance of youthfulness. This growing acceptability of difference should not, however, necessarily be seen as a sign of social progress, for it brings with it its own problems: ontological insecurity because of the unreality of the identities; the possibility of conflict between groups (in fact, conflict may be more likely if the old dominations—and the respect for authority which went with them (Albrow 1999)—are breaking down); and castigation and disadvantage for people who cannot buy into the favoured lifestyles. Thus even without the improvements in life expectancy, social ageing is changing and our central question must be to do with the impact of postmodernity or advanced modernity on ageing and how it can be interpreted.

This immediately raises the problem of whether a postmodern society needs different kinds of explanatory theory from those which applied to modern society. For sociologists are often considered to be adherents of the 'grand narrative', that is: belief in the dominance of one particular set of explanatory social forces, supported by a belief in an underlying reality, and in the possibility of social progress. In leaving behind the notion of social progress (which was one of the hallmarks of 'modern' society), sociological theory itself has undergone considerable change in adapting to postmodern society.

Explanatory social theories

It is certainly the case that, along with the undisputed social changes, we have developed different ways of explaining social life, and therefore also of conceiving the future. Theories have moved away from the Descarteian rationalism of modernism towards poststructuralist theory in which:

> the idea of the individual as a self-reflecting, rational, unified, fixed subject is rejected in favour of a dislocated, contradictory, fragmented subjectivity which is not fixed but reconstituted in language on each and every occasion we speak. (Thomas and Walsh 1998, p. 367)

Under the rationalistic theories of the founding fathers of sociology—Karl Marx, Max Weber, and Emile Durkheim—there was a belief in an underlying reality. For Marx of course, and to some extent Weber, the key explanatory force was the economic substructure of a society, with power vested in those who controlled the means of production, and with social institutions and culture (superstructure) developing to support this power structure. Power makes for inequality and divides society into groupings or classes of those with greater or lesser control. Durkheim put greater explanatory emphasis on the superstructure, which was seen as holding an increasingly differentiated society together through a common culture purveyed through social institutions such as the church, family, and education. In studying older people such theorists asked about, and sought to explain, their socially disadvantaged position (e.g. their lack or loss of power or social roles). Indeed, inequality has for many years been a guiding theme in the sociology of ageing. Those who placed the emphasis on the economic base explained the social position of older people as being a direct consequence of their current and former position in relation to economic production. Those who focused more on knowledge, values, beliefs, or social institutions saw older people as being necessarily marginalized to allow for the development and implementation of new ideas and skills, particularly within the economy but also in other social institutions.

To more recent theorists there is no single reality but only multiple and changing meanings. Therefore there can be no such thing as social progress, liberation, or emancipation because we can have no immutable standards against which to judge it. For example, the old sexual restrictions of the nineteenth century were thought by believers in social progress to have been discarded in favour of the sexual liberation of the twentieth, until the theorist Michel Foucault (1979), argued that the so-called liberation is itself only another form of repression (in that nowadays we are obliged to be defined by our sexuality). Foucault showed that power is incorporated within prevailing forms of knowledge, purporting to be the 'truth', and operates not just through the class system (as emphasized by Marx) but as a general force in society distinct from any agents. To oppose it therefore means to 'critique' it: to reveal it through reason, the way it works, and what it does to people. This view has provoked some very interesting arguments. Some take a very conservative position, believing that it is impossible to see beyond the forms of knowledge which constrain us. Others might say that there is no point in attempting to understand the social position of older people so that one may help to improve it, because any such 'improvement' would only be another form of repression. However, not all agree, seeing poststructuralism as undermined by its own stance: if there is no truth, then poststructuralism is not true either; and many believe there is much of value in Foucauldian analysis, not excluding the fact that Foucault himself could, by comparative analysis, see beyond the strictures of prevailing knowledge. In fact, sociology could not continue to exist if it took the conservative poststructuralist view.

Adherents of 'critical theory' (or for ageing, 'critical gerontology') agree with the philosopher and theorist Jurgen Habermas about the possibility of emancipation, and with Foucault and others about the need to examine current practices in order to show the partial nature of the 'truths' they claim to embody. Current (or Habermasian) critical theory is basically optimistic, seeing emancipation as possible through critiquing rather than opposing the forces of power. Power is seen as embodied in culture—i.e. knowledge, values, tastes, and images—as well as in economic relations and structures, and separate from any agencies which may administer it, so therefore opposition to agents of power is unlikely to be successful. Making people aware of the way in which things are defined and ordered liberates them from their repression and enables them to see other ways of being. For Habermas 'emancipatory interest, the desire to be freed of all oppression' and 'the interest in understanding one another' (Cuff *et al.* 1990) are fundamental human interests, and he believed that they will allow us to reach an agreement about the nature of the social world not dominated by one set of instrumental interests.

This debate between the optimists and conservatives is emotional as well as contentious. Although it can only be touched on briefly here, it is important to bear it in mind because of the enormous emphasis that 'sociology of ageing' research places on the drive to improve the social position of older people. Thus some researchers still believe in the possibility of social progress. For example, Johnson (1998) says that the public policy and labour-market systems which have developed over the last 50 years have had a profound and largely beneficial effect on the lives of older people in the UK, whose 'command over resources and their political and social standing appear to have been unmatched in past societies' (p. 224). In the main however, although the social theories of today still lead sociologists of ageing to ask questions about repression and disadvantage, they seek the answers in different areas: for example, in the understandings, views, and images presented about older people through cultural representations that may influence the way they are treated and the social roles which they occupy. These theories also suggest the need to examine social differences and divisions: not just in the old 'grand narrative' tradition of economic structures and general social status, but in relation to the many spheres of differentiation now accepted as conveying the partial and manifold realities of social life. These theories now acknowledge that social change is brought about not just through major upheavals in the economy or scientific advances, but also through the interactions of individuals and groups of individuals in the fluidity of discourse. That is to say, we all help to bring about change. From this theoretical perspective arises the need to examine these individual interactions at even the most basic levels of social life. Although emancipation may be an unattainable goal, none the less the difficult task of exploring social constraints and the ways in which they operate, remains the sociological aim.

Old age in postmodern society

The individual or social actor

Individuals possess some relatively enduring traits. Many of these (e.g. colour of eyes) may not be particularly significant as defining or explanatory factors for social behaviour, but others are highly significant. Most important as key defining traits (apart from social class) are gender, ethnicity, and age. Of course, age is constantly changing but it is an enduring trait in the sense that one carries one's chronological age in a predictable way (59 never follows 60) throughout life. A person's generation too is important, that is—to use one definition—the stratum of people who were born at around the same time and have therefore shared some of the same cultural and social experiences at about the same age. Many might argue that age is less important than the other enduring traits, because the inequalities due to age (or generation) are smaller and less important than those resulting from gender, class position, or ethnic group (Attias-Donfut and Arber 2000); none the less, age plays a highly significant part. Some argue that the postmodern world allows us, as never before, flexibility over these traits. Gender used to be seen as assigned at birth and unchanging, but now we acknowledge both that people may change their sex, and that they can conceal it or minimize the differences between the sexes. The same is true of age to some extent. Through dress, diet, exercise, and body manipulation, age has become less visible. For this reason some have said that the postmodern age 'could lead to the liberation of elderly people' (Abbott and Wallace 1997). However, this is a highly contentious proposition. This section asks in what sense age influences people's socially constructed sense of identity, and the impact on them of postmodern trends. Later sections examine how the institutions of the economy, family, biomedicine, and the state define and treat older people.

Individuals can be said to consist of constellations of social roles which adhere to form a particular type of *social identity* (for example, elderly–female–spouse–carer). Individuals also have a deeper sense of self or *personal identity*, formed through social interaction and maintained as a *sine qua non* within our culture. One of the abiding topics for sociologists of ageing has been the change with age in this constellation of social roles. For many years it was assumed that as people age they lose social roles, and even today this view can often be found. But the emphasis on roles identified with economic production (and the accompanying family roles of maintaining the health and well-being of the workers and of rearing the next generation)—vital though they are—neglects the other roles that make up a social identity. Even before older people's role as consumers was recognized, they had many other social roles which did not disappear with retirement from paid employment. For example, it is now acknowledged that the role of parent continues into the child's adult life, and likewise for grandparents' and other kin relationships. In addition, there are the roles of care recipient or patient, caregiver, friend and neighbour, association member, voluntary worker, pet owner, television viewer, voter, home owner or tenant, leisure pursuer. Some of these roles will take up as much time as paid work (if not more), some will be a more important part of the person's conception of herself. Each will similarly involve a moral element, with expectations of how that role should be executed, and be a means whereby a person imbibes or expresses some of the key values of his or her community or society. Being a pensioner or retiree is often not seen as a social role in itself (though this could be disputed, since there are some expectations about how such people should and should not behave). But, although the key defining role of paid employee may have been lost, people continue to demonstrate their class and status position in the way in which they fulfil these other roles. So, although in one sense identity may change as the constellation of social roles one inhabits changes with age, much of what underlies these roles is likely to remain the same.

Considering the deeper sense of personal identity, sociologists have also asked whether this also changes as people age, and if so why. Perhaps the most obvious contributor to a person's sense of self, and which changes with age, is the body. As Giddens says:

> 'The body' sounds a simple notion, particularly as compared to concepts like 'self' or 'self-identity.' The body is an object in which we are all privileged, or doomed, to dwell, the source of feelings of well-being and pleasure, but also the site of illnesses and strains.

> However...the body is not just a physical entity which we 'possess', it is an action-system, a mode of praxis, and its practical immersion in the interactions of day-to-day life is an essential part of the sustaining of a coherent sense of self-identity. (Giddens 1991, p. 99)

Thus the way people feel about their bodies, and the way other people react to them, will influence the way they see themselves; and this may be increasingly the case in postmodern society when the body has become a more important part of the sense of identity. Since aged bodies and minds are considered neither beautiful nor efficient in our society (nor in most), and since our culture provides largely negative images of ageing, one would expect older people to have lowered self-esteem and sense of self, and to be finding it increasingly difficult to maintain a preferred sense of self. But there appear to be various ways in which they avoid this, despite a counterproductive social environment (Biggs 1997). For example, they may deny or hold back ageing (and perhaps increasingly are able to do this in postmodern society), or they may see their ageing bodies as a mere mask or adjunct that conceals their real selves, using the more traditional mind–body split (Featherstone and Hepworth 1991). As one woman said in a study of people's experience of growing older: 'I don't feel my age. It's just my legs that feel old, not me head. I don't feel nearly eighty' (Thompson *et al.* 1990). Or they may emphasize the continuity of their lives through particular enduring themes, traits, or values which give meaning to their life (Kaufman 1986). Or they may focus on social settings which are less inimical, such as age-segregated communities. With increasing post-modern trends, where 'self-identity becomes a reflexively organized endeavour' (Giddens 1991) and is continuously revised, one would expect the first method to be increasingly adopted and for there to be growing uncertainty about identity in later life. Indeed Phillipson (1998) has argued that the breaking down of some of the old certainties which defined old age or the old—such as the institution of retirement—has produced a crisis, leading both to increased scapegoating of the old and more fundamentally to uncertainty about identity, and doubt about 'the meaning and purpose of growing old'. (Phillipson 1998, p. 3) (However, it should be noted that this is a somewhat masculine proposition; retirement has not been a clear marker for older women. They have been socially defined by more variable transitions, such as the cessation of childbearing and rearing, rather than by fixed transitions such as retirement.) More broadly, Phillipson accepts that these changes, whilst producing positive outcomes for privileged older people, may have no such advantage for the less privileged. It will also of course be likely that the postmodern changes are advantageous to younger older people but disadvantageous for the very old when, as Biggs (1997) says, 'the project of maintaining multiple options for identity hits the buffers of ageing as a physical process'. However, it should be said that so far the research evidence about what happens to the self in later life in the postmodern era is very sparse, and some of it does not support the kind of reflexivity assumed to exist among older people today (Riggs and Turner 1997).

Optimism about the future identities of older people may also be shaken if we adapt the views of Edward Said, analyst of colonialism, on the opposition between the West and the Orient. Said wrote that 'European culture gained strength and identity by setting itself off against the Orient as sort of surrogate or even underground self'. (Said 1978, p. 3). In other words, it needed its distorted ideas about the East to confirm its own sense of the West. In a similar way, youth or middle adulthood needs a certain conception of old age. Things are only defined by what surrounds them (like clearings in woods). Only when youth ceases to dominate can there be any real chance of a change in the place of older people in society.

Finally, what about the 'increased scapegoating of the old' as suggested by Phillipson (1998)? In this area, concerning attitudes of others towards the old, or how old age is conceptualized and defined in postmodern culture, we are also on tricky ground for identifying ongoing changes. Research suggests that we still live in an ageist society (Bytheway 1995). This is confirmed not just by the position of older people as far as the major social institutions are concerned, but by the discourses of popular culture, even though that culture includes many of the newer images of later life and the interests of postmodern older people

(Blaikie 1999). The kind of language we use, and the way in which we use it, expresses our attitudes towards older people rather better than public opinion surveys. For example, a sign indicating that one should give up one's seat to 'an elderly or disabled person' tells us into which category an older person should be placed. In the same way discriminatory practices in economic, state, health, and social care institutions tell us how to value older people (see below). Asked to give a one- or two-word answer to a question about whether pensions should be increased, or whether people over 50 years of age should be encouraged to leave the workforce, or older people made a lower priority for health services than younger people, the majority of adults in sample surveys come down on the non-discriminatory side. But that does not mean that we are not an ageist society (Walker and Maltby 1997), it merely means that such methods of investigation are not adequate to the task.

Key social institutions

Individuals and their social relationships are embedded within a huge variety of social institutions. Institutions are sets of standardized practices, with accompanying rules and values, designed to achieve certain outcomes. A crucial part of the work of sociology is uncovering the *latent features* of institutions. It is these latent features which determine how the institutions really work: they may make some of the desired outcomes more likely but through unexpected means; or make some outcomes less likely even though the expected means are used.

The key institution emphasized by sociologists has always been the economic institution of work; but almost equally important as subjects of study have been the institutions of the family, the state, education, religion, and health care. All these domains have generated their own sociologies (though some of declining focus, such as the sociology of religion). Some of them have been particularly affected by postmodern changes, no longer carrying the certainty and authority which used to be theirs; and some have paid more attention to ageing than others. We will therefore concentrate more on the latter. Of course, this chapter cannot hope to cover all relevant fields. The institutions discussed below play a major role in helping to define us, unite and separate us, confirm our well-being and sense of self, or their absence. Before this discussion, however, other institutions should be mentioned. For any relatively enduring pattern of expectations and relationships will help to structure the lives of older as well as of younger people. In particular, this chapter gives very little space to dying and death, or to housing and the built environment, both of which have been convincingly described as key social institutions; for example, 'those writing about postmodernity have noted the importance of the 'spatiality' of social life, a key theme in Foucault's work' (Laws 1995). 'Living arrangements' mean more than the housing and household structures of older people, though they have often been studied in this very instrumental way. In particular—as with the institution of retirement—not only must we consider how standard patterns have been conceptualized, and are now being seen as breaking down, but also how ageism operates within housing, as well as the meanings that older people themselves give to their living arrangements. As Laws (1995) says:

> The construction of self and other reflected in built environments is all part of the transition to postmodernity, where universal images are destabilized and local cultures create their own images to challenge the hegemonic paradigms of the status quo. (p. 117)

The way our society structures and constrains how older people die is also of key importance, but less weighty institutions like religious or cultural festivals (such as birthdays or Christmas), how we take our leisure and holidays, shopping, and transportation are also significant. They too help to reinforce an identity, a set of roles, a distinct social position for older people, and they too are changing.

Producers and consumers

As described above, the economic sphere has traditionally been seen as the centrally important area for understanding the nature of society: the fundamental source of power, values, and social distinctions. For individuals—particularly men—it determines how they spend much of their time, provides the source of their expenditure, sense of identity, social networks, and social standing (Kohli 1988). Sociologists of ageing have paid particular attention to the trends over time in economic activity, retirement rates, and income of older people. Whilst these figures in themselves are not sociology (though they are part of a sociological process, and some would argue that clarifying and making them public helps to empower older people), the attempt to explain trends and inequalities both between older and younger adults and within the older population itself in recent years, is indeed sociology.

Sociologists of ageing might conclude that it would be relatively easy to identify the disadvantaged position of older people and to link it to their position within the economic system (which has indeed been a key part of the definition of being old). However, the argument has not been straightforward, partly because of the complexity of the social trends at the societal level and partly because of the complexity of the outcomes of work and retirement for individuals. It must not be forgotten that there are key differences within the older population, particularly those between men and women (Arber and Ginn 1991). Of course, in many ways a system for permitting workers to retire, with a continuing income, must be seen as a sign of social progress. But ignoring those who have not been part of the workforce, or obliging people to retire into conditions that have adverse effects on them, and in financial circumstances which disadvantage them is not social progress.

In the United Kingdom (and other Western nations) since the 1950s or thereabouts there have been three economic phases relevant to older people. These phases are conceptually fairly distinct, though temporally and in practice very much overlapping. From the first to the third we move from the 'modern' into the 'postmodern' era. To consider the benefits and disadvantages for older people it is important to distinguish them. The first phase can be placed from around 1950 until about 1970. In this phase, retirement for men aged 65 and over became institutionalized, accepted as the norm, and reinforced by employer and state policies. It was accepted that most men would work until they were around 65 and thereafter most would receive a state pension. But the level of the state pension was low, and poverty among pensioners high. As a consumer market they were insignificant, partly as a result of their small numbers but also because they had little surplus spending power. To some extent this phase was beneficial to older people in that it legitimized retirement, and income in retirement, as a right. It was also seen by some sociologists as beneficial to society, allowing for the orderly withdrawal of people from the labour market and their replacement by younger workers with more up-to-date skills and knowledge. However, it did not take long for the overriding negative side to be identified as far as older people were concerned: it deprived them of the opportunity to work, it lowered their incomes often to critical levels (except for a minority), decreased their social status, and took away (for men largely) their friendship networks and sense of identity. There was not much sign of social progress here, but considerable evidence of the powerlessness of those older people unable to sell their labour or retain some other hold on the economic institutions of society.

The second phase can be linked to the period from the mid-1960s to about the mid-1980s. During this phase there was a continuing downward trend in the employment of older men and an increasing trend towards early retirement from the age of 55 or thereabouts. The movement for women is harder to assess because of some competing trends (such as the general increase in female employment); however, it looks as though the underlying trend was similar. Along with this move towards spending more years in retirement there was also an improvement in pension provision, partly through an increase in state pension in the earlier part of this period but also through the growth in personal or occupational pensions (mainly the latter). This phase saw a marked and growing inequality *within* the older population as far as the decision to retire and income in retirement were concerned, which complicates any attempt to explain what was happening. For some analysts (see Johnson 1998, cited above) the ability to choose earlier retirement and to have a better standard of living than pensioners in former times was a sign of the growing power of older people and of social progress. For others there was more pessimism, with the emphasis being on the pressure exerted by government and employers to extrude older workers in order to streamline and modernize the economic base and to lower unemployment in a time of recession. Although some pensioners were well off, poverty remained for many, particularly women, those in former manual occupations, and the very old. And although a 'third age' giving time for fulfilment and leisure had dawned for some, it became increasingly apparent that this was only for a small minority. This was because (i) even those in relatively comfortable financial circumstances were often tied by continuing responsibilities such as caregiving for sick or disabled relatives, voluntary work, or grandchild care (Disney *et al.* 1997), and (ii) although some people had 'chosen' to retire early, this was not the case for the majority, many of whom had been forced into it by age-discrimination among employers or by ill-health or disability. For example, in a 1988/9 survey of people aged 55–69 who were reinterviewed in 1994, it was concluded that only about one-third of early retirements were 'the result of individual choice' and 'close to another third...were reported to be due to ill-health' (Disney *et al.* 1997). The lack of power of older people in this sphere is indicated not only directly by their disadvantaged retirement and pension position, but also in the related ideas prevailing about them. For example, age discrimination in employment results partly from pure economic factors—e.g. a desire to employ cheaper labour—but it is also due to 'deep-seated but quite erroneous, beliefs that the productivity of workers declines after 40' (Johnson 1998, p. 218).

This second phase shades into the third from the 1980s onwards, as it began to be recognized that work was becoming more unstable and careers more changeable and that the transition between work and retirement was also fragmenting. As an example of the former we can cite a national survey of people aged 16 to 69 years carried out in 1994/5 in Britain, which showed that men and women over 60 had had fewer job changes in their working lives than the changes *already* experienced by those in their late forties and fifties (McKay and Middleton 1998). It is also the case nowadays that, with the greater concern about population ageing, some older workers may be encouraged to remain in the workforce for as long as possible. For instance, male employment rates have been growing in the 50 to 64 age group in the United Kingdom since 1993, following an earlier decline, while for women there has been a consistent upward trend (EOT 1999) (though this move will continue to compete with that which emphasizes jobs for younger people). The sphere of work has become much more flexible, and therefore the distinction between those in work and those who are retired is much less clear-cut. There has been an increase in unpredictable or insecure work careers in middle and later working life, an increase in working from home, an increase in self-employment, particularly among older workers; and an increase in the numbers of people who see themselves as not economically active but also as not retired. For example, the survey mentioned above showed that of people aged 60–64 in Britain who were not employed, only about two-thirds considered themselves retired (McKay and Middleton 1998).

Since the previous stable pattern was one that helped to define old age, these recent changes have affected the very nature and meaning of old age. Aside from the growing diversification of older people on the basis of employment status, income inequality within the older population is also widening, and is likely to go on increasing as the value of the state pension declines and as well-resourced occupational pensions continue to be available only to some workers (EOT 1999). As a recent report from the House of Commons Social Security Committee stated:

> ...the overall growth in pensioner incomes conceals serious and growing inequalities among pensioner households...Although the incomes of all pensioners have grown, the gap between the richest and poorest pensioners has also increased dramatically. (Social Security Committee 2000)

Again some analysts have seen this situation very optimistically. Poverty among older people has gone on decreasing, and increasing proportions of retired people have incomes above the average. Projections for 25 years' time suggest that older people will be better off financially (Evandrou and Falkingham 2000). They are also increasingly likely to own some capital in the form of homes and savings. Johnson (1998) also says that the increasing existence of pensions shows a weakening of the historic association between work and income, and that this is part of:

> ...a more fundamental restructuring of the value system of modern society, a restructuring which has seen consumption and consumerism challenge production and the world of work as the indicator by which social standing is measured. This change permits retirees today to define themselves not by what they do or produce, but by where they travel, how they spend their time, with whom they associate. (p. 223)

However, retired people are still more likely to be poor than adults below retirement age, (Attias-Donfut and Arber 2000), and this is particularly true of older women. Thus while older people are being empowered by their growing importance as consumers and by the increasingly blurred distinction between them and the working population, their increasing diversity leaves many in financial hardship and still deprives them of the freedom to work and the security of a long-term job.

Family relationships

In the 'modern', production-oriented society the family was seen as relatively stable and providing fairly efficiently not only for the health and well-being of the workers and the socialization of the next generation of workers, but also for the support and care of ex-workers. In 'postmodern' society however, the family is seen as fragmenting, in the sense that no longer is there only one acceptable form of family, endorsed by powerful religious and state institutions. Variants on the traditional form of family, such as consensual unions, same sex couples, single-parent families, or step-families are all increasingly evident. Greater flexibility in the labour market changes role relationships in the family—with more women working, men are more likely to share household tasks and childcare, but only on a flexible and unstable basis. Although some argue that the state is engaged in more surveillance of what goes on in the private world of the family, conversely the welfare state can provide less in the way of financial support to families than in the past. Probably at no time in the past has the family been thought to be improving in the way it carried out its role (i.e. there has been no period when the general notion of social progress was applied to the family). But in a 'postmodern' society the family (whatever that now means) comes under constant criticism, even though it is still expected to provide for the health and well-being of adults and children, and to play an important role as a consumption unit and as the socialization agent of the next generation of consumers.

The distinction between the 'modern' and 'postmodern' eras is very helpful in considering ageing and the family. For example, sociologists of the 'modern' family spent a good deal of time and energy scotching myths about the 'traditional' family, to show that the family had not changed as much as popular imagination thought between these two eras. Thus popular imagination saw a traditional picture of a preindustrial society in which elderly people were a respected and central part of their children's households in which they were supported with affection. 'Modern' sociology showed that though in premodern times the family had been supportive to its members, co-residence had not been the typical reality. It went on to argue that 'modern' times had seen no decline in the strength and supportiveness of the family. Interestingly, this is still largely the stance taken today by sociologists of ageing and the family. For example, as recently as 1996 three of the doyens of American sociology of ageing were stating what they saw as the popular myth and arguing against it:

> That the family is no longer the important institution it once was in American society has become the orthodox view of many pundits and politicians. That many elderly Americans are isolated from, or abandoned by, the families they have created is a frequent corollary to this view. (Bengtson *et al.* 1996, p. 254)

Bengtson *et al.* went on to say that, although they agree that the family is changing, research evidence does not support the claim of family decline, indeed that there is persuasive evidence concerning intergenerational support today, 'especially in crisis situations such as 'surrogate parenting' by grandparents and great grandparents'. (p. 273)

In Britain too there has been a good deal of research on older people and their families over the last 50 years. Again the key issue for investigation was—and still is—whether the family is breaking up, and the bonds between older and younger members loosening. A recent study by a social historian of ageing (Thane 1998) argues that the research all points towards older people remaining well connected to their families and not isolated—even when they do not live in the same household. Despite the increase in separation of households between the generations (e.g. in Wolverhampton in 1945 51% of people aged 60/65+ lived in households containing at least one of their children, whereas the comparable figure for 1995 was only 20%; Bernard *et al.* 2000), older and younger family members are said to have remained close. In fact, in attempting to explain this, some have argued that the increasing uncertainty which marks postmodern life has drawn the family closer and made intimate relationships more, rather than less, important to them (Giddens 1992). Therefore—so the argument goes—there is no need to worry about older people in the future; their families will go on caring for them. But this is a very blinkered view. Sociologists seem to be part of the myth enterprise as far as family life is concerned. Just because they were able to scotch the myth of a traditional 'golden age' for family care they may not be able to prove that the belief that family care in the postmodern age is now becoming more problematic, is also a myth.

Although researching the postmodern is acknowledged to be difficult, when we are still in the middle of experiencing the changes which it brings, it is important to begin to explore the emerging trends. For the changes that accompany postmodernization are affecting the family lives of older people, even though they are taking longer to affect older cohorts than younger people. First, older people are increasingly likely to choose to live either on their own or just with a spouse; and although, compared with 20 years ago, there has been an increase in the proportion of older people who are married (Bridgwood 2000), in 20 years time the picture will look very different, with more older people living on their own, and more who have no children or grandchildren (Shaw 1999; Evandrou and Falkingham 2000). For example, the divorced population has been growing steadily, with divorced women outnumbering divorced men (Haskey 1999). This is projected to continue and the differential to widen, with more women than men remaining divorced into old age. Second, there is evidence that independence between parents and adult children has grown; although the expressed emotional attachment and sense of mutual obligation remain strong (Wertheimer and McCrae 1999), contacts between them are less locally based and less likely to be face to face. Indeed, nowadays one in ten adults never sees his/her father (McGlone *et al.* 1996), and '60% of people aged 70 and over who live alone do not have a child or grandchild living within half an hour's journey time of their home' (Grundy *et al.* 1999). Third, with more women working and not living nearby it is becoming increasingly difficult for them to provide extensive support to their parents. A recent survey also showed that family-centredness was related to religious observance; since the latter is falling the former is likely to do so too (McGlone *et al.* 1996). Fourth, although older people are sometimes involved in family roles through providing grandchild care, this does not always happen nor is it always unproblematic. For example, a recent survey (Dench *et al.* 1999) showed that the highest rates of dissatisfaction with the grandparent role were expressed by those grandparents who had a greater caring role for grandchildren (following the parents' divorce or separation).

Since growing diversity and the acceptance of diversity marks postmodern society, there is no straightforward answer to the question whether family members experience growing independence and separation from each other, or continuing ties between them; or whether responsibility for each other is increasing or decreasing. Probably, both are happening. It is certainly not the job of sociology to assert that all is well with the family, to claim that it is not subject to strain, or that role relationships within it are not oppressive to the individuals involved. Instead it must be to reveal these problematic issues, for example the conflicts that arise when too much is demanded of families, sometimes resulting in elder abuse (see Chapter 37), the role overload experienced particularly by women, and the isolation or loneliness particularly experienced by elderly men living on their own.

The state

We have already noted that one of the so-called postmodern trends is the decline of the nation state, through two opposing moves. On the one hand is the growing importance of global political issues, powerful international economic enterprises, increasing transnational collaboration; on the other are issues of regionalism, identification with ethnic groupings, and growing individualism, together with the desire of citizens to retain more personal control over their spending power. Alongside these trends it is said that individuals have become more global in outlook as communications across the world improve, travel becomes more widespread, and consumer goods more international; and that they have lost deference for, interest, and even confidence in the state. However, the state has been and remains to a large extent a key institution as far as ageing and older people are concerned (Estes 1999). For in harness with the economic institutions the state plays an important role in defining old age, in maintaining the social status, dependence, or autonomy of older people, and the divisions between groups in the population. None the less, postmodern changes cannot be ignored.

First, through legislation and public policies the state sets age markers that help to define old age, and these have tended to reinforce the negative images of later life. This is particularly the case when the age marker dictates when someone becomes *in*eligible to do something; for example, people over the age of 70 in Britain cannot serve as jurors; or a person over 65 may in some areas not be eligible for local authority services. For example:

> ...a woman with physical disabilities discovered that the weekly swimming trip available to her as a younger adult with physical disabilities aged 18–64 ceased on her 65th birthday. She was simply told: 'We don't do swimming for the elderly.' However, she failed to see—and the social services department failed to convince her—that her needs had changed so radically (and literally) overnight. (Age Concern England 1998)

But age markers also reinforce negative stereotypes when they dictate at what age people become eligible for certain benefits, etc. The most obvious example is the age at which one may receive the retirement pension, but there are many others—e.g. free television licenses from the age of 75, free prescriptions and eyesight tests from the age of 60 (suggesting that there is something about being old which makes one unable to pay for ones own tests or license and therefore a worthy recipient of charity). Age markers are of course used in health service provision also, such as the age at which one may be offered the influenza vaccine (Tinker 1994). Of course there are sensible reasons for this, given our understanding of the age-related risks of contracting the disease; none the less such markers also have the effect of defining what it means to be old.

Over the past 50 years state policies have contributed to the dependent status of older people. For example, in the early welfare state legislation 'there continued to be complete reliance on residential care as the solution to the needs of older people' (Bernard and Phillips 1998), with its attendant transmission of ideas about the dependency of the aged. Even by the end of the 1970s:

> ...older people were still seen, in policy terms, as primarily a dependent group in need of care. Their own views and voices were unheard, and issues about autonomy, privacy and dignity in residential care, together with ideas about what older people at home might need to bolster their independence, had yet to be addressed in policy debates. (Bernard and Phillips 1998, p. 8)

Gradually that view changed—in part because of research carried out by sociologists, which showed convincingly that institutional care was not only in practice often inhumane, but could not by its very nature maintain the autonomy and independence of the inmates (Dalley 1998). However, it is not only residential care which helps to enforce the dependency of the old. More recent changes emphasizing the targeting of services on the very frail or disabled, and their assessment and means-testing by professional care managers, continues to enforce this dependency.

However, legislation has also helped in the redistribution of resources from younger to older citizens. This was especially true in Britain following the introduction of the National Health Service after the Second World War, with older people benefiting equally with younger people from the NHS. But, through its policies, the state also affects the relative position of different groups of older people and thereby helps to maintain divisions and differences (Walker 1996; Evandrou 1997). For example, the pension scheme it implements or endorses will affect the extent of income disadvantage experienced by older women compared with older men. In Britain, for example, the government's emphasis in recent years on personal or occupational pensions, and the reduction in the universal state pension, has disadvantaged women because of their more chequered employment careers. It has also disadvantaged those in low earning occupations, or others with disrupted employment careers, who are least likely to have a private pension. Some have argued that these pension policy changes are due to the increasing individualism in postmodern society; and its effect of disadvantaging those who care for others rather than taking long-term, full-time employment 'may lead to a society in which no one can afford to care for others'. (Ginn and Arber 2000).

But the institution of the state can be said to have been undermined in recent years and it now plays a more detached or circumscribed role. For example, it has retreated from pension provision in the United Kingdom, with much greater emphasis being given to private personal or occupational pensions. It has placed increasing emphasis on the family and independent sector as providers of residential care and community services (Dalley 1998), with a withdrawal of the statutory sector from the direct provision of such services. Recipients of services are referred to as consumers, with rights to choose and to complain if services are inadequate. But this change of emphasis does not mean that older people have become empowered: rights to services have been withdrawn, as they become targeted on specific groups, but choice has not increased for those older people who are deemed to need them. And as Gilleard and Higgs (1996) say, in a discussion of the impact of broad social changes on the position of older people vis-à-vis the state:

> Those falling within the eligible or targeted group form a sub-class of elderly consumers too weak to choose but who because of this self-same weakness are the only ones entitled to be treated as consumers of the health and social care resources which the state is prepared to purchase on their behalf. (p. 87)

Some have argued that postmodernity's consumer consciousness (as well as their growing numbers) is encouraging older people to be more politically active (Walker 1996). However, there is comparatively little evidence of this, and one could equally well argue that the growing individualism of postmodernity is having the opposite effect, especially in the light of the acknowledged general decline in political activism in the United Kingdom.

Health and care services

Along with retirement, the medical institutions of Western society have over the past 50 years helped to define old age, medicalizing and colonizing it (Estes and Binney 1989), and thus reinforcing its negative conceptualization, despite the fact that most older people describe themselves as healthy. This has had three serious consequences: first, it leads to the belief that if you are not sick you are not old (leading to the development of the concept of 'the third age' (healthy old age) before infirmity sets in the 'fourth age' (Laslett 1996). This is fine for those who are not sick, but disadvantageous for those who are, since they become even more negatively perceived. Second, lest such colonization put unmanageable pressure on medical science, the view is encouraged that to a large extent cure is not possible, but only symptom treatment and care services ('care' rather than 'cure' is the usual discourse for many of the health concerns involving older people). Third, there is the propagation of the view that it is up to older people to foster their own well-being (hence the surge of emphasis on health promotion in recent years).

Perhaps because of the medicalization of old age, sociology has until recently paid relatively little attention to older people and health care, beyond extrapolating from research focused mainly on younger people about inequalities in morbidity or mortality. Such research has been useful in countering notions that to be old is to be sick, and it has emphasized that social factors influence health in old age. Such factors include experiences within the medical and other social institutions—particularly the economy and the family—both in old age and, more importantly, at earlier points in people's lives.

For inequalities in health are found to persist into later life. For example, a recent British study showed that 'for the middle-aged and those entering retirement, chronic illness is more prevalent among the manual socioeconomic groups than the non-manual groups' (Dunnell and Dix 2000). Of course the impact of the economic institutions has been found to be hugely important, both from earlier periods of life as well as from current factors such as low income, poor housing, and environment (shown, for example, in a Norwegian study by Dahl and Birkelund 1997). Indeed it has been found that quite fine-grained differences make a difference to life expectancy, such as between those who have a car and a garden or only the former (Bartley *et al.* 1998). It is not just the direct influence of economic institutions but also of the differential culture that develops around differences in status or class. For example, it has been found that 'middle class' older people are more likely to consult doctors than those from working class backgrounds (Victor 1991).

The educational institutions may also affect the health of older people. Along with the family, the educational institutions foster knowledge about health and illness, and yet older people have until comparatively recently had very little access to education (and not a great deal now). We still tend to take it for granted that education is for the young. Research shows what a large part the family plays in caring for older people (see above), but we know much less about how family members influence older people's ideas about health and how to keep healthy. There is some evidence that marriage is more beneficial in health terms to older men than older women because wives help to maintain husbands' good health behaviours, whereas women do not appear to need marriage in order to maintain healthy behaviours. Social relationships with family and friends also have an effect on health, through buffering against stress as well as deterring the older people from engaging in unhealthy practices, helping them to comply with treatments, and encouraging positive health self images (Lewis *et al.* 1994). However, such relationships do not necessarily have positive benefits: Lewis *et al.* (1994) found in one of their studies that '19% of the older adults...reported that network members had tried to influence them to engage in unhealthy and unwanted behaviours. Such results suggest that peer pressure still operates in late adulthood' (p. 205). In general, however, the benefits of family relationships are clear, and they are independent of economic position.

Postmodern social changes have begun to encourage a new set of questions. Although economic position may continue to be important, could it be that increasing diversity and greater control over resources is giving older people more power over their health and their receipt of health care? The traditional view was that ill health was something one had to accept as one grew older, and that the health services could not be expected to treat illness as actively in old age as they would the ailments of younger people. This was a view that encouraged—or turned a blind eye to—age discrimination in health care, but it is giving way to considerable interest in, and evidence about, the extent to which older patients are discriminated against simply because they are old. For example, in the United Kingdom routine breast screening is not as yet offered to women over the age of 65 even though the incidence of breast cancer is higher at the older ages; older people are often omitted from clinical trials; they may be denied access to the best treatment for cancer or end-stage renal failure; and so on.

There is a growing research interest in how age discrimination operates in practice, through medical discourse and in the interaction between service providers and patients. For example, a study of stroke patient care in the USA showed that it was only after undertaking long-term treatment of their patients that doctors began to take a more holistic and less medicalized view, to be more optimistic about their patients, and to concentrate more on prevention (Kaufman and Becker 1991). Research in this country has shown how older patients may be infantilized and controlled in their encounters with health service staff (Clark 1996). Similar evidence has been found from research on social care; for example, researchers in New Zealand showed how social work organizations are influenced by 'dominant Western discourses of ageing, where loneliness, isolation and withdrawal from the social have been defined as part of the condition of ageing' (Opie 1996).

An end to such discrimination also has popular support, suggesting that older people are becoming more powerful. However, it remains a very problematic issue given the increased numbers of older people in the population, the growing pressure on the health service, and the unwillingness of people to vote for parties that will increase taxation to fund greater resources for the health service.

The complexity of the issue is evidenced by the fact that in some quarters the increasing size of the older population is considered to give them greater power (as a pressure group or as voters). It is also suggested that some recent policy developments, such as the move to quasi-markets and purchaser-provider relationships in health and social care, which may have been introduced to curtail public expenditure, also have the effect of giving older people more power. For instance, it has been suggested that the emphasis on community care may empower service recipients. As Fox (1993) says in discussing younger disabled people:

> Legislation in the UK has been constituted so as to generate a consumer-like relationship between cared-for and carers. The formulation of care plans on the basis of economics, with those needing care receiving—in effect—a sum of money which they can spend on care as they wish, or at least with a degree of flexibility, places those needing care in a more powerful position than when dependent either on central services or upon goodwill in informal care relationships. The creation of a 'market in care' may, in this sense, enable people who need care to make choices...to choose to have the 'health' they wish inscribed upon them. (Fox 1993, p. 118)

But the extent to which community-care policies allow older people—as consumers—to take more control over their care has been much debated. They may be beginning to benefit from the increased empowerment of younger disabled people, who managed to obtain the right to pay directly for care services, a situation which is now being extended to older people in Britain under recent legislation. But if care professionals still retain the power to define older people's 'needs' and to control their access to services, then their full empowerment is some way off (Higgs 1995). The postmodern trends of increasing uncertainty, choice, and individual reflexivity, which are expected to diminish the power of the medical profession and encourage the empowerment of lay people, have come under some scrutiny and may not in fact do so. For example, in studying screening for genetic disorders Kerr and Cunningham-Burley (2000) found that 'professionals and policy-makers are still powerful managers of lay ambivalence' (p. 294).

Indeed, not only is there evidence about the continuing control by medical and social care professionals over decision-making on behalf of older people, there is also continuing evidence of the relatively passive views older people themselves hold about their health, with the traditional models still being much in evidence. For instance, older people are more likely to see health as a state of good social functioning, whereas young people are more likely to see it as either being physically active or as not being ill (Victor 1991). There is also a good deal of research showing that older people are stoical about health, having low expectations, seeing ill-health as inevitable, and not necessarily as a crisis when placed in the context of their long experience of other life events (Williams 1990; Bury and Holme 1991;

Coupland and Coupland 1994; Pound *et al.* 1998; Russell *et al.* 1996). As far as postmodern trends in health and social care are concerned, therefore, no clear influences are yet emerging for older people. This is hardly surprising, given the complexity of the issues and the fact that health in people's old age is partly dependent on behaviour which may have occurred 60 or more years ago.

Conclusions

There has never been a more interesting time in which to grow old, or to study ageing. Because we are in the midst of phenomenal social change, sociological research has few answers to the questions about the implications of these changes for ageing and older people. But over the past 50 years sociology has contributed much to the understanding of the subject. Most importantly, it has highlighted the social and cultural specificity of ageing and of our views about it; for example, clarifying how the concept of 'successful ageing' is value-laden. Sociology has therefore been able to show the way in which social structural and cultural factors combine in the construction of the concept of ageing. Yet, though the meaning of old age varies from society to society and culture to culture, 'in virtually no society is old age defined as one of the most desirable parts of life' (Fry 1996). Sociology has also shown how later life varies within a society or community, drawing particular attention to the differential experiences of people from different socioeconomic groups, and of men and women, identifying the greater disadvantage of the latter, in economic resources, health, ageist attitudes, and, to some extent, family resources. The life course itself has also been shown to be part of the differential experience, and the fallacy of generalizing to all older people, whatever their age and previous experiences, has been emphasized.

Now, however, one of the main questions preoccupying sociologists of ageing today is whether older people benefit or suffer from postmodernization. This chapter has shown that there can of course be no unambiguous answer to this question (and probably no answer at all in certain areas for some time). Much of the social experience of old age remains firmly 'modern' rather than 'postmodern.' However, certain trends are evident, and the dynamism of postmodern society, the differentiation and flexibility of identities, and the decline of the key institutions can be seen as both detrimental and advantageous to older people. On the one hand Phillipson argues that older people need a 'secure anchorage' (Phillipson 1998, p. 136) in stable social institutions that allow them to know who they are and what the future is likely to bring. This seems unlikely he says, because of the unravelling of the key institutions that support old age. The growing social importance of the body as a part of identity is also in the long run a disadvantage to older people, since their bodies will in the end let them down. Increasing diversity and the emphasis upon consumption will disadvantage those who have low command over resources in a society of growing inequality of income. The retreat of the state in the face of a rising older population also disadvantages those who cannot afford to provide for their own pensions and care services (particularly women and those who were employed in low-status manual occupations). The declining influence of religious and educational institutions, leading to decreasing respect for authority, may also depress the standing of older people, whilst changes in the institution of the family will in time increase the number of older people living alone and without available children to help care for them should they need it.

But on the other hand new institutions are emerging, which may be more fragile, of shorter duration, and less dominant, but may be well adapted to the needs of today's (and tomorrow's) older people. And, anyway, it may be that our need for support of the kind provided by the institutions of the welfare state and retirement is changing. The flexibility of identities, which enable older people to hold the ageing process at bay, and the blurring of the distinction between the retired and the non-retired, are advantageous in helping them to avoid the label of 'old'; while the increasing number of identities—especially that of consumer—accorded to them also offers higher status and increased control over their lives. Their greater command over resources may improve their political and social standing; they may eventually be able to wield more power over their health care; and family relationships may become closer as a result of the uncertainties of postmodern life. Only time and further sociological research will tell.

References

Abbott, P. and Wallace, C. (1997). *An introduction to sociology: feminist perspectives* (2nd edn). Routledge, London.

Age Concern England (1998). *Age concern briefings*, Ref. 1298. Age Concern England, London.

Albrow, M. (1999). *Sociology: the basics*. Routledge, London.

Arber, S. and Ginn, J. (1991). *Gender and later life: a sociological analysis of resources and constraints*. Sage, London.

Attias-Donfut, C. and Arber, S. (2000). Equity and solidarity across the generations. In *The myth of generational conflict* (ed. S. Arber and C. Attias-Donfut), pp. 1–21. Routledge, London.

Bartley, M., Blane, D., and Davey Smith, G. (1998). *The sociology of health inequalities*. Blackwell, Oxford.

Beck, U. (1992). *Risk society: towards a new modernity*. Sage, London.

Bengtson, V., Rosenthal, C., and Burton, L. (1996). Paradoxes of families and aging. In *Handbook of aging and the social sciences* (4th edn) (ed. R. Binstock and L. George), pp. 253–82. Academic Press, California.

Berger, P. (1963). *Invitation to sociology*. Doubleday, New York.

Bernard, M. and Phillips, J. (1998). Social policy and the challenge of old age. In *The social policy of old age* (ed. M. Bernard and J. Phillips), pp. 1–19. Centre for Policy on Ageing, London.

Bernard, M., Phillips, J., Phillipson, C., and Ogg, J. (2000). Continuity and change: the family life of older people in the 1990s. In *The myth of generational conflict* (ed. S. Arber and C. Attias-Donfut), pp. 209–27. Routledge, London.

Biggs, S. (1997). Choosing not to be old? Masks, bodies and identity management in later life. *Ageing and Society*, **17**, 553–70.

Blaikie, A. (1999). *Ageing and popular culture*. Cambridge University Press. Cambridge.

Bridgwood, A. (2000). *People aged 65 and over*. Government Statistical Service, Office for National Statistics, London.

Bury, M. and Holme, A. (1991). *Life after ninety*. Routledge. London.

Bytheway, B. (1995). *Ageism*. Open University Press, Buckingham.

Clark, P. (1996). Communication between provider and patient: values, biography and empowerment in clinical practice. *Ageing and Society*, **16**, 747–74.

Coupland, J. and Coupland, N. (1994). Old age doesn't come alone: discursive representations of health-in-ageing in geriatric medicine. *International Journal of Aging and Human Development*, **39**, 81–95.

Cuff, E., Sharrock, W., and Francis, D. (1990). *Perspectives in sociology* (3rd edn). Routledge, London.

Dahl, E. and Birkelund, G. (1997). Health inequalities in later life in a social democratic state. *Social Science and Medicine*, **44**, 6.

Dalley, G. (1998). Health and social welfare policy. In *The social policy of old age* (ed. M. Bernard and J. Phillips), pp. 20–39. Centre for Policy on Ageing, London.

Dench, G., Ogg, J., and Thomson, K. (1999). The role of grandparents. In *British social attitudes: the 16th Report* (ed. R. Jowell, J. Curtice, A. Park and K. Thomson) pp. 135–56. SCPR/Dartmouth, Aldershot.

Disney, R., Grundy, E., and Johnson, P. (ed.) (1997). *The dynamics of retirement*. DSS Research Report 72. HMSO, London.

Dunnell, K. and Dix, D. (2000). Are we looking forward to a longer and healthier retirement?' *Health Statistics Quarterly*, Summer, 18–25.

EOT (1999). Older workers on the labour market. *Employment Observatory Trends*, **33**, 1–27 Winter.

Estes, C. (1999). Critical gerontology and the new political economy of aging. In *Critical gerontology: perspectives from political and moral economy* (ed. M. Minkler and C. Estes), pp. 17–36. Baywood, New York.

Estes, C. and Binney, E. (1989). The biomedicalization of aging: dangers and dilemmas. *The Gerontologist*, **29**, 587–98.

Evandrou, M. (1997). Introduction. In *Baby boomers: ageing into the 21st century* (ed. M. Evandrou), pp. 8–14. Age Concern England, London.

Evandrou, M. and Falkingham, J. (2000). Looking back to look forward: lessons from four birth cohorts for ageing in the 21st century. *Population Trends*, **99**, Spring, 27–36.

Featherstone, M. (1988). In pursuit of the post-modern: an introduction. *Theory, Culture and Society*, **5**, 2/3, 195–216.

Featherstone, M. and Hepworth, M. (1991). The mask of ageing and the post-modern lifecourse. In *The body: social processes and cultural theory* (ed. M. Featherstone, M. Hepworth, and B. Turner), pp. 371–89. Sage, London.

Foucault, M. (1979). *The history of sexuality*. Penguin, Harmondsworth.

Fox, N. (1993). *Post-modernism, sociology and health*. Open University Press, Buckingham.

Fry, C. (1996). Age, aging and culture. In *Handbook of aging and the social sciences* (ed. R. Binstock and L. George), pp. 117–36. Academic Press, New York.

Giddens, A. (1991). *Modernity and self identity*. Polity Press, Cambridge.

Giddens, A. (1992). *The transformation of intimacy*. Stanford University Press, Stanford, CA.

Gilleard, C. and Higgs, P. (1996). Cultures of ageing: self. citizen and the body. In *Sociology of aging: international perspectives* (ed. V. Minichiello, N. Chappell, H. Kendig, and A. Walker), pp. 82–92. International Sociological Association, Research Committee on Aging, Melbourne, Australia.

Ginn, J. and Arber, S. (2000). Gender, the generational contract and pension privatization. In *The myth of generational conflict* (ed. S. Arber and C. Attias-Donfut), pp. 133-53. Routledge, London.

Grundy, E., Murphy, M. and Shelton, N. (1999). Looking beyond the household: intergenerational perspectives on living kin and contacts with kin in Great Britain. *Population Trends,* **97**, Autumn, pp. 19–27.

Habermas, J. (1987). *The theory of communicative action.* Vol. 2 Lifeworld and system (transl. T. McCarthy). Polity Press, Cambridge.

Haskey, J. (1999). Divorce and remarriage in England and Wales. *Population Trends*, Spring, 18–22.

Higgs, P. (1995). Citizenship and old age: the end of the road? *Ageing and Society,* **15**, 535–50.

Holmes, E. and Holmes, L. (1995). *Other cultures, elder years* (2nd edn). Sage, London.

Johnson, P. (1998). Parallel histories of retirement in modern Britain. In *Old age from antiquity to post-modernity* (ed. P. Johnson and P. Thane), pp. 211–25. Routledge, London.

Kaufman, S. (1986). *The ageless self: sources of meaning in late life.* University of Wisconsin Press, Wisconsin.

Kaufman, S. and Becker, G. (1991). Content and boundaries of medicine in long-term care: physicians talk about stroke. *The Gerontologist,* **31**, 238–45.

Kerr, A. and Cunningham-Burley, S. (2000). On ambivalence and risk: reflexive modernity and the new human genetics. *Sociology*, **34**, 283–304.

Kohli, M. (1988). Ageing as a challenge to sociological theory. *Ageing and Society*, **8**, 367–95.

Laslett, P. (1989). The Third Age: *a fresh map of life.* Weidenfeld and Nicholson, London.

Laws, G. (1995). Understanding ageism: lessons from feminism and post-modernism. *The Gerontologist*, **35**, 112–18.

Lewis, M., Rook, K., and Schwarzer, R. (1994). Social support, social control and health among the elderly. In *Health psychology: a lifespan perspective* (ed. G. Penny, P. Bennett, and M. Herbert), pp. 191–211. Harwood Academic Publishers, Chur, Switzerland.

McGlone, F., Park, A., and Roberts, C. (1996). Relative values: kinship and friendship. *British social attitudes: the 13th Report.* SCPR/Dartmouth, Aldershot.

McKay, S. and Middleton, S. (1998). *Characteristics of older workers.* Department for Education and Employment Research Report RR45. HMSO, London.

Minois, G. (1989). *History of old age.* Polity Press, Cambridge.

Opie, A. (1996). Discourses at work: organisational policies and the effectiveness of social work services for caregivers and people with dementia. In *Sociology of aging: international perspectives* (ed. V. Minichiello, N. Chappell, H. Kendig, and A. Walker), pp. 415–29. International Sociological Association, Research Committee on Aging, Melbourne, Australia.

Phillipson, C. (1998). *Reconstructing old age: new agendas in social theory and practice.* Sage, London.

Pound, P., Gompertz, P., and Ebrahim, S. (1998). Illness in the context of old age: the case of stroke. *Sociology of Health and Illness*, **20**, 489–506.

Riggs, A. and Turner, B. (1997). The sociology of the postmodern self: intimacy, identity and emotions in adult life. *Australian Journal on Ageing,* **16**, 229–32.

Russell, C., Hill, B., and Basser, M. (1996). Identifying needs among 'at risk' older people: does anyone here speak health promotion? In Sociology of aging: international perspectives (ed. V. Minichiello, N. Chappell, H. Kendig, and A. Walker), pp. 378–93. International Sociological Association, Research Committee on Aging, Melbourne, Australia.

Said, E. (1978). *Orientalism: Western conceptions of the Orient.* Routledge and Kegan Paul, London.

Shaw, C. (1999). 1996-based population projections by legal marital status for England and Wales. *Population Trends*, **95**, Spring, 23–32.

Social Security Committee (2000). *Social Security Seventh Report, pensioner poverty.* House of Commons, London.

Thane, P. (1998). The family lives of old people. In *Old age from antiquity to post-modernity* (ed. P. Johnson and P. Thane), pp. 180–210. Routledge, London.

Thomas, H. and Walsh, D. (1998). Modernity/post-modernity. In *Core sociological dichotomies* (ed. C. Jenks), pp. 363–90. Sage, London.

Thompson, P., Itzin, C., and Abendstern, M. (1990). *I don't feel old.* Oxford University Press, Oxford.

Tinker, A. (1994). Elderly people, discrimination and some implications for interprofessional work. *Journal of Interprofessional Care*, **8**, 193–201.

Victor, C. (1991). *Health and health care in later life.* Open University Press, Buckingham.

Walker, A. (1996). From acquiescence to dissent? A political sociology of population aging in the United Kingdom. In *Sociology of aging: international perspectives* (ed. V. Minichiello, N. Chappell, H. Kendig, and A. Walker), pp. 31–46. International Sociological Association, Research Committee on Aging, Melbourne, Australia.

Walker, A. and Maltby, T. (1997). *Ageing Europe.* Open University Press, Buckingham.

Wertheimer, A. and McCrae, S. (1999). *Family and household change in Britain: a summary of findings from projects in the ESRC population and household change programme.* Centre for Family and Household Research. Oxford Brookes University, Oxford.

Williams, R. (1990). *A Protestant legacy: attitudes to death and illness among older Aberdonians.* Clarendon Press, Oxford.

3 Cognitive change in old age

Elizabeth Milwain and Susan Iversen

The scientific methods of the twentieth century have ratified the belief, held for centuries, that intellectual powers fade in old age (for a review of how the scientific study of intellectual change in old age developed, see Woodruff-Pak 1997). Cognitive research shows that most people experience a decline in intellectual ability that begins during their late sixties or early seventies (Schaie 1996). The first part of this paper describes the patterns of cognitive loss and preservation typical in old age, whilst the second part considers the most influential cognitive theories advanced to explain these patterns. The strengths and weaknesses of these theories are briefly evaluated before presenting a synthesis which incorporates recent evidence from functional imaging paradigms. The final part of the chapter covers important, but less well understood, issues concerning first, the causes of intellectual change in old age, second, variation in the degree of decline experienced from one individual to the next, and finally the question of whether there is any distinction between 'normal ageing' and dementia, particularly DAT (dementia of the Alzheimer type).

Patterns of cognitive change in old age

Before beginning a brief review of the now considerable body of literature addressing the question, 'How does ageing affect cognition?', a few words about the organization of cognition within the brain will be helpful. Prior to the latter decades of the last century, a debate had raged for over 100 years as to whether the brain acted as an undifferentiated whole to produce intellectual functions or whether the brain was divided into different parts being specialized to perform specific cognitive functions (see introductory chapters in Kandel *et al.* 1995 and Kolb and Whishaw 1995 for discussion). Advances during the twentieth century led to agreement that intelligent behaviour is a combination of specialized functions interacting with some general factor, captured by the layman's notion of intelligence or, more formally, by either Spearman's concept of 'g' (Spearman 1927) or the cognitive psychologists' notion of 'general processing capacity' (see pp. 55–6 for further discussion). Early studies of cognitive ageing focused on quantifying changes in overall intelligence, whilst more recent research has tended to investigate changes to specific domains of cognitive function, particularly memory and language. It is difficult to integrate findings from these different frameworks because most research has confined itself to a single domain, without considering relationships with findings from other domains. Given that there has been this segmentation in how evidence has been gathered, this review will be structured according to these same divisions. However, it is hoped that the discussion will illustrate that a similar pattern emerges from each domain, namely, that there is little evidence for age-related decline in the specialized cognitive functions, but that when a test is made difficult by requiring active manipulation of information, age-related deficits occur in all the cognitive domains. The idea that the primary effect of old age upon cognition is to leave the fundamental architecture of cognition unchanged but to reduce overall 'processing capacity' is an old one (Welford 1958) that is well-expressed by this quotation from Craik and Rabinowitz 1984:

> ...many age-related decrements appear to reflect inefficiencies of processing, or to be strategic in nature,

rather than to be reflections of broken or lost components. (Craik and Rabinowitz 1984, p. 472)

The idea has been often criticized during the development of the literature, but it will be argued that the pervasive pattern of preserved abilities under simple situations with impaired abilities under complex situations supports the essence of the idea. The major challenge, which has been the basis for most criticism against the idea, is to provide a theoretical definition of exactly what makes a test 'complex' and to define 'processing capacity'. At present it is not possible to answer this challenge, but these controversial issues will be followed up in the section entitled 'Theories of cognitive change in old age' (see below), with a focus upon how future research could capitalize on the development of functional imaging technologies to answer the challenge.

Changes in intelligence and problem-solving

The notion of intelligence is linked to the activities of the psychometric psychologists who were dedicated to producing simple tests that could predict how well a person would perform in a variety of real-life situations, such as at school, in a given job, in the army, and so forth. Much of the early work on cognition and ageing used these psychometric tests (for reviews see Stuart-Hamilton 1994; Schaie 1996; and Woodruff-Pak 1997). However, it soon became apparent that whilst some intelligence tests showed clear age effects, others did not, or even found better performance amongst the elderly. Doppelt and Wallace (1955), for example, reported that the Performance IQ subtests from the WAIS (Wechsler Adult Intelligence Scale; Wechsler 1955, 1981) were more sensitive to age than the Verbal IQ subtests. By age 60, average performance in all five of the Performance IQ subtests fell below 1 standard deviation of the average performance of young adults. In contrast, by age 75, the average performance in four of the six Verbal IQ subtests remained within 1 standard deviation of young adults' performance levels. The finding of Doppelt and Wallace has been replicated so frequently that it has become known as the 'classic ageing pattern' (Botwinick 1977) and considerable effort has been directed at explaining why there should be this discrepancy between intelligence tests that use verbal and non-verbal materials.

The most widely accepted explanation derives from Horn and Cattell's (1967) theory that there are two sources of intelligent behaviour. The first, which Horn and Cattell refer to as 'fluid intelligence', is that typically associated with the concept of intelligence, whereby a person relies on his own reasoning powers to identify structure in the problem and apply appropriate strategies to reach a solution. However, intelligent behaviour can also be developed through education and practice. Horn and Cattell refer to this as 'crystallized intelligence'. Crystallized intelligence is determined to some extent by fluid intelligence, in that those with greater fluid intelligence will benefit more rapidly from education and experience, but it also depends upon an individual's opportunity and motivation to learn. Horn and Cattell argue that fluid intelligence deteriorates in old age, but that crystallized intelligence is robust. The insensitivity of Verbal IQ subtests to old age is attributed to the fact that performance in these tests is determined by the size of a person's general knowledge and vocabulary, paradigm examples of crystallized intelligence. In the Performance IQ subtests, on the other hand, the materials presented are novel and must be actively manipulated, usually within a stringent time limit. In these tests prior knowledge is of little value, and fluid intelligence becomes dominant in determining success.

The notion that fluid intelligence is vulnerable to old age is supported by studies of problem-solving. These studies have shown the elderly to be less strategic and flexible in their thought processes relative to the young. For example, several studies have examined strategic behaviour using the '20 questions' game whereby the experimenter thinks of an item and the subject's task is to ask questions which lead to the rapid identification of that item. The best strategy is to begin by asking constraint-seeking questions such as, 'Is it an animal?', 'Is it a mammal?', 'Is it a pet?', to narrow down the set of possibilities.

Once the set is sufficiently small, the subject should switch to asking identity-seeking questions such as, 'Is it a dog?' Investigations show that the elderly spend less time asking constraint-seeking questions, switching to identity-seeking questions when the number of possibilities remains too high (see Denney and Denney 1973, 1974 for reviews).

The elderly have also been found to be poor at abstracting structure from problems. A classic test of abstraction is to present stimuli that vary along a number of dimensions, such as colour, size, and shape, one of which dictates sorting (for example, all stimuli of the same colour should be grouped together). The subject tries various sorting rules and is required to use the experimenter's feedback to work out the correct rule. A number of studies have shown that the elderly are impaired at using feedback to abstract concepts and rules (for reviews see Reese and Rodeheaver 1985 and Woodruff-Pak 1997). It has been argued that the problem may arise because the materials used in these tests are abstract and less familiar to the elderly, whose educational days are in the distant past. However, Arenberg (1982) used problems in which logical deductions were presented in the framework of everyday scenarios, for example by listing a series of meals, following which hypothetical diners either lived or died, and then requiring subjects to use this information to identify the poisoned food. Arenberg found that even when the problems were given this practical presentation, the elderly experienced difficulty in determining the solution.

Whilst these studies show that the elderly are poor at solving novel problems, it should be noted that problem-solving skills relating to well-practised activities are maintained in old age. Charness (1981*a*), for example, has studied chess playing skills in young and old experts. Charness's experiments revealed that whilst the elderly chess players were impaired at the immediate recall of board positions, they matched the performance of young players in problem-solving tasks requiring the selection of the best next move. Indeed, the results showed that the elderly were able to select the best move more quickly than the young. Charness (1989) suggests that this is because their knowledge base is better organized through practice and experience, meaning that moves the young may evaluate and reject are not even considered by elderly players. Salthouse (1984) reached a similar conclusion in a study of typing experts. In this series of studies the elderly typists showed equivalent speed and accuracy in their typing, even though their basic perceptuomotor skills, measured by tapping speed and reaction time, were impaired. The elderly maintained their typing speed because they were able to look further ahead to prepare for the coming text. It seems probable that this preservation of problem-solving skills and techniques relating to familiar activities mitigates the consequences of declining fluid intelligence in old age, allowing most elderly people to maintain active, independent, and fulfilling lives.

In conclusion, it appears that skills and knowledge acquired during youth and practised extensively during life are resistant to the effects of old age. However, the elderly are at a clear disadvantage when presented with novel situations which require active problem-solving strategies, and are also slower to learn and retain new skills (Salthouse and Somberg 1982; Wright and Payne 1985; Moscovitch *et al.* 1986; Charness 1987).

Changes in memory

Most psychologists maintain that memory refers to a set of independent but interacting functions, rather than a unitary cognitive function. However, there is considerable disagreement as to how memory should be divided, with some experimental psychologists arguing that there are no true divisions (for an introductory text see Baddeley 1996, and for more advanced discussion see Schacter 1994; Squire and Knowlton 1995; and Tulving 1995). Given that this controversy continues, the most straightforward division between primary and secondary memory will be adopted for the purposes of this review (for discussions of ageing with reference to more advanced theories of memory see Mitchell 1989; Light 1991, 1996; Craik and Jennings 1992; and Schacter *et al.* 1997). This framework is based on a simple information-processing model of memory, in which information is thought to pass through a series of stages on its way to long-term retention. Information is first encountered via perceptual processes, which hold information long enough for the information to be recognized and for the system to decide whether the information is important and requires further processing. Information selected for further processing enters primary memory, a fixed-capacity storage space that can maintain a limited amount of information in consciousness for a short time. If it is decided that the new information may be required at a later date then the information needs to be transferred to secondary memory, conceived as a long-term store with effectively unlimited capacity. In early models, it was thought that information could only enter secondary memory from primary memory (Atkinson and Shiffrin 1968). Within these models, the main purpose of primary memory was to hold information until it was no longer needed, or was passed on to secondary memory for permanent storage. However, it is now clear that new information can proceed directly from perception to secondary memory (Shallice and Warrington 1970), and that the storage aspects of primary memory do not define its function (see Baddeley 1996, Chapter 3 therein). Rather, the purpose of primary memory is to hold information so that it can be actively processed during a variety of cognitive activities, such as comprehension, learning, and reasoning (Baddeley 1986). When this processing function is added to the concept of primary memory it becomes 'working memory', a concept now central to cognitive theory that will be discussed in greater detail below in the section entitled 'Theories of cognitive change in old age'.

Although the storage aspects of primary memory do not define its function, it is none the less the case that primary memory has a limited storage capacity and this is most commonly measured using span tasks in which the number of unrelated items (usually words or numbers) a person can hold in mind for a few seconds following a single presentation is determined. Most studies show a minimal decline in the capacity of primary memory in old age. Young subjects can hold an average of six or seven items in mind at one time, whilst in elderly subjects the average falls slightly to five or six items (Botwinick and Storandt 1974; Parkinson 1982). However, the extent of the deficit in primary memory depends critically upon how primary memory is used. Whenever a requirement to process or manipulate the information is introduced, making the test a working memory test, age-decrements reliably appear. For example, Bromley (1958) found that although the forward-digit span item from the WAIS was not subject to an age effect, there was an age-related deficit in the backward-digit span test, in which the numbers have to be repeated in the reverse order. Gick and Craik (reported in Craik 1986) found similar results using a span task in which the words had to be mentally rearranged and repeated back in alphabetical order. A meta-analysis by Babcock and Salthouse (1990) revealed that in 19 out of 20 of studies which had compared active and passive-span tasks, the age effect was significantly greater in the active-span task.

The minimal and inconsistent age deficits in the storage of information in primary memory also contrast with the reliable and sizeable age differences found in tests requiring the use of secondary memory (Craik 1977; Burke and Light 1981; Poon 1985; Light 1991; Craik and Jennings 1992). However, the processes involved in successfully getting new information into and out of secondary memory are complex, and an individual's general processing capacity is an important determinant of secondary memory performance. This is because most failures of secondary memory arise from failures to access information rather than failures of storage (see Chapter 8 in Baddeley 1996). The chances of successful access are determined by how much supporting information is encoded with the target information during the initial learning experience; the greater the amount of contextual detail, the greater the chances of finding a route back to the target information when it is required. Strategies that promote the encoding of such detail, such as the use of imagery and the rearranging of information to enhance coherence, have been proven to be very effective in boosting memory performance, but have also been shown to be very demanding of processing resources (Hasher and Zacks 1979, Rabinowitz *et al.* 1982). Although studies of memory impairment in old age have yielded inconsistent findings (see reviews by Craik and Jennings 1992 and Light 1991), there is sufficient evidence to support the view that reduced processing capacity is at the root of the problems the elderly experience with establishing new material in secondary memory. This review will focus on elaborating this evidence, but reference will be made to studies in which phenomena have not been replicated. A brief note on why it might be that ageing and memory phenomena are so difficult to replicate is included at the end of this subsection.

Investigations of text recall have found the elderly to be more impaired at remembering details, such as names, places, and other incidental information, than at remembering the main points of a story (Byrd 1981 quoted in Dixon *et al.* 1984; and see Spilich 1983; Craik and Rabinowitz 1984, Dixon *et al.* 1984; Zelinski *et al.* 1984; Byrd 1985; Holland and Rabbitt 1990). Subjects of all ages are known to prioritize the extraction of the main argument, and these results suggest that there is no change to this practice in old age. However, it is proposed that because processing resources are reduced in old age (see the section entitled 'Theories of cognitive change in old age' below), there are insufficient resources available for encoding extraneous details which do not fundamentally affect the meaning of the text. Cohen (1979) and Meyer and Rice (1981) have found the reverse pattern, of age-impairments in memory for main points being greater than memory for detail, but see Meyer and Rice (1989) for an explanation of how the type of material and the intelligence of the subject interact with the availability of processing resources to produce these apparently contradictory findings.

The problem with encoding detail is not restricted to verbal information. In experiments equating the ability of the old and young to recognize items from the learning list, the elderly are less likely to detect subtle perceptual changes, such as a change in right/left orientation (Bartlett *et al.* 1983), additions or deletions (Pezdek 1987), or a change in colour (Park and Puglisi 1985). Deficits in remembering the format in which the information was presented have also been found, such as whether words were presented in a spoken or written format (Lehmann and Mellinger 1984), in upper or lower case (Kausler and Puckett 1981*a*), or in a male or female voice (Kausler and Puckett 1981*b*). The elderly also have difficulty remembering actions performed on material to be learnt. Cohen and Faulkener (1989), Guttentag and Hunt (1988), and Hashtroudi *et al.* (1990) conducted studies in which subjects were asked to learn a list of actions. The subjects performed half of these actions and imagined the other half. All three studies found that the elderly were impaired relative to the young at remembering whether they performed the action or merely imagined it. Johnson *et al.* (1989) and Rabinowitz (1989*a*) presented learning material in which the subject either read the material (e.g. HOT–COLD) or generated the material (HOT–C__D). Both studies again found that the elderly were impaired at remembering whether they had read or generated words. However, Mitchell *et al.* (1986) found that variation in memory for this judgement was considerable in their elderly group, and that if the data for three particularly poor subjects was removed the age difference became non-significant.

Overall, there is considerable evidence to suggest that the memory traces created by elderly subjects are lacking in detail and this is likely to reduce the chances of later access. However, there have been numerous demonstrations that if the elderly are given appropriate guidance during learning then this difficulty can be ameliorated. In most memory tests the subject is given no guidance concerning how to approach learning. Under such conditions the elderly are less likely to engage in strategies which promote elaborative encoding (for reviews see Craik 1977 and Burke and Light 1981). If, however, the elderly are explicitly instructed to use such strategies, their memory performance improves and the size of the age-related deficit decreases (Hulicka and Grossman 1967; Canestrari 1968; Hultsch 1974; Treat and Reese 1976; Perfect *et al.* 1995). In 1972, Craik and Lockhart performed experiments with young subjects, which suggested that the key to successful mnemonic strategy is to attend to the meaning of material to be learnt (technically termed as engaging in semantic processing). Semantic processing can be enforced by asking subjects appropriate questions about each item in the learning set (such as to categorize it, to rate is pleasantness, or to think of an associate). When elderly subjects are asked such orienting questions at learning, the size of the age difference in later memory performance is usually found to reduce (White, quoted in Craik 1977; see also Perlmutter 1978, 1979; Craik and Simon 1980; West and Boatwright 1983; Rankin and Collins 1986), although some studies have not replicated this result (see Craik and Jennings 1992 and Light 1991 for reviews). Age differences in memory for spatial materials can also be reduced by presenting the material in an integrated and meaningful framework (Waddell and Rogoff 1981; Sharps and Gollin 1987, 1988; Park *et al.* 1990; Sharps 1991).

Just as procedures that compensate for the strategic imbalance between the old and the young reduce age deficits, procedures which exacerbate the strategic difference increase the size of the age deficit. For example, Rabinowitz (1989*b*) provided subjects with unlimited time during the learning phase and allowed subjects to make notes in order to boost their memory performance. However, there were no instructions relating to how to make best use of this additional time. Rabinowitz found greater age differences in this condition than in a condition where the experimenter controlled the pace of learning and note-making was not allowed. Craik and Rabinowitz (1985) compared the utility of structured versus unstructured study periods and found that it was indeed the case that only the former are of help to the elderly. Erber *et al.* (1980) found that when subjects were asked to make judgements at encoding which hinder memory, the young were better able to engage in additional and meaningful encoding operations to compensate against the inappropriate strategy.

There is little doubt that unless considerable support is provided during learning, the elderly do not encode information into secondary memory as efficiently as the young. Poor performance in secondary memory tests, however, is only partially attributable to encoding deficits. The hypothesized reduction in processing capacity also has implications for the efficiency of the retrieval processes that search secondary memory when information is required. Self-initiated retrieval processes are recognized to be demanding of general processing capacity (Macht and Buschke 1983; Craik and McDowd 1987; Whiting and Smith 1997). However, not all memory tests demand such processes to the same degree and age effects vary according to the requirement for self-initiated retrieval (Rabinowitz 1984, 1986). Self-initiated retrieval is most important in free recall tests in which the subject is given only the instruction, 'Remember that information'. Cued recall tests provide partial support by providing a clue, such as, 'What was the animal?', whilst recognition testing eliminates the need for search processes because stimuli are re-presented and all that is required is verification of the presence or absence from the learning list. Age deficits in memory performance systematically decline in passing from free recall memory tests to cued recall tests to recognition tests (Schonfield and Robertson 1966; Craik 1977; Perlmutter 1978, 1979; Ceci and Tabor 1981; Spilich and Voss 1983; Craik and McDowd 1987; Fell 1992; Whiting and Smith 1997). Indeed, many studies have found no age deficits in recognition tests. It has been objected that this is due to the ceiling effects which frequently occur in recognition tests, but there are several examples of no age differences in tests where the majority of subjects did not perform with 100% accuracy (Perlmutter 1979; Craik and McDowd 1987; Fell 1992). None the less, age differences in recognition are found when the difficulty of the test is increased, either by providing inadequate guidance during learning (Craik and Simon 1980) or by using lures that are very similar to the presented items (Till *et al.* 1982; Bartlett and Leslie 1986). There is also evidence that the elderly rely to a greater extent on feelings of familiarity in making recognition judgements than on true retrieval of the material (Fell 1992; Perfect *et al.* 1995). For example, the elderly are better at recognizing typical rather than atypical incidents from a scenario (Hess 1985; Hess *et al.* 1989) and are more likely to be misled by plausibility in making recognition judgements (Reder *et al.* 1986; Cohen and Faulkener 1989; but see Light and Anderson 1983; Zelinski 1988). This plausibility effect has also been noted in the free recall of texts or incidents where the elderly sometimes 'remember' plausible but absent information (Spilich 1983; Cohen *et al.* 1994). It is suggested that this over-reliance on plausibility represents another effect of the reduction in processing resources because access to well-established and general information is considered to be automatic, whilst specific retrieval of presented material is considered demanding (Rabinowitz and Ackerman 1982; Reder *et al.* 1986; Hess *et al.* 1989).

The evidence reviewed supports the notion that deficits in secondary memory in old age do not spring from a fundamental disruption to the memory system, but rather from a processing reduction that prevents the memory system from being used with maximal efficiency. However, as noted at the outset, the body of evidence is inconsistent (compare, for example, the review of Craik and Jennings 1992 with that of Light 1991). With such a large body of conflicting findings it is almost certainly the case that many variables are interacting in ways that are not understood. Variations across studies in the characteristics of the subjects, the type of learning material used, the amount of learning material used, the similarity of the targets and lures used in recognition tests, and the types of manipulation used to support the learning process are all likely to have an effect upon the outcome. Add to this the facts that variation in memory ability increases in elderly populations and that statistical procedures do not always provide the right answer—particularly when second-order effects are being sought (differences between age differences) and practical constraints require that subject groups are smaller than theoretical power calculations would recommend—and the degree of inconsistency is perhaps not so surprising. Until the influence of these factors has been systematically investigated it is impossible to draw firm conclusions from the existing body of evidence. But it is felt that the phenomenon of reducing age differences in the context of increasing support and structure has been demonstrated a sufficient number of times for the phenomenon to be regarded as genuine.

Up to this point, the review of secondary memory has been concerned with the encoding of new material into secondary memory. With respect to information that has been learnt during earlier life, evidence suggests there is no significant loss during old age. In the discussion on intelligence it has already been noted that the elderly are not impaired in tests of vocabulary and general knowledge (Botwinick 1977, Perlmutter 1979, Salthouse 1988). Furthermore, there appears to be no change to the organization of information within secondary memory (see Light 1992 for a detailed review). Nebes and Brady (1988) presented old and young subjects with a list of objects and asked them to generate either an action related to the object, a feature of the object, or a common associate of the object. It was found that the associations generated by the elderly were very similar to those generated by the young, suggesting against any disorganization of knowledge in old age (see also Lovelace and Cooley 1982; Burke and Peters 1986). Other studies have examined the understanding of common events and activities. Hess (1985) gave subjects a list of events relating to 10 everyday activities (such as washing the car or going to a restaurant) and asked the subjects to rate how typical each event was with respect to the 10 activities. The ratings of the young and the old were found to be highly congruent (see also Light and Anderson 1983; List 1986; Hess *et al.* 1989). Hess and Tate (1991), Hess *et al.* (1987), and Hochman *et al.* (1986) found no differences in the stereotypes of different types of people held by the young and the old, suggesting that abstractions relating to people are also represented in the same way in the memories of the old and the young.

A technique that has been used extensively to examine the organization of established information in secondary memory is priming, whereby the presentation of priming information facilitates the processing of any subsequent information related to the priming material. For example, subjects are quicker to decide that 'doctor' is a word if they have recently encountered the word 'nurse'. A number of experiments have shown that although the elderly are always slower to make lexical decisions, they none the less benefit to the same degree as the young from the presentation of related words (Howard *et al.* 1981; Howard 1983; Burke and Yee 1984). Equivalent priming effects have been found using material related through category membership (BIRD–SPARROW; LION–MOUSE), descriptive relationships (RAIN–WET), functional relationships (BROOM–SWEEP) and association (HEARTS–FLOWERS) (see Burke and Harrold 1988 and Light 1992 for detailed reviews of priming phenomena in old age). The fact that such a variety of priming materials produce equivalent benefits for the young and the old suggests again that the organization of information in secondary memory is not disrupted by old age.

However, although a variety of paradigms point towards no loss of established information from secondary memory, the retrieval difficulties which apply to newly learnt information appear to apply equally to well-established information (Reder *et al.* 1986; Holland and Rabbitt 1990). Although the elderly are accurate when making semantic judgements about material in secondary memory, they are slower to make these judgements (Meuller *et al.* 1980; Petros *et al.* 1983; Byrd 1984; Hertzog *et al.* 1986). Furthermore, access is not only slower but also less reliable. When asked to generate members of a category, the elderly typically generate less category members than the young (Howard 1980; Obler and Albert 1985; McCrae *et al.* 1987; Brown and Mitchell 1991; Schaie and Parham 1977). The elderly also show deficits in picture naming tests, particularly for items encountered only infrequently, such as 'trellis' or 'sextant' (Bowles *et al.* 1987; Albert *et al.* 1988; La Rue 1992). Analysis of picture naming errors reveals that the elderly are prone to circumlocutions ('an artistic thing for flowers' for 'trellis', Nicholas *et al.* 1985), nominalizations ('ringer' for 'bell', La Rue 1992), and comments that indicate knowledge of the concept but not the name ('I have one of these on my porch but I cannot think of its name', Bowles *et al.* 1987). These error types suggest that the conceptual information remains in secondary memory but that the transmission of information from secondary memory to the lexicon is unreliable (Bowles *et al.* 1989, Kempler and Zelinski 1994). This interpretation of the naming problem is supported by several studies reporting an increase in the number of 'tip of the tongue' (TOT) experiences in old age, particularly with respect to rare words and proper nouns (Cohen and Faulkener 1986; Maylor 1990*a*; Burke *et al.* 1991). When the elderly find themselves in a TOT state they are less able than the young to provide partial information, such as the first letter or number of syllables (Cohen and Faulkener 1986; Maylor 1990*b*), but the rate at which TOT states spontaneously resolve is equivalent (Burke *et al.* 1991). This again suggests a temporary access problem rather than loss of the concept.

Access to established information also appears to be less flexible in old age. For example, in a standard vocabulary where the subject is given the word and must indicate its definition the elderly do not show impairments. However, the elderly are impaired in the less familiar task of providing the word in response to the definition (Rissenberg and Glanzer 1987; Bowles 1989; Maylor 1990*b*). This reduced flexibility is reflected in Holland and Rabbitt's (1990) finding that although there is little impairment in retrieving general themes from past experiences, both the recent and remote reminiscences of the old are impoverished in detail relative to those of the young (see Cohen and Faulkener 1987; Fitzgerald 1988; and Craik and Jennings 1992 for further discussion of remote memories in old age). Rabbitt (1989) found that elderly people who had lived in Oxford for at least 30 years reported fewer landmarks on a mental walk down the high street than middle-aged people who had lived in Oxford for the same amount of time. When the subjects were cued for missing landmarks the size of the age deficit was significantly reduced, although not eliminated. This finding again reveals impaired access to well-established information in old age, particularly when retrieval is unsupported.

In conclusion, although there are many inconsistencies in the body of evidence concerning memory and ageing, there is substantial evidence to show that, as in the domain of intelligence, the extent of age deficits in memory tests varies according to demands of the test. Optimal new learning requires active manipulation of information during learning. Under conditions where no support is provided, age-related deficits with encoding new information have been extensively documented. However, it seems probable that these deficits can be reduced by structuring the learning episode and supporting retrieval. There appears to be no loss of well-established information from secondary memory in old age and no disruption to the organization of this knowledge. However, as with newly learnt information, access to well-established information is impaired when the difficulty of retrieval is increased, either because self-initiated search strategies must be used, the information or the mode of access is less familiar, or the potential for interference is increased (Reder *et al.* 1986).

Changes in language

In general it is not difficult to communicate with elderly people, and formal studies demonstrate the essential preservation of the semantic and syntactic processes which associate meaning with the symbols and structures of language. The preservation of vocabulary has already been noted, whilst the previous subsection reviewed evidence that the organization of knowledge remains unchanged in old age. One powerful technique used to investigate the organization of knowledge was priming, and evidence showed that exposure to words will prime related words in the old as they do in the young. Priming effects can also be elicited by ideas presented in sentences, an application useful for investigating whether the elderly can extract meaning from linguistic structures as well as from individual words. For example, Burke and Harrold (1988) used a paradigm in which sentences were used to facilitate responses to questions such as, 'Is a diamond hard?' The participants were quicker to answer this question when they had previously read the sentence, 'The man cut the glass with the diamond', than when they had previously read the sentence 'The woman wore a diamond'. Burke and Harrold report that the response times of the elderly subjects were slower overall, but that the degree of facilitation created by the priming sentences was equivalent in the young and old groups. A variety of other paradigms using sentences to facilitate the processing of subsequent verbal material has also revealed equivalent effects in young and old subjects (see Light 1992 for a review). This body of evidence suggests that the processes that parse and interpret sentential structures remain intact during old age. Indeed, it seems that the elderly can use their powers of comprehension to overcome some perceptual difficulties associated with their declining sensory powers (Stine *et al.* 1989; Tun and Wingfield 1993). Cohen and Faulkener (1983) requested participants to listen to a series of target words and write down each word as it occurred. The words occurred either alone, or at the end of a short sentence that provided a predictable context for the word, against varying levels of background noise. When the words were presented in isolation the elderly were impaired at perceiving the words relative to the young, with the size of the deficit increasing with the amount of background noise. However, presentation of the context sentences enhanced the ability of the elderly to perceive the target words and reduced the size of the age difference. Wingfield *et al.* (1985) have shown that the elderly are also able to use linguistic information to counteract difficulties in registering rapid speech.

A study by Stine *et al.* (1989) of the processes used to comprehend longer passages of discourse suggests that the old and young segment speech according to the same principles. In this experiment the subjects were required to segment running speech into recallable segments by stopping the speech periodically and repeating what had just been said. Stine *et al.* found that although the elderly selected shorter segments, both the old and the young demonstrated a strong tendency to stop the speech at a syntactic boundary (84% of stops for the young and 81% for the old, a non-significant difference). The results also revealed that both young and old subjects were equally accurate in recalling the segments, demonstrating that the elderly were as capable at monitoring their comprehension. However, although from moment to moment the comprehension processes used by the young and the old appear to be equivalent, comprehension studies, which present the text as a whole and then test comprehension by either asking questions or requiring recall, have generally found impairments (Cohen 1979; Till and Walsh 1980; Spilich 1983; Till 1985). It seems more probable, however, that these impairments reflect problems with secondary memory rather than problems with the comprehension processes that integrate text into a meaningful representation (Light and Albertson 1988). Other studies demonstrating that the elderly experience particular difficulty in retrieving the information once a comprehension has decayed from primary memory, will be described later in this subsection.

The previous studies have all shown that with respect to comprehension, the linguistic capacities of the elderly are essentially preserved. Studies of language production have led to the same conclusions. There is no evidence for a restriction in the range of vocabulary used in old age; moreover, discourse remains meaningful and grammatical in structure (Kempler and Zelinski 1994). Studies examining the high-level structure of discourse have produced mixed findings, probably because it is difficult to derive objective and reliable measures for what constitutes good structure. Kemper (1987), Kemper *et al.* (1990), and Pratt and Robins (1991) report that the stories told by the elderly have clear beginnings, middles, and ends and that the elderly are competent at introducing new themes and characters into the narrative. However, whilst some authors have argued that discourse is less coherent in old age (Critchley 1984; Glosser and Deser 1992), others have found that the stories of the elderly are rated as being better formed and more entertaining than those of the young (Mergler *et al.* 1985; Kemper *et al.* 1990).

However, the elderly do encounter some problems with the use and comprehension of language. 'Tip of the tongue' experiences and naming difficulties increase in old age, as discussed in the last subsection, and the elderly can also experience difficulty in following conversations when many participants are involved and the topic of the conversation is unfamiliar. In light of what has gone before, the reader will perhaps not be surprised to discover that cognitive research has revealed deficits in the processing of language when the demands upon the cognitive system are increased. The previous paragraph, for example, has noted that the speech of the elderly remains free of syntactic error, but several studies have noted a decrease in the range and complexity of syntactic constructions used by elderly subjects both in spoken (Kynette and Kemper 1986) and written (Kemper 1987, quoted in Stuart-Hamilton 1994) discourse. The effect of syntactic complexity is also apparent in the comprehension performance of the elderly, as indexed by disproportionately poor performance relating to sentences with a complex syntactic structure relative those with a simple structure (Kemper 1987; Davis and Ball 1989; Norman *et al.* 1991; Obler *et al.* 1991).

Another area in which complexity is seen to influence the performance of the elderly concerns the ability to make inferences from verbal material. A number of studies again suggest that the elderly do not have a fundamental problem with using their knowledge of language and the world to make appropriate inferences. Zelinski and Miura (1986, quoted in Zelinski 1988) used a paradigm in which the making of an inference was indexed by the increase in reading speed for sentences whose comprehension depended upon inference. For example, participants were slower to read the second sentence in this pair:

1. We bought a new appliance for our church.
2. The refrigerator will be much appreciated there.

than in this pair, where no matching of terms is required:

1. We bought a new refrigerator for our church.
2. The refrigerator will be much appreciated there.

Zelinski and Miura found that the elderly read more slowly overall, but did not find that their reading speed increased disproportionately in the inference condition. They concluded, therefore, that the elderly did not encounter any specific difficulty with making the inference required. Light and Capps (1986) examined the use of inference for matching pronouns with their referents. In this study a typical pair of sentences would be:

1. Henry spoke at the meeting whilst John went to the beach.
2. He lectured on administration.

Light and Capps found that the elderly were able to use the content of the first sentence to determine that 'he' was Henry rather than John in this example. However, Light and Capps also found that the elderly were likely to misattribute 'he' to being John if irrelevant material was inserted between the first and second sentences. Other studies suggest that it is not the insertion of additional material *per se* which causes the problem, but specifically the insertion of material which instigates a shift in topic. Light and Albertson (1988) investigated the capacity of the elderly to detect anomalies in written material (using a paradigm first used by Cohen 1979). They compared short stories in which the material intervening between the two bits of conflicting information involved a shift of topic (example 1), with stories in which the intervening material maintained attention to the key facts (example 2):

1. Next door to us there's an old man who's completely blind. He lives with his unmarried sister who works as housekeeper for a banker. She works long hours and rarely seems to get any time off to be with her brother. We often see him sitting on his porch reading his newspaper.
2. Next door to us there's an old man who's completely blind. He lives quite alone and nobody ever goes to visit him, but he seems to manage quite well. He has a guide dog and goes out every day to do his shopping. We often see him sitting on his porch reading his newspaper.

Light and Albertson replicated Cohen's finding that the elderly are impaired in detecting the anomaly in examples of the first kind, but they found no differences between the young and old in examples of the second kind. Further results suggest that the problem with maintaining comprehension over more than one topic relates to a problem with retrieving information relating to the earlier topic. Light and Albertson (1988) repeated the earlier Light and Capps paradigm, but tested not only whether participants could determine whether 'he' was John or Henry, but also whether they could recall the initial sentence that contained the key information. When the inference was conditionalized on recalling the first sentence, there was no difference between the performance of the old and the young. Similarly, when the elderly fail to detect the anomaly in the examples above, they also fail to answer the more straightforward question 'What handicap did the old man have?' Thus, it seems that the elderly can use their knowledge of language and the world to make appropriate inferences, but that problems with secondary memory can lead to difficulties with remembering what is what and who is who when reading or listening to long passages of material.

The elderly are also compromised in making inferences when the inference is made difficult by requiring that the information presented be mentally transformed and manipulated (see Cohen 1988 for detailed review). Cohen (1981) and Light *et al.* (1982), for example, found that the elderly are impaired at making a variety of logical deductions from verbal information. The problem persists when the written information remains present during the inferential processing, showing that this is a problem with the reasoning required, and not a problem with secondary memory (Cohen 1981). Salthouse (1982) reported that although the elderly are not impaired in WAIS Verbal IQ subtests such as Vocabulary and Information, in which the answer simply has to be produced, they are impaired in Similarities in which two concepts are given and the participant must work out the higher level category connecting them (ranging from 'BANANA–APPLE'—fruits, to 'PRAISE–PUNISHMENT'—methods for encouraging good behaviour). Other examples of impairments with problem-solving inferences are Riegel's (1959) demonstration that the elderly are impaired at making verbal analogies, and Light and Albertson's (1988) finding that the elderly show a disproportionate deficit when answering questions presented in a double-negative format.

In conclusion, the elderly show basic preservation of the semantic and syntactic processes which parse and extract meaning from language. They are also able to make use of their knowledge of language and the world to make inferences. However, their capacity to make inferences can be impaired under two situations, both of which are associated with a high demand for general processing resources. The first is when earlier information is required from secondary memory and the second is when the inference requires problem-solving. Thus, the phenomenon observed with respect to intelligence and memory appears again with respect to language skills: there is preservation of the fundamental abilities, but these abilities become compromised under demanding situations.

Changes in spatial cognition

The study of spatial skills in old age has been neglected relative to that of memory and language, but studies of everyday usages of spatial information suggest minimal change to the fundamentals of spatial cognition (see Kirasic 1989 for a review). This supports the informal opinion one would form based on the fact that elderly people do not get lost in their homes or neighbourhood and are able to manipulate clothes, household objects, appliances, and tools appropriately (assuming their are no motoric difficulties). A small-scale diary study by Kirasic (1989) documenting one week in the lives of three elderly women confirms that problems with orientation within the home and travel within the locality do not occur. All difficulties reported by these women related to problems with memory rather than spatial cognition, such as losing things in the home, entering rooms to discover that the purpose of the visit was forgotten, and remembering where the car was parked in large car parks.

Most evidence on spatial performance has been generated indirectly through studies of intelligence. Intelligence subtests involving a component of spatial manipulation have been found to be very sensitive to age (Meudell and Greenhalgh 1987; Koss *et al.* 1991; Schaie 1996). It has already been mentioned that most elderly people over the age of 60 perform more than 1 standard deviation below the average performance of the young in the Performance IQ subtests from the WAIS (Doppelt and Wallace 1955). Salthouse (1982) also reports a decline of 5% to 10% per decade in those WAIS subtests involving spatial manipulations (Object assembly, Block design, Picture completion, and Picture arrangement). Both these studies are cross-sectional, and thus are likely to overestimate age effects due to cohort effects (see Schaie 1996 and Woodruff-Pak 1997, and also Chapter 15 in this volume for discussion of the methodological issues associated with cross-sectional research), but Schaie's extensive longitudinal study of different generational cohorts using the Primary Mental Abilities tests (Thurstone 1938; Thurstone and Thurstone 1962) confirms that individuals begin to show decline in the Space test of this battery after age 50.

The particular sensitivity of psychometric tests with a spatial component has been interpreted as indicating the greater vulnerability of the right hemisphere of the brain relative to the left (Schaie and Schaie 1977; Klisz 1978; Goldstein and Shelly 1981), but there is no evidence to suggest that the right hemisphere ages more rapidly than the left. It seems more likely that the sensitivity of spatial psychometric tests is due to dependence upon 'fluid intelligence' (Horn and Cattell 1967; Ardila and Rosselli 1989), as explained above in the 'Changes in intelligence and problem-solving' section. This position is supported by experimental studies of spatial competence, which suggest that age deficits in spatial cognition are pronounced in tasks that require internal manipulation of information. Cerella *et al.* (1981) found that the elderly are slower to rotate stimuli mentally and are also less accurate in deciding whether two rotated stimuli are the same or mirror-images. Bruce and Herman (1983) took photographs of a variety of environmental features from a number of different perspectives. Subjects were shown a feature and then asked to imagine it from a different angle. By probing recognition with the appropriate photographs, Bruce and Herman demonstrated that the elderly were impaired at anticipating what something would look like from an unseen perspective.

However, as within the other cognitive domains examined, age deficits in spatial cognition can be ameliorated by increasing the familiarity of the task or the material. Kirasic (1980, quoted in Kirasic 1989) demonstrated that the elderly are poor at generating internal perspectives relating to a mock-town (which they were required to learn in an earlier phase of the experiment), but are less impaired with reference to their home town. In a subsequent study, Kirasic (1981, quoted in Kirasic 1989) found the elderly to be impaired when completing shopping tasks in an unfamiliar supermarket, but not when shopping in their own supermarket. Scheidt and Schaie (1978) found that the everyday spatial tasks which created most concern for the elderly were those involving unfamiliar environments in which little help was available. Driving in heavy traffic and moving into a new home were paradigm examples of the types of activity that caused low confidence and anxiety in the elderly, whilst shopping in a familiar supermarket was not approached with fear or apprehension. The studies of Charness (1981*a*,*b*) and Salthouse (1984) examining chess and typing performance, respectively, also show that when people have expertise relating to particular forms of spatial cognition, old age does not affect their competence (see p. 45).

In summary, although most psychometric tests of spatial cognition reveal dramatic age impairments, it seems likely this is because such tests demand the high-level manipulation of unfamiliar and abstract information, rather than because spatial cognition *per se* is vulnerable to the ageing process. As in the other cognitive domains reviewed, when the familiarity of the material or the task is increased, the observed age deficits in spatial cognition are reduced. The findings from laboratory studies are supported by investigations into the everyday activities of the elderly, which suggest that problems with spatial cognition are only prominent if there is a memory demand or if the situation is unfamiliar and complex.

Theories of cognitive change in old age

The evidence reviewed in the previous section suggests that age deficits appear in all cognitive domains, but only when the demands made upon cognition are high. This is consistent with the view expressed by Craik and Rabinowitz (1984) that old age does not affect the structure of specific cognitive components, but rather affects processing efficiency throughout the cognitive system. It was noted earlier that the problem of defining what, in cognitive terms, makes a task difficult has so far proven intractable, but at a descriptive level it can be said that the elderly show impairments in tests when one or more of the following apply:

- the material and the task are unfamiliar;
- internal (mental) manipulation of the material is required;
- optimal performance depends upon the generation of strategies.

This section describes the most influential theories advanced to define 'processing capacity', and explains what it is that differentiates the 'difficult' tasks in which the elderly are impaired from the 'easy' tasks in which they are not impaired. These theories divide into two main types, attentional theories and speed theories.

Attentional theories derive from the information-processing models of the mind developed by cognitive psychologists between the late 1950s and the 1970s (Broadbent 1958; Kahneman 1973; Norman and Bobrow 1975; Schneider and Shiffrin 1977). Within such models it is assumed that perceptual processes can simultaneously extract large amounts of information from the environment and process it to a low level, but that the amount of information which can be processed to a high level at one time (for example, to determine identity, consider implications, perform transformations, or memorize information) is strictly limited. It is further assumed that the cognitive system contains a central attentional component which selects the information that will be processed and filters out irrelevant information. The central attentional component is thought to possess a limited quantity of processing resources that can be deployed to undertake the high-level processing of the selected information. The notion of the central attentional component is essentially synonymous with the concept of working memory which evolved from the concept of primary memory (see the section entitled 'Changes in memory'). Working memory is usually conceived as including the mental space within which all high level cognitive processing occurs, the limited pool of processing resources required for high-level processing, and the mechanism that selects what will be processed and controls how it is processed.

Attentional theories of cognitive ageing converge in assuming that old age has a deleterious effect upon the working memory system. The evidence that old age has a marked effect upon the ability to perform active-span tasks, thought to provide the best measures of working memory capacity, has already been reviewed above. There is also a wealth of evidence showing that these active-span tasks correlate with performance in a wide range of cognitive tasks typical of those which show age effects (see Engle 1996 for a review). Different theories, however, have focused on different aspects of the working memory system as being critically affected in old age. Parkinson and colleagues have argued that size of the mental space in which cognitive processing occurs contracts, restricting the amount of information which can be processed at any one time (Parkinson 1982; Inman and Parkinson 1983; Parkinson *et al.* 1985). However, although the passive-span studies reviewed earlier show a mild reduction in the basic storage capacity of working memory, the deficit is markedly exacerbated when processing is required. These passive-span measures are also poor predictors of ability in higher cognitive tests (Daneman and Carpenter 1980; Turner and Engle 1989). This suggests that the changes in working memory are more likely to represent a restriction in processing capacity than a reduction in storage capacity (Craik and Rabinowitz 1984; Gick *et al.* 1988).

However, the validity of the notion of limited capacity, whether expressed in terms of storage or processing, has frequently been questioned (Allport 1980; Navon 1984; Hasher and Zacks 1988). There are three key objections, which are clearly set out by Stoltzfus *et al.* (1996). First, there are no measures available that provide an unambiguous index of the amount of processing resources present in working memory. Second, it is not clear whether there is one central working memory system shared between all types of cognitive processing (Engle *et al.* 1992) or whether there are separate working memory systems dedicated for language processing, arithmetic, spatial analysis and so forth (Daneman and Tardif 1987). Third, the notion of capacity is not sufficiently well specified to allow for predictions that could advance the development of the theory. The capacity of working memory has been defined with sufficient looseness to tempt researchers into advancing circular arguments when experiments yield data that do not support a prediction. That is, explanations to the effect that although it was expected a task would demand processing resources, the task was too easy and did not require processing resources after all, are common within the literature.

These problems with the notion of limited capacity have led other theorists to view cognitive decline in old age as stemming from changes to the control function of working memory (Welford 1958; Taub 1968; Rabbitt 1981). An example of such a theory, which has captured considerable interest, is Hasher and Zacks' (1988) proposal that the apparent limitations in working memory capacity are caused by interference or 'cross-talk' between the various bits of information present in working memory at any one time. Efficient performance of a task requires that only information relevant to the task in hand be present within working memory. The most effective way in which relevant information can be sifted from irrelevant information is through a combination of facilitatory processes and inhibitory processes (Houghton and Tipper 1994). Hasher and Zacks propose that ageing has a specific impact upon the efficiency of inhibitory processes. Thus, whilst the elderly do not have difficulties with the facilitatory processes which first bring information into working memory, they do have difficulty with the removal of irrelevant information that has either entered working memory accidentally or that has already been processed and needs to be dismissed. The contents of the elderly working memory, therefore, are more likely to contain a mixture of both relevant and irrelevant information, leading to contradictory trains of thought and causing slowness and error in a wide variety of cognitive tests. Hasher and Zacks' theory has stimulated a wealth of experiments examining the inhibitory powers of the elderly. These have shown that the elderly are more susceptible to a wide variety of distractions than the young (for a review see Zacks and Hasher 1997). However, conflicts within the body of evidence have prompted McDowd (1997) to argue that the three objections raised against the notion of the limited capacity apply equally to the idea of inhibitory processes. Specifically, first, there is no agreement upon how to measure an individual's inhibitory power; second, different measures of inhibition do not always correlate with one another, raising controversy as to whether there is one central inhibitory mechanism or a number of specialized inhibitory mechanisms; and, third, these uncertainties have led to imprecision in the theory, again allowing for circular arguments such that when a prediction fails, it is argued that the test did not, after all, tap the expected type of inhibitory mechanism.

The major attraction of *speed theories* of cognitive ageing is that, set against this background of controversy within attentional theory, it appears to be refreshingly simple. Speed theorists argue that the many problems which have beset the definition of working memory spring from the fact that there is no such component within the cognitive system. They argue that limitations in human thought can be explained with reference only to the basic speed with which information can be processed, making the postulation of such a component unnecessary. It is suggested that in old age the basic speed of processing reduces, causing generalized inefficiency throughout the cognitive system (this is called the generalized slowing hypothesis). It is certainly the case that the reaction times of the elderly are slower than those of the young, regardless of the task performed (Cerella 1985; Hale *et al.* 1991), and thus there is evidence for a general slowing of processing in old age. The generalized slowing hypothesis predicts that when there is a general slowing of processing, difficult tasks will reveal larger impairments than simple tasks. This is because difficult tasks contain more component operations than simple tasks, and so the effects of the slowing are multiplicative. If the elderly are slower than the young by x amount, then in a task with one cognitive operation they will be x amount slower, but in a task with two operations they will be $2x$ slower, and $3x$ slower in a task with three components, and so on. Support for this multiplicative function comes from a technique first used by Brinley (1965) who examined the reaction times (RT) of the young and the old in two series of tests that involved matching stimuli. In one series, attentional demands were minimal because the matching feature was kept constant, whilst in the other series attentional demands were high because the subjects had to monitor several aspects of the stimuli to detect the match. Brinley found that both the young and old were slower in the attentional than the non-attentional tests, and also that the absolute difference in RT between the old and the young was greatest in the attentional tasks. At first sight this may suggest a specific difficulty with attentional operations, but when the results were plotted, such that for each task the x coordinate was the average RT for the young and the y coordinate was the average RT of the old, all the points lay along a straight line, regardless of whether the test had included an attentional component or not. This is interpreted as showing that the elderly are not specifically penalized in tests which have a strong attentional component, but rather are slowed by a constant factor relative to the young, that factor being measurable by the slope of the line (this phenomenon has been replicated several times, see Rabbitt 1996 for a review).

A simple objection to the generalized slowing hypothesis is that although the evidence suggests that, in any reaction time task, the average RT of the elderly can be predicted by multiplying the average RT of the young by the critical factor, the scope of the hypothesis is limited because the elderly often fail in tasks which have no time limit. However, many acts of cognition require integrating the outcomes of earlier processes into ongoing processes. If these cognitive products are not available at the right time, due to slowing of the earlier cognitive operations, it may be impossible to achieve a solution. This point is supported by partial correlation analyses, which show that measures of speed can account for most of the age-related variance in a wide variety of higher cognitive tests, regardless of whether those tests have a time limit or not (Salthouse 1993, 1996). Calculations show that around 90–99% of the variance shared between age and higher cognition is also shared with speed measures (Salthouse 1993). This is taken to provide evidence that age effects upon higher cognition are not direct, but are mediated primarily through a loss of speed. Indeed, Salthouse and Babcock (1991) report that whilst partialling out speed can account for nearly all the age-related variance in working memory tests, partialling out working memory performance has little impact upon the relationship between age and speed. They interpret this asymmetry as indicating that it is speed, and not working memory, which is the fundamental resource affected by ageing.

The generalized slowing hypothesis undoubtedly has the virtue of parsimony relative to attentional theories, but it is only possible to be parsimonious when the evidence permits and, despite the findings reviewed above, it is not clear that the evidence does permit. Although the Brinley plot technique has proven highly reliable, it has been argued that the method is not sensitive enough for drawing conclusions concerning the effects of normal ageing upon cognition (Fisk and Fisher 1994; Perfect 1994; Rabbitt 1996). There is also no question as to the reliability of Salthouse's partial correlation analyses, but it is important to recognize that the speed measures used by Salthouse and colleagues are only assumed, and not proven, to measure basic processing speed. Salthouse emphasizes the simplicity of his speeded measures, but if the speeded task becomes too simple then the power is lost. A paradigm example of an effective task, widely used by Salthouse and colleagues, is the Digit symbol subtest from the WAIS. In this test the subject is given a key which associates seven abstract symbols with the numbers 1–7. The subject is also given a page containing rows of numbers and is instructed to use the key to draw the appropriate symbol under each number. The subject's score is the number of numbers decoded into symbols in the time allowed. Simpler speed tests, such as simple reaction time or copying rather than decoding symbols, are much less effective in explaining age-related variance in cognitive performance (Milwain 1999). Salthouse does not seem unduly concerned by this fact, and even seems to believe it promotes his theory stating that:

> The discovery that there was more attenuation of the relations between age and cognition after statistical control of perceptual speed measures involving comparison or transformation operations than after motor speed measures requiring *little or no cognitive operations* suggests that the speed of primary interest in the mediation of relations between age and cognition is perceptual or cognitive in nature rather than motoric. (Salthouse 1993, p. 736 (italics added by author))

However, this admission that the content or type of processing is critical is in direct opposition to the spirit of the generalized slowing hypothesis, which states that there are no different 'types' of speed but only a global slowing of all processes, regardless of their nature. Whilst it can be held that cognitive speed (usually termed 'perceptual speed' by Salthouse, to maintain the illusion that the type of speed in question is fundamental and does not require a theoretical definition) varies independently of the speed of sensorimotor processing, the fact that cognitive and sensorimotor processes all occur within the same central nervous system means that any global change would be expected to affect cognitive and sensorimotor processes equally. In other words, there is no *a priori* reason to suppose that neurons involved in cognition age more rapidly than those involved in sensation and action. Furthermore, even if evidence were to reveal that they do, there would then be reason to suppose that some populations of 'cognitive' neurons may age more rapidly than others, and the foundations of the generalized slowing hypothesis would collapse. A more systematic explanation is required as to what differentiates cognitive processing from sensorimotor processing, and this requirement leads back to attentional theories in which cognitive processing and sensorimotor processing are distinguished by the degree to which they need high-level control.

A more thorough evaluation of the evidence suggests in favour of attentional theories, but it is necessary to align this with Salthouse and Babcock's (1991) finding that speeded measures, comparable to Digit symbol, are more effective in explaining age-related variance than the measures used by working memory theorists. Although simple on the surface, Digit symbol in fact involves coordination of a large number of component processes. The subject must scan the grid to find the next number to be decoded, maintain this number in working memory, scan the key to find the appropriate symbol, hold this symbol in working memory, re-scan the test grid to find his place, and coordinate his motoric functions to write the correct symbol in the correct place. Once completed this whole operation must be deleted from working memory in order to focus on the next symbol in the grid. Speed in this task requires maintaining a strong focus to prevent distraction from other symbols in the grid and from extraneous sources. In other words, it may be that Digit symbol is the most successful measure of the resource lost during normal ageing because it a highly structured task that everyone can perform accurately and which does not allow for idiosyncratic approaches, but which also requires a high level of attentional control. Working memory theorists, by contrast, have attempted to capture attentional control through the use of accuracy-based measures which are less constraining and do allow for idiosyncracity of approach, introducing noise into the measures and reducing their sensitivity. Indeed, accuracy measures are inherently blunter than speeded measures because they do not distinguish between those who can achieve accuracy quickly and those who are accurate but slow. Equally, when a subject gets a problem wrong, there is no indication as to how close he was to getting it right. Thus, although the Salthouse phenomenon is highly reliable, and is often used to support the generalized slowing hypothesis, the phenomenon may reveal only that 'perceptual speed' tests are more sensitive measures of attentional function than the accuracy-based tests which have traditionally been used to assess aspects of working memory. Overall, it seems that an attentional explanation of ageing is more plausible than a speed-based explanation, and the problems of poor predictive power and circularity which have beset attentional explanations must continue to be tackled. The remainder of this section attempts to address this challenge.

The attempt begins by considering the relationship between the hypothesized attentional control function and the specialized cognitive functions or modules. Evidence from cognitive neuropsychology demonstrates that the cognitive system is divided into specialized components which operate with some degree of independence from one another (see Kolb and Whishaw 1995 and Shallice 1988 for discussion). However, within the 'systems' philosophy of cognition, currently emerging from cognitive neuroscience, areas of the brain are seen to be specialized for a particular function, but can only produce behaviour when integrated into a distributed system (see, for example, Mesulam 1990; Posner and Petersen 1990; Tulving 1995). Thus, any act of cognition, no matter how simple, requires that the relevant modules be integrated into an effective system. It is possible that individuals vary according to their ability to effectively channel information from perception (primary sensory cortex) through cognition (association cortex) to action (primary motor cortex). In other words, 'intelligence' or 'attentional control' may be equivalent to the ability of the individual to organize particular modules (sensory, cognitive, and motor) into an appropriate system.

The problems associated with defining working memory may arise because the concept derives from hierarchical models of the mind, in which it is assumed that information passes through an ordered set of stages from perception to selection to apprehension. Findings from neuroscience and neuroimaging suggest that this one-way hierarchy is too simplistic. More recent theories see high-level control as operating not upon advanced forms of representation, but rather upon original perceptions, as illustrated by these quotations from Posner and Raichle (1994):

> Attention can amplify computations within particular areas, but often appears to do so by reentering the same area that initially performed the computations, not by activating new higher-level association areas. (Posner and Raichle 1994, p. 147)
>
> Computer models of neural networks whose computations require closely coordinated cooperative activity among many areas also suggest the importance of information being fed back to sensory-specific areas for additional computation. (Posner and Raichle 1994, p. 144)
>
> In general one thinks of brain circuitry as formed of fixed anatomical connections between brain areas or between neurons within an area. However, it is well known that any brain area can be anatomically connected to any other area by either direct or indirect routes. In higher cognition, the act of attending organizes the circuitry between brain areas. (Posner and Raichle 1994, p. 147)

Posner and Raichle localize this controlling function, whereby activation in specialized brain areas in the posterior of the brain is modulated according to the demands of the current situation, to a network of areas in the front of the brain, specifically within the anterior cingulate and dorsolateral prefrontal cortex. This hypothesis suggests that, in complex situations, the appropriate use of function-specific brain regions depends upon the efficiency of a network located in the frontal lobe. Thus, the conclusions concerning cognition in old age—namely that although there is no direct damage to cognitive modules, there is an impairment in the ability to use them flexibly—could be explained by a disruption to the anterior cingulate/dorsolateral prefrontal network.

Functional imaging paradigms have revealed particular involvement of these frontal areas in a variety of circumstances under which the elderly are known to be impaired. Several studies, for example, have found activation in these areas in working memory tests that require active processing, but not in passive 'storage-only' tasks (Owen *et al.* 1998, Smith *et al.* 1998). There is also evidence that the dorsolateral prefrontal cortex and anterior cingulate are activated by novel tasks which cannot be supported by either habits or expertise. Petrides *et al.* (1993) contrasted the brain activity associated with the generation of the numbers 1–10 in their usual order with that associated with the generation of the numbers 1–10 in a random order without repetition. The PET (positron emission tomography) scan data revealed significant activation of the dorsolateral prefrontal cortex in the random task, but not in the habitual task. Raichle *et al.* (1994) investigated the effects of practice upon the brain activations associated with a verb-generation task, and found that the involvement of the dorsolateral prefrontal cortex and anterior cingulate diminished as practice increased (see also Passingham 1996 for similar findings using a motor coordination task). Functional imaging techniques have also been used to localize areas involved in inhibitory functions, and the dorsolateral prefrontal cortex and anterior cingulate have again found to be implicated. Jonides *et al.* (1998) presented subjects with a set of target letters to be held in working memory until a probe letter appeared 3 seconds later. The task was to decide whether the probe was one of the target letters. Jonides compared a condition that required inhibition of a prepotent response with one that made no inhibitory demands. In the non-inhibitory condition the probe was not a target and, in addition, had not been a target for at least two trials, allowing its association with a positive response to decay away. In the inhibitory condition the probe was not a target for the current trial, but had been a target in one of the two preceding trials, meaning that the letter remained associated with a positive response which had to be suppressed. Jonides *et al.* found significant activation of the left prefrontal cortex in the inhibitory condition but not in the non-inhibitory condition. Pardo *et al.* (1990) examined the pattern of brain activation associated with the Stroop task, the classic inhibitory test in which the subject is presented with the name of a colour written in an ink of a conflicting colour which must be named, necessitating suppression of the natural tendency to read the word. When Pardo *et al.* compared this test with a control test that had no inhibitory requirement (naming coloured bars) a strong activation in the anterior cingulate was observed.

It appears, therefore, that the anterior cingulate and dorsolateral prefrontal cortex are implicated in several situations where the elderly are known to experience particular difficulty. There have only been a few studies where functional imaging technology has been applied to study the effects of old age upon cognition directly, but the findings are again consistent with the proposal that there may be a problem in the anterior cingulate/dorsolateral prefrontal network. Grady *et al.* (1995) used PET imaging to study brain activity in young and old adults during the encoding phase of a face-recognition memory test. It was found that the old did not remember as many faces as the young, and that a key feature which differentiated the pattern of brain activation in the elderly subjects during encoding was failure to activate the anterior cingulate. Furthermore, in the young, it was found that, during encoding, activity in the hippocampus (known to be critical for memory performance) was augmented relative to a non-mnemonic face-matching task, and that hippocampal activity correlated with anterior cingulate activity (r = 0.94). By contrast, hippocampal activity during encoding in the old was not augmented relative to the face-matching task (bar one exception) and there was no correlation with anterior cingulate activity (r = 0.02). Grady *et al.* concluded that:

> ...older people employ no particular strategy, beyond that used in perception, in their attempt to memorize the faces. (Grady *et al.* 1995, p. 220)

This conclusion directly parallels that drawn by Craik and colleagues on the basis of the evidence reviewed in the section above on changes in memory. With respect to Craik's work, it is relevant that Grady *et al.* told their subjects simply to 'study the faces'. This is the type of undirected learning condition that Craik identifies as being likely to lead to inefficient memory performance in the old. Craik's work suggests that an age effect in the face-recognition task would have been less likely had the subjects been asked to make some kind of judgement concerning each face. It would be interesting to investigate how these types of guiding instructions alter the pattern of brain activation during encoding.

A study by Schacter *et al.* (1996) also led to the conclusion that the differences between the old and young in memory performance are due to inefficiencies within prefrontal areas and not within the hippocampus. In this study, subjects were scanned whilst completing three-letter word stems. In the first scan, the subjects were instructed to complete each stem with the first word that came to mind (baseline). Following this, the subjects were shown a list of 40 words which they were required to learn. Memory for 20 of these words ('easy recall' condition) was promoted by asking the subjects to make a semantic judgement about each word and by the interviewer presenting each word four times. Memory for the remaining 20 words ('hard recall' condition) was hampered by asking the subjects to make a perceptual judgement about each word and by the interviewer presenting each word only once. After this learning phase, the subjects were presented with word stems and asked to remember a word from the list of 40 that would complete the stem. Schacter *et al.* found that when the activation in the easy recall condition was compared with either the baseline condition (in which no recall was attempted by the subjects), or the hard recall condition (in which recall was largely unsuccessful), both old and young groups showed significant activation in the hippocampus. The increase in hippocampal blood flow under the easy recall condition was equivalent in both groups. Schacter *et al.* concluded that when memory is successful there is no difference in the pattern of brain activation between old and young. However, comparison of the hard recall condition with the baseline condition revealed increased activation in the anterior regions of the prefrontal cortex and in the anterior cingulate in the young subjects, but not in the elderly subjects. These areas have been shown in previous studies to be important for the initiation of retrieval processes (see Buckner and Petersen 1996 for a review). Schacter *et al.* therefore concluded that following non-optimal learning conditions, the elderly did not engage the appropriate retrieval processes for searching memory and that this is an important factor in explaining the difficulty the elderly experience in memory tests.

In summary, Posner and Raichle (1994) have proposed the existence of an attentional network in the anterior cingulate and dorsolateral prefrontal cortex, which has the function of coordinating activation throughout the brain so that the chances of achieving goals are maximized. It is proposed that the cognitive changes associated with old age are those that would be expected were the efficiency of this proposed network to decline. Functional imaging studies provide preliminary evidence for this proposal, in that it has been shown that the dorsolateral prefrontal cortex and anterior cingulate are involved in many of the cognitive tasks identified as being particularly sensitive to old age. It has previously been claimed that ageing may be a form of dysexecutive function (Albert and Kaplan 1980; Dempster 1992; West 1996; Parkin 1997; Woodruff-Pak 1997). However, these dysexecutive hypotheses have been criticized, on the same basis as the earlier working memory theories, for being underspecified. The purpose of the prefrontal cortex has been summarized as underpinning 'executive functions', these functions being implicated in a diverse collection of activities, ranging from sustaining attention, holding and processing information in working memory, setting goals, developing plans, evaluating and selecting strategies, monitoring plans, adapting to unexpected occurrences, inhibiting inappropriate behaviours, and underpinning socially acceptable behaviour. It is not clear what definition of 'executive function' would unite all these different functions. Furthermore, both the reliability and the validity of tests designed to measure 'executive function' are questionable (Phillips 1997; Rabbitt 1997). It is thought that one reason for the current confusion of what is meant by 'executive function' is that the prefrontal cortex, which occupies a large volume of the cortical mantle, is not undifferentiated but contains a number of functionally separable subsystems (Goldman-Rakic 1996; Robbins 1996; Shallice and Burgess 1996). It is probable that not all these subsystems are equally vulnerable to the effects of ageing. Thus, development of the ideas outlined in the final passages of this section depend upon the identification of these separable subsystems, followed by examination of which are sensitive to age. The critical question would then be whether deterioration of the sensitive subsystems could explain all the results reviewed in the previous section. This is a considerable task, but the development of increasingly sensitive brain-imaging technologies is leading to rapid advancement in the understanding of how cognition is organized within the brain. So long as these advances are incorporated into the study of cognitive ageing, there can be optimism that rapid advance will also occur in the understanding of the relationship between age and cognition.

What causes cognitive change in old age?

The review in the previous section shows that theoretical approaches to cognitive decline in old age continue to generate controversy, but two speculative conclusions have been drawn. First, that old age affects processing efficiency throughout the cognitive system, but does not cause fundamental damage to the specialized cognitive components which underpin memory, language, and visuospatial functions. Second, that it seems more likely that this loss of efficiency springs from disruption to an attentional function rather than a generalized slowing of processing. Assuming that these conclusions are correct, the next question to arise concerns the cause of the reduction in efficiency of the attentional network. The most direct hypothesis would be a selective loss of neurons from the frontal lobe in old age. Haug and colleagues have reported, on the basis of postmortem findings, that whilst the volume of the temporal, parietal, and occipital lobes reduces by only 1% in old age, the volume of the frontal lobe reduces by between 8% and 17% (Haug *et al.* 1983; Haug and Eggers 1991), although the loss of volume is thought to be due to the shrinkage, rather than loss, of neurons (Terry *et al.* 1987; Haug and Eggers 1991). Time-of-life studies, using structural MRI (magnetic resonance imaging), have also concluded that the frontal lobe shows the greatest volume reduction in old age (Coffey *et al.* 1992; Raz *et al.* 1997). The cause behind the shrinkage of cells remains unknown, but it is probable there is a loss of synaptic density in the frontal cortex. Adams (1987) noted a 50% reduction in synaptic density in the precentral gyrus, but no change in synaptic density in the postcentral gyrus, whilst Gibson (1983) found evidence for a loss of synapses in the frontal cortex with no loss of synapses in the temporal cortex. Studies by Huttenlocher (1979) and Masliah *et al.* (1993) provide additional evidence for synaptic loss in the frontal cortex, although these investigators did not examine other areas of cortex, so the differential pattern is not addressed by these studies. Conclusions based upon neuronal and synaptic change in elderly brains, however, need to be viewed with caution because the number of studies remains small and the technologies for investigation are currently undergoing rapid evolution (West 1996; Wickelgren 1996). There is considerable debate concerning methodology and it is difficult to be certain what constitutes evidence and what does not. It is likely that a clearer picture will emerge as interest in the ageing brain grows and methodological practice becomes sufficiently well established for agreement to develop.

At first sight, functional imaging evidence, which shows greater hypometabolism in the frontal areas of the brain relative to posterior areas in old age (Kuhl *et al.* 1984; Shaw *et al.* 1984; Warren *et al.* 1985; Gur *et al.* 1987), would appear to support the conclusions based on volume change and synaptic densities reviewed above. However, both this metabolic change and the cognitive changes discussed in the previous section could result from indirect causes that affect the functioning of the frontal network without damaging neurons or their connections. Indeed, old age is associated with a number of changes outside the brain which could be expected to have an influence on brain functions. First, most elderly people experience a deterioration in the sensitivity of their sensory organs. Cognitive studies require that subjects can see and hear, with or without the use of aids, but this requirement may not be sufficient to balance the sensory capabilities of the young and the old. Rabbitt (1968) found that a group of young subjects who heard a list of words presented against a background of noise could repeat the words as accurately as those who heard the words in silence, but had impaired memory for the words. In an investigation of elderly subjects with very mild hearing impairments, Rabbitt (1991) found a similar pattern of results. Dickinson and Rabbitt (1991) undertook an analogous experiment for vision in which one group of young subjects were asked to wear lenses that induced mild astigmatism. These subjects showed no impairment in their reading speed, but were found to have impaired comprehension for the material relative to a group whose vision was undistorted. It is possible that the increasingly impoverished information provided by the senses in old age means that basic perception requires increased input from the frontal attentional network, leaving less resources available for higher cognitive processes (for more detailed discussion of the relationship between sensory loss and higher cognition in old age see Salthouse *et al.* 1996 and Baltes and Lindenberger 1997).

Older people also have more physical health problems than the young, some of which, together with the medications used to treat them, could have an impact upon cognitive function. Cardiovascular disease, in particular, restricts blood supply to the brain and increases the risk of pathological changes occurring within the brain (see Mann 1997 for a review). Several studies have noted that the cognitive performance of those with subclinical signs of cardiovascular disease is impaired relative to those of an equivalent age with no signs of cardiovascular disease (Manton *et al.* 1986; Elias *et al.* 1990, 1995; Sands and Meredith 1992). Furthermore, the hypometabolism revealed by functional imaging is exacerbated by the presence of cardiovascular disease, even at very mild levels. Indeed, when elderly people are thoroughly screened for signs of cardiovascular dysfunction, this hypometabolism is sometimes not found (for reviews see Shaw *et al.* 1984; Creasey and Rapaport 1985; Smith 1985). Many elderly people also suffer from subclinical problems with carbohydrate and glucose metabolism, which, again, may affect energy supply to the brain (see Kuhl *et al.* 1984; Smith 1985; Rowe and Kahn 1987 for reviews). It is worth noting that cognitive activities requiring central attentional control have been described as 'effortful' (Hasher and Zacks 1979), implicitly acknowledging that such operations are tiring, and implying that they will be the first to suffer should there be a restriction on energy supply to the brain.

In addition to these physiological changes, a number of psychosocial changes associated with old age could affect cognitive ability. As people age and become frail, their autonomy is often reduced. The extent of this loss ranges from a total removal of responsibility, associated with entering a nursing home, to the help provided by well-meaning relatives who take over many of the more difficult tasks in life. Studies have consistently demonstrated that the restriction of control and responsibility has negative effects upon cognitive and behavioural performance, as well as wider implications for reducing subjective well-being and general health (see Rowe and Kahn 1987 for a review). It is a harsh reality that many elderly people do require more help from other people, but these studies show unambiguously that, whenever possible, this help should consist of encouragement and support to maintain independence rather than direct assistance and assumption of responsibilities. Unfortunately it is much quicker and easier for carers to do things themselves, and restraints on time and resources means that the removal of responsibilities from the elderly is common. Other lifestyle changes which can affect the cognitive and emotional well-being of the elderly include retirement, bereavement, relocation, and reduced access to social support and activities.

The previous three paragraphs highlight the fact that many of the cognitive changes associated with old age may not be caused by old age *per se*, but rather by a multitude of other changes which often occur in old age. Whether these other changes are sufficient to account for all cognitive decline in old age is controversial. The balance of evidence, although at present somewhat sparse and unsystematic, suggests that whilst these factors undoubtedly have an effect, there remains an effect attributable to age itself (Kuhl *et al.* 1984; Shaw *et al.* 1984; Smith 1985; Perlmutter and Nyquist 1990; Hultsch *et al.* 1993; but see Creasey and Rapaport 1985 and Rowe and Kahn 1987 for the alternative view). The importance of these extrinsic factors associated with old age, however, should not be underestimated, because they are probably relevant to the fact that whilst some elderly people experience significant cognitive decline, others experience very little change (Albert 1988; Welford 1993). In essence, growing old may have an inevitable impact upon cognition, just as it does upon the quality of the skin, but the extent to which cognition is affected is almost certainly multifactorial. Moreover, it is important to be aware that when studying 'normal ageing' it is not a homogenous phenomenon that is being investigated. Future studies of cognitive change in old age need to take more care in monitoring important background variables, such as those discussed above, so that it can be established whether old age itself does have an effect upon cognition, and if so, what particular aspects of cognitive change are caused by age itself and what aspects are attributable to other causes. The matter is important because many of these factors associated with old age are modifiable. Public health policy changes could reduce the likelihood of these elements occurring in old age and thereby protect people's cognition (Khaw 1994). This should help more elderly people to maintain an active role in the community, and may also reduce the incidence of dementia, as will be discussed further in the remainder of this chapter.

The term 'normal ageing' has become widespread of late because of a perceived need to distinguish between benign cognitive changes and more serious forms of cognitive decline that lead to dementia. The traditional view is that dementia is a disease state that is qualitatively different from the mild cognitive decline associated with old age. However, given that there is this evidence for considerable variation in the extent to which people can suffer from 'normal' ageing, it has been asserted that dementia is on a continuum with these changes and represents the most extreme form of the cognitive ageing process. Efforts to find markers which can distinguish between 'normal ageing' and early dementia have been intensified during the past decade due to the rapid increase in the number of people surviving into advanced old age, and, hence, the rapid increase in the number of people suffering from dementia. However, when cognitive ability in both demented and non-demented people is measured using the Mini-Mental State Examination (Folstein *et al.* 1975), or an equivalent instrument, there is no sign of bimodality in the distribution of scores to suggest that elderly people divide into two separate populations: those who have dementia and those who are merely growing old (Brayne and Calloway 1988). Neither has it proven possible to find a biological or physiological marker which can distinguish those with dementia from those without (see Huppert and Brayne 1994 for a review). Dementia is most commonly caused by either Alzheimer's disease or cerebrovascular disease, but subclinical signs of both types of pathology are frequently found in the brains of individuals known not to have been demented at the time of their death. Combining this evidence for a pathological continuum with the evidence for a cognitive continuum, it is suggested that the mild cognitive loss observed in the 'normal elderly' has the same cause as the more severe cognitive loss seen in the demented elderly. In other words, it is argued that it is only the quantity of pathology, and not the type of pathology, which differentiates between the two groups.

The failure to find a qualitative difference between demented and non-demented people has undoubtedly made the continuum hypothesis persuasive, but here it will be argued that the continuum hypothesis encourages perspectives that misrepresent the relationship between pathological and non-pathological causes of cognitive decline in old age. Proponents of the continuum hypothesis often cite evidence that dementia can be caused by a multitude of different factors as evidence against the traditional 'disease model' of dementia. However, the fact that the continuum hypothesis is usually discussed with reference to 'the continuum' means that this hypothesis implies more strongly that all cognitive decline in old age is attributable to a single cause. With Alzheimer's disease being the most common cause of dementia in old age, this single cause is often assumed to be the quantity of Alzheimer's pathology within the brain, and so the continuum model of dementia is often viewed as being interchangeable with the question, 'Is Alzheimer's disease a true disease or accelerated ageing?'

With respect to this question, the continuum view is correct in asserting that fulfilment of the criteria for dementia does not demarcate between those who have Alzheimer's disease and those who do not. Alzheimer's disease is a pathological process which develops slowly but inexorably, with symptoms showing a parallel worsening in which there are no points of precipitous decline but rather a gradual sinking into the demented state. This is the accepted progression following the diagnosis of dementia, and yet the transition from normality to dementia has traditionally been treated as an all-or-none phenomenon. Proponents of the continuum hypothesis have correctly identified this position as being untenable. Given there is a wide gulf between normal cognition and the symptoms of dementia, it seems almost certain that Alzheimer's disease begins long before the criteria for dementia are fulfilled, and this explains why Alzheimer's pathology is frequently found in the brains of the non-demented elderly. Such instances represent people who had developed Alzheimer's disease but who died before the pathology had become severe enough to cause dementia. The problem is that during a patient's life, clinicians are unable to reliably distinguish between the subtle cognitive changes associated with predementia Alzheimer's disease and those caused either by age alone or the age-related, but non-pathological, factors discussed at the outset of this section. Thus, the concept of dementia remains important in clinical practice today because it is only once the criteria for this condition are fulfilled that the clinician can be confident that something abnormal is occurring.

However, although the continuum hypothesis is correct in asserting that the onset of dementia does not mark the boundary between Alzheimer's disease and normality, the implication often drawn from the hypothesis, that all age-related cognitive change is caused by subclinical Alzheimer's disease, is wrong. Alzheimer's dementia is associated with a particular (although only partially understood) set of processes whose presence is detected at postmortem by the existence of plaques and tangles within the brain. Other dementias that are not caused by this pathology are not considered to be the same disease. If not all dementias are caused by Alzheimer's disease then it is most unlikely that all 'normal ageing' is caused by Alzheimer's disease. This reveals that the question, 'Is Alzheimer's disease accelerated ageing?', does not make sense because the question implies that 'ageing' refers to a single process when, in fact, it does not. Cognitive decline is a common outcome of many possible underlying causes, and the challenge, when presented with an elderly person complaining about declining cognition, is to decide whether the decline is likely to continue into dementia. Maintenance of the traditional disease model within which certain causes, such as Alzheimer's disease or cerebrovascular disease, are viewed as pathological, whilst others, such as simply growing old or loss of autonomy, are viewed as non-pathological, is likely to prove most useful in learning to answer this challenge. Public health policies that encourage a healthy lifestyle and address psychosocial changes could improve cognitive function and allow certain sections of the elderly population to maintain their independence for longer, but attention must not be deflected from the fact that there are pathological causes of cognitive decline for which effective treatments are required urgently. If an individual develops Alzheimer's disease, dementia will follow. Endeavours on the part of the individual to maintain their intellectual powers and general health, and on the part of the community to provide support, may delay the onset of dementia, but such interventions will not prevent the dementia.

However, although essentially sound, the traditional medical model does need to change its assumption that fulfilment of the criteria for dementia differentiates between the 'normal elderly' and those who have Alzheimer's disease (or other pathological causes of cognitive decline). As mentioned above, the number of studies addressing the issue of how Alzheimer's disease can be diagnosed earlier has been rapidly increasing during the past decade, but as yet no reliable methods have been found. The evidence that both old age and Alzheimer's disease affect the higher cognitive functions of memory, language, visuospatial functions, and attention has been used to support the continuum hypothesis. It is argued that although the deficits within each domain are more serious in Alzheimer's disease, this simply represents the greater accumulation of pathology in those with a diagnosis. However, the review in the first section of this chapter led to the conclusion that memory, language, and visuospatial functions are essentially unaffected by old age, deficits arising only under circumstances which require attentional control. The evidence regarding Alzheimer's disease, however, suggests there is direct damage to these specialized functions. Neuropathological evidence shows that Alzheimer pathology develops and spreads through the brain in a systematic manner (Brun and Englund 1981; Pearson *et al.* 1985; Lewis *et al.* 1987; Esiri *et al.* 1990; Arnold *et al.* 1991; Braak and Braak 1991; Guela and Mesulam 1994). Knowledge of the functions of different regions of the brain reveals a parallel between the order in which specific brain areas are damaged by Alzheimer's disease and the development of specific cognitive symptoms. This parallel suggests that in Alzheimer's disease deficits in specific cognitive functions represent direct damage, each function being affected when the pathology begins to erode its biological substrate. In the vast majority of cases, the pathology first develops within the structures of the limbic system, particularly the entorhinal cortex and the hippocampus. These structures are critical components in the system that allows for the development of new memories (with reference to pp. 45–6, this type of memory is equivalent to establishing new information in secondary memory, but at a theoretical level it has been defined as either 'declarative memory' or 'episodic memory', see Squire and Zola-Morgan 1991 and Tulving 1985, respectively, for further discussion). A large number of longitudinal studies have now shown that people who develop dementia of the Alzheimer type (DAT) are characterized by a disproportionate memory deficit during the years prior to the onset of the dementia (Bondi *et al.* 1994; Masur *et al.* 1994; Jacobs *et al.* 1995; Linn *et al.* 1995; Howieson *et al.* 1997; Hodges 1998; Elias *et al.* 2000). These results strongly suggest that Alzheimer's disease does have a predementia phase, which lasts several years, during which the loss of memory is the dominant and often only symptom.

As Alzheimer's disease develops, the pathology spreads from the limbic system to affect the neocortex, affecting particularly the highest order association cortices in the temporal, parietal, and frontal lobes. These areas support the higher cognitive functions of 'semantic memory' (the store of knowledge which makes perception and language meaningful, equivalent to what has been referred to as well-established information in secondary memory, see Tulving 1985 for further explanation of the term), spatial cognition, and attentional functions, respectively. When the pathology begins to spread from the limbic system to the neocortex, it affects the association cortex of the temporal lobe before developing within the parietal and frontal association cortices (Rossor and Iversen 1986; Van Hoesen and Damasio 1987; Esiri *et al.* 1990; Arnold *et al.* 1991; Guela and Mesulam 1994), with the possibility that the frontal areas are the last to be affected (Brun and Englund 1981). Semantic memory deficits do not occur with the consistency of episodic memory deficits during the predementia phase of Alzheimer's disease, but there is evidence to suggest that up to 70% of subjects are impaired in the most sensitive semantic memory tests during the predementia phase (Hodges and Patterson 1995; Hodges *et al.* 1996; but see Perry *et al.* 2000). Furthermore, several longitudinal studies have shown that when predicting who will develop Alzheimer's disease it is a combination of poor episodic memory with poor semantic memory that is most predictive (Storandt and Hill 1989; Flicker *et al.* 1991, 1993; Masur *et al.* 1994, Jacobs *et al.* 1995; Locascio *et al.* 1995). Once dementia is established, problems with spatial cognition are frequent in Alzheimer's disease, but longitudinal studies have found that impairments in tests of praxis are not typical at the baseline evaluation of those who later develop dementia (Morris *et al.* 1991; Welsh *et al.* 1992; Bondi *et al.* 1994). It has also been shown that these tests do not have the predictive value of episodic and semantic memory tests (Storandt and Hill 1989; Flicker *et al.* 1991, 1993; Masur *et al.* 1994; Jacobs *et al.* 1995; Locascio *et al.* 1995), consistent with evidence that the parietal association cortex is not damaged until a later stage of the disease.

Impairments in certain attentional tests, on the other hand, are common in predementia Alzheimer's disease (Lafleche and Albert 1995; Perry and Hodges 1999; Perry *et al.* 2000) and, at first sight, the parallel between the probable sites of pathology and symptoms of early Alzheimer's disease appears to break down here. However, at present, the most influential explanations for this attentional deficit do not focus upon direct damage to the frontal lobe, but rather upon damage to the basal forebrain cholinergic system (Albert 1996; Perry and Hodges 1999) or the indirect consequences of the loss of connectivity within the posterior association cortices (Parasuraman and Haxby 1993; Morris 1996; Spinnler 1999). Furthermore, although many of the attentional tests that are exquisitely sensitive to normal ageing (such as Digit symbol) are also likely to reveal impairments in predementia Alzheimer patients, the relationship between this attentional impairment and the deficits in the specialized cognitive functions appears to be different in the two conditions. This is most easily illustrated with respect to episodic memory because this function has been extensively studied in both normal ageing and in Alzheimer's disease. Sliwinski and Buschke (1997) applied the Salthouse method of partialling out performance in tests like Digit symbol to examine the residual relationships between age and memory and between dementia and memory. Sliwinski and Buschke found, consistent with the results of Salthouse, that after controlling for processing speed, the effects of age upon episodic memory were much reduced, usually to non-significance. The demented patients were slower at processing than the elderly subjects, but when this excessive slowing was statistically controlled, the relationship between dementia and performance in all four episodic memory tests none the less remained significant. The results show that, in contrast to normal ageing, dementia impairs episodic memory function beyond the level associated with losses of processing speed (or attention if the arguments articulated earlier are correct), implying that episodic memory itself is damaged in Alzheimer's disease. Further evidence comes from the fact that the size of the memory deficit observed in Alzheimer patients relative to non-demented controls cannot be reduced by procedures that engender the strategic encoding of new material (see pp. 46–8; and Corkin 1982; Butters *et al.* 1983; Martin *et al.* 1985; Mitchell *et al.* 1986; Grober and Buschke 1987; Bäckman and Herlitz 1990). Indeed, it has been suggested that because these procedures benefit the normal elderly to a greater degree than those with Alzheimer's disease, tests employing such procedures have potential as diagnostic tools (Grober *et al.* 1988; Buschke *et al.* 1997). The fact that Alzheimer patients continue to perform near floor levels in memory tests which limit the need for strategic or controlled processing (Strauss *et al.* 1985; Grafman *et al.* 1990; Milwain 1999), also implies that it is the memory system itself that is damaged in Alzheimer's disease.

With respect to semantic memory and spatial functions, the evidence again suggests that in Alzheimer's disease, unlike in normal ageing, there is fundamental damage to the cognitive components. Both old age and Alzheimer's disease are associated with a naming deficit, but most researchers believe that in Alzheimer's disease the problem is one of semantic breakdown, rather than unreliable access to the lexicon (see p. 50; and Hodges *et al.* 1992; Kempler and Zelinski 1994; Salmon and Fennema-Notestine 1996; but see Nebes 1989 and Bayles *et al.* 1991 for an alternative viewpoint). As with episodic memory, semantic memory performance cannot be improved by providing strategic aids (Randolph *et al.* 1993), suggesting again that the deficit is fundamental and not an indirect consequence of attentional loss. This conclusion is further bolstered by the fact that the appearance of semantic memory deficits during early Alzheimer's disease is not correlated with attentional deficits (Binetti *et al.* 1996; Phillips *et al.* 1996; Perry *et al.* 2000). Similarly, many of the visuospatial problems that Alzheimer patients experience (such as dressing apraxia and the inability to copy simple shapes) would appear to represent a fundamental breakdown in spatial cognition, rather than a problem with attentional control or 'fluid intelligence' (see p. 44 and p. 55).

These considerations lead to the conclusion that enterprises to distinguish between predementia Alzheimer's disease and normal ageing are valid. It has been learnt that the most telling sign of incipient Alzheimer's disease is a memory deficit. This means that memory loss in the elderly needs to be taken more seriously, but it is important to appreciate that a memory deficit alone does not identify those with predementia Alzheimer's disease. Memory loss can occur for a variety of reasons, of which Alzheimer's disease is only one. There is some evidence that memory tests which do not depend heavily upon the attentional function that is damaged in normal ageing provide a better separation between normal ageing and predementia Alzheimer's disease (Grober *et al.* 1988; Buschke *et al.* 1997; Milwain 1999), but such tests are only a partial solution and additional investigations will be required to detect predementia Alzheimer's disease. Longitudinal follow-up of non-demented subjects with memory loss is likely to be of particular use, given that a key feature of the memory loss caused by Alzheimer's disease is that it worsens over time and, according to the evidence reviewed above, should become accompanied by deficits in certain semantic memory tests (Hodges and Patterson 1995; Hodges *et al.* 1996; Milwain 1999) and attentional tests (Lafleche and Albert 1995; Perry *et al.* 2000) during the following few years.

Progress in learning to detect predementia Alzheimer's disease requires that the issue is not obscured by recent controversy concerning the status of various categories of subclinical cognitive decline in the elderly, the most influential being age-associated memory impairment (AAMI; Crook *et al.* 1986) and mild cognitive impairment (MCI; Petersen *et al.* 1999) (see Ritchie and Touchon 2000 for a detailed review of these and other similar categories). These categories have been treated as separate diagnostic entities, but it is important to recognize that these categories cannot be diagnostic entities. The essence of all the categories cited above is a memory impairment in the absence of any other symptoms of dementia. In other words, the characteristics that define these diagnoses are the same as those associated with predementia Alzheimer's disease. Indeed, of people who fulfil the criteria for these categories, between 10% and 15% develop DAT each year (Petersen *et al.* 1995; Tierney *et al.* 1996), with 50% of such people having dementia within 4 years (Bowen *et al.* 1997; Petersen *et al.* 1999). In the years prior to the diagnosis of DAT these subjects do not have a different disease called 'mild cognitive impairment' which then changes into Alzheimer's disease once the criteria for dementia are fulfilled. They had Alzheimer's disease throughout. Categories such as MCI have been influential in drawing attention to the important fact that isolated memory impairment carries a high risk for the imminent development of DAT, but it is critical not to be misled into thinking that MCI is a diagnostic category, distinguishable from both normal ageing and Alzheimer's disease, as suggested by Petersen *et al.* (1999). Rather, of people who fulfil the criteria for MCI, approximately 50% are in a very early stage of Alzheimer's disease whilst the other 50% have a memory impairment for some other reason. The key question is how to identify the 50% who do have Alzheimer's disease. As discussed above, this can only be achieved by the longitudinal investigation of subjects with an isolated memory impairment to find the additional signs that predict the development of DAT. To achieve this it is imperative that the current practice of dismissing memory loss as a normal part of growing old should stop, but the practice should not be replaced by diagnostic entities whose status is not merely unproven (Ritchie and Touchon 2000) but is proven to be invalid (Milwain 2000).

Conclusions

The review in the first section of this chapter revealed that the majority of people can expect to experience some deterioration in their cognitive powers during old age. Next it was hypothesized that this is due to a reduction in the efficiency of an attentional network, centred in the anterior cingulate and dorsolateral prefrontal cortex. However, the third section revealed that the cause of this putative change is far from clear. There is evidence for a disproportionate change within frontal regions of the cortex, but it is equally possible that the efficiency of the network is affected by remote causes. Consideration of potential remote causes, such as sensory decline, deteriorating health, and changing psychosocial circumstances, revealed that it cannot be concluded with certainty that old age itself has any negative implications for cognition, although it is probable that it does. Systematic study of these other factors is urgently required because they almost certainly contribute to the great variation in the degree of cognitive loss experienced by different people during old age. Acknowledgement of the broad variation within the 'normal' range of cognitive decline inevitably leads to the continuum hypothesis, which asserts there is no real difference between 'normal ageing' and dementia. The continuum hypothesis has raised awareness of two important facts. First, that fulfilment of the criteria for dementia does not mark the boundary between benign and pathological cognitive decline, and second, that cognition is affected by factors which, although not pathological, could none the less be manipulated to improve the cognitive health of the elderly. However, the implication that there is no distinction between pathological and non-pathological causes of cognitive decline is incorrect. Some elderly people will develop pathological conditions, such as Alzheimer's disease, which will lead to dementia. There is a clear need to understand Alzheimer's disease, and other pathological processes that cause dementia, so that effective treatments can be developed. It is also necessary to develop procedures that can detect these processes as early as possible so that future treatments can be applied at the time when the chances of success are highest. At present it is not possible to detect Alzheimer's disease with reliability before the onset of dementia. However, evidence suggests that the dementia is preceded by a phase, which can last as long as 10 years, during which the only symptom is a memory impairment. Unlike the memory impairment associated with non-pathological ageing, it appears that in predementia Alzheimer's disease there is direct damage to memory. However, at a practical level, it is very difficult to distinguish between these two causes of memory impairment. More longitudinal studies of individuals with isolated memory impairment are required to identify the additional symptoms which signal that Alzheimer's disease is causing the memory deficit. There have been a number of longitudinal studies of such people in the recent past, but the utility of the findings is being obscured by the debate over whether categories such as MCI represent diagnostic entities. It is argued that MCI and similar categories cannot be diagnostic entities, and thus they should either be avoided altogether—or researchers should make clear that the category is being used only for convenience so that other researchers can understand the criteria used to select participants for the study.

References

Adams, I. (1987). Plasticity of the synaptic contact zone following loss of synapses in the cerebral cortex of aging humans. *Brain Research*, **424**, 343–51.

Albert, M. S. (1988). Cognitive function. In *Geriatric neuropsychology* (ed. M. S. Albert and M. B. Moss), pp. 33–53. Guilford Press, New York.

Albert, M. S. (1996). Cognitive and neurobiologic markers of early Alzheimer's disease. *Proceedings of the National Academy of Science, USA*, **93**, 13547–51.

Albert, M. S. and Kaplan, E. (1980). Organic implications of neuropsychological deficits in the elderly. In *New directions in memory and aging: Proceedings of the George A. Talland Memorial Conference* (ed. L. W. Poon), pp. 403–32. Lawrence Erlbaum, Hillsdale, NJ.

Albert, M. S., Heller, H. S., and Milberg, W. (1988). Changes in naming ability with age. *Psychology and Aging*, **3**, 173–8.

Allport, D. A. (1980). Attention and performance. In *Cognitive psychology: new directions* (ed. G. Claxton), pp. 26–64. Routledge and Kegan Paul, London.

Ardila, A. and Rosselli, M. (1989). Neuropsychological characteristics of normal aging. *Developmental Neuropsychology*, **5**, 307–20.

Arenberg, D. (1982). Changes with age in problem solving. In *Aging and cognitive processes* (ed. F. I. M. Craik and A. S. Trehub), pp. 221–35. Plenum, New York.

Arnold, S. E., Hyman, B. T., Flory, J., *et al.* (1991). The topographic and neuroanatomical distribution of neurofibrillary tangles and neuritic plaques in the cerebral cortex of patients with Alzheimer's disease. *Cerebral Cortex*, **1**, 103–16.

Atkinson, R. C. and Shiffrin, R. M. (1968). Human memory: a proposed system and its control processes. In *The psychology of learning and motivation: advances in research and theory* (ed. K. W. Spence), pp. 89–195. Academic Press, New York.

Babcock, R. L. and Salthouse, T. A. (1990). Effects of increased processing demands on age differences in working memory. *Psychology and Aging*, **5**, 421–8.

Bäckman, L. and Herlitz, A. (1990). The relationship between prior knowledge and face recognition memory in normal aging and Alzheimer's disease. *Journal of Gerontology: Psychological Sciences*, **45**, 94–100.

Baddeley, A. D. (1986). *Working memory*. Oxford University Press, Oxford.

Baddeley, A. D. (1996). *Human memory: theory and practice*. Psychology Press, Hove, Sussex.

Baltes, P. B. and Lindenberger, U. (1997). Emergence of a powerful connection between sensory and cognitive functions across the adult life span: a new window to the study of cognitive aging? *Psychology and Aging*, **12**, 12–21.

Bartlett, J. C. and Leslie, J. E. (1986). Aging and memory for faces versus single views of faces. *Memory and Cognition*, **14**, 371–81.

Bartlett, J. C., Till, R. E., Gernsbacher, M., *et al.* (1983). Age-related differences in memory for lateral orientation of pictures. *Journal of Gerontology*, **38**, 439–46.

Bayles, K. A., Tomoeda, C. K., Kasniak, A. W., *et al.* (1991). Alzheimer's disease effects on semantic memory: loss of structure or impaired processing? *Journal of Cognitive Neuroscience*, **3**, 166–82.

Binetti, G., Magni, E., Padovani, A., *et al.* (1996). Executive dysfunction in early Alzheimer's disease. *Journal of Neurology, Neurosurgery and Psychiatry*, **60**, 91–3.

Bondi, M. W., Monsch, A. U., Galasko, D., *et al.* (1994). Preclinical cognitive markers of dementia of the Alzheimer type. *Neuropsychology*, **8**, 374–84.

Botwinick, J. (1977). Intellectual abilities. In *Handbook of the psychology of aging* (ed. J. E. Birren and K. W. Schaie), pp. 580–605. Van Nostrand Reinhold, New York.

Botwinick, J. and Storandt, M. (1974). *Memory related functions and age*. Charles C. Thomas, Springfield, IL.

Bowen, J., Teri, L., Kukull, W., *et al.* (1997). Progression to dementia in patients with isolated memory loss. *Lancet*, **349**, 763–5.

Bowles, N. L. (1989). Age and semantic inhibition in word retrieval. *Journal of Gerontology: Psychological Sciences*, **44**, P88–90.

Bowles, N. L., Obler, L. K., and Albert, M. L. (1987). Naming errors in healthy aging and dementia of the Alzheimer type. *Cortex*, **23**, 519–24.

Bowles, N. L., Obler, L. K., and Poon, L. W. (1989). Aging and word retrieval: naturalistic, clinical and laboratory data. In *Everyday cognition in adulthood and late life* (ed. L. W. Poon, D. C. Rubin and B. A. Wilson), pp. 244–64. Cambridge University Press, Cambridge.

Braak, H. and Braak, E. (1991). Neuropathological staging of Alzheimer-related changes. *Acta Neuropathologica*, **82**, 238–59.

Brayne, C. and Calloway, P. (1988). Normal ageing, impaired cognitive function and senile dementia of the Alzheimer's type: a continuum? *Lancet*, **ii**, 1265–7.

Brinley, J. F. (1965). Cognitive sets, speed and accuracy of performance in the elderly. In *Behavior, aging and the nervous system* (ed. A. T. Welford and J. E. Birren), pp. 191–216. Charles C. Thomas, Springfield, IL.

Broadbent, D. E. (1958). *Perception and communication*. Pergamon, Oxford.

Bromley, D. B. (1958). Some effects of age on short-term learning and memory. *Journal of Gerontology*, **13**, 398–406.

Brown, A. S. and Mitchell, D. B. (1991). Age differences in retrieval consistency and response dominance. *Journal of Gerontology: Psychological Sciences*, **46**, P332–9.

Bruce, P. R. and Herman, J. F. (1983). Spatial knowledge of young and elderly adults: scene recognition from familiar and novel perspectives. *Experimental Aging Research*, **9**, 169–73.

Brun, A. and Englund, E. (1981). Regional pattern of degeneration in Alzheimer's disease: neuronal loss and histopathological grading. *Histopathology*, **5**, 549–64.

Buckner, R. L. and Petersen, S. E. (1996). What does neuroimaging tell us about the role of prefrontal cortex in memory retrieval? *Seminars in the Neurosciences*, **8**, 47–55.

Burke, D. M. and Harrold, R. M. (1988). Automatic and effortful semantic processes in old age: experimental and naturalistic approaches. In *Language, memory and aging* (ed. L. L. Light and D. M. Burke), pp. 100–16. Cambridge University Press, Cambridge.

Burke, D. M. and Light, L. L. (1981). Memory and aging: the role of retrieval processes. *Psychological Review*, **90**, 513–46.

Burke, D. M. and Peters, L. (1986). Word associations in old age: evidence for consistency in semantic encoding during adulthood. *Psychology and Aging*, **1**, 283–92.

Burke, D. M. and Yee, P. L. (1984). Semantic priming during sentence processing by young and older adults. *Developmental Psychology*, **20**, 903–10.

Burke, D. M., MacKay, D. G., Worthley, J. S., *et al.* (1991). On the tip of the tongue: what causes word finding failures in young and older adults? *Journal of Memory and Language*, **30**, 542–79.

Buschke, H., Sliwinski, M. J., Kuslansky, G., *et al.* (1997). Diagnosis of early dementia by the Double Memory Test: encoding specificity improves diagnostic sensitivity and specificity. *Neurology*, **48**, 989–97.

Butters, N., Albert, M. S., Sax, D. S., *et al.* (1983). The effect of verbal mediators on the pictorial memory of brain damaged patients. *Neuropsychologia*, **21**, 307–32.

Byrd, M. (1984). Age differences in the retrieval of information from semantic memory. *Experimental Aging Research*, **10**, 29–33.

Byrd, M. (1985). Age differences in the ability to recall and summarise text information. *Experimental Aging Research*, **11**, 87–91.

Canestrari, R. E. (1968). Age changes in acquisition. In *Human aging and behavior* (ed. G. A. Talland), pp. 169–88. Academic Press, New York.

Ceci, S. J. and Tabor, L. (1981). Flexibility and memory: are the elderly really less flexible? *Experimental Aging Research*, **7**, 147–58.

Cerella, J. (1985). Information processing rates in the elderly. *Psychological Bulletin*, **98**, 67–83.

Cerella, J., Poon, L. W. and Fozard, J. L. (1981). Mental rotation and age reconsidered. *Journal of Gerontology*, **36**, 620–4.

Charness, N. (1981*a*). Aging and skilled problem solving. *Journal of Experimental Psychology: General*, **110**, 21–38.

Charness, N. (1981*b*). Search in chess: aging and skill differences. *Journal of Experimental Psychology: Human Perception and Performance*, **7**, 467–76.

Charness, N. (1987). Component processes in bridge bidding and novel problem solving tasks. *Canadian Journal of Psychology*, 41, 223–43.

Charness, N. (1989). Age and expertise: responding to Talland's challenge. In *Everyday cognition in adulthood and late life* (ed. L. W. Poon, D. C. Rubin, and B. A. Wilson), pp. 437–56. Cambridge University Press, Cambridge.

Coffey, C. E., Wilkinson, W. E., Parashos, L. A., *et al.* (1992). Quantitative cerebral anatomy of the aging human brain: a cross-sectional study using magnetic resonance imaging. *Neurology*, **42**, 527–36.

Cohen, G. (1979). Language comprehension in old age. *Cognitive Psychology*, **11**, 412–29.

Cohen, G. (1981). Inferential reasoning in old age. *Cognition*, **9**, 59–72.

Cohen, G. (1988). Age differences in memory for texts: production deficiency or processing limitations? In

Language, memory and aging (ed. L. L. Light and D. M. Burke), pp. 171–90. Cambridge University Press, Cambridge.

Cohen, G. and Faulkener, D. (1983). Word recognition: age differences in contextual facilitation effects. *British Journal of Psychology*, **74**, 239–51.

Cohen, G. and Faulkener, D. (1986). Memory for proper names: age differences in retrieval. *British Journal of Developmental Psychology*, **4**, 187–97.

Cohen, G. and Faulkener, D. (1987). Life span changes in autobiographical memory. In *Practical aspects of memory: current research and issues* (ed. M. M. Gruneberg, P. E. Morris and R. N. Sykes), pp. 277–82. John Wiley, Chichester.

Cohen, G. and Faulkener, D. (1989). Age differences in source forgetting: effects on reality monitoring and on eyewitness testimony. *Psychology and Aging*, **4**, 10–17.

Cohen, G., Conway, M. A., and Maylor, E. A. (1994). Flashbulb memory in young and older adults. *Psychology and Aging*, **9**, 454–63.

Corkin, S. (1982). Some relationships between global amnesias and the memory impairments in Alzheimer's disease. In *Alzheimer's disease: a report of progress in research* (ed. S. Corkin, K. L. Davis, J. H. Growdon *et al.*), pp. 149–64. Raven Press, New York.

Craik, F. I. M. (1977). Age differences in human memory. In *Handbook of the psychology of aging* (ed. J. E. Birren and K. W. Schaie), pp. 384–420. Van Nostrand Reinhold, New York.

Craik, F. I. M. (1986). A functional account of age differences in memory. In *Human memory and cognitive capabilities, mechanisms and performances* (ed. F. Klix and H. Hagendorf), pp. 409–22. Elsevier, North Holland.

Craik, F. I. M. and Jennings, J. M. (1992). Human memory. In *Handbook of aging and cognition* (ed. F. I. M. Craik and T. Salthouse), pp. 51–110. Lawrence Erlbaum, Hillsdale, NJ.

Craik, F. I. M. and Lockhart, R. S. (1972). Levels of processing: a framework for memory research. *Journal of Verbal Learning and Verbal Behavior*, **11**, 671–84.

Craik, F. I. M. and McDowd, J. M. (1987). Age differences in recall and recognition. *Journal of Experimental Psychology: Learning, Memory and Cognition*, **13**, 474–9.

Craik, F. I. M. and Rabinowitz, J. C. (1984). Age differences in the acquisition and use of verbal information: a tutorial review. In *Attention and performance X: control of language processes* (ed. H. Bouma and D. G. Bouwhuis), pp. 471–99. Lawrence Erlbaum, Hillsdale, NJ.

Craik, F. I. M. and Rabinowitz, J. C. (1985). The effects of presentation rate and encoding task on age-related memory deficits. *Journal of Gerontology*, **40**, 309–15.

Craik, F. I. M. and Simon, E. (1980). Age differences in memory: the roles of attention and depth of processing. In *New directions in memory and aging* (ed. L. W. Poon, J. L. Fozard, L. S. Cermak, *et al.*), pp. 95–112. Lawrence Erlbaum, Hillsdale, NJ.

Creasey, H. and Rapaport, S. I. (1985). The aging human brain. *Annals of Neurology*, **17**, 2–10.

Critchley, M. (1984). And all the daughters of musick shall be brought low. *Archives of Neurology*, **41**, 1135–9.

Crook, T., Bartus, R. T., Ferris, S. H., *et al.* (1986). Age-associated memory impairment: proposed diagnostic criteria and measures of clinical change—report of a National Institute of Mental Health Work Group. *Developmental Neuropsychology*, **2**, 261–76.

Daneman, M. and Carpenter, P. A. (1980). Individual differences in working memory and reading. *Journal of Verbal Learning and Verbal Behavior*, **19**, 450–66.

Daneman, M. and Tardif, T. (1987). Working memory and reading skill re-examined. In *Attention and performance XII: the psychology of reading* (ed. M. Coltheart), pp. 491–508. Erlbaum, Hove, Sussex.

Davis, G. A. and Ball, H. E. (1989). Effects of age on comprehension of complex sentences in adulthood. *Journal of Speech and Hearing Research*, **32**, 143–50.

Dempster, F. N. (1992). The rise and fall of the inhibitory mechanism: toward a unified theory of cognitive development and aging. *Developmental Review*, **12**, 45–75.

Denney, D. R. and Denney, N. W. (1973). The use of classification for problem solving: a comparison of middle and old age. *Developmental Psychology*, **9**, 275–8.

Denney, N. W. and Denney, D. R. (1974). Modelling effects on the questioning strategies of the elderly. *Developmental Psychology*, **10**, 458.

Dickinson, C. M. and Rabbitt, P. M. A. (1991). Simulated visual impairment: effects on text comprehension and reading speed. *Clinical Vision Science*, **6**, 301–8.

Dixon, R. A., Hultsch, D. F., Simon, E. W., *et al.* (1984). Verbal ability and text structure effects on adult age differences in text recall. *Journal of Verbal Learning and Verbal Behavior*, **23**, 569–78.

Doppelt, J. W. and Wallace, W. L. (1955). Standardization of the Wechsler Adult Intelligence Scale for older persons. *Journal of Abnormal and Social Psychology*, **51**, 312–30.

Elias, M. F., Elias, J. W., and Elias, P. K. (1990). Biological health influences on behavior. In *Handbook of the psychology of aging* (ed. J. E. Birren and K. W. Schaie), pp. 79–102. Academic Press, San Diego, CA.

Elias, M. F., Elias, P. K., Cobb, J., *et al.* (1995). Blood pressure affects cognitive functioning: the Framingham studies revisited. In *Quality of life in behavioral medicine* (ed. J. Dimsdale and A. Baum), pp. 121–43. Lawrence Erlbaum, Hillsdale, NJ.

Elias, M. F., Beiser, A., Wolf, P. A., *et al.* (2000). The preclinical phase of Alzheimer disease. *Archives of Neurology*, **57**, 808–13.

Engle, R. W. (1996). Working memory and retrieval: an inhibition-resource approach. In *Working memory and human cognition* (ed. J. T. Richardson, R. W. Engle, L. Hasher, *et al.*), pp. 89–119. Oxford University Press, Oxford.

Engle, R. W., Cantor, J., and Carullo, J. J. (1992). Individual differences in working memory and comprehension: a test of four hypotheses. *Journal of Experimental Psychology: Learning, Memory and Cognition*, **18**, 972–92.

Erber, J. T., Herman, T. G., and Botwinick, J. (1980). Age differences in memory as a function of depth of processing. *Experimental Aging Research*, **6**, 341–8.

Esiri, M. M., Pearson, R. C. A., Steele, J. E., *et al.* (1990). A quantitative study of the neurofibrillary tangles and the choline acetyltransferase activity in the cerebral cortex and the amygdala in Alzheimer's disease. *Journal of Neurology, Neurosurgery and Psychiatry*, **53**, 161–5.

Fell, M. (1992). Encoding, retrieval and age effects on recollective experience. *Irish Journal of Psychology*, **13**, 62–78.

Fisk, A. D. and Fisher, D. L. (1994). Brinley plots and theories of aging: the explicit, muddled and implicit debates. *Journal of Gerontology: Psychological Sciences*, **49**, P81–9.

Fitzgerald, J. M. (1988). Vivid memories and the reminiscence phenomenon: the role of a self narrative. *Human Development*, **31**, 261–73.

Flicker, C., Ferris, S. H., and Reisberg, B. (1991). Mild cognitive impairment in the elderly: predictors of dementia. *Neurology*, **41**, 1006–9.

Flicker, C., Ferris, S. H., and Reisberg, B. (1993). A two-year longitudinal study of cognitive function in normal aging and Alzheimer's disease. *Journal of Geriatric Psychiatry and Neurology*, **6**, 85–96.

Folstein, M. F., Folstein, S. E., and McHugh, P. R. (1975). Mini-mental state: a practical method for grading the cognitive state of patients for the clinician. *Journal of Psychiatric Research*, **12**, 189–98.

Gibson, P. H. (1983). EM study of the numbers of cortical synapses in the brains of aging people and people with Alzheimer-type dementia. *Acta Neuropathologica*, **62**, 127–33.

Gick, M. L., Craik, F. I. M., and Morris, R. G. (1988). Task complexity and age differences in working memory. *Memory and Cognition*, **16**, 353–61.

Glosser, G. and Deser, T. (1992). A comparison of changes in macrolinguistic and microlinguistic aspects of discourse production in normal aging. *Journal of Gerontology*, **35**, 722–8.

Goldman-Rakic, P. S. (1996). The prefrontal landscape: implications of functional architecture for understanding human mentation and the central executive. *Philosophical Transactions of the Royal Society of London: Biological Sciences*, **351**, 1445–54.

Goldstein, G. and Shelly, C. H. (1981). Does the right hemisphere age more rapidly than the left? *Journal of Clinical Neuropsychology*, **3**, 65–78.

Grady, C. L., McIntosh, A. R., Horwitz, B., *et al.* (1995). Age-related reductions in human recognition memory due to impaired encoding. *Science*, **269**, 218–21.

Grafman, J., Weingartner, H., Lawlor, B., *et al.* (1990). Automatic memory processes in patients with dementia-Alzheimer-type (DAT). *Cortex*, **26**, 361–71.

Grober, E. and Buschke, H. (1987). Genuine memory deficits in dementia. *Developmental Neuropsychology*, **3**, 13–36.

Grober, E., Buschke, H., Crystal, H., *et al.* (1988). Screening for dementia by memory testing. *Neurology*, **38**, 900–3.

Guela, C. and Mesulam, M. M. (1994). Cholinergic systems and related neuropathological predilection patterns in Alzheimer's disease. In *Alzheimer disease* (ed. R. D. Terry, R. Katzman, and K. L. Bick), pp. 263–91. Raven Press, New York.

Gur, R. C., Gur, R. E., Orbist, W. D., *et al.* (1987). Age and regional cerebral blood flow at rest and during cognitive activity. *Archives of General Psychiatry*, **44**, 617–21.

Guttentag, R. E. and Hunt, R. R. (1988). Adult age differences in memory for imagined and performed actions. *Journal of Gerontology: Psychological Sciences*, **43**, P107–8.

Hale, S., Lima, S. D., and Myerson, J. (1991). General cognitive slowing in the nonlexical domain: an experimental validation. *Psychology and Aging*, **6**, 512–21.

Hasher, L. and Zacks, R. T. (1979). Automatic and effortful processes in memory. *Journal of Experimental Psychology: General*, **108**, 356–88.

Hasher, L. and Zacks, R. T. (1988). Working memory, comprehension and aging: a review and a new view. In *The psychology of learning and motivation* (ed. G. H. Bower), pp. 193–225. Academic Press, San Diego, CA.

Hashtroudi, S., Johnson, M. K., and Chrosniak, L. D. (1990). Aging and quantitative characteristics of memories for perceived and imagined complex events. *Psychology and Aging*, **5**, 119–26.

Haug, H. and Eggers, R. (1991). Morphometry of the human cortex cerebri and corpus striatum during aging. *Neurobiology of Aging*, **12**, 336–8.

Haug, H., Barnwater, U., Eggers, R., *et al.* (1983). Anatomical changes in aging brain: morphometric analysis of the human prosencephalon. In *Brain aging: neuropathology and neuropharmacology* (ed. J. Cervois-Navarro and H. I. Sarkander), pp. 1–12. Raven Press, New York.

Hertzog, C., Raskind, C. L., and Cannon, C. J. (1986). Age-related slowing in semantic information processing speed: an individual differences analysis. *Journal of Gerontology*, **41**, 500–2.

Hess, T. M. (1985). Aging and context influences on recognition memory for typical and atypical script actions. *Developmental Psychology*, **21**, 1139–51.

Hess, T. M. and Tate, C. S. (1991). Adult age differences in explanations and memory for behavioral information. *Psychology and Aging*, **6**, 86–92.

Hess, T. M., Vandermaas, M. O., Donley, J., *et al.* (1987). Memory for sex-role consistent and inconsistent actions in young and old adults. *Journal of Gerontology*, **42**, 505–11.

Hess, T. M., Donley, J., and Vandermaas, M. O. (1989). Aging-related changes in the processing and retention of script information. *Experimental Aging Research*, **15**, 89–96.

Hochman, L. O., Storandt, M., and Rosenberg, A. M. (1986). Age and its effects on perceptions of psychopathology. *Psychology and Aging*, **1**, 337–8.

Hodges, J. R. (1998). The amnestic prodrome of Alzheimer's disease. *Brain*, **121**, 1601–2.

Hodges, J. R. and Patterson, K. (1995). Is semantic memory consistently impaired early in the course of

Alzheimer's disease? Neuroanatomical and diagnostic implications. *Neuropsychologia*, **33**, 441–59.

Hodges, J. R., Salmon, D. P., and Butters, N. (1992). Semantic memory impairment in Alzheimer's disease: failure of access or degraded knowledge? *Neuropsychologia*, **30**, 301–14.

Hodges, J. R., Patterson, K., Graham, N., *et al.* (1996). Naming and knowing in dementia of the Alzheimer type. *Brain and Language*, **54**, 302–25.

Holland, C. A. and Rabbitt, P. M. A. (1990). Autobiographical and text recall in the elderly: an investigation of a processing resource deficit. *The Quarterly Journal of Experimental Psychology*, **42A**, 441–70.

Horn, J. L. and Cattell, R. B. (1967). Age differences in fluid and crystallized intelligence. *Acta Psychologica*, **26**, 107–29.

Houghton, G. and Tipper, S. P. (1994). A model of inhibitory mechanisms in selective attention. In *Inhibitory processes in attention, memory and language* (ed. D. Dagenbach and T. H. Carr), pp. 53–112. Academic Press, San Diego, CA.

Howard, D. V. (1980). Category norms: a comparison of the Battig and Montague (1969) norms with the responses of adults between the ages of 20 and 80. *Journal of Gerontology*, **35**, 225–31.

Howard, D. V. (1983). The effects of aging and degree of association on the semantic priming of lexical decisions. *Experimental Aging Research*, **9**, 145–51.

Howard, D. V., McAndrews, M. P., and Lasaga, M. I. (1981). Semantic priming of lexical decisions in young and old adults. *Journal of Gerontology*, **36**, 707–14.

Howieson, D. B., Dame, A., Camicioli, R., *et al.* (1997). Cognitive markers preceding Alzheimer's dementia in the healthy oldest old. *Journal of the American Geriatrics Society*, **45**, 584–9.

Hulicka, I. and Grossman, J. L. (1967). Age-group comparisons for the use of mediators in paired-associate learning. *Journal of Gerontology*, **22**, 46–51.

Hultsch, D. F. (1974). Learning to learn in adulthood. *Journal of Gerontology*, **29**, 302–8.

Hultsch, D. F., Hammer, M., and Small, B. J. (1993). Age differences in cognitive performance in later life: relationships to self-reported health and activity lifestyle. *Journal of Gerontology*, **48**, 1–11.

Huppert, F. A. and Brayne, C. (1994). What is the relationship between dementia and normal aging? In *Dementia and normal aging* (ed. F. A. Huppert, C. Brayne, and D. W. O'Connor), pp. 3–14. Cambridge University Press, Cambridge.

Huttenlocher, P. R. (1979). Synaptic density in human frontal cortex: developmental changes and effects of aging. *Brain Research*, **163**, 195–205.

Inman, V. W. and Parkinson, S. R. (1983). Differences in Brown–Petersen recall as a function of age and retention interval. *Journal of Gerontology*, **38**, 58–64.

Jacobs, D. M., Sano, M., Dooneief, G., *et al.* (1995). Neuropsychological detection and characterization of preclinical Alzheimer's disease. *Neurology*, **45**, 957–62.

Johnson, M. M. S., Schmitt, F. A., and Pietrukowicz, M. (1989). The memory advantages of the generation effect: age and process differences. *Journal of Gerontology: Psychological Sciences*, **44**, P91–4.

Jonides, J., Smith, E. E., Marshuetz, C., *et al.* (1998). Inhibition in working memory revealed by brain activation. *Proceedings of the National Academy of Science, USA*, **95**, 8410–13.

Kahneman, D. (1973). *Attention and effort*. Prentice-Hall, Englewood Cliffs, NJ.

Kandel, E. R., Schwartz, J. H., and Jessell, T. M. (1995). *Essentials of neural science and behavior*. Prentice Hall International, Englewood Cliffs, NJ.

Kausler, D. H. and Puckett, J. M. (1981*a*). Adult age differences in memory for modality attributes. *Experimental Aging Research*, **7**, 117–25.

Kausler, D. H. and Puckett, J. M. (1981*b*). Adult age differences in memory for sex of voice. *Journal of Gerontology*, **36**, 44–50.

Kemper, S. (1987). Life-span changes in syntactic complexity. *Journal of Gerontology*, **42**, 323–8.

Kemper, S., Rash, S. R., Kynette, D., *et al.* (1990). Telling stories: the structure of adults' narratives. *European Journal of Cognitive Psychology*, **2**, 205–28.

Kempler, D. and Zelinski, E. M. (1994). Language in dementia and normal aging. In *Dementia and normal aging* (ed. F. A. Huppert, C. Brayne, and D. W. O'Connor), pp. 331–65. Cambridge University Press, Cambridge.

Khaw, K.-T. (1994). Public health implications of a continuum model of dementia. In *Dementia and normal aging* (ed. F. A. Huppert, C. Brayne, and D. W. O'Connor), pp. 552–60. Cambridge University Press, Cambridge.

Kirasic, K. C. (1989). Acquisition and utilization of spatial information by elderly adults: implications for day-to-day situations. In *Everyday cognition in adulthood and late life* (ed. L. W. Poon, D. C. Rubin, and B. A. Wilson), pp. 265–83. Cambridge University Press, Cambridge.

Klisz, D. (1978). Neuropsychological evaluation in older persons. In *The clinical psychology of aging* (ed. M. Storandt, I. Siegler, and M. F. Elias), pp. 71–95. Plenum Press, New York.

Kolb, B. and Whishaw, I. Q. (1995). *Fundamentals of human neuropsychology*. W. H. Freeman, New York.

Koss, E., Haxby, J. V., DeCarli, C., *et al.* (1991). Patterns of performance preservation and loss in healthy aging. *Developmental Neuropsychology*, **7**, 99–113.

Kuhl, D. E., Metter, E. J., Riege, W. H., *et al.* (1984). The effect of normal aging on patterns of local cerebral glucose utilization. *Annals of Neurology*, **15** (Suppl.)., S133–7.

Kynette, D. and Kemper, S. (1986). Aging and the loss of grammatical forms: a cross-sectional study of language performances. *Language and Communication*, **6**, 65–72.

La Rue, A. (1992). *Aging and neuropsychological assessment*. Plenum Press, New York.

Lafleche, G. and Albert, M. S. (1995). Executive function deficits in mild Alzheimer's disease. *Neuropsychology*, **9**, 313–20.

Lehmann, E. B. and Mellinger, J. C. (1984). Effects of aging on memory for presentation modality. *Developmental Psychology*, **20**, 1210–17.

Lewis, D. A., Campbell, M. J., Terry, R. D., *et al.* (1987). Laminar and regional distributions of neurofibrillary tangles and neuritic plaques in Alzheimer's disease: a quantitative study of visual and auditory cortices. *Journal of Neuroscience*, **7**, 1799–808.

Light, L. L. (1991). Memory and aging: four hypotheses in search of data. *Annual Review of Psychology*, **42**, 333–76.

Light, L. L. (1992). The organization of memory in old age. In *Handbook of aging and cognition* (ed. F. I. M. Craik and T. A. Salthouse), pp. 111–65. Lawrence Erlbaum, Hillsdale, NJ.

Light, L. L. (1996). Memory and aging. In *Memory* (ed. E. L. Bjork and R. A. Bjork), pp. 443–90. Academic Press, San Diego, CA.

Light, L. L. and Albertson, S. A. (1988). Comprehension of pragmatic implications in young and older adults. In *Language, memory and aging* (ed. L. L. Light and D. M. Burke), pp. 133–53. Cambridge University Press, Cambridge.

Light, L. L. and Anderson, P. A. (1983). Memory for scripts in young and older adults. *Memory and Cognition*, **11**, 435–44.

Light, L. L. and Capps, J. L. (1986). Comprehension of pronouns in young and older adults. *Developmental Psychology*, **22**, 580–5.

Light, L. L., Zelinski, E. M., and Moore, M. (1982). Adult age differences in reasoning from new information. *Journal of Experimental Psychology: Learning, Memory and Cognition*, **8**, 435–47.

Linn, R. T., Wolf, P. A., Bachman, D. L., *et al.* (1995). The 'preclinical phase' of probable Alzheimer's disease. *Archives of Neurology*, **52**, 485–90.

List, J. A. (1986). Age and schematic differences in the reliability of eyewitness testimony. *Developmental Psychology*, **22**, 50–7.

Locascio, J. J., Growdon, J. H., and Corkin, S. (1995). Cognitive test performance in detecting, staging and tracking Alzheimer's disease. *Archives of Neurology*, **52**, 1087–99.

Lovelace, E. A. and Cooley, S. (1982). Free associations of older adults to single words and conceptually related word triads. *Journal of Gerontology*, **37**, 432–7.

McCrae, R. R., Arenberg, D., and Costa, P. T. (1987). Declines in divergent thinking with age: cross-sectional, longitudinal and cross-sequential analyses. *Psychology and Aging*, **2**, 130–7.

Macht, M. L. and Buschke, H. (1983). Age differences in cognitive effort in recall. *Journal of Gerontology*, **38**, 695–700.

McDowd, J. M. (1997). Inhibition in attention and aging. *Journal of Gerontology: Psychological Sciences*, 52B, P265–73.

Mann, D. M. A. (1997). *Sense and senility: the neuropathology of the aged human brain*. R. G. Landes, Austin, TX.

Manton, K. G., Siegler, I. C., and Woodbury, M. A. (1986). Patterns of intellectual development in later life. *Journal of Gerontology*, **41**, 486–9.

Martin, A., Brouwers, P., Cox, C., *et al.* (1985). On the nature of the verbal memory deficit in Alzheimer's disease. *Brain and Language*, **25**, 323–41.

Masliah, E., Mallory, B. S., Hansen, L., *et al.* (1993). Quantitative synaptic alterations in the human neocortex during normal aging. *Neurology*, **43**, 192–7.

Masur, D. M., Sliwinski, M., Lipton, R. B., *et al.* (1994). Neuropsychological prediction of dementia and the absence of dementia in healthy elderly persons. *Neurology*, **44**, 1427–32.

Maylor, E. A. (1990*a*). Recognizing and naming faces: aging, memory retrieval and the tip of the tongue state. *Journal of Gerontology: Psychological Sciences*, **45**, P215–26.

Maylor, E. A. (1990*b*). Age, blocking and the tip of the tongue state. *British Journal of Psychology*, **81**, 123–34.

Mergler, N., Faust, M., and Goldstein, M. (1985). Storytelling as an age-dependent skill. *International Journal of Aging and Human Development*, **20**, 205–28.

Mesulam, M.-M. (1990). Large-scale neurocognitive networks and distributed processing for attention, language and memory. *Annals of Neurology*, **28**, 597–613.

Meudell, P. R. and Greenhalgh, M. (1987). Age related differences in left and right hand skill and in visuo-spatial performance: their possible relationships to the hypothesis that the right hemisphere ages more rapidly than the left. *Cortex*, **23**, 431–45.

Meuller, J. H., Kausler, D. H., and Faherty, A. (1980). Age and access time for different memory codes. *Experimental Aging Research*, **6**, 445–9.

Meyer, B. J. F. and Rice, G. E. (1981). Information recalled from prose by young, middle and old adults. *Experimental Aging Research*, **7**, 253–68.

Meyer, B. J. F. and Rice, G. E. (1989). Prose processing in adulthood: the text, the reader and the task. In *Everyday cognition in adulthood and late life* (ed. L. W. Poon, D. C. Rubin, and B. A. Wilson), pp. 157–94. Cambridge University Press, Cambridge.

Milwain, E. J. (1999). An evaluation of memory loss in old age and Alzheimer's disease. Unpublished D.Phil. thesis, Department of Experimental Psychology, University of Oxford.

Milwain, E. J. (2000). Mild cognitive impairment: further caution. *Lancet*, **355**, 1018.

Mitchell, D. B. (1989). How many memory systems? Evidence from aging. *Journal of Experimental Psychology: Learning, Memory and Cognition*, **15**, 31–49.

Mitchell, D. B., Hunt, R. R., and Schmitt, F. A. (1986). The generation effect and reality monitoring: evidence from dementia and normal aging. *Journal of Gerontology*, **41**, 79–84.

Morris, J. C., McKeel, D. W., Storandt, M., *et al.* (1991). Very mild Alzheimer's disease: informant-based clinical, psychometric and pathologic distinction from normal aging. *Neurology*, **41**, 469–78.

Morris, R. G. (1996). Neurobiological correlates of cognitive dysfunction. In *The cognitive neuropsychology of Alzheimer-type dementia* (ed. R. G. Morris), pp. 223–54. Oxford University Press, Oxford.

Moscovitch, M., Winocur, G., and McLachlan, D. (1986). Memory as assessed by recognition and reading time in normal and memory-impaired people with Alzheimer's disease and other neurological disorders. *Journal of Experimental Psychology: General*, **115**, 331–47.

Navon, D. (1984). Resources—a theoretical soup stone? *Psychological Review*, **91**, 216–34.

Nebes, R. D. (1989). Semantic memory in Alzheimer's disease. *Psychological Bulletin*, **106**, 377–94.

Nebes, R. D. and Brady, C. B. (1988). Integrity of semantic fields in Alzheimer's disease. *Cortex*, **24**, 291–9.

Nicholas, M., Obler, L., Albert, M., *et al.* (1985). Lexical retrieval in healthy aging. *Cortex*, **21**, 595–606.

Norman, D. A. and Bobrow, D. G. (1975). On data-limited and resource-limited processes. *Cognitive Psychology*, **7**, 44–64.

Norman, S., Kemper, S., Kynette, D., *et al.* (1991). Syntactic complexity and adult's running memory span. *Journal of Gerontology: Psychological Sciences*, **46**, P346–51.

Obler, L. K. and Albert, M. L. (1985). Language skills across adulthood. In *Handbook of the psychology of aging* (ed. J. E. Birren and K. W. Schaie), pp. 463–73. Van Nostrand Reinhold, New York.

Obler, L. K., Fein, D., Nicholas, M., *et al.* (1991). Auditory comprehension and aging: decline in syntactic processing. *Applied Psycholinguistics*, **12**, 433–52.

Owen, A. M., Stern, C. E., Look, R. B., *et al.* (1998). Functional organization of spatial and non-spatial working memory processing within the human lateral frontal cortex. *Proceedings of the National Academy of Science, USA*, **95**, 7721–6.

Parasuraman, R. and Haxby, J. V. (1993). Attention and brain function in Alzheimer's disease: a review. *Neuropsychology*, **7**, 242–72.

Pardo, J. V., Pardo, P. J., Janer, K. W., *et al.* (1990). The anterior cingulate cortex mediates processing selection in the Stroop attentional conflict paradigm. *Proceedings of the National Academy of Science, USA*, **87**, 256–9.

Park, D. C. and Puglisi, J. T. (1985). Older adults' memory for the color of pictures and words. *Journal of Gerontology*, **40**, 198–204.

Park, D. C., Smith, A. D., Morrell, R. W., *et al.* (1990). Effects of contextual integration on recall of pictures by older adults. *Journal of Gerontology: Psychological Sciences*, **45**, P52–7.

Parkin, A. J. (1997). Normal age-related memory loss and its relation to frontal lobe dysfunction. In *Methodology of frontal and executive function* (ed. P. M. A. Rabbitt), pp. 177–90. Psychology Press, Hove, Sussex.

Parkinson, S. R. (1982). Performance deficits in short term memory tasks: a comparison of amnesic Korsakoff patients and the aged. In *Human memory and amnesia* (ed. L. S. Cermak), pp. 77–96. Lawrence Erlbaum, Hillsdale, NJ.

Parkinson, S. R., Inman, V. W., and Dannenbaum, S. E. (1985). Adult age differences in short-term forgetting. *Acta Psychologica*, **60**, 83–101.

Passingham, R. E. (1996). Attention to action. *Philosophical Transactions of the Royal Society of London: Biological Sciences*, **351**, 1473–82.

Pearson, R. C. A., Esiri, M. M., Hiorns, R. W., *et al.* (1985). Anatomical correlates of the distribution of the pathological changes in the neocortex in Alzheimer's disease. *Proceedings of the National Academy of Science, USA*, **82**, 4531–4.

Perfect, T. J. (1994). What can Brinley plots tell us about cognitive aging? *Journal of Gerontology: Psychological Sciences*, **49**, P60–4.

Perfect, T. J., Williams, R. B., and Anderton-Brown, C. (1995). Age differences in reported recollective experience are due to encoding effects, not response bias. *Memory*, **3**, 169–86.

Perlmutter, M. (1978). What is memory aging the aging of? *Developmental Psychology*, **14**, 330–45.

Perlmutter, M. (1979). Age differences in adults' free recall, cued recall and recognition. *Journal of Gerontology*, **34**, 533–9.

Perlmutter, M. and Nyquist, L. (1990). Relationships between self-reported physical and mental health and intelligence performance across adulthood. *Journal of Gerontology: Psychological Sciences*, **45**, P145–55.

Perry, R. J. and Hodges, J. R. (1999). Attention and executive deficits in Alzheimer's disease: a critical review. *Brain*, **122**, 383–404.

Perry, R. J., Watson, P., and Hodges, J. R. (2000). The nature and staging of attentional dysfunction in early (minimal and mild) Alzheimer's disease: relationship to episodic and semantic memory impairment. *Neuropsychologia*, **38**, 252–71.

Petersen, R. C., Smith, G. E., Ivnik, R. J., *et al.* (1995). Apolipoprotein E status as a predictor of the development of Alzheimer's disease in memory-impaired individuals. *Journal of the American Medical Association*, **273**, 1274–8.

Petersen, R. C., Smith, G. E., Waring, S. C., *et al.* (1999). Mild cognitive impairment: clinical characterization and outcome. *Archives of Neurology*, **56**, 303–8.

Petrides, M., Alivisatos, B., Meyer, E., *et al.* (1993). Functional activation of the human frontal cortex during the performance of verbal working memory tasks. *Proceedings of the National Academy of Science, USA*, **90**, 878–82.

Petros, T. V., Zehr, H. D., and Chabot, R. J. (1983). Adult age differences in accessing and retrieving information from long-term memory. *Journal of Gerontology*, **38**, 589–92.

Pezdek, K. (1987). Memory for pictures: a lifespan study of memory for visual detail. *Child Development*, **58**, 807–15.

Phillips, L. H. (1997). Do 'frontal tests' measure executive function?: issues of assessment and evidence from fluency tests. In *Methodology of frontal and executive function* (ed. P. M. A. Rabbitt), pp. 191–214. Psychology Press, Hove, Sussex.

Phillips, L. H., Della Sala, S., and Trivelli, C. (1996). Fluency deficits in patients with Alzheimer's disease and frontal lobe lesions. *European Journal of Neurology*, **3**, 102–8.

Poon, L. W. (1985). Differences in human memory with aging: nature, causes and clinical implications. In *Handbook of the psychology of aging* (ed. J. E. Birren and K. W. Schaie), pp. 427–62. Van Nostrand Reinhold, New York.

Posner, M. I. and Petersen, S. E. (1990). The attention system of the human brain. *Annual Review of Neuroscience*, **13**, 25–42.

Posner, M. I. and Raichle, M. E. (1994). *Images of mind.* Scientific American Library, New York.

Pratt, M. W. and Robins, S. W. (1991). That's the way it is: age differences in the structure and quality of adults' personal narratives. *Discourse Processes*, **14**, 73–85.

Rabbitt, P. M. A. (1968). Channel-capacity, intelligibility and immediate memory. *Quarterly Journal of Experimental Psychology*, **20**, 241–8.

Rabbitt, P. M. A. (1981). Human ageing and disturbances of memory control processes underlying 'intelligent' performance of some cognitive tasks. In *Intelligence and learning* (ed. M. P. Friedman, J. P. Das, and N. O'Connor), pp. 427–39. Plenum Press, New York.

Rabbitt, P. M. A. (1989). Inner-city decay? Age changes in structure and process in recall of familiar topographical information. In *Everyday cognition in adulthood and late life* (ed. L. W. Poon, D. C. Rubin, and B. A. Wilson), pp. 284–99. Cambridge University Press, Cambridge.

Rabbitt, P. M. A. (1991). Mild hearing loss can cause apparent memory failures which increase with age and reduce with IQ. *Otolaryngologica*, **Suppl. 476**, 167–76.

Rabbitt, P. M. A. (1996). Do individual differences in speed reflect 'global' or 'local' differences in mental abilities? *Intelligence*, **22**, 69–88.

Rabbitt, P. M. A. (1997). Introduction: methodologies and models in the study of executive function. In *Methodology of frontal and executive function* (ed. P. M. A. Rabbitt), pp. 1–38. Psychology Press, Hove, Sussex.

Rabinowitz, J. C. (1984). Aging and recognition failure. *Journal of Gerontology*, **39**, 65–71.

Rabinowitz, J. C. (1986). Priming in episodic memory. *Journal of Gerontology*, **41**, 203–13.

Rabinowitz, J. C. (1989*a*). Judgments of origin and generation effects: comparisons between young and elderly adults. *Psychology and Aging*, **4**, 259–68.

Rabinowitz, J. C. (1989*b*). Age deficits in recall under optimal study conditions. *Psychology and Aging*, **4**, 378–80.

Rabinowitz, J. C. and Ackerman, B. P. (1982). General encoding of episodic events by elderly adults. In *Aging and cognitive processes* (ed. F. I. M. Craik and A. S. Trehub), pp. 145–54. Plenum, New York.

Rabinowitz, J. C., Craik, F. I. M., and Ackerman, B. P. (1982). A processing resource account of age differences in recall. *Canadian Journal of Psychology*, **36**, 325–44.

Raichle, M. E., Fiez, J. A., Videen, T. O., *et al.* (1994). Practice-related changes in human brain functional anatomy during nonmotor learning. *Cerebral Cortex*, **4**, 8–26.

Randolph, C., Braun, A. R., Goldberg, T. E., *et al.* (1993). Semantic fluency in Alzheimer's, Parkinson's and Huntington's disease: dissociation of storage and retrieval failures. *Neuropsychology*, **7**, 82–8.

Rankin, J. L. and Collins, M. (1986). The effects of memory elaboration on adult age differences in incidental recall. *Experimental Aging Research*, **12**, 231–4.

Raz, N., Gunning, F. M., Head, D., *et al.* (1997). Selective aging of human cerebral cortex observed *in vivo*: differential vulnerability of the prefrontal gray matter. *Cerebral Cortex*, **7**, 268–82.

Reder, L. M., Wible, C., and Martin, J. (1986). Differential memory changes with age: exact retrieval versus plausible inference. *Journal of Experimental Psychology: Learning, Memory and Cognition*, **12**, 72–81.

Reese, H. W. and Rodeheaver, D. (1985). Problem solving and complex decision making. In *Handbook of the psychology of aging* (ed. J. E. Birren and K. W. Schaie), pp. 474–99. Van Nostrand Reinhold, New York.

Riegel, K. F. (1959). A study of verbal achievements of older persons. *Journal of Gerontology*, **14**, 453–6.

Rissenberg, M. and Glanzer, M. (1987). Free recall and word finding ability in normal aging and dementia of the Alzheimer's type: the effect of item concreteness. *Journal of Gerontology*, **42**, 318–22.

Ritchie, K. and Touchon, J. (2000). Mild cognitive impairment: conceptual basis and current nosological status. *Lancet*, **355**, 225–8.

Robbins, T. W. (1996). Dissociating executive functions of the prefrontal cortex. *Philosophical Transactions of the Royal Society of London: Biological Sciences*, **351**, 1463–72.

Rossor, M. and Iversen, L. L. (1986). Non-cholinergic neurotransmitter abnormalities in Alzheimer's disease. *British Medical Bulletin*, **42**, 70–4.

Rowe, J. W. and Kahn, R. L. (1987). Human aging: usual and successful. *Science*, **237**, 143–9.

Salmon, D. P. and Fennema-Notestine, C. (1996). Implicit memory. In *The cognitive neuropsychology of Alzheimer-type dementia* (ed. R. G. Morris), pp. 105–27. Oxford University Press, Oxford.

Salthouse, T. A. (1982). *Adult cognition.* Springer, New York.

Salthouse, T. A. (1984). Effects of age and skill in typing. *Journal of Experimental Psychology: General*, **113**, 345–71.

Salthouse, T. A. (1988). Effects of aging on verbal abilities: Examination of the psychometric literature. In *Language, memory and aging* (ed. L. L. Light and D. M. Burke), pp. 17–35. Cambridge University Press, Cambridge.

Salthouse, T. A. (1993). Speed mediation of adult age differences in cognition. *Developmental Psychology*, **29**, 722–38.

Salthouse, T. A. (1996). The processing-speed theory of adult age differences in cognition. *Psychological Review*, **103**, 403–28.

Salthouse, T. A. and Babcock, R. L. (1991). Decomposing adult age differences in working memory. *Developmental Psychology*, **27**, 763–76.

Salthouse, T. A. and Somberg, B. L. (1982). Time–accuracy relationships in young and old adults. *Journal of Gerontology*, **37**, 349–53.

Salthouse, T. A., Hancock, H. E., Meinz, E. J., *et al.* (1996). Interrelations of age, visual acuity and cognitive functioning. *Journal of Gerontology: Psychological Sciences*, **51B**, P317–30.

Sands, L. P. and Meredith, W. (1992). Blood pressure and intellectual functioning in late midlife. *Journal of Gerontology*, **47**, P81–4.

Schacter, D. L. (1994). Priming and multiple memory systems: perceptual mechanisms of implicit memory. In *Memory Systems 1994* (ed. D. L. Schacter and E. Tulving), pp. 233–68. MIT Press, Cambridge, MA.

Schacter, D. L., Savage, C. R., Alpert, N. M., *et al.* (1996). The role of hippocampus and frontal cortex in age-related memory changes: a PET study. *NeuroReport*, **7**, 1165–9.

Schacter, D. L., Koutstaal, W., and Norman, K. A. (1997). False memories and aging. *Trends in Cognitive Sciences*, **1**, 229–36.

Schaie, K. W. (1996). Intellectual development in adulthood. In *Handbook of the psychology of aging* (ed. J. E. Birren and K. W. Schaie), pp. 266–86. Academic Press, San Diego, CA.

Schaie, K. W. and Parham, I. A. (1977). Cohort-sequential analyses of adult intellectual development. *Developmental Psychology*, **13**, 649–53.

Schaie, K. W. and Schaie, J. P. (1977). Clinical assessment and aging. In *Handbook of the psychology of aging* (ed. J. E. Birren and K. W. Schaie), pp. 692–723. Van Nostrand Reinhold, New York.

Scheidt, R. J. and Schaie, K. W. (1978). A taxonomy of situations for an elderly population: generating situational criteria. *Journal of Gerontology*, **33**, 848–57.

Schneider, W. and Shiffrin, R. M. (1977). Controlled and automatic human information processing: 1. detection, search and attention. *Psychological Review*, **84**, 1–66.

Schonfield, D. and Robertson, B. A. (1966). Memory storage and aging. *Canadian Journal of Psychology*, **20**, 228–36.

Shallice, T. (1988). *From neuropsychology to mental structure*. Cambridge University Press, Cambridge.

Shallice, T. and Burgess, P. (1996). The domain of supervisory processes and temporal organization of behaviour. *Philosophical Transactions of the Royal Society of London: Biological Sciences*, **351**, 1405–12.

Shallice, T. and Warrington, E. K. (1970). Independent functioning of verbal memory stores: a neuropsychological study. *Quarterly Journal of Experimental Psychology*, **22**, 261–73.

Sharps, M. J. (1991). Spatial memory in young and elderly adults: the category structure of stimulus sets. *Psychology and Aging*, **6**, 309–12.

Sharps, M. J. and Gollin, E. S. (1987). Memory for object locations in young and elderly adults. *Journal of Gerontology*, **42**, 336–41.

Sharps, M. J. and Gollin, E. S. (1988). Aging and free recall for objects located in space. *Journal of Gerontology: Psychological Sciences*, **43**, P8–11.

Shaw, T. G., Mortel, K. F., Meyer, J. S., *et al.* (1984). Cerebral blood flow changes in benign aging and cerebrovascular disease. *Neurology*, **34**, 855–62.

Sliwinski, M. and Buschke, H. (1997). Processing speed and memory in aging and dementia. *Journal of Gerontology: Psychological Sciences*, **52B**, P308–18.

Smith, C. B. (1985). Aging and changes in cerebral energy metabolism. *Trends in Neurosciences*, **7**, 203–8.

Smith, E. E., Jonides, J., Marshuetz, C., *et al.* (1998). Components of verbal working memory: evidence from neuroimaging. *Proceedings of the National Academy of Science, USA*, **95**, 876–82.

Spearman, C. (1927). *The abilities of man*. Macmillan, New York.

Spilich, G. J. (1983). Life-span components of text processing: structural and procedural differences. *Journal of Verbal Learning and Verbal Behavior*, **22**, 231–44.

Spilich, G. J. and Voss, J. F. (1983). Contextual effects upon text memory for young, aged-normal and aged-impaired individuals. *Experimental Aging Research*, **9**, 45–9.

Spinnler, H. (1999). Alzheimer's disease. In *Handbook of clinical and experimental neuropsychology* (ed. G. Denes and L. Pizzamuglio), pp. 699–746. Psychology Press, Hove, Sussex.

Squire, L. R. and Knowlton, B. J. (1995). Memory, hippocampus and brain systems. In *The cognitive neurosciences* (ed. M. S. Gazzaniga), pp. 825–37. MIT Press, Cambridge, MA.

Squire, L. R. and Zola-Morgan, S. (1991). The medial temporal lobe memory system. *Science*, **253**, 1380–6.

Stine, E. L., Wingfield, A., and Poon, L. W. (1989). Speech comprehension and memory through adulthood: the roles of time and strategy. In *Everyday cognition in adulthood and late life* (ed. L. W. Poon, D. C. Rubin, and B. A. Wilson), pp. 195–221. Cambridge University Press, Cambridge.

Stoltzfus, E. R., Hasher, L., and Zacks, R. T. (1996). Working memory and aging: current status of the inhibitory view. In *Working memory and human cognition* (ed. J. T. E. Richardson, R. W. Engle, L. Hasher *et al.*), pp. 66–88. Oxford University Press, Oxford.

Storandt, M. and Hill, R. D. (1989). Very mild senile dementia of the Alzheimer type II: psychometric test performance. *Archives of Neurology*, **46**, 383–6.

Strauss, M. E., Weingartner, H., and Thompson, K. (1985). Remembering words and how often they occurred in memory-impaired patients. *Memory and Cognition*, **13**, 507–10.

Stuart-Hamilton, I. (1994). *The psychology of ageing: an introduction*. Jessica Kingsley Publishers, London.

Taub, H. A. (1968). Age differences in memory as a function of rate of presentation, order of report and stimulus organization. *Journal of Gerontology*, **23**, 159–64.

Terry, R. D., DeTeresa, R., and Hansen, L. A. (1987). Neocortical cell counts in normal human adult aging. *Annals of Neurology*, **12**, 530–9.

Thurstone, L. L. (1938). *Primary mental abilities*. University Chicago Press, Chicago.

Thurstone, L. L. and Thurstone, T. G. (1962). *Primary mental abilities—revised*. Science Research Associates, Chicago.

Tierney, M. C., Szalai, J. P., Snow, W. G., *et al.* (1996). Prediction of probable Alzheimer's disease in memory impaired patients: a prospective longitudinal study. *Neurology*, **46**, 661–5.

Till, R. E. (1985). Verbatim and inferential memory in young and elderly adults. *Journal of Gerontology*, **40**, 316–23.

Till, R. E. and Walsh, D. A. (1980). Encoding and retrieval factors in adult memory for implicational sentences. *Journal of Verbal Learning and Verbal Behavior*, **19**, 1–16.

Till, R. E., Bartlett, J. C., and Doyle, A. H. (1982). Age differences in picture memory with resemblance and discrimination tasks. *Experimental Aging Research*, **8**, 179–84.

Treat, N. J. and Reese, H. W. (1976). Age, pacing and imagery in paired-associate learning. *Developmental Psychology*, **12**, 119–24.

Tulving, E. (1985). How many memory systems are there? *American Psychologist*, **40**, 385–98.

Tulving, E. (1995). Organization of memory: quo vadis? In *The cognitive neurosciences* (ed. M. S. Gazzaniga), pp. 839–47. MIT Press, Cambridge, MA.

Tun, P. A. and Wingfield, A. (1993). Is speech special? Perception and recall of spoken language in complex environments. In *Adult information processing: limits on loss* (ed. J. Cerella, J. Rybash, W. Hoyer, *et al.*), pp. 425–57. Academic Press, San Diego, CA.

Turner, M. L. and Engle, R. W. (1989). Is working memory capacity task dependent? *Journal of Memory and Language*, **28**, 127–54.

Van Hoesen, G. W. and Damasio, A. R. (1987). Neural correlates of cognitive impairment in Alzheimer's disease. In *The handbook of physiology* (ed. V. B. Mountcastle, F. Plum, and S. R. Geiger), pp. 871–98. American Physiological Society, Bethesda, MD.

Waddell, K. J. and Rogoff, B. (1981). Effect of contextual organization on spatial memory of middle-aged and older women. *Developmental Psychology*, **17**, 878–85.

Warren, L. R., Butler, R. W., Katholi, C. P., *et al.* (1985). Age differences in cerebral blood flow during rest and during mental activation measurements with and without incentive. *Journal of Gerontology*, **40**, 53–9.

Wechsler, D. (1955). *WAIS manual.* The Psychological Corporation, New York.

Wechsler, D. (1981). *WAIS-R manual.* The Psychological Corporation, New York.

Welford, A. T. (1958). *Aging and human skill.* Oxford University Press, Oxford.

Welford, A. T. (1993). The gerontological balance sheet. In *Adult information processing: limits on loss* (ed. J. Cerella, J. Rybash, W. Hoyer, *et al.*), pp. 3–10. Academic Press, San Diego, CA.

Welsh, K. A., Butters, N., Hughes, J. P., *et al.* (1992). Detection and staging of dementia in Alzheimer's disease: use of the neuropsychological measures developed for the Consortium to Establish a Registry for Alzheimer's Disease. *Archives of Neurology*, **49**, 448–52.

West, R. L. (1996). An application of prefrontal cortex function theory to cognitive aging. *Psychological Bulletin*, **120**, 272–92.

West, R. L. and Boatwright, L. K. (1983). Age differences in cued recall and recognition under varying encoding and retrieval conditions. *Experimental Aging Research*, **9**, 185–9.

Whiting, W. L. and Smith, A. D. (1997). Differential age-related processing limitations in recall and recognition tasks. *Psychology and Aging*, **12**, 216–24.

Wickelgren, I. (1996). For the cortex, neuron loss may be less than thought. *Science*, **273**, 48–50.

Wingfield, A., Poon, L. W., Lombardi, L., *et al.* (1985). Speed of processing in normal aging: effects of speech rate, linguistic structure and processing time. *Journal of Gerontology*, **40**, 579–85.

Woodruff-Pak, D. S. (1997). *The neuropsychology of aging*. Blackwell, Oxford.

Wright, B. M. and Payne, R. B. (1985). Effects of aging on sex differences in psychomotor reminiscence and tracking proficiency. *Journal of Gerontology*, **40**, 179–84.

Zacks, R. T. and Hasher, L. (1997). Cognitive gerontology and attentional inhibition: a reply to Burke and McDowd. *Journal of Gerontology: Psychological Sciences*, **52B**, P274–83.

Zelinski, E. M. (1988). Integrating information from discourse: do older adults show deficits? In *Language, memory and aging* (ed. L. L. Light and D. M. Burke), pp. 117–32. Cambridge University Press, Cambridge, UK.

Zelinski, E. M., Light, L. L., and Gilewski, M. J. (1984). Adult age differences in memory for prose: the question of sensitivity to passage structure. *Developmental Psychology*, **20**, 1181–92.

4 Epidemiology

Martin Prince

What is epidemiology?

Last's dictionary of epidemiology defines epidemiology as:

> The study of the distribution and determinants of health-related states or events in specified populations, and the application of this study to the control of health problems. (Last 2001)

Epidemiology is concerned with the health states of populations, communities, and groups, whereas the health states of individuals is the concern of clinical medicine. Epidemiology may simply describe the distribution of health states (extent, type, severity) within a population—this is *descriptive epidemiology*.

Alternatively, it may try to explain the distribution of health states—termed *analytical epidemiology* (Fig. 4.1). The basic strategy is to compare the distribution of disease between groups or between populations, looking for *associations* between hypothesized *risk factors* (genes, behaviours, lifestyles, environmental exposures) and *health states*. These associations may or may not indicate that the hypothesized risk factor has caused the disease.

What do epidemiologists do?

Epidemiological studies are generally not controlled experiments. Observations are made on individuals living freely in the 'real world'; these non-experimental studies are referred to as 'observational'. There is much background 'noise' in these types of studies, so it is difficult to make clear-cut inferences from the resulting data. Observed associations between risk factors and diseases may represent the effects of chance (random error), or bias, or confounding factors (non-random error). Occasionally the apparent risk factor may be a consequence rather than a cause of the disease—this is called 'reverse causality'. It is important to note that a valid association may or may not be causal.

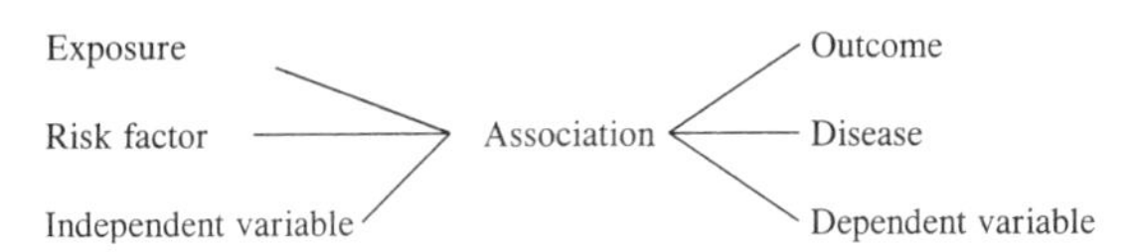

Fig. 4.1 Some terminology used in analytical epidemiology.

Two key functions for epidemiologists are therefore to design and analyse their studies in such a way as to maximize the *precision* and *validity* of their findings.

Maximizing precision reduces random error, the two main sources of random error being sampling error and measurement error. Precision may be increased by ensuring an adequate sample size and by maximizing the accuracy of the measures.

Maximizing validity implies the avoidance of non-random error, which arises from bias and confounding (these concepts will be dealt with in more detail later in this chapter). The error is non-random because its effects are unequal (differential) between the two or more groups being compared.

If precision and validity of epidemiological studies are adequate, and the effects of chance, bias, confounding, and reverse causality can be confidently excluded, then, and only then, can tentative causal inferences be made from observed associations. The identification of causal factors may lead to strategies for prevention.

For ethical reasons, it is generally not possible to study the effects of factors thought likely to increase the risk of disease in human populations under experimental conditions. However, causal inferences made from observational (non-experimental) studies can be assessed further by testing the disease-preventing effects of reducing or eliminating exposure to potential risk factors under experimental conditions. Thus epidemiologists have tested the effects of:

- laying babies on their backs on sudden infant death syndrome (cot death);
- reducing dietary fat on coronary heart disease;
- iodine supplementation on cretinism.

The optimal experimental design is the randomized controlled trial, in which the allocation to either the active intervention or the control or placebo arms is randomly determined.

Epidemiology has been described as the basic science of public health medicine; in reality these are complementary disciplines. Without epidemiology there can be no evidence-based direction to public health policy. Without public health medicine, epidemiological findings cannot be prioritized and converted into practical policies.

Context

Mental health in an ageing world

Some 6 per cent of the world's population comprises those aged 65 years or over. However, this proportion varies according to region—17% in the United Kingdom (one of the world's 'oldest' countries), 14% in the rest of Europe, 13% in the United States, but only 3% in African countries, and 5% in Latin America and SE Asia. In many developing countries, children account for around half of the total population. Given these indices, it is perhaps surprising to learn that at present approximately two-thirds of the world's older citizens live in the developing world. This preponderance is set to increase further, with three-quarters residing in developing countries by the year 2020. The apparent paradox is explained by the vast size of some of the developing country populations; India alone has a population of one billion, of whom 4%, or 40 million, are aged 65 or over. The rapid increase in the absolute and relative numbers of older persons in the developing world is explained by the phenomenon of demographic ageing. The proportion of older persons in the population increases partly as a result of increasing life expectancy, but more particularly because of falling fertility rates in response to declining child mortality, education, and economic development; in classical demographic theory this is the third and final 'demographic transition' before the achievement of population stability. The rates of demographic ageing currently seen in China, India, and parts of Latin America are completely unprecedented in world history, and will have far-reaching consequences for the health and welfare needs of their populations. The hope is that economic growth will match the growing needs for care of dependent older persons, but there is as yet little evidence of relevant policy development or service planning.

The consequences in terms of the predicted rise in numbers of persons with dementia by world region are illustrated in Fig. 4.2.

The final demographic transition now underway in most developing countries (other than sub-Saharan Africa) is largely complete in Great Britain and in Western Europe. Warnes (1989) points out that the ageing of these populations has been neither very recent, nor particularly rapid. What is new is the public awareness of these changes. Over the last 100 years annual mortality rates have declined from 3% to 1%, and the expectation of life has nearly doubled. The increase over the last 100 years in the proportion of the British population aged over 65, from approximately 5% to approximately 16%, has been gradual and relatively painless in economic terms. However, there may be a 'sting in the tail' of demographic ageing. By 2040 in the UK, the proportion of those aged 60 and over will have increased from 21% to 26%. Moreover, the proportion of the oldest old will have nearly doubled, i.e. from 6% to 11%, in 2040 (OPCS 1991; Table 4.1). It is this increase in the numbers and relative proportions of the oldest old which accounts for the continuing projected increase in the numbers of persons with dementia in the world's developed regions (see Fig. 4.2).

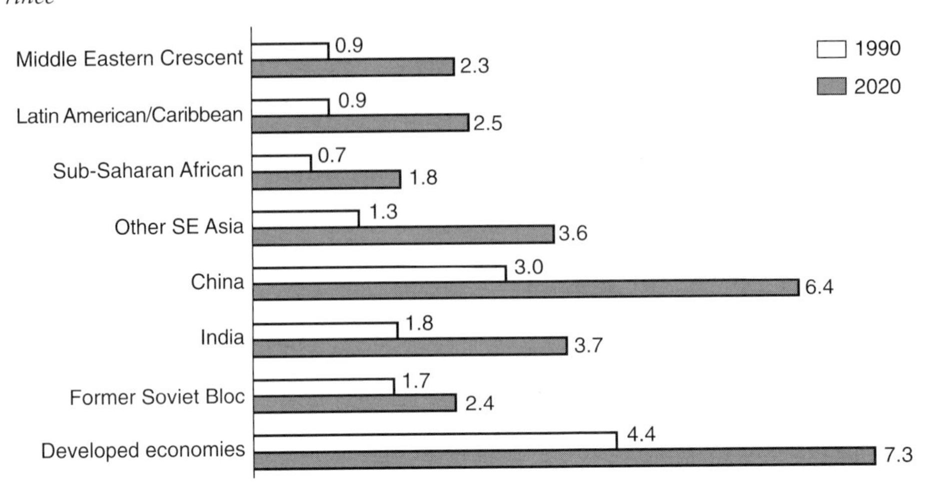

Fig. 4.2 Projected changes in the absolute numbers of those with dementia by world region.

Table 4.1 UK population trends (standard projection assumptions)[a]

Age band (years)	Sex	Year 2001	2011	2021	2041
60–64	m	1.4	1.8	1.8	1.5
	f	1.4	1.9	1.9	1.5
65–74	m	2.2	2.4	2.8	2.9
	f	2.6	2.7	3.2	3.2
75–84	m	1.3	1.3	1.5	1.9
	f	2.0	1.9	2.0	2.7
85+	m	0.3	0.4	0.4	0.6
	f	0.8	0.9	0.9	1.1
All 60+	m	5.2	5.9	6.5	6.9
	f	6.8	7.4	8.0	8.5
Whole population	m	29.0	29.3	29.6	29.2
	f	30.0	30.1	30.3	29.9

[a]Numbers in millions of population.
Taken from OPCS (1991) with permission.

Epidemiological methods

Measurement in psychiatric epidemiology

The science of the measurement of mental phenomena, termed 'psychometrics', is central to quantitative research in psychiatry. Without appropriate, accurate, stable, and unbiased measures, research is doomed to fail. Most measurement strategies are based on eliciting symptoms, either by asking the subject to complete a self-report questionnaire or by using an interviewer to question the subject. Some are long, detailed, and comprehensive clinical diagnostic assessments. Others are much briefer, designed either to screen for probable cases or as scaleable measures in their own right of a trait or dimension such as depression, neuroticism, or cognitive function. Researchers in other medical disciplines sometimes criticize psychiatric measures for being vague or 'woolly', because they are not based on biological markers of pathology. For this very reason, psychiatry was among the first medical disciplines to develop internationally recognized, operationalized diagnostic criteria. At the same time the research interview has become progressively refined, such that the processes of eliciting, recording, and distilling symptoms into diagnoses or scaleable traits are now also highly standardized. These criticisms are therefore mainly misplaced.

Epidemiologists' confidence in these measures is based on an understanding of their psychometric properties, principally their *validity* and *reliability*. Validity refers to the extent to which a measure really does measure what it sets out to measure. Reliability refers to the consistency of a measure when applied repeatedly under similar circumstances. Put simply, a measure is reliable if it is used twice to measure the same thing and if both give the same answer. A measure is valid if the same thing is measured twice using two different measures, one known to be valid, and the same answer results. The reliability and validity of all measures needs to be cited in research grant proposals and research publications. If they have not been adequately established, particularly if the measure is new, then the investigators need to do this themselves in a pilot investigation. A resource guide to commonly used and well-validated measures, with an emphasis upon those validated upon older populations, is given in Appendix 4.1 at the end of this chapter.

Domains of measurement

Measures in common use in psychiatric epidemiology can be thought of as covering six main domains:

1. *Demographic status*—takes in age, gender, marital status, household circumstances, and occupation.
2. *Socioeconomic status*—comprises social class, income, wealth, debt.
3. *Social circumstances*—involve social network and social support.
4. *Activities, lifestyles, behaviours*—this is a very broad area, its contents being dictated by the focus of the research—examples would include tobacco and alcohol consumption, substance use, diet, and exercise. Some measures, such as recent exposure to positive and negative life events, may be particularly relevant to psychiatric research.
5. *Opinions and attitudes*—is an area of measurement initially restricted to market research organizations, but increasingly is being adopted by social science and biomedical researchers.
6. *Health status*—measures of which can be further grouped into:
   (a) specific measures of 'caseness' in dichotomous diagnoses such as schizophrenia, or of dimensions used for continuously distributed traits such as mood, anxiety, neuroticism, and cognitive function;
   (b) global measures, e.g. subjective or objective global health assessment, disablement (impairment, activity, and participation), and health-related quality of life; and
   (c) measures reflecting the need for, or use of, health services.

Caseness and dimensions

Measures of 'caseness'

At first sight, the concept of psychiatric caseness can seem arbitrary, confusing, and possibly even unhelpful. For example, a recent review of 40 community-based studies of the prevalence of late-life depression concluded there was wide variation in reported prevalence, but that the most important source of variation seemed to be the diagnostic criteria used to identify the cases (Beekman *et al.* 1999). Thus the 15 studies that measured DSM major depression had a weighted average prevalence of 2% (range 0–3%). However, 25 studies using other criteria gave a weighted average prevalence of 13% (range 9%-18%). Is the correct prevalence of late-life depression 2% or 13%? Surely both these contrasting estimates cannot be 'right'. In our confusion, we are led to ask the question, 'What is a case of depression?' The answer will depend always on the purpose for which the measurement is being made. The question should therefore not be 'What is a case?' so much as 'A case for what?'

Diagnostic criteria can be classified as broad or narrow, and as more or less operationalized. Broader criteria will embrace diffuse and less severe forms of the disorder, narrow criteria exclude all but the most clear-cut and severe cases. Operationalized criteria make explicit a series of unambiguous rules, according to which people either qualify or do not qualify as cases. DSM-IV major depression criteria (American Psychiatric Association 1994) are both narrow and strictly operationalized. In the other studies included in the review, late-life depression was both more broadly and more loosely defined. Operationalized criteria were not used; for these studies the threshold was defined in terms of the concept of 'clinical significance', a level of depression that a competent clinician would consider merited some kind of active therapeutic intervention.

The narrow criteria for major depression define a small proportion of persons with an unarguably severe form of depressive disorder, implying strong construct validity. Since the criteria are strictly operationalized they can also be applied reliably. This might then be a good case definition for the first studies investigating the efficacy of a new treatment for depressive disorder. Major depression might also be a good 'pure' case definition for a genetic linkage study, aiming to identify gene loci predisposing to depression in a multiply affected family pedigree. However, these criteria will not suit all purposes. One cannot presume, for instance, that the findings from the drug efficacy studies will generalize to the broader group of depressed patients whom clinicians typically diagnose and treat, but who do not meet the criteria for major depression. Also, major depression criteria arguably miss much of the impact of depressive disorder within a community population. Depressed persons are known to be heavy users of health and social services. However, the very small number of cases of major depression account for a tiny proportion of this excess, which is mainly made up of cases of 'common mental disorder'.

Measures of dimensions

The idea of a psychiatric disorder as a dimension can be difficult for psychiatrists to grasp. They are used to making a series of dichotomous judgements in their clinical practice. Is this patient depressed? Does he need treatment? Should he be admitted? Does he have insight? Is he a danger to himself? As Pickering commented (when arguing that hypertension was better understood as a dimensional rather than a dichotomous disorder) 'doctors can count to one but not beyond'. It is important to recognize that a dimensional concept need not contradict a categorical view of a disorder. As with the relativity of the concept of 'a case', it may be useful under some circumstances to think categorically and in others dimensionally. There is, for instance, a positive correlation between the number of symptoms of depression experienced by a person and:

- the impairment of their quality of life;
- the frequency with which they use general practitioner (GP; i.e. primary care) services; and
- the number of days they take off work in a month.

Thus a dimensional perspective, even more so than broadly based diagnostic criteria, can offer useful insights into the way in which the consequences of mental disorder are very widely distributed in the community.

From a technical point of view, continuous measures of dimensional traits such as depression, anxiety, neuroticism, and cognitive function offer some advantages over their dichotomous equivalents: major depression, generalized anxiety disorder, personality disorder, and dementia. These diagnoses tend to be rather rare—collapsing a continuous trait into a dichotomous diagnosis may mean that the investigators are in effect throwing away informative data; the net effect may be loss of statistical power to demonstrate an important association with a risk factor or a real benefit of a treatment.

Validity

Construct validity

This refers to the extent to which the construct that the measure seeks to address is real and coherent, and then also to the relevance of the measure to that construct. Construct validity cannot be demonstrated empirically, but evidence can be sought to support it. For example, the scope and content of the construct can be identified in open-ended interviews and focus-group discussions with experts or key informants. These same informants can review the proposed measure and comment on the appropriateness of the items (face validity).

Concurrent validity

Concurrent validity is tested by the extent to which the new measure relates, as hypothesized, to other measures taken at the same time (hence concurrent). There are four main variants: criterion, convergent, divergent, and known group validity.

Criterion validity

This is tested by comparing measures obtained with the new instrument to those obtained with an existing *criterion* measure. The criterion is the current 'gold standard' measure and is usually more complex, lengthier, or more expensive to administer, otherwise there would be little point in developing the new measure! In psychiatry there are generally no biologically based criterion measures as, for example, bronchoscopy and biopsy for carcinoma of the bronchus. The first measures developed for psychiatric research were compared with the criterion or 'gold standard' of a competent psychiatrist's clinical diagnosis. More recently, detailed standardized clinical interviews such as SCAN (schedules for assessment of negative symptoms) have taken the place of the psychiatrist's opinion.

Convergent and divergent validity

These validity measures should be tested in relation to each other. A measure will be more closely related to an alternative measure of the same construct than it will be to measures of different constructs. Thus the general health questionnaire (GHQ—a measure of psychiatric morbidity) should correlate more strongly with the Beck Depression Scale than with a physical functioning scale, or with a measure of income.

Known group validity

This can be assessed where no established 'gold standard' external criterion exists. Thus a new questionnaire measuring the amount of time parents spend in positive joint activities with their children could be applied to two groups of parents, identified by their health visitors or teachers as having contrasting levels of involvement with their children.

Predictive validity

Predictive validity assesses the extent to which a new measure can predict future variables. Thus depression may predict time off work, or use of health services; cognitive impairment may predict dementia.

Reliability

Test–retest reliability (intrameasurement reliability)

This tests the stability of a measure over time. The measure is administered to a subject, and then after an interval is administered again to the same subject, under the same conditions (e.g. by the same interviewer). The selection of the time interval is a matter of judgement. Too short and the subject may simply recall and repeat their response from the first testing. Too long, and the trait that the measure was measuring may have changed, e.g. the subject may have recovered from their depression.

Interobserver reliability

In contrast, this tests the stability of the measure when administered or rated by different investigators. Administering the measure to the same subject under the same conditions by first one and then the other interviewer tests inter-interviewer reliability. Having the same interview rated by two or more investigators tests inter-rater reliability.

Measuring reliability

Intrameasurement and interobserver reliability are assessed using measures of agreement. For a continuous scale measure the appropriate statistic would be the intraclass correlation. For a categorical measure the appropriate statistic is Cohen's kappa; this takes into account the agreement expected by chance, and is independent of the prevalence of the condition in the test population.

The internal consistency of a measure indicates the extent to which its component parts (in the case of a scale, the individual items) address a common underlying construct. This is conventionally considered a component of reliability. For a scale it is usually measured using Cronbach's coefficient alpha, which varies between 0 and 1. A coefficient alpha of 0.6 to 0.8 is moderate but satisfactory, above 0.8 it indicates a highly internally consistent scale. Another measure of internal consistency is the split-half reliability, a measure of agreement between subscales derived from two randomly selected halves of the scale.

Study designs

As with the plots of Hollywood movies, there have only ever been a limited number of epidemiological designs in general use. However, the details of the study designs, and the conduct and analysis of these studies have become increasingly refined and sophisticated. Studies may be experimental or non-experimental (observational). Observational studies may use observations made on individuals or aggregated data from groups or populations. They may be descriptive or analytical in purpose and design. Figure 4.3 summarizes the main types of study design.

On the following pages, the essentials of these basic types of study design are illustrated with

Non-experimental					Experimental
Descriptive		Analytical			
1. Population prevalence/ incidence (a) Geographical variation (b) Temporal ('secular') variation	2. Ecological correlation	3. Cross-sectional survey	4. Case-control study	5. Cohort study	6. Randomized controlled trial

Fig. 4.3 The main types of epidemiological study design.

reference to their application to the epidemiology of mental health conditions in late-life.

Descriptive studies

Prevalence is defined as the proportion of persons in a defined population that has the disease under study at a defined time. This may be point prevalence (prevalence at the instant of the survey), one-month prevalence (prevalence at any time over the month before the study), and so on. The prevalence of dementia (and of the common subtype, Alzheimer's disease) increases exponentially with increasing age, and is therefore generally quoted in the form of age-specific rates in 5-year age bands. Thus the EURODEM (dementia in Europe) consortium meta-analysis (Hofman *et al.* 1991) for European population-based studies applying DSM-III dementia criteria reported the following rates—1% (65–69 years), 4% (70–74), 6% (75–79), 13% (80–84), 22% (85–89), 32% (90–94). The overall prevalence for those aged 65 years and over is in the region of 6%.

Incidence risk is defined as the probability of occurrence of disease in a disease-free population (population at risk) during a specified period. The annual incidence risk for dementia again typically increases exponentially with increasing age. The overall incidence risk for those aged 65 years and over has been reported to lie between 1% and 2%. Note that the prevalence of dementia is approximately three to six times greater than the annual incidence risk. Prevalence (P) is approximately equal to the product of incidence (I) and disease duration (T), i.e. $P = I \times T$. Disease is terminated either by death or recovery. For conditions with high short-term mortality rates (lung cancer) or short-term recovery rates (common cold), the prevalence and incidence rates are similar. Dementia is a more chronic condition.

Most functional mental illnesses, including depression, do not fit the classical incidence model in that they are typically relapsing and remitting disorders. Some authors prefer, therefore, to talk of onset rates rather than incidence. Typically around 12% of those not suffering from depression will have experienced an onset at follow-up 1 year later (Prince *et al.* 1998). However, much may have occurred in the intervening year. Few population-based studies have assessed the natural course of the disorder in the community with frequent repeated assessments. In a small, Dutch community-based sample (Beekman *et al.* 1995), older participants were assessed using a postal questionnaire on five occasions over 1 year. Some 48% of the older population met CES-D (Center for Epidemiological Studies of Depression) criteria for 'depression of clinical significance' at one time or another over the course of the year. Most followed a variable, or relapsing and remitting, course. While half of all incident episodes were brief and self-limiting, 43% of prevalent cases at baseline remained depressed at each assessment throughout the subsequent year.

The cross-sectional survey

The cross-sectional survey is the basic descriptive study. All members of a population, or a representative sample of the population, are surveyed simultaneously for evidence of the disease under study (the outcome) and for exposure to potential risk factors.

Cross-sectional surveys can be used to measure the point prevalence of a disorder within a population. This may be useful for:

- planning services—identifying need, both met and unmet;
- drawing public and political attention to the extent of a problem within a community;
- making comparisons with other populations or regions (in a series of comparable surveys conducted in different populations);
- charting trends over time (in a series of comparable surveys of the same population).

They can also be used to compare the characteristics of those in the population with and without the disorder, thus:

- identifying cross-sectional associations with potential risk factors for the disorder; and
- identifying suitable (representative) cases and controls for population-based, case-control studies.

Findings from population-based, cross-sectional surveys can be generalized to the base population for that survey, and, to some extent, to other populations with similar characteristics. The main drawback of cross-sectional surveys for analytical as opposed to descriptive epidemiology, is that they can only give clues about aetiology. Because exposure (potential risk factor) and outcome (disease or health condition) are measured simultaneously one can never be sure, in the presence of an association, which led to which. The technical term is 'direction of causality'.

Cross-sectional surveys are generally inefficient designs for the study of rare disorders, such as, for example, late-onset schizophrenia. All participants in the survey need to be screened for the presence of the disorder. However, with a population prevalence of less than 1%, non-cases of late-onset schizophrenia will outnumber cases by more than 100 to 1. If all the true cases are to be identified, many false-positives will also have to be processed. Cases will be over-represented in inpatient facilities, in residential, and nursing-home settings. These populations may be difficult to access by standard community-survey techniques. In the community sufferers often live alone and may be unlikely to open their doors or consent to interview. Unless special attempts are made to sample these subpopulations there is a clear risk that an unrepresentative sample of cases would be identified, leading to bias.

Cross-sectional surveys survey a defined base population. This could be, for instance:

- all inpatients in a hospital;
- all hospital inpatients in a given country;
- all residents of a city borough aged 65 and over;
- all residents of a country (aged 18–60).

First, it is necessary to identify a sampling frame of all eligible persons. Criteria for eligibility need to be thought through carefully, but usually include a place of residence criterion and a period criterion; thus all residents of a defined area, resident on a particular day or month. Participants may (rarely) need to be excluded from the survey because of health or other circumstances that render their participation difficult or impossible. These exclusion criteria should ideally be specified in advance. Every effort should be made to be as inclusive as possible, to maximize the potential for generalization of the survey findings. Sampling frames for population-based surveys require an accurate register of all eligible participants in the base population. In most countries, such registers are drawn up and updated regularly for general population censuses, for taxation, and other administrative purposes, and for establishing voting entitlement in local and national elections. However, there are problems associated with using such registers. Some may not contain all the information (e.g. age, sex, and address) that is needed to identify and contact a sample of older adults. Many governments will either not allow researchers to have access to these registers, or will set limits on the information that can be gleaned from them, or will limit the way in which the data are used. Also many administrative registers are surprisingly inaccurate. This is particularly the case for older people who may have moved address without informing the relevant agency, or have moved or died in the interval between regular updates of the register. Because of these deficiencies, some population-based surveys draw up their own register by carrying out a 'door-knock' census of the area to be surveyed. While this is practical for a small catchment-area survey, a survey of a larger base population, such as the population of a whole country, would need a different strategy. Investigators often draw a random sample of households, which are then visited by researchers who interview either all eligible residents or individuals selected at random from among the eligible residents in the household.

Descriptive studies of disease frequency can be used to generate hypotheses about disease aetiology, particularly where the prevalence and incidence of a disease varies by geographical region (geographical variation) or over time (secular variation).

Geographical variation

The EURODEP consortium estimated the prevalence of late-life depression in a series of European population-based studies of those aged 65 years and over (Copeland *et al.* 1999*a*). They

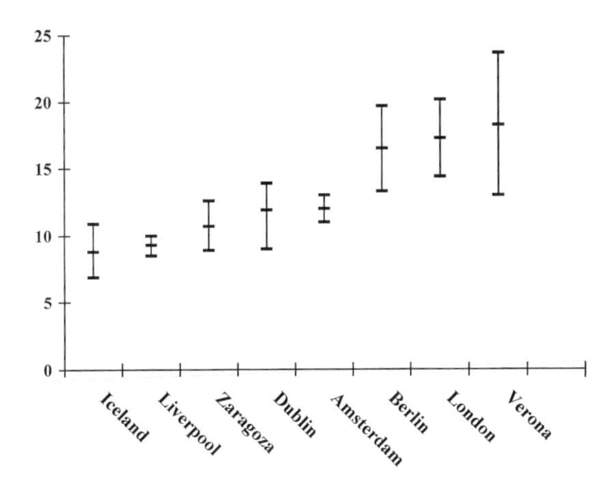

Fig. 4.4 The EURODEP consortium—the prevalence (%) of late-life depression in Europe. (Taken from Copeland *et al.* with permission.)

reported considerable (over twofold) variation in the prevalence of the disorder (see Fig. 4.4). The studies had all used the same semistructured clinical assessment interview, the Geriatric Mental State, and had used similar sampling strategies. Regional clusters of low or high prevalence for a disorder are of great interest to epidemiologists, as they may give important clues about its aetiology. The relationship between sun exposure and melanoma was established in this way, it was found that the prevalence of the disease in light-skinned persons increased as one approached the equator. The high prevalence of motor neurone type diseases in Guam, and the rarity of multiple sclerosis in Southern Africa are other examples of regional differences that have led to theories about the aetiology of those diseases. In the EURODEP consortium study, there was no clear pattern discernible to explain the origins of the differences in the prevalence of depression, and this remains an important area for further study. Identification of large differences in social or environmental characteristics of the low-and high-prevalence populations could lead to further hypothesis-driven research, or to attempts at community-level intervention.

The consensus until recently has been that there are no important regional differences in the frequency of dementia or Alzheimer's disease (AD). Jorm (1987) reviewed 47 studies of the prevalence of dementia published between 1945 and 1985. Much of the variability in prevalence between studies was explained by the different methods used by the investigators, involving principally sampling, inclusion, and exclusion criteria, research instruments, and diagnostic criteria. Corrada (1995) reviewed AD prevalence surveys published between 1984 and 1993, with a very similar pattern of findings. Since then the research methods for these investigations have been increasingly refined and standardized. The EURODEM consortium found that among European studies using similar methodologies and diagnostic criteria, there were only trivial differences in the age-specific prevalence of dementia (12 studies) (Hofman *et al.* 1991) and AD (six centres) (Rocca *et al.* 1991), concluding that 'ecological comparisons were unlikely to be informative about aetiology'. However, the large majority of these studies have been carried out in urban, developed-country settings. Other evidence suggests that AD may be less common in rural than urban areas, and in developing compared with developed regions

A recent review of population-based dementia prevalence studies in the developing world (10/66 Dementia Research Group 2000) identified a large variation in the age-adjusted prevalence of dementia, from 1.3% to 5.3% for all those aged 60 or over and from 1.7% to 5.2% for all those aged 65 and over. This may represent genuine differences in dementia prevalence, or may simply be an artefact of the methodological differences between the studies. Two of the developing-country studies (Chandra *et al.* 1998; Hendrie *et al.* 1995a) reported a strikingly low prevalence of dementia (Figs 4.5(a), (b)). These are also the two developing country studies with the most rigorously developed culture- and education-fair dementia diagnostic procedures, which had furthermore been harmonized for use in US–Nigeria and US–India transnational studies. The Nigerian study supported earlier observations on the rarity of AD in Ibadan, and on the absence of amyloid plaques and neurofibrillary tangles in an unselected brain autopsy series (Osuntokun *et al.* 1992). Quite apart from these two studies, there

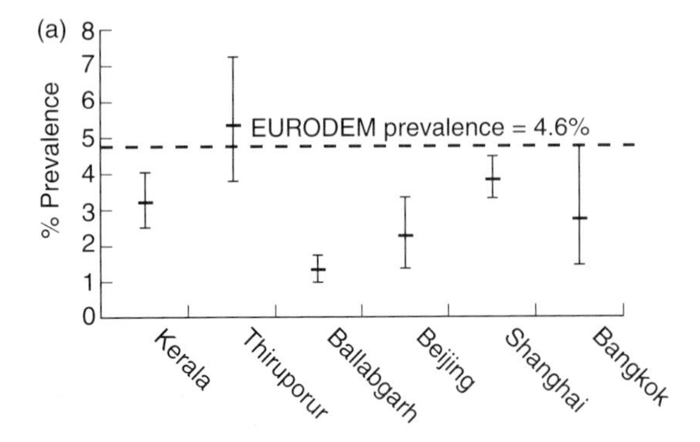

Fig. 4.5(a) The prevalence (95% confidence intervals) of dementia (for those aged 60 and over) in six developing-country studies. Prevalence adjusted for age and sex (Ballabgarh and Beijing) or for age (Thiruporur, Ibadan, Shanghai, Bangkok, and EURODEM), using the Kerala population as standard.

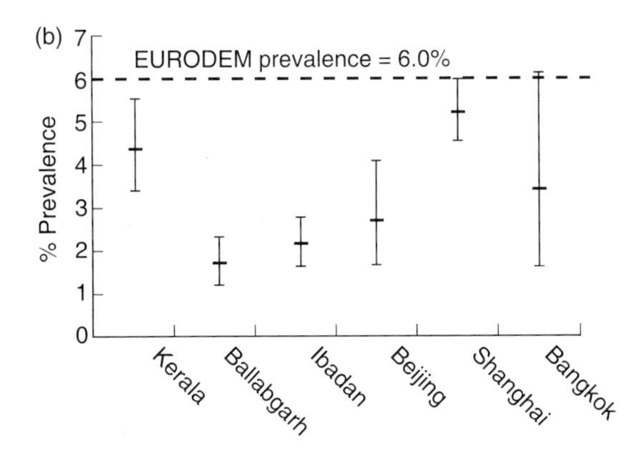

Fig. 4.5(b) The prevalence (95% confidence intervals) of dementia (for those aged 65 and over) in six developing-country studies. Prevalence adjusted for age and sex (Ballabgarh and Beijing) or for age (Thiruporur, Ibadan, Shanghai, Bangkok, and EURODEM), using the Kerala population as standard.

seems to be a general trend for the dementia prevalence estimates from the developing world, age-adjusted, to be lower than those for EURODEM.

However, it is important to understand that even striking differences in disease frequency between studies and populations may have mundane explanations:

1. Diagnostic procedures for psychiatric disorders that have been standardized in one setting may not be applied indiscriminately to another. They may turn out to be culturally biased, giving a misleadingly high or low estimate of the prevalence of the disease.
2. Other methodological differences between studies, for example in sampling procedures and in inclusion and exclusion criteria, may have important effects on prevalence estimates.
3. Low prevalence may be accounted for either by selective out-migration of susceptible persons, or by in-migration of those unlikely to develop the disorder, and vice versa for high prevalence.
4. As prevalence is the product of incidence and duration, low prevalence rates may indicate a high recovery rate or a low survival rate for those with the disorder, rather than a true difference in incidence. One obvious explanation for the low prevalence of dementia and AD seen in Nigeria and in India is that it is simply reflects a particularly high mortality rate among people with dementia in developing countries. Thus the incidence rate for dementia may be similar between the two settings, but survival with the disease may be longer in developed countries thus allowing cases to accumulate, and resulting in higher point prevalence estimates. Several factors may be implicated. Intercurrent illnesses are probably less likely to be treated. Diagnoses of dementia are unlikely to be forthcoming, as is access to the full range of specialist dementia services available in most developed countries, including formal support for caregivers, and provision for residential and nursing-home care. Thus, only longitudinal studies, with their capacity for disaggregating the frequency of new cases and their duration, will suffice to understand and explore geographical variation in dementia.

Temporal (secular) variation

Secular trends (changes over time in disease frequency) may help to generate or support aetiological hypotheses. Doll's and Hill's studies into the association between smoking and lung cancer were preceded by the observation that by the mid-twentieth century the United Kingdom faced a rapidly growing epidemic of the disease among males. This was temporally related, with a time lag for the cancer to develop, to the rise in cigarette smoking during and after World War I. In the field of mental health, it is rare for data on disease frequency to have been collected and collated in a reliable way over long periods, such as to allow valid secular comparisons to be made. One example is that of schizophrenia, where, it has been suggested, falling first-admission rates may reflect an underlying progressive fall in disease incidence (Der *et al.* 1990)

The USA Epidemiological Catchment Area (ECA) survey (Weissman *et al.* 1988) reported a decline in the prevalence of major depression with increasing age, not only for prevalence over the past year, but also for lifetime diagnoses (see Table 4.2).

These data could be interpreted as providing evidence of a cohort effect. Those born later in the twentieth century might be more prone to major depression (perhaps as a consequence of having had more adverse early life experiences). However, these cross-sectional findings need not even imply that the frequency of depression is increasing over time. Alternative explanations include a selective tendency for older people not to recall earlier undiagnosed yet significant episodes of depression (Giuffra and Risch. 1994), and a selective mortality of those most vulnerable to repeated severe episodes of depression (Ernst and Angst 1995; van Ojen *et al.* 1995). A broad review of this area reported similar findings for most psychiatric diagnoses, including schizophrenia, and concluded that cohort trends cannot be safely extrapolated from cross-sectional data (Simon and Von Korff. 1992).

Table 4.2 Lifetime prevalence (%) of major depression by age and gender: United States epidemiological catchment area (ECA) survey[a]

Age band (years)	Men	Women
18–29	6.4	10.6
30–44	6.6	15.3
45–64	3.6	9.3
65+	1.6	3.3

[a]Taken from Weissman *et al.* (1986) with permission.

Two epidemiological programmes have continued to survey the residents of the same area over long periods, and are therefore in the unusual position of being able to comment on the trends in the prevalence of dementia over time. The Lundby study in Sweden (Rorsman *et al.* 1986) reported no significant change in the prevalence or incidence of either multi-infarct dementia or what was described at the time as 'senile dementia' over the period from 1947 to 1972. In Rochester in the US (Beard *et al.* 1991), the meticulously maintained health care register suggested no change in the prevalence of either AD or dementia between 1975 and 1980. However, despite the recent stability of prevalence rates we cannot exclude the possibility that dementia is a more common disease nowadays than say 100 or even 50 years ago, at a time when developed countries were still developing. Accounts of typical cases of AD are to be found in historical sources, centuries before Alois Alzheimer's description of early-onset cases. However, up to the last 20–30 years, we lack any kind of hard data on prevalence that would allow valid comparison with modern studies. The recent findings of a substantial prospective association between both established vascular disease and its risk factors and the risk for AD and dementia, suggest that, in so far as vascular disease is preventable, incidence rates for dementia and AD may also fall. Changes in vascular risk exposures, particularly the reduction in smoking together with improvements in the treatment of hypertension and established vascular disease, have led to a reduction in cardiovascular and cerebrovascular morbidity and mortality in many developed-world populations. It will be both interesting and important in the future to monitor whether these changes have a discernible effect on the age-specific incidence of dementia and AD. Recent standardization of research methods and the establishment of precise baseline estimates in large population-based samples will assist such future secular comparisons. Any reductions in age-specific incidence rates are likely still to be accompanied by an increase in the absolute numbers of those with dementia, because of the continuing ageing of the population in developed- and, particularly, developing-country populations.

Analytical studies

Analytical studies differ from descriptive studies in that they are designed to address one or more specific hypotheses regarding the aetiology of a health condition. The basic strategy involves a comparison of the distribution of disease between groups or between populations, looking for associations between hypothesized risk factors and health experiences. There are two common types of study: the case-control and cohort study.

Case-control studies

Case-control studies are relatively quick and cheap to perform, and are useful for the initial investigation of the aetiology of rare conditions. As such, they would be particularly appropriate for the study of a condition such as late-onset schizophrenia. Surprisingly, there are few examples in the literature, and these are in effect clinical case series with small and potentially biased control comparison groups (Prager and Jeste 1993; Phillips *et al.* 1997; Brodaty *et al.* 1999). In the field of old age psychiatry the case-control study has been used primarily for studying the aetiology of dementia.

Case-control studies aim to recruit, from a notional base population, a random sample of all persons with the disease under study (cases) and a random sample of persons without the disease (controls). The odds of being exposed for cases is compared with the odds of being exposed for controls. The resulting measure of effect, an odds ratio (OR; Table 4.3), will approximate to the relative risk (RR) if the disease is rare. The OR begins to depart significantly from the RR when the prevalence of the disease in the population reaches 10%.

Table 4.3 Case-control studies

	Cases	Controls
Exposure	*a*	*b*
Not exposed	*c*	*d*

Odds of being exposed if a case = a/c
Odds of being exposed if a control = b/d
Odds ratio = $(a/c)/(b/d) = ad/bc$

Bias can be a particular problem in case-control studies unless great care is taken with the study design. The selection of subjects is crucial. The chances of being selected as a case or as a control must not depend on exposure, as this would lead to *selection bias*. An example of this problem occurred in an Australian case-control study reporting on the association between arthritis and AD (Broe *et al.* 1990). Cases were referred from primary care to a secondary-care dementia service. Controls were selected from among *attenders* at the same primary-care practice. Of course, the controls would have required a reason to attend the practice, and arthritis is a common pathology in older people. Hence, the selection procedures would have been likely to produce a spurious, biased, inverse association between arthritis and risk of AD. The authors themselves highlighted this difficulty.

In case-control studies, since people have already developed the disease, any enquiry into exposure to risk factors is generally retrospective. The methods used to ascertain exposure must be applied symmetrically to both cases and controls to reduce *information bias* (observer bias or recall bias). It has been suggested that recall bias might have accounted for the often reported association between head injury with loss of consciousness and AD (Mortimer *et al.* 1991). Histories are taken from informants for both case and control subjects. However, the informant for the case subject may be more likely to recall and report the head injury that occurred many years before than the informant for the control, because they had been seeking a plausible explanation for their relative's decline into dementia; this phenomenon is sometimes referred to as making an 'effort after meaning'. Thus, the fact that the outcome has already occurred at the time when the exposure (risk factor) is ascertained can lead to bias. This facet of the case-control design also limits the inferences to be drawn from positive findings, in that it is usually impossible to determine direction of causality for the association. Thus for an association between depression and AD, has the depression caused the AD or the AD caused the depression (Jorm *et al.* 1991)?

Given the inherent limitations of the case-control design, research into the aetiology of dementia has now largely progressed to the use of the cohort-study design. However, the efficiency of the case-control study means that examples continue to appear in the literature. There is a particular vogue for a variant of the case-control study, the 'nested case-control study'. In this design, recently incident cases recruited from an ongoing cohort study are compared with suitable controls from the same cohort, for exposures that would be prohibitively expensive or impractical to have measured on all participants at the outset of the study. Thus Bots *et al.* (1998) has reported an association between the thrombin–antithrombin complex (TAT) and dementia, having compared 277 cases and 298 controls recruited from within the larger Rotterdam longitudinal survey, suggesting that increased thrombin generation may have a role to play in the aetiology of dementia. Future case-control studies may also have a role in the elucidation of gene–environment interactions. The detection of such interactions requires very large numbers of cases, the logistics of which might be managed more effectively in a case-control design.

Cohort studies

Cohort studies compare the incidence of new cases of the disease under study in groups of persons free of the disease at the outset, but who are (1) exposed and (2) not exposed to a hypothesized risk factor. The ratio of the incidence risk between the two groups gives a RR, which is the measure of effect for a cohort study (Table 4.4).

Table 4.4 Cohort studies

	Cases	Non-cases	Total
Exposed	a	b	$a + b$
Not exposed	c	d	$c + d$

Incidence risk in exposed = $a/(a + b)$
Incidence in non-exposed = $c/(c + d)$

Risk ratio = $[a/(a + b)]/[c/(c + d)]$

Cohort studies have two principal advantages over case-control studies. First, the longitudinal perspective allows the direction of causality to be established. Since the exposed and unexposed cohorts are both free of the disease at the outset of the study, an increased risk of disease onset among those exposed implies that the exposure has led to the disease rather than vice versa. Second, information bias is limited, for at the time when the exposure is ascertained neither the participant nor the investigator should be influenced by the disease outcome, which has not yet occurred. However, cohort studies can be lengthy and costly, as the sample size needs to be large enough, and the period of follow-up long enough to accumulate sufficient numbers of incident cases of the disease to make a statistically meaningful comparison between the two groups. For these reasons they are not the first choice of study design for rare conditions.

The defining characteristics, the advantages and disadvantages of case-control and cohort studies are described and compared in Table 4.5.

Table 4.5 Case-control and cohort studies—characteristics, advantages, and disadvantages

	Case-control	Cohort
Subjects selected according to:	Caseness	Exposure
Perspective:	Retrospective	Prospective (usually)
(subjects' recall exposure)	(observers attend outcome)	
Sources of bias:	Selection; information	Information (observer only)
(recall and observer)	Non-response	
Resources:	Quick; relatively cheap	Lengthy; relative expensive
Useful for:	Rare outcomes; single outcomes;	Rare exposures; single exposures;
multiple exposures	multiple outcomes	
Measure of effect:	Odds ratio	Relative risk

There is little doubt that the longitudinal perspective of the cohort study can clarify and sometimes change the interpretation of findings from cross-sectional or retrospective (e.g. case-control study) research. In the first instance, factors associated cross-sectionally with prevalent cases may be differentially associated with the incidence and chronicity of disease episodes. Thus in one community-based study, disablement arising from health conditions was associated with the onset of episodes of depression, but not with their duration, which was predicted rather by social support and social engagement at baseline (Prince *et al.* 1998). Second, in case-control studies, selection effects or prevalence bias can give misleading results. In aetiological research into AD, the consensus from the earlier case-control studies was that smoking appeared to be a protective factor reducing the risk for AD, and with a negative dose-response effect; the more one smoked, the lower the risk of AD (Graves *et al.* 1991). The first findings from a major cohort study suggest that the opposite may be true, that smoking increases the risk for AD, particularly in men (Ott *et al.* 1998). Factors found to be associated with case outcomes in case-control studies may be factors predicting survival with the disease, rather than the onset of the disease itself. Doubt has also now been cast upon the consistent finding from case-control studies of an association between head injury with loss of consciousness and AD (Mortimer *et al.* 1991). This has not been borne out in a large cohort study (Mehta *et al.* 1999). Recall bias may have explained the positive association from case-control studies.

Many of the obstacles associated with cohort studies can be removed where the outcome may be cheaply and conveniently ascertained in an existing cohort, in which appropriate baseline exposure measures have already been ascertained for another purpose. Thus Jones (1994) used data on child development gathered during the UK National Survey of Health and Development, based on a representative sample of all babies born in one week in 1946, and related it to the subjects' future risk of developing schizophrenia. The continuing regular surveillance of the birth cohort helped to identify those who had developed the disorder. In the UK there is no national register of schizophrenia cases, but the 1946 cohort could also be cross-linked with the Mental Health Enquiry, a central register of all admissions to psychiatric hospitals, with ICD (International classification of diseases) diagnoses on discharge. There is growing interest in the notion that mental health conditions of late life, particularly dementia, may have their antecedents in early life. Such associations across the entire lifespan can only feasibly be studied using historical cohort designs. One fascinating example of such a study is the Nuns' study (Snowdon *et al.* 1996). This study assessed verbal ability by analysing the autobiographies for density of ideas and grammatical complexity that the nuns had written as young adults. Cognitive function was assessed approximately 58 years later, and those nuns who subsequently died had a neuropathological examination. Low idea density and low grammatical complexity in young adulthood were associated with poorer cognitive functioning in old age. More surprising was the finding, among the nuns who had died and consented to postmortem, that low idea density at age 18 was strongly correlated with AD pathology.

Randomized controlled trials

Randomized controlled trials (RCTs) are often seen as the prerogative of clinical and health services researchers, rather than epidemiologists. However, epidemiologists are commonly involved in this area of research.

1. Randomized controlled trials are, in a sense, a special variant of the cohort study, in which the exposure has been allocated at random, instead of recruiting participants who happen, for whatever reasons, to be exposed or not exposed. Therefore the design is particularly attractive to epidemiologists, in that, when it can be used, it effectively eliminates the problem of confounding. Since, when randomization has been effective, all potential confounding variables should be evenly distributed between the intervention and control conditions, then any observed difference in outcome can safely be

assumed to be causally associated with the randomized variable. Thus, where the condition of equipoise is met, when there is genuine uncertainty as to the balance of risks and benefits associated with the randomized condition, the randomized controlled trial is the best design for assessing the effect of a protective factor identified in observational epidemiology.

2. These conditions apply particularly to the testing of apparent protective effects of medications identified in case-control and cohort studies. Thus, there is a body of evidence from observational epidemiology suggesting around a 40% risk reduction for Alzheimer's disease in those older people using non-steroidal, anti-inflammatory drugs (NSAIDs) (Stewart *et al.* 1997), and in postmenopausal women prescribed hormone-replacement therapy (HRT) (Tang *et al.* 1996). The consistency and strength of these protective associations argues for a causal association. However, there is a substantial and insuperable problem with all these observational studies. The dementia syndrome is known to have a long preclinical prodrome, therefore, even in cohort studies, there is the possibility that older people who are developing Alzheimer's disease may be less likely to present to doctors in such a way as would elicit a prescription. Alternatively, their general health status may be sufficiently impaired that their doctor would perceive a contraindication to the prescription of these medications. This methodological trap has been neatly termed 'confounding by indication and contraindication (Andersen *et al.* 1995). The question can only be settled in a large, well-designed, randomized controlled trial in which the prescription is allocated at random, rather than on the presentation of the patient and by the clinical decision-making of the doctor. Such randomized controlled trials are currently underway in the USA and UK to test the hypothesis that HRT reduces the risk for dementia and limits the extent of cognitive decline. Interestingly, each of these studies involves the opportunistic 'piggy-backing' of cognitive outcomes on to trials designed primarily to test other outcomes: cardiovascular disease and stroke. A randomized controlled trial of the potential preventive effects of NSAIDs has also recently been funded in the USA.

3. Certain risk exposures identified in observational studies may not be amenable to clinical intervention. Thus, it would be unethical to increase blood pressure levels in a randomized controlled trial as a definitive test of the hypothesis that hypertension is associated with an increased risk for AD or cognitive decline. However, it is possible to include AD and cognitive decline as outcomes in an RCT which is designed primarily to test the hypothesis that lowering blood pressure levels may reduce their incidence. In fact, cognitive outcomes are usually incorporated as secondary end-points in trials primarily designed to evaluate the effect of antihypertensives on cardio- and cerebrovascular disease outcomes. Two RCTs of this kind have suggested no effect of antihypertensive treatment on cognitive decline (Systolic Hypertension in the Elderly Program (SHEP) Cooperative Research Group 1991; Prince *et al.* 1996), while one RCT has suggested a protective effect for dementia (Forette *et al.* 1998). Another trial, involving older participants with a higher absolute risk of developing dementia, is currently in the field.

4. Older persons are commonly excluded from RCTs, often for no good reason. Thus, the evidence base for the efficacy and effectiveness of commonly available therapies can often not be extended to older people, in whom the balance of risks and benefits may be somewhat different. Gerson, reviewing double-blind, placebo-controlled, antidepressant drug trials, focusing on older subjects and reported between 1964 and 1986, located 25 studies, many of which were 'plagued with methodological difficulties' (Gerson *et al.* 1988). The studies were small, and in total only 746 subjects aged 60 and over were involved.

5. Most RCTs are conducted in secondary-care settings. Thus, in the case of depression, those who are recruited generally have more severe forms of the disorder, and the evidence base for non-major depression, accounting for around 90% of cases of depression of clinical significance in population-based studies, has scarcely been studied. This restriction of the evidence base is compounded when RCTs in clinical settings

address the efficacy of treatments under ideal conditions (recruiting unusually fit older people, lacking comorbidity), rather than their effectiveness under more routine clinical conditions. This process is particularly evident in the evidence base for the effectiveness of procholinergic therapies for dementia, where the exclusion criteria clearly do not reflect the profile of the patients for whom the drug may be prescribed in routine clinical practice (Table 4.6). Epidemiologists, with their focus upon the representativeness of the populations they recruit, and the consequent generalizability of findings, clearly have something to contribute to the design of trials that assess effectiveness rather than efficacy.

Genetic epidemiology studies

Association studies

Dementia epidemiologists are currently in a unique position. The discovery in 1992 of the association between the *APOE* gene and the risk for both the dementia syndrome and Alzheimer's disease (Saunders *et al.* 1993) has ushered in a new phase in epidemiological research that will undoubtedly serve as a model for research into other chronic conditions. However, as yet, despite extensive research, the *APOE* dementia association remains the only locus that has been reliably identified as having a major effect on risk for a common chronic disorder. The finding of the association with the *APOE* gene is now among the most replicated findings in biomedicine, with over 1000 positive reports in the literature. Research has now moved on to second-order considerations:

Table 4.6 Exclusion criteria for a procholinergic drug trial in patients with Alzheimer's disease

- Over 85 years of age
- Unable to walk freely with help
- Visual/hearing impairment
- Psychiatric or neurological impairment
- Past or present active disease (gastrointestinal, cardio vascular, renal, hepatic, endocrine)
- Any diabetes
- Obstructive lung disease
- Oncology, haematology onset in last 2 years
- Vitamin B_{12} or folate deficiency
- Alcohol or drug abuse
- Anticonvulsant medication
- Anticholinergic medication
- Antidepressant medication
- Antipsychotic medication
- Other drugs with CNS activity

1. The association appears to be modified by age (decreasing effect size with increasing age) and by race (lower effect sizes in Africans and Asians, compared with Caucasians (Farrer *et al.* 1997). The age effect is most likely to be explained by differential mortality; those who survive to a great age despite the APOE ε4 allele may have other genetic or constitutional characteristics that protect against neurodegeneration.

2. The apparent effect of race is more interesting. One striking finding is the apparent lack of an association in Nigeria and Kenya (Osuntokun *et al.* 1995; Kalaria *et al.* 1997), despite a higher than usual prevalence of the ε4 allele in Africa, and typically robust associations in an African–American sample (Hendrie *et al.* 1995*b*). As we have seen, the prevalence of AD in the Nigerian sample was only about a quarter of that in Europe and the USA. These findings are strongly suggestive of a gene–environment interaction, in which the *APOE* gene is not a direct risk factor for AD, but modifies the effect of one or more environmental factors that are common exposures in the developed world, but very rare exposures in sub-Saharan Africa. The USA/Nigerian researchers are currently investigating the role of vascular disease and its risk factors that are common in African–Americans and rare in Nigerians. Other researchers, employing a similar model, have suggested that widely differing levels of exposure to cholesterol (Chandra and Pandav 1998) or toxic effects on the developing brain (Prince 1998) may have been responsible both for the difference in disease frequency and the differences in level of association with *APOE*.

3. Observational epidemiology has already suggested that *APOE* may interact with a variety of environmental exposures that have the capacity to insult the brain at different stages over the life

course. Thus *APOE* seems to modify mortality after stroke (Corder *et al.* 2000), the association between atherosclerosis and both cognitive decline (Slooter 1998) and dementia (Hofman 1997), the association between white-matter lesions and dementia (Skoog 1998), and the association between head injury (Mayeux 1995) and boxing (Jordan 1997) and Alzheimer's disease. These findings suggest a mechanism for the operation of the *APOE* gene product as a neuroprotective factor influencing the growth and regeneration of peripheral and central nervous system tissues in normal development and in response to injury (Prince 1998).

Conclusion

One thing that is certain is that there is a continuing need for further epidemiological research into the mental health problems of ageing populations. Priorities will include:

(1) descriptive studies of the extent and distribution of both functional illness and dementia in the developing world—very few reliable studies have been conducted, and awareness of the extent of the problem posed by demographic ageing in these regions is very limited;
(2) comparative epidemiological studies validating and then further exploring possible differences in the prevalence and incidence of late-life mental disorders between different geographical regions and populations;
(3) monitoring age-specific incidence rates for dementia in the developed world for evidence of possible reductions in incidence in response to striking health improvements in a population (e.g. nutrition, education, and vascular health);
(4) further large-scale, population-based, cohort and case-control studies focusing on interactions between genetic and environmental risk factors. At present, the focus is upon *APOE* and dementia, but it is likely in the next few years that further genes for dementia, and also perhaps genes for functional disorders, will be identified, thus revolutionizing and energizing the study of these disorders too;
(5) pragmatic trials of the effectiveness of common therapies for dementia and late-life depression in the settings where, and among the patient groups to whom, they are typically administered.

Appendix 4.1—A resource guide to measures in common use in psychiatric epidemiology

This is a selection of the more rigorously constructed, best validated, and most widely used measures.* To some extent, the choice reflects the author's bias towards briefer measures.

Scaleable measures with validated screening properties

Measuring psychiatric disorder

GHQ General Health Questionnaire

Self-administered (5 minutes)

Goldberg, D. P., Gater, R., Sartorius, N., Ustun, T. B., *et al.* (1997). The validity of two versions of the GHQ in the WHO study of mental illness in general health care. *Psychological Medicine*, **27**, 191–7.

Goldberg, G. and Williams, P. (1988). *A user's guide to the General Health Questionnaire*. NFER-Nelson, Windsor, Berks.

CIS-R Clinical Interview Schedule—revised

Interviewer or self (computer) administered (20–30 minutes)

(**NB** not specifically validated in older persons)

Lewis, G., Pelosi, A. J., Araya, R., and Dunn, G. (1992). Measuring psychiatric disorder in the community: a standardized assessment for use by lay interviewers. *Psychological Medicine*, **22**, 465–86.

Measuring depression

CES-D Center for Epidemiological Studies—depression

Self-administered (5–10 minutes)

Radloff, L. S. (1977). The CES-D scale: a self-report depression scale for research in the general population. *Applied Psychological Measurement*, **1**, 385–401.

ZDS Zung Depression Scale
Self-administered (5–10 minutes)

Zung, W. W. K. (1965). A self-rating depression scale. *Archives of General Psychiatry*, **12**, 62–70.

GDS Geriatric Depression Scale (over 65-year-olds)
Self-administered (5–10 minutes)

Yesavage, J., Rose, T., and Lum, O. (1983). Development and validation of a Geriatric Depression Screening Scale: a preliminary report. *Journal of Psychiatric Research*, **17**, 43–9.

Measuring cognitive function (and screening for dementia)

MMSE Mini-Mental State Examination
Interviewer administered (10–15 minutes)

Folstein, M. F., Folstein, S. E., and McHugh, P. R. (1975). 'Mini-mental State': a practical method for grading the cognitive state of patients for clinicians. *Journal of Psychiatric Research*, **12**, 189–98.

TICS-m Telephone Interview for Cognitive Status
Interviewer administered (over the telephone—10–15 minutes)

Brandt, J., Spencer, M., and Folstein, M. (1988). The Telephone Interview for Cognitive Status. *Neuropsychiatry, Neuropsychology and Behavioral Neurology*, **1**, 111–17.

CSI-D Cognitive Screening Instrument for Dementia
Interviewer administered to subject (5–10 minutes) and informant (10 minutes)

Hall, K. S., Hendrie, H. H., Brittain, H. M., Norton, J. A., *et al.* (1993). The development of a dementia screening interview in two distinct languages. *International Journal of Methods in Psychiatric Research*, **3**, 1–28.

IQ-CODE The Informant Questionnaire of Cognitive Decline in the Elderly
Interviewer administered to informant (10 minutes)

Jorm, A. F. (1994). A short form of the Informant Questionnaire on Cognitive Decline in the Elderly (IQCODE): development and cross-validation. *Psychological Medicine*, **24**, 145–53.

Instruments generating diagnoses according to established algorithms

Assessing a comprehensive range of clinical diagnoses

CIDI Composite International Diagnostic Interview
Interviewer administered (2 hours in its full form, although shorter versions, CIDI-PC and UM-CIDID, have also been developed)

(**NB** not specifically validated in older persons)

WHO (1990). *Composite International Diagnostic Interview (CID, version I)*. WHO, Geneva.

Wittchen, H. U. (1994). Reliability and validity studies of the WHO-Composite International Diagnostic Interview (CIDI): a critical review. *Journal of Psychiatric Research*, **28**, 57–84.

SCAN and PSE Schedules for Assessment of Negative Symptoms; Present State Examination
Clinician administered (1_–2 hours)

Wing, J. (1983). Use and misuse of the PSE. *British Journal of Psychiatry*, **143**, 117–17.

Wing, J. (1996). SCAN and the PSE tradition. *Social Psychiatry and Psychiatric epidemiology*, **31**, 50–4.

GMS Geriatric Mental State (over-65s)
Interviewer administered (25–40 minutes)

Copeland, J. R. M., Dewey, M. E., and Griffith-Jones, H. M. (1986). A computerised psychiatric diagnostic system and case nomenclature for the elderly subjects: GMS and AGECAT. *Psychological Medicine*, **16**, 89–99.

CAMDEX Cambridge Examination for Mental Disorders in the Elderly (over-65s)
Interviewer administered to subject and informant (1 hour)

Roth, M., Tym, E., Mountjoy, C. Q., Huppert, F. A., *et al.* (1986). CAMDEX. A standardised instrument for the diagnosis of mental disorder in the elderly with special reference to the early detection of dementia. *British Journal of Psychiatry*, **149**, 698–709.

Assessing personality disorder

SAP Standardized Assessment of Personality
Interviewer administered to informant (20–30 minutes)

Pilgrim, J. A. and Mann, A. H. (1990). Use of the ICD-10 version of the Standardized Assessment of

Personality to determine the prevalence of personality disorder in psychiatric in-patients. *Psychological Medicine*, **20**, 985–92.
Pilgrim, J. A., Mellers, J. D., Boothby, H. A. and Mann, A. H. (1993). Inter-rater and temporal reliability of the Standardized Assessment of Personality and the influence of informant characteristics. *Psychological Medicine*, **23**, 779–86.

Measures of other variables, relevant to mental disorder

Measuring stable traits

EPQ Eysenck Personality Questionnaire (neuroticism/extroversion/introversion)

Self or interviewer administered (5–10 minutes)

Eysenck, H. J. (1959). The differentiation between normal and various necrotic groups on the Maudsley Personality Inventory. *British Journal of Psychology*, **50**, 176–7.

Measuring life events

LTE The List of Threatening Events

Self or interviewer administered (5–10 minutes)

Brugha, T. S., Bebbington, P., Tennant, C., and Hurry, J. (1985). The list of threatening experiences: a subset of 12 life events categories with considerable long-term contextual threat. *Psychological Medicine*, **15**, 189–94.

Measuring social support

SPQ The Social Problems Questionnaire

Self or interviewer administered (5–10 minutes)

Corney, R. H. and Clare, A. W. (1985). The construction, development and testing of a self-report questionnaire to identify social problems. *Psychological Medicine*, **15**, 637–49.

CPQ The Close Persons Questionnaire

Interviewer administered (10–20 minutes)

Stansfeld, S. and Marmot, M. (1992). Deriving a survey measure of social support: the reliability and validity of the Close Persons Questionnaire. *Social Science and Medicine*, **35**, 1027–35.

Describing social network

Social Network Assessment Instrument

Self or interviewer administered (5–10 minutes)

Wenger, G. C. (1989). Support networks in old age: constructing a typology. In *Growing old in the twentieth century* (ed. M. Jeffreys), Routledge, London.

Quality of life

WHOQOL BREF World Health Organization Quality of Life

Self-report or interviewer administered (10–15 minutes)

WHO (1997). Measuring quality of life. The World Health Organization Quality of Life Instruments (The WHOQOL—100 and the WHOQOL-BREF). WHO/MNH/PSF/97.4. WHO, Geneva. (e-mail: whoqol@who.ch)

Global health/disablement

LHS The London Handicap Scale

Self or interviewer administered (5–10 minutes)

Harwood, R. H., Gompertz, P., and Ebrahim, S. (1994). Handicap one year after a stroke: validity of a new scale. *Journal of Neurology, Neurosurgery and Psychiatry*, **57**, 825–9.

SF-12 Short Form-12 (reduced version of MOS SF-36)

Self or interviewer administered (5–10 minutes)

Jenkinson, S. and Layte, R. (1998). Development and testing of the UK SF-12. *Journal of the Health Services Research Policy*, **2**, 14–18.

*A fuller account of validated health measures, with particular reference to older subjects, is contained in:

Prince, M. J., Harwood, R., Thomas, A., and Mann, A. H. (1997). Gospel Oak V. Impairment, disability and handicap as risk factors for depression in old age. *Psychological Medicine*, **27**, 311–21.

References

10/66 Dementia Research Group. (2000). Dementia in developing countries. A consensus statement from the 10/66 Dementia Research Group. *International Journal of Geriatric Psychiatry*, **15**, 14–20
American Psychiatric Association. (1994) *Diagnostic and statistical manual of mental disorders* (4th edn). AMA, Washington, DC.
Andersen, K., Launer, L. J., Ott, A., Hoes, A. W., Breteler, M. M., and Hofman, A. (1995). Do nonsteroidal anti-inflammatory drugs decrease the risk for Alzheimer's disease? The Rotterdam study. *Neurology*, **45**, 1441–5.
Beard, C. M., Kokmen, E., Offord, K., and Kurland, L. T. (1991). Is the prevalence of dementia changing? *Neurology*, **41**, 1911–14.
Beekman, A. T. F., Deeg, D. J. H., Smit, J. H., and Van Tilburg, W. (1995). Predicting the course of depression in the older

population: results from a community-based study in the Netherlands. *Journal of Affective Disorders*, **34**, 41–9.

Beekman, A. T. F., Copeland, J. R. M., and Prince, M. J. (1999). Review of community prevalence of depression in later life. *British Journal of Psychiatry*, **174**, 307–11.

Bots, M. L., Breteler, M. M., van Kooten, F., Haverkate, F., Meijer, P., Koudstaal, P. J., *et al.* (1998). Coagulation and fibrinolysis markers and risk of dementia. The Dutch Vascular Factors in Dementia Study. *Haemostasis*, **28**(3–4), 216–22.

Brodaty, H., Sachdev, P., Rose, N., Rylands, K., and Prenter, L. (1999). Schizophrenia with onset after age 50 years. I: Phenomenology and risk factors. *British Journal of Psychiatry*, **175**, 410–15.

Broe, G. A., Henderson, A. S., Creasey, H., *et al.* (1990). A case-control study of Alzheimer's disease in Australia. *Neurology*, **40**, 1698–707.

Chandra, V. and Pandav, R. (1998). Gene–environment interaction in Alzheimer's disease: a potential role for cholesterol. *Neuroepidemiology*, **17**, 225–32.

Chandra, V., Ganguli, M., Pandav, R., Johnston, J., Belle, S., and DeKosky, S. T. (1998). Prevalence of Alzheimer's disease and other dementias in rural India. The Indo–US study. *Neurology*, **51**, 1000–8.

Copeland, J. R. M., Hooijer, C., Jordan, A., Lawlor, B., Lobo, A., Magnusson, H., *et al.* (1999). Depression in Europe: geographical distribution among older people. *British Journal of Psychiatry*, **174**, 312–21.

Corder, E. H., Basun, H., Fratiglioni, L., Guo, Z., Lannfelt, L., Viitanen, M., *et al.* (2000). Inherited frailty. ApoE alleles determine survival after a diagnosis of heart disease or stroke at ages 85+. *Annals of the New York Academy of Sciences*, **908**, 295–8.

Corrada, M., Brookmeyer, R., and Kawas, C. (1995). Sources of variability in prevalence rates of Alzheimer's disease. *International Journal of Epidemiology*, **24**, 1000–5.

Der, G., Gupta, S., and Murray, R. M. (1990). Is schizophrenia disappearing? *Lancet*, **335**, 513–16.

Ernst, C. and Angst, J. (1995). Depression in old age. Is there a real decrease in prevalence? A review. *European Archives of Psychiatry and Clinical Neuroscience*, **245**, 272–87.

Farrer, L. A., Cupples, L. A., Haines, J. L., *et al.* (1997). Effects of age, sex, and ethnicity on the association between apolipoprotein E genotype and Alzheimer disease. A meta-analysis. APOE and Alzheimer Disease Meta Analysis Consortium. *Journal of the American Medical Association*, **278**, 1349–56.

Forette, F., Seux, M. L., Staessen, J. A., Thijs, L., Birkenhager, W. H., Babarskiene, M. R., *et al.* (1998). Prevention of dementia in randomised double-blind placebo-controlled Systolic Hypertension in Europe (Syst-Eur) trial *Lancet*, **352**, 1347–51.

Gersson, S., Plotkin, D., and Jarvik, L. (1998). Antidepressant drug studies, 1964–1986: empirical evidence for ageing patients. *Clinical Psychopharmacology*, **8**, 311–22.

Giuffra, L. A. and Risch, N. (1994). Diminished recall and the cohort effect of major depression: a simulation study. *Psychological Medicine*, **24**, 375–83.

Graves, A. B., van Duijn, C. M., Chandra, V., *et al.* (1991). Alcohol and tobacco consumption as risk factors for Alzheimer's disease: a collaborative re-analysis of case-control studies. EURODEM Risk Factors Research Group. *International Journal of Epidemiology*, **20** (Suppl. 2), S48–S57.

Hendrie, H. C., Osuntokun, B. O., Hall, K. S., *et al.* (1995*a*). Prevalence of Alzheimer's disease and dementia in two communities: Nigerian Africans and African Americans. *American Journal of Psychiatry*, **152**, 1485–92.

Hendrie, H. C., Hall, K. S., Hui, S., Unverzagt, F. W., Yu, C. E., Lahiri, D. K., *et al.* (1995*b*). Apolipoprotein E genotypes and Alzheimer's disease in a community study of elderly African Americans. *Annals of Neurology*, **37**, 118–20.

Hofman, A., Rocca, W. A., Brayne, C., *et al.* (1991). The prevalence of dementia in Europe: a collaborative study of 1980–1990 findings. Eurodem Prevalence Research Group. *International Journal of Epidemiology*, **20**, 736–48.

Hofman, A., Ott, A., Breteler, M. M. B., *et al.* (1997). Atherosclerosis, apolipoprotein E, and prevalence of dementia and Alzheimer's disease in the Rotterdam Study. *Lancet*, **349**, 151–4.

Jones, P., Rodgers, B., Murray, R. and Marmot, M. (1994). Child development risk factors for adult schizophrenia in the British 1946 birth cohort. *Lancet*, **344**, 1398–402.

Jordan, B. D., Relkin, N. R., Ravdin, L. D., Jacobs, A. R., Bennett, A., and Gandy, S. (1997). Apolipoprotein E epsilon4 associated with chronic traumatic brain injury in boxing. *Journal of the American Medical Association*, **278**, 136–40.

Jorm, A. F., Korten, A. E., and Henderson, A. S. (1987). The prevalence of dementia: a quantitative integration of the literature. *Acta Psychiatrica Scandinavica*, **76**, 465–79.

Jorm, A. F., van Duijn, C. M., Chandra, V., *et al.* (1991). Psychiatric history and related exposures as risk factors for Alzheimer's disease: a collaborative re-analysis of case-control studies. EURODEM Risk Factors Research Group. *International Journal of Epidemiology*, **20** (Suppl. 2), S43–7.

Kalaria, R. N., Ogeng'o, J. A., Patel, N. B., *et al.* (1997). Evaluation of risk factors for Alzheimer's disease in elderly east Africans. *Brain Research Bulletin*, **44**, 573–7.

Last, J. M. (2001). *A Dictionary of Epidemiology*, 4th edition. Oxford University Press, Oxford.

Mayeux, R., Ottman, R., Maestre, G., Ngai, C., Tang, M.-X., Ginsberg, H., *et al.* (1995). Synergistic effects of traumatic head injury and apolipoprotein-*ge4 in patients with Alzheimer's disease. *Neurology*, **45**, 555–7.

Mehta, K. M., Ott, A., Kalmijn, S., Slooter, A. J., van Duijn, C. M., Hofman, A., *et al.* (1999). Head trauma and risk of dementia and Alzheimer's disease: The Rotterdam Study. *Neurology*, **53**, 1959–62.

Mortimer, J. A., van Duijn, C. M., Chandra, V., *et al.* (1991). Head trauma as a risk factor for Alzheimer's disease: a collaborative re-analysis of case-control studies. EURODEM Risk Factors Research Group. *International Journal of Epidemiology*, **20** (Suppl. 2), S28–35.

OPCS (Office of Population Censuses and Surveys) (1991). *National population projections: mid 1989 based.* OPCS Monitor PP 2 91.1. HMSO, London.

Osuntokun, B. O., Ogunniyi, A. O., and Lekwauwa, U. G. (1992). Alzheimer's disease in Nigeria. *African Journal of Medicine and Medical Science*, **21**, 71–7.

Osuntokun, B. O., Sahota, A., Ogunniyi, A. O., Gureje, O., Baiyewu, O., Adeyinka, A., *et al.* (1995). Lack of an association between apolipoprotein E epsilon 4 and Alzheimer's disease in elderly Nigerians. *Annals of Neurology*, **38**, 463–5.

Ott, A., Slooter, A. J. C., Hofman, A., *et al.* (1998). Smoking and risk of dementia and Alzheimer's disease in a population-based cohort study: the Rotterdam Study. *Lancet*, **351**, 1841–3.

Phillips, M. L., Howard, R., and David, A. S. (1997). A cognitive neuropsychological approach to the study of delusions in late-onset schizophrenia. *International Journal of Geriatric Psychiatry*, **12**, 892–901.

Prager, S. and Jeste, D. V. (1993). Sensory impairment in late-life schizophrenia. *Schizophrenia Bulletin*, **19**, 755–72.

Prince, M. (1998). Is chronic low-level lead exposure in early life an aetiological factor in Alzheimer's disease? *Epidemiology*, **9**, 618–21.

Prince, M. J., Bird, A. S., Blizard, R. A., and Mann, A. H. (1996). Is the cognitive function of older patients affected by antihypertensive treatment? Results from 54 months of the Medical Research Council's treatment trial of hypertension in older adults. *British Medical Journal*, **312**, 801–5.

Prince, M. J., Harwood, R., Thomas, A., and Mann, A. H. (1998). A prospective population-based cohort study of the effects of disablement and social milieu on the onset and maintenance of late-life depression. Gospel Oak VII. *Psychological Medicine*, **28**, 337–50.

Rocca, W. A., Hofman, A., Brayne, C., *et al.* (1991). Frequency and distribution of Alzheimer's disease in Europe: a collaborative study of 1980–1990 prevalence findings. The EURODEM-Prevalence Research Group. *Annals of Neurology*, **30**, 381–90.

Rorsman, B., Hagnell, O., and Lanke, J. (1986). Prevalence and incidence of senile and multi-infarct dementia in the Lundby Study: a comparison between the time periods 1947–1957 and 1957–1972. *Neuropsychobiology*, **15**, 122–9.

Saunders, A. M., Strittmatter, W. J., Schmechel, D., St.George-Hyslop, P. H., Pericak-Vance, M. A., Joo, S. H., *et al.* (1993). Association of apolipoprotein E allele e4 with late-onset familial and sporadic Alzheimer's disease. *Neurology*, **43**, 1467–72.

SHEP Cooperative Research Group. (1991). Prevention of stroke by antihypertensive drug treatment in older persons with isolated systolic hypertension. Final results of the systolic hypertension in the elderly program (SHEP). *Journal of the American Medical Association*, **265**, 3255–64.

Simon, G. E. and Von Korff, M. (1992). Reevaluation of secular trends in depression rates. *American Journal of Epidemiology*, **135**, 1411–22.

Skoog, I., Hesse, C., Aevarsson, O., Landahl, S., Wahlstrom, J., Fredman, P., *et al.* (1998). A population study of apoE genotype at the age of 85: relation to dementia, cerebrovascular disease, and mortality. *Journal of Neurology, Neurosurgery and Psychiatry*, **64**, 37–43.

Slooter, A. J., van Duijn, C. M., Bots, M. L., Ott, A., Breteler, M. B., De Voecht, J., *et al.* (1998). Apolipoprotein E genotype, atherosclerosis, and cognitive decline: the Rotterdam Study. *Journal of Neural Transmission. Supplementum*, **53**, 17–29.

Snowdon, D. A., Kemper, S. J., Mortimer, J. A. *et al.* (1996). Linguistic ability in early life and cognitive function and Alzheimer's disease in late life. *Journal of the American Medical Association*, **275**, 528–32.

Stewart, W. F., Kawas, C., Corrada, M., and Metter, E. J. (1997). Risk of Alzheimer's disease and duration of NSAID use. *Neurology*, **48**, 626–32.

Tang, M. X., Jacobs, D., Stern, Y., *et al.* (1996). Effect of oestrogen during menopause on risk and age at onset of Alzheimer's disease. *Lancet*, **348**, 429–32.

Van Ojen, R., Hooijer, C., Jonker, C., Lindeboom, J., *et al.* (1995). Late-life depressive disorder in the community: early onset and the decrease of vulnerability with increasing age. *Journal of Affective Disorders*, **33**, 159–66.

Warnes, A. M. (1989). Elderly people in Great Britain: variable projections and characteristics. *Care of the Elderly*, **1**, 7–10.

Weissman, M. M., Leaf, P. J., Tischler, G. L., Blazer, D. G., *et al.* (1988). Affective disorders in five United States communities. *Psychological Medicine*, **18**, 141–53.

5 Neuropathology

Margaret Esiri and Zsuzsanna Nagy

Introduction

This chapter commences with a review of the changes that are found to accompany normal ageing in the human brain. This is followed by an account of the neuropathology of Alzheimer's disease, vascular dementia, dementia with Lewy bodies, and other less common causes of dementia in old age. Anatomical diagrams of the parts of the brain referred to in this chapter are provided in Figs 5.1–5.3.

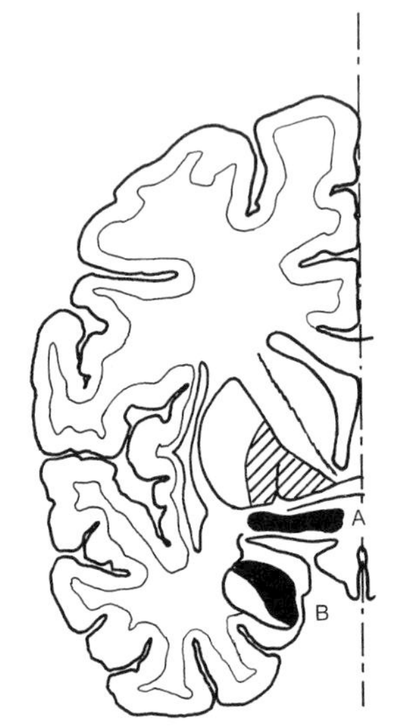

Fig. 5.1 Low-power view of a coronal section through the left cerebral hemisphere to show the position of the nucleus basalis (A), lying ventral to the globus pallidus and close to the amygdala (B).

Normal ageing and the brain

Changes in nerve cells

The cellular constituents of the brain are, on the one hand, nerve cells in their enormous variety in terms of size, shape, length, and number of processes, and the type, distribution, and number of synapses made; and, on the other hand, the glial and vascular components that support them. Hardly any nerve cell division takes place after birth, though details of synaptic connections are certainly added later; however, individual nerve cells grow, as the body grows, during childhood. Some changes to nerve cells have been documented in early life—for example, the first readily detectable accumulation of neuromelanin in pigmented cells of the brainstem occurs during early childhood, but in this chapter it is more appropriate to consider ways in which young and old adult brains differ. The reasons for the changes that occur in the brain with ageing are not well understood. There are probably many factors involved. Among these, two have attracted particular attention recently: the influence of oxygen and other free radicals which are generated as a by-product particularly in metabolically active cells such as neurons, and the toxic effects of the excitatory neurotransmitter, glutamate (Beal 2000; Perry *et al.* 2000). Another concept that colours contemporary views on the causes of age-related changes in the nervous system is that of programmed cell death or apoptosis, an active process that plays an important part in normal nervous system development. There are reasons for thinking that a similar process underlies neuronal loss in ageing. There are four aspects concerning nerve cells that are considered below: change in numbers, change in size, changes in cytoplasmic constituents, and changes in nerve cell processes and connections. Changes in glial cells, consisting

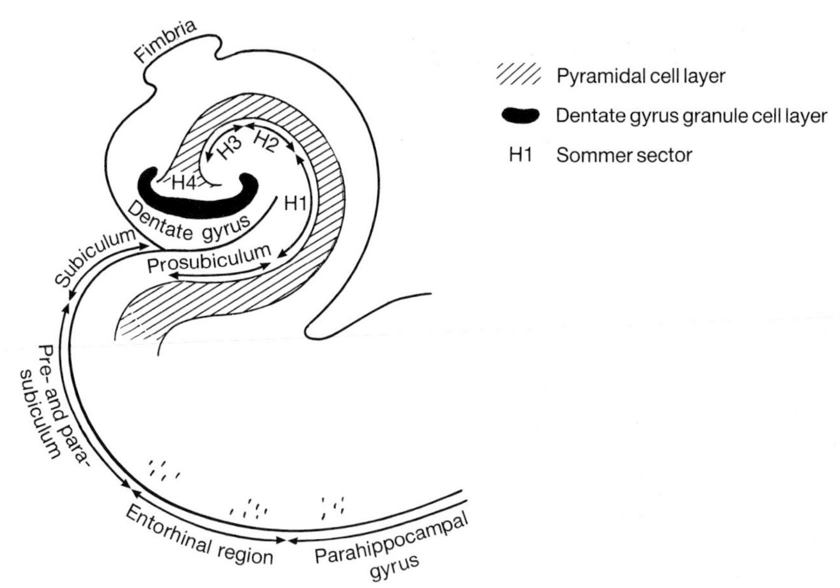

Fig. 5.2 Diagram of a coronal section of the right hippocampus showing the main anatomical features of the region and the subdivision of the pyramidal cell layer into regions CA1–4. The positions of large stellate neurons in the entorhinal region that are highly susceptible to neurofibrillary tangle formation in old age and Alzheimer's disease are indicated as dots.

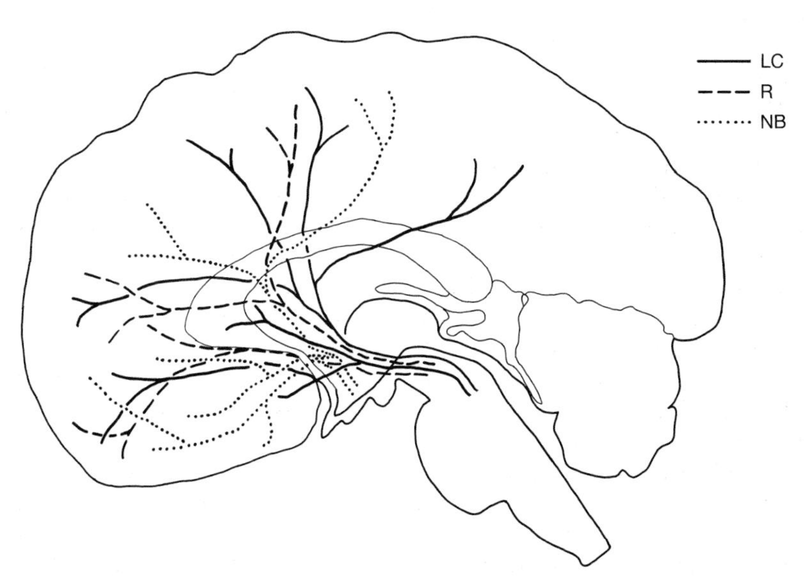

Fig. 5.3 Diagram of a sagittal section through the brain to show the origins and widespread cortical distribution of axonal processes of nerve cells situated in the nucleus basalis (NB) (cholinergic), raphe nuclei (R) (serotonergic), and locus coeruleus (LC) (noradrenergic).

mainly of an increase in astrocytes and microglia, accompany these neuronal changes.

Number of nerve cells

Several populations of nerve cells are known to become depleted in their old age. This depletion does not necessarily result in impaired function, because in most nuclei there seems to be an overprovision of neurons, providing a generous reserve.

Examples of sites where neuron loss has been documented in old age include various parts of the cerebral cortex, hippocampus (subiculum and dentate hilus), substantia nigra, and Purkinje cells of the cerebellum. The extent of the nerve cell loss is variable but may be small, for example 1% of cells lost each year in the inferior frontal gyrus after the age of 70 years (Anderson *et al.* 1983). However, higher figures with loss of 37% of neurons in the hilus and 43% of neurons in the subiculum of the hippocampus between the ages of 13 and 101 years (West *et al.* 1994) and 2.5% per decade of Purkinje cells of the cerebellum throughout adult life have also been found (Hall *et al.* 1975). Nerve cell loss does not seem to be an inevitable consequence of ageing; for example, certain cranial nerve nuclei and the dentate nuclei of the cerebellum show no significant loss in nerve cells even in extreme old age.

Size of nerve cells

Many of the sites from which nerve cells are lost in old age also show some reduction in nerve cell size from the age of 85 years onwards (Meier-Ruge 1988). This change can confound attempts to estimate cell numbers, since large nerve cells become smaller nerve cells and small nerve cells tend to shrink to the size of neuroglia and may seem to have been lost. Shrinkage of nerve cells is studied by measuring the size of their cell bodies, but it is likely, though difficult to demonstrate, that the cell processes may also be reduced in calibre or length, with all that that implies for the maintenance of connections between them. Shrinkage of nerve cells in old age has been shown to occur in the cerebral cortex and putamen. Using an antibody to synaptophysin as a marker for synaptic terminals, immunocytochemical studies indicate a reduction in frontal cortex synapses of 15–25% between the ages of 16 and 98 years (Masliah *et al.* 1993).

Change in brain size

The normal weight of an adult brain varies—between 1240 and 1680 g in men, and between 1130 and 1510 g in women.

From about 50 years of age, the loss and shrinkage of nerve cells is accompanied by a slow, steady, but modest fall in the volume and weight of the brain itself. As the brain shrinks, the ventricles and subarachnoid space enlarge to fill the intracranial space, which remains constant. Thus, the ratio of the brain volume to cranial cavity volume is reduced from 92% earlier in adult life to 83% by the ninth decade. The meninges surrounding the brain show slight thickening due to collagen deposition.

Changes in cytoplasmic constituents of nerve cells

The most obvious change to constituents of nerve cells in old age is the accumulation in their cytoplasm of the granular pigment lipofuscin. This process starts early in life and progresses into old age. Lipofuscin is a complex of substances including lysosomal enzymes and lipids, which are probably contributed to by partially degraded and defunct cellular components. Nuclei of the brain vary in the extent of their lipofuscin accumulation. Lipofuscin-rich nuclei in old age include the inferior olives, lateral geniculate bodies, other thalamic nuclei, and anterior-horn motor neurons. Neuromelanin is related to lipofuscin chemically and also accumulates with age.

There are important changes in components of the proteinaceous neuronal cytoskeleton in old age. The cytoskeleton forms the internal framework of the nerve cells and is responsible for maintaining their shapes. It also serves an important transport function, assisting in the transfer of substances, such as enzymes and other proteins, produced in the cell body to the nerve dendrites and axonal endings, and return transport of synaptic substances to the cell body.

Components of the cytoskeleton themselves move at a slow rate from the centre to the periphery. There are three main components of the cytoskeleton: microfilaments, intermediate filaments (neurofilaments), and microtubules. The microfilaments are composed principally of actin, neurofilaments of at least three different neurofilament proteins, and microtubules of tubulin. Additional proteins are required to help maintain links between these components and with the cell membrane and the extracellular matrix. One such protein, tau, is involved in links between neurofilaments and microtubules. Tau accumulates to form ultrastructurally detectable abnormal, helically wound, paired filaments that form *neurofibrillary tangles* (NFT) in some old nerve cells. Pyramidal neurons in the hippocampus and large stellate cells in superficial layers of the entorhinal cortex are susceptible to this change, though it usually affects only a small proportion of the cells present (Fig. 5.4). Accompanying this alteration is the formation of argyrophilic or *senile plaques* (SP), i.e. abnormal deposits of β-amyloid protein in a roughly spherical formation, in some cases with a core at the centre. SP lacking a core are sometimes referred to as 'primitive' or 'diffuse' and those with one as 'mature' (Figs 5.5(a), (b)). SP have a wider distribution than NFT in normal brains, occurring in the neocortex (cortex outside the hippocampus and entorhinal cortex) and amygdala as well as in the hippocampus and entorhinal cortex. There is no clearly defined and widely agreed cut-off between the numbers and distribution of SP in normal ageing and those in patients with Alzheimer's disease (AD). But of particular importance for higher mental function is the accumulation of plaques with abnormal, tau-positive neuritic components. These may be present, but only in small numbers, in normal ageing. Criteria have been put forward for making a distinction between normal ageing and AD based on a requirement for more numerous neuritic SP to be found in the neocortex of patients with AD (Mirra *et al.* 1991) (see also Alzheimer's disease below).

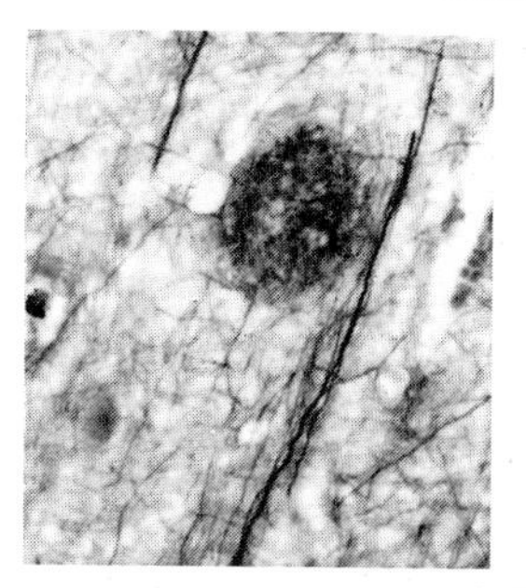

Fig. 5.5(a) Example of an immature argyrophilic plaque in the cerebral cortex of a case of Alzheimer's disease. (Von Braunmühl silver stain, × 200)

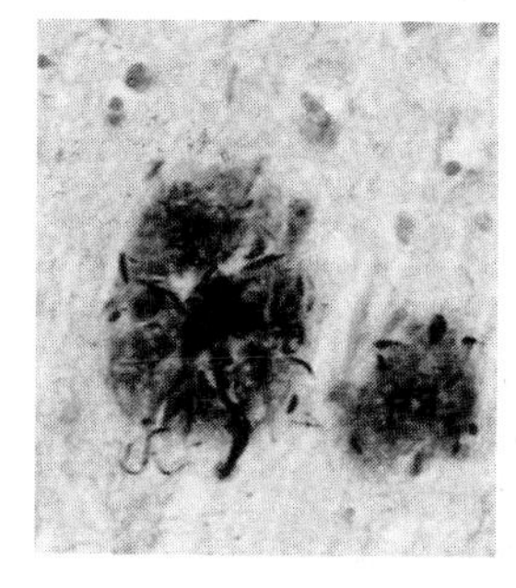

Fig. 5.5(b) Example of a mature plaque in the cerebral cortex of an undemented elderly subject. There is a well-defined core at the core and condensation of surrounding neuritic processes to form a corona. (Von Braunmühl silver stain, × 200)

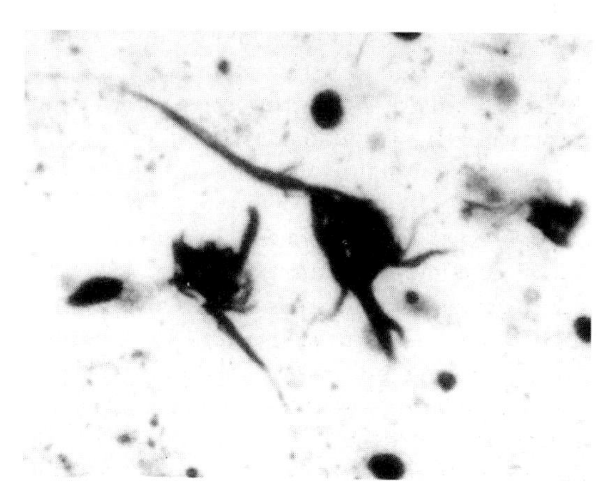

Fig. 5.4 Neurofibrillary tangles in a few remaining large stellate neurons in entorhinal cortex from a case of Alzheimer's disease. (Von Braunmühl silver stain, × 400)

Another cytoskeletal abnormality that occurs to a mild degree in normal ageing is the development of *Hirano bodies*, eosinophilic rod-shaped or carrot-shaped structures in or close to pyramidal nerve cells in the hippocampus. These contain large amounts of the microfilament protein actin. Like NFT and SP, they are much more numerous in AD. Their presence there is frequently accompanied by *granulovacuolar degeneration*, which appears in pyramidal nerve cells as a cluster of vacuoles containing dense granules (Fig. 5.6). This also is much more common in AD but occurs to a slight extent in normal ageing.

Lewy bodies (LB), like NFT, are abnormal intracellular inclusions. They are found in small numbers in the substantia nigra and locus coeruleus in a small proportion of the brains of normal old subjects, but are much more numerous and associated with severe neuron loss in the brains of patients with Parkinson's disease. LB take the form of a spherical single body, or small cluster of bodies, in the cytoplasm of a nerve cell, and have a laminated appearance with a dense core of mainly granular material at the centre and radiating fibrillary material in the outer corona (Fig. 5.7). A major component of Lewy bodies is formed by a protein, *α-synuclein*. The gene on chromosome 4 coding for this protein has recently been recognized as the site of mutation in rare, dominantly inherited, early-onset Parkinson's disease (Polymeropoulos *et al.* 1997).

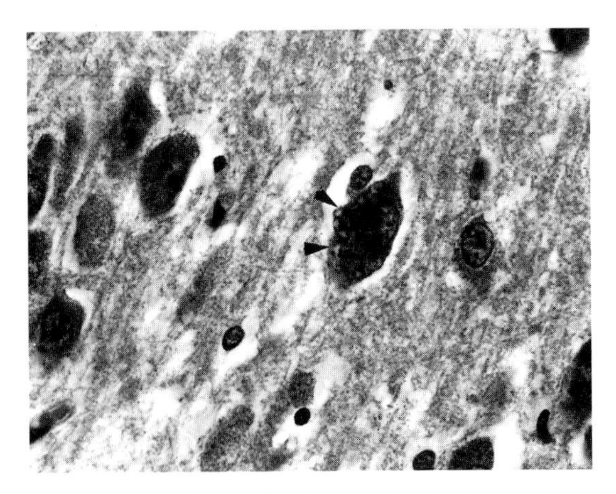

Fig. 5.6 Granulovacuolar degeneration in the cytoplasm of a hippocampal pyramidal cell from a case of Alzheimer's disease. Note granules of differing size occupying pale vacuoles (arrowheads). (Haematoxylin and eosin stain, × 1000)

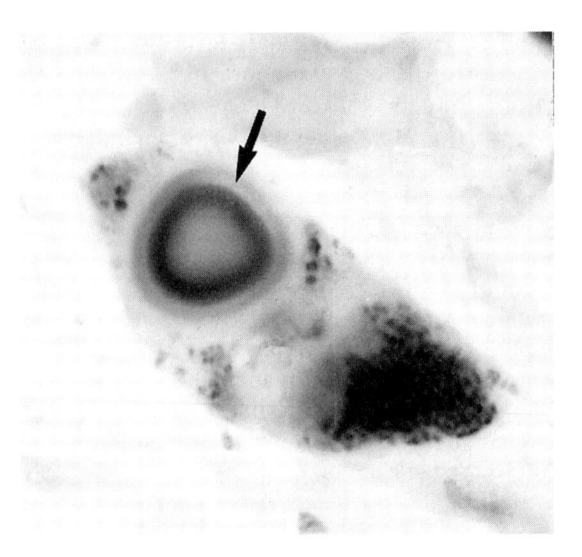

Fig. 5.7 Lewy body (arrow) forming a laminated intracytoplasmic inclusion in a melanin-containing neuron in the substantia nigra from a case of Parkinson's disease. (× 800)

Finally, in about 30% of old people's brains some foci of *amyloid deposition* in the walls of leptomeningeal and cortical blood vessels can be found. This deposition shows up as a positive reaction with a Congo red stain, which also causes the material to show an apple-green birefringence under polarized light. In normal old people's brains in which such deposits are present, the foci are usually only small, very frequently widespread, and present in superficial cortex and leptomeninges overlying all the main cerebral lobes. Occasionally they occur in leptomeninges over the cerebellum, but the hippocampus tends to be spared. The nature of the amyloid deposited in blood vessels is the same as that found in SP and it is described in more detail below. It is termed A4, or beta amyloid, to distinguish it from amyloid of quite different origin deposited at different sites in various circumstances, for example light chains of immunoglobulins. In addition to being present in blood vessels and SP, A4/beta amyloid protein is also deposited in the form of more irregular patches—some small and granular and others larger and more fibrillary—in cerebral cortex in normal ageing. It can be demonstrated by immunostaining using an antiserum to the protein. The quantity of deposits is much less in normal ageing subjects than in those with AD.

A further biochemical alteration in ageing brains, which can be shown up by immunostaining, is the occurrence of deposits of *ubiquitin*, particularly in the hippocampus. These take the form of small granules or threads in the white and grey matter. Ubiquitin, as its name implies, is a protein that is found to be widespread in animal cells. It becomes complexed to proteins destined for degradation, though that is not its only role. In addition to forming granular deposits of unknown significance in normal old people's brains, ubiquitin is also found as a constituent in SP, NFT, LB, Pick bodies (see page 117), Hirano bodies, fibrillary inclusions in motor neurons in motor neuron disease, and the granules of granulovacuolar degeneration.

Changes in nerve cell processes and connections

Much less is known about changes in nerve cell processes and connections in nervous system ageing than about the biochemical alterations, but there are indications from Golgi impregnation studies that cortical nerve cells have a reduced number of spines in old age. Other dendrites show excessive, branched extensions, as if in compensation for the loss of others. Loss of synapses in old age has been referred to above.

Changes in glial cells

In old age, most attention to the alterations of glial cells has been directed towards astrocytes. These are cells that enlarge and increase their processes to assist the healing of damaged central nervous tissue and the formation of scars. Thus, dense focal collections of astrocytic processes accompany any local damage to the CNS. More diffuse and less conspicuous gliosis occurs, particularly in subpial and subependymal layers, in normal ageing. Another very familiar change that occurs with ageing is the accumulation of *corpora amylacea,* most commonly in subpial perivascular and subependymal regions. These are spherical bodies 20–50 μm across, sometimes laminated, and stain strongly by Periodic acid–Schiff. Ultrastructural examination has shown that they are mostly situated in astrocyte processes, though similar bodies can also be found in axons.

Pathological changes in dementia

In large, published autopsy series of cases of adult dementia, there is general agreement that the commonest cause of this condition is AD (Esiri *et al.* 1997*a*; Jellinger *et al.* 1990). There is, however, considerable variation in the proportion of cases that are attributed to AD. In most series the proportion lies between a half and three-quarters. Differences in the referral pattern of cases included in these studies may partly account for the variation. For example, of cases of dementia diagnosed in Oxford and referred for autopsy during the last decade, 50% of those from geriatric psychiatrists were diagnosed neuropathologically as suffering from AD. Causes of dementia that give rise to physical disability, particularly Parkinson's disease and cerebrovascular disease, are more represented, perhaps not surprisingly, in the physicians' series. To obtain a true indication of the relative importance of different causes of dementia, community-based, prospectively assessed subjects needed to be studied and followed to autopsy.

The cause of death in most cases of dementia, regardless of the cause of dementia, is bronchopneumonia or pulmonary embolism. In the terminal stages of the condition, subjects may become quite severely wasted.

Alzheimer's disease (AD)

The pathology of AD defies precise definition at present. This is because its individual components all occur to some extent in normal ageing. The key distinction between changes that can be dismissed as normal ageing and those of AD is that the changes are all more numerous and, for some of them, more widely distributed in AD than in normal ageing. Thus, the characteristic features of AD are the following:

1. The presence of numerous SP, particularly neuritic SP, in cerebral cortex, hippocampus, and certain subcortical nuclei, particularly the amygdala, nucleus basalis, locus coeruleus, and hypothalamus. Suggestions have been made about how many SP in cerebral cortex need to be found in order for a neuropathological diagnosis of AD to be made (CERAD—Mirra *et al.* 1991). This CERAD diagnosis is based on a semiquantitative estimate of neuritic SP, using picture-matching, of the most severely affected foci in neocortex of each of three lobes. The frequencies of SP required to make a diagnosis of AD rise with age and whether or not the patient was clinically demented. The protocol allows the neuropathologist to make a diagnosis of definite, probable, or possible AD, and it has had wider acceptance than the earlier criteria suggested by Khachaturian (1985), or Tierney *et al.* (1988) (Fig 5.8).
2. Some NFT, particularly those in the hippocampus and transentorhinal cortex, occur as extracellular structures, the nerve cells that contained them having degenerated. NFT are also commonly present in AD in the amygdala, nucleus basalis, some hypothalamic nuclei, raphe nuclei of the brainstem, locus coeruleus of the pons (see Figs 5.1–5.3 for the positions of these nuclei). Brains from elderly subjects with only mild AD-related pathology have NFT confined to the transentorhinal cortex, those with slightly more pathology also show NFT in the hippocampus, and those with the most severe pathology and clinical AD show extension of NFT to neocortical and subcortical sites (Braak and Braak 1991). Recognition of this progression has led to the development of the Braak staging of Alzheimer pathology, which recognizes entorhinal (stages 1 and 2), limbic (stages 3 and 4), and neocortical (stages 5 and 6) stages. Symptoms of dementia tend to develop in the limbic stages. A4/beta protein deposits in the form of amyloid occur in small leptomeningeal and cortical blood vessel walls in almost all cases of AD (Fig. 5.9): their extent is variable, from very slight to extensive. If extensive, the vessels may show secondary changes such as occlusion and recanalization of the lumen or slight haemorrhage around them (Fig. 5.9).

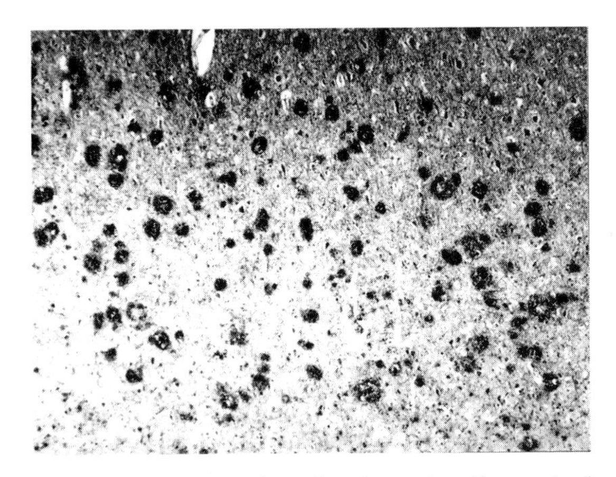

Fig. 5.8 Low-power view of methenamine silver-stained area of association cortex in a case of Alzheimer's disease showing the abundance of plaques that is characteristic of this disease. (× 12)

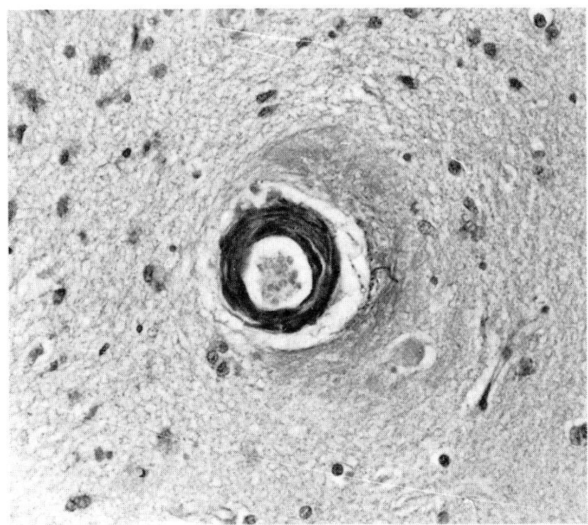

Fig. 5.9 Cortical arteriole containing amyloid deposit in its wall from a case of Alzheimer's disease. (Congo red stain, × 100)

3. Frequent granulovacuolar degeneration and abundant Hirano bodies occur in the hippocampus.

Accompanying these changes, a substantial loss of nerve cells (30% or more) has been demonstrated among populations susceptible to NFT formation, such as pyramidal cells of the neocortex and hippocampus (Mountjoy 1988), though this has been disputed (Regeur *et al.* 1994). Cell loss is accompanied by an increase in astrocytes and a microglial cell reaction in the cortex and white matter. In prospective studies, correlations with the severity of dementia have been shown most convincingly for NFT counts and nerve cell loss in the cerebral cortex and hippocampus (Wilcock and Esiri 1982; Arriagada *et al.* 1992; Nagy *et al.* 1995). More recent studies indicate that the main determinants of cognitive deficit are the accumulation of hyperphosphorylated tau protein and neuritic plaques (Smith *et al.* 2000).

Behavioural abnormalities, in contrast to cognitive decline, correlate best with changes associated with subcortical pathology (Esiri 1996). Excessive wandering and overactivity correlate with a reduction in the level of cortical choline-acetyltransferase activity, reflecting damage to basal forebrain cholinergic nuclei (Minger *et al.* 2000). Depression in patients with Alzheimer's disease correlates with reductions in the density of 5-hydroxytryptamine (5-HT) endings in the cortex, reflecting raphe pathology (Chen *et al.* 1996) or with locus coeruleus cell loss (Förstl *et al.* 1992). In another study, rostral locus coeruleus cell loss correlated with aggressive behaviour in patient's with Alzheimer's disease (Matthews *et al.* 2001), while in a further study aggression correlated with the preservation of nigral neurons (Victoroff *et al.* 1996).

The weight and volume of the brain, particularly the cerebral hemispheres, are reduced in AD, though there is much overlap in individual cases with the normal range (Fig. 5.10). Figures of about a 7–8% reduction in brain weight in series of brains from AD compared with normal have been described. Occasionally there is severe generalized cortical atrophy in AD, usually in the relatively young patients. The volumes of white matter and of deep grey matter are also reduced in AD, and the amygdala, hippocampus, and parahippocampal gyrus may be selectively affected and the inferior horns of the ventricles compensatorily dilated (Fig. 5.11). The volume reduction in the hippocampus and amygdala can be detected during life using temporal lobe-oriented CT scans or MRI (Jobst *et al.* 1992; Kesslak *et al.* 1991; respectively). The cortical ribbon in coronal slices of the brain may appear marginally narrowed in some cases.

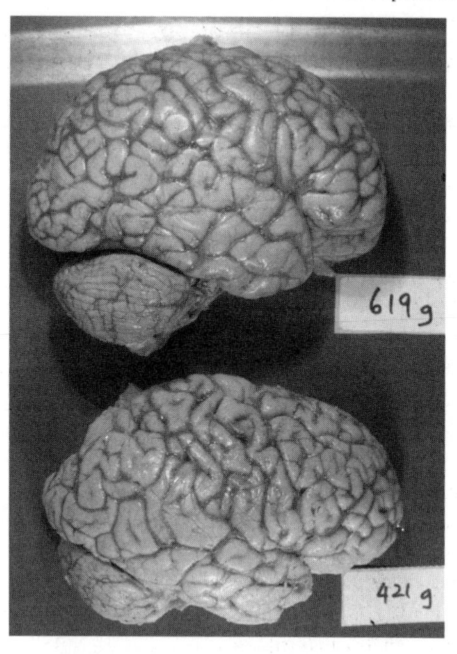

Fig. 5.10 Right lateral views of the brain from an elderly undemented subject (above) and a case of Alzheimer's disease (below). The cerebrum is slightly smaller, and the cortical sulci slightly wider in the case of Alzheimer's disease. The weights given to the right are for the respective cerebral hemispheres.

Anatomical considerations

As indicated above, SP and NFT are much more numerous and widely distributed in AD than in normal ageing. However, they are not randomly scattered throughout the cortex and subcortical nuclei, but show a distribution that is closely

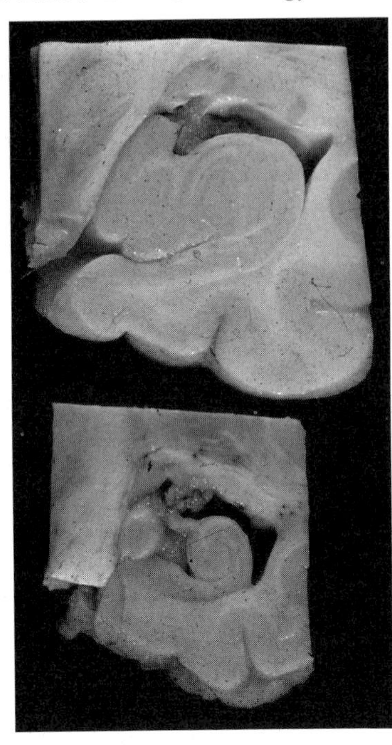

Fig. 5.11 Coronal section of the hippocampus from an elderly undemented subject (above) and a case of Alzheimer's disease (below). Note atrophy of the hippocampus and adjacent temporal lobe cortex in Alzheimer's disease.

linked to neuroanatomical connections. This is particularly true of NFT. In general, areas of association cortex that are closely linked, with no or only one intervening synapse, to the entorhinal cortex, are severely affected, whereas those that are separated by more synapses are little affected. Thus, primary motor and somatosensory cortices far removed from entorhinal cortex are relatively spared, while areas of association cortex more directly linked to entorhinal cortex are severely affected. The primary olfactory cortex, unlike other sensory cortex, is severely affected, in keeping with its relatively close anatomical links to entorhinal cortex. It is of interest that more peripheral parts of the olfactory system are also affected in AD, with pathological changes even being documented in primary olfactory nasal mucosa (Harrison and Pearson 1989). It is of interest that olfactory deficits have heen documented in dementia, although these are a more marked feature of dementia with LB (p. 113) than of AD (McShane *et al.* 2001). Regarding the involvement of subcortical nuclei in the pathological changes of AD, it is generally the case that nuclei receiving a heavy input of afferent fibres *from* the cortex develop SP, while those that have many fibres projecting *to* the cortex develop NFT (Pearson and Powell 1989). Those basal forebrain and brainstem nuclei diffusely innervating the cortex and hippocampus are among the nuclei that develop tangles and lose nerve cells in AD: the nucleus basalis (cholinergic), raphe nuclei (serotonergic), and locus coeruleus (noradrenergic). Loss of pigmented cells in the locus coeruleus is usually sufficiently severe to impart abnormal pallor to this nucleus, which is visible to the naked eye. Loss of transmitters released by these nuclei in the cortex are among the most prominent neurochemical effects of AD.

Relationship of senile plaques (SP) to neurofibrillary tangles (NFT) in Alzheimer's disease

The paired helical filaments that compose NFT are also detectable ultrastructurally in the abnormal neuritic processes which participate in SP; and the most prominent protein antigen detectable in NFT, tau, is detectable also in the neuritic corona of SP in cases of AD that have plentiful NFT. This suggests that nerve cells with NFT in the perinuclear cytoplasm also participate, at their endings, in SP. This relationship between SP and NFT is borne out by studies of the hippocampus, in which it is possible to show that when there are NFT-bearing neurons in the entorhinal cortex, then SP are also found where the axons of these neurons terminate in the dentate fascia of the hippocampus (Hyman *et al.* 1986). Evidence from subjects with Down's syndrome, in whom AD pathology almost invariably develops by late middle age, suggests that diffuse SP develop first, followed by neuritic SP and NFT (Mann and Esiri 1989).

However, the presence of diffuse amyloid deposits, unaccompanied by neurofibrillary pathology, in the brain of healthy elderly individuals indicates that amyloid deposition on its own is not sufficient to trigger the development of Alzheimer's disease and related dementia. Although several hypotheses have been put forward, the link between the development of the different features of Alzheimer's disease (i.e. amyloid deposition, neurofibrillary degeneration, and neuronal death) has remained elusive. However, recent evidence from sporadic Alzheimer's disease and Down's syndrome patients raised the possibility that these features may be the end-result of a common mechanism triggered in the brain by age- or damage-related loss of synapses. It has been hypothesized that synaptic loss, and/or the loss of the synaptic remodelling ability in the brain, may result in the loss of the differentiated phenotype of neurons. These cells, although unable to complete cell division, attempt to re-enter the cell cycle. As a consequence of this aberrant cell-cycle re-entry, and a subsequent regulatory failure, neurons may either develop Alzheimer-type pathology or die via an apoptotic mechanism (Nagy *et al.* 1998). The factors responsible for this aborted attempt of neurons to divide are to yet be elucidated.

Alzheimer's disease and other pathology

Evidence of Alzheimer's disease may be found in conjunction with evidence of other CNS disease, most commonly Parkinson's disease or cerebrovascular disease. The relationship of Parkinson's disease to AD is discussed on p. 113. The relationship to vascular disease is probably partly due to chance (both conditions being common in old age), partly to the effects of amyloid deposition in blood vessels, and partly to the fact that AD and atheromatous vascular disease share common risk factors, such as elevated plasma homocysteine levels (Clarke *et al.* 1998) and the apolipoprotein E genotype $\varepsilon 4$ (Strittmatter *et al.* 1993) (see Chapter 7).

Amyloid deposition in blood vessel walls in AD is usually mild and not associated with local ischaemic or haemorrhagic lesions. However, occasionally it is severe and widespread and may then be associated with thrombotic occlusion of small leptomeningeal and cortical blood vessels, leading to the formation of multiple small cortical infarcts or ischaemic damage to subcortical white matter. Occasionally, leakage of blood from amyloid-infiltrated superficial vessels results in small or massive intracerebral and subarachnoid haemorrhage. Small haemorrhages may be asymptomatic, but are evidenced at autopsy by the presence of focal areas of rusty discoloration of the leptomeninges, where haemoglobin has been processed to the brown pigment haemosiderin. The massive haemorrhages may be fatal. Their position, relatively peripherally situated in one cerebral lobe (lobar haemorrhage), distinguishes them from the common major haemorrhages due to hypertension and the rupture of short, penetrating arterioles which are generally centred on the basal ganglia . Cerebral amyloid angiopathy accounts for about 10% of major intracerebral haemorrhages in the elderly. They usually occur in subjects who are not known to have been demented previously, but whose brains nevertheless show at least some of the pathology of AD at autopsy. Possession of the apolipoprotein E $\varepsilon 2$ genotype increases the risk of haemorrhage from congophilic angiopathy (Nicoll *et al.* 1997).

Cerebrovascular dementia

Ischaemic dementia is the next most common cause of adult dementia after AD. Ischaemic brain lesions often coexist with those of AD. Even when the severity of AD-type pathology is insufficient to diagnose AD they may summate with multiple small vascular lesions to give rise to symptoms of dementia. Recent evidence indicates that the presence of even minimal cerebrovascular pathology lowers the threshold for cognitive deficit and results in clinical dementia in patients with preclinical Alzheimer-related pathology (Esiri *et al.* 1999).

Lesions in grey matter

One of the important underlying processes for causing ischaemic dementia is atheromatous arterial degeneration, causing narrowing of the lumen of arteries or ulceration of their surface, thereby predisposing to mural thrombus formation and embolization. This disease commonly predisposes to embolization of the brain. The internal carotid, vertebral, basilar, and other large cerebral arteries can be affected, leading to embolic or thrombotic occlusion of small arterial branches. Less commonly, thrombosis may occur in the small vessels themselves. This gives rise to multiple small cortical infarcts, which may be widely distributed but are particularly common in territory supplied by middle and posterior cerebral arteries. (Occlusion of larger vessels is likely to lead to larger infarcts which give a stroke-like illness rather than dementia.) In studies of dementia associated with stroke, multiple infarcts, including bilateral infarcts and recurrent infarcts, distinguished demented from non-demented subjects at autopsy (Del Ser *et al.* 1990; Pohjasvaara *et al.* 1998; Schmidt *et al.* 2000). Since emboli derived from mural thrombus in the vertebrobasilar vasculature can become distributed in both posterior cerebral artery territories (including the hippocampus), infarction or hypoxia may develop in both hippocampi and give rise to a severe deficit of short-term memory (Fig. 5.12). Bilateral infarction in boundary-zone territories in both cerebral hemispheres is liable to develop following a precipitate fall in blood pressure, for example during cardiac arrest. Infarcts (lacunae) may be found in deep grey matter as well as cortex.

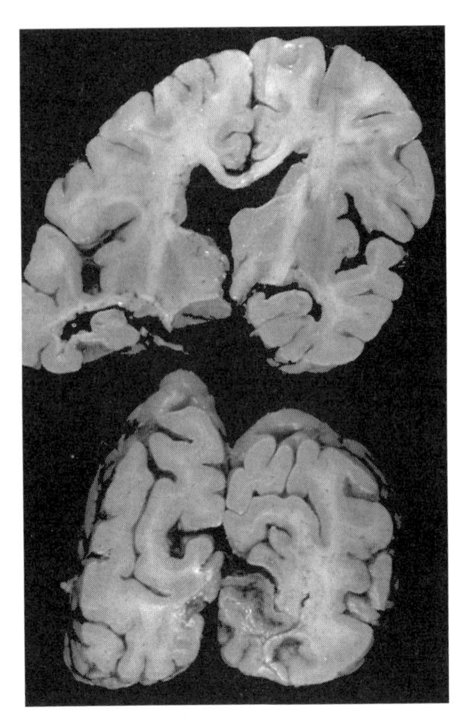

Fig. 5.12 Coronal slices through the cerebral hemispheres at mid-thalamic level (above) and in the parieto-occipital region (below). Infarcts in posterior cerebral artery territory are present on both sides, in the hippocampus on the left in the top slice and in the right calcarine cortex on the right in the lower slice. The right hippocampus was included in the damage in an intermediate slice. The patient was an 84-year-old female with a 5-year history of confusion and memory loss with some episodes of aggression.

Other causes of multiple small infarcts in grey and white matter, resulting in dementia in old age, include various forms of vasculitis such as polyarteritis nodosa, systemic lupus erythematosus, and granulomatous arteritis. These are all conditions that are only rarely encountered. A common condition that may exacerbate damage produced when the circulation is compromised, for whatever reason, is iron-deficiency anaemia.

Lesions in white matter

Well-defined infarcts are less common in white matter than in grey matter, but white matter frequently suffers from more diffuse ischaemic hypoxic damage. Frequently, the basis of this type of damage is longstanding hypertension, which leads to hyalinization of the walls of arterioles in white matter and deep grey matter and increased tortuosity of vessels. Rarefaction of white matter around these arterioles follows, possibly from the high pulse pressure inside the vessels. The resulting condition of the brain, sometimes referred to as 'cribriform state' (*état cribré*), resembles a fine sponge to naked-eye examination, with each tiny vessel being surrounded by a widened perivascular space in which there are likely to be a few pigment-containing macrophages, and beyond that a zone of poorly myelinated, loosened white matter (Fig. 5.13). These changes may be maximal in temporal lobe white matter or basal ganglia and thalamus, or

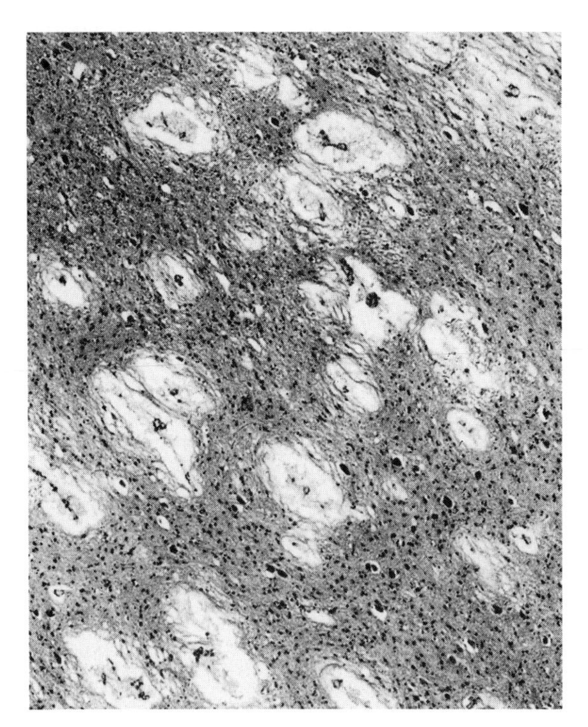

Fig. 5.13 Low-power view of a section from the cerebrum from a case of *état cribré* in which there is dilation of the perivascular spaces and rarefaction of adjacent tissue (× 80).

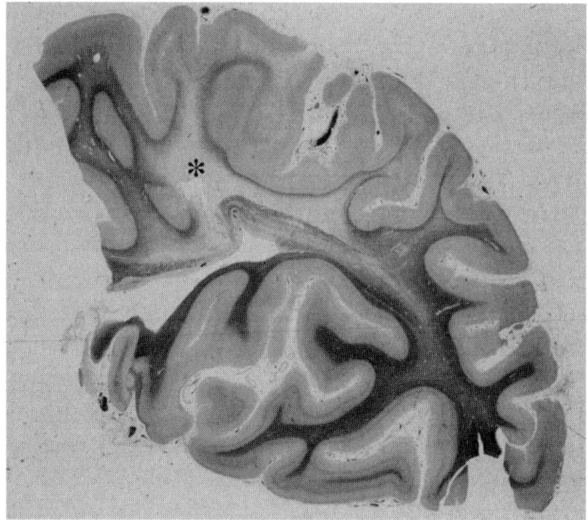

Fig. 5.14 Low-power view of a section through the parieto-occipital region of the left cerebral hemisphere from a case of progressive dementia complicating longstanding hypertension. The section has been stained for myelin, and shows loss of myelin in inferior parietal and occipital white matter (*) with sparing only of the immediately subcortical myelin. The damage to white matter was attributable to occlusion and narrowing by intimal proliferation of many small arterioles in white matter. (× 1)

may be widespread in cerebral white matter. The white matter volume is then correspondingly reduced and lateral ventricles enlarged. The vessels themselves show reduplication of the intimal lining and collagenous deposition in the media. The internal elastic lamina may show reduplication and there may be two or three small vascular channels replacing a normal single one, indicating thrombosis with recanalization or tortuosity. Although these changes are classically seen in elderly subjects with longstanding hypertension, they may also occur in the sixth to tenth decades in the absence of a strong history of hypertension. There is reason to believe that this type of vascular disease is the commonest form of vascular dementia (Esiri *et al.* 1997*b*, 2001). Such lesions may be the only ones demonstrable in the brains of subjects with a history of progressive dementia, or they may be combined with grey matter infarcts and/or AD pathology. In some cases, the white matter rarefaction may be unusually diffuse and widespread. The pathology is then appropriately referred to as that of Binswanger's disease (Fig. 5.14). Many cases of this sort will also be shown at autopsy to have an enlarged heart with a hypertrophied left ventricle.

Parkinson's disease and dementia with Lewy bodies

There is a substantial minority of patients with idiopathic Parkinson's disease (PD) who are demented and a similar minority of patients with AD who have symptoms of parkinsonism (see Chapter 24iv). There has therefore been considerable interest in discovering a possible relationship between these two diseases and in clarifying the reasons for the development of dementia in PD and of symptoms of parkinsonism in AD. It is worth noting that both PD and AD produce pathological changes in the nucleus basilis which may have additive effects. It must also be borne in mind that both AD and PD are common and may therefore occur together in the same patient by chance.

An additional factor that needs to be considered is that in PD, Lewy bodies (LBs) may be found beyond those nuclei conventionally recognized to be regularly affected in PD, and may occur in large numbers in cerebral cortex, particularly in demented subjects. The resulting condition is known as diffuse or cortical Lewy body disease or dementia with Lewy bodies (DLB). The detection of widespread LBs has been made easier by immunostaining with antibodies to ubiquitin or α-synuclein, with which LBs react. It has been suggested that, in the past, some cases of diffuse LB disease may have gone undetected and that diffuse LB disease is not rare, as was supposed a few years ago, but is as common, or nearly as common, as vascular disease in causing dementia (Lennox *et al.* 1989).

Most patients with PD, although they may have worse cognitive function than age- and education-matched controls, do not suffer from true dementia, and in such cases the pathology (consisting of LB formation, neuron loss, and gliosis) occurs predominantly in subcortical and brainstem nuclei, particularly in nuclei containing melanized neurons. Thus, the naked-eye lesion characteristic of PD is pallor of (normally pigmented) brainstem nuclei, the substantia nigra, and locus coeruleus. Studies of demented PD subjects have found a variety of pathologies that might explain the dementia:

1. More cell loss is seen in the nucleus basalis than in undemented PD subjects.
2. Cortical LBs are often combined with the presence of diffuse SP (but not always neuritic SP, hence the CERAD criteria for AD may not be met) (Hurtig *et al.* 2000). Patients suffering from cortical Lewy body disease, with many cortical Lewy bodies, frequently develop severe dementia and earlier on may show a fluctuating course to their illness. They are also likely to suffer from persistent (usually visual) hallucinations (Byrne *et al.* 1990; McKeith *et al.* 1994), and are unusually sensitive to the effect of neuroleptic drugs (McKeith *et al.* 1992; McShane *et al.* 1997). Cortical Lewy bodies are particularly numerous in cingulate, insular, and parahippocampal cortices. They have a less distinctive appearance than Lewy bodies in the substantia nigra, showing less clear lamination (Fig. 5.15). A constant accompaniment of cortical Lewy bodies is the presence of many abnormal α-synuclein immunoreactive neurites. These are particularly numerous in the hippocampus in the CA_{2-3} region where they have been correlated in some reports with dementia severity (Churchyard and Lees 1997).
3. In classical AD pathology with classical subcortical PD pathology, there are usually a few cortical Lewy bodies present in such cases.
4. Some cases show only the expected subcortical PD pathology, with or without a few cortical Lewy bodies and with or without some ischaemic vascular pathology.

Most subjects, but not all, with many cortical LBs have clinical features of parkinsonism, though dementia may be the presenting complaint. A quantitative correlation between the severity of dementia and the density of cortical LBs has been demonstrated (Lennox *et al.* 1989; Hurtig *et al.* 2000). The LBs in diffuse cortical LB disease are found to be most numerous in entorhinal, temporal, insular, and cingulate cortex, where they occur mainly in small- and medium-sized pyramidal cells in the deeper cortical layers. They are rare in the hippocampus but common in the amygdala. Cases with cortical LBs almost invariably also show cell loss and LBs in the substantia nigra.

Because some cases of diffuse LB disease show many diffuse SP and because LBs can be difficult to detect in cerebral cortex unless they are specifically looked for or immunostained with an antibody to ubiquitin or α-synuclein, it is possible that some cases considered as cases of AD with SP predominating are actually cases of diffuse cortical LB disease (Hansen *et al.* 1993).

Brain damage due to alcohol

There is a wide spectrum of neuropathological changes that may be found in the brains of subjects with a prolonged high intake of alcohol.

(a)

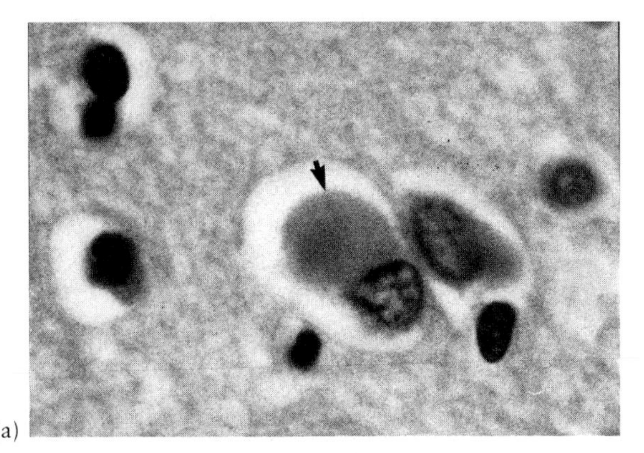

(b)

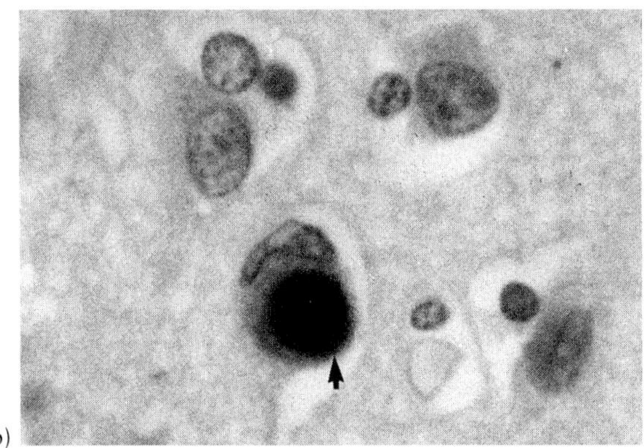

Fig. 5.15 Cerebral cortex from a case of diffuse Lewy body disease (a) stained with H&E and (b) stained with antibody to ubiquitin (arrows) (×400).

Features of Wernicke's encephalopathy are common, as is cerebellar cortical degeneration (Victor 1976). Those who have developed cirrhosis of the liver and terminal liver failure may have features of acute hepatic encephalopathy. Since alcoholics are prone to repeated falls, they commonly develop brain damage, due to head injury, such as cortical contusions and subdural haematomas. Cerebrovascular disease is also common in alcoholics. Exceptionally, the pathological features of Marchiafava–Bignami disease or central pontine myelinolysis may be found. Recent studies indicate that the brain shrinkage due to uncomplicated alcoholism is mainly due to white matter loss, which, to some extent, appears to be reversible (Harper 1998). While alcohol-related neuronal loss has been well documented in the superior frontal cortex (Harper and Kril 1987), hypothalamus (Harper 1998), and cerebellum (Victor 1976), findings in the hippocampus and amygdala are more controversial (Harper 1998).

Wernicke's encephalopathy and cerebellar degeneration in alcoholics

The lesions of Wernicke's encephalopathy have been found in 1.7–2.7% of unselected autopsies and are probably frequently undetected unless they are specifically sought. They are due to a deficiency of vitamin B_1 (thiamine). The lesions chiefly affect the grey matter around the third ventricle and aqueduct and in the floor of the fourth ventricle. The mamillary bodies are particularly liable to be affected . The appearance of the lesions depends on how acute they are. In the initial stages there are petechial haemorrhages, but more commonly the pathology is seen at a chronic stage when there is brown discoloration and atrophy of the areas affected. The lesions cannot be reliably detected by naked-eye examination alone. Microscopy shows, in the acute stage, prominent enlargement of the endothelial cells of capillaries and some red blood cells and macrophages in perivascular tissue. Surrounding astrocytes are enlarged, but neurons are usually relatively well preserved. In the chronic stage, there is an increased content of reticulin in perivascular spaces and some prominence of endothelium with a few scattered haemosiderin-containing macrophages. The dorsal medial thalamic nuclei, as well as the mamillary bodies, are at risk for developing these lesions and their involvement may explain the prominence of memory disturbances in such patients. Although alcoholic patients with Wernicke's syndrome develop neurofibrillary pathology in the nucleus basalis, the loss of cholinergic cells in this region is minor and is not related to the profound memory disorder (Cullen *et al.* 1997).

The cerebellar degeneration seen in alcoholics is distinctive for its relatively selective involvement of the superior vermis. To the naked eye, the affected cerebellar folia appear shrunken; microscopically they show severe loss of Purkinje cells, patchy loss of granule cells, and gliosis of the Bergmann glia (astrocytes) extending into the molecular layer of the cortex. Cerebellar cortical degeneration in alcoholics may occur in conjunction with Wernicke's encephalopathy, but it is not clearly due to thiamine deficiency. Similarly, the cortical degeneration and cognitive deficits seen in Korsakoff's syndrome cannot be explained by thiamine deficiency alone (Homewood *et al.* 1999). It has recently been found that the ApoE genotype has a significant role in determining whether patients suffering from Korsakoff's syndrome will develop a global cognitive deficit or not (Muramatsu *et al.* 1997).

Hydrocephalus

A small number of demented patients are found at autopsy to have marked dilation of the lateral ventricles without significant cerebral atrophy (Fig. 5.16). The third ventricle may also be dilated. The appearances suggest an obstructive hydrocephalus, and this impression may be borne out by the presence of defects in the septum. Rarely, there is an obvious tumour mass obstructing the flow of cerebrospinal fluid, for example a non-functioning pituitary adenoma, but this is exceptional. In some cases, there may be thickening of the leptomeninges, providing an explanation for obstruction to cerebrospinal fluid circulation in the subarachnoid space, but most cases show no clear evidence of such an obstruction to flow. Alternatively, there may be signs of old intracerebral or subarachnoid haemorrhage, or head injury, perhaps sufficient to have impaired the uptake of cerebrospinal fluid (CSF) at the arachnoid villi. These cases usually lack classical clinical features of raised intracranial pressure but show the triad of dementia, incontinence, and ataxia that characterize normal pressure (or more correctly, intermittently raised pressure) hydrocephalus (Chapter 24vi). It may be significant that a high percentage of such cases display small foci of deep cerebral vascular damage, which may result in transient obstruction to CSF flow by haemorrhage into the ventricles (Esiri 1997).

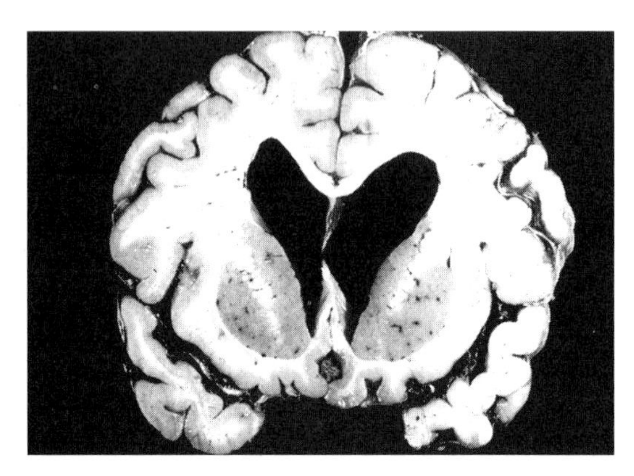

Fig. 5.16 Coronal slice across the frontal lobes of a case of dementia due to hydrocephalus in a 76-year-old male. The frontal horns of the ventricles are markedly dilated. This is not due to compensatory dilatation following atrophy, because the cortical gyri are well preserved and the sulci are narrow, while the corpus callosum is of good width. The appearance is typical of that seen in 'normal pressure' hydrocephalus.

Pick's disease

Pick's disease is a rare, autosomal dominant disease, though occasional apparently sporadic cases can also be encountered. It is sometimes called *lobar atrophy* because of the distinctive naked-eye atrophy of the cortex that characterizes the brain in most cases of this disease. The atrophy usually affects most prominently the frontal and/or temporal poles of the cerebral hemispheres. In the temporal lobes, the posterior two-thirds of the superior temporal gyrus are relatively spared. There may be asymmetry, with one cerebral hemisphere more affected than the other. The degree of atrophy present in the most severely affected parts of the cortex is usually more marked than that seen in AD. The overlying leptomeninges are usually considerably thickened. On slicing the brain, the deep grey matter, particularly the caudate nuclei, and the white matter can be seen to be included in the atrophic process. The lateral ventricles, particularly the frontal and inferior horns, are grossly dilated to compensate for this atrophy and the corpus callosum is thin (Fig. 5.17).

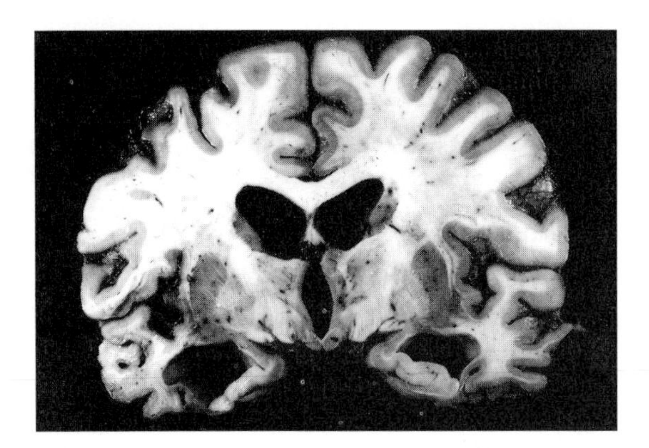

Fig. 5.17 Coronal slice across the brain at the level of the mamillary bodies from a case of Pick's disease. In this case the atrophy is confined to the temporal lobes, in which the cortex is narrowed and the sulci are widened. The inferior horns of the ventricles are correspondingly grossly dilated, while the main body of the lateral ventricles and third ventricle are only mildly dilated. The corpus callosum and frontal cortex are relatively well preserved.

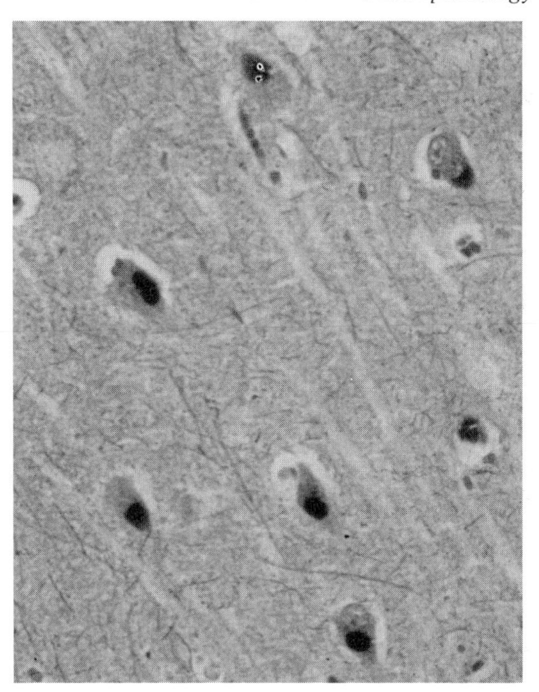

Fig. 5.18 Neurons containing condensed, rounded Pick bodies immunoreactive with antibody to tau protein (× 200).

On microscopy, neuron loss in the affected parts of the cortex is usually obvious, or even gross, with few surviving large pyramidal neurons. This cell loss is accompanied by marked astrocytosis in both grey and white matter. Myelin staining in atrophic white matter is poor, reflecting a diffuse loss of myelinated fibres. Some remaining cortical neurons show expansion and enlargement by argyrophilic bundles of neurofilaments that immunostain for tau. Expanded cells of this sort are called Pick cells; rounded, perinuclear condensations of such filaments are called Pick bodies (Fig. 5.18). These can frequently be detected in the dentate fascia of the hippocampus as well as scattered in the cortex, though here their numbers may be low if most cells have disappeared. Pick bodies give immunocytochemical reactions for neurofilaments and ubiquitin as well as tau. Some microscopic features of AD, particularly granulovacuolar degeneration, may be found in Pick's disease.

Dementia of frontal lobe type

Such a description (Chapter 24v) is primarily a clinical diagnosis. These patients typically present with an alteration in their personality, disinhibited behaviour, neglect of personal appearance, loss of social awareness, and impulsive or ill-considered actions. The condition encompasses several different pathological conditions. Some cases are cases of typical or atypical Pick's disease (Brun *et al.* 1994). Atypical Pick's disease has macroscopic appearances in the brain of Pick's disease but it lacks Pick cells or Pick bodies. Other cases are categorized as cases of '*non-specific frontal lobe dementia*', and have less marked frontal and/or temporal lobe atrophy than in Pick's disease. Microscopically, such cases usually have a characteristic microvacuolation of layer 2 of the cortex of frontal and temporal lobes, together with some shrinkage and loss of cortical pyramidal neurons in these lobes, and astrocytosis of deep cortex and subcortical white matter. They do not show Pick cells or Pick bodies. Subcortical nuclei including the substantia nigra, striatum, and medial thalamus, may show neuron loss and gliosis. Non-specific frontal lobe dementia shows neuropathological similarities in the cerebral cortex to rare cases of dementia associated with motor neuron disease (Kew and Leigh 1992), but in these cases there are, in addition, neuropathological features of motor neuron disease, with degeneration of upper and lower motor neurons.

Frontal lobe dementia associated with mutations in the tau gene located on chromosome 17

Recent reports have documented 20 or so different mutations in the gene encoding microtubule-associated protein tau on chromosome 17, which are linked to frontotemporal dementia and parkinsonism (Poorkaj *et al.* 1998; Spillantini *et al.* 1998). Many of these mutations lead to a reduced ability of tau to interact with microtubules (Arawaka *et al.* 1999; Sahara *et al.* 2000) and an abundance of tau pathology in the form of neurofibrillary tangles in both neuronal and glial cells and neuropil threads in the brains of those affected. The ultrastructure of the filaments that accumulate differs somewhat from that of classical Alzheimer tangles, in that there is an abundance of straight filaments and wide twisted ribbons in isolated material (Heutink 2000). Although most reported cases have presented primarily with dementia, some have had a clinical and pathological phenotype more akin to progressive supranuclear palsy or corticobasal degeneration. The reasons for the widely variable phenotypic expression remain unexplained at present, but the recognition of these tau gene mutations represents an important new development in the understanding of neurodegeneration.

Huntington's disease (HD)

Huntington's disease is an autosomal dominant disease determined by a gene on chromosome 4. Recent research on the genetics and biology of the disease has been reviewed by Reddy *et al.* (1999). Although symptoms of fidgetiness progressing to chorea, and alterations in mood or behaviour progressing to dementia, characteristically occur in the middle decades of adult life, some cases present later and come under the care of geriatric psychiatrists.

By the time of death, the brain is usually small, although external evidence of cortical atrophy is rarely severe. The characteristic pathology is seen when the brain is sliced, i.e. selective atrophy of the caudate nucleus and putamen (Fig. 5.19). Somewhat similar atrophy may be seen in Pick's disease, but in that disease the atrophy of the cortex is much more marked than in HD. The globus pallidus may also be atrophic, particularly in its external segment. Microscopy shows severe loss of small neurons and gliosis in the caudate nucleus and putamen, with relative sparing of large- and medium-sized neurons. The neurons most at risk contain gamma aminobutyric acid (GABA). Neuron loss in the basal ganglia is most severe in cases showing advanced chorea (Vonsattel *et al.* 1985). Dementia, which has been described as subcortical in its pattern of deficits, may also be related to cell loss in the frontal cortex which can be documented using quantitative methods, though it may not be evident on inspection. Some cases show a more widespread neuron loss, for example in certain thalamic and hypothalamic nuclei, substantia nigra (zona reticularis), and dentate nuclei of the cerebellum.

Symptoms in Huntington's disease may become treatable or preventable in the future. This

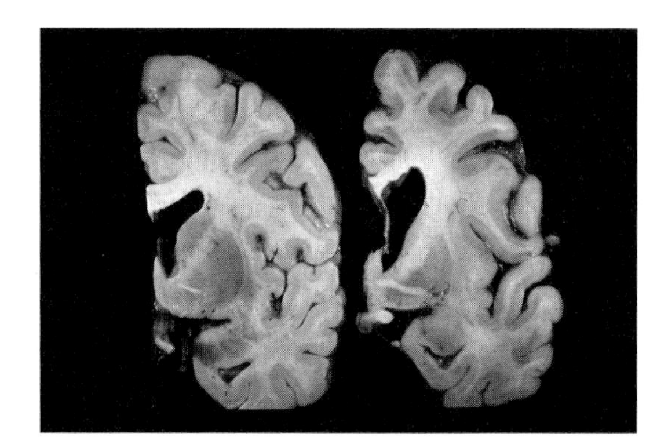

Fig. 5.19 Coronal slices through the frontal and temporal lobes from a case of Huntington's disease (right) and control (left). Note dilated ventricle and reduced volume of caudate nucleus in Huntington's disease.

optimism has been generated by the report that in a mouse model of Huntington's disease pathological features and symptoms can be reversed by switching off the activation of the mutant gene (Yamamoto *et al.* 2000).

Progressive supranuclear palsy and corticobasal degeneration

Progressive supranuclear palsy is a rare, sporadic disease occurring in the fifth to seventh decades and characterized clinically by ataxia, dysarthria, nuchal rigidity, and slowly progressive loss of upward gaze. Some patients have impaired cognitive abilities, though these are different from those in AD and suggestive of a subcortical dementia (Snowden *et al.* 1987). The most obvious pathological changes are found in the globus pallidus, subthalamic nucleus, substantia nigra, red nucleus, and dentate nucleus of the cerebellum. In these areas there is atrophy, loss of neurons, and gliosis. Some remaining neurons contain NFT in their cell bodies, as do some glial cells in a similar distribution. At the ultrastructural level these tangles differ from those in AD in being composed predominantly of straight, 15 nm-diameter filaments but, like NFT, they contain tau and ubiquitin antigens.

Corticobasal degeneration has only recently emerged as a distinct disease entity. Clinically, it represents a heterogeneous group of 'Parkinson's plus' syndromes with features of cortical and basal ganglionic dysfunction. However, it has emerged that some patients present with a dementia syndrome alone. Pathologically, corticobasal degeneration is characterized by neuronal loss and gliosis in the frontal and parietal cortices and in the basal ganglia (Gras *et al.* 1994). The same areas are affected by abundant cytoplasmic inclusions of the hyperphosphorylated form of the microtubule associated protein tau, similar to that found in Alzheimer's disease (Li *et al.* 1998).

Paraneoplastic syndrome

Rapidly progressive dementia may form the presenting clinical picture in some forms of paraneoplastic syndrome. In this syndrome, various neurological deficits result from a probable autoimmune attack against neural antigens, this response being triggered by the presence of a carcinoma, which is often occult. The commonest form of carcinoma to be associated with this syndrome is small-cell (or oat-cell) carcinoma of the lung, and the neurological involvement can occur at any level of the neuraxis, from the cerebral cortex to peripheral nerves. In cases with dementia, the pathological changes are those of an encephalitis involving the temporal lobe and hippocampus, though other areas may also be affected such as the basal ganglia, thalamus, and brainstem. In these areas there are perivascular lymphocytic infiltrates, microglial proliferation, astrocytosis, and variable, but usually patchy, loss of nerve cells. Some cases have a circulating antibody that reacts with nuclei of a variety of neurons, but it remains to be shown that these have an aetiological role in the syndrome (Darnell 1996).

Creutzfeldt–Jakob disease

Sporadic Creutzfeldt–Jakob disease (CJD) is a very rare cause of rapidly progressive dementia, occasionally presenting in an elderly person but more characteristically in the fifth or sixth decade. A few cases are familial (probably fewer than 10%). In most cases death occurs within 6–12 months of the onset of symptoms. Neurological deficits, particularly ataxia, are likely to be present in addition to dementia.

At autopsy, the brain usually appears normal to naked-eye inspection. With microscopy, the characteristic feature is a spongy or vacuolar change in the neuropil of grey matter, particularly in cerebral and cerebellar cortex (Fig. 5.20). The vacuoles measure 50–200 μm across, and occur in the processes of nerve cells. Accompanying this change there is loss of nerve cells and reactive astrocytosis in similar distribution. These pathological changes resemble those of similar spongiform encephalopathies in animals, such as scrapie in sheep and bovine spongiform encephalopathy (BSE). All these diseases are experimentally transmissible to laboratory

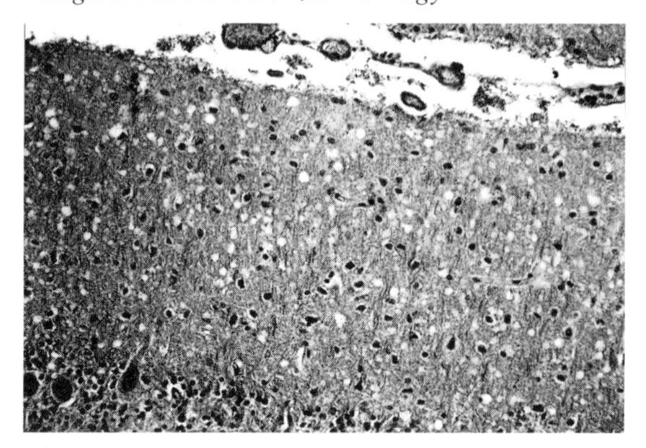

Fig. 5.20 Low-power view of the microscopy of the cerebellar cortex in Creutzfeldt–Jakob disease. There is a loosening of the neuropil and a spongy appearance particularly in the molecular layer. (Haematoxylin and eosin stain, × 100)

animals, with similar symptoms developing months or years after intracerebral inoculation of affected brain homogenates. The infective agent of scrapie, the most extensively studied of the spongiform encephalopathies, has several unusual properties, such as resistance to normal agents that inactivate bacteria and viruses, failure to provoke an immune response, and no well-characterized ultrastructure. No nucleic acid has been unequivocally demonstrated in the agent and the high infectivity fraction of the brain homogenates has been found to consist largely of a protein. This observation has led to the suggestion that the agent may itself be a protein, termed prion protein, the amino-acid sequence of which is identical to a normal cellular membrane-associated protein of unknown function (De Armond and Prusiner 1995). An important difference between the two proteins derives from the fact that only the disease version is resistant to degradation by certain cellular proteases and it tends to polymerize to form minute amyloid fibrils. Much active research is engaged in defining more of the properties of prions and their normal cellular counterparts. There are other human diseases related to CJD: Kuru, a now almost extinct cerebellar degeneration occurring in a remote tribe in Papua New Guinea, and the inherited Gerstmann–Sträussler syndrome, in which cerebellar ataxia forms a prominent clinical feature. In this disease, amyloid plaques containing prion protein (PrP) antigen are found in the brain, and the gene coding for the cellular, prion-like protein is abnormal, resulting in a protein with an abnormal sequence. A different prion gene mutation is associated with a condition known as fatal familial insomnia. Recently a new form of human prion disease has emerged in the United Kingdom, known as variant (v; or new variant, nv) CJD. This is closely linked to the recent epidemic there of bovine spongiform encephalopathy (Will *et al.* 1996). This condition, in which prominent, protease-resistant, PrP-containing plaques as well as spongiform change and gliosis occur in the brain has now been described in a male in the 8th decade (Lorains *et al.* 2001).

Human immunodeficiency virus (HIV-type 1), AIDS, and dementia

HIV-1 causes neurological symptoms in a significant proportion of cases of AIDS, though this is reduced if antiretroviral treatment is given. Dementia is one of the most prominent features of AIDS encephalopathy, a degenerative condition of the brain which appears to be related to HIV-1 infection itself rather than to other CNS complications of immunodeficiency such as other infections or lymphoma. In Western countries most cases of HIV-1 encephalopathy occur in young or middle aged male homosexuals or intravenous drug abusers, but some cases occur in elderly males. In developing countries millions of cases have occurred in heterosexuals. Blood transfusions as well as sexual contact can transmit the disease.

The pathology of HIV-1 encephalopathy is found mainly in the white matter of the cerebral and cerebellar hemispheres and in deep grey matter (Esiri and Kennedy 1997). These areas show a diffuse lack of the normal staining quality of myelin (Fig. 5.21), sometimes with patchy axonal, as well as myelin, damage. These changes are associated with an infiltrate of macrophages and increased microglial cells as well as reactive astrocytosis. In the most severely affected cases,

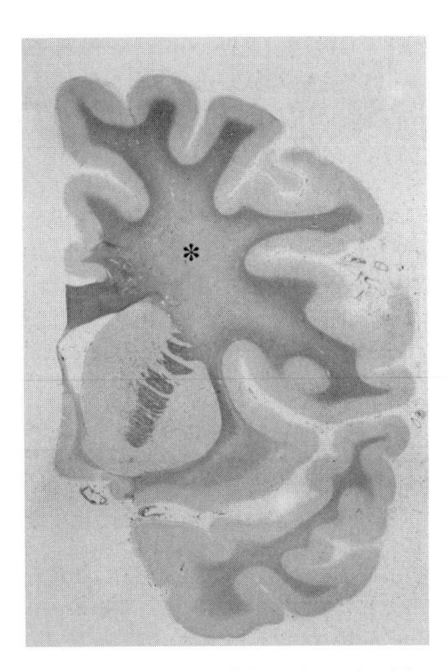

Fig. 5.21 Coronal section of the left cerebral hemisphere from a case of HIV encephalopathy. The section has been stained to show myelin and there is a diffuse deficiency of myelin in the deep white matter (*).

multinucleated giant cells of macrophage origin are found in affected white matter and basal ganglia. These cells and other macrophages and microglia contain productive infection with HIV-1. Exactly how this infection causes the white matter damage is still uncertain, but there are two mechanisms thought likely to play a part. First, some protein products coded for by the virus and shed from infected cells, particularly the envelope protein gp120, are known to have toxic effects on cultured nerve cells *in vitro*. When expressed in astrocytes in transgenic mice, gp120 produced neuropathological changes similar to those seen in human HIV encephalopathy (Toggas *et al.* 1994). Second, HIV-infected macrophages, microglia, and multinucleated cells secrete cytokines, such as tumour necrosis factor alpha (TNF-α), that are capable of damaging neurons and myelin. In addition to white matter damage due to HIV infection, there is also a loss of cortical neurons and a reduction in dendritic spines and synapses in those that remain (Everall *et al.* 1993). However, the extent of the contribution of damage to the clinical state, which seems mainly a reflection of subcortical dysfunction (Peavy *et al.* 1994), is unclear.

The problem of dementia of uncertain aetiology

In most large autopsy series of dementia there is a small percentage of cases in which no definite cause for the dementia can be ascertained, despite careful examination of the brain. It is likely that some other causes for dementia will be identified if postmortem studies are extended. Examples of relatively recently described diseases which can present with dementia are progressive supranuclear palsy, non-specific frontal lobe dementia, diffuse Lewy body disease, the chromosome 17 tau mutations, and AIDS. It is therefore important that clinicopathological studies should continue to be carried out on cases of dementia. This calls for frank discussion with relatives about the importance of autopsy examination of the brain in unusual cases of dementia, so that their informed consent can be gained.

Other neuropathological conditions associated with dementia in the elderly

There are a number of other conditions that may occasionally give rise to dementia in the elderly. All the following have been known to do so in the authors' personal experience: metachromatic leucodystrophy, damage due to head injuries or herpes simplex encephalitis, and tumours (particularly gliomas and meningiomas) or cerebral metastases. Consideration of the pathology of these varied conditions is beyond the scope of this chapter but can be found in Graham and Lantos (1997) and other similar textbooks.

Recommended further reading

Esiri, M. M. and Morris, J. H. (ed.) (1997). *The neuropathology of dementia*. Cambridge University Press.

Graham, D. I. and Lantos, P. L. (1997). *Greenfield's neuropathology* (6th edn). Arnold, London.

Markesbery, W. R. (ed.) (1998). *Neuropathology of dementing disorders*. Arnold, London.

References

Anderson, J. M., Hubbard, B. M., Coghill, G. R., and Slidders, W., *et al.* (1983). The effect of advanced old age on the neurone content of the cerebral cortex. Observations with an automatic image analyser point counting method. *Journal of the Neurological sciences*, **58**, 235–46.

Arawaka, S., Usami, M., Sahara, N., Schellenberg, G.D., Lee, G., and Mori, H. (1999). The tau mutation (val337met) disrupts cytoskeletal networks of microtubules. *Neuroreport*, **10**, 993–7.

Arriagada, P. V., Growdon, J. H., Hedley-Whyte, T. E., and Hyman, B. T. (1992). Neurofibrillary tangles but not senile plaques parallel duration, and severity of Alzheimer's disease. *Neurology*, **45**, 631–9.

Beal, M. F. (2000). Energetics in the pathogenesis of neurodegenerative diseases (2000). *Trends in Neuroscience*, **23**, 298–304.

Braak, H. and Braak, E. (1991). Neuropathological staging of Alzheimer-related changes. *Acta Neuropathologica*, **82**, 239–59.

Brun, A., Englund, B., Gustafson, L., Passant, W., Mann, D. M. A., Neary, D., *et al.* (1994). Clinical and neuropathological criteria for frontotemporal dementia. *Journal of Neurology, Neurosurgery and Psychiatry*, **57**, 416–18.

Byrne, E. J., Lennox, G., Lowe J., and Reynolds, G. (1990). Diffuse Lewy body disease: the clinical features. *Advances in Neurology*, **53**, 283–6.

Chen, C. P. L-H., Alder, J. T., Bowen, D. M., Esivi, M. M., McDonald, B., Hope, T. *et al.* (1996). Presynaptic serotonergic markers in community-acquired cases of Alzheimer's disease: correlations with depression, and neuroleptic medication. *Journal of Neurochemistry*, **66**, 1592–8.

Clarke, R., Smith, A.D., Jobst, K. A., Refsum, H., Sutton, L., and Ueland, P. M. (1998). Folate, vitamin B**12**, and serum total homocysteine levels in confirmed Alzheimer disease. *Archives of Neurology*, **55**, 1449–55. [See comments.]

Churchyard, A. and Lees, A. J. (1997). The relationship between dementia and direct involvement of the hippocampus and amygdala in Parkinson's disease. *Neurology*, **49**, 1570–6.

Cullen, K. M., Halliday, G. M., Caine, D., and Kril, J. J. (1997). The nucleus basalis (Ch4) in the alcoholic Wernicke–Korsakoff syndrome: reduced cell number in both amnesic and non-amnesic patients. *Journal of Neurology, Neurosurgery and Psychiatry*, **63**, 315–20.

Darnell, R. B. (1996). Onconeural antigens and the paraneoplastic neurological disorders: at the intersection of cancer, immunity, and the brain (Review). *Proceedings of the National Academy of Sciences, USA*, **93**, 4529–36.

De Armond, J. S. and Prusiner, S. B. (1995). Etiology, and pathogenesis of prion diseases. *American Journal of Pathology*, **146**, 785–811.

Del Ser, T., Bermejo, F., Portera, A., Arredondo, J. M., Bouras, C. and Constantinides, J. (1990). Vascular dementia: a clinico-pathological study. *Journal of Neurological Science*, **96**, 1–17.

Esiri, M. M.(1996). The basis of behavioural disturbances in dementia. *Journal of Neurology, Neurosurgery and Psychiatry*, **61**, 127–30. [Editorial]

Esiri, M. M.(1997). Hydrocephalus. In *Neuropathology of dementia* (ed. M. M. Esiri and J. H. Morris), pp. 332–43. Cambridge University Press.

Esiri, M. M. and Kennedy, P. G. E. (1992). Virus diseases of the nervous system. In *Greenfield's neuropathology* (5th edn) (ed. J. H. Adams and L. W. Duchen), pp. 335–99. Arnold, London.

Esiri, M. M. and Kennedy, P. G. E. (1997). Viral diseases. In *Greenfield's neuropathology* (6th edn) (ed. D. I. Graham and P. L. Lantos), Vol. **2**, pp. 3–63. Arnold, London.

Esiri, M. M., Hyman, B., Beyreuther, K., and Masters, C. (1997*a*). Ageing and the dementias. In *Greenfield's neuropathology* (6th edn) (ed. D. I. Graham and P. L. Lantos), Vol. **2**, pp. 153–233. Arnold, London.

Esiri, M. M., Wilcock, G. K., and Morris, J. H. (1997*b*). Neuropathological assessment of the lesions of significance in vascular dementia. *Journal of Neurology, Neurosurgery and Psychiatry*, **63**, 749–53.

Esiri, M. M., Nagy, Z., Joachim, C., Barnetson, L., and Smith, A. D. (1999). Cerebrovascular disease lowers the threshold for dementia in the early stages of Alzheimer's disease. *Lancet*, **354**, 919–20.

Esiri, M. M., Matthews, F., Brayne, C., and Ince, P. (2001). Pathological correlates of late onset dementia in a multicentre community-based population in England and Wales. *Lancet*. (In press.)

Everall, I. P., Luthert, P. J., and Lantos, P. T. (1993). A review of neuronal damage in human immunodeficiency virus infection: its assessment, possible mechanism and relationship to dementia. *Journal of Neuropathology and Experimental Neurology*, **52**, 561–6.

Förstl, H., Burns, A., Luthert, P., Cairns, N., Lantos, P. and Levy, R. (1992). Clinical and neuropathological correlates of depression in Alzheimer's disease. *Psychological Medicine*, **22**, 877–84.

Graham, D. I. and Lantos, P. L. (ed.) (1997). *Greenfield's neuropathology* (6th edn). Arnold, London.

Gras, P., Creisson, E., Giroud, M., Dumas, R., and Didier, J. P. (1994). Cortico-basal degeneration: a new entity. *Presse Medicale*, **23**, 1772–4.

Hall, T. C., Miller, A. K. H., and Corsellis, J. A. N. (1975). Variations in the human Purkinje cell population according to age and sex. *Neuropathology and Applied Neurobiology*, **1**, 267–92.

Hansen, L. A., Masliah, E., Terry, R. D., and Mirra, S. S. (1993). Plaque-only Alzheimer disease is usually the Lewy body variant. *Journal of Neuropathology and Experimental Neurology*, **52**, 648–54.

Harper, C. (1998). The neuropathology of alcohol-specific brain damage, or does alcohol damage the brain? *Journal of Neuropathology and Experimental Neurology*, 57, 101–10.

Harper, C. and Kril, J. (1987). Are we drinking our neurones away? *British Medical Journal*, **294**, 534–6.

Harrison, P. J. and Pearson, R. C. A. (1989). Olfaction and psychiatry. *British Journal of Psychiatry*, **155**, 822–8.

Heutink, P. (2000). Untangling tau-related dementia. *Human Molecular Genetics*, **9**, 979–86.

Homewood, J. and Bond, N. W. (1999). Thiamin deficiency, and Korsakoff's syndrome: failure to find memory impairments following nonalcoholic Wernicke's encephalopathy. *Alcohol*, **19**, 75–84.

Hurtig, H. I., Trojanowski, J. Q., Galvin, J., Ewbank, D., Schmidt, M. L., Lee, V. M. *et al.* (2000). Alpha-synuclein cortical Lewy bodies correlate with dementia in Parkinson's disease. *Neurology*, **54**, 1916–21.

Hyman, B. T., van Hoesen, G. N., Kromer, L. J., and Damasio, A. R. (1986). Perforant pathway changes and the memory impairment of Alzheimer's disease. *Annals of Neurology*, **20**, 472–81.

Jellinger, K., Danielczyk, K. W., Fischer, P., and Gabriel, E. (1990). Clinicopathological analysis of dementia disorders in the elderly. *Journal of the Neurological Sciences*, **95**, 239–58.

Jobst, K. A., Smith, A. D., Szatmari, M., Molyneux, A., Esiri, M. M., King, E., *et al.* (1992). Detection in life of confirmed Alzheimer's disease using a simple measurement of medial temporal lobe atrophy by computed tomography. *Lancet*, **340**, 1179–83.

Kesslak, J. P., Nalcioglu, O., and Cotman, C. W. (1991). Quantification of magnetic resonance scans for hippocampus and parahippocampal atrophy in Alzheimer's disease. *Neurology*, **41**, 51–4.

Kew, J. and Leigh, N. (1992). Dementia with motor neuron disease. In *Unusual dementias* (ed. M. N. Rossor). Baillière's clinical neurology, Vol. 1, pp. 611–26. Baillière Tindall, London.

Khachaturian, Z. S. (1985). Diagnosis of Alzheimer's disease. *Archives of Neurology*, **42**, 1097–104.

Lennox, G., Lowe, J., Landon, M., Byrne, E. J., Mayer, R. J., and Goodwin-Austen, R. B. (1989). Diffuse Lewy body disease: correlative neuropathology using anti-ubiquitin immunocytochemistry. *Journal of Neurology, Neurosurgery and Psychiatry*, **52**, 1236–47.

Li, F., Iseki, E., Odawara, T., Kosaka, K., Yagishita, S., and Amano, N. (1998). Regional quantitative analysis of tau-positive neurons in progressive supranuclear palsy: comparison with Alzheimer's disease. *Journal of Neurological Science*, **159**, 73–81.

Lorains, J. W., Henry, C., Agbamu, D. A., Rossi, M., Bishop, M., Will, R. G. *et al.* (2001). Variant Creutzfeldt–Jakob disease in an elderly patient. *Lancet*, **357**, 1339–40.

McKeith, I. G., Perry, R. H., Fairbairn, A. F., Jabeen, S., and Perry, E. K. (1992). Operational criteria for senile dementia of Lewy body type (SDH). *Psychological Medicine*, **22**, 911–22.

McKeith, I. G., Fairbairn, A. F., Perry, R. H., and Thompson, P. (1994). The clinical diagnosis, and misdiagnosis of senile dementia of Lewy body type. *British Journal of Psychiatry*, **165**, 324–32.

McShane, R., Keene, J., Gedling, K., Fairburn, C., Jacoby, R. and Hope, T. (1997). Do neuroleptic drugs hasten cognitive decline in dementia? Prospective study with necropsy follow-up. *British Medical Journal*, **314**, 211–12.

McShane, R., Nagy, Zs., Esiri, M. M., King, E., Joachim, C., Sullivan, N. *et al.* (2001). Anosmia in dementia is associated with Lewy bodies rather than Alzheimer's pathology. *Journal of Neurology Neurosurgery and Psychiatry*, **70**, 739–43.

Mann, D. M. A. and Esiri, M. M.(1989). The pattern of acquisition of plaques and tangles in the brains of patients under 50 years of age with Down's syndrome. *Journal of Neurological Sciences*, **89**, 169–79.

Masliah, E., Mallory, M., Hansen, L., DeTeresa, R., and Terry, R. D. (1993). Quantitative synaptic alterations in the human neocortex during normal ageing. *Neurology*, **43**, 192–7.

Matthews, K. L., Chen, C. P. L-H., Esiri, M. M., Keene, J., Minger, S. and Francis, P. T. (2001). Relationship between noradrenergic changes and aggressive behaviour in patients with dementia. *Neurology*. (In press.)

Meier-Ruge, W. (1988). Morphometric methods and their potential value for gerontological brain research. In *Histology and histopathology of the ageing brain, Interdisciplinary topics in gerontology*, Vol. 25 (ed. J. Ulrich), pp. 90–100. Karger, Basel.

Minger, S. L., Esivi, M. M., McDonald, B., Keene, J., Carter, J., Hope, T., *et al.* (2000). Cortical cholinergic deficits contribute to behavioural disturbances in prospectively assessed patients with dementia. *Neurology*, **55**, 1460–7.

Mirra, S. M., Heyman, A., McKeel, D., Sumi, S. M., Crain, B. J., Brownlee, L. M., *et al.* (1991). The consortium to establish a registry of Alzheimer's disease (CERAD). Pt II: Standardisation of the neuropathologic assessments of Alzheimer's disease. *Neurology*, **41**, 479–86.

Mountjoy, C. Q. (1988). Number of plaques and tangles, loss of neurons: their correlation with deficient neurotransmitter synthesis and the degree of dementia. In *Histology and histopathology of the ageing brain, Interdisciplinary topics in gerontology*, Vol. 25 (ed. J. Ulrich), pp. 74–89. Karger, Basel.

Muramatsu, T., Kato, M., Matsui, T., Yoshimasu, H., Yoshino, A., Matsushita, S., *et al.*(1997). Apolipoprotein E epsilon 4 allele distribution in Wernicke–Korsakoff syndrome with or without global intellectual deficits. *Journal of Neural Transmission*, **104**, 913–20.

Nagy, Zs., Esiri, M. M., Jobst, K. A., Morris, J. H., King, E. M-F., McDonald, B., *et al.* (1995). Relative roles of tangles in the dementia of Alzheimer's disease: correlations using three sets of neuropathological criteria. *Dementia*, **6**, 21–31.

Nagy, Zs., Esiri, M. M., and Smith, A. D. (1998). The cell division cycle and the pathophysiology of Alzheimer's disease. *Neuroscience*, **84**, 731–9.

Nicoll, J. A., Burnett, C., Love, S., Graham, D. I., Dewar, D., Ironside, J. W. *et al.* (1997). High frequency of apolipoprotein E epsilon 2 allele in haemorrhage due to cerebral amyloid angiopathy. *Annals of Neurology*, **41**, 716–21.

Pearson, R. C. A. and Powell, T. P. S. (1989). The neuroanatomy of Alzheimer's disease. *Reviews in Neuroscience*, **1**, 101–21.

Peavy, G., Jacobs, D., Salmon, D. P., Butters, N., Delis, D. C., Taylor, M., *et al.* (1994). Verbal memory performance of patients with human immune deficiency virus infection: evidence of subcortical dysfunction. *Journal of Clinical and Experimental Neuropsychology*, **16**, 508–23.

Perry, G., Nunomura, A., and Hirai, K. (2000). Oxidative damage in Alzheimer's disease: the metabolic dimension. *International Journal of Developmental Neuroscience*, **18**, 417–21.

Pohjasvaara, T., Erkinjuntti, T., Ylikoski, R., Hietanen, M., Vataja, R. and Kaste, M. (1998). Clinical determinants of post-stroke dementia. *Stroke*, **29**, 75–81.

Polymeropoulos, M. H., Lavedan, C., Leroy, E., Ide, S. E., Dehejia, A., Dutra, A. *et al.* (1997). Mutation in the α-synuclein gene identified in families with Parkinson's disease. *Science*, **276**, 2045–7.

Poorkaj, P., Bird, T. D., Wijsman, E., Nemens, E., Garruto, R. M., Anderson, L. *et al.* (1998). Tau is a candidate gene for chromosome 17 frontotemporal dementia. *Annals of Neurology*, **43**, 815–25.

Reddy, P. H., Williams, M., and Tagle, D. A. (1999). Recent advances in understanding the pathogenesis of Huntington's disease. *Trends in Neuroscience*, **22**, 248–55.

Regeur, L., Jensen, G. B., Pakkenberg, H., Evans, S. M., and Pakkenberg, B. (1994). No global neocortical nerve cell loss in brains from patients with senile dementia of Alzheimer's type. *Neurobiology of Aging*, **15**, 347–52.

Sahara, N., Tomiyama, T., and Mori, H. (2000). Missense point mutations of tau to segregate with FTDP-17 exhibit site-specific effects on microtubule structure in COS cells: a novel action of R406W mutation. *Journal of Neuroscience Research*, **60**, 380–7.

Schmidt, R., Schmidt, H., and Fazekas, F. (2000). Vascular risk factors in dementia. *Journal of Neurology*, **247**, 81–7.

Smith, M. Z., Nagy, Zs., Barnetson, L., King, E. M-F., and Esiri, M. M.(2000). Coexisting pathologies in the brain: influence of vascular disease and Parkinson's disease on Alzheimer's pathology in the hippocampus. *Acta Neuropathologica (Berlin)*, **100**, 87–94.

Snowden, J. S., Northern, B., and Neary, D. (1987). The subcortical dementias. In *Degenerative neurological disease in the elderly* (ed. R. A. Griffiths and S. T. McCarthy), pp. 157–68. Wright, Bristol.

Spillantini, M. G., Murrell, J. R., Goedert, M., Farlow, M. R., Klug, A., Ghetti, B. *et al.* (1998). Mutation in the tau gene in familial multiple system tauopathy with presenile dementia. *Proceedings of the National Academy of Sciences USA*, **95**, 7737–41.

Strittmatter, W. J., Saunders, A. M., Schmechel, D., Pericak, Vance M., Enghild, J., Salvesen, G. S., *et al.* (1993). Apolipoprotein E: high-avidity binding to beta-amyloid and increased frequency of type 4 allele in late-onset familial Alzheimer disease. *Proceedings of the National Academy of Sciences USA*, **90**, 1977–81.

Tierney, M. C., Fisher, R. H., Lewis, A. J., Zorzitto, M. L., Snow, W. G., Reid, D. W., *et al.* (1988). The NINCDS-ADRDA work group criteria for the clinical diagnosis of probable Alzheimer's disease: a clinicopathological study of 57 cases. *Neurology*, **38**, 359–64.

Toggas, S. M., Masliah, E., Rockenstein, E. M., Rall, G. F., Abraham, C. R., and Mucke, L. (1994). Central nervous system damage produced by expression of the HIV-1 coat protein gp120 in transgenic mice. *Nature*, **367**, 188–93.

Victor, M. (1976). The Wernicke–Korsakoff syndrome. In *Handbook of clinical neurology*, Vol. 28 (ed. P. J. Vinken and G. W. Bruyn), pp. 243–70. Elsevier, Amsterdam.

Victoroff, J., Zarow, C., Mack, W. J., *et al.* (1996). Physical aggression is associated with preservation of substantia nigra pars compacta in Alzheimer's disease. *Archives of Neurology*, **48**, 619–24.

Vonsattel, J-P., Myers, R. H., Stevens, T. J., Ferrante, R. J., Bird, E. D., and Richardson Jr, E. P. (1985). Neuropathologic classification of Huntington's disease. *Journal of Neuropathology and Experimental Neurology*, **44**, 559–77.

West, M. J., Coleman, P. D., Flood, D. G., and Troncoso, J. C. (1994). Differences in the pattern of hippocampal neuron loss in normal ageing and Alzheimer's disease. *Lancet*, **344**, 769–72.

Wilcock, G. K. and Esiri, M. M.(1982). Plaques, tangles and dementia. *Journal of the Neurological Sciences*, **56**, 343–56.

Will, R. G., Ironside, J. W., Zeidler, M., Cousens, S. N., Estibeiro, K., Alperovitch, A. *et al.* (1996). A new variant of Creutzfeldt–Jakob disease in the UK. *Lancet*, **347**, 921–5.

Yamamoto, A., Lucas, J. J., and Hen, R. (2000). Reversal of neuropathology and motor dysfunction in a conditional model of Huntington's disease. *Cell*, **101**, 57–66.

6 Neurochemical pathology of neurodegenerative disorders in old age

Andrew W. Procter

Introduction

The introduction of rational neurotransmitter-based therapies for Alzheimer's disease (AD) in recent years (see Wilkinson 2000 for review) has only occurred after more than two decades of the neurobiological study of this condition. The impetus to this work was the greater understanding of the monoamine and other neurotransmitter systems and the description of the neurochemical pathology of Parkinson's disease which occurred in the 1960s and led to the therapy for this common neurodegenerative condition.

Around that time it also became accepted that the cognitive impairment frequently associated with ageing was due to disorders with specific histological features, rather than being an inevitable part of the ageing process (Corsellis 1962). Furthermore, two conditions appeared to account for the majority of cases of dementia among the elderly: one characterized by cerebral vascular disease, and the other with similar histological features to those described in a patient in her fifties by Alzheimer early in the twentieth century. AD therefore became recognized as a major cause of dementia rather than a relatively rare neurodegenerative disorder causing presenile dementia, and it was one of the first conditions subjected to intensive neurochemical study.

These neurochemical studies have not only been used to provide information about neurotransmitter function, but also about other metabolic processes. The main source of this information in neurodegenerative conditions, including AD, is the study of brain tissue obtained postmortem. However, such studies need to be interpreted carefully and conducted in such a way as to take account of potential artefacts and epiphenomena. The interpretation of studies in AD has been complicated by such confounding factors, and AD therefore provides a model of how the effects of these factors may be taken into account.

The neurochemical study of postmortem brains

Selection of cases

Postmortem neurochemical studies are generally based on a relatively small number of AD subjects. Yet conclusions are drawn from these about patients in general. For such conclusions to be accepted with confidence it is essential that the characteristics of these patients represent those of patients with AD as a whole. This may not always be the case.

Many biochemical studies have been made of patients previously resident in institutions, therefore these studies may have been subject to the inadvertent selection of subjects with prominent behavioural symptoms. For example, the behavioural symptoms of AD are frequently a source of distress to carers and may determine whether patients come to medical attention and the care they subsequently require, so that these patients may be over-represented in hospital postmortem studies. This in turn may well have influenced the apparent biochemical features of the condition (see below and Procter and Bowen 1988; Procter *et al.* 1992). For example, a lowered serotonin (5-HT, 5-hydroxytryptamine) concentration in the frontal cortex at postmortem has been considered a characteristic feature of AD (e.g. Palmer *et al.* 1987*a*). More detailed analysis indicates that this is an oversimplification, and that loss of presynaptic measures of 5-HT innervation may be confined to those subjects who had prominent behavioural disorders in life, such as depression (Chen *et al.* 1996), aggression (Palmer *et al.* 1988), or those who had undergone drug treatment of these disorders (Chen *et al.* 1996). Similar considerations apply to the widespread reduction in 5-HT_2 receptors (Procter *et al.* 1992).

Studies which have been based upon more epidemiologically sound samples (such as that by Hope *et al.* 1997), from subjects assessed during life for the range of clinical features of AD, are likely to be able to resolve these issues and demonstrate which biochemical features are characteristic of AD, and which are those of subsets with particular behavioural syndromes.

Selection of controls

Just as the AD cases examined must represent typical subjects, so the controls must definitely be free of the condition. While it may be relatively easy to ensure they are free from advanced disease, it may be harder to be confident they are free of an early or presymptomatic disorder. If neurochemical changes occurring early in the course of the disease, which may be of possible pathogenic significance, are to be detected, it may be necessary to screen potential control subjects before death to confirm they are genuinely asymptomatic.

Antemortem factors

Studies of many aspects of the biochemistry of human brain have demonstrated an apparent inherent variability compared to the situation in experimental animals. While factors such as age and sex, or drug treatment, must be taken into account, the mode of the patient's death is a factor of particular note, indicated by measures such as the duration of terminal coma (Harrison *et al.* 1991). The precise details of this are rarely available to the biochemist working with postmortem samples, but the pH value of brain tissue homogenates (Yates *et al.* 1990; Kingsbury *et al.* 1995) may be a valid index. Some of the first studies which carefully controlled for some of these factors include those of O'Neill (1991) and Reinikainen (1988) and their colleagues (see also Burke *et al.* 1991).

Cerebral atrophy

Tissue atrophy may confound the interpretation of biochemical data, because the usual practice of reporting results relative to unit mass does not make allowance for any reduction in the volume of brain structure. Therefore, shrinkage or loss of some structures but not of others may lead to reports of an increase in the markers in unaffected structures, such as an increased γ-aminobutyric acid (GABA) content of frontal cortex from Alzheimer biopsy tissue (Lowe *et al.* 1988).

This potentially confounding factor only applies to those studies performed on tissue homogenates. When discrete subcortical nuclei are examined histochemically, biochemical parameters may be related to the total number of cells in the nucleus (Chen *et al.* 2000).

Stage of disease

Although AD is a progressive disorder, this is rarely acknowledged in postmortem studies, which almost invariably examine patients dying at an advanced stage of disease, often after suffering for many years.

It has been possible to study samples removed earlier in the course of the disease, as neocortical tissue is occasionally removed surgically for diagnostic purposes. These samples have been compared with comprehensive control data obtained from neurosurgical procedures in which the removal of neocortical tissue of normal appearance was a necessary part of the surgical procedure (Table 6.1). In general, postmortem studies reveal more extensive and severe neurochemical pathology than is found in biopsy material.

Neurochemical pathology of Alzheimer's disease

In this review the results of studies of tissue obtained by neurosurgery early in the course of the disease will be emphasized and compared to corresponding evidence from postmortem studies, conducted where possible in such a way as to make allowance for some of the other potentially confounding factors discussed above. While the functional activity of any particular transmitter is dependent upon intact postsynaptic effector mechanisms, the results of studies of postsynaptic neurotransmitter receptors will not be described in detail here.

The premise on which the interpretation of studies is based is that if any particular neurochemical finding is to be considered of primary importance in AD, then it should meet two

Table 6.1 Summary of corticopetal and cortical interneuron transmitter pathology (% control values) in Alzheimer's disease

	Temporal cortex		Frontal cortex		Source
	Biopsy	Autopsy	Biopsy	Autopsy	
Acetylcholine					
Synthesis	41	—	47	—	Sims *et al.* 1983
ChAT activity	35	40	36	50	Palmer *et al.* 1987*a*
Choline uptake	57	—	—	—	Sims *et al.* 1983
Serotonin					
Turnover	—	160	—	n.s.	Palmer *et al.* 1987*c*
Release	—	—	51	—	Palmer *et al.* 1987*a*
Concentration	31	51	n.s.	65	Palmer *et al.* 1987*a,c*
Uptake	39	—	—	—	Palmer *et al.* 1987*a*
5-HIAA concentration	44	n.s.	63	n.s.	Palmer *et al.* 1987*a,c*
Carrier index*	—	82	—	—	Bowen *et al.* 1983
Noradrenaline					
Turnover	1700	353	—	n.s.	Palmer *et al.* 1987*b,c*
Release	—	—	n.s.	—	Palmer *et al.* 1987*b*
Concentration	32	48	—	67	Palmer *et al.* 1987*b,c*
Uptake	47	—	—	—	Palmer *et al.* 1987*b*
MHPG concentration	n.s.	n.s.	—	161	Palmer *et al.* 1987*b,c*
Dopamine					
Release	—	—	n.s.	—	Palmer *et al.* 1987*b*
Concentration	n.s.	n.s.	n.s.	n.s.	Palmer *et al.* 1987*b,c*
DOPAC concentration	n.s.	n.s.	n.s.	n.s.	Palmer *et al.* 1987*b,c*
HVA concentration	n.s.	n.s.	n.s.	141	Palmer *et al.* 1987*b,c*
γ-Aminobutyric acid					
Release	n.s.	—	—	—	Smith *et al.* 1983
Concentration	n.s.	n.s.†	145	n.s.†	Lowe *et al.* 1988
GAD activity	n.s.	n.s.†	—	n.s.†	Lowe *et al.* 1988
Somatostatin					
Release	—	—	n.s.	—	Francis *et al.* 1987
Concentration	n.s.	61	n.s.	n.s.	Francis *et al.* 1987

Percentages are given only for values significantly different from controls; n.s. indicates not significant $p > 0.05$; —indicates not determined. *Using [^{3}H]imipramine binding; †matched for agonal status; DOPAC and HVA are dopamine metabolites.

key criteria: first, that it be present in the early stages of the disease; and, second, that the magnitude of that change be correlated with the severity of some clinical or pathological hallmark of the disorder.

The neocortical cholinergic system

The cerebral cortex receives two major distally projecting cholinergic pathways (as reviewed by Mesulam 1995). One pathway originates in the basal forebrain, comprising the nuclei of the septum, diagonal band, and Meynert. This terminates in all areas of the cortex, with particularly dense innervation of the hippocampus, as well as the amygdala. The other pathway originates in the brainstem; and while it particularly innervates the thalamus, it also terminates in selected areas of the cortex, notably the frontal and occipital cortex. This cholinergic projection is thought to have a major role in processes such as attention and arousal. The basal forebrain cholinergic system is thought to have a role in regulating the activity of the entire cerebral cortex and to maintain the cortex in its operative mode (Mesulam 1995; Wenk 1997). The practical manifestation of this is that acetylcholine is thought to have a role in the control of selective attention (Voytko 1996), through affecting discriminatory processes, the reception and evaluation of stimuli, and the modification of cortical responsiveness. Cholinergic mechanisms therefore appear to govern many brain functions associated with different cortical regions such as perception, learning, cognition, and judgement.

In view of what is now known about the role of cholinergic systems in the brain, it is not surprising that the early demonstrations of substantial losses of the enzyme for the synthesis of acetylcholine (choline acetyltransferase, ChAT) from the brains of patients with AD postmortem (Bowen *et al.* 1976; Davies and Maloney 1976; Perry *et al.* 1977*a,b*; Davies 1979; Table 6.1) and antemortem (Bowen *et al.* 1982; Table 6.1) stimulated much subsequent research into this neurotransmitter.

Other evidence has also established a cholinergic deficit as one of the most prominent features of AD. Neuropathological studies have shown that there is usually a considerable loss of the neurons which give rise to cortical cholinergic innervation, the neurons of the nucleus basalis of Meynert (nbM) (Whitehouse *et al.* 1982; Mann and Yates 1982; Nagai *et al.* 1983; Mann *et al.* 1984; Arendt *et al.* 1985), which is associated with a loss in the nucleolar volume of the cells (Mann *et al.* 1984). The observations of neurofibrillary tangle formation in the nbM (Ishii 1966) and cholinergic neurites in senile plaques (Struble *et al.* 1982) suggested a link between the cholinergic system and the pathological features of AD.

Biochemical measures of cholinergic function have shown consistent and extensive losses of those biochemical activities associated with cholinergic terminals. In particular, ChAT activity seems to be reduced postmortem in all areas of the cerebral cortex of patients with AD (Bowen *et al.* 1976; Davies and Maloney 1976; Perry *et al.* 1977*a,b*; Davies 1979; Mountjoy *et al.* 1984). Neurosurgical specimens taken early in the course of the disease confirm this loss of activity and a reduced ability of the tissue to synthesize acetylcholine (Bowen *et al.* 1982; Sims *et al.* 1983).

It is generally accepted that there is probably little alteration in the M_1 subtype of the postsynaptic receptor, at least until late in the disease; and that the M_2 subtype is, at most, only moderately affected (Roberson and Harrell 1997; Perry 2000). However, a consistent finding is the loss of nicotinic receptors (Aubert *et al.* 1992; Perry *et al.* 1995), which has led to the proposition that this may be an early and important aetiological event (Perry 2000).

The magnitude of the cholinergic dysfunction is correlated with the severity both of the cognitive impairment assessed on global measures of cognitive function (Perry *et al.* 1978; Neary *et al.* 1986; Palmer *et al.* 1987*b*) and of the neuropathological changes, including senile plaque formation (Perry *et al.* 1978, 1981; Mountjoy *et al.* 1984) and loss of neurons (Mountjoy *et al.* 1984) especially pyramidal cells (Neary *et al.* 1986). Considerable emphasis has been placed on the significance of this cholinergic deficit, and it has been suggested that this is the primary cause of the dementia in AD (Coyle *et al.* 1983). Other conditions associated with cognitive impairment are also associated with cholinergic pathology, and these include Parkinson's disease, progressive supranuclear palsy, cerebrovascular dementia head injury (Murdoch *et al.* 1998), and dementia with Lewy bodies (DLB) (Samuel *et al.* 1997), independently of the severity of any Alzheimer pathology found incidentally in these cases..

However, doubts have been raised as to the validity of the view that AD is solely a disorder of the cholinergic system. Subsets of patients with dementia have been reported with the typical neuropathological features, yet cortical ChAT activity was not selectively reduced (Palmer *et al.* 1986). Other patients with AD, particularly the elderly, had, at most, only a minimal loss of cholinergic neurons from the nucleus basalis of Meynert (Perry, R. H. *et al.* 1982; Pearson *et al.* 1983). A reduction in the numbers of these basal forebrain neurons which innervate the neocortex and a reduction in cortical ChAT activity of similar magnitude occur in another neurodegenerative condition, i.e. olivopontocerebellar atrophy, yet cognitive impairment in this condition is not prominent (Kish *et al.* 1988). Thus the neocortical cholinergic deficit probably only explains a part of the cognitive decline, as has been suggested by neuropsychological studies into the effects of cholinergic antagonists (e.g. Kopelman and Corn 1988).

The clinical syndrome of AD comprises more than just cognitive impairment, and frequently includes behavioural and psychiatric symptoms such as wandering, aggression, and depression. Although the extent to which these disorders of conduct and personality have been found in AD could be an overestimate, especially in the presenium, these symptoms are almost certainly related to non-cholinergic transmitter pathologies. However, some non-cognitive symptoms may have a cholinergic basis. Visual hallucinations are related to the severity of the cholinergic deficits in DLB (Perry *et al.* 1994), a condition in which the cholinergic deficits are generally more severe and visual hallucinations more common than in AD (Perry *et al.* 1993).

Other corticopetal neurotransmitters

In addition to cholinergic innervation, the cortex receives inputs from at least three other populations of subcortical neurons, each using a different transmitter. Of these, the inputs using noradrenaline and dopamine are relatively unaffected, whereas the situation regarding 5-HT is complex.

Serotonin (5-HT)

As a result of its presence in various structures of the central nervous system, 5-HT plays a role in a great variety of behaviours such as food intake, activity rhythms, sexual behaviour, and emotional states. The serotonergic system is also thought to play a significant role in learning and memory (Meltzer *et al.* 1998; Buhot *et al.* 2000), in particular by interacting with the cholinergic, glutamatergic, dopaminergic, or GABAergic systems.

Biochemical determinations of neurons containing 5-HT in AD have mostly relied on determinations of the concentrations of 5-HT and its major metabolite, 5-hydroxy-indoleacetic acid (5-HIAA), in postmortem samples. The content of these may be reduced in many areas of the neocortex of AD subjects (Cross *et al.* 1983; Gottfries *et al.* 1983; Arai *et al.* 1984; Reinikainen *et al.* 1988), and neurofibrillary degeneration and neuronal loss in the raphe nucleus has been reported (Palmer *et al.* 1988). However, this is by no means a consistent finding, and even in AD brains at autopsy half of the cortical areas may show no selective reduction of presynaptic 5-HT activity.

As discussed above, this discrepancy between studies may partly be explained by the inadvertent selection of cases for which institutional care had been necessary because of their behavioural symptoms. Many of these studies have been based on predominantly hospitalized patients. In an attempt to examine this in an epidemiologically representative sample of AD patients, using a standardized and evaluated method, Chen and colleagues (2000) have studied the frontal and temporal cortex of 20 community-acquired cases of AD and 16 controls matched for age, sex, postmortem delay, and storage. Clinical assessments, including behavioural symptoms, of the AD cases were made once every 4 months during life. Presynaptic serotonergic markers, 5-HT uptake sites (measured by [^{3}H]paroxetine binding), and concentrations of 5-HT and its metabolite, 5-HIAA, were measured in this tissue.

Presynaptic cortical markers of 5-HT neurons were not uniformly affected in AD. Thus, while the density of 5-HT uptake sites in the temporal cortex was significantly reduced (61% of control), there was no significant alteration in the frontal cortex. Similarly, concentrations of 5-HT and 5-HIAA were not significantly reduced in either region. However, the 5-HIAA/5-HT ratio in both regions was increased in AD cases compared with controls. As individual dorsal raphe nuclei (DRN) neurons project diffusely to several areas of the brain and no significant loss of $[^3H]$paroxetine binding was found in frontal cortex, this may provide evidence for some plasticity in the system by the sprouting of remaining serotonergic innervation in a region less affected by the pathological process of AD. Concentrations of 5-HT were unchanged in either area; and, as has been found in other series, the ratio of 5-HIAA to 5-HT was significantly increased in both areas. This has been interpreted as evidence for the increased turnover of 5-HT in surviving serotonergic terminals.

The study of patients assessed for the presence of a behavioural disorder in life by a retrospective review of case notes, indicates that patients judged to be aggressive during life had both a more severe reduction in 5-HT concentration and loss of postsynaptic receptors (Palmer *et al.* 1988; Procter *et al.* 1992). The assessment of behavioural symptoms in this way is potentially unreliable, but compatible results were obtained when patients were assessed prospectively (Chen *et al.* 1996). The number of 5-HT uptake sites, assessed by B_{max} values for $[^3H]$paroxetine binding, was significantly reduced in the frontal and temporal cortex of those AD cases with persistent depression, anxiety, and overactivity. Stepwise multiple regression analysis, including all three behavioural symptoms, revealed that of these, only depression significantly predicted variability of the number of uptake sites. There was no association between 5-HT or 5-HIAA concentrations and any behavioural symptom.

When postsynaptic markers of serotonergic innervation were assessed in the same patients, the density of 5-HT_{1A} receptors was not significantly altered in AD, while the density of 5-HT_{2A} receptors was significantly reduced in both cortical areas compared to controls. This finding is in keeping with the *in vivo* assessment of the integrity of these receptors (Meltzer *et al.* 1999). Postmortem this reduction correlated with dementia severity, and AD cases with severe and persistent symptoms of anxiety were found to have significantly higher 5-HT_{2A} receptor densities compared to non-anxious AD cases.

On the basis of these results it is difficult to assign particular symptoms to pathology in the serotonergic system (Table 6.2), as patients with aggression, depression, and overactivity all showed a loss of $[^3H]$paroxetine binding of comparable magnitude; and antemortem antipsychotic drug treatment was associated with lower concentrations of 5-HT in frontal cortex. In other studies, aggressive behaviour has been linked to more advanced disease (Procter *et al.* 1992), compatible with the view that a loss of 5-HT_2 receptors is a feature of more extensive pathology found towards the endstage of the disorder. Positron emission tomographic (PET) studies of 5-HT_{2A} receptors show these to be unaffected in elderly depressed patients, but reduced in patients with AD whether they are depressed or not (Meltzer *et al.* 1999). Such brain imaging studies potentially offer a method for differentiating the serotonergic basis of non-cognitive symptoms of AD from that of late-life depression (Meltzer *et al.* 1998).

Thus it appears that only at a late stage of the disease is prominent *structural* pathology of the serotonergic neurons found in the cerebral cortex. While earlier, an increased turnover of transmitter within remaining serotonergic terminals may effectively maintain serotonergic activity.

Catecholamines

There are only two postmortem studies of dopamine-β-hydroxylase activity: one indicating reduced activity (Perry *et al.* 1981), and the other finding no change (Davies and Maloney 1976). All other postmortem biochemical studies of catecholaminergic neurons have focused on the concentrations of dopamine and noradrenaline and their respective principal metabolites,

Table 6.2 Summary of relationships between behavioural symptoms and measures of serotonergic innervation in Alzheimer's disease

Measure	Change	Behavioural symptom	Source
Presynaptic			
5-HT concentration	↓	Aggression	Palmer *et al.* 1998
	→	Depression	Chen *et al.* 1996
	→	Anxiety	Chen *et al.* 1996
	→	Overactivity	Chen *et al.* 1996
5-HIAA concentration	→	Depression	Chen *et al.* 1996
	→	Anxiety	Chen *et al.* 1996
	→	Overactivity	Chen *et al.* 1996
Uptake sites	↓*	Depression	Chen *et al.* 1996
	↓	Anxiety	Chen *et al.* 1996
	↓	Overactivity	Chen *et al.* 1996
Postsynaptic			
5-HT_{2A} receptors	↓	Aggression	Procter *et al.* 1992
	↑	Anxiety	Chen *et al.* 1996
	→	Depression	Chen *et al.* 1996
	→	Overactivity	Chen *et al.* 1996
5-HT_{1A} receptors	→	Anxiety	Chen *et al.* 1996
	→	Depression	Chen *et al.* 1996
	→	Overactivity	Chen *et al.* 1996

*Indicates only behavioural symptom to significantly predict variability when other symptoms included in multiple regression analysis.

homovanillic acid and 3-methoxy-4-hydroxyphenylglycol (MHPG). The concentration of dopamine is not reduced (Gottfries *et al.* 1983; Arai *et al.* 1984; Table 6.1), but dopamine metabolite concentrations are reported to be lower in some regions and elevated in others (Gottfries *et al.* 1983; Arai *et al.* 1984; Table 6.1). Not surprisingly therefore there seems to be little relationship between these measures of dopamine innervation and the clinical features of the syndrome (Bierer *et al.* 1993).

The locus coeruleus (LC) is the major nucleus of the origin of noradrenergic fibres in the mammalian brain. Rostral and dorsal LC neurons innervate forebrain and cortical structures, whilst the caudal and ventral neurons project to the cerebellum and spinal cord (Loughlin *et al.* 1982; Waterhouse *et al.* 1983). It has been proposed that this noradrenergic system together with other sympathetic systems yield rapid adaptive responses to urgent stimuli (Aston-Jones *et al.* 1995), although other proposed roles of LC-noradrenaline (NA) neurons include those in sleep, attention, memory, and vigilance.

The LC is known to be significantly damaged in AD (Mann *et al.* 1980; Bondareff *et al.* 1981, 1982; Chan-Palay and Asan 1989), and as a result NA content in the cerebral cortex is decreased (Adolfsson *et al.* 1979; Gottfries *et al.* 1983; Arai *et al.* 1984; Francis *et al.* 1985; Palmer *et al.* 1987*c*). Concentrations of MHPG are unaltered or even elevated (Cross *et al.* 1983; Gottfries *et al.* 1983; Arai *et al.* 1984; Reinikainen *et al.* 1988; Table 6.1), probably reflecting an increased turnover of NA. In the LC itself, alterations in neuronal morphology, neurofibrilliary tangle (NFT) formation, and loss of pigmented NA neurons in topographically distinct regions have been observed (Iversen *et al.* 1983; Chan-Palay and Asan 1989).

The clinical significance of changes in the NA system in AD is not at all clear. Relatively few studies have sought clinical correlates of the LC neuron loss, but the extent of this loss has been reported to relate to disease duration (German *et al.* 1992) and the severity of cognitive decline (Bondareff *et al.* 1981, 1982). Some studies have also found greater LC neuron loss in depressed subjects with AD (Zubenko and Moossy 1988;

Zweig *et al.* 1988; Förstl *et al.* 1992), though this was not confirmed by others (Hoogendijk *et al.* 1999). Preservation of tyrosine hydroxylase-immunoreactive nerve fibres in the cerebellum and an increase in noradrenergic receptors in the cerebellum have been correlated in recent studies to aggressive behaviour in AD (Russo-Neustadt and Cotman 1997; Russo-Neustadt *et al.* 1998).

Cortical interneurons

γ-Aminobutyric acid

Within the cortex there are large numbers of interneurons containing the inhibitory transmitter γ-aminobutyric acid (GABA), often colocalized with one or more of a variety of neuropeptides. The balance of evidence indicates that loss of these substances is not a fundamental characteristic of AD. Postmortem assessment of GABA-releasing neurons has been complicated by artefacts and epiphenomena (Lowe *et al.* 1988). Thus, no change in the activity of the enzyme responsible for GABA synthesis, namely GLU decarboxylase (GAD, glutamic acid decarboxylase), was found in a careful study where AD and control subjects were matched for the nature of the terminal illness (Reinikainen *et al.* 1988). Normal GAD activity and GABA content have been confirmed in cortical biopsy tissue (Table 6.1). Another presynaptic measure of GABA innervation, the GABA transporter GAT-1, was similarly unaltered in AD (Nagga *et al.* 1999). Perhaps not surprisingly, an attempt at treating AD with a GABA agonist was unsuccessful (Mohr *et al.* 1986).

Somatostatin

Many studies have demonstrated that somatostatin-like immunoreactivity (SLIR) is reduced, but this was not confirmed in biopsy samples (Table 6.1). Larger reductions of SLIR and GABA content have been reported in postmortem studies that included only subjects displaying severe histopathology rather than in those where no such selection criteria were employed (Lowe *et al.* 1988). These data have been interpreted as showing that a loss of SLIR is not a hallmark of the disease process; however, other studies have shown a reduction in SLIR, even when other neuropeptides are unaffected (Gabriel *et al.* 1996; Davis *et al.* 1999). The loss of SLIR correlates with the severity of cognitive impairment and may be influenced by apolipoprotein E (Apo-E) (Minthon *et al.* 1997; Grouselle *et al.* 1998). The results of clinical trials with the synthetic somatostatin analogue octreotide are inconclusive: one failed to show improvement in the cognition of AD patients (Mouradian *et al.* 1991), while another demonstrated such an effect (Craft *et al.* 1999).

Other amino acids and neuropeptides

Glycine and taurine are also thought to function as inhibitory neurotransmitters. Their content is unchanged in AD, based on both postmortem and biopsy tissue (Lowe *et al.* 1988, 1990). Cholecystokinin, vasoactive intestinal polypeptide, and neuropeptide Y content are unchanged in AD as are galanin (Beal *et al.* 1988; Gabriel *et al.* 1996) and, possibly, neurons containing corticotropin-releasing factor (DeSouza *et al.* 1986). A difference in selection criteria may also explain why reduced concentrations of neuropeptide Y have been found in some studies but not in others (Beal *et al.* 1986). These discrepancies between studies do seem to be related to the criteria used for selecting postmortem cases, including the severity of the pathological changes, and they emphasize the value of information obtained from studies on biopsy specimens.

Cortical pyramidal neurons

Histological studies

Examination of AD brains almost invariably shows moderate to severe atrophy of the temporal, parietal, and frontal lobes, with ventricular enlargement and sulcal widening, although this is not always accompanied by generalized atrophy (Brun 1983; Esiri 1991). Deep cortical areas within the medial temporal lobe are most markedly atrophied. These include the hippocampus, entorhinal and uncal cortices, parahippocampal gyrus, and the corticomedial amygdala. Primary sensory areas, for example visual cortex (BA 17), and motor cortex are relatively unaffected. The intervening association areas of the parieto-temporal and prefrontal cortex are involved to an intermediate degree (for reviews see Pearson and Powell 1989; Esiri *et al.* 1990). The involvement of an area appears to be related to the closeness of its connection to the entorhinal cortex. Thus those areas with no or only one intervening synapse are severely affected, whereas those separated by more synapses are relatively spared (Esiri 1991). Another observation regarding the regional vulnerability to cell loss and tangle formation, is that those areas of cortex which demonstrate the greatest synaptic plasticity also show the most marked pathological changes (Arendt *et al.* 1998). Within any single cortical area, the distribution of histopathological hallmarks of AD also supports a dependency on connectivity. Cell loss from the frontal and temporal association cortex in AD is primarily a disappearance of pyramidal neurons (Terry *et al.* 1991), and remaining neurons of layer III and V, mainly pyramidal neurons, are sites of tangle formation (Braak and Braak 1985; Pearson *et al.* 1985; Lewis *et al.* 1987). The cells that are lost together with those subject to tangle formation form the majority of cortical efferents (Jones 1984).

An attempt has been made to describe the earliest stages of the disease using autopsy samples (83 brains, but only 32 from patients with a clinical history of dementia). The entorhinal cortex (in particular the transentorhinal region) was considered to be the first area to be affected by neurofibrillary tangles and senile plaques, the histopathological hallmarks of AD (Braak and Braak 1991). Pre-α-neurons were thought to be the first cells to develop neurofibrillary tangles, subsequently the CA1 region of the hippocampus and regions of the temporal neocortex showed the hallmarks. The next stage was considered to be characterized by extensive tangle formation in entorhinal cortex and CA1, with increasing involvement of CA4, subiculum, neocortical association areas, cortical medial nuclei of the amygdala and putamen. Three independent studies indicated that the severity of dementia correlates with degeneration of corticocortical pyramidal neurons in association areas (Neary *et al.* 1986; Palmer *et al.* 1987a; DeKosky and Scheff 1990; Terry *et al.* 1991).

Neurochemistry and histochemistry of glutamatergic neurons

There are difficulties in separating that glutamate (GLU) which subserves a neurotransmitter function from the large metabolic pools. However, a combination of techniques, including histochemistry for GLU and its putative synthetic enzyme and retrograde transport of radiolabelled GLU, has provided strong evidence for a transmitter role for GLU in a number of pathways (Ottersen 1991).

This has been most convincingly demonstrated for corticofugal fibres. Layer V pyramidal neurons, which typically form these pathways, are subject to tangle formation and are lost in AD (Neary *et al.* 1986; Hof *et al.* 1990). There is other evidence that there is some degeneration of the corticostriatal pathway in AD, since [^{3}H]GLU-binding in the striatum was found to increase with tangle count in the temporal cortex (Pearce *et al.* 1984). This was interpreted as indicating denervation supersensitivity.

There is less definitive evidence available to establish a role for GLU as a transmitter of other cortical pyramidal neurons, in particular the corticocortical association and transcallosal fibres (typically found in cortical layers II and III). However, results obtained using a variety of techniques are consistent with GLU being the major neurotransmitter of these groups of neurons.

The temporal and parietal lobes of AD patients may be major and early sites of pathological changes—when assessed by PET these regions showed reductions in glucose metabolism, a measurement in living brain which is sensitive to atrophy (Chawluk *et al.* 1987). Neuropsychological test scores correlated with the PET data (Cutler *et al.* 1985; Miller *et al.* 1987; see also Gustafson *et al.* 1987; Neary *et al.* 1987), with the pyramidal cell counts in layer III (Neary *et al.* 1986), and with the number of synapses in layer III (DeKosky and Scheff 1990). Thus, it is probable that a clinically relevant shrinkage or loss of association fibres occurred from circumscribed (i.e. parietotemporal) areas and that this contributed to an overall reduction in glucose metabolism as assessed by scanning. This view is supported by the finding of prominent cell loss and tangle formation in layer III in postmortem samples of association cortex, but not in primary sensory areas (Braak and Braak 1985; Pearson *et al.* 1985; Hof *et al.* 1990).

Synaptosomal, Na^+-dependent, D-[^{3}H]aspartate uptake (ASP uptake) has been used as a marker of the relative density of GLU nerve terminals. ASP uptake may be reliably measured in tissue from promptly performed autopsies, and in such specimens was found to be reduced by 50% in the temporal cortex of AD patients (Procter *et al.* 1988*b*) thus indicating a loss of GLU synapses. The most likely interpretation is that this reflects a loss of synapses of corticocortical fibres since loss of the cells of origin of these fibres is the major pathology. However, this may be an oversimplification, as a K^+-stimulated release of GLU from tissue prisms of neurosurgical samples obtained early in the course of the disease was not decreased (Smith *et al.* 1983). Later in the disease, tissue atrophy may confound the interpretation of biochemical data expressed relative to unit mass without taking into account the reduction in volume of the brain structure. Thus the release studies in AD are compatible with a coexistent reduced activity of ASP uptake processes *at a neuronal level.*

Both high- and low-affinity uptake systems for GLU and other dicarboxylic amino acids have been demonstrated in brain. The high-affinity mechanisms are thought to be relevant to synaptic function and are temperature-dependent, regionally distributed, enriched in synaptosomal fractions, and driven by a transmembrane sodium gradient. However, uptake systems for GLU are present on both neurons and glia. Molecular characterization of these excitatory amino acid transporter (EAAT) proteins is now possible (Danbolt *et al.* 1990; Arriza *et al.* 1994); distinct cDNAs encoding structurally related EAATs have been identified in the rat, and those expressed in glia appear to be distinct from those in neurons (Shashidharan and Plaitakis 1993; Shashidharan *et al.* 1994*a,b*). Human sequences analogous to those expressed in neurons of other animals (Arriza *et al.* 1994) provide a potential index of glutamatergic cell bodies, free of the effect of glia. Studies of the EAAT proteins and their mRNA have however failed to demonstrate a consistent loss of the neuronal component in AD (Li *et al.* 1997; Beckstrom *et al.* 1999), in contrast to the glial transporter (Li *et al.* 1997).

Studies in human and animal hippocampus have indicated that all the major input and output pathways (except the septohippocampal cholinergic pathway) use GLU as a transmitter (Ottersen 1991). Cell loss and tangle formation in the entorhinal cortex and in CA1 was found in AD patients at postmortem. Indeed, recent evidence from *in vivo* imaging suggests that atrophy of the hippocampus had occurred by the midpoint of the disease process (Kesslak *et al.* 1991). Hyman and colleagues (1987) measured the concentration of GLU in the terminal zone of the perforant pathway and found an 80% decrease in AD specimens. Consistent with this, decreased GLU staining was observed in the molecular layer of the dentate gyrus (Kowall and Beal 1991). Although this latter study did not examine the entorhinal cortex, they noted that GLU and glutaminase immunoreactive pyramidal neurons in the CA fields were decreased in number and that the remaining neurons showed irregular shortening and disorganized dendritic fields. Many also showed tangle formation. These data imply that if the glutamatergic pathways are considered to be involved in memory (see Hyman *et al.* 1990), it follows that the loss of glutamatergic function may contribute to the memory dysfunction in AD. It should be noted that since AD is a slowly progressive disorder these changes seen at autopsy represent the final stages of the disease (see also Braak and Braak 1991).

In summary, there is now accumulating evidence that GLU is the principal transmitter of the corticocortical association fibres and the major hippocampal pathways. Histological and some neurochemical studies indicate that these pathways degenerate quite early in AD. However, the role of glutamate metabolism in glia cells in AD must be clarified before the results of studies of the neurotransmitter function (e.g. Cacabelos *et al.* 1999; Robinson 2000) can be confidently interpreted.

Putative links between neuronal pathology and aberrant protein metabolism

Neurobiological research has emphasized two cardinal features of AD: amyloid deposition, exemplified by senile plaque formation; and tangle formation within, or loss of, subpopulations of cortical pyramidal neurons. No direct link between these features has been established (see Neary *et al.* 1986; Braak and Braak 1991). The distribution of pathology does, however, support the idea that the disease spreads along anatomically well-defined cortical pathways (Pearson *et al.* 1985; Pearson and Powell 1989; Esiri *et al.* 1990) which may share the common property of synaptic plasticity (Arendt *et al.* 1998). Reduced glutamatergic activity may promote the formation of senile plaques (see Bowen *et al.* 1994).

Tau

Hyperphosphorylation of tau protein probably accounts for its abnormal transformation into paired helical filament (PHF) tau, a key constituent of tangles, but the mechanism(s) is not well understood. Activation of a protein kinase that can generate PHF tau may thereby promote tangle formation (Yang *et al.* 1994). Hypoactivity of glutamatergic neurons is also implicated in aberrant mechanisms of tau hyperphosphorylation, since primary cultures of fetal rat cortical neurons contained much lower amounts of PHF-like tau identified with antibody AT8 (Brion *et al.* 1993) when treated with a high (1 mM) concentration of glutamate (Davis *et al.* 1994). It is possible that agents which increase the activity of pyramidal cells (e.g. by stimulating the M_1 receptor) may lead to tangle formation. However, there is little evidence that this is the case: protein kinase C has been demonstrated to phosphorylate tau, but this does not lead to the characteristic shift in electrophoretic mobility associated with PHF tau. Moreover, another kinase implicated in the formation of PHF tau (Brion *et al.* 1993) may be downregulated and inactivated by protein kinase C activation (Goode *et al.* 1992).

Amyloid precursor protein

Protein kinase C-regulated protein phosphorylation almost certainly affects the metabolism of the major component of the extracellular amyloid, the 4-kDa β-amyloid protein (βA4). This is encoded within a much larger protein, the amyloid precursor protein (APP). APP comprises a family of glycoproteins, including APP_{695} and other isoforms with a serine protease inhibitory domain or KPI (APP_{751} and APP_{770}), all derived by alternative splicing. At least two pathways have been described for the processing of APPs. The first is a secretory pathway dependent on protein kinase C, which involves phosphorylation and insertion of APP into the cell membrane followed by cleavage of a large N-terminal fragment (Esch *et al.* 1990; Sambamurti *et al.* 1992). The second is a lysosomal/endosomal pathway which yields small C-terminal fragments, some of which contain the βA4 sequence (Golde *et al.* 1992). The secretory pathway does not appear to yield intact βA4, as the cleavage site is within that sequence (Esch *et al.* 1990; Sambamurti *et al.* 1992). By contrast, the secreted βA4 found in cerebrospinal fluid and conditioned culture medium is considered to be derived by lysosomal/endosomal processing of APPs (Haass *et al.* 1992; Seubert *et al.* 1992). It is not yet clear whether the secreted βA4 forms the characteristic β-pleated sheet amyloid found in senile plaques following changes in the extracellular environment (Barrow and Zagorski 1991), or if aberrant intracellular handling or catabolism of APP is responsible (Golde *et al.* 1992). Although various groups have proposed that the mismetabolism of APP and deposition of βA4 is the seminal pathogenic event in AD (Hardy and Higgins 1992), no association has been found between senile plaque formation and dementia score (Neary *et al.* 1986; Terry *et al.* 1991).

Glial cells in culture have been shown to express APP, but do not appear to secrete large amounts of the soluble form (as reviewed by Haass *et al.* 1992). However, pyramidal neurons of both rat and human brain appear to be a major source of APP, and this is localized in granular structures which, at the electron microscope level, appear to be the Golgi apparatus and lysosomes or other secretory granules (as reviewed by Shigematsu *et al.* 1992).

Concentrations of the major species of APP and a protein species putatively identified as a homologous protein, APLP2 (Webster *et al.* 1994), have been determined in two membrane fractions and a soluble fraction of brain tissue from demented patients, collected using techniques designed to minimize autolysis (Procter *et al.* 1990, 1994). These tissue samples were also subjected to an assessment of GABA activity in interneurons (Lowe *et al.* 1988) and of ASP uptake (Procter *et al.* 1988*b*), and ChAT activity in pyramidal neurons. Intercorrelation of all these indices were determined. Allowance could be made for the potentially confounding factors of age, postmortem delay, and duration of terminal coma by the use of multiple regression analysis.

The main finding (Procter *et al.* 1994) is that measures of the integrity of neurons rather than of astrocytes most closely reflect the amount of APP detected. Astrocyte numbers did not correlate with any measure of APP. Measures of APP did show correlations with markers of interneurons; the concentration of GABA was correlated only with APP_{695}. The pyramidal cell indices showed correlations with measures of APP species. In the temporal cortex there were significant correlations between ChAT activity and APP_{695} both in the soluble fraction and in the low-density membranes.

The secretion of APP from pyramidal cells appears to be regulated by neuronal activity, in particular by transmitter transduction mechanisms. Notably this includes muscarinic cholinergic (M_1 and probably M_3) receptor activation (Nitsch 1996), and possibly others which use products of phosphatidylinositol bisphosphate (PIP_2) hydrolysis as second messengers. While there are no drugs presently in routine clinical use that would be expected to *increase* APP secretion, drugs such as lithium or antidepressants are likely either to interfere with PIP_2 recycling or to inhibit neuronal activity by other, possibly similar, mechanisms. Treatment with such drugs would be expected to be associated with lower APP concentrations in ventricular CSF, a finding borne out when this can be examined (Clarke *et al.* 1993). It has been suggested that nicotinic receptor activation may cause increased activity of the secretory pathway and thereby minimize amyloid deposition (Perry 2000), a suggestion supported by postmortem studies (Ulrich *et al.* 1997; Court *et al.* 1998).

The concentration of APP_{751} and APP_{770} was high in the soluble fraction of brain tissue, when the number of pyramidal neurons was low. A loss of pyramidal neurons is likely to reduce excitatory input into the remaining neurons, and, as a consequence, will almost certainly reduce the secretion of APP since this is positively modulated by neuron depolarization (Nitsch *et al.* 1992). This would be compounded by reduced receptor-mediated phosphorylation of APP linked to cholinergic hypoactivity (Bowen *et al.* 1992; Buxbaum *et al.* 1992; Nitsch *et al.* 1992; Webster *et al.* 1993), as occurs in AD. The finding of high concentrations of APP_{695} in the soluble fraction when ChAT activity is low is compatible with this hypothesis.

In subjects with severe pathology, indicated by fewer pyramidal neurons or a low index of interneurons, there are also lower concentrations of APP_{695} in membrane fractions (Webster *et al.* 1994). This is compatible with the hypothesis that the *increase* of APP_{751} and APP_{770} in the soluble fraction in subjects with severe pathology may be due to *functional* changes in APP secretion, as it occurs in spite of an apparent fall in these other measures.

While the precise nature of the neurotoxic process in AD remains to be identified, further work is required to establish whether the intracellular accumulation of soluble APP is toxic or whether the lack of one or both of the secreted forms (Seubert *et al.* 1993) so disrupts normal neuronal integrity as to be the pathogenic agent. Any hypothetical pathological process must address the distribution of lesions and the apparent differential vulnerability of subpopulations of neurons.

Neurotransmitter modulation of cortical neuron activity

The preceding discussion has emphasized that in the cerebral cortex reduced excitatory glutamatergic transmission is due to the loss of some pyramidal neurons and their synapses forming circumscribed association pathways. This reduced transmission may be compounded by reduced excitatory cholinergic modulation. Underactivity of the remaining pyramidal neurons may be directly related to the pathological process by an influence upon APP processing. Drugs that affect neurotransmitter function may be effective in AD, if they enhance the activity of the remaining pyramidal neurons.

Receptor regulation of cortical pyramidal neurons

The excitability of pyramidal neurons of the neocortex is affected by many transmitters, according to *in vitro* electrophysiological studies (as reviewed by McCormick and Williamson 1989). However, such studies have consistently shown that only a proportion of cells respond to a particular drug, which suggests that there is a substantial degree of heterogeneity with respect to the transmitter receptors on pyramidal neurons.

Unilateral intrastriatal injections of volkensin, a retrogradely transported toxic lectin, selectively destroys subpopulations of cortical and hippocampal pyramidal neurons distant from the site of injection (reviewed by Wiley 1992). This leads to a loss of large, infragranular, pyramidal neurons of the rat frontal cortex with preservation of glutamic acid decarboxylase (GAD) mRNA-positive interneurons (Pangalos *et al.* 1991). Intracortical injections cause a subpopulation of corticocortical pyramidal neurons (those with contralateral transcallosal projections) to be selectively destroyed.

The receptors present on cortical pyramidal cells can be identified by the use of such volkensin-induced lesions (Chessell *et al.* 1994). Table 6.3 summarizes the receptor localization based on the radioligand-binding changes demonstrated autoradiographically in rats.

These studies emphasize the potential importance of M_1 receptors for regulating the activity of both corticofugal and corticocortical pyramidal neurons. This is based on the small but *consistent* reductions in the binding of $[^3H]$pirenzipine to M_1 receptors in areas of neocortex that showed pyramidal neuron loss. This work shows that the most selective marker of the subpopulation of corticofugal neurons is the 5-HT_{1A} receptor. Although this does not appear to be true for corticocortical neurons in the rat, an important species difference should be emphasized. In rats 5-HT_{1A} receptors are found in the lower cortical layers, whilst in primates (including man) there is an additional high density in upper layers. This observation suggests that the receptor is enriched on ipsilateral-projecting

Table 6.3 Summary of receptor localization on cortical pyramidal neurons

Receptor	Pyramidal neurons Corticofugal Medial	Lateral	Corticocortical
5-HT_{1A}	++	++	–
M_1	+	±	+
Nicotinic	++	±	+
Kainate	+	–	n.d.
NMDA	+	–	n.d.
$GABA_A$	–	–	n.d.
5-HT_2	–	–	–
Adenosine A_1	–	–	–
$a_{1\ total}$	–	–	n.d.
a_{1b}	–	–	n.d.

Data taken with permission from Chessell *et al.* 1994.
++, Obvious enrichment; +, enriched; ±, some evidence of enrichment; –, no enrichment; n.d. not determined.

corticocortical pyramidal neurons (Francis *et al.* 1993*b*). The receptors present in the greatest numbers are the obvious drug targets for normalizing the activity of these neurons. The most suitable receptors by other criteria are those linked to protein kinase C, and which may avoid the possibility of excitotoxicity. Hence, positive modulation of impulse flow by the M_1 receptor, perhaps in combination with an antagonist of the 5-HT_{1A} receptor-induced hyperpolarization, may represent a promising therapeutic strategy.

Drug effects on pyramidal neuron activity

The action of drugs on pyramidal cell activity may be determined by measuring the release of glutamate by intracerebral microdialysis in anaesthetized rats (Dijk *et al.* 1994*a*). From pyramidal neurons forming the corticostriatal pathway such studies may be used to test the hypotheses described above: i.e. that a selective 5-HT_{1A} antagonist would block the hyperpolarizing effect of endogenous 5-HT on pyramidal neurons in layer V of the rat cortex, and would potentiate the effect of a depolarizing agent such as *N*-methyl-D-aspartate (NMDA). Topically applied NMDA causes a rise in both aspartate and glutamate, which is dependent on coapplied tetrodotoxin. This suggests that depolarization of layer V cortical pyramidal neurons, which form the corticostriatal pathway, underlies this phenomenon. The simplest explanation for this effect is that the compound reduces the resting potential of cortical pyramidal neurons by blocking the action of an endogenous hyperpolarizing transmitter (5-HT), thereby increasing the likelihood that a given cell is depolarized by NMDA. These results indicate that, in the rats, selective 5-HT_{1A} antagonists can potentiate the effect of a depolarizing agent (NMDA) on the activity of glutamatergic pyramidal neurons, as well as facilitate endogenous neurotransmission. These antagonists may therefore be useful for the symptomatic treatment of patients with AD.

An ability to increase glutamate release in this paradigm might indicate a common mode of action of antidementia agents. Physostigmine increased extracellular glutamate, but not aspartate concentrations, in the rat striatum. In contrast, physostigmine added to the perfusion fluid did not affect amino acid concentrations. To obtain evidence that the action of acetylcholine was to positively modulate cortical pyramidal neuron activity via the M_1 receptor, the selective M_1 agonist PD142505–0028 was topically applied to the frontal cortex. Like physostigmine, PD142505–0028 rapidly increased glutamate release in the striatum, whereas telenzepine (an M_1 antagonist) blocked the effect of physostigmine (Dijk *et al.* 1995).

The most likely explanation for the increase in glutamate concentrations in the striatum after peripheral administration of physostigmine is that increased concentrations of acetylcholine in the cortex facilitates neurotransmission in the corticostriatal pathway, resulting from an increased likelihood that a given cortical pyramidal neuron is depolarized by endogenous excitatory amino acids. Although the receptor(s) which mediate this effect need to be characterized in more detail, the observation that PD142505–0028 had an effect not dissimilar from physostigmine indicates that the M_1 receptor mediates at least part of this effect. This is supported by the observation that M_1 receptor activation produces a prolonged facilitation of cortical neurons (McCormick and Prince 1985), rendering them more likely to depolarize following excitatory application of glutamatergic agonists.

One theoretical side-effect of such cognition-enhancing drugs could be excitotoxicity, although this is usually considered in the context of ischaemia, where a massive release of excitatory amino acids may be followed by neuronal degeneration. Moreover, while an increase in glutamate might be viewed as potentially excitotoxic in normal individuals, cholinomimetics would be acting to ameliorate *decreased* glutamate release in AD. In addition, the role of glucose in glutamate excitotoxicity has to be considered. Studies using the PET technique indicate that glucose utilization is relatively more impaired than oxygen metabolism in AD (e.g. Fukuyama *et al.* 1994), and the quantity of the glucose transporter in Alzheimer's brains is reported to be reduced compared with normal controls (Simpson *et al.* 1994). Experimental studies in the rat indicate that glutamate loses most of its excitotoxic capability when glucose concentrations in the brain are reduced to low physiological concentrations (Francis *et al.* 1993*b*; Dijk *et al.* 1994*b*).

Conclusions about AD

Studies of the neurochemical pathology of AD have indicated that abnormalities of relatively few neurotransmitters are obvious early in the course of the disease. This is in contrast to the situation late in the disease, which is usually examined in postmortem tissue. Thus the most reliable and consistent changes are those seen in the cholinergic innervation of the cortex and the cortical pyramidal neurons. Clinically, these changes are generally linked to some aspects of the cognitive dysfunction characteristic in AD. However, it is most likely that it is disorders of other transmitters, especially monoamine neurotransmitters, which cause most of the behavioural and other non-cognitive symptoms.

The likely consequence of the loss of cortical cholinergic innervation and pyramidal cell influences is a functional underactivity of the remaining cortical pyramidal neurons. This is accentuated by the loss of excitatory inputs (such as terminals of cholinergic neurons acting via the M_1 receptor), and by the functional preservation of inhibitory inputs such as serotonergic neurons (acting via 5-HT_{1A} receptors).

Well-designed trials with adequate numbers of subjects showed that cholinesterase inhibitors benefit some patients, expressed either as an improvement in the core deficits of AD, or as a reduced rate of deterioration (Francis *et al.* 1995; Wilkinson 2000). However, as only few patients benefit greatly, another approach to supplement the deficit in acetylcholine in the AD brain has been to use M_1 agonists such as xanomeline. The results from *in vitro* studies suggest that, in terms of increasing the excitability of cortical pyramidal neurons, selective M_1 agonists could be at least as useful as any improved cholinesterase inhibitor. However, the functional status of the M_1 receptor in AD needs to be clarified (as reviewed by Bowen *et al.* 1995). In view of this it may transpire that the most effective treatment requires polypharmacy. One possible combination would be an M_1 agonist in combination with a 5-HT_{1A} antagonist.

While this strategy is essentially aimed at providing a symptomatic treatment, a serendipitous consequence of enhancing the activity of pyramidal neurons might be to affect the disease process itself by altering the deranged protein metabolism which appears to be at the core of the disease.

Neurochemical pathology of lobar atrophy

As discussed above, AD represents a neurodegenerative disorder with a characteristic clinical syndrome, histological features, and an increasingly well-understood neurochemical pathology. Although the cortical changes are prominent, there are, as has been described above, consistent and important changes in subcortical structures. Any hypothesis as to aetiology must explain the characteristic topographic distribution of the pathology across the cortex, and the apparent selective vulnerability of temporal and parietal regions. It has been suggested that the subcortical changes are secondary to the cortical pathology. If this is the case, comparisons with Pick's disease, where the lesions are primarily frontal and temporal, will indicate the extent to which the corticofugal neurotransmitters are also lost.

Pick's disease was described at the beginning of the twentieth century. It has a characteristic histopathological appearance of swollen neurons with ubiquitin- and/or tau-positive inclusions, as well as widespread and abundant gliosis. There are other forms of frontal lobe degeneration which are not always accompanied by such Pick cells and Pick bodies. In 1987, Brun reported a postmortem study of 158 demented patients, of whom 10% constituted a group without characteristic Pick's or Alzheimer's histopathology, but showing spongiform degeneration with minimal gliosis and no neuronal swellings or inclusions. This group has been termed 'dementia of frontal lobe type' (DFT; Mann *et al.* 1993).

These conditions have not been the subject of as intensive systematic neurochemical study as AD, and initial studies indicate that the neurochemical pathology is distinct (Francis *et al.* 1993*a*; Qume *et al.* 1994, 1995*a,b*; Procter *et al.* 1999). Furthermore, those patients with Pick-type pathology and those with DFT-type pathology may exhibit some neurochemical differences (Qume *et al.* 1995*a,b*; Procter *et al.* 1999).

In a recent study (Procter *et al.* 1999) measures of cholinergic, serotonergic, and glutamatergic innervation were made in frontal, temporal, and parietal cerebral cortex from 10 subjects with Pick pathology, 6 subjects with DFT, and 9 subjects with AD, as well as 28 matched controls.

The most marked difference between the conditions was observed in the cholinergic system (Fig. 6.1). The postsynaptic cholinergic M_1 receptor index ([^{3}H]pirenzepine binding) was unaffected in any of the conditions, whereas ChAT activity was significantly reduced in all areas of the cortex in AD but unaltered in both DFT and Pick's disease.

Both serotonergic 5-HT_{1A} and 5-HT_{2A} receptor indices were significantly reduced in the temporal lobes of all disease groups; and in the frontal lobe in Pick's disease. The 5-HT_{2A} receptor index alone was significantly reduced in the frontal lobes of DFT and parietal lobe of AD (Fig. 6.2).

The kainate receptor index was preserved in all three conditions in the areas studied. This is in contrast to the α-amino-3-hydroxy-5-methyl-4-isoxazole propionic acid (AMPA) and NMDA receptor, both of which were reduced in frontal and temporal cortex of Pick's disease. The AMPA receptor alone was reduced in these areas in DFT. In AD both the NMDA and AMPA receptors

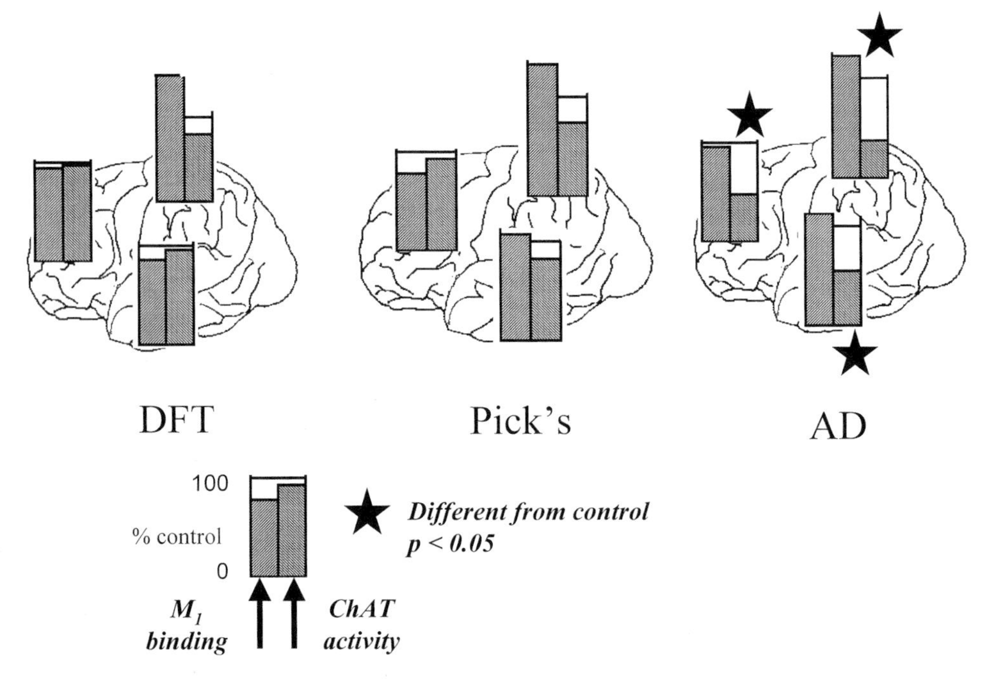

Fig. 6.1 Cholinergic neurochemical measurements in frontal, parietal, and temporal cerebral cortex of subjects with dementia of frontal type (DFT), Pick's disease (Pick's), and Alzheimer's disease (AD). Muscarinic M_1 receptor was determined using 1 nM [^{3}H]pirenzipine displaced by 0.1 mM atropine (Qume *et al.* 1995*a*; Procter *et al.* 1999). Histobars indicate mean percentage of control values. Statistical significant results are indicated as shown. In frontal, temporal, and parietal cortex, ChAT values for the control group were 97 ± 5, 143 ± 9, 93 ± 7 pmol/mg protein/min, respectively, and M_1 receptor-binding values were 9.5 ± 0.9, 13.6 ± 1.1, 9.5 ± 1.2 fmol/mg protein.

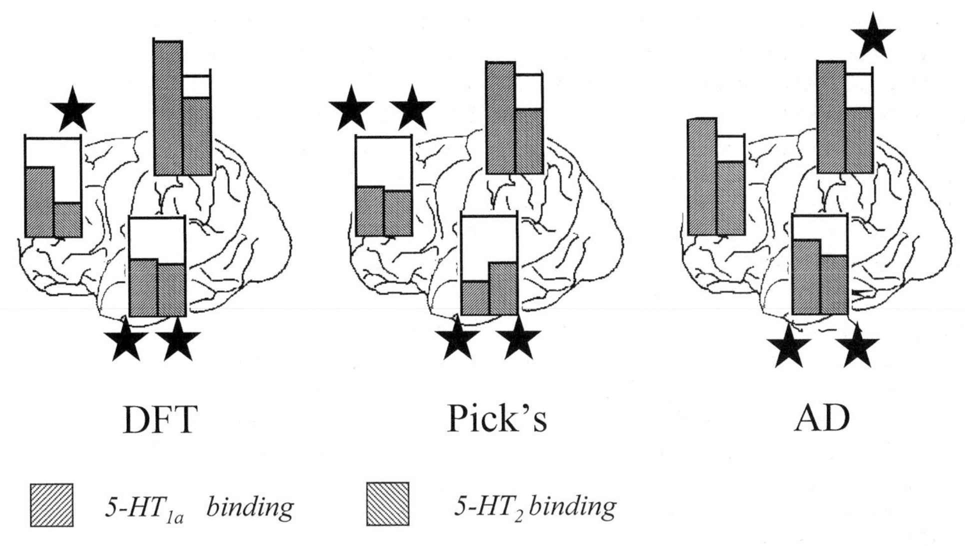

Fig. 6.2 Serotonergic receptor binding in frontal, parietal, and temporal cerebral cortex of subjects with dementia of frontal type (DFT), Pick's disease (Pick's), and Alzheimer's disease (AD), from (Procter *et al.* 1999). 5-HT_{1A} receptors were determined using 2 nM [^{3}H]8-hydroxy-*N*,*N*-dipropyl-2-aminotetraline (8-OH-DPAT), displaced by 10 mM 5-HT (Middlemiss *et al.* 1986); and 5-HT_{2A} receptors using 2 nM [^{3}H]ketanserin, displaced by 10 mM mianserin (Procter *et al.* 1988*a*). Histobars indicate mean percentage of control values with statistical significant results indicated as shown as in Fig. 6.1. In frontal, temporal, and parietal cortex, 5-HT_{1A} receptor-binding values for the control group were 34 ± 4, 44 ± 4, 50 ± 3 pmol/mg protein/min, respectively, and 5-HT_{2A} receptor-binding values were 74 ± 8, 64 ± 5, 92 ± 7 fmol/mg protein.

were reduced in the parietal lobe, the NMDA receptor alone in the temporal lobe and the AMPA receptor alone in the frontal lobe (Figure 6.3).

This study, like the vast majority of neurochemical studies of neurodegenerative conditions, has employed the technique of expressing results relative to unit mass of tissue. The effect of loss of brain tissue may therefore complicate the interpretation of results, whereby shrinkage or loss of some structures but not others may lead to the apparent increase in markers of unaffected structures. Where apparent losses of a marker are observed from a region of brain, that reduction may be an underestimate of the true extent of loss. This argument assumes, however, that the relationship between the cell and its marker remains constant.

The most striking difference is in the cholinergic system. Neither presynaptic innervation indicated by ChAT activity, nor the postsynaptic receptor measured were altered in Pick's disease. This argues that there is unlikely to be a role of cholinergic deficiency in the pathogenesis of the cognitive features of Pick's disease or DFT. In AD, where the histological lesions are most severe in the temporal and parietal lobes, the loss of serotonergic receptors reflects this distribution of pathology. The situation with the glutamate receptors is less clear as there is loss of the AMPA receptor from frontal cortex. Clinically, the parietal lobes are relatively unaffected in the lobar atrophies. As would therefore be expected, these present neurochemical studies show that few measures are altered in the parietal cortex in Pick's disease.

Histological and clinical studies of Pick's disease show lesions of the frontal and temporal cortices associated with a loss of pyramidal neurons. These neurochemical studies also indicate this distribution of pathology. It has previously been proposed that glutamate receptors and 5-HT_{1A} receptors are enriched on pyramidal cells (see above and Pangalos *et al.*

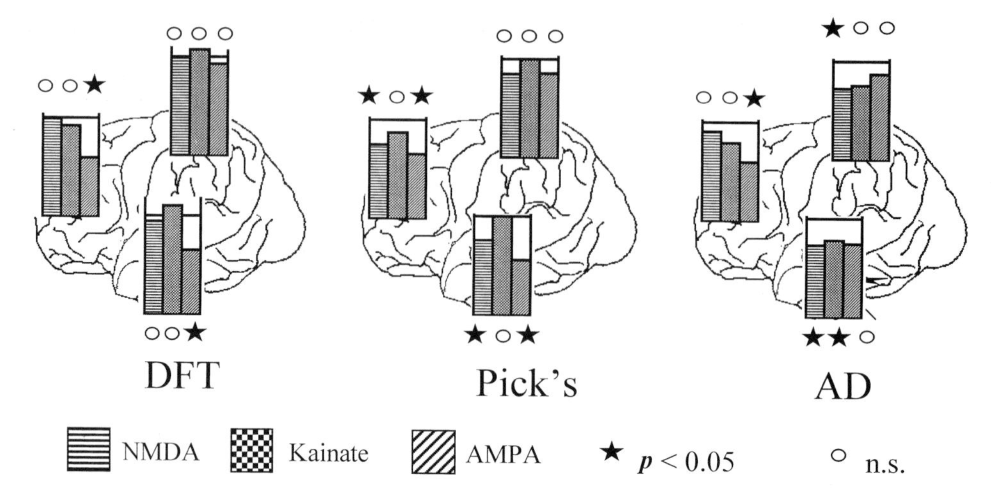

Fig. 6.3 Glutamatergic receptor binding in frontal, parietal, and temporal cerebral cortex of subjects with dementia of frontal type (DFT), Pick's disease (Pick's), and Alzheimer's disease (AD) (Procter *et al.* 1999). NMDA receptors were determined using 5 nM [^{3}H]dizocilpine, displaced with 10 mM dizocilpine (Procter *et al.* 1988*a*); AMPA receptors using 2 nM [^{3}H]6-cyano-7-nitroquinoxaline-2,3-dione (CNQX), displaced with 0.7 mM glutamate (Qume *et al.* 1995*a*); and kainate receptors using 2.5 nM [^{3}H]kainic acid, displaced by 100 mM kainic acid (Qume *et al.* 1995*a*). Histobars indicate mean percentage of control values with statistical significant results indicated as shown as in Fig. 6.1. In frontal, temporal, and parietal cortex NMDA receptor-binding values for the control group were 213 ± 11, 286 ± 16, 318 ± 12 pmol/mg protein/min, respectively; kainate receptor-binding values were 39 ± 3, 19 ± 2, 15 ± 1 fmol/mg protein and AMPA receptor-binding values were 67 ± 6, 94 ± 7, 84 ± 2 fmol/mg protein.

1991, 1992) and thus represent a neurochemical marker for these cells. These receptors are reduced in these areas in both conditions. However, loss of the NMDA receptor is a feature of only Pick-type lobar atrophy. This may be due to a selective loss of only a subpopulation of cells in the DFT, and suggests that there may be more scope for remedial treatments to enhance the activity of the remaining cells

A serotonergic basis for aspects of the behavioural symptoms of lobar atrophy has been suggested (Anderson *et al.* 1995; Miller *et al.* 1997). Preliminary data on presynaptic measures of 5-HT innervation indicate there is no loss (Qume *et al.* 1995*b*), thus any role of this transmitter in the pathogenesis of these symptoms has to be by way of loss of the postsynaptic elements—most probably pyramidal cells. As has been described above, this is in marked contrast to the situation in AD where serotonergic pathology appears to be associated with behavioural disturbance.

Conclusions

It is generally assumed that the neurochemical study of postmortem brain tissue reveals information of relevance to the understanding of that condition in life. However, many factors need to be considered for this to be a valid assumption. It is probably true to say that the rigorous demonstration of reliability and validity normally expected in many other areas of psychiatry are rarely applied to biological measures. When these are applied, studies of the neurochemical pathology of AD have indicated that early in the course of the disease relatively few neurotransmitters show obvious abnormalities. This is in contrast to the situation late in the disease, which is usually examined in postmortem tissue. Thus the most reliable and consistent changes are those seen in the cholinergic innervation of the cortex and the cortical pyramidal neurons. However, by the time of death, there is usually considerable involvement of other neurons.

The likely consequence of this is that early in the disease there may be a functional underactivity of the remaining cortical pyramidal neurons and excitatory inputs due to loss of excitatory inputs, such as terminals of cholinergic neurons acting via the M_1 receptor. In addition, there may be functional preservation of inhibitory inputs such as serotonergic neurons acting via 5-HT_{1A} receptors.

The state of knowledge about lobar atrophy is rudimentary compared to that of AD. However, confounding factors which confused the interpretation of studies of AD can be addressed in lobar atrophy, and initial studies of this latter condition indicate a relatively selective lesion of cortical pyramidal neurons. The basis of the usually severe behavioural symptoms in this condition does not appear to be associated with a serotonergic lesion—in distinction to the apparent situation in AD. However, in both conditions the precise nature of the pathogenic process and the mechanism whereby the lesion remains apparently confined to selected populations of pyramidal neurons is unknown.

Acknowledgements

I am grateful to many colleagues for helpful discussions during the preparation of this chapter. In particular Professor D. M. Bowen and Drs P. T. Francis, M. Qume, and C. Chen. I also wish to thank Professor D. Neary, and Drs B. Doshi, M. Esiri, T. Hope, B. McDonald, D. Mann, and J. Snowden for the collection and classification of samples.

References

Adolfsson, R., Gottfries, C. G., Roos, B. E., and Winblad, B. (1979). Changes in brain catecholamines in patients with dementia of Alzheimer type. *British Journal of Psychiatry*, **135**, 216–23.

Anderson, I. M., Scott, K., and Harborne, G. (1995). Serotonin and depression in frontal lobe dementia. *American Journal of Psychiatry*, **152**, 645.

Arai, H., Kosaka, K., and Iizuka, R. (1984). Changes of biogenic amines and their metabolites in postmortem brains from patients with Alzheimer-type dementia. *Journal of Neurochemistry*, **43**, 388–93.

Arendt, T., Bigl, V., Tennstedt, A., and Arendt, A. (1985). Neuronal loss in different parts of the nucleus basalis is related to neuritic plaque formation in cortical target areas in Alzheimer's Disease. *Neuroscience*, **14**, 1–14.

Arendt, T., Bruckner, M. K., Gertz, H. J., and Marcova, L. (1998). Cortical distribution of neurofibrillary tangles in Alzheimer's disease matches the pattern of neurons that retain their capacity of plastic remodelling in the adult brain. *Neuroscience*, **83**, 991–1002.

Arriza, J. L., Fairman, W. A., Wadiche, J. I., Murdoch, G. H., Kavanaugh, M. P., and Amara, S. G. (1994). Functional comparisons of three glutamate transporter subtypes cloned from human motor cortex. *Journal of Neuroscience*, **14**, 5559–69.

Aston-Jones, G., Shipley, M. T., and Grazanna, R. (1995). The locus coeruleus, A5 and A7 noradrenergic cell groups. In *The rat nervous system* (ed. G. Paxinos), pp. 183–213. Academic Press, Sydney.

Aubert, I., Araujo, D. M., Cecyre, D., Robitaille, Y., Gauthier, S., and Quirion, R. (1992). Comparative alterations of nicotinic and muscarinic binding sites in Alzheimer's and Parkinson's diseases. *Journal of Neurochemistry*, **58**, 529–41.

Barrow, C. J. and Zagorski, M. G. (1991). Solution structures of beta-peptide and its constituent fragments: relation of amyloid deposition. *Science*, **253**, 179–82.

Beal, M. F., McAllister, V. L., Chattha, G. K., Svendsen, C. N., Bird, E. D., and Martin, J. B. (1986). Neuropeptide Y immunoreactivity is reduced in cerebral cortex in Alzheimer's disease. *Annals of Neurology*, **20**, 282–8.

Beal, M. F., Clevens, R. A., Chatta, G. K., MacGarvey, M. U., Mazurek, M. F., and Gabriel, S. M. (1988). Galanin-like immunoreactivity is unchanged in Alzheimer's disease. *Journal of Neurochemistry*, **51**, 1935–41.

Beckstrom, H., Julsrud, L., Haugeto, O., Dewar, D., Graham, D. I., Lehre, K. P., *et al.* (1999). Interindividual differences in the levels of the glutamate transporters GLAST and GLT, but no clear correlation with Alzheimer's disease. *Journal of Neuroscience Research*, **55**, 218–29.

Bierer, L. M., Knott, P. J., Schmeidler, J. M., Marin, D. B., Ryan, T. M., Haroutunian, V., *et al.* (1993). Post-mortem examination of dopaminergic parameters in Alzheimer's disease: relationship to noncognitive symptoms. *Psychiatry Research*, **49**, 211–17.

Bondareff, W., Mountjoy, C. Q., and Roth, M. (1981). Selective loss of neurones of origin of adrenergic projection to cerebral cortex (nucleus locus coeruleus) in senile dementia. *Lancet*, **i**, 783–4.

Bondareff, W., Mountjoy, C. Q., and Roth, M. (1982). Loss of neurons of origin of the adrenergic projection to cerebral cortex (nucleus locus coeruleus) in senile dementia. *Neurology*, **32**, 164–8.

Bowen, D. M., Smith, C. B., White, P., and Davison, A. N. (1976). Neurotransmitter-related enzymes and indices of hypoxia in senile dementia and other abiotrophies. *Brain*, **99**, 459–96.

Bowen, D. M., Benton, J. S., Spillane, J. A., Smith, C. C., and Allen, S. J. (1982). Choline acetyltransferase activity and histopathology of frontal neocortex from biopsies of demented patients. *Journal of the Neurological Sciences*, **57**, 191–202.

Bowen, D. M., Allen, S. J., Benton, J. S., Goodhardt, M. J., Haan, E. A., Palmer, A. M. *et al.* (1983). Biochemical assessment of serotonergic and cholinergic dysfunction and cerebral atrophy in Alzheimer's disease. *Journal of Neurochemistry*, **41**, 266–72.

Bowen, D. M., Francis, P. T., Sims, N. R., and Cross, A. J. (1992). Protection from dementia. *Science*, **258**, 1422–3.

Bowen, D. M., Francis, P. T., Chessell, I. P., and Webster, M.-T. (1994). Neurotransmission—the link integrating Alzheimer's research. *Trends in Neurosciences*, **17**, 149–50.

Bowen, D. M., Francis, P. T., Chessell, I. P., Webster, M.-T., Procter, A. W., Chen, C. P. L., *et al.* (1995). Alzheimer's disease: is the improvement of cholinergic transmission the correct strategy ? In *Alzheimer's disease: clinical and treatment aspects* (ed. N. R. Cutler, C. G. Gottfries, and K. R. Siegfried), pp. 89–116. Wiley, Chichester.

Braak, H. and Braak, E. (1985). On areas of transition between entorhinal allocortex and temporal isocortex in the human brain. Normal morphology and lamina-specific pathology in Alzheimer's disease. *Acta Neuropathologica*, **68**, 325–32.

Braak, H. and Braak, E. (1991). Neuropathological stageing of Alzheimer's disease. *Acta Neuropathologica*, **82**, 239–59.

Brion, J., Smith, C., Couck, A., Gallo, J., and Anderton, B. H. (1993). Developmental changes in tau phosphorylation: fetal tau is transiently phosphorylated in a manner similar to paired helical filament-tau characteristic of Alzheimer's disease. *Journal of Neurochemistry*, **61**, 2071–80.

Brun, A. (1983). An overview of light and electron microscopic changes. In *Alzheimer's disease: the standard reference* (ed. B. Reisberg), pp. 37–47. Free Press, New York.

Brun, A. (1987). Frontal lobe degeneration of non-Alzheimer type 1. Neuropathology. *Archives of Gerontology and Geriatrics*, **6** 193–208.

Buhot, M. C., Martin, S., and Segu, L. (2000). Role of serotonin in memory impairment. *Annals of Medicine*, **32**, 210–21. [Review] [125 refs]

Burke, W. J., Omalley, K. L., Chung, H. D., Harmon, S. K., Miller, J. P., and Berg, L. (1991). Effect of pre-mortem and post-mortem variables on specific messenger RNA levels in human brain. *Molecular Brain Research*, **1**, 37–41.

Buxbaum, J. D., Oishi, M., Chen, H. I., Pinkas-Kramarski, P., Jaffe, E. A., Gandy, S. E., *et al.* (1992). Cholinergic agonists and interleukin 1 regulate processing and secretion of the Alzheimer beta/A4 amyloid protein. *Proceedings of the National Academy of Science USA*, **89**, 10075–8.

Cacabelos, R., Takeda, M., and Winblad, B. (1999). The glutamatergic system and neurodegeneration in dementia: preventive strategies in Alzheimer's disease. *International Journal of Geriatric Psychiatry*, **14**, 3–47. [Review] [228 refs]

Chan-Palay, V. and Asan, E. (1989). Alterations in catecholaminergic neurones of the locus coeruleus in senile dementia of the Alzheimer type and in Parkinson's disease and amyotropic lateral sclerosis. *Journal of Comparative Neurology*, **287**, 373–92.

Chawluk, J. B., Alavi, A., Dann, R., Hurtig, H. I., Bais, S., Kushner, M. J., *et al.* (1987). Positron emission tomography in aging and dementia: effect of cerebal atrophy. *Journal of Nuclear Medicine*, **28**, 431–7.

Chen, C. P. L., Alder, J. T., Bowen, D. M., Esiri, M. M., McDonald, B., Hope, T., *et al.* (1996). Presynaptic serotonergic markers in community-acquired cases of Alzheimer's disease: correlations with depression and neuroleptic medication. *Journal of Neurochemistry*, **66**, 1592–8.

Chen, C. P., Eastwood, S. L., Hope, T., McDonald, B., Francis, P. T., and Esiri, M. M. (2000). Immunocytochemical study of the dorsal and median raphe nuclei in patients with Alzheimer's disease prospectively assessed for behavioural changes. *Neuropathology and Applied Neurobiology*, **26**, 347–55.

Chessell, I. P., Francis, P. T., Webster, M.-T., Procter, A. W., Heath, P. R., Pearson, R. C. A., *et al.* (1994). An aspect of Alzheimer neuropathology after suicide transport damage. *Journal of Neural Transmission Supplement*, **44**, 231–43.

Clarke, N. A., Webster, M.-T., Francis, P. T., Procter, A. W., Hodgkiss, A. D., and Bowen, D. M. (1993). Beta-amyloid precursor protein-like immunoreactivity can be altered in humans by drugs affecting neurotransmitter function. *Neurodegeneration*, **2**, 243–8.

Corsellis, J. A. N. (1962). *Mental illness and the aging brain.* Oxford University Press, Oxford:

Court, J. A., Lloyd, S., Thomas, N., Piggott, M. A., Marshall, E. F., Morris, C. M., *et al.* (1998). Dopamine and nicotinic receptor binding and the levels of dopamine and homovanillic acid in human brain related to tobacco use. *Neuroscience*, **87**, 63–78.

Coyle, J. T., Price, D. L., and DeLong, M. R. (1983). Alzheimer's disease: a disorder of cortical cholinergic innervation. *Science*, **219**, 1184–90.

Craft, S., Asthana, S., Newcomer, J. W., Wilkinson, C. W., Matos, I. T., Baker, L. D., *et al.* (1999). Enhancement of memory in Alzheimer disease with insulin and somatostatin, but not glucose. *Archives of General Psychiatry*, **56**, 1135–40.

Cross, A. J., Crow, T. J., Johnson, J. A., Joseph, M. H., Perry, E. K., Perry, R. H., *et al.* (1983). Monoamine metabolism in senile dementia of Alzheimer type. *Journal of the Neurological Sciences*, **60**, 383–92.

Cutler, N. R., Haxby, J. V., Duara, R., Grady, C. L., Kay, A. D., Kessler, R. M., *et al.* (1985). Clinical history, brain metabolism, and neuropsychological function in Alzheimer's disease. *Annals of Neurology*, **18**, 298–309.

Danbolt, N. C., Pines, G., and Kanner, B. I. (1990). Purification and reconstitution of the sodium- and potassium-coupled glutamate transport glycoprotein from rat brain. *Biochemistry*, **29**, 6734–40.

Davies, P. (1979). Neurotransmitter-related enzymes in senile dementia of the Alzheimer type. *Brain Research*, **171**, 319–27.

Davies, P. and Maloney, A. J. F. (1976). Selective loss of central cholinergic neurons in Alzheimer's disease. *Lancet*, **ii**, 1403.

Davis, D. R., Brion, J., Couck, A., and Other, A. N. (1994). Glutamate and colchicine cause dephosphorylation of the microtubule associated protein tau and a change in perikaryal tau immunoreactivity. *Brain Research Association*, **11**, 38 (abstract).

Davis, K. L., Mohs, R. C., Marin, D. B., Purohit, D. P., Perl, D. P., Lantz, M., *et al.* (1999). Neuropeptide abnormalities in patients with early Alzheimer disease. *Archives of General Psychiatry*, **56**, 981–7. [See comments.]

DeKosky, S. and Scheff, S. W. (1990). Synapse loss in frontal cortex biopsies in Alzheimer's disease: correlation with cognitive severity. *Annals of Neurology*, **27**, 457–64.

DeSouza, E. B., Whitehouse, P. J., Kuhar, M. J., Price, D. L., and Vale, W. V. (1986). Reciprocal changes in corticotropin releasing factor (CRF)-like immunoreactivity and CRF receptors in cerebral cortex of Alzheimer's disease. *Nature*, **319**, 593–5.

Dijk, S. N., Francis, P. T., and Bowen, D. M. (1994*a*). NMDA-induced glutamate release from rat cortical pyramidal neurones is potentiated by a 5-HT_{1a} antagonist. *British Journal of Pharmacology*, **112**, 10P (abstract).

Dijk, S. N., Krop-Van Gastel, W., Obrenovitch, T. P., and Korf, J. (1994*b*). Food deprivation protects the rat striatum against hypoxia-ischaemia despite high extracellular glutamate. *Journal of Neurochemistry*, **62**, 1847–51.

Dijk, S. N., Francis, P. T., Stratmann, G. C., and Bowen, D. M. (1995). Cholinomimetics increase glutamate outflow by action of the corticostriate pathway: implications for Alzheimer's disease. *Journal of Neurochemistry*, **115**, 1169–74.

Esch, F. S., Keim, P. S., Beattie, E. C., Blacher, R. W., Culwell, A. R., Oltersdorf, T., *et al.* (1990). Cleavage of amyloid beta peptide during constitutive processing of its precursor. *Science*, **248**, 1122–4.

Esiri, M. M. (1991). Neuropathology. In *Psychiatry in the elderly* (ed. R. Jacoby and C. Oppenheimer), pp. 113–47. Oxford University Press, Oxford.

Esiri, M. M., Pearson, R. C., Steele, J. E., Bowen, D. M., and Powell, T. P. (1990). A quantitative study of the neurofibrillary tangles and the choline acetyltransferase activity in the cerebral cortex and the amygdala in Alzheimer's disease. *Journal of Neurology, Neurosurgery and Psychiatry*, **53**, 161–5.

Förstl, H., Burns, A., Luthert, P., Cairns, N., Lantos, P., and Levy, R. (1992). Clinical and neuropathological correlates of depression in Alzheimer's disease. *Psychological Medicine*, **22**, 877–84.

Francis, P. T., Palmer, A. M., Sims, N. R., Bowen, D. M., Davison, A. N., Esiri, M. M., *et al.* (1985). Neurochemical studies of early-onset Alzheimer's disease. Possible influence on treatment. *New England Journal of Medicine*, **313**, 7–11.

Francis, P. T., Bowen, D. M., Lowe, S. L., Neary, D., Mann, D. M., and Snowden, J. S. (1987). Somatostatin content and release measured in cerebral biopsies from demented patients. *Journal of the Neurological Sciences*, **78**, 1–16.

Francis, P. T., Holmes, C., Webster, M.-T., Stratmann, G. C., Procter, A. W., and Bowen, D. M. (1993*a*). Preliminary neurochemical findings in non-Alzheimer dementia due to lobar atrophy. *Dementia*, **4**, 172–7.

Francis, P. T., Sims, N. R., Procter, A. W., and Bowen, D. M. (1993*b*). Cortical pyramidal neurone loss may cause glutamatergic hypoactivity and cognitive impairment in Alzheimer's disease: investigative and therapeutic perspectives. *Journal of Neurochemistry*, **60**, 1589–603.

Francis, P. T., Chessell, I. P., Webster, M.-T., Clarke, N. A., Procter, A. W., Alder, J. T., *et al.* (1995). Is improvement of cholinergic transmission the correct strategy in Alzheimer's disease? In *Recent advances in Alzheimer's disease and related disorders* (ed. K. Iqbal, J. A. Mortimer, and B. Winblad), pp. 273–81. Wiley, Chichester.

Fukuyama, H., Ogawa, M., Yamauchi, H., Yamaguchi, S., Kimura, J., Yonekura, Y., *et al.* (1994). Altered cerebral energy metabolism in Alzheimer's disease: a PET study. *Journal of Nuclear Medicine*, **35**, 1–6.

Gabriel, S. M., Davidson, M., Haroutunian, V., Powchik, P., Bierer, L. M., Purohit, D., *et al.* (1996). Neuropeptide deficits in schizophrenia vs. Alzheimer's disease cerebral cortex. *Biological Psychiatry*, **39**, 82–91. [See comments.]

German, D. C., Manaye, K. F., White, C. L., 3rd, Woodward, D. J., McIntire, D. D., Smith, W. K., *et al.* (1992). Disease-specific patterns of locus coeruleus cell loss. *Annals of Neurology*, **32**, 667–76.

Golde, T. E., Estus, S., Younkin, L. H., Selkoe, D. J., and Younkin, S. G. (1992). Processing of the amyloid protein precursor to potentially amyloidogenic derivatives. *Science*, **255**, 728–30.

Goode, N., Hughes, K., Woodgett, J. R., and Parker, P. J. (1992). Differential regulation of glycogen synthase kinase-3 beta by protein kinase C isotypes. *Journal of Biological Chemistry*, **267**, 16878–82.

Gottfries, C. G., Adolfsson, R., Aquilonius, S. M., Carlsson, A., Eckernas, S-A., Nordberg, A., *et al.* (1983). Biochemical changes in dementia disorders of Alzheimer type (AD/SDAT). *Neurobiology of Aging*, **4**, 261–71.

Grouselle, D., Winsky-Sommerer, R., David, J. P., Delacourte, A., Dournaud, P., and Epelbaum, J. (1998). Loss of somatostatin-like immunoreactivity in the frontal cortex of Alzheimer patients carrying the apolipoprotein epsilon 4 allele. *Neuroscience Letters*, **255**, 21–4.

Gustafson, L., Edvinsson, L., Dahlgren, N., Hagberg, B., Risberg, J., Rosen, I., *et al.* (1987). Intravenous physostigmine treatment of Alzheimer's disease evaluated by psychometric testing, regional cerebral blood flow (rCBF) measurement and EEG. *Psychopharmacology*, **93**, 31–5.

Haass, C., Schlossmacher, M. G., and Hung, A. Y. (1992). Amyloid beta peptide is produced by cultured cells during normal metabolism. *Nature*, **359**, 322–5.

Hardy, J. and Higgins, G. A. (1992). Alzheimer's disease: the amyloid cascade hypothesis. *Science*, **256**, 184–5.

Harrison, P. J., Procter, A. W., Barton, A. J. L., Lowe, S. L., Bertolucci, P. H. F., Bowen, D. M., *et al.* (1991). Terminal coma affects messenger RNA detection in post mortem human brain tissue. *Molecular Brain Research*, **9**, 161–4.

Hof, P. R., Cox, K., and Morrison, J. H. (1990). Quantitative analysis of a vulnerable subset of pyramidal neurones in Alzheimer's disease: I. Superior frontal and inferior temporal cortex. *Journal of Comparative Neurology*, **30**, 44–54.

Hoogendijk, W. J., Sommer, I. E., Pool, C. W., Kamphorst, W., Hofman, M., Eikelenboom, P., *et al.* (1999). Lack of association between depression and loss of neurons in the locus coeruleus in Alzheimer disease. *Archives of General Psychiatry*, **56**, 45–51.

Hope, T., Keene, J., Gedling, K., Cooper, S., Fairburn, C., and Jacoby, R. (1997). Behaviour changes in dementia. 1: Point of entry data of a prospective study. *International Journal of Geriatric Psychiatry*, **12**, 1062–73.

Hyman, B. T., Van Hoesen, G. W., and Damasio, A. R. (1987). Alzheimer's disease: glutamate depletion in the hippocampal perforant pathway zone. *Annals of Neurology*, **22**, 37–40.

Hyman, B. T., Van Hoesen, G. W., and Damasio, A. R. (1990). Memory related neural systems in Alzheimer's disease: an anatomic study. *Neurology*, **40**, 1721–30.

Ishii, T. (1966). Distribution of Alzheimer's neurofibrillary changes in the brain stem and hypothalamus of senile dementia. *Acta Neuropathologica*, **6**, 181–7.

Iversen, L. L., Rossor, M. N., Reynolds, G. P., Hills, R., Roth, M., Mountjoy, C. Q., *et al.* (1983). Loss of pigmented dopamine-β-hydroxylase positive cells from locus coeruleus in senile dementia of Alzheimer's type. *Neuroscience Letters*, **39**, 95–100.

Jones, E. G. (1984). Laminar distribution of cortical efferent cells. In *Cerebral cortex: Volume 1, Cellular components of the cerebral cortex* (ed. A. Peters and E. G. Jones), pp. 521–53. Plenum Press, New York.

Kesslak, J. P., Nalcioglu, O., and Cotman, C. W. (1991). Quantification of magnetic resonance scans for hippocampal and parahippocampal atrophy in Alzheimer's disease. *Neurology*, **41**, 51–4.

Kingsbury, A. E., Foster, O. J. F., Nisbet, A. P., Cairns, N., Bray, L., Eve, D. J., *et al.* (1995). Tissue pH as an indicator of mRNA preservation in human post mortem brain. *Molecular Brain Research*, **28**, 311–18.

Kish, S. J., Munir, E., Schut, L., Leach, L., Oscar-Berman, M., and Freedman, M. (1988). Cognitive deficits in olivopontocerebellar atrophy: implications for the cholinergic hypothesis of Alzheimer's dementia. *Annals of Neurology*, **24**, 200–6.

Kopelman, M. D. and Corn, T. H. (1988). Cholinergic 'blockade' as a model for cholinergic depletion. *Brain*, **111**, 1079–10.

Kowall, N. W. and Beal, M. F. (1991). Glutamate-, glutaminase- and taurine-immunoreactive neurons develop neurofibrillary tangles in Alzheimer's disease. *Annals of Neurology*, **29**, 162–7.

Lewis, D. A., Campbell, M. J., Terry, R. D., and Morrison, J. H. (1987). Lamina and regional distribution of neurofibrillary tangles and neuritic plaques in Alzheimer's disease: a quantitative study of visual and auditory cortices. *Journal of Neuroscience*, **7**, 1799–809.

Li, S., Mallory, M., Alford, M., Tanaka, S., and Masliah, E. (1997). Glutamate transporter alterations in Alzheimer disease are possibly associated with abnormal APP expression. *Journal of Neuropathology and Experimental Neurology*, **56**, 901–11.

Loughlin, S. E., Foote, S. L., and Fallon, J. H. (1982). Locus coeruleus projections to cortex: topography, morphology, and collateralisation. *Brain Research Bulletin*, **9**, 1–16.

Lowe, S. L., Francis, P. T., Procter, A. W., Palmer, A. M., Davison, A. N., and Bowen, D. M. (1988). Gamma-aminobutyric acid concentration in brain tissue at two stages of Alzheimer's disease. *Brain*, **111**, 785–99.

Lowe, S. L., Bowen, D. M., Francis, P. T., and Neary, D. (1990). Ante mortem cerebral amino acid concentrations indicate selective degeneration of glutamate-enriched neurons in Alzheimer's disease. *Neuroscience*, **38**, 571–7.

McCormick, D. A. and Prince, D. A. (1985). Two types of muscarininc responses to acetyl choline in mammalian cortical neurones. *Proceedings of the National Academy of Science USA)*, **82**, 6344–8.

McCormick, D. A. and Williamson, A. (1989). Convergence and divergence of neurotransmitter action in human cerebral cortex. *Proceedings of the National Academy of Science USA*, **86**, 8098–102.

Mann, D. M. A. and Yates, P. O. (1982). Is the loss of cerebral cortical choline acetyltransferase activity in Alzheimer's disease due to degeneration of ascending cholinergic nerve cells. *Journal of Neurology, Neurosurgery and Psychiatry*, **45**, 936.

Mann, D. M. A., Lincoln, J., Yates, P. O., Stamp, J. E., and Toper, S. (1980). Changes in the monoamine containing neurones of the human CNS in senile dementia. *British Journal of Psychiatry*, **136**, 533–41.

Mann, D. M., Yates, P. O., and Marcyniuk, B. (1984). Presenile Alzheimer's disease, senile dementia of Alzheimer type and Down's syndrome of middle age all form an age related continuum of pathological changes. *Neuropathology and Applied Neurobiology*, **10**, 185–207.

Mann, D. M. A., South, P. W., Snowden, J. S., and Neary, D. (1993). Dementia of frontal lobe type: neuropathology and immunohistochemistry. *Journal of Neurology, Neurosurgery and Psychiatry*, **56**, 605–14.

Meltzer, C. C., Smith, G., DeKosky, S. T., Pollock, B. G., Mathis, C. A., Moore, R. Y., *et al.* (1998). Serotonin in aging, late-life depression, and Alzheimer's disease: the emerging role of functional imaging. *Neuropsychopharmacology*, **18**, 407–30. [See comments.] [Review] [230 refs]

Meltzer, C. C., Price, J. C., Mathis, C. A., Greer, P. J., Cantwell, M. N., Houck, P. R., *et al.* (1999). PET imaging of serotonin type 2A receptors in late-life neuropsychiatric disorders. *American Journal of Psychiatry*, **156**, 1871–8.

Mesulam, M. M. (1995). The cholinergic contribution to neuromodulation in the cerebral cortex. *The Neurosciences*, 7, 297–307.

Middlemiss, D. N., Palmer, A. M., Edel, N., and Bowen, D. M. (1986). Binding of the novel serotonin agonist 8-hydroxy-2-(di-*n*-propylamino)tetralin in normal and Alzheimer brain. *Journal of Neurochemistry*, **46**, 993–6.

Miller, B. L., Darby, A., Benson, D. F., Cummings, J. L., and Miller, M. H. (1997). Aggressive, socially disruptive and antisocial behaviour associated with fronto-temporal dementia. *British Journal of Pharmacology*, **170**, 150–5.

Miller, J. D., De Leon, M. J., Ferris, S. H., Kluger, A., George, A. E., Reisberg, B., *et al.* (1987). Abnormal temporal lobe response in Alzheimer's disease during cognitive processing as measured by ^{11}C-2-deoxy-D-glucose and PET. *Journal of Cerebral Blood Flow and Metabolism*, 7, 248–51.

Minthon, L., Edvinsson, L., and Gustafson, L. (1997). Somatostatin and neuropeptide Y in cerebrospinal fluid: correlations with severity of disease and clinical signs in Alzheimer's disease and frontotemporal dementia. *Dementia and Geriatric Cognitive Disorders*, **8**, 232–9.

Mohr, E., Bruno, G., Foster, N., Gillespie, M., Cox, C., Fedio, P., *et al.* (1986). GABA-agonist therapy for Alzheimer's disease. *Clinical Neuropharmacology*, **9**, 257–63.

Mountjoy, C. Q., Rossor, M. N., Iversen, L. L., and Roth, M. (1984). Correlation of cortical cholinergic and GABA deficits with quantitative neuropathological findings in senile dementia. *Brain*, **107**, 507–18.

Mouradian, M. M., Biln, J., Giuffra, M., Heuser, I. J. E., Baronti, F., Ownby, J., *et al.* (1991). Somatostatin replacement therapy of Alzheimer disease. *Annals of Neurology*, **30**, 610–30.

Murdoch, I., Perry, E. K., Court, J. A., Graham, D. I., and Dewar, D. (1998). Cortical cholinergic dysfunction after human head injury. *Journal of Neurotrauma*, **15**, 295–305.

Nagai, R., McGeer, P. L., Peng, J. H., McGeer, E. G., and Dolman, C. E. (1983). Choline acetyltransferase immunohistochemistry in brains of Alzheimer's disease patients and controls. *Neuroscience Letters*, **36**, 195–9.

Nagga, K., Bogdanovic, N., and Marcusson, J. (1999). GABA transporters (GAT-1) in Alzheimer's disease. *Journal of Neural Transmission (Budapest)*, **106**, 1141–9.

Neary, D., Snowden, J. S., Mann, D. M. A., Bowen, D. M., Sims, N. R., Northen, B., *et al.* (1986). Alzheimer's disease: a correlative study. *Journal of Neurology, Neurosurgery and Psychiatry*, **49**, 229–37.

Neary, D., Snowden, J. S., Shields, R. A., Burjan, A. W. I., Northen, B., Macdermott, N., *et al.* (1987). Single photon emission tomography using ^{99m}Tc-HM-PAO in the investigation of dementia. *Journal of Neurology, Neurosurgery and Psychiatry*, **50**, 1101–9.

Nitsch, R. M. (1996). From acetylcholine to amyloid: neurotransmitters and the pathology of Alzheimer's disease. *Neurodegeneration*, 5, 477–82. [Review] [44 refs]

Nitsch, R. M., Slack, B. E., Wurtman, R. J., and Growdon, J. H. (1992). Release of Alzheimer amyloid precursor stimulated by activation of muscarinic acetylcholine receptors. *Science*, **258**, 304–7.

O'Neill, C., Cowburn, R. F., Wiehager, B., Alafuzoff, I., Winblad, B., and Fowler, C. J. (1991). Preservation of 5-hydroxytryptamine 1a receptor–G protein interactions in the cerebral cortex of patients with Alzheimer's disease. *Neuroscience Letters*, **133**, 15–19.

Ottersen, O. P. (1991). Excitatory amino acid neurotransmitters: anatomical systems. In *Excitatory amino acid antagonists* (ed. B. S. Meldrum), pp. 14–38. Blackwell Scientific, Oxford.

Palmer, A. M., Procter, A. W., Stratmann, G. C., and Bowen, D. M. (1986). Excitatory amino acid-releasing and cholinergic neurones in Alzheimer's disease. *Neuroscience Letters*, **66**, 199–204.

Palmer, A. M., Francis, P. T., Benton, J. S., Sims, N. R., Mann, D. M., Neary, D., *et al.* (1987*a*). Presynaptic serotonergic dysfunction in patients with Alzheimer's disease. *Journal of Neurochemistry*, **48**, 8–15.

Palmer, A. M., Francis, P. T., Bowen, D. M., Benton, J. S., Neary, D., Mann, D. M., *et al.* (1987*b*). Catecholaminergic neurones assessed ante-mortem in Alzheimer's disease. *Brain Research*, **414**, 365–75.

Palmer, A. M., Wilcock, G. K., Esiri, M. M., Francis, P. T., and Bowen, D. M. (1987*c*). Monoaminergic innervation of the frontal and temporal lobes in Alzheimer's disease. *Brain Research*, **401**, 231–8.

Palmer, A. M., Stratmann, G. C., Procter, A. W., and Bowen, D. M. (1988). Possible neurotransmitter basis of behavioral changes in Alzheimer's disease. *Annals of Neurology*, **23**, 616–20.

Pangalos, M. N., Francis, P. T., Pearson, R. C. A., Middlemiss, D. N., and Bowen, D. M. (1991). Selective destruction of a sub-population of cortical neurones by suicide transport of volkensin, a lectin from *Adenia volkensia*. *Journal of Neuroscience Methods*, **40**, 17–29.

Pangalos, M. N., Francis, P. T., Foster, A. C., Pearson, R. C. A., Middlemiss, D. N., and Bowen, D. M. (1992). NMDA receptors assessed by autoradiography with [3H] L-689,560 are present but not enriched on corticofugal-projecting pyramidal neurones. *Brain Research*, **596**, 223–30.

Pearce, B. R., Palmer, A. M., Bowen, D. M., Wilcock, G. K., Esiri, M. M., and Davison, A. N. (1984). Neurotransmitter dysfunction and atrophy of the caudate nucleus in Alzheimer's disease. *Neurochemical Pathology*, **2**, 221–32.

Pearson, R. C. and Powell, T. P. (1989). The neuroanatomy of Alzheimer's disease. *Reviews in Neurosciences*, **2**, 101–23.

Pearson, R. C. A., Sofroniew, M. V., Cuello, A. C., Powell, T. P. S., Eckenstein, F., Esiri, M. M., *et al.* (1983). Persistence of cholinergic neurones in the basal nucleus in a brain with senile dementia of the Alzheimer's type demonstrated by immunohistochemical staining for choline acetyltransferase. *Brain Research*, **289**, 375–9.

Pearson, R. C. A., Esiri, M. M., Hiorns, R. W., Wilcock, G. K., and Powell, T. P. S. (1985). Anatomical correlates of the distribution of the pathological changes in the neocortex in Alzheimer's disease. *Proceedings of the National Academy of Science USA*, **82**, 4531–4.

Perry, E. K. (2000). The cholinergic system in Alzheimer's disease. In *Dementia* (ed. J. O'Brien, D. Ames, and A. Burns), pp. 417–32. Arnold, London.

Perry, E. K., Gibson, P. H., Blessed, G., Perry, R. H., and Tomlinson, B. E. (1977*a*). Neurotransmitter enzyme abnormalities in senile dementia. Choline acetyltransferase and glutamic acid decarboxlyase activities in necropsy brain tissue. *Journal of the Neurological Sciences*, **34**, 247–65.

Perry, E. K., Perry, R. H., Blessed, G., and Tomlinson, B. E. (1977*b*). Necropsy evidence of central cholinergic deficits in senile dementia. *Lancet*, **i**, 189.

Perry, E. K., Tomlinson, B. E., Blessed, G., Bergmann, K., Gibson, P. H., and Perry, R. H. (1978). Correlation of cholinergic abnormalities with senile plaques and mental test scores in senile dementia. *British Medical Journal*, **2**, 1457–9.

Perry, E. K., Blessed, G., Tomlinson, B. E., Perry, R. H., Crow, T. J., Cross, A. J., *et al.* (1981). Neurochemical activities in human temporal lobe related to aging and Alzheimer-type changes. *Neurobiology of Aging*, **2**, 251–6.

Perry, E. K., Marshall, E., Thompson, P., McKeith, I. G., Collerton, D., Fairbairn, A. F., *et al.* (1993). Monoaminergic activities in Lewy body dementia: relation to hallucinosis and extrapyramidal features. *Journal of Neural Transmission—Parkinsons Disease & Dementia Section*, **6**, 167–77.

Perry, E. K., Haroutunian, V., Davis, K. L., Levy, R., Lantos, P., Eagger, S., *et al.* (1994). Neocortical cholinergic activities differentiate Lewy body dementia from classical Alzheimer's disease. *Neuroreport*, **5**, 747–9.

Perry, E. K., Morris, C. M., Court, J. A., Cheng, A., Fairbairn, A. F., McKeith, I. G., *et al.* (1995). Alteration in nicotine binding sites in Parkinson's disease, Lewy body dementia and Alzheimer's disease: possible index of early neuropathology. *Neuroscience*, **64**, 385–95.

Perry, R. H., Candy, J. M., Perry, E. K., Irving, D., Blessed, G., Fairbairn, A. F., *et al.* (1982). Extensive loss of choline acetyltransferase activity is not reflected by neuronal loss in the nucleus of Meynert in Alzheimer's disease. *Neuroscience Letters*, **33**, 311–15.

Procter, A. W. and Bowen, D. M. (1988). Ageing, the cerebral neocortex and psychiatric disorder. In *Banbury Report 27: Molecular neuropathology of aging* (ed. C. E. Finch and P. Davies), pp. 3–20. Cold Spring Harbor Laboratory, Cold Spring Harbor.

Procter, A. W., Lowe, S. L., Palmer, A. M., Francis, P. T., Esiri, M. M., Stratmann, G. C., *et al.* (1988*a*). Topographical distribution of neurochemical changes in Alzheimer's disease. *Journal of the Neurological Sciences*, **84**, 125–40.

Procter, A. W., Palmer, A. M., Francis, P. T., Lowe, S. L., Neary, D., Murphy, E., *et al.* (1988*b*). Evidence of glutamatergic denervation and possible abnormal metabolism in Alzheimer's disease. *Journal of Neurochemistry*, **50**, 790–802.

Procter, A. W., Doshi, R., Bowen, D. M., and Murphy, E. (1990). Rapid autopsy brains for biochemical research: experiences in establishing a programme. *International Journal of Geriatric Psychiatry*, **5**, 287–94.

Procter, A. W., Francis, P. T., Stratmann, G. C., and Bowen, D. M. (1992). Serotonergic pathology is not widespread in Alzheimer patients without prominent aggressive symptoms. *Neurochemistry Research*, **17**, 917–22.

Procter, A. W., Francis, P. T., Holmes, C., Webster, M.-T., Qume, M., Stratmann, G. C., *et al.* (1994). Beta-amyloid precursor protein isoforms show correlations with neurones but not with glia of demented subjects. *Acta Neuropathologica*, **88**, 545–52.

Procter, A. W., Qume, M., and Francis, P. T. (1999). Neurochemical features of fronto-temporal dementia. *Dementia*, (In press.)

Qume, M., Zeman, S., Stratmann, G. C., Wort, C., Francis, P. T., Procter, A. W., *et al.* (1994). A neurochemical study of non-Alzheimer dementia. *British Journal of Pharmacology*, **116**, S237 (abstract).

Qume, M., Misra, A., Zeman, S., Boddy, J. L., Cross, A. J., Francis, P. T., *et al.* (1995*a*). Non-serotonergic profiles of lobar atrophies. *Biochemical Society Transactions*, **23**, 601S (abstract).

Qume, M., Misra, A., Zeman, S., Muthu, J., Cross, A. J., Francis, P. T., *et al.* (1995*b*). Serotonergic profiles of lobar atrophies. *Biochemical Society Transactions*, **23**, 600S (abstract).

Reinikainen, K. J., Paljarvi, L., Huuskonen, M., Soininen, H., Laasko, M., and Reikkinen, P. J. (1988). A post mortem study of noradrenergic serotonergic and GABAergic neurons in Alzheimer's disease. *Journal of the Neurological Sciences*, **84**, 101–16.

Roberson, M. R. and Harrell, L. E. (1997). Cholinergic activity and amyloid precursor protein metabolism. *Brain Research—Brain Research Reviews*, **25**, 50–69. [Review] [184 refs]

Robinson, S. R. (2000). Neuronal expression of glutamine synthetase in Alzheimer's disease indicates a profound impairment of metabolic interactions with astrocytes. *Neurochemistry International*, **36**, 471–82.

Russo-Neustadt, A. and Cotman, C. W. (1997). Adrenergic receptors in Alzheimer's disease brain: selective increases in the cerebella of aggressive patients. *Journal of Neuroscience*, **17**, 5573–80.

Russo-Neustadt, A., Zomorodian, T. J., and Cotman, C. W. (1998). Preserved cerebellar tyrosine hydroxylase-immunoreactive neuronal fibers in a behaviorally aggressive subgroup of Alzheimer's disease patients. *Neuroscience*, **87**, 55–61.

Sambamurti, K., Shioi, J., Anderson, J. P., Pappolla, M. A., and Robakis, N. K. (1992). Evidence for intracellular cleavage of the Alzheimer's amyloid precursor in PC12 cells. *Neuroscience Research*, **33**, 319–29.

Samuel, W., Alford, M., Hofstetter, C. R., and Hansen, L. (1997). Dementia with Lewy bodies versus pure Alzheimer disease: differences in cognition, neuropathology, cholinergic dysfunction, and synapse density. *Journal of Neuropathology and Experimental Neurology*, **56**, 499–508.

Seubert, P., Vigo-Pelfrey, C., Esch, F. S., Lee, M., Dovey, H., Davis, D., *et al.* (1992). Isolation and quantification of soluble Alzheimer's beta-peptide from biological fluids. *Nature*, **359**, 325–7.

Seubert, P., Oltersdorf, T., Lee, M. G., Barbour, R., Blomquist, C., Davis, D. L., *et al.* (1993). Secretion of beta-amyloid precursor protein cleaved at the amino terminus of the beta-amyloid peptide. *Nature*, **361**, 260–3.

Shashidharan, P. and Plaitakis, A. (1993). Cloning and characterisation of a glutamate transporter cDNA from human cerebellum. *Biochimica et Biophysica Acta*, **1216**, 161–4.

Shashidharan, P., Huntley, G. W., Meyer, T., Morrison, J. H., and Plaitakis, A. (1994*a*). Neuron-specific human glutamate transporter: molecular cloning, characterisation and expression in human brain. *Brain Research*, **662**, 245–50.

Shashidharan, P., Wittenberg, I., and Plaitakis, A. (1994*b*). Molecular cloning of human brain glutamate/aspartate transporter II. *Biochimica et Biophysica Acta*, **1191**, 393–6.

Shigematsu, K., McGeer, P. L., and McGeer, E. G. (1992). Localisation of amyloid precursor protein in selective postsynaptic densities of rat cortical neurons. *Brain Research*, **592**, 353–7.

Simpson, I. A., Koteswara, R., Chundu, M. D., Davis-Hill, T., Honer, W. G., and Davies, P. (1994). Decreased concentrations of GLUT1 and GLUT3 glucose transporters in the brains of patients with Alzheimer's disease. *Annals of Neurology*, **35**, 546–51.

Sims, N. R., Bowen, D. M., Allen, S. J., Smith, C. C. T., Neary, D., Thomas, D. J., *et al.* (1983). Presynaptic cholinergic dysfunction in patients with dementia. *Journal of Neurochemistry*, **40**, 503–9.

Smith, C. C., Bowen, D. M., Sims, N. R., Neary, D., and Davison, A. N. (1983). Amino acid release from biopsy samples of temporal neocortex from patients with Alzheimer's disease. *Brain Research*, **264**, 138–41.

Struble, R. G., Cork, L. C., Whitehouse, P. J., and Price, D. L. (1982). Cholinergic innervation in neuritic plaques. *Science*, **216**, 413–15.

Terry, R. D., Masliah, E., Salmon, D. P., Butters, N., DeTeresa, R., Hill, R., *et al.* (1991). Physical basis of cognitive alterations in Alzheimer's disease: synapse loss is the major correlate of cognitive impairment. *Annals of Neurology*, **30**, 572–80.

Ulrich, J., Johannson-Locher, G., Seiler, W. O., and Stahelin, H. B. (1997). Does smoking protect from Alzheimer's disease? Alzheimer-type changes in 301 unselected brains from patients with known smoking history. *Acta Neuropathologica*, **94**, 450–4.

Voytko, M. L. (1996). Cognitive functions of the basal forebrain cholinergic system in monkeys: memory or attention?. *Behavioural Brain Research*, **75**, 13–25. [Review] [123 refs]

Waterhouse, B. D., Lin, C. S., Burne, R. A., and Woodward, D. J. (1983). The distribution of neocortical projections neurones in the locus coeruleus. *Journal of Comparative Neurology*, **217**, 418–31.

Webster, M.-T., Vekrellis, K., Francis, P. T., Pearce, B. R., and Bowen, D. M. (1993). Factors affecting the beta-amyloid precursor in PC12 cells. *Biochemical Society Transactions*, **21**, 239S.

Webster, M.-T., Francis, P. T., Procter, A. W., Stratmann, G. C., Doshi, R., Mann, D. M. A., *et al.* (1994). Post-mortem brains reveal similar but not identical amyloid precursor protein-like immunoreactivity in Alzheimer compared with other dementias. *Brain Research*, **644**, 347–51.

Wenk, G. L. (1997). The nucleus basalis magnocellularis cholinergic system: one hundred years of progress. *Neurobiology of Learning and Memory*, **67**, 85–95. [Review] [119 refs]

Whitehouse, P. J., Price, D. L., Struble, R. G., Clark, A. W., Coyle, J. T., and DeLong, M. R. (1982). Alzheimer's disease and senile dementia: loss of neurons in the basal forebrain. *Science*, **215**, 1237–9.

Wiley, R. G. (1992). Neural lesioning with ribosome-inactivating proteins: suicide transport and immunolesioning. *Trends in Neurosciences*, **15**, 285–90.

Wilkinson, D. (2000). How effective are cholinergic therapies in improving cognition in Alzheimer's disease ? In *Dementia* (ed. J. O'Brien, D. Ames, and A. Burns), pp. 549–58. Arnold, London.

Yang, S., Yu, J., Shiah, S., and Huang, J. (1994). Protein kinase F_A/glycogen synthase kinase 3alpha after heparin potentiation phosphorylates tau sites abnormally phosphorylated in Alzheimer's disease. *Journal of Neurochemistry*, **63**, 1416–25.

Yates, C. M., Butterworth, J., Tennant, M. C., and Gordon, A. (1990). Enzyme activities in relation to pH and lactate in post mortem brain in Alzheimer type and other dementias. *Journal of Neurochemistry*, **55**, 1624–30.

Zubenko, G. S. and Moossy, J. (1988). Major depression in primary dementia. Clinical and neuropathologic correlates. *Archives of Neurology*, **45**, 1182–6.

Zweig, R. M., Ross, C. A., Hedreen, J. C., Steele, C., Cardillo, J. E., Whitehouse, P. J., *et al.* (1988). The neuropathology of aminergic nuclei in Alzheimer's disease. *Annals of Neurology*, **24**, 233–42.

7 Molecular genetics and molecular biology of dementia

Simon Lovestone

Molecular genetics of dementia

Introduction

The unravelling of the molecular biology and genetics of Alzheimer's disease (AD) and the related dementias has been one of the most exciting and productive scientific developments of recent years. The pathology of AD provided a route map to understanding pathogenesis, but it has been the identification of genes that has been the compass allowing use of this map and, hopefully, has identified the path to drug discovery. And this is why genetic studies are performed—to understand the aetiopathogenesis in order to intervene; in order to develop disease modification strategies. In fact the precedents for such planned drug discovery programmes leading to useful therapies are not many, anti-HIV treatments being one of the few, albeit outstanding, examples of the success of modern molecular medicine. None the less, there is confidence that the power of molecular approaches is such that the only doubts sustained are ones of timing—will the process yield drugs this decade or next? It is this combination of identifying mutations in genes causing early-onset AD together with the presence of well-defined pathological lesions that has ensured that the speed of progress in AD has been so rapid. For all other psychiatric and even many neurological disorders these 'handles', i.e. pathological lesions and genetic defects, are not present and there is little information to begin molecular research. However, despite the promises of understanding pathogenesis and of developing treatments, it is not these aspects that result first from developments in genetics. First comes testing, together with the clinical, ethical, and practical dilemmas that always accompany this Pandora's box of a discipline.

Genes affect the dementias in two clearly distinct ways. Although both involve DNA, there the similarity ends. Early-onset familial dementias can be inherited as autosomal dominant disorders. These are usually, but not always, single-gene disorders with a clear-cut Mendelian inheritance pattern apparent from the family tree. The early-onset familial dementias include those where the genes are known, such as AD and some frontotemporal dementias (FTD), other disorders where the gene is known but where dementia is a secondary syndrome in most cases, such as Huntington's disease, and yet other disorders where the gene remains to be found such as FTD linked to chromosome 3 (Poduslo *et al.* 1999) and familial British Dementia (Ghiso *et al.* 1995). In marked contrast to these are the late-onset dementias, such as AD and dementia with Lewy bodies (DLB) where the inheritance is unclear, where there are multiple genes involved, and where the genes themselves are by and large unknown (Table 7.1).

Early-onset familial dementia

Early-onset AD is not common, but early-onset familial AD is rare. Unfortunately the definition of late onset usually adopted is one developed in response to services rather than biology. The often-used cut-off of 60–65 years of age is inappropriate for early-onset familial Alzheimer's disease (FAD) where the onset is most often

Table 7.1 Genetically linked disorders

Disorder	Gene	Chromosome
Autosomal dominant, primary degenerative dementias		
Familial early-onset AD (FAD)	*PS-1*	14
	PS-2	1
	APP	21
Familial British dementia, familial Danish dementia	*BRI*	13
Familial frontotemporal dementias including FTDP-17 (frontotemporal dementia with Parkinson's disease linked to chromosome 17)	*tau*	17
Atypical progressive supranuclear palsy (PSP)	*tau*	17
Familial prion disorders (e.g. Creutzfeld–Jakob disease (CJD) and Gerstmann–Straussler–Scheinker syndrome (GSS)	*PrP*	20
Autosomal dominant neurodegeneration with dementia as a secondary syndrome		
Huntington's disease	*huntingtin*	4
Dentato-rubro-pallido-luysian atrophy (DRPLA)	*DRPLA*	12
Hereditary cerebral haemorrhage with amyloidosis—Dutch type (HCHWA-D)	*APP*	21
Cerebral autosomal dominant arteriopathy with subcortical infarcts and leucoencephalopathy (CADASIL)	*Notch3*	19
Autosomal dominant dementia—gene unidentified		
Alzheimer's disease (some familial AD kindreds)		
Dementia linked to chromosome 3		3
Progressive supranuclear palsy (some families)		
Non-autosomal dominant dementia with an undoubted genetic contribution to aetiology		
Alzheimer's disease	APOE	19
Dementia with Lewy bodies		
Progressive supranuclear palsy (PSP)	*tau*	17

before the age of 55 years. In fact, there is no cut-off in age that fully separates early-onset FAD from other forms of the condition as some very infrequent cases do have an onset of autosomal dominant AD after the age of 60. Campion *et al.* (1999) determined the prevalence of early-onset AD, both familial and non-familial, in the city of Rouen, France, and found the frequency of the former to be 5.3, and the latter to be 41.2 per 100 000 persons at risk. Thus FAD is about as rare as HD, which has a prevalence of 6.4/100 000 (Morrison *et al.* 1995). Among these cases with clear-cut, early-onset FAD the gene mutation was identified in over 70% (Campion *et al.* 1999), being either *PS-1* or *APP* in most cases and *PS-2* in some families. Others estimate the frequency of these gene mutations in early-onset AD to be less, implying that there are other FAD genes waiting to be discovered.

Amyloid precursor-protein (APP) gene genetics

The *APP* gene was associated with AD before mutations were found, when it was shown that the amyloid that forms the core of plaques is derived from the protein product of the gene. Furthermore, as *APP* is carried on chromosome 21 and all patients with trisomy 21 (Down's syndrome) suffer from the pathological lesions of AD and often dementia as well, *APP* was an obvious candidate. The early studies failed to find a linkage between *APP* and FAD, but in retrospect this was only because they included families subsequently shown to have mutations in other genes. This genetic heterogeneity delayed the identification of genes for dementia. However, subsequently the research group of Hardy and colleagues in London identified a mutation causing a valine to isoloeucine amino acid change at position 717 in the *APP* gene in a single family (Goate *et al.* 1991). Later, other mutations were identified at this site, which has become known as the 'London' mutation. Yet other mutations have been found at other sites in the *APP* gene, including the double mutation in a Swedish family at position 670/671 and mutations at positions 692 and 693 (reviewed in Price and Sisodia 1998). These mutations have different consequences for the metabolism of the *APP* gene as described in the next section. Interestingly, however, the mutation at position 693 causes not AD but a disorder with amyloid deposition in vessel walls causing early and profound cerebral haemorrhage (Haan *et al.* 1991). The genotype (gene) influences the phenotype (clinical syndrome) in a very profound way, with mutations in the same gene and very close to each other causing very different disorders. This correlation between genotype and phenotype is seen for other dementias, albeit in a less dramatic fashion.

The pathological examination of individuals harbouring the val717ile mutation demonstrated the lesions of AD, with not only a high density of both plaques and tangles but also with many cortical and subcortical Lewy bodies (Lantos *et al.* 1992). Other families with the *APP* mutation do not show Lewy body pathology (Ghetti *et al.* 1992). The onset of AD in *APP* families is most often in the sixth decade, compared to an onset a decade earlier in the families with the presenilin gene (Mullan *et al.* 1993). In other respects the clinical phenotype of *APP* families is similar to that of other FADs.

Presenilin genes

The presenilin-1 (*PS-1*) gene on chromosome 14 was found by positional cloning just a few years after the linkage was first described (Schellenberg *et al.* 1992*a*; Sherrington *et al.* 1995). Having discovered *PS-1* a search for homologous or similar genes was performed. A nearly identical gene, now known as *PS-2*, was found on chromosome 1 (Levy-Lahad *et al.* 1995). Linkage of FAD to chromosome 1 had already been found in some families, and mutations were described in these families shortly after the mutations in *PS-1* were found. Computing power accelerated the search for genes, not for the first time, and now that the first draft of the human genome is completed, certainly not for the last either.

The genetics of *PS-1* FAD differs from that of *APP* FAD in one important respect. Whereas in *APP* a few mutations only (less than 12) are found in a limited number of positions, in *PS-1* many mutations (more than 70) are scattered through the length of a moderately large gene. This has important consequences for clinical genetics, as it is a formidable task to screen for mutations in *PS-1* and many families have unique mutations. When a change in the gene is found in an affected person it can be difficult to determine if the change is a normal variant not previously discovered, or a pathogenic mutation. This complicates clinical genetic counselling.

The onset of *PS-1*, early-onset, familial Alzheimer's disease (EOFAD) is, on average, a decade before that of *APP* families and there is clustering of the age of onset within families (Mullan *et al.* 1993). However, non-penetrance has been reported, with a family member carrying an undoubted pathogenic mutation remaining free of dementia beyond the age of onset for that family (Rossor *et al.* 1996). This is uncommon and might relate to other genetic factors in this family, but such non-penetrance must be borne in mind when advising families of risk. On the other hand, the *PS-2* families have an onset later than those with *APP* mutations and one which overlaps with late-onset AD. Mutations in *PS-2* are the least common cause of FAD and are confined largely, but not entirely, to the Volga German people who originated in Germany, emigrated to the Volga basin, where many contributed to the productive agriculture of the region, before emigrating again to the United States at the turn of the twentieth century. A founder individual from this community almost certainly harboured the first mutation, and that it has not spread more widely is due to the close-knit nature of the community rendered self-reliant by sequential emigrations (Bird *et al.* 1988).

Tau gene

The mechanism of effect of the mutations in the gene for tau on the brain is discussed below, but all mutations in *tau* result in aggregation of tau protein into highly phosphorylated inclusion bodies similar to those found in AD. Like APP, tau was of interest to AD molecular biologists long before genetic evidence was provided of its role in dementia. APP was of interest as it provides the peptide that constitutes plaques, while tau was of interest as it is the protein that constitutes tangles. However, as with *APP*, it was the discovery of mutations in *tau* that secured its undoubted role as an aetiological agent (as opposed to inconsequential epiphenomenon) in dementia. Interestingly, *tau* mutations were found not in AD but in frontal lobe dementia. The frontal lobe dementias are a collection of disorders rather than a single disease with a common aetiology. Autosomal dominant forms of the disorders have been noted for many years and many individuals with FTD also have diverse motor disorders (Mann 1998). One group of families have frontal lobe dementia, early prominent aphasia, and parkinsonism. These families were grouped together as FTDP-17 (frontotemporal dementia with Parkinson's), the 17 referring to linkage to chromosome 17 demonstrated in some of these families (Foster *et al.* 1997). The *tau* gene is present on chromosome 17, and mutations in the *tau* gene segregating with disease were demonstrated in some families by a number of groups simultaneously (Heutink 2000). Mutations in *tau* are not confined to individuals with the full FTDP-17 clinical syndrome; they are also found in other cases of FTD, including cases with pathological features of Pick's disease (Murrell *et al.* 1999). Other disorders, such as corticobasal degeneration, are also caused by mutations in *tau* and on neuropathological examination have similar intraneuronal tau-containing lesions (Gibb *et al.* 1989; Mori *et al.* 1994).

The mechanism of effect of the *tau* mutations on the brain is discussed below, but all mutations in the *tau* gene result in aggregation of tau into highly phosphorylated inclusion bodies similar to those found in AD. These are present not only in neurons (as in AD) but also in glia. This is interesting, as tau is normally expressed predominantly, if not exclusively, in neurons. The mutations in *tau* fall into two types. First, missense mutations (changes in DNA that alter the reading of a DNA codon and hence alter the protein product produced by one or more amino acids) in the coding region are found in and around the microtubule binding domains, which are essential for the normal function of tau. Second, non-coding mutations occur that alter the splicing of *tau*. A single *tau* gene is responsible for all the six isoforms of tau expressed in the central nervous system (CNS), this diversity being achieved by differential splicing (Goedert *et al.* 1989). Differential splicing is the process whereby multiple isoforms of a protein can be generated from a single gene. A gene contains introns and exons, the exons being the sequences of DNA that are transcribed into mRNA and then translated into protein. When the *tau* gene is transcribed, some exons are skipped and hence not translated into protein, thus resulting in a diversity of protein isoforms from the same gene. A critical splicing of the *tau* gene occurs with inclusion, or not, of exon 10 in the final protein product of the gene. Inclusion results in tau with four imperfect repeat domains that bind to microtubules; splicing out of exon 10 results in only three such domains. At the splicing site at the exon 10 boundary, the DNA molecule loops in on itself, and this physical structure of the DNA prevents binding of the translation apparatus and results in exclusion of exon 10 from the protein. Normally some, but not all, the DNA molecules result in exon 10 exclusion in this way. Mutations associated with FTDP-17 were found in this area, suggesting that a splicing abnormality might result, and in line with this the tau protein present in the tangles that occur in FTDP-17 is predominantly, possibly entirely, 4-repeat tau (Grover *et al.* 1999). If this suggested mechanism is correct, it would be predicted that other mutations resulting in altered splicing would also give rise to disease. Quite remarkably every single nucleotide in the splicing region was subsequently found to be mutated in one affected family or another (Hutton 2000).

Another condition also associated with changes in the *tau* gene, albeit tentatively, is progressive supranuclear palsy (PSP) or Steele–Richardson–Olszewski syndrome, a disorder characterized by a gait difficulty, vertical gaze palsy, and generalized severe akinesia. Dementia, if it occurs, is a late syndrome in PSP, although executive function difficulties are seen early in the disease process on psychometric assessment. PSP was thought until recently to be a sporadic disorder, but this is almost certainly because the range of phenotypes led to under-recognition of the disorder (Rojo *et al.* 1999). Neuropathologically, the disease is characterized by atrophy, pallor of the substantia nigra, shrinkage of the globus pallidus, gliosis, neuronal loss, and, most importantly, a high density of tau-positive neurofibrillary tangles and neuropil threads in subcortical regions (Lees 1987; Probst *et al.* 1988). As in FTDP-17, these pathological inclusions are predominantly 4-repeat tau (Buee and Delacourte 1999). Not surprisingly PSP has also been associated with *tau* gene changes: a set of polymorphisms linked together (a haplotype) is commoner in PSP than in age-matched controls (Baker *et al.* 1999). Also, just as with FTDP-17, a splice-site mutation in the *tau* gene results in PSP in one family. This causes an increase in exon-10 splicing resulting in an increase in 4-repeat tau (Stanford *et al.* 2000).

Other genes and familial dementias

British familial dementia (BFD) is an autosomal dominant disorder with an onset most often in the sixth decade, characterized by dementia, progressive spastic paresis, and cerebellar ataxia (Mead *et al.* 2000). The pathological features include an abundant amyloidopathy, with plaques (in contrast to AD these are non-neuritic) and vessel wall deposits together with neurofibrillary tangles (Revesz *et al.* 1999). However, in BFD the amyloid is not derived from APP but from an entirely different protein the gene of which shares no homology with *APP*, although both code for a single-pass, membrane-associated protein. Mutations in the *BRI*[1] gene are associated with BFD just as *APP* mutations are associated with AD (Vidal *et al.* 1999). To add to the increasing complexity another disorder, Familial Danish dementia (FDD), also known as heredopathia ophthalmo-oto-encephalica, a disease with cataracts, deafness, ataxia, and dementia, is also caused by mutations in the *BRI* gene. There are, therefore, three disorders (AD, FBD, FDD), caused by two different genes (*BRI*, *APP*), but with one common pathological process (amyloid deposition).

CADASIL (central autosomal dominant arteriopathy with subcortical infarcts and leucoencephalopathy) rarely presents with dementia, but dementia can occur as a result of the vascular lesions that are typical of the disorder (Davous 1998). Mutations in a gene, *Notch3*, are a cause of this autosomal dominant disorder. Interestingly, Notch is itself metabolized by *PS-1*, one of the AD genes. It is not known whether this is an interesting coincidence or whether it is evidence of common mechanisms between these disorders.

The prion disorders can be inherited in an autosomal dominant form as well as being acquired. Familial Creutzfeldt–Jakob disease (CJD), caused by mutations in the prion protein (PrP) gene, is rare but can be confused with AD and other dementias (Collinge and Palmer 1993). Point missense mutations in the *PrP* gene are thought to favour protein folding of the gene product into a form that is insoluble, and acts as a nidus to convert other prion protein into the aggregates that are found in the plaques at postmortem. The molecular biology of prion disorders is reviewed by Wadsworth *et al.* (1999). Distressingly, given the bovine spongiform encephalopathy (BSE) epidemic in the UK and elsewhere, external prions can also precipitate this change and result in the disease termed variant CJD (vCJD) (Collinge 1997). Here too genetics plays a role, as evidence suggests that a common methionine/valine polymorphism at codon 129 within *PrP* gene alters susceptibility to vCJD (methionine homozygosity increasing risk), although it does not result in disease itself (Windl *et al.* 1996).

Finally, Huntington's disease also has dementia as a feature, albeit usually late in the disease process. HD shows the phenomenon of anticipation—the disease becomes more virulent (earlier onset or more severe) with each generation, and is also more severe if inherited through the father. Both observations were explained by the fact that HD is a triplet-repeat disorder (Paulson and Fischbeck 1996). The genetics of HD are reviewed by Walling *et al.* (1998). The normal gene contains a CAG nucleotide repeat sequence that varies in size between individuals. At the upper end of this normal size distribution, however, the repeat becomes unstable and can expand in gametes (ova or sperm). If an expanded CAG repeat is inherited then that individual will develop HD. Moreover, once expanded into the disease range, the DNA is unstable and has a tendency to expand with each generation, thus explaining the increase in severity in offspring. Expansion in sperm is greater than that in ova, explaining the tendency to a more aggressive form of the disease if inherited from a father. As other neurological disorders such as myotonic dystrophy and fragile X are also triplet-repeat disorders and also show anticipation, it follows that this may be a common mechanism in brain disease. This underlies the search currently taking place for anticipation as a phenomenon in psychiatric disorders as well (McInnis *et al.* 1999).

Late-onset non-familial dementia

Apolipoprotein E

Determining the genetic contribution to early-onset AD and identifying the genes has been a far from trivial task. However, the situation for late-onset Alzheimer's disease (LOAD) is even more difficult. Because of attrition due to other causes before the age of onset of LOAD, pedigree analysis of individual families is rarely useful in determining patterns of inheritance. However, studies of siblings of affected patients show a substantially increased risk—greater than 50% by the age of 90 years in many studies (Breitner *et al.* 1988; Huff *et al.* 1988; Farrer *et al.* 1989; Korten *et al.* 1993). Chromosome 19 was implicated in LOAD in studies showing an association with a region containing the apolipoprotein *CII* locus (Schellenberg *et al.* 1992*b*). This locus is adjacent to a related gene—the apolipoprotein E (*APOE*) gene. In the general population, three common variants of this gene are found that differ by an arginine/cysteine substitution at positions 112 and 158 in the protein. Although there are some differences between populations, the E3 isoform is the commonest, followed by the E4 isoform, and with the E2 isoform being relatively rare. (ApoE2–4 refers to the protein isoforms and *APOE ε2–4* refers to the genetic alleles corresponding to the different proteins. Both the ApoE phenotype and *APOE ε* genotype can be easily determined.) Other isoforms, including E1, E5, and E3 prime, are found but are rarer still. ApoE is produced by astrocytes in the brain and had been independently implicated in AD as it had been shown to be a constituent of senile plaques.

The profile of this protein was raised very considerably in AD research when it was demonstrated that the frequency of the *APOE ε4* allele was very much greater in AD subjects than in controls (reviewed by Rubinsztein 1995). This finding was rapidly replicated using familial and sporadic, autopsy and clinically diagnosed, AD in populations from around the world. Carrying the *APOE ε*4 allele increases the risk of AD. Possibly it decreases the age of onset—it has been claimed that APOE affects *when*, not if, one gets AD (Meyer *et al.* 1998). In addition the *ε2* allele is possibly protective, showing an influence in decreasing risk and increasing the age of onset (Corder *et al.* 1994; Talbot *et al.* 1994). The relationship between *APOE* and late-onset AD is now beyond doubt in many different populations, the only anomalous studies being those in the Black population in America where the relationship between *APOE* and AD is not fully determined. In a meta-analysis of different ethnic populations the effect of *APOE* on African-Americans was present but was weaker than for Caucasians, and there were significant differences between studies (Farrer *et al.* 1997). The anomalous results are most likely due to other risk factors confounding the studies.

The degree of risk associated with *APOE* is difficult to determine and is likely to be different at different ages. Combining data from studies comparing nearly 6000 patients with AD and nearly 9000 controls without dementia demonstrated that the risk of AD was significantly increased for people with genotypes *ε2/ε4* (odds ratio (OR) = 2.6), *ε3/ε4* (OR = 3.2), and *ε4/ε4* (OR = 14.9); but was decreased for those with genotype *ε2/ε2* (OR = 0.6) (Farrer *et al.* 1997). However, an important consideration is that carrying the *ε4* allele is neither necessary nor a sufficient condition for AD since many individuals are found with AD and no *ε4* allele, and conversely *ε4*/*ε4* homozygous individuals can reach late age without evidence of dementia. Although the *APOE ε4* effect holds true for all ages between 40 and 90 years, it diminishes in size after age 70 years.

APOE has been found to be associated in some studies with other dementia disorders, including vascular dementia (Hébert *et al.* 2000), CJD (Amouyel *et al.* 1995), age of onset of frontal lobe dementias (Farrer *et al.* 1995*a*), and DLB (Kawanishi *et al.* 1996). In fact, at the present time it is difficult to be certain that there is a dementia *not* associated with *APOE*. However, most of these studies are deeply and intrinsically flawed and other studies (equally flawed) fail to find an association with these conditions. Take for example DLB. There is no doubt that clinically diagnosed DLB is associated with increased *APOE ε4*. However, clinically diagnosed DLB is also associated with neuritic plaques and, to a lesser extent, with tangles as well—evidence of both the amyloid and tau pathologies of AD. A proportion of DLB, possibly the majority of DLB, is present as mixed AD and DLB. It is important to remember that genetics is blind to clinical definitions of disease—genes alter the risk of pathological processes and not of the, ultimately artificial, disease constructs. If therefore Lewy body and AD pathologies frequently occur together and if *APOE ε4* increases the risk of AD pathology, then it is not surprising that *APOE ε4* is increased in clinically diagnosed DLB.

Other genes and association studies

However, *APOE* is not the only gene. Of the genetic risk it has been calculated that *APOE* contributes approximately half—there are other genes yet to be discovered, let alone other risk factors (Owen *et al.* 1994). The list of genes associated with AD in some, but invariably not all, studies is long—over 25 such genes at the beginning of the year 2000. None of these putative genetic factors can be reliably refuted or confirmed. Of the more promising, the gene for angiotensin converting enzyme (ACE) has been associated with a number of different studies and different populations, although the results are not entirely consistent (R. Alvarez *et al.* 1999; Hu *et al.* 1999; Kehoe *et al.* 1999*a*; Crawford *et al.* 2000; Farrer *et al.* 2000). This is interesting as ACE has been associated previously with hypertension (although again the results are not entirely consistent), and so the ACE finding links AD to vascular factors through genes. The gene for *α*2-macroglobulin (interesting, as it is another ligand for ApoE receptors) is also associated with AD in some, but not all, studies (Blacker *et al.* 1998; Crawford *et al.* 1999; Korovaitseva *et al.* 1999; Wavrant-DeVrièze *et al.* 1999).

Why are these inconsistent results obtained from association studies? Two important confounding factors are population admixture and false-positive results. The importance of population admixture is not known and this is a largely theoretical objection to case-control type association studies. If the control population differs in some substantive way from the proband population, then the results will be contaminated—the association might be with the confounder rather than the disease. For genetic studies the most obvious confounder would be some ethnic, or more subtle, genetic difference between cases and controls. For this reason some researchers advocate the use of family-based association strategies—comparing individuals to their own siblings (Collins and Morton 1998). Another intrinsic problem lies in multiple testing. Few studies properly adjust for multiple testing as only one or two genes are analysed. However, as a study of 2–300 individuals at one gene can be conducted in a matter of weeks, and as there are many laboratories conducting such analyses at any one time, and as many stratify their results by both gender and *APOE* genotype, it is easy to see how hundreds of studies are conducted each year. Given this it is perhaps surprising that there are so few positive findings reported. The net effect of all this, however, is that any association study should be treated with extreme caution until it has been replicated many times.

Other strategies

An alternative and more systematic approach is linkage—looking for genome regions associated with disease. In addition to linkage in large 'Mendelian' families, linkage can be performed in affected sibling pairs. In effect, the genome is scanned at regular intervals for sharing of polymorphic markers. If many affected sibling pairs share the same markers then this suggests a gene in the same general region. By analysing many such markers spaced out at as small a distance along the genome as possible, a map indicating likely sites or 'hot-spots' is generated. Such a map lacks resolution and a 'hot-spot' might contain hundreds of genes, not all of which will be recognized as such. Nonetheless, in this way a number of studies have identified regions of the genome, including chromosomes 10, 12, 19, and 21, as sites associated with AD (Pericak-Vance *et al.* 1998; Zubenko *et al.* 1998; Kehoe *et al.* 1999*b*). The next task will be to identify the genes in these regions, to find variation in these genes, to demonstrate which variability in which gene is associated with AD, and then to confirm the findings. This is a considerable undertaking, but it is only when this is done that the promise of genetics—in particular, the exciting prospects of genetic epidemiology—can get off the ground.

Genotype and phenotype in Alzheimer's disease

Little is known as to why there is so much clinical heterogeneity in AD, including the age of onset, rate of progression, and pattern of cognitive and non-cognitive symptoms. However, some evidence suggests that this phenotypic variability reflects genotypic variability. The clearest association between genotype and phenotype is with age of onset—different families with autosomal dominant AD have different ages of onset that remain constant within a family (Mullan *et al.* 1993). In LOAD, as discussed above, variability at the *APOE* locus influences age of onset, with the $\varepsilon 4$ allele advancing, and the $\varepsilon 2$ allele delaying the age of onset (Meyer *et al.* 1998). Clustering of non-cognitive symptoms also occurs in siblings affected by non-autosomal dominant AD (Tunstall *et al.* 2000). Affected sibling pairs with AD were more likely to share age of onset, current mood state, and agitation. As these elderly siblings have relatively little shared environment over a lifetime it is almost certain that such trait-sharing reflects gene-sharing. Two genes have already been identified that might account for some of this trait-sharing. Polymorphic variation in serotonin receptor genes was associated with visual hallucinations in a dose-dependent manner (Holmes *et al.* 1998) and variability in the dopamine receptors has been associated with delusions in AD (Sweet *et al.* 1998). These findings strongly point towards genetic variations as being trait-markers in AD—*APOE* as a marker of age of onset and neurotransmitter receptors as markers of non-cognitive symptoms. A model of non-cognitive symptoms or behavioral and psychological symptoms of dementia (BPSD) in AD then might be that individuals differ in their personal susceptibility to, for example, psychotic features. A very severe personal vulnerability might underlie certain personality traits which when combined with other insults, birth trauma for example, might result in psychotic illness. Alternatively, a milder vulnerability, although lowering the threshold for psychosis, might have no discernible effects until combined with very severe insult—the onset of AD for example. There may, after all, be some truth behind the links suspected by Emil Kraepelin and Alois Alzheimer between dementia senilis and dementia praecox.

Clinical implications of the genetics of dementia

Finding genes associated with AD raises the possibility of genetic testing. Some three types of testing might be envisaged—predictive, diagnostic, and risk assessment. Diagnostic genetic testing is performed on an individual with a given condition to determine the precise aetiology. This already makes substantial contributions to the diagnostic process in many areas of medicine. In dementia, diagnostic testing is now a distinct possibility for all the early-onset, autosomal dominant conditions listed in Table 7.1. A definitive diagnosis, in life, can now be made for most FAD, familial FTD, familial CJD, and other disorders. The same is not true for late-onset AD and it is apparent that genetic testing will never supplant clinical diagnosis. Although probably contributing the greatest amount to the risk of LOAD, *APOE* is neither sensitive nor specific enough to make an absolute diagnosis. However, it is possible that *APOE* genotyping could be used as an adjunctive test in the diagnostic work-up. In a large, multicentre, postmortem study, Mayeux *et al.* found that adding in *APOE* genotyping to the diagnostic process did increase specificity considerably, but at the expense of sensitivity (Mayeux *et al.* 1998). The sensitivity of 61% for combined clinical and genetic diagnosis in this study falls considerably below the 'gold standard' of 80% set for biomarkers of AD (Alzheimer's Association and the National Institute for Aging 1998). Although promoted as a diagnostic adjunctive test, the use of *APOE* in clinical diagnosis remains controversial.

Predictive testing is performed on relatives of patients to determine whether they too will suffer from the disorder. Such an endeavour is fraught with ethical problems. Huntington's disease (HD) has probably most to teach us about AD. Protocols for predictive testing have been adopted in many countries and considerable experience gained in counselling families (Simpson and Harding 1993). Contrary to the expectations of many, most individuals receiving predictive testing do not have significant psychological side-effects and report an increased feeling of well-being even after receiving bad news (Wiggins *et al.* 1992). Some, however, do show increased psychological problems at follow-up a year after receiving even a good test result—probably because of survivor guilt and the change in life that follows such momentous information being given (Huggins *et al.* 1992). This, and the high frequency of problems encountered in the course of genetic counselling (Tyler *et al.* 1992; Scourfield *et al.* 1997), strongly supports the notion that predictive testing is best performed by clinical geneticists and their teams. Predictive testing for early-onset AD is now technically possible and, despite some differences between the conditions, the HD guidelines have been suggested for use in early-onset AD (Lennox *et al.* 1994). There is international consensus that predictive testing for late-onset AD (or more accurately risk assessment) based upon genotyping at the *APOE* locus is not possible as the information yielded by this test is neither sensitive nor specific to AD (Farrer *et al.* 1995*b*; Tunstall and Lovestone 1999; Panegyres *et al.* 2000).

Molecular biology of dementia

Alzheimer's disease and the amyloid cascade hypothesis

Alzheimer described two critical lesions in the brain of his patient, Auguste D. Progress towards understanding the process whereby plaques and tangles are formed has been remarkable, and has led to strategies for disease modification now undergoing detailed assessment at all stages from laboratory to clinical trial. The aetiopathogenesis of AD is best understood in terms of the amyloid cascade hypothesis, first proposed by John Hardy but which has seen many modifications as the data accumulate (Hardy and Higgins 1992). It is testimony, however, to the hypothesis that almost every new major discovery in AD molecular research fits with the amyloid cascade model. In its most essential form the cascade hypothesis proposes that amyloid pathology precedes tau pathology. The hypothesis derived originally from the observation that mutations in the amyloid precursor protein are a cause of AD, and that these individuals have not only amyloid pathology but also tangle pathology. As the mutations were in the gene that gives rise to the amyloid protein it would have been surprising if these mutations did not directly cause the increased amyloid production which must therefore be the primary event. Subsequently, this was shown biochemically—the mutations in *APP* do in fact give rise to increased amyloid protein (Aβ), and moreover other mutations in other genes causing FAD also alter the metabolism of APP. The definitive proof of the amyloid cascade hypothesis came with the discovery that mutations in *tau*, the protein of tangles, gives rise to tangle-only disease, placing tau pathology 'downstream' of amyloid pathology. Many questions regarding the hypothesis remain. Not least of these concerns the biochemical basis of a link between amyloid and tau. Is it plaques that are the problem, or the amyloid that makes them; and is it possible that there is some third 'cause' in late-onset AD that gives rise, independently, to plaques and tangles? All these questions will be answered in due course, but in the meantime the amyloid cascade hypothesis underpins work accelerating towards finding a disease-modifying therapy.

Amyloid plaques and the metabolism of amyloid precursor protein

Amyloid plaques, large extracellular structures with a central core of amyloid material surrounded by degenerating neurons, are perhaps the most striking neuropathological change described by Alzheimer. Amyloid, this 'peculiar substance in the cerebral cortex' (Alzheimer 1907) is deposited in plaque cores as 9–10-nm fibrils and shows birefringent green/red staining when viewed under polarized light. This is a common property of all amyloid proteins and results from the secondary structure adopted by the polypeptide *in vivo*. In addition to accumulations within plaques, amyloid fibrils are also deposited in the walls of small cortical blood vessels in AD cortex, and these vessels are also birefringent under polarized light. Amyloid protein (Aβ) was first isolated from AD meningeal blood vessel walls (Glenner and Wong 1984) and soon after from plaques themselves (Masters *et al.* 1985). This 39–43 amino acid peptide is derived from a larger membrane-bound protein—amyloid precursor protein (APP; Kang *et al.* 1987). The development of antibodies to Aβ revealed, for the first time, large diffuse amorphous structures in cortex that are invisible under conventional haematoxylin–eosin or silver impregnation staining of the brain. These lesions, known as diffuse plaques, are commonly found in young Downs' syndrome patients before the appearance of widespread plaque and tangle formation, giving rise to the suggestion that they are an early progenitor of the senile plaques found in AD (Mann *et al.* 1989).

APP is widely expressed in many tissues, and *in situ* assumes a transmembranous location with a small amino-terminus within the cell and a large carboxy-terminus projecting into the extracellular space. The Aβ fragment is located in the region of the protein anchored within the external cell membrane. The exact function of APP is still not determined, and in any case is likely to differ in different tissues. A general or housekeeping function is suggested by the observation that the protein shows considerable evolutionary conservation with cross-species similarities, and by the fact that it is part of a family of homologous proteins. Soluble forms of APP containing the KPI (Kunitz-type protease inhibitor) domain are identical to a protein previously recognized as protease nexin 2, the known functions of which suggest, by analogy, a role for APP in promoting stable cell-to-cell interaction. Further evidence suggesting that APP acts as a mediator of cellular contacts comes from evidence that it can influence adhesion and the growth properties of neuronal cells in culture (Schubert *et al.* 1989). As APP is expressed in the synapse it has been suggested that the putative cell-to-cell interaction role of APP might be involved with neuronal activity and, in line with this, mice with absent or disrupted APP show behavioural abnormalities and seizures (Muller *et al.* 1996; Steinbach *et al.* 1998).

As it is only a proportion of APP that is deposited in plaques and vessel walls in AD, it was immediately obvious that it was necessary to understand the metabolism of this protein (reviewed in Storey and Cappai 1999; Wilson *et al.* 1999). APP is cleaved by at least three putative peptidases—α-, β-, and γ-secretase (Fig. 7.1). Cleavage at the α-secretase site yields a large secreted molecule, sAPPα, which may have a role in neuroprotection, and a smaller carboxy-terminus stub which is degraded. As the cleavage site is within the Aβ part of APP then no amyloid is produced and this pathway is termed non-amyloidogenic. Combined β- and γ-secretase cleavage, on the other hand, generates the Aβ peptide. The site for γ-secretase is somewhat variable and Aβ peptides varying in length from 39 to 42 amino acids are produced. It is the longer form, Aβ42, that is most pathogenic, being more

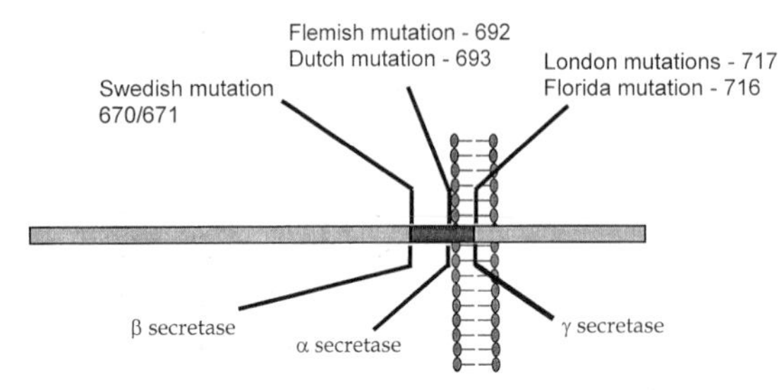

Fig. 7.1 Amyloid precursor protein. Amyloid precursor protein straddles the cell membrane with the larger amino-terminus being extracellular. The central, darker bar of the molecule is the amyloid moiety (Aβ39–42) which is deposited in amyloid plaques and blood vessel walls. Mutations in APP causing familial Alzheimer's disease and hereditary cerebral haemorrhage occur close to the sites of cleavage of APP.

liable to aggregate into insoluble fibrils and being the predominant species in plaques (Jarrett *et al.* 1993). Both amyloidogenic and non-amyloidogenic metabolism occur in normal cells; one important adaptation of the amyloid cascade hypothesis would postulate that increased Aβ42 is the key to aetiopathogenesis (Fig. 7.2).

The protein kinase C (PKC) stimulation of the α-secretase metabolism of APP may be important in disease modification, both because α-secretase cleavage precludes Aβ generation, and because the product of α-secretase cleavage (sAPPα) may be neuroprotective. PKC is a second messenger of many cell receptors, including certain members of the muscarinic acetylcholine group (M_1 and M_3). It follows that muscarinic agonism should increase sAPPα production and reduce amyloid formation. This appears to be the case in model systems, including those for muscarinic agonists being developed for clinical use as symptomatic treatments in AD (Eckols *et al.* 1995). As discussed below these compounds might also protect against some of the processes thought to underlie tangle formation. It has been suggested that this might have some aetiological importance in AD (Francis *et al.* 1999). Loss of cholinergic neurons would lead to decreased activity at postsynaptic receptors, decreased non-amyloidogenic metabolism of APP, increased tau phosphorylation (see below), and death of that neuron. In turn the cholinergic output of this neuron would be diminished, leading to an accelerating spread of pathology along neuroanatomical circuits and not purely to geographically adjacent cells. The pathological process of AD does seem to follow this course.

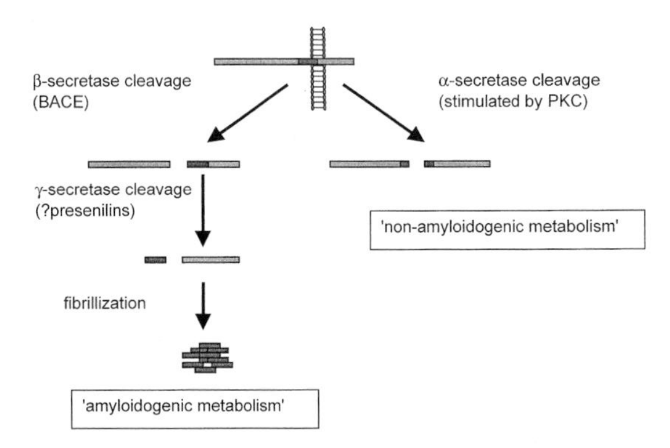

Fig. 7.2 The metabolism of amyloid precursor protein. APP is metabolized by the combined activities of BACE and γ-secretase to generate Aβ39–42 peptides. Aβ42 peptides have a tendency to fibrillize and form the nidus of amyloid plaques. An alternative metabolism of APP by α-secretase, stimulated by PKC, cleaves in the Aβ moiety itself, precluding the generation of amyloid.

The molecular genetics of the dementias have provided a stunning endorsement of the amyloid cascade hypothesis. Mutations in *APP* closely mirror the secretase sites in the molecule, and in cells mutated *APP* shows altered metabolism, generating more total Aβ (Haass *et al.* 1995) or more Aβ42 (Suzuki *et al.* 1994) depending on the mutation (Fig. 7.1). The other genes mutated in FAD are the two highly homologous presenilin genes, encoding multipass, membrane-bound proteins. As they are essential for the metabolism of APP, these proteins probably possess γ-secretase activity or possibly tightly regulate γ-secretase. Loss of presenilin activity in neurons from transgenic animals reduces or abolishes γ-secretase cleavage of APP without affecting α- or β-secretase activity (De Strooper *et al.* 1998). Unfortunately, in terms of therapy for AD, the same enzymatic activity of presenilin also cleaves Notch. Loss of Notch cleavage, a protein essential for the normal growth of neurons and other tissues, renders genetically modified mice lacking

Notch unviable from an early embryonic stage. Notch is also present in adult brain and is involved in haemopoeisis, and so the role of γ-secretase or presenilin inhibition in future disease-modification strategies is uncertain. The other enzyme responsible for amyloidogenic metabolism of APP: β-secretase, or beta-site APP-cleaving enzyme (BACE), has been identified and inhibitors of this protein are under development as potential therapeutic strategies in AD (Vassar *et al.* 1999).

If the amyloid cascade hypothesis is correct then transgenic animals overexpressing amyloidogenic proteins should have plaques, tangles, and dementia. The observation that they do not have all three of these features of AD does not disprove the hypothesis, but it demonstrates that it is only a framework for understanding and that the actual molecular biology of AD is complex. A number of animal models have been generated that overexpress human APP with different disease-causing mutations, and these animals do display plaques and some cognitive abnormalities, and in some cases some minor changes in tau protein (Games *et al.* 1995; Hsiao *et al.* 1995; Moechars *et al.* 1999). None, however, have full AD-like tangles. Mice with *PS-1*-mutation overexpression have increased Aβ42 generation but no amyloid deposition; mice with both mutant *PS-1* and mutant *APP* overexpression have the most severe amyloid deposition and an acquired cognitive impairment syndrome (Holcomb *et al.* 1998). Even so, they do not have tangles. Clearly the connection between plaques and tangles is one of the most challenging puzzles remaining in AD molecular research.

Preventing the formation of amyloid thorough presenilin or BACE inhibition is one obvious strategy for tackling the plaque pathology of AD. An alternative would be to reduce the aggregation of amyloid peptides (Lansbury 1999) and compounds that prevent or delay fibrillogenesis are under development. However, perhaps the most startling development has been the discovery that active immunization (against Aβ peptide) or even passive immunization (with antibody) reverses the pathology in transgenic mice. Transgenic mice expressing human mutant *APP* have amyloid deposits and plaques in brain. When Aβ42 protein was injected peripherally it either prevented the formation of this pathology or prevented its progression, depending upon the time of injection (Schenk *et al.* 1999). Subsequently it was demonstrated that both active immunization with peptide and passive immunization with antibody reduced amyloid deposition, and that the acquired cognitive impairment seen in some of the animal models was prevented (Janus *et al.* 2000). These studies demonstrate that the brain is not the immunologically preserved organ it was once thought to be, and suggest that 'amyloid vaccination' might be a therapeutic strategy in AD. It remains to be seen whether a similar immune response can be generated in humans, whether there are adverse consequences of such a response (Aβ42 is generated in small quantities in normal brain), and, importantly, whether the effects on cognition and amyloid seen in mice will extrapolate to effects on dementia in humans. The absence of tangles in the transgenic mice models may be a limiting factor in interpreting the animal studies. Also, at present, it is difficult to reconcile the finding that an immune response delays disease progression with those observations from epidemiology that anti-inflammatory treatment might be protective. None the less, this approach will be the most important test of the amyloid cascade hypothesis and the first disease-modifying treatment to be tested in humans.

Tau protein and the importance of tangles

The second characteristic neuropathological lesion described by Alzheimer was the neurofibrillary tangle, visible in the cortex on silver-impregnation staining. Neurofibrillary tangles are intracellular fibrillar structures with a typical flame-shaped morphology, frequently observed as the tangle accumulates within the neuronal cell body and gradually assumes that shape. Round or globular tangles are also seen, as are 'ghost' or 'tombstone' tangles that remain in the neuropil after neuronal death. Whilst the debate regarding the pathogenicity of plaques continues, it is clear that tangles most certainly do cause disease as they result in neuronal death. It is probable that the function of neurons is compromised long before loss of the neuron itself; and, in line with this, neurofibrillary tangle counts correlate well with the degree of cognitive impairment (Nagy *et al.* 1995).

Ultrastructural analysis of tangles demonstrates that their fibrillar structure comes from multiple paired helical filaments. These paired helical filaments (PHF) are found not only in tangles but also in the degenerating neurites surrounding senile plaques and scattered throughout the cortex and in neuropil threads. Direct biochemical analysis of the PHFs of tangles was made possible by extraction procedures that utilized detergents to solubilize the relatively resistant tangle-containing preparations. By direct sequencing and by immunochemical methods, these studies unequivocally demonstrated that the central component of PHFs was the microtubule-associated protein tau (Lee *et al.* 1991; Goedert *et al.* 1992*a*).

Microtubules are a major component of the cellular cytoskeleton, present in all cells, but assuming a very different structure and function in the highly specialized neuron. In non-neuronal cells, microtubules appear like the spokes of a wheel radiating out from a central hub—the centrosome—to the periphery of the cells. These microtubules, composed of polymers of the protein tubulin, are intimately involved in cell division and contribute to the arrangement of organelles and chromosomes during mitosis and meiosis. The neuron is a postmitotic, non-dividing cell, so this function of microtubules in cell division is therefore redundant. Instead, in neurons, microtubules are arranged in parallel with neurofilaments, along the axis of the axon, and they have a role in facilitating transport between the cell body and the synapse. Tubulin polymerizes *in vitro* into microtubule-like structures, but this process is facilitated by a group of proteins known as microtubule-associated proteins (MAPs). A number of these are common to all cells; but of neuronal specific MAPS, MAP2 predominantly assumes a dendritic location whereas tau is present in axons. Thus tau has a specialized role in neurons in maintaining the neuronal, and indeed axonal, specific structure and function of microtubules.

The tau accumulated into PHFs in AD is highly phosphorylated and can be distinguished from normal adult tau by antibodies specific to phosphorylated epitopes and by a change in apparent molecular weight on electrophoresis (reviewed in Lovestone and Reynolds 1997). Initially it was assumed that this phosphorylation was abnormal and specific to AD, but subsequently it has been recognized that highly phosphorylated tau is present during development and is also present in normal adult brains (Garver *et al.* 1994; Matsuo *et al.* 1994). This realization that PHF-like tau is not specific to AD brain, mirrors to some extent the development of amyloid research described above. The deposits of Aβ in plaques and highly phosphorylated tau in tangles are, it turns out, pathological deposits of normal proteins as opposed to accumulations of pathological proteins. In retrospect, this might have been predicted in such a late-onset disorder as AD—if pathologically abnormal proteins were constitutively produced then an onset much earlier in life would have been expected. With AD a subtle increase in the proportion of Aβ42 or highly phosphorylated tau produced might result in a neurodegenerative process. Alternatively, the pathogenetic factor might be an abnormal process of fibrillogenesis of both amyloid and tau.

The binding of microtubule-associated proteins to tubulin, and hence their functional ability to promote microtubule stability, is modified by changes in phosphorylation. Highly phosphorylated PHF-like tau is less effective at polymerizing tubulin *in vitro*. It can be predicted therefore that as the proportion of highly phosphorylated tau in neurons is increased then microtubules will become less stable. Changes in the stability of the microtubules and subsequent cytoskeletal disruption would certainly result in functional changes in affected neurons, and the symptoms of AD might well result from this cytoskeletal-associated functional impairment as much as from actual neuronal loss.

The recognition that PHFs are composed of highly phosphorylated tau promoted an intensive search for kinases and phosphatases responsible for regulating tau phosphorylation. *In vitro* studies suggested that a number of proline-directed kinases would phosphorylate tau at PHF epitopes including mitogen-activated protein kinases (MAP kinases), cyclin-dependent kinases (Cdk), glycogen synthase kinase-3 (GSK-3) and others. However, *in vitro* studies do not necessarily reflect the *in vivo* situation, and in intact mammalian cells it was shown that GSK-3, but not MAP kinases, phosphorylate tau at PHF epitopes (Lovestone *et al.* 1994). In neurons, inhibition of GSK-3 activity results in a decrease in the phosphorylation of tau, and in transgenic mice increasing GSK-3 activity increases tau phosphorylation (Hong *et al.* 1997; Hong and Lee 1997). There can be little doubt that GSK-3 is an important, if not the only, tau-kinase in neurons. This does not imply that GSK-3 alone is responsible for changes in the phosphorylation in AD, as it might be that the disease results from an underactivity of phosphatases rather than an overactivity of kinases (Goedert *et al.* 1992*b*).

As tau phosphorylation is a critical factor in the regulation of the normal function of the cytoskeleton in neurons, the regulation of GSK-3 is likely to be important in other contexts. Of interest to psychiatry then is the finding that lithium is a potent inhibitor of GSK-3. Lithium also inhibits inositol monosphosphatase, but increasingly it seems that this function of lithium does not underlie its therapeutic function in the affective disorders (Manji *et al.* 1999). Lithium inhibits GSK-3, it does so at therapeutic concentrations and in doing so alters tau phosphorylation in neurons in intact animals, and alters tau function (Hong *et al.* 1997; Muñoz-Montaño *et al.* 1997; Lovestone *et al.* 1999; Leroy *et al.* 2000). Sodium valproate also inhibits GSK-3 (Chen *et al.* 1999), offering some support for the idea that inhibition of GSK-3 may be therapeutic in affective disorders, although still not ruling out the possibility that it is this function of lithium that may underlie its neurotoxicity (Kores and Lader 1997). With respect to AD, it has been suggested that GSK-3 is the missing link between amyloid plaque and tangle pathology, as Aβ increases GSK-3 activity (Takashima *et al.* 1998) and lithium protects neurons from Aβ toxicity (G. Alvarez *et al.* 1999). It follows that inhibition of GSK-3 might be therapeutic.

GSK-3 is normally regulated via two main pathways—one involving insulin, PI3-kinase, and protein kinase B (PKB); and the other involving PKC. PKB and PKC both result in the inhibition of GSK-3 activity. As discussed above in the context of APP metabolism, PKC is activated by M_1 and M_3 acetylcholine muscarinic receptors and it follows that muscarinic agonists would be predicted to inhibit the GSK-3-mediated phosphorylation of tau. This has now been shown to be the case (Sadot *et al.* 1996; Forlenza *et al.* 2000). In cell models, muscarinic agonists favourably alter both APP metabolism and tau phosphorylation, suggesting that any strategy to increase muscarinic activity (including both the muscarinic agonists and the acetylcholinesterase inhibitors) might be disease-modifying (Lovestone 1997). This hypothesis deserves testing in human trials.

Whilst tau in PHF is relatively stably phosphorylated, it is not yet determined whether this is a primary or secondary event. Some studies have suggested there is a redistribution of tau to PHFs in AD, as a primary event, that reduces the amount of tau available for stabilizing microtubules (Mukaetova-Ladinska *et al.* 1993). Such a redistribution would be predicted to occur as a result of an increase in phosphorylation, but might also occur as a result of mutations in *tau* that cause FTDP-17 and related disorders. Splice-site mutations increase the proportion of tau with 4-microtubule-binding repeat domains, and the proportion of 3- and 4-repeat tau may be critical in ensuring maximal tau–tubulin binding (Buee and Delacourte 1999). The missense mutations in *tau* reduce the binding of tau to tubulin and reduce the ability of tau to promote microtubule extensions *in vitro* and in cells. The best working model of tau pathology at present is that, in AD, amyloid production somehow alters the phosphorylation of tau, perhaps mediated through GSK-3, whereas in FTDP-17 mutations in *tau* either result in a disruption of the proportion of 3- and 4-repeat tau and increase the amount of unbound tau, or directly reduce tau binding to microtubules. Increase in phosphorylation, decrease in binding to microtubules, or a change in the normal proportion of 3- and 4-repeat tau all result in an abnormal accumulation of tau in the cell body, allowing tau to aggregate into PHFs which form tangles and hence result in neuronal death.

Synuclein and Lewy bodies

Amyloid plaques contain other proteins, and one major non-amyloid component was found to be a normal presynaptic protein called synuclein (Brookes and St Clair 1994; Iwai *et al.* 1995). Unexpectedly, identical mutations in one of the synuclein genes (α-synuclein) were found in apparently unrelated families with autosomal dominant Parkinson's disease (PD) (M. Farrer *et al.* 1999). Subsequently it was shown that antibodies to α-synuclein labelled Lewy bodies in both sporadic dementia with Lewy bodies (DLB) and PD (Spillantini *et al.* 1997). In Lewy bodies, α-synuclein accumulates in an aggregated fibrillized and insoluble form (Baba *et al.* 1998) and *in vitro* the mutations causing PD enhance α-synuclein fibrillization (Conway *et al.* 1998).

Moves are afoot to redefine the neurodegenerative conditions not in clinical diagnostic categories but in aetiological or at least pathogenetic categories. Thus the tauopathies include the frontal lobe dementias and progressive supranuclear palsy (Van Slegtenhorst *et al.* 2000), the synucleinopathies include dementia with Lewy bodies, Parkinson's disease, and multiple system atrophy (Farrer *et al.* 1999), and the amyloidopathies include familial British dementia and hereditary cerebral haemorrhage with amyloidosis. Alzheimer's disease straddles these categories, being in some respects simultaneously an amyloidopathy, a tauopathy, and a synucleinopathy. Understanding the interplay of these pathological processes in AD remains a considerable challenge.

Apolipoprotein E and the pathogenesis of AD

Although the association between the *APOE* gene and AD was demonstrated unequivocally in 1993, the pathogenesis of this link is not understood. Two main hypotheses have attempted to account for the association of AD with *APOE* genotype by implicating ApoE isoforms in the generation of either amyloid plaques or neurofibrillary tangles. Alternatively, it might be that the effect of ApoE variation is mediated through some other, and more general, mechanism such as one associated with its known function in lipid and cholesterol transport. *In vitro* studies have attempted to examine the association of ApoE with both Aβ and tau. ApoE does show an isoform-specific effect in binding to Aβ, but the direction of effect is unclear (Strittmatter *et al.* 1993; LaDu *et al.* 1997). *In vitro* studies have also suggested that there are ApoE isoform differences in binding to tau protein, with non-E4 isoforms showing a greater binding avidity (Strittmatter *et al.* 1994; Huang *et al.* 1995). This led to the hypothesis that ApoE2 or -E3 isoforms bind to tau and hence protect it from stable hyperphosphorylation (Roses *et al.* 1996). In line with this suggestion is the observation that some strains of transgenic mice lacking ApoE protein have increased tau phosphorylation, as do mice expressing only human ApoE4 (Genis *et al.* 1995; Tesseur *et al.* 2000). The different ApoE isoforms also have differential effects on neurons in culture, with ApoE3 increasing and ApoE4 reducing neurite outgrowth (Bellosta *et al.* 1995). Whether this is through the cytoskeleton and tau or some other mechanism, such as altering local cholesterol transport, remains to be seen. Finally, a role for ApoE peripherally cannot be discounted, as ApoE clearly alters the risk of cardiac disease and cardiac risk factors alter the risk of diverse dementias (Shi *et al.* 2000). However, in a direct epidemiological study of this potential interaction between cardiovascular risk factors and incident dementia this supposition was not confirmed: the presence of the *APOE* $\varepsilon 4$ allele increased the risk for dementia independently of its effect on dyslipidaemia and atherogenesis, as measured by blood pressure and electrocardiography (ECG) (Prince *et al.* 2000).

Integrating molecular science and epidemiology

One of the great challenges of modern science is that of integrating molecular research with large-scale clinical research. This is being achieved most notably in the course of the human genome project, and it is now routine for epidemiological studies of dementia to include, for example, *APOE* genotyping in addition to assessments of environmental risks. Even here, however, there are challenges of scale—genetic association studies ideally involve many hundreds of affected subjects and within-study replications are becoming mandatory. Accessing suitably large, selected populations with prevalent dementia is an achievable challenge. The resources required to obtain similarly sized populations of incident dementia are considerably greater. However, in addition to the challenge of genetics, increasing attempts are being made to integrate epidemiological findings into molecular research. One example is that of diabetes. Increasing evidence suggests that non-insulin diabetes is a risk factor for AD (Ott *et al.* 1999; Stewart and Liolitsa 1999). It might be that diabetes simply increases the vascular risk factors of dementia, but the fact that insulin resistance also increases the risk of AD (Kuusisto *et al.* 1997) suggests instead that the relationship is more direct.

This relationship between insulin and the pathogenesis of AD has been approached in many different ways. Insulin signalling involves protein kinase C (PKC) and, as discussed above, PKC increases the non-amyloidogenic metabolism of APP. In cells, insulin has been shown to increase the non-amyloidogenic fragment sAPPα (Solano *et al.* 2000) and in patients it also alters APP protein in serum (Craft *et al.* 2000). Insulin acts to downregulate the activity of GSK-3, and in neurons insulin reduces tau phosphorylation (Hong and Lee 1997). In animals, hypoglycaemia does the same (Yanagisawa *et al.* 1999). Mutations in *PS-1* that cause AD reduce the activity of protein kinase B (PKB)—an even more important insulin signalling intermediary than PKC (Weihl *et al.* 1999). Finally, insulin-degrading enzyme reduces the available insulin and also degrades amyloid (Kurochkin and Goto 1994; Qiu *et al.* 1998; Vekrellis *et al.* 2000). One hypothesis therefore to explain the link between AD and non-insulin-dependent diabetes mellitus (NIDDM) is that a failure of normal insulin signalling results in an increase in amyloid formation and tau phosphorylation, whilst a loss of normal activity of insulin-degrading enzyme would result in an increase in amyloid deposition. Whilst not yet able to explain the association between NIDDM and AD, such studies are attempting to bridge the gap between molecular and epidemiological sciences, and such attempts will become increasingly important.

Molecular biology and molecular markers

Molecular biology is also being used to try and identify a molecular marker of AD that might be used as a test—either for diagnosis or to follow the course of the condition. No such test is yet available although progress is being made. The neuropathology of AD starts many years, probably decades, before the onset of clinical symptoms, with some of the earliest changes being the appearance of phosphorylated tau epitopes and then the accumulation of neurofibrillary tangles (Braak and Braak 1995). It was therefore logical to determine if tau protein is present in the cerebrospinal fluid (CSF) of patients with AD, and examine whether this constitutes a biomarker (Vandermeeren *et al.* 1993; Mori *et al.* 1995). Measuring tau in CSF has been performed in over 25 studies—including more than 1100 patients with AD. One finding is remarkably consistent—in almost every study comparing AD and normal elderly people the amount of tau is significantly and substantially elevated in AD (the early studies were reviewed by the Alzheimer's Association and the National Institute for Aging (1998). However, the discriminant power with other neurological disorders (and hence specificity) is less certain (Tapiola *et al.* 1998). For example, elevated levels of tau also occur in CJD (Otto *et al.* 1997), normal-pressure hydrocephalus (Arai *et al.* 1997*a*), B_{12} deficiency encephalopathy (Arai *et al.* 1997*a*), frontotemporal dementia (Green *et al.* 1999), dementia with Lewy bodies (DLB) (Arai *et al.* 1997*b*), and corticobasal degeneration (Urakami *et al.* 1999). Some studies show significant discrimination between AD and vascular dementia (Arai *et al.* 1998), whereas others do not (Skoog *et al.* 1995). Also, it is unclear whether tau levels correlate with dementia severity; some studies have reported that an increase in tau levels is associated with increased severity (Skoog *et al.* 1995; Tato *et al.* 1995), whereas others do not find such a correlation (Riemenschneider *et al.* 1996; Galasko *et al.* 1997; Green *et al.* 1999; Sunderland *et al.* 1999). Thus whilst the evidence that CSF tau is increased in AD is robust, it also appears to be increased in other disorders and shows no clear relation with disease severity.

Other studies of CSF in AD provide evidence that metabolic products of amyloid precursor protein (APP) are also altered in AD. Thus, soluble APP is decreased in symptomatic carriers of pathogenic *APP* mutations and in sporadic AD, but it is also low in spongiform encephalopathies (Farlow *et al.* 1992, 1994; Lannfelt *et al.* 1995). The Aβ1–42 peptide, and in some but not all studies the Aβ1–40 peptide as well, is also decreased in dementia (Tamaoka *et al.* 1997; Galasko *et al.* 1998; Samuels *et al.* 1999). However, the specificity of the reduction in metabolites of APP relative to other non-AD dementias has not yet been determined (Galasko *et al.* 1998).

Whilst neither levels of tau nor APP metabolites alone appear to meet the requirements for a diagnostic test, their combined sensitivity and specificity is better (Galasko *et al.* 1998; Kanai *et al.* 1998), but this has not been fully assessed for important diagnostic distinctions (i.e. mild cognitive impairment vs. AD; AD vs. other similar dementias). Examining tau and Aβ in CSF was an obvious first step in searching for protein changes in AD, but other proteins have also been found to be altered in CSF—including cholinesterases (Appleyard *et al.* 1987; Appleyard and McDonald 1992; Sáez-Valero *et al.* 1999), monoamines (Blennow *et al.* 1992), apolipoprotein E (Blennow *et al.* 1994), interleukins (Blum-Degen *et al.* 1995), and insulin (Craft *et al.* 1998). However, few of these studies have been replicated.

It seems unlikely that CSF will ever be useful in routine clinical testing for AD, but these studies provide promise that molecular biology insights might one day lead to such a test.

Molecular biology and non-AD dementias

Molecular biology is also making inroads into other, non-AD dementias. Two illustrate very different mechanisms from the tauopathy, synucleinopathy, or amyloidopathy disorders discussed above. A small but significant proportion of dementia results from HD and related disorders, although the onset is usually in midlife. HD is caused by a genetic mechanism that appears to be exclusive to the neurological systems, causing also dentato-rubro-pallido-luysian atrophy, myotonic dystrophy, Kennedy's motor neuron disorder, fragile X, and other conditions. A number of these rarer conditions also result in dementia. The genetic mechanism underlying all these conditions is an expansion of a region of repeats of a triplet nucleotide sequence in different genes (see Zoghbi and Orr 2000 for a review). For HD, for example, in the upstream, non-coding region of the huntingtin gene, a sequence of DNA contains a repeating CAG triplet, coding for glutamine. The number of repeats varies from individual to individual, but HD results when the triplet is expanded. As transgenic mice overexpressing only this non-coding polyglutamine repeat sequence have many of the characteristics of HD, this suggests that the mutation causes a novel and toxic gain of function as opposed to the loss of the normal function of the huntingtin gene (Mangiarini *et al.* 1996). When these transgenic mice were characterized, intraneuronal inclusions were observed that prompted a successful search for similar inclusions in HD brain (Davies *et al.* 1997). Huntingtin protein containing polyglutamine expansions forms fibrils *in vitro*, which probably underlie the aggregation of the protein (Scherzinger *et al.* 1997). However, the role of these aggregates in nuclei remained a mystery until it was demonstrated that huntingtin containing polyglutamine repeat sequences binds to, and interferes with, proteins involved with CREB (cAMP responsive-element binding protein) mediated gene transcription. This nuclear event is of critical importance in many neuronal processes, not least of which is the formation of memory (Frank and Greenberg 1994). It appears as if in HD the normal polyglutamine repeat sequence encoded by a CAG triplet acquires, when mutated by expansion, the pathological characteristics of suppressing normal neuronal gene activation including those specific genes involved in cognition. It remains to be seen whether other triplet-repeat disorders act in the same way.

Perhaps the strangest contribution to the molecular biology of dementia comes from work on the spongiform encephalopathies—Creutzfeldt–Jakob disease (CJD), Gerstmann–Sträussler–Scheinker Disease (GSS), and kuru. Like scrapie in sheep and a host of similar disorders, including bovine spongiform encephalopathy (BSE), these disorders can be transmitted to laboratory animals. The transmissible agent, in material from the central nervous system, is resistant to ultraviolet irradiation and high temperatures and was stylishly named 'The Prion Particle'—a proteinaceous infectious agent distinct from viruses and bacteria (reviewed in Prusiner 1991).

In human forms of these disorders, prion diseases occur as familial and sporadic forms. Familial spongiform encephalopathy is associated with mutations in the prion protein (PrP) gene (reviewed in Collinge and Palmer 1993). The *PrP* gene codes for a protein normally expressed by neurons and present on the cell surface, possibly having a role in synaptic transmission (Collinge *et al.* 1994). In CJD and GSS this protein accumulates and is deposited in plaques as amyloid (not the AD amyloid but prion-amyloid which shows some of the same physical characteristics). It is this protein that in the prion diseases becomes resistant to proteolysis and is itself infectious.

Normal cellular protein is designated PrP^{c} and the disease-associated protein as PrP^{sc}. Astonishingly, direct analysis of PrP^{c} and PrP^{sc} from cases of sporadic spongiform encephalopathy have shown these proteins to have an identical amino acid sequence. One model that has been developed to explain these findings is that PrP^{c} undergoes a conformational or post-translational modification and is thereby converted to PrP^{sc}. In the process PrP^{sc} becomes resistant to proteolysis and to other processes such as UV-irradiation, formaldehyde treatment, and high temperatures. This PrP^{sc} protein acts as a pathological molecular chaperone—a protein that causes another protein, in this case PrP^{c}, to undergo conformational change. In this way PrP^{sc} is able to catalyse the conversion of further PrP^{c} molecules to PrP^{sc} resulting in an accelerating process of PrP^{sc} accumulation and deposition into plaques. The rapid clinical deterioration would result from this stage with an accompanying and ever-accelerating neurodegeneration. The initial event converting PrP^{c} to PrP^{sc} is unknown, but might be exogenous PrP^{sc} from nervous tissue of an infected individual in the sporadic form, or it may result from the mutations in the *PrP* gene in familial forms.

Transgenic animal models have gone some way to confirming this hypothesis. Mice with *PrP* mutations analogous to familial *GSS* mutations succumb to an encephalopathy (Hsiao *et al.* 1990). Mice carrying the hamster prion gene are susceptible to hamster exogenous prions, whereas those carrying excess mice prion genes are not (Prusiner *et al.* 1990). In a fascinating extension of this work it has also been shown that mice with no prion gene are normal but resistant to infectious prions. When hamster genes are introduced to this prion-deficient transgenic line, the mice become susceptible to hamster but not to mice prions (Prusiner *et al.* 1993). These experiments clearly confirm the unique nature of prion disease—an infectious condition caused by exogenous protein or by mutations, but where susceptibility to the disease is a host as well as a donor property.

This host–donor relationship is of critical importance in the pathogenicity of the prion protein. Where the agent jumps species barriers, the pathogenicity is altered and the agent then appears capable of infecting a wider host range. This has been dramatically and tragically illustrated with the jump of bovine spongiform encephalopathy (BSE) to humans in the form of new variant CJD (vCJD). BSE spread through the UK cattle herd resulting in an epidemic (Hope *et al.* 1989). The cause is not fully understood, but almost certainly results from the practice of using cattle feeds containing processed animal protein, including that from sheep and cows. New variant CJD is a form of the disorder that was recognized as having a particularly virulent course, and affecting young people with a prodromal period characterized by neuropsychiatric symptoms including depression followed by dementia (Zeidler *et al.* 1997). Transgenic animal experiments and strain analysis suggested that this disorder was, in effect, human BSE (Bruce *et al.* 1997) and there is now very little doubt remaining that vCJD has resulted from BSE-infected cattle entering the human food chain (Collinge 1997). Whether this results in an epidemic of human CJD or is limited to a moderate number of affected people will be one of the more tragic and worrying pieces of data to come. Detection of presymptomatic vCJD by the glycation pattern of prion protein in tissue (including, for example, tonsils) is possible, and may give some idea of the numbers of people likely to be affected (Ironside *et al.* 2000). Equally, differential diagnosis may be helped by the finding that 14–3–3 proteins in CSF are altered in CJD (Poser *et al.* 1999; Wiltfang *et al.* 1999). For some considerable while to come, however, countries affected by BSE and with cases of vCJD, most obviously the UK, but also possibly other European countries such as France (Streichenberger *et al.* 2000), will live under a terrible shadow.

Conclusions

Huge progress has been made in understanding the diverse aetiopathogenesis of the dementias. Throughout these various and sometimes surprising findings, the amyloid cascade hypothesis stands firm. The genes causing much early-onset FAD have been found, and progress is being made with the monumental task of finding the genes altering susceptibility to late-onset AD. The metabolism of APP underlying the formation of amyloid is pretty much understood, and the process of tangle formation is unravelling itself. These advances in molecular biology and genetics have altered our understanding of the dementias to such an extent that the molecular biologists have become confident enough to suggest a reformulation of the classification of the neurodegenerative diseases into the tauopathies, the synucleinopathies, and the amyloidopathies. Disorders with very different clinical appearances—Pick's disease and corticobasal degeneration, for example—are now seen to have a similar pathogenesis. But reclassification of disease is not the goal of molecular biology and genetics. Nor is the molecular diagnosis of autosomal dominant dementias, although that is now possible, nor is finding molecular tests for other diseases, although progress here is also being made. The true goal of the molecular biology of the dementias is to find a therapy that will modify, delay, prevent, or even reverse the pathology of the condition. It is a testament to the power of the approach that the first such putative treatments started to be tested in patients just 15 years after the molecular biology and genetics of dementia really got going.

Notes

1. The name *BRI* gene derives from the peptide that forms the amyloid in this condition—British amyloid, or Abri for short.

References

Alvarez, G., Muñoz-Montaño, J. R., Satrústegui, J., Avila, J., Bogónez, E., and Díaz-Nido, J. (1999). Lithium protects cultured neurons against β-amyloid-induced neurodegeneration. *FEBS Letters*, **453**, 260–4.

Alvarez, R., Alvarez, V., Lahoz, C. H., Martinez, C., Pena, J., Sanchez, J. M., *et al.* (1999). Angiotensin converting enzyme and endothelial nitric oxide synthase DNA polymorphisms and late onset Alzheimer's disease. *Journal of Neurology, Neurosurgery and Psychiatry*, **67**, 733–6.

Alzheimer, A. (1907). Über eine eigenartige Erkrankung der Hirnrinde. *Zentralblatt für Nervenheilkunde und Psychiatrie*, **30**, 177–9.

Alzheimer's Association, National Institute for Aging. (1998). Consensus report of the Working Group on: 'Molecular and Biochemical Markers of Alzheimer's Disease'. *Neurobiology of Aging*, 19, 109–16.

Amouyel, P., Alpérovitch, A., Delasnerie-Lauprêtre, N., and Laplanche J-L. (1995). Apolipoprotein E in Creutzfeldt–Jakob disease. *Lancet*, **345**, 595–6.

Appleyard, M. E. and McDonald, B. (1992). Acetylcholinesterase and butyrylcholinesterase activities in cerebrospinal fluid from different levels of the neuraxis of patients with dementia of the Alzheimer type. *Journal of Neurology, Neurosurgery and Psychiatry*, **55**, 1074–8.

Appleyard, M. E., Smith, A. D., Berman, P., Wilcock, G. K., Esiri, M. M., Neary, D., *et al.* (1987). Cholinesterase activities in cerebrospinal fluid of patients with senile dementia of Alzheimer type. *Brain*, **110** (Pt 5), 1309–22.

Arai, H., Higuchi, S., and Sasaki H. (1997*a*). Apolipoprotein E genotyping and cerebrospinal fluid tau protein: implications for the clinical diagnosis of Alzheimer's disease. *Gerontology*, **43**(Suppl. 1), 2–10.

Arai, H., Morikawa, Y., Higuchi, M., Matsui, T., Clark, C. M., Miura, M., *et al.* (1997*b*). Cerebrospinal fluid tau levels in neurodegenerative diseases with distinct tau-related pathology. *Biochemical and Biophysical Research Communications*, **236**, 262–4.

Arai, H., Satoh-Nakagawa, T., Higuchi, M., Morikawa, Y., Miura, M., Kawakami, H., *et al.* (1998). No increase in cerebrospinal fluid tau protein levels in patients with vascular dementia. *Neuroscience Letters*, **256**, 174–6.

Baba, M., Nakajo, S., Tu, P. H., Tomita, T., Nakaya, K., Lee, V. M. Y., *et al.* (1998). Aggregation of α-synuclein in Lewy bodies of sporadic Parkinson's disease and dementia with lewy bodies. *American Journal of Pathology*, **152**, 879–84.

Baker, M., Litvan, I., Houlden, H., Adamson, J., Dickson, D., Perez-Tur, J., *et al.* (1999). Association of an extended haplotype in the tau gene with progressive supranuclear palsy. *Human Molecular Genetics*, **8**, 711–15.

Bellosta, S., Nathan, B. P., Orth, M., Dong, L-M., Mahley, R. W., and Pitas, R. E. (1995). Stable expression and secretion of apolipoproteins E3 and E4 in mouse neuroblastoma cells produces differential effects on neurite outgrowth. *Journal of Biological Chemistry*, **270**, 27063–71.

Bird, T. D., Lampe, T. H., Nemens, E. J., Miner, G. W., Sumi, S. M., and Schellenberg, G. D. (1988). Familial Alzheimer's disease in American descendants of the Volga Germans: probable genetic founder effect. *Annals of Neurology*, **23**, 25–31.

Blacker, D., Wilcox, M. A., Laird, N. M., Rodes, L., Horvath, S. M., Go, R. C. P., *et al.* (1998). Alpha-2 macroglobulin is genetically associated with Alzheimer disease. *Nature Genetics*, 19, 357–60.

Blennow, K., Wallin, A., Gottfries, C. G., Lekman, A., Karlsson, I., Skoog, I. *et al.* (1992). Significance of decreased lumbar CSF levels of HVA and 5-HIAA in Alzheimer's disease. *Neurobiology of Aging*, **13**, 107–13.

Blennow, K., Hesse, C., and Fredman, P. (1994). Cerebrospinal fluid apolipoprotein E is reduced in Alzheimer's disease. *Neuroreport*, **5**, 2534–6.

Blum-Degen, D., Müller, T., Kuhn, W., Gerlach, M., Przuntek, H., and Riederer P. (1995). Interleukin-1β and interleukin-6 are elevated in the cerebrospinal fluid of Alzheimer's and *de novo* Parkinson's disease patients. *Neuroscience Letters*, **202**, 17–20.

Braak, H. and Braak E. (1995). Staging of Alzheimer's disease-related neurofibrillary changes. *Neurobiology of Aging*, **16**, 271–8.

Breitner, J. C., Silverman, J. M., Mohs, R. C., and Davis, K. L. (1988). Familial aggregation in Alzheimer's disease: comparison of risk among relatives of early- and late-onset cases, and among male and female relatives in successive generations. *Neurology*, **38**, 207–12.

Brookes, A. J. and St Clair, D. (1994). Synuclein proteins and Alzheimer's disease. *Trends in Neuroscience*, **17**, 404–5.

Bruce, M. E., Will, R. G., Ironside, J. W., McConnell, I., Drummond, D., Suttie, A., *et al.* (1997). Transmissions to mice indicate that 'new variant' CJD is caused by the BSE agent. *Nature*, **389**, 498–501.

Buee, L. and Delacourte, A. (1999). Comparative biochemistry of tau in progressive supranuclear palsy, corticobasal degeneration, FTDP-17 and Pick's disease. *Brain Pathology*, **9**, 681–93.

Campion, D., Dumanchin, C., Hannequin, D., Dubois, B., Belliard, S., Puel, M., *et al.* (1999). Early-onset autosomal dominant Alzheimer disease: prevalence, genetic heterogeneity, and mutation spectrum. *American Journal of Human Genetics*, **65**, 664–70.

Chen, G., Huang, L. D., Jiang, Y. M., and Manji, H. K. (1999). The mood-stabilizing agent valproate inhibits the activity of glycogen synthase kinase-3. *Journal of Neurochemistry*, **72**, 1327–30.

Collinge J. (1997). Human prion diseases and bovine spongiform encephalopathy (BSE). *Human Molecular Genetics*, **6**, 1699–705.

Collinge, J. and Palmer, M. S. (1993). Prion diseases in humans and their relevance to other neurodegenerative diseases. *Dementia*, **4**, 178–85.

Collinge, J., Whittington, M. A., Sidle, K. C. L., Smith, C. J., Palmer, M. S., Clarke, A. R., *et al.* (1994). Prion protein is necessary for normal synaptic function. *Nature*, **370**, 295–7.

Collins, A. and Morton, N. E. (1998). Mapping a disease locus by allelic association. *Proceedings of the National Academy of Sciences USA.*, **95**, 1741–5.

Conway, K. A., Harper, J. D., and Lansbury, P. T. (1998). Accelerated *in vitro* fibril formation by a mutant α-synuclein linked to early-onset Parkinson disease. *Nature Medicine*, **4**, 1318–20.

Corder, E. H., Saunders, A. M., Risch, N. J., Strittmatter, W. J., Schmechel, D. E., Gaskell, P. C. Jr., *et al.* (1994). Protective effect of apolipoprotein E type 2 allele for late onset Alzheimer disease. *Nature Genetics*, **7**, 180–4.

Craft, S., Peskind, E., Schwartz, M. W., Schellenberg, G. D., Raskind, M., and Porte, D. Jr. (1998). Cerebrospinal fluid and plasma insulin levels in Alzheimer's disease—relationship to severity of dementia and apolipoprotein E genotype. *Neurology*, **50**, 164–8.

Craft, S., Asthana, S., Schellenberg, G., Baker, L., Cherrier, M., Boyt, A. A., *et al.* (2000). Insulin effects on glucose metabolism, memory, and plasma amyloid precursor protein in Alzheimer's disease differ according to apolipoprotein-E genotype. *Annals of the New York Academy of Sciences*, **903**, 222–8.

Crawford, F., Town, T., Freeman, M., Schinka, J., Gold, M., Duara, R., *et al.* (1999). The alpha-2 macroglobulin gene is not associated with Alzheimer's disease in a case-control sample. *Neuroscience Letters*, **270**, 133–6.

Crawford, F., Abdullah, L., Schinka, J., Suo, Z., Gold, M., Duara, R., *et al.* (2000). Gender-specific association of the angiotensin converting enzyme gene with Alzheimer's disease. *Neuroscience Letters*, **280**, 215–19.

Davies, S. W., Turmaine, M., Cozens, B. A., DiFiglia, M., Sharp, A. H., Ross, C. A., *et al.* (1997). Formation of neuronal intranuclear inclusions underlies the neurological dysfunction in mice transgenic for the HD mutation. *Cell*, **90**, 537–48.

Davous, P. (1998). CADASIL: a review with proposed diagnostic criteria. *European Journal of Neurology*, **5**, 219–33.

De Strooper, B., Saftig, P., Craessaerts, K., Vanderstichele, H., Guhde, G., Annaert, W., *et al.* (1998). Deficiency of presenilin-1 inhibits the normal cleavage of amyloid precursor protein. *Nature*, **391**, 387–90.

Eckols, K., Bymaster, F. P., Mitch, C. H., Shannon, H. E., Ward, J. S., DeLapp, N. W. (1995). The muscarinic M1 agonist xanomeline increases soluble amyloid precursor protein release from Chinese hamster ovary-m1 cells. *Life Sciences*, **57**, 1183–90.

Farlow, M., Ghetti, B., Benson, M. D., Farrow, J. S., Van Nostrand, W. E., and Wagner, S. L. (1992). Low cerebrospinal-fluid concentrations of soluble amyloid beta-protein precursor in hereditary Alzheimer's disease. *Lancet*, **340**, 453–4.

Farlow, M., Ghetti, B., Dlouhy, S., Giaccone, G., Bugiani, O., Tagliavini, F., *et al.* (1994). Cerebrospinal fluid levels of amyloid β-protein precursor are low in Gerstmann–Sträussler–Scheinker disease: Indiana kindred. *Neurology*, **44**, 1508–10.

Farrer, L. A., O'Sullivan, D. M., Cupples, L. A., Growdon, J. H., and Myers, R. H. (1989). Assessment of genetic risk for Alzheimer's disease among first-degree relatives. *Annals of Neurology*, **25**, 485–93.

Farrer, L. A., Abraham, C. R., Volicer, L., Foley, E. J., Kowall, N. W., McKee, A. C., *et al.* (1995*a*). Allele $\varepsilon 4$ of apolipoprotein E shows a dose effect on age at onset of pick disease. *Experimental Neurology*, **136**, 162–70.

Farrer, L. A., Brin, M. F., Elsas, L., Goate, A., Kennedy, J., Mayeux, R., *et al.* (1995*b*). Statement on use of apolipoprotein E testing for Alzheimer disease. *Journal of the American Medical Association*, **274**, 1627–9.

Farrer, L. A., Cupples, L. A., Haines, J. L., Hyman, B., Kukull, W. A., Mayeux, R., *et al.* (1997). Effects of age, sex, and ethnicity on the association between apolipoprotein E genotype and Alzheimer disease—a meta-analysis. *Journal of the American Medical Association*, **278**, 1349–56.

Farrer, L. A., Sherbatich, T., Keryanov, S. A., Korovaitseva, G. I., Rogaeva, E. A., Petruk, S., *et al.* (2000). Association between angiotensin-converting enzyme and Alzheimer disease. *Archives of Neurology*, **57**, 210–14.

Farrer, M., Gwinn-Hardy, K., Hutton, M., and Hardy J. (1999). The genetics of disorders with synuclein pathology and parkinsonism. *Human Molecular Genetics*, **8**, 1901–5.

Forlenza, O., Spink, J., Anderton, B. H., Olesen, O. F., and Lovestone, S. (2000). Muscarinic agonists reduce tau phosphorylation via GSK-3 inhibition. *Journal of Neural Transmission*, **107**, 1201–12.

Foster, N. L., Wilhelmsen, K., Sima, A. A., Jones, M. Z., D'Amato, C. J., and Gilman, S. (1997). Frontotemporal dementia and parkinsonism linked to chromosome 17: a consensus conference. *Annals of Neurology*, **41**, 706–15.

Francis, P. T., Palmer, A. M., Snape, M., and Wilcock, G. K. (1999). The cholinergic hypothesis of Alzheimer's disease: a review of progress. *Journal of Neurology, Neurosurgery and Psychiatry*, **66**, 137–47.

Frank, D. A. and Greenberg, M. E. (1994). CREB: a mediator of long-term memory from mollusks to mammals. *Cell*, **79**, 5–8.

Galasko, D., Clark, C., Chang, L., Miller, B., Green, R. C., Motter, R., *et al.* (1997). Assessment of CSF levels of tan protein in mildly demented patients with Alzheimer's disease. *Neurology*, **48**, 632–5.

Galasko, D., Chang, L., Motter, R., Clark, C. M., Kaye, J., Knopman, D., *et al.* (1998). High cerebrospinal fluid tau and low amyloid $\beta 42$ levels in the clinical diagnosis of Alzheimer disease and relation to apolipoprotein E genotype. *Archives of Neurology*, **55**, 937–45.

Games, D., Adams, D., Alessandrini, R., Barbour, R., Berthelette, P., Blackwell, C., *et al.* (1995). Alzheimer-type neuropathology in transgenic mice overexpressing V717F β-amyloid precursor protein. *Nature*, **373**, 523–7.

Garver, T. D., Harris, K. A., Lehman, R. A., Lee, V. M., Trojanowski, J. Q., and Billingsley, M. L. (1994). Tau phosphorylation in human, primate, and rat brain: evidence that a pool of tau is highly phosphorylated *in vivo* and is rapidly dephosphorylated *in vitro*. *Journal of Neurochemistry*, **63**, 2279–87.

Genis, I., Gordon, I., Sehayek, E., and Michaelson, D. M. (1995). Phosphorylation of tau in apolipoprotein E-deficient mice. *Neuroscience Letters*, **199**, 5–8.

Ghetti, B., Murrell, J., Benson, M. D., and Farlow, M. R. (1992). Spectrum of amyloid beta-protein immunoreactivity in hereditary Alzheimer disease with a guanine to thymine missense change at position 1924 of the APP gene. *Brain Research*, **571**, 133–9.

Ghiso, J., Plant, G. T., Revesz, T., Wisniewski, T., and Frangione B. (1995). Familial cerebral amyloid angiopathy (British type) with nonneuritic amyloid plaque formation may be due to a novel amyloid protein. *Journal of Neurological Science*, **129**, 74–75.

Gibb, W. R., Luthert, P. J., and Marsden, C. D. (1989). Corticobasal degeneration. *Brain*, **112**, 1171–92.

Glenner, G. G. and Wong, C. W. (1984). Alzheimer's disease: initial report of the purification and characterization of a novel cerebrovascular amyloid protein. *Biochemical and Biophysical Research Communications*, **120**, 885–90.

Goate, A., Chartier-Harlin, M. C., Mullan, M., Brown, J., Crawford, F., Fidani L., *et al.* (1991). Segregation of a missense mutation in the amyloid precursor protein gene with familial Alzheimer's disease. *Nature*, **349**, 704–6.

Goedert, M., Spillantini, M. G., Jakes, R., Rutherford, D., and Crowther, R. A. (1989). Multiple isoforms of human microtubule-associated protein tau: sequences and localization in neurofibrillary tangles of Alzheimer's disease. *Neuron*, **3**, 519–26.

Goedert, M., Spillantini, M. G., Cairns, N. J., and Crowther, R. A. (1992*a*). Tau proteins of Alzheimer paired helical filaments: abnormal phosphorylation of all six brain isoforms. *Neuron*, **8**, 159–68.

Goedert, M., Cohen, E. S., Jakes, R., and Cohen P. (1992*b*). p42 Map kinase phosphorylation sites in microtubule-associated protein tau are dephosphorylated by protein phosphatase $2A_1$: implications for Alzheimer's disease. *FEBS Letters*, **312**, 95–9.

Green, A. J. E., Harvey, R. J., Thompson, E. J., and Rossor, M. N. (1999). Increased tau in the cerebrospinal fluid of patients with frontotemporal dementia and Alzheimer's disease. *Neuroscience Letters*, **259**, 133–5.

Grover, A., Houlden, H., Baker, M., Adamson, J., Lewis, J., Prihar G., *et al.* (1999). 5' splice site mutations in tau associated with the inherited dementia FTDP-17 affect a stem-loop structure that regulates alternative splicing of exon 10. *Journal of Biological Chemistry*, **274**, 15134–43.

Haan, J., Hardy, J. A., and Roos, R. A. (1991). Hereditary cerebral hemorrhage with amyloidosis–Dutch type: its importance for Alzheimer research. *Trends in Neuroscience*, **14**, 231–4.

Haass, C., Lemere, C. A., Capell, A., Citron, M., Seubert, P., Schenk D., *et al.* (1995). The Swedish mutation causes early-onset Alzheimer's disease by β- secretase cleavage within the secretory pathway. *Nature Medicine*, **1**, 1291–6.

Hardy, J. A. and Higgins, G. A. (1992). Alzheimer's disease: the amyloid cascade hypothesis. *Science*, **256**, 184–5.

Heutink, P. (2000). Untangling tau-related dementia. *Human Molecular Genetics*, **9**, 979–86.

Hébert, R., Lindsay, J., Verreault, R., Rockwood, K., Hill, G., and Dubois, M. F. (2000). Vascular dementia—incidence and risk factors in the Canadian Study of Health and Aging. *Stroke*, **31**, 1487–93.

Holcomb, L., Gordon, M. N., McGowan, E., Yu, X., Benkovic, S., Jantzen P., *et al.* (1998). Accelerated Alzheimer-type phenotype in transgenic mice carrying both mutant *amyloid precursor protein* and *presenilin 1* transgenes. *Nature Medicine*, **4**, 97–100.

Holmes, C., Arranz, M. J., Powell, J. F., Collier, D. A., and Lovestone, S. (1998). $5\text{-}HT_{2A}$ and $5\text{-}HT_{2C}$ receptor polymorphisms and psychopathology in late onset Alzheimer's disease. *Human Molecular Genetics*, **7**, 1507–9.

Hong, M. and Lee, V. M. Y. (1997). Insulin and insulin-like growth factor-1 regulate tau phosphorylation in cultured human neurons. *Journal of Biological Chemistry*, **272**, 19547–53.

Hong, M., Chen, D. C., Klein, P. S., and Lee, V. M. (1997). Lithium reduces tau phosphorylation by inhibition of glycogen synthase kinase-3. *Journal of Biological Chemistry*, **272**, 25326–32.

Hope, J., Ritchie, L., Farquhar, C., Somerville, R., and Hunter N. (1989). Bovine spongiform encephalopathy: a scrapie-like disease of British cattle. *Progress in Clinical and Biological Research*, **317**, 659–67.

Hsiao, K. K., Scott, M., Foster, D., Groth, D. F., DeArmond, S. J., and Prusiner, S. B. (1990). Spontaneous neuro-degeneration in transgenic mice with mutant prion protein. *Science*, **250**, 1587–90.

Hsiao, K. K., Borchelt, D. R., Olson, K., Johannsdottir, R., Kitt, C., Yunis W., *et al.* (1995). Age related CNS disorder and early death in transgenic FVB/N mice overexpressing Alzheimer amyloid precursor proteins. *Neuron*, **15**, 1203–18.

Hu, J., Miyatake, F., Aizu, Y., Nakagawa, H., Nakamura, S., Tamaoka A., *et al.* (1999). Angiotensin-converting enzyme genotype is associated with Alzheimer disease in the Japanese population. *Neuroscience Letters*, **277**, 65–7.

Huang, D. Y., Weisgraber, K. H., Goedert, M., Saunders, A. M., Roses, A. D., and Strittmatter, W. J. (1995). ApoE3 binding to tau tandem repeat I is abolished by tau $serine_{262}$ phosphorylation. *Neuroscience Letters*, 192, 209–12.

Huff, F. J., Auerbach, J., Chakravarti, A., and Boller F. (1988). Risk of dementia in relatives of patients with Alzheimer's disease. *Neurology*, **38**, 786–90.

Huggins, M., Bloch, M., Wiggins, S., Adam, S., Suchowersky, O., Trew, M., *et al.* (1992). Predictive testing for Huntington disease in Canada: adverse effects and unexpected results in those receiving a decreased risk. *American Journal of Medical Genetics*, **42**, 508–15.

Hutton, M. (2000). 'Missing' tau mutation identified. *Annals of Neurology*, **47**, 417–18.

Ironside, J. W., Head, M. W., Bell, J. E., McCardle, L., and Will, R. G. (2000). Laboratory diagnosis of variant Creutzfeldt–Jakob disease. *Histopathology*, **37**, 1–9.

Iwai, A., Masliah, E., Yoshimoto, M., Ge, N., Flanagan, L., Rohan de Silva, H. A., *et al.* (1995). The precursor protein of non-Aβ component of Alzheimer's disease amyloid is a presynaptic protein of the central nervous system. *Neuron*, **14**, 467–75.

Janus, C., Pearson, J., McLaurin, J., Mathews, P. M., Jiang, Y., Schmidt, S. D., *et al.*(2000). A beta peptide immunization reduces behavioural impairment and plaques in a model of Alzheimer's disease. *Nature*, **408**, 979–82.

Jarrett, J. T., Berger, E. P., and Lansbury, P. T. Jr. (1993). The carboxy terminus of the β amyloid protein is critical for the seeding of amyloid formation: implications for the pathogenesis of Alzheimer's disease. *Biochemistry*, **32**, 4693–7.

Kanai, M., Matsubara, E., Isoe, K., Urakami, K., Nakashima, K., Arai H., *et al.* (1998). Longitudinal study of cerebrospinal fluid levels of tau, Aβ1–40, and Aβ1–42(43) in Alzheimer's disease: a study in Japan. *Annals of Neurology*, **44**, 17–26.

Kang, J., Lemaire, H. G., Unterbeck, A., Salbaum, J. M., Masters, C. L., Grzeschik, K. H., *et al.* (1987). The precursor of Alzheimer's disease amyloid A4 protein resembles a cell-surface receptor. *Nature*, **325**, 733–6.

Kawanishi, C., Suzuki, K., Odawara, T., Iseki, E., Onishi, H., Miyakawa T., *et al.* (1996). Neuropathological evaluation and apolipoprotein E gene polymorphism analysis in diffuse Lewy body disease. *Journal of Neurological Science*, **136**, 140–2.

Kehoe, P. G., Russ, C., McIlroy, S., Williams, H., Holmans, P., Holmes C., *et al.* (1999*a*). Variation in *DCP1*, encoding ACE, is associated with susceptibility to Alzheimer disease. *Nature Genetics*, **21**, 71–2.

Kehoe, P., Wavrant-De Vrieze, F., Crook, R., Wu, W. S., Holmans, P., Fenton I., *et al.* (1999*b*). A full genome scan for late onset Alzheimer's disease. *Human Molecular Genetics*, **8**, 237–45.

Kores, B. and Lader, M. H. (1997). Irreversible lithium neurotoxicity: an overview. *Clinical Neuropharmacology*, **20**, 283–99.

Korovaitseva, G. I., Premkumar, S., Grigorenko, A., Molyaka, Y., Galimbet, V., Selezneva N., *et al.* (1999). Alpha-2 macroglobulin gene in early- and late-onset Alzheimer disease. *Neuroscience Letters*, **271**, 129–31.

Korten, A. E., Jorm, A. F., Henderson, A. S., Broe, G. A., Creasey, H., and McCusker, E. (1993). Assessing the risk of Alzheimer's disease in first-degree relatives of Alzheimer's disease cases. *Psychological Medicine*, **23**, 915–23.

Kurochkin, I. V. and Goto, S. (1994). Alzheimer's β-amyloid peptide specifically interacts with and is degraded by insulin degrading enzyme. *FEBS Letters*, **345**, 33–7.

Kuusisto, J., Koivisto, K., Mykkänen, L., Helkala, E. L., Vanhanen, M., Hänninen T., *et al.* (1997). Association between features of the insulin resistance syndrome and Alzheimer's disease independently of apolipoprotein E4 phenotype: cross sectional population based study. *British Medical Journal*, **315**, 1045–9.

LaDu, M. J., Lukens, J. R., Reardon, C. A., and Getz, G. S. (1997). Association of human, rat, and rabbit apolipoprotein E with β-amyloid. *Journal of Neuroscience Research*, **49**, 9–18.

Lannfelt, L., Basun, H., Wahlund, L-O., Rowe, B. A., and Wagner, S. L. (1995). Decreased α-secretase-cleaved amyloid precursor protein as a diagnostic marker for Alzheimer's disease. *Nature Medicine*, **1**, 829–32.

Lansbury, P. T. Jr. (1999). Evolution of amyloid: what normal protein folding may tell us about fibrillogenesis and disease. *Proceedings of the National Academy of Sciences USA*, **96**, 3342–4.

Lantos, P. L., Luthert, P. J., Hanger, D., Anderton, B. H., Mullan, M., and Rossor M. (1992). Familial Alzheimer's disease with the amyloid precursor protein position 717 mutation and sporadic Alzheimer's disease have the same cytoskeletal pathology. *Neuroscience Letters*, **137**, 221–4.

Lee, V. M., Balin, B. J., Otvos, L. J., and Trojanowski, J. Q. (1991). A68: a major subunit of paired helical filaments and derivatized forms of normal Tau. *Science*, **251**, 675–8.

Lees, A. J. (1987). The Steele–Richardson–Olszewski syndrome (progressive supranuclear palsy). In *Movement Disorders* (ed. S. Fahn and C. D. Marsden), pp. 272–87. Butterworths, London.

Lennox, A., Karlinsky, H., Meschino, W., Buchanan, J. A., Percy, M. E., and Berg, J. M. (1994). Molecular genetic predictive testing for Alzheimer's disease: deliberations and preliminary recommendations. Alzheimer Disease and Associated Disorders, **8**, 126–47.

Leroy, K., Menu, R., Conreur, J. L., Dayanandan, R., Lovestone, S., Anderton, B. H., *et al.* (2000). The function of the microtubule-associated protein tau is variably modulated by graded changes in glycogen synthase kinase- 3β activity. *FEBS Letters*, **465**, 34–8.

Levy-Lahad, E., Wasco, W., Poorkaj, P., Romano, D. M., Oshima, J., Pettingell, W. H., *et al.* (1995). Candidate gene for the chromosome 1 familial Alzheimer's disease locus. *Science*, **269**, 973–7.

Lovestone, S. (1997). Muscarinic therapies in Alzheimer's disease: from palliative therapies to disease modification. *International Journal of Psychiatry in Clinical Practice*, **1**, 15–20.

Lovestone, S. and Reynolds, C. H. (1997). The phosphorylation of tau: a critical stage in neurodevelopmental and neurodegenerative processes. *Neuroscience*, **78**, 309–24.

Lovestone, S., Reynolds, C. H., Latimer, D., Davis, D. R., Anderton, B. H., Gallo, J-M., *et al.* (1994). Alzheimer's disease-like phosphorylation of the microtubule-associated protein tau by glycogen synthase kinase-3 in transfected mammalian cells. *Current Biology*, **4**, 1077–86.

Lovestone, S., Davis D. R., Webster, M-T., Kaech, S., Brion, J-P., Matus, A., *et al.* (1999). Lithium reduces tau phosphorylation—effects in living cells and in neurons at therapeutic concentrations. *Biological Psychiatry*, **45**, 995–1003.

McInnis, M. G., McMahon, F. J., Crow, T., Ross, C. A., and Delisi, L. E. (1999). Anticipation in schizophrenia: a review and reconsideration. *American Journal of Medical Genetics*, **88**, 686–93.

Mangiarini, L., Sathasivam, K., Seller, M., Cozens, B., Harper, A., Hetherington C., *et al.* (1996). Exon 1 of the HD gene with an expanded CAG repeat is sufficient to cause a progressive neurological phenotype in transgenic mice. *Cell*, **87**, 493–506.

Manji, H. K., McNamara, R., Chen, G., and Lenox, R. H. (1999). Signalling pathways in the brain: cellular transduction of mood stabilisation in the treatment of manic-depressive illness. *Australian and New Zealand Journal of Psychiatry*, **33**(Suppl.), S65–S83.

Mann, D. M. (1998). Dementia of frontal type and dementias with subcortical gliosis. *Brain Pathology*, **8**, 325–38.

Mann, D. M., Brown, A., Prinja, D., Davies, C. A., Landon, M., Masters, C. L., *et al.* (1989). An analysis of the morphology of senile plaques in Down's syndrome patients of different ages using immunocytochemical and lectin histochemical techniques. *Neuropathology and Applied Neurobiology*, **15**, 317–29.

Masters, C. L., Simms, G., Weinman, N. A., Multhaup, G., McDonald, B. L., and Beyreuther, K. (1985). Amyloid plaque core protein in Alzheimer disease and Down syndrome. *Proceedings of the National Academy of Sciences USA*, **82**, 4245–9.

Matsuo, E. S., Shin, R-W., Billingsley, M. L., Van DeVoorde, A., O'Connor, M., Trojanowski, J. Q., *et al.* (1994). Biopsy-derived adult human brain tau is phosphorylated at many of the same sites as Alzheimer's disease paired helical filament tau. *Neuron*, **13**, 989–1002.

Mayeux, R., Saunders, A. M., Shea, S., Mirra, S., Evans, D., Roses, A. D., *et al.* (1998). Utility of the apolipoprotein E genotype in the diagnosis of Alzheimer's disease. *New England Journal of Medicine*, **338**, 506–11.

Mead, S., James-Galton, M., Revesz, T., Doshi, R. B., Harwood, G., Pan, E. L., *et al.* (2000). Familial British dementia with amyloid angiopathy: early clinical, neuropsychological and imaging findings. *Brain*, **123**, 975–91.

Meyer, M. R., Tschanz, J. T., Norton, M. C., Welsh-Bohmer, K. A., Steffens, D. C., Wyse, B. W., *et al.* (1998). *APOE* genotype predicts when—not whether—one is predisposed to develop Alzheimer disease. *Nature Genetics*, 19, 321–2.

Moechars, D., Dewachter, I., Lorent, K., Reverse, D., Baekelandt, V., Naidu, A., *et al.* (1999). Early phenotypic changes in transgenic mice that overexpress different mutants of amyloid precursor protein in brain. *Journal of Biological Chemistry*, **274**, 6483–92.

Mori, H., Nishimura, M., Namba, Y., and Oda M. (1994). Corticobasal degeneration: a disease with widespread appearance of abnormal tau and neurofibrillary tangles, and its relation to progressive supranuclear palsy. *Acta Neuropathologica (Berlin)*, **88**, 113–21.

Mori, H., Hosoda, K., Matsubara, E., Nakamoto, T., Furiya, Y., Endoh, R., *et al.* (1995). Tau in cerebrospinal fluids: establishment of the sandwich ELISA with antibody specific to the repeat sequence in tau. *Neuroscience Letters*, **186**, 181–3.

Morrison, P. J., Johnston, W. P., and Nevin, N. C. (1995). The epidemiology of Huntington's disease in Northern Ireland. *Journal of Medical Genetics*, **32**, 524–30.

Mukaetova-Ladinska, E. B., Harrington, C. R., Roth, M., and Wischik, C. M. (1993). Biochemical and anatomical redistribution of tau protein in Alzheimer's disease. *American Journal of Pathology*, **143**, 565–78.

Mullan, M., Houlden, H., Crawford, F., Kennedy, A., Rogues, P., and Rossor M. (1993). Age of onset in familial early onset Alzheimer's disease correlates with genetic aetiology. *American Journal of Medical Genetics*, **48**, 129–30.

Muller, U., Cristina, N., Li, Z. W., Wolfer, D. P., Lipp, H. P., Rulicke, T., *et al.* (1996). Mice homozygous for a modified beta-amyloid precursor protein (beta APP) gene show impaired behavior and high incidence of agenesis of the corpus callosum. *Annals of the New York Academy of Sciences*, 777, 65–73.

Muñoz-Montaño, J. R., Moreno, F. J., Avila, J., and Díaz-Nido J. (1997). Lithium inhibits Alzheimer's disease-like tau protein phosphorylation in neurons. *FEBS Letters*, **411**, 183–8.

Murrell, J. R., Spillantini, M. G., Zolo, P., Guazzelli, M., Smith, M. J., Hasegawa, M., *et al.* (1999). *Tau* gene mutation G389R causes a tauopathy with abundant Pick body-like inclusions and axonal deposits. *Journal of Neuropathology and Experimental Neurology*, **58**, 1207–26.

Nagy, Z., Esiri, M. M., Jobst, K. A., Morris, J. H., King, E. M., McDonald, B., *et al.* (1995). Relative roles of plaques and tangles in the dementia of Alzheimer's disease: correlations using three sets of neuropathological criteria. *Dementia*, **6**, 21–31.

Ott, A., Stolk, R. P., van Harskamp, F., Pols, H. A. P., Hofman, A., and Breteler, M. M. B. (1999). Diabetes mellitus and the risk of dementia—The Rotterdam Study. *Neurology*, **53**, 1937–42.

Otto, M., Wiltfang, J., Tumani, H., Zerr, I., Lantsch, M., Kornhuber J., *et al.* (1997). Elevated levels of tau-protein in cerebrospinal fluid of patients with Creutzfeldt–Jakob disease. *Neuroscience Letters*, **225**, 210–12.

Owen, M., Liddell, M., and McGuffin P. (1994). Alzheimer's disease. *British Medical Journal*, **308**, 672–3.

Panegyres, P. K., Goldblatt, J., Walpole, I., Connor, C., Liebeck, T., and Harrop K. (2000). Genetic testing for Alzheimer's disease. *Medical Journal of Australia*, **172**, 339–43.

Paulson, H. L. and Fischbeck, K. H. (1996). Trinucleotide repeats in neurogenetic disorders. *Annual Review of Neuroscience*, 19, 79–107.

Pericak-Vance, M. A., Bass, M. L., Yamaoka, L. H., Gaskell, P. C., Scott, W. K., Terwedow, H. A., *et al.* (1998). Complete genomic screen in late-onset familial Alzheimer's disease. *Neurobiology of Aging*, 19(Suppl.), S39–S42.

Poduslo, S. E., Yin, X., Hargis, J., Brumback, R. A., Mastrianni, J. A., and Schwankhaus, J. (1999). A familial case of Alzheimer's disease without tau pathology may be linked with chromosome 3 markers. *Human Genetics*, **105**, 32–7.

Poser, S., Mollenhauer, B., Krauss, A., Zerr, I., Steinhoff, B. J., Schroeter, A., *et al.* (1999). How to improve the clinical diagnosis of Creutzfeldt–Jakob disease. *Brain*, **122**, 2345–51.

Price, D. L. and Sisodia, S. S. (1998). Mutant genes in familial Alzheimer's disease and transgenic models. *Annual Review of Neuroscience*, **21**, 479–505.

Prince, M., Lovestone, S., Cervilla, J., Joels, S., Powell, J., Russ C., *et al.* (2000). The association between *APOE* and dementia does not seem to be mediated by vascular factors. *Neurology*, **54**, 397–402.

Probst, A., Langui, D., Lautenschlager, C., Ulrich, J., Brion, J. P., and Anderton, B. H. (1988). Progressive supranuclear palsy: extensive neuropil threads in addition to neurofibrillary tangles. Very similar antigenicity of subcortical neuronal pathology in progressive supranuclear palsy and Alzheimer's disease. *Acta Neuropathologica (Berlin)*, 77, 61–8.

Prusiner, S. B. (1991). Molecular biology and transgenetics of prion diseases. *Critical Reviews in Biochemistry and Molecular Biology*, **26**, 397–438.

Prusiner, S. B., Groth, D., Serban, A., Koehler, R., Foster, D., Torchia, M., *et al.* (1993). Ablation of the prion protein (PrP) gene in mice prevents scrapie and facilitates production of anti-PrP antibodies. *Proceedings of the National Academy of Sciences USA*, **90**, 10608–12.

Prusiner, S. B., Scott, M., Foster, D., Pan, K. M., Groth, D., Mirenda, C., *et al.* (1990). Transgenetic studies implicate interactions between homologous PrP isoforms in scrapie prion replication. *Cell*, **63**, 673–86.

Qiu, W. Q., Walsh, D. M., Ye, Z., Vekrellis, K., Zhang, J. M., Podlisny, M. B., *et al.* (1998). Insulin-degrading enzyme regulates extracellular levels of amyloid β-protein by degradation. *Journal of Biological Chemistry*, **273**, 32730–8.

Revesz, T., Holton, J. L., Doshi, B., Anderton, B. H., Scaravilli, F., and Plant, G. T. (1999). Cytoskeletal pathology in familial cerebral amyloid angiopathy (British type) with non-neuritic amyloid plaque formation. *Acta Neuropathologica (Berlin)*, **97**, 170–6.

Riemenschneider, M., Buch, K., Schmolke, M., Kurz, A., and Guder, W. G. (1996). Cerebrospinal protein tau is elevated in early Alzheimer's disease. *Neuroscience Letters*, **212**, 209–11.

Rojo, A., Pernaute, R. S., Fontan, A., Ruiz, P. G., Honnorat, J., Lynch T., *et al.* (1999). Clinical genetics of familial progressive supranuclear palsy. *Brain*, **122**, 1233–45. [Published erratum appears in *Brain*, 2000, **123** (Pt 2), 419.]

Roses, A. D., Einstein, G., Gilbert, J., Goedert, M., Han, S. H., Huang D., *et al.* (1996). Morphological, biochemical, and genetic support for an apolipoprotein E effect on microtubular metabolism. *Annals of the New York Academy of Sciences*, **777**, 146–57.

Rossor, M. N., Fox, N. C., Beck, J., Campbell, T. C., and Collinge, J. (1996). Incomplete penetrance of familial Alzheimer's disease in a pedigree with a novel presenilin-1 gene mutation. *Lancet*, **347**, 1560.

Rubinsztein, D. C. (1995). Apolipoprotein E: a review of its roles in lipoprotein metabolism, neuronal growth and repair and as a risk factor for Alzheimer's disease. *Psychological Medicine*, **25**, 223–9.

Sadot, E., Gurwitz, D., Barg, J., Behar, L., Ginzburg, I., and Fisher, A. (1996). Activation of m1 muscarinic acetylcholine receptor regulates tau phosphorylation in transfected PC12 cells. *Journal of Neurochemistry*, **66**, 877–80.

Sáez-Valero, J., Sberna, G., McLean, C. A., and Small, D. H. (1999). Molecular isoform distribution and glycosylation of acetylcholinesterase are altered in brain and cerebrospinal fluid of patients with Alzheimer's disease. *Journal of Neurochemistry*, **72**, 1600–8.

Samuels, S. C., Silverman, J. M., Marin, D. B., Peskind, E. R., Younki, S. G., Greenberg, D. A., *et al.* (1999). CSF beta-amyloid, cognition, and APOE genotype in Alzheimer's disease. *Neurology*, **52**, 547–51.

Schellenberg, G. D., Bird, T. D., Wijsman, E. M., Orr, H. T., Anderson, L., Nemens, E., *et al.* (1992*a*). Genetic linkage evidence for a familial Alzheimer's disease locus on chromosome 14. *Science*, **258**, 668–71.

Schellenberg, G. D., Boehnke, M., Wijsman, E. M., Moore, D. K., Martin, G. M., and Bird, T. D. (1992*b*). Genetic association and linkage analysis of the apolipoprotein CII locus and familial Alzheimer's disease. *Annals of Neurology*, **31**, 223–7.

Schenk, D., Barbour, R., Dunn, W., Gordon, G., Grajeda, H., Guido T., *et al.* (1999). Immunization with amyloid-beta attenuates Alzheimer-disease-like pathology in the PDAPP mouse. *Nature*, **400**, 173–7.

Scherzinger, E., Lurz, R., Turmaine, M., Mangiarini, L., Hollenbach, B., Hasenbank, R., *et al.* (1997). Huntingtin-encoded polyglutamine expansions form amyloid-like protein aggregates *in vitro* and *in vivo*. *Cell*, **90**, 549–58.

Schubert, D., Jin, L. W., Saitoh, T., and Cole, G. (1989). The regulation of amyloid beta protein precursor secretion and its modulatory role in cell adhesion. *Neuron*, **3**, 689–94.

Scourfield, J., Soldan, J., Gray, J., Houlihan, G., and Harper, P. S. (1997). Huntington's disease: psychiatric practice in molecular genetic prediction and diagnosis. *British Journal of Psychiatry*, **170**, 146–9.

Sherrington, R., Rogaev, E. I., Liang, Y., Rogaeva, E. A., Levesque, G., Ikeda, M., *et al.* (1995). Cloning of a gene bearing missense mutations in early-onset familial Alzheimer's disease. *Nature*, **375**, 754–60.

Shi, J., Perry, G., Smith, M. A., and Friedland, R. P. (2000). Vascular abnormalities: the insidious pathogenesis of Alzheimer's disease. *Neurobiology of Aging*, **21**, 357–61.

Simpson, S. A. and Harding, A. E. (1993). Predictive testing for Huntington's disease: after the gene. The United Kingdom Huntington's Disease Prediction Consortium. *Journal of Medical Genetics*, **30**, 1036–8.

Skoog, I., Vanmechelen, E., Andreasson, L. A., Palmertz, B., Davidsson, P., Hesse, C., *et al.* (1995). A population-based study of tau protein and ubiquitin in cerebrospinal fluid in 85-year-olds: relation to severity of dementia and cerebral atrophy, but not to the apolipoprotein E4 allele. *Neurodegeneration*, **4**, 433–42.

Solano, D. C., Sironi, M., Bonfini, C., Solerte, S. B., Govoni, S., and Racchi, M. (2000). Insulin regulates soluble amyloid precursor protein release via phosphatidyl inositol 3 kinase-dependent pathway. *FASEB Journal*, **14**, 1015–22.

Spillantini, M. G., Schmidt, M. L., Lee, V. M., Trojanowski, J. Q., Jakes, R., and Goedert, M. (1997). Alpha-synuclein in Lewy bodies. *Nature*, **388**, 839–40. [Letter]

Stanford, P. M., Halliday, G. M., Brooks, W. S., Kwok, J. B. J., Storey, C. E., Creasey, H., *et al.* (2000). Progressive supranuclear palsy pathology caused by a novel silent mutation in exon 10 of the *tau* gene—expansion of the disease phenotype caused by *tau* gene mutations. *Brain*, **123**, 880–93.

Steinbach, J. P., Muller, U., Leist, M., Li, Z. W., Nicotera, P., and Aguzzi, A. (1998). Hypersensitivity to seizures in beta-amyloid precursor protein deficient mice. *Cell Death Differentiation*, **5**, 858–66.

Stewart, R. and Liolitsa, D. (1999). Type 2 diabetes mellitus, cognitive impairment and dementia. *Diabetic Medicine*, **16**, 93–112.

Storey, E. and Cappai, R. (1999). The amyloid precursor protein of Alzheimer's disease and the Aβ peptide. *Neuropathology and Applied Neurobiology*, **25**, 81–97.

Streichenberger, N., Jordan, D., Verejan, I., Souchier, C., Philippeau, F., Gros, E., *et al.* (2000). The first case of new variant Creutzfeldt–Jakob disease in France: clinical data and neuropathological findings. *Acta Neuropathologica (Berlin)*, **99**, 704–8. [In Process Citation.]

Strittmatter, W. J., Weisgraber, K. H., Huang, D. Y., Dong, L-M., Salvesen, G. S., Pericak-Vance, M., *et al.* (1993). Binding of human apolipoprotein E to synthetic amyloid β peptide: isoform-specific effects and implications for late-onset Alzheimer disease. *Proceedings of the National Academy of Sciences USA*, **90**, 8098–102.

Strittmatter, W. J., Saunders, A. M., Goedert, M., Weisgraber, K. H., Dong, L. M., Jakes, R., *et al.* (1994). Isoform-specific interactions of apolipoprotein E with microtubule-associated protein tau: implications for Alzheimer disease. *Proceedings of the National Academy of Sciences USA*, **91**, 11183–6.

Sunderland, T., Wolozin, B., Galasko, D., Levy, J., Dukoff, R., Bahro, M., *et al.* (1999). Longitudinal stability of CSF tau levels in Alzheimer patients. *Biological Psychiatry*, **46**, 750–5.

Suzuki, N., Cheung, T. T., Cai, X-D., Odaka, A., Otvos, L. Jr, Eckman, C., *et al.* (1994). An increased percentage of long amyloid β protein secreted by familial amyloid β protein precursor (βAPP_{717}). mutants. *Science*, **264**, 1336–40.

Sweet, R. A., Nimgaonkar, V. L., Kamboh, M. I., Lopez, O. L., Zhang, F., and DeKosky, S. T. (1998). Dopamine receptor genetic variation, psychosis, and aggression in Alzheimer disease. *Archives of Neurology*, **55**, 1335–40.

Takashima, A., Honda, T., Yasutake, K., Michel, G., Murayama, O., Murayama, M., *et al.* (1998). Activation of tau protein kinase I glycogen synthase kinase-3β by amyloid β peptide (25–35) enhances phosphorylation of tau in hippocampal neurons. *Neuroscience Research*, **31**, 317–23.

Talbot, C., Lendon, C., Craddock, N., Shears, S., Morris, J. C., and Goate, A. (1994). Protection against Alzheimer's disease with apoE $\varepsilon 2$. *Lancet*, **343**, 1432–3.

Tamaoka, A., Sawamura, N., Fukushima, T., Shoji, S., Matsubara, E., Shoji, M., *et al.* (1997). Amyloid β protein 42(43) in cerebrospinal fluid of patients with Alzheimer's disease. *Journal of Neurological Science*, **148**, 41–5.

Tapiola, T., Lehtovirta, M., Ramberg, J., Helisalmi, S., Linnaranta, K., Riekkinen, P., Sr.., *et al.* (1998). CSF tau is related to apolipoprotein E genotype in early Alzheimer's disease. *Neurology*, **50**, 169–174.

Tato RE, Frank, A., Hernanz A. (1995). Tau protein concentrations in cerebrospinal fluid of patients with dementia of the Alzheimer type. *Journal of Neurology, Neurosurgery and Psychiatry*, **59**, 280–283.

Tesseur, I., Van Dorpe, J., Spittaels, K., Van Den Haute, C., Moechars, D., Van Leuven F. (2000). Expression of human apolipoprotein E4 in neurons causes hyperphosphorylation of protein tau in the brains of transgenic mice. *American Journal of Pathology*, **156**, 951–964.

Tunstall, N. and Lovestone, S. (1999). UK Alzheimer's disease genetics consortium. *International Journal of Geriatric Psychiatry*, **14**, 789–91.

Tunstall, N., Owen, M. J., Williams, J., Rice, F., Carty, S., Lillystone, S., *et al.* (2000). Familial influence on variation in age of onset and behavioural phenotype in Alzheimer's disease. *British Journal of Psychiatry*, **176**, 156–9.

Tyler, A., Morris, M., Lazarou, L., Meredith, L., Myring, J., and Harper, P. (1992). Presymptomatic testing for Huntington's disease in Wales 1987–90. *British Journal of Psychiatry*, **161**, 481–8.

Urakami, K., Mori, M., Wada, K., Kowa, H., Takeshima, T., Arai, H., *et al.* (1999). A comparison of tau protein in cerebrospinal fluid between corticobasal degeneration and progressive supranuclear palsy. *Neuroscience Letters*, **259**, 127–9.

Vandermeeren, M., Mercken, M., Vanmechelen, E., Six, J., Van de Voorde, A., Martin, J-J., *et al.* (1993). Detection of τ proteins in normal and Alzheimer's disease cerebrospinal fluid with a sensitive sandwich enzyme-linked immunosorbent assay. *Journal of Neurochemistry*, **61**, 1828–34.

Van Slegtenhorst, M., Lewis, J., and Hutton, M. (2000). The molecular genetics of the tauopathies. *Experimental Gerontology*, **35**, 461–71.

Vassar, R., Bennett, B. D., Babu-Khan, S., Kahn, S., Mendiaz, E. A., Denis, P., *et al.* (1999). Beta-secretase cleavage of Alzheimer's amyloid precursor protein by the transmembrane aspartic protease BACE. *Science*, **286**, 735–41.

Vekrellis, K., Ye, Z., Qiu, W. Q., Walsh, D., Hartley, D., Chesneau, V., *et al.* (2000). Neurons regulate extracellular levels of amyloid β-protein via proteolysis by insulin-degrading enzyme. *Journal of Neuroscience*, **20**, 1657–65.

Vidal, R., Frangione, B., Rostagno, A., Mead, S., Revesz, T., Plant, G., *et al.* (1999). A stop-codon mutation in the BRI gene associated with familial British dementia. *Nature*, **399**, 776–81.

Wadsworth, J. D., Jackson, G. S., Hill, A. F., and Collinge, J. (1999). Molecular biology of prion propagation. *Current Opinion in Genetics and Development*, **9**, 338–45.

Walling, H. W., Baldassare, J. J., and Westfall, T. C. (1998). Molecular aspects of Huntington's disease. *Journal of Neuroscience Research*, **54**, 301–8.

Wavrant-DeVrièze, F., Rudrasingham, V., Lambert, J. C., Chakraverty, S., Kehoe, P., Crook, R., *et al.* (1999). No association between the alpha-2 macroglobulin I1000V polymorphism and Alzheimer's disease. *Neuroscience Letters*, **262**, 137–9.

Weihl, C. C., Ghadge, G. D., Kennedy, S. G., Hay, N., Miller, R. J., and Roos, R. P. (1999). Mutant Presenilin-1 induces apoptosis and downregulates Akt/PKB. *Journal of Neuroscience*, 19, 5360–9.

Wiggins, S., Whyte, P., Huggins, M., Adam, S., Theilmann, J., Bloch, M., *et al.* (1992). The psychological consequences of predictive testing for Huntington's disease. Canadian Collaborative Study of Predictive Testing. *New England Journal of Medicine*, **327**, 1401–5. [See comments.]

Wilson, C. A., Doms, R. W., and Lee, V. M. Y. (1999). Intracellular APP processing and Aβ production in Alzheimer disease. *Journal of Neuropathology and Experimental Neurology*, **58**, 787–94.

Wiltfang, J., Otto, M., Baxter, H. C., Bodemer, M., Steinacker, P., Bahn, E., *et al.* (1999). Isoform pattern of 14–3–3 proteins in the cerebrospinal fluid of patients with Creutzfeldt–Jakob disease. *Journal of Neurochemistry*, **73**, 2485–90.

Windl, O., Dempster, M., Estibeiro, J. P., Lathe, R., De Silva, R., Esmonde, T., *et al.* (1996). Genetic basis of Creutzfeldt–Jakob disease in the United Kingdom: a systematic analysis of predisposing mutations and allelic variation in the PRNP gene. *Human Genetics*, **98**, 259–64.

Yanagisawa, M., Planel, E., Ishiguro, K., and Fujita, S. C. (1999). Starvation induces tau hyperphosphorylation in mouse brain: implications for Alzheimer's disease. *FEBS Letters*, **461**, 329–33.

Zeidler, M., Stewart, G. E., Barraclough, C. R., Bateman, D. E., Bates, D., Burn, D. J., *et al.* (1997). New variant Creutzfeldt–Jakob disease: neurological features and diagnostic tests. *Lancet*, **350**, 903–7.

Zoghbi, H. Y. and Orr, H. T. (2000). Glutamine repeats and neurodegeneration. *Annual Review of Neuroscience*, **23**, 217–47.

Zubenko, G. S., Hughes, H. B., Stiffler, J. S., Hurtt, M. R., and Kaplan, B. B. (1998). A genome survey for novel Alzheimer disease risk loci: results at 10-cM resolution. *Genomics*, **50**, 121–8.

8 The economics of health care provision for elderly people with dementia

Jane Wolstenholme and Alastair Gray

Introduction

Although increases in the longevity and the ageing of the population have been a medical triumph, they also represent a major challenge for medical and social services and for families in the provision of care. To some, they represent a financial burden on society, a situation exacerbated by funding restrictions on health and social services worldwide. The projection for the year 2025 is that the number of people aged 65 and over will then form one-quarter of the population, compared to the current proportion of one in six people (World Bank 1993). Given the consistent age-specific prevalence rates for Alzheimer's disease (AD), dementia, cognitive impairment, and general disability (Rocca *et al.* 1991*a,b*), the expectation is that the numbers of individuals requiring treatment and/or care will continue to increase steeply worldwide. This increase in ageing-related diseases has been accompanied by an expanding literature on the health economics of AD, dementia, and cognitive impairment in the elderly. This chapter will introduce the reader to the concepts and techniques of health economics that have been used in published studies of these diseases of the elderly, and will go on to summarize the published literature on the economics of AD, cognitive impairment, and dementia.

Methodology used by health economists

This section gives the reader a brief introduction to health economic tools used for analysis and evaluation. Detailed information can be gained from reading textbooks on economic evaluation (Gold *et al.* 1996; Drummond *et al.* 2000).

Types of studies

Descriptive studies of the costs of a particular intervention, disease process, or patient group can be split into cost analyses, which aim to measure per patient costs, and cost-of-illness (COI) or burden of disease (BOD) studies, which estimate the societal burden of a disease in monetary terms. These studies can provide useful information—for example, cost-of-illness studies may help in prioritizing research expenditure—but as they provide no information on the association between costs and likely effects or outcomes, they are of limited usefulness to decision makers and policy makers. What is required to make decisions about resource allocation concerning treatment is information on both the costs and effects of available interventions. Economic evaluation involves the comparison of the incremental costs and benefits of one intervention with those of the next best alternative.

Formally, cost-effectiveness analyses (CEA) explore the relationship between the costs (resources used) and effects (health benefits) of an intervention compared with an alternative strategy. The incremental cost-effectiveness ratio (ICER) reports the difference in mean per patient cost (C) divided by the difference in benefits (E) of the alternatives being assessed:

$$\frac{C_A - C_B}{E_A - E_B} \leq M$$

The left-hand side of the above equation is the incremental cost-effectiveness ratio (ICER). *M* represents the maximum amount a decision maker is willing (and able) to pay for an extra unit of effectiveness. Where the effects of alternative therapies are of proven equivalence it is possible to perform a study known as a cost-minimization analysis (CMA), in which the focus of the analysis is on identifying the least costly alternative. However, this should be performed only where there is positive evidence of equivalence, and not where there is simply an absence of evidence on effect differences.

Almost any meaningful measure of outcome or process can be used to calculate a cost-effectiveness ratio, including, for example, symptom-free days, adverse events averted, endpoint-free time, mm Hg reductions in blood pressure, or scale-point improvements in cognition. However, economists generally favour outcome measures that are less specific to any particular intervention, so that comparison across a range of different therapeutic areas is possible. Hence many cost-effectiveness studies report a cost per life-year saved, or use a composite measure of survival and quality of life to estimate the cost per quality-adjusted life year (QALY). As the process of adjusting survival to take account of quality of life requires measurement and valuation of the *utility* derived from different health states, such studies are sometimes referred to as cost–utility analyses.

Finally, cost–benefit analysis (CBA) is a form of evaluation in which all costs and all benefits are expressed in monetary terms, in order to assess whether the costs exceed the benefits or vice-versa. Advantages of this approach are that it is firmly based in economic theory, and that the decision rule is straightforward: as long as benefits exceed costs the project should be adopted. However, because of the methodological and empirical difficulties of making monetary valuations of different health states and of life, cost–benefit analysis is less frequently used in the health sector than in other fields such as environmental and transport economics. Indeed, the majority of health sector evaluations that describe themselves as cost–benefit analyses are misnamed, as they do not attempt to monetize the benefits of an intervention but simply compare costs incurred against costs reduced.

Perspective

The perspective or viewpoint of an economic analysis influences the choice of which costs to include (Luce and Elixhauser 1990; Davidoff and Powe 1996; Drummond *et al.* 1997). This perspective is partly dependent on the target audience. Perspectives range from the very specific viewpoints of the patient or clinician, to the intermediary viewpoints of purchaser, decision maker, health authority, provider unit, or government, to the wider perspective of society as a whole. The costs a patient incurs when a treatment decision is made—such as transport costs to attend a clinic, lost earnings, or child-care costs—are very different from those incurred by the National Health Service (NHS). Similarly, only the societal perspective takes account of any costs associated with production loss. The societal approach relies on the collection and valuation of all costs, regardless of who incurs them. The societal approach has been recommended as the standard perspective for costing, as it allows the analysis to be carried out from a number of viewpoints (CCOHTA 1994; Johannesson 1995; Gold *et al.* 1996).

The choice of perspective is particularly important for economic studies of dementia. For example, a policy of home support for people with dementia may reduce hospital costs (NHS costs) and institutional care costs (social services and patients) but increase the burden of informal care provided by relatives. This process of cost-shifting may transfer costs from one sector or budget to another, but may not reduce the total cost to society as a whole. Therefore when evaluating these types of programmes, one should be careful to take a broad societal perspective that includes the costs incurred by non-health care sectors such as social services and unpaid caregivers.

Costs—which costs?

In economic terms, costs are thought of as the value of resources consumed as a consequence of a medical intervention. These are valued in terms of their opportunity cost (the value of the resource in its next best alternative use to society). An overview of the types of costs to be considered for inclusion is provided below. It is useful to consider these costs under the headings of direct health care costs, direct non-health care costs, informal care costs, and productivity costs.

Direct health care costs

Direct health care costs are defined as the 'organizing and operating costs within the health care sector' (Drummond *et al.* 1997), including the cost of prevention, diagnosis, treatment, rehabilitation, therapeutic and continuing care, and terminal care. They include: variable costs such as staff time, general practitioner (GP) services, drugs, and other medical supplies; fixed costs such as medical equipment and building use; and overheads such as laundry, electricity, portering, etc. They also include the number of inpatient bed days, outpatient visits, clinic visits as well as general practitioner, psychiatrist, and nurse visits.

Some economists have also argued that, where an intervention extends life expectancy, the resulting future use of health care for any reason should also be included. For example, Weinstein *et al.* (1980) argue that:

> ...if treatment results in a prolonged life because a condition has been cured or early disease has been avoided, then the cost of treating later disease that would not otherwise have arisen must be considered. [Weinstein *et al.* 1980, p. 240]

However, other analysts have countered this, suggesting that:

> ...if the purpose of the analysis is to determine whether the programme is a good investment, only the costs of the preventive program should be counted. Added years of life involve added expenditures to food, clothes and housing as well as medical care. None...is relevant to deciding whether the program is a good investment... [Russell 1986, pp. 35–6]

In the face of this lack of consensus, most studies at present include future related health care costs but exclude unrelated future health care costs from their analysis (Meltzer 1997). (See also Hodgson and Meiners 1982; Mushlin and Fintor 1992; Gold *et al.* 1996; Garber and Phelps 1997; Johannesson *et al.* 1997; Johnston *et al.* 1999.)

Direct non-health care costs

Direct non-health care costs may include the costs of care to other agencies such as social service departments providing day care or home helps, as well as the out-of-pocket costs incurred by the patient, relatives, and friends, for example in making home adaptations, buying over-the-counter medications, or travelling to and from hospitals or surgeries for treatment and incurring train, bus, or taxi fares, petrol costs, and parking fees. Patients' time costs are calculated as the opportunity cost of having to take time off work or from normal activities to attend treatment. They are particularly important in screening programmes, where if the opportunity cost is perceived to be too high it may deter attendance (Sculpher and Buxton 1993; Torgerson *et al.* 1994; Bryan *et al.* 1995; Frew *et al.* 1999).

Informal care costs

Informal care costs consist primarily of the time provided by relatives and friends in caring for someone whose condition impairs their independence. All the evidence indicates that the volume of time thus provided is very substantial, but for economists the problem lies in trying to place a valuation on it. The approach typically adopted has been to assess the opportunity costs of informal care: if informal care was not provided in this way, what would the informal carer be doing instead, and what care would the patient receive instead? However, this raises some difficult issues: informal carers are often the elderly partners of elderly patients, and it may be hard to define and measure what they would otherwise be doing, and harder still to place a value on this. Similarly, while some of the time provided by informal carers might otherwise be provided by formal carers, it seems unlikely that substitution could occur except at the margin.

Productivity costs

Productivity costs of disease may occur as a result of reduced productivity at work, absence from work, disability, and premature mortality attributable to the disease of interest (Luce *et al.* quoted in Gold *et al.* 1996). Several studies have debated the issue surrounding the measurement of productivity costs (Koopmanschap and van Inveld 1992; Koopmanschap and Rutten 1993, 1996*a,b*, Koopmanschap *et al.* 1995, 1997; Posnett and Jan 1996; Brouwer *et al.* 1997*a,b*; Johannesson and Karlsson 1997). Koopmanschap and colleagues (1995) argue that productivity costs are only relevant where the disease or intervention brings about significant changes in productivity. They have contested the idea that production is directly affected by illness and absenteeism, putting forward the idea of *friction* costs: even if patients take time off work, actual production may be unaffected because other workers can take on the patient's work in the short term, or because the patient makes up lost production on return to work. In the long run, if the patient is unable to return to work, they will be replaced by another employee, and so the cost to society in terms of lost production is close to zero. However, this argument is very much dependent on the perspective of the analysis. When a patient perspective is taken, productivity loss to the patient due to absenteeism or the inability to continue working and carrying out everyday activities may well be a cost, depending on the patient's employment conditions and loss of earnings during sickness absence.

Others have argued that the measures used to value productivity costs are unreliable and unrealistic and therefore productivity costs should be excluded from the analysis. Gerard and Mooney (1993) have proposed that, since the outcome measures in economic evaluations are health specific, the opportunity cost of resources should be defined in terms of health and therefore productivity costs should be excluded. However, Meltzer (1997) has argued that, if the health care budget has to compete with other public sector budgets to maximize utility, future consumption costs need to be included.

Ethical reasons for excluding productivity costs from economic evaluations are also sometimes invoked. For example, it is argued that their inclusion will mean the allocation of resources in favour of those of productive age, biasing against the economically inactive and elderly. However, the ethical arguments are not clear-cut: resource allocation decisions do sometimes explicitly take into account the productive potential of individuals, both in health care treatment decisions and in other areas such as court settlements in personal injury cases.

Even if the debate as to whether productivity costs should be included could be resolved, and a decision made as to how to value these productivity costs, there remains a debate as to whether they should be treated as a cost (the numerator in a cost-effectiveness ratio (CER)), or a health effect (the denominator of the CER) (Brouwer *et al.* 1997*a,b*).

Identification of cost events

Although the literature has described the types of cost available for inclusion in an economic analysis and the factors influencing which costs to include, it rarely specifies how to identify the events that generate these costs. Detailed identification of the costs requires knowledge of the different care pathways for the particular disease or intervention under scrutiny. This can be obtained from a number of different sources.

- literature on specific diseases/illnesses or interventions and treatments;
- previous studies, which may highlight the parameters that are the main determinants of cost;
- clinicians' and experts' advice on the treatment and care of particular diseases;
- pilot studies using a small sample of the medical notes of patients known to have the disease or to have received the intervention in question;
- trials or routinely collected databases;
- observations of practice.

If the key cost-generating events can be identified in advance, time and money will be saved by collecting data only on these events. It will also limit any burden placed on the patients themselves if questionnaires are involved. Knapp and Beecham (1993) and Whynes and Walker (1995) have presented two studies identifying key cost-generating events in mental health care and cancer care, respectively. However, it remains difficult to predict these key cost-generating events. Moreover, since the average total patient cost varied widely in these studies, simply looking at a reduced list of cost-generating events conceals the important cost variation between patients (Whynes and Walker 1995).

Measuring resource-use

When the cost-generating events have been recognized and identified, they have to be measured and quantified in some format.

Direct health care costs

Direct health care resource-use is usually measured in physical units, for example the number of outpatient/GP/inpatient visits, number of days spent in hospital, staff time, dosage of drugs administered, or time spent in an operating theatre. These elements of resource-use can be measured in varying degrees of detail, ranging between what Gold and colleagues call 'gross costing' and 'micro costing' (Gold *et al.* 1996). Gross costing measures the resource-use at an aggregated level, then multiplies through by an appropriate unit cost. For example, the cost of an individual's inpatient stay can be estimated from the number of days they spent as an inpatient multiplied by a unit cost (here, the cost of a 'standard' inpatient day, averaged across all inpatients). Micro-costing involves breaking down the hospital stay into its resource components, such as staff time, equipment used, ward space used, overheads such as electricity, portering, and laundry and multiplying each of these measures by their corresponding unit costs. This may require information on staff earnings, the replacement cost of equipment with an allowance for depreciation, the replacement cost of ward space, and hospital overhead costs. It may also be necessary to consider the time spent by nursing staff or medical staff with specific patients, for example if the level of dependency of patients is relevant to the study (see also below).

Luce and Elixhauser (1990) illustrate the varying levels of detail that can be involved in measuring costs. They cite two studies. One employed crude methods to assess the change in health care resources brought about by changes in the use of cholesterol-lowering drugs (Oster and Epstein 1987). The other used a detailed time-and-motion study to assess the resource implications of changing the methods for administering antibiotics in secondary care (Eisenberg *et al.* 1984).

Direct non-health care costs

The measurement of direct non-health care costs, such as time and travel costs and out-of-pocket payments made by the patient and their family/carers, is usually achieved by administering questionnaires to patients or carers (Sculpher and Buxton 1993; Bryan *et al.* 1995; Frew *et al.* 1999). The measurement issues relating to costs pertaining to other public-sector budgets have been explored by researchers at the PSSRU (Personal Social Services Research Unit, University of Kent) and CEMH (Centre for the Economics of Mental Health), leading to the development of a questionnaire to abstract cost information: the 'Client Service Receipt Interview' (CSRI) (Beecham *et al.* 1992, 1994).

Informal care

In collecting information on caregivers' time, techniques such as direct observation, retrospective estimation, and diary keeping are used. Standardized instruments have been developed for the collection of resource-use information in studies of dementia, for example the Caregiver Activities Time Survey (CATS; see Moore and Clipp 1994; Clipp and Moore 1995), the Caregiver Activity Survey (CAS; see Davis *et al.* 1997), and the Resource Utilization in Dementia (RUD; see Wimo *et al.* 1998). Measurement of informal care has been discussed by Smith and Wright (1994).

Productivity costs

The measurement of the impact of illness on productivity has been well documented (Koopmanschap and Rutten 1996a). A questionnaire has been designed to collect data on the relationship between illness, treatment, and performance at work (van Roijen *et al.* 1996).

Valuing resource-use measurement

Direct costs

The valuation of resource-use is dependent on data availability and time constraints. Micro-costing involves estimating a unit cost for each level of resource-use to be measured: for example, unit costs are estimated for staff time, capital (equipment and land), overheads, drugs, etc. If resource-use has been measured using the gross-costing approach, then the unit cost (daily cost) will invariably include all capital, overhead, and staff costs (Donaldson and Shackley 1997; Drummond *et al.* 1997). In practice, unit costs are obtained from a variety of sources. In rare cases they are estimated in minute detail by collecting the following data and information:

(1) staff time and salaries, ascertained from personnel departments or pay-review bodies;
(2) equipment and its useful lifetime, replacement costs, and maintenance costs (from the supplier or hospital finance department);
(3) overheads including portering, general administration, electricity, cleaning, catering, and laundry, costed by assessing time, salaries, and actual market cost (from hospital finance and accounts departments).

For the more aggregated costing methods, data from previously published studies or more formalized published cost information (for example, PSSRU costing guidelines (Netten and Dennett 1999) or Department of Health Reference Costs) may be used. The accounts/finance departments of hospitals can also offer a source of unit-cost data. The availability and relevance of UK accounts data differs, however, from the US where charge data is readily available and relevant to evaluations.

Direct non-health care costs

For direct non-health care costs such as travel, the measurement is in miles travelled, which can be equated with the Automobile Association car mileage rate if private transport was used, along with the charges for car parking at the hospital. If buses, taxis, or trains were used the actual market price, i.e. the fares, can be used to value the travel cost (Sculpher and Buxton 1993; Bryan *et al.* 1995; Frew *et al.* 1999).

Informal care costs

Two techniques have been used for valuing caregivers' time. The first is the opportunity-cost approach, which estimates the opportunity cost of foregone activities using the market wage rate as a proxy value for lost work-time and leisure-time. The second approach is the replacement-cost approach, which uses an imputed value for the unpaid caregiver of payment at the national wage level for similar care provided in the marketplace.

Productivity costs

The most influential and widely debated approach to evaluating production gains from improvements in health care is the human capital approach (Weisbrod 1961; Rice 1967; Hodgson 1983), which focuses on the economic consequences of a disease. In practice, if productivity costs are included at all, the typical approach would be to attach an average earnings figure to the estimated time lost.

Discounting

Different interventions have different time profiles of costs and benefits. This has to be taken into account when conducting an economic evaluation. This is achieved by discounting future costs and benefits to present values by attaching smaller weights to future events. The weights are equal to $(1 + r)^{-t}$, where r = the discount rate and t is the number of years ahead in which the event occurs. Different rates have been applied, but are generally between 1.5% and 10% (Weinstein and Stason 1977; Parsonage and Neuberger 1992; Krahn and Gafni 1993; HM Treasury 1997; Cairns and van der Pol 2000).

Handling uncertainty

Uncertainty is inherent in economic evaluation. It exists in the data inputs, methods, and assumptions used in the analysis, and in the extrapolation and generalizability of the results (Briggs *et al.* 1994). The two main methods for handling uncertainty in the results of a cost-effectiveness analysis are statistical analysis and sensitivity analysis. Where patient-specific, cost-and-effect data have been collected it is possible to examine uncertainty in the point-estimate ICER using confidence intervals. The estimation of these confidence intervals around such a ratio statistic is not straightforward. The parametric approach based on Fieller's theorem (van Hout *et al.* 1994; Willan and O'Brien 1996) or the non-parametric approach of bootstrapping (Manning *et al.* 1996; Briggs *et al.* 1997) should be used.

In practice, many economic evaluations do not use patient-specific data, but instead use data from a number of sources (literature reviews, clinical judgement), where statistical methods cannot be used. Even in studies where statistical analysis has been performed, an examination of the extent of uncertainty in certain point estimates (e.g. discount rate or unit-cost data) should be undertaken. This is done by a process known as sensitivity analysis (Briggs and Sculpher 1995), which involves the systematic investigation of how changes in the uncertain parameters affect the overall results. Briggs and colleagues (1994) have specified four types of sensitivity analysis: simple; threshold; analysis of extremes; and probabilistic sensitivity analysis. For a review of handling uncertainty in economic evaluations see Briggs and Gray (1999).

Effects/benefits

Trials of new drugs for Alzheimer's disease (AD) and dementia have frequently used intermediate measures of effectiveness such as the Mini-Mental State Examination (MMSE) (Folstein *et al.* 1975). The results of a cost-effectiveness analysis are then reported as the cost per unit change in MMSE. However, as noted earlier, this way of expressing cost-effectiveness is limited. First, the cost per unit change in MMSE is difficult to interpret as the scale is not linear; a change from a score of 5 to 9 does not mean the same as a change from 25 to 29. Second, the use of MMSE as a measure of effectiveness does not allow for comparisons with interventions in other disease areas. For example, the cost per unit change in MMSE cannot be compared with the cost per cancer detected. Policy makers require standardized information on the cost-effectiveness of interventions in order to make decisions about what competing treatments or interventions should be funded from a limited budget.

One standardized method is to report the results of cost-effectiveness analyses in terms of the cost per life year gained, using information on the effect of the intervention on life expectancy. However, this approach takes no account of the quality of these life years gained. For example, using this measure, an added month with severe AD would be valued equally with an added month with mild AD. The use of QALYs attempts to overcome this problem. This measure of benefit incorporates length of life with a measure of the quality of the extended life, and reflects the value attributed to different health outcomes. The results of this type of CEA are reported as cost per QALY, and have been classified as cost-utility analyses (CUA). They have advantages over other forms of CEA in that they allow for direct comparisons across diverse interventions. The quality-weights represent the desirability or utility of being in a health state, ranging from 0 (equivalent to death) to 1 (equivalent to perfect health), although it is possible to define health states considered worse than death and therefore having values of less than 0.

A variety of different methods have been used to arrive at such valuations of different states of health or disease. One approach uses direct preference-elicitation methods, such as the 'visual analogue scale' (VAS), 'standard gamble' (SG), 'time trade-off' (TTO), or 'person trade-off' (PTO) approaches (Torrance 1986; Nord 1995).

All these methods rest on obtaining the views and preference of respondents. These are usually not people suffering from the disease in question, but healthy people working out their preferences for hypothetical situations. The VAS involves asking respondents to value health states by indicating a point along a line drawn on a page with well defined end-points, with the most preferred health state at one end and the least preferred health state at the other end.

The SG involves respondents making a choice between alternative health states, where one involves a lottery in which the possible outcomes are full health or death. They are asked how much they would be willing to accept in terms of the risk of death (or some health state worse than the one being valued) to be certain of avoiding the health state being valued. The expected value of the gamble at this point is the utility for the health state.

The TTO asks the respondents to choose between two alternatives: a number of years in full health (x) versus a number of years in the health state being evaluated (t). The respondent is asked to trade a health improvement against a reduction in the length of life. Time x is varied until the respondent claims to be indifferent between the two alternatives, at which point the health state is valued as x/t, i.e. the fraction of healthy years equivalent to a year in the health state being evaluated. The PTO asks respondents to indicate how many people in one health state they would need to be able to treat to make them indifferent to treating a stated number in another health state.

The other approach to obtaining quality weights is by using generic health-state questionnaires also known as 'multi-attribute utility scales' (MAUS), which describe patients' health using a number of dimensions such as mobility, anxiety, pain, cognition, emotion, etc. Each dimension can be subdivided into a number of severity levels. These dimensions and levels combine to form a number of health states, for which utility/quality weights have been obtained using one of the direct preference-elicitation methods outlined above. The patient is assigned to one of the health states, either by self-completing a questionnaire or by asking a clinician or family member to complete the generic health-state questionnaire or interview. A total of six MAUS exist for use as weights in QALYs: the Rosser classification (Rosser and Kind 1978), the Quality of Well-being Scale (QWB) (Patrick *et al.* 1973; Kaplan *et al.* 1976; Kaplan and Anderson 1988), the Health Utility Index (HUI) Mark I, Mark II, and Mark III (Torrance 1982; Feeny *et al.* 1997; Torrance *et al.* 1995; Torrance *et al.* 1996; Feeny *et al.* 1998), the 15D (Sintonen 1981), and the EuroQol (EQ-5D) (EuroQol Group 1990; Dolan 1997). Neumann and colleagues (1998) provide an excellent review of the use of QALYs in dementia.

'Willingness to pay' (WTP) and 'conjoint analysis' are two relatively new techniques for measuring benefits in health economics. Neither has been used in the health-economics literature of Alzheimer's disease or dementia. WTP is based on the assumption that the maximum amount of money an individual is willing to pay for a commodity is an indicator of the utility (satisfaction) to them of that commodity. This benefit value encompasses all the attributes of the intervention, not just the health gains. Diener and colleagues (1998) provide a review of the methods involved in WTP. Conjoint analysis is another method that can be used to elicit utilities (for health and non-health outcomes) and WTP values indirectly. Ryan (1996) provides a review of the application of conjoint analysis in health care.

Modelling

In economic evaluations of drug interventions for AD and dementia, data are often limited due to the short-term nature of many clinical trials. This results in uncertainty about long-term costs and outcomes related to the treatment. In many CEAs, mathematical models have been developed to address this problem. In fact the US Panel on Cost-Effectiveness Analysis upheld the use of models when direct primary or secondary analyses are not possible (Gold *et al.* 1996). The Markov model is a particular type of model frequently used in economic evaluation. The time component of this type of model makes it well suited to modelling disease progression and the related costs and effects (Briggs and Sculpher 1998). Markov models have been used in economic evaluations of treatments for AD and dementia where the disease progresses through well-defined states such as mild, moderate, and severe dementia as measured by Mini-Mental State Examination (MMSE) or Clinical Dementia Rating (CDR) (O'Brien *et al.* 1999; Stewart *et al.* 1998; Fenn and Gray 1999; Neumann *et al.* 1999).

Review of the literature on the economics of AD, dementia, and cognitive impairment in the elderly

Having briefly considered some of the main methodological issues that arise in conducting economic evaluations, we now review published studies on the economics of AD, dementia, and cognitive impairment in the elderly. To ensure that all relevant methodological studies, cost and cost-effectiveness analyses, and modelling exercises were identified, a broad semi-structured literature review was performed, involving an initial search of Medline, Embase, Cinahl, and Econlit databases (using search terms: #1 COST, #2 ECONOM*, #3 DEMENT*, #4 ALZHEIM*; #5 #1 or #2; #6 #3 or #4; #7 #5 and #6). This search was supplemented by a secondary search of the reference lists.

Reviews

A number of methodology reviews (Neumann *et al.* 1997, 1998; Whitehouse 1997; Winblad *et al.* 1997; Meek *et al.* 1998; Dinusson and Knopman 1999) and reviews of the literature on the economics of AD, dementia, and cognitive impairment in the elderly have been undertaken (e.g. see Keen 1993; Ernst and Hay 1997; Fox 1997; Alloul *et al.* 1998; Kanowski 1998; Schumock 1998; Whitehouse 1998; Trabucchi 1999), mostly over the last decade.

Cost-of-illness studies

A number of cost-of-illness studies undertaken in the US, UK, Sweden, Ireland, Canada, and The Netherlands have provided estimates of the burden of dementia and AD (Hay and Ernst 1987; Huang *et al.* 1988; Gray and Fenn 1993; Ernst and Hay 1994; Ostbye and Crosse 1994; Wimo *et al.* 1997b; Meerding 1998; O'Shea and O'Reilly 2000).

Huang and colleagues (1988) estimated the cost impact of all senile dementias in the US. Formal medical care, social services, and nursing-home care costs were estimated to be $13.3 billion, informal care and patient lost productivity costs were estimated to be $31.5 and $43.2 billion, respectively (1985 $US).

A UK-based study concluded that the total cost of AD in England in 1990/91 was £1.039 million (1990/91 £UK), 66% of which was due to the costs of residential and nursing-home care. This study only included the direct costs of care; the authors made no estimate of the informal care costs (Gray and Fenn 1993).

Ernst and Hay (1994) estimated the burden of AD in the US for 1991, updating estimates from a previous study reporting direct and indirect costs of AD in the US for 1983 (Hay and Ernst

1987). Direct care costs, unpaid caregiver costs, and lost productivity costs amounted to $20.6 billion, $33.3 billion, and $13.4 billion, respectively (1991 $US).

Another study conducted in Canada by Ostbye and Crosse (1994) calculated the societal burden of AD to be $3.9 billion (1991 $Canadian), $1.25 billion was estimated to be due to community care, $636 million due to unpaid care.

Wimo and colleagues (1997b) undertook a cost-of-illness study for dementia in Sweden in 1991. The estimated cost was 20–36 billion SEK.

Meerding and colleagues (1998) in a COI study estimating the health care costs for all diseases in The Netherlands, reported the costs of dementia to be ranked third highest across all age groups (ranked first for age 65 years and over). Dementia accounted for 5.6% of the total health care costs.

O'Shea and O'Reilly (2000) estimated the total costs of dementia in the Irish Republic. They included costs of inpatient acute care, inpatient psychiatric care, residential long-stay care, informal care by the family, medical and social services in the community, and mortality. They estimated the average cost per patient for dementia care to be £8261, amounting to a total cost of £248 million in the Irish Republic (1998 £IR). Inpatient acute and psychiatric care account for 8% of the total, family care accounts for 50%, community care for 10%, and residential care for 33% of the total care costs.

Allowing for the variations in the settings, currencies, and dates of these studies, it is clear that there remain wide variations in the values cited. Reasons for the variation are: first, the distribution of patients between institutional and community care varies with the severity of illness and reflects national care trends and availability of services; and, second, a diversity in the methodologies employed. Informal care/unpaid caregiver time and lost productivity have been included in some of the above studies and excluded in others. There are also wide variations in how these values have been imputed.

Cost analyses

Coughlin and Liu (1989) used data from the 1981–1982 US National Long-Term Care Channeling Demonstration Project to estimate the mean annual per patient cost for home and institutional care in the United States. The average annual cost was $18 500 (1981/82 $US) for the cognitively impaired, and $16 650 for those with no cognitive problems. A pre- and postnursing-home admission analysis indicated that for the cognitively impaired the annual cost of community care was $11 700, whereas the cost of nursing-home care was $22 300.

Rice and colleagues (1993) prospectively collected resource-use data for 93 community- and 94 institution-based patients and their caregivers in northern California. They estimated the average total cost of caring for a patient with Alzheimer's disease to be approximately $47 000 per year (1990 $US). The annual cost of formal care for patients residing in the community was $12 572, while the cost for those in institutional care was $42 049. For community-based patients, 75% of the total cost represents an imputed value for unpaid informal care compared with 12% for institutionalized patients (Table 8.1). Over 60% of the services provided to patients in either care setting were paid out of pocket.

Weinberger and colleagues (1993), from prospectively completed interviews and the diaries of 141 primary caregivers, examined both formal and informal services and the associated costs of dementia. Expenditure incurred over 6 months was extensive for both formal ($6986) and informal ($786) services (1990 $US). Multivariate analyses indicated that patients with more severe symptoms of dementia and families with higher incomes reported significantly higher expenditures.

Shapiro and Tate (1997) estimated the average annual per patient direct cost related to care of the elderly with no cognitive impairment (n = 74, $1102), with cognitive impairment but no dementia (n = 94, $1882), and with dementia (n = 58, $2343) ($Canadian, price base not reported) using data from the Manitoba Study of Health and Aging. The costs for the cognitively impaired were almost twice those for the unimpaired, while the costs for those with dementia were 25% higher than those for the cognitively impaired.

Table 8.1 Average annual costs of care for persons with Alzheimer's disease by type of cost, location of residence, and severity—Northern California, 1990 ($US)

Location of residence	Total costs	Formal costs	Informal costs
Community	47 083	12 572	34 517
Severe dementia (n = 51)	52 667	16 278	36 389
Mild/moderate dementia (n = 42)	39 558	7 621	31 937
Institution	47 591	42 049	5 542
Severe dementia (n = 89)	48 201	42 477	5 728
Mild/moderate dementia (n = 5)	37 729	34 828	2 901

Data taken from Rice *et al.* 1993 with permission.

A study of non-institutionalized patients in the Lombardy region of Italy used questionnaire responses from 423 patients to estimate the non-medical care costs of AD. The annual average non-medical costs (for example, paid caregivers) were estimated to be L13 388 000, while the corresponding costs for unpaid caregiver time (valued using the replacement cost approach) were estimated to be L86 265 000 (1995 Italian Lira) (Cavallo and Fattore 1997).

Menzin and colleagues (1999) used administrative claims' data from a 10% random sample of recipients of the Medi-Cal program in California, USA. The average annual Medicaid payments (incorporating the costs of medication, hospital and nursing-home care) for AD patients compared to a control cohort were $14 488 (inter quartile range $12 528–17 725) and $6799 (inter quartile range $3371–8478) (1995 $US).

A similar study conducted by Gutterman and colleagues explored the cost of AD and related dementia for 677 Medicare enrollees from four regions of the USA in a managed-care organization. Mean total costs were significantly higher ($p < 0.001$) for patients with AD and related dementia compared to the matched controls ($13 487 vs. $9276; $US, no price base reported) (Gutterman *et al.* 1999).

Holmes *et al.* (1999) reported on the costs of AD in Scotland. They used responses from a postal survey of 655 caregivers from an initial random sample of 1847. Their direct-cost estimates included institutional care, health and social services, and out-of-pocket expenditure made by the patients and caregivers. The indirect costs were calculated using estimates of loss of earnings for the working-age patients and caregivers (the opportunity-cost approach), and loss of leisure time for the caregivers. The average total cost of care increased from £21 000 (1996 £UK) per annum in the first 3 years to £29 700 per annum after 9 years. The average direct cost of care increased from £12 600 per annum in the first 3 years to £22 400 per annum after 9 years. Within these direct costs, 62% was due to long-term institutional care, 20% due to medical and social services, and 18% due to out-of-pocket expenditure.

During the 1980s there was a considerable amount of research on the costs and outcomes of care for the elderly. In most developed countries the key question is whether community or institutional care is the best option for care of the elderly suffering from dementia. The economist's approach is to explore the relative costs and outcomes of the care options for the patient and caregiver. A comprehensive study by Schneider and colleagues (1993) investigated the mean per patient weekly costs of various care packages for elderly people with advanced cognitive impairment in England. The reported mean weekly costs were £169.38 for people living alone in private households, £209.99 for people in private households living with others, £309.02 for local authority residential homes, £212.12 for non-statutory residential homes, £310.00 for non-statutory nursing homes, and £729.44 for NHS hospitals (1991/92 £UK).

Home-based care

Caregiver burden is one of the most important determinants of the institutional care of patients with AD, and a caregiver support programme can delay institutionalization (Mittleman *et al.* 1996).

Huang and colleagues (1988) estimated the imputed costs of care at home to be $14 308 for severely demented people and $5732 for mild/moderate cases (1985 $US).

A Canadian-based economic evaluation of a caregiver support programme (CSP) compared with community nursing for elderly demented patients at home was undertaken by Drummond and colleagues (1991). The CSP involved regular visits from a support nurse to provide respite for the caregiver and to allow attendance at a self-support group. Outcome in terms of the carer's quality of life was measured using the Caregiver Quality of Life Instrument. Over a 6-month period the average health care cost per caregiver was $3562 (1988 $Canadian) for the CSP group and $2897 for the control group, with a 20% difference in caregiver quality of life in favour of the intervention group.

An Australian-based study explored the cost-effectiveness of an intensive 10-day, residential-based, training programme for caregivers of patients with dementia. The programme resulted in patients staying longer at home before institutionalization, with those whose carers had been on the programme having higher adjusted rates of survival at home (53% versus 13%); the associated cost savings were estimated to be $7967 ($Australian, price base not reported) (Brodaty and Peters 1991).

However, a study by Donaldson and Gregson (1989) found that a scheme for home-residing, elderly dementia patients and their carers was almost three times more costly than normal care services, although it was beneficial in terms of delayed admission to residential care.

Souetre *et al.* (1995) estimated the annual cost of care for community-dwelling AD patients. The assessment was based on a 3-month, follow-up study of 51 probable AD patients living in France. Data on demographic, clinical (including actual Mini-Mental State Examination scores), and economic variables were collected. Total costs included actual expenditures, such as direct medical costs and direct non-medical costs, as well as indirect costs (loss of earnings due to loss of productivity). They found that indirect costs represented a significant portion of total costs (36–40%) and found a positive and significant correlation between disease severity and costs.

Nursing-home care

The principal form of institutional care for people suffering from dementia is the nursing home. Nursing-home costs account for a significant proportion of the total burden of AD costs (Gray and Fenn 1993). Donaldson and Bond (1991), reported that NHS nursing-home care costs are comparable to hospital care. In a prospective cohort study of 126 AD patients in the US, only four patients at the start of the study were in nursing homes; by the end of the study 75% of the cohort were nursing-home residents (Welch *et al.* 1992). The median length of stay for these residents was 2.75 years, over 10 times the national median length of stay for all diagnoses. Total nursing-home charges for the cohort were estimated to be approximately $4.3–6.4 million (1991 $US).

Group-living

Wimo and colleagues (1995) used a Markov model to compare three modes of residency: group or sheltered accommodation; home; and institutionalized. On the basis of cost per QALY estimates, it appeared that the group-living or sheltered accommodation option was the most cost-effective, with an average 8-year cost of $172 852 (1987 $US) and an average QALY of 3.27. Home care and institutional care resulted in higher average costs of $215 022 and $272 855 and reduced average QALYs of 2.99 and 2.89, respectively.

Informal care

The costs of unpaid caregiver time account for a large proportion (approximately half to two-thirds) of the total costs of dementia care. This is due to the immense time burden placed on informal caregivers, especially if the patient is being cared for in a community setting.

Weinberger and colleagues (1993) estimated the cost of caring for patients with dementia at home to be approximately $52 000 (1990 $US), with most of the costs borne by patients and their families.

Stommel and colleagues (1994) report on the costs of dementia care incurred by families from a retrospective analysis of their resource-use 3 months prior to the interview. They found that among 182 such families, average care costs for the 3-month period amounted to $4564 (1989 $US). Average cash expenditures amounted to 29% of total care costs, with unpaid labour accounting for 71% of the family care costs. Total care costs rise by $1158 for each additional dependency in an activity of daily living (ADL).

Max *et al.* (1995) estimated the cost of informal care provided to patients with Alzheimer's disease living in Northern California. Data were collected from 93 community-residing and 94 institutionalized patients and their caregivers over a 12-month period. The annual cost of informal care was $34 517 (1990 $US) for the community sample and $5 542 for the institutionalized sample. They also examined the determinants of informal caregiving. Informal costs are positively related to cognitive impairment no matter what the residential setting. In an institutional setting, patient and caregiver age was inversely related to costs. If the caregiver was not a spouse, higher informal care costs were also found.

Correlating cost with disease severity

An important cost factor in dementia is the progression of the disease through mild, moderate, and severe stages. The balance between formal and informal costs of care is highly dependent on the stage of the disease. In the early, mild and moderate stages patients tend to be cared for at home and the burden of care is on the informal caregiver, thus the costs are predominantly informal care costs and indirect costs. As cognitive function declines, the costs shift to direct medical care costs in the form of respite care and institutionalization. Establishing a link between cost and disease severity (measured for example by the MMSE) is useful in evaluating drug interventions for AD and related dementias. If the drug has an impact on MMSE scores it is possible to estimate the related cost savings.

A number of studies have established a positive association between increasing disease severity and increasing care costs (Hu *et al.* 1986; Rice *et al.* 1993 (Table 8.1); Ernst *et al.* 1998; Leon *et al.* 1998; Leon and Neumann 1999 in the USA; Hux *et al.* 1998 in Canada; Kronborg Andersen *et al.* 1999 in Holland; Fagnani *et al.* 1999 in France; Jonsson *et al.* 1999b in Sweden; Souetre *et al.* 1999 in the UK).

Economic evaluation of cholinesterase inhibitors

The introduction of cholinesterase inhibitors used to treat AD has resulted in an increase in the number of studies into the economic costs and benefits of such treatment. The economic studies are based on the results of clinical trials, although this presents problems in that the trials are often of short duration, and modelling and extrapolation of short-term costs and effects must be undertaken. Many of the above studies relating costs to disease severity have been used as a basis for evaluations of these new drugs. In Europe, three main cholinesterase inhibitors are currently used for the treatment of AD: tacrine (Cognex), donepezil (Aricept), and rivastigmine (Exelon).

Results of studies on tacrine

Tacrine was the first drug approved (in 1993) by the US Food and Drug Administration (FDA) for the treatment of AD. However, it is not widely prescribed due to hepatotoxicity, which requires regular monitoring and therefore adds to the total cost of the drug use. A number of pharmacoeconomic studies have been published on the use of tacrine. Lubeck and colleagues (1994) conducted a CEA based in the US. They estimated that in those patients taking the highest doses (160 mg/day) of tacrine, institutionalization would be delayed by 12.1 months. The estimated savings as a result of tacrine use were reported to be $4052 per patient per annum (1993 $US). However, informal care costs were not included in the cost estimate and therefore any potential cost-shifting from institutional care costs to informal care costs was excluded from the analysis. Wimo and colleagues used a similar modelling approach correlating MMSE score and levels of care (Wimo *et al.* 1997a). It was calculated that tacrine improved MMSE and delayed progression to a nursing home, resulting in a cost saving equivalent to approximately 1.3% of total costs, corresponding to an annual benefit per patient of 2900 SEK (1991 Swedish Kronor (SEK)).

Henke and Burchmore (1997), using a decision-analytical model to estimate formal care costs (community and nursing-home care) and survival, also found that drug use was related to a reduction in institutionalization, resulting in an average lifetime cost saving of $9250 (1994 $US). Moreover, for AD patients who took the higher doses of tacrine (80–160 mg/day) formal costs decreased by 25% ($36 500) over 5 years compared to the no-treatment group. Limitations of this study include the use of a very simple model that assumed only two states—residence in a nursing home and not residing in a nursing home—when in fact other studies have shown that costs increase in home-dwelling patients as they move from mild to moderate to severe disease states (Wimo *et al.* 1997a; Leon *et al.* 1998). The model was also dependent on data from an uncontrolled study of the effect of tacrine on the delay to nursing-home residency (Knopman *et al.* 1996). Ernst and Hay (1997) questioned the benefit to the patient and caregiver in terms of quality of life. They estimated the incremental cost-effectiveness of tacrine treatment compared to placebo in terms of cost per QALY to be $US 48 333.

Results of studies on donepezil

Donepezil is a second-generation cholinesterase inhibitor with proven efficacy in treating cognitive and functional symptoms of dementia. It was approved for use in the US in 1996. A number of studies have published their cost-effectiveness results on the use of donepezil.

Using the results of a 30-week clinical trial of donepezil and the costing exercise by Hux *et al.* (1998), O'Brien *et al.* used the 30-week MMSE scores in a Markov model of AD progression to calculate the associated cost savings extrapolated to 5 years. The study found that patients treated with 5 mg/day of donepezil endured 2.41 years out of 5 with non-severe AD compared with 2.21 years for untreated patients. The Markov model predicted a net saving of $882 (1996 $Canadian) per patient; a saving in direct medical costs of $929, and an increase in informal care costs of $48 per patient (O'Brien *et al.* 1999).

Stewart and colleagues also used a Markov model to estimate the costs related to the impact of donepezil on disease progression. They found that donepezil was approximately cost-neutral, as the increased drug costs were balanced by lower costs of care due to treated patients not declining as rapidly as those untreated (Stewart *et al.* 1998).

Small and colleagues (1998) conducted a cost analysis using data collected on two matched groups of patients (one group receiving donepezil, the other receiving nothing) over a 6-month period. The mean 6-month direct medical cost for a patient receiving donepezil was $3443, whereas the mean cost for the comparison group was $3476 per patient ($US, price base not reported). As with the study by Stewart *et al.*, although the patients receiving donepezil spent more on prescription drugs, these costs were offset by a slower rate of institutionalization.

Jonsson *et al.* (1999*a*) used a Markov model to explore the cost-effectiveness of 5 and 10 mg of donepezil compared to no treatment, in terms of cost per patient year in the non-severe state over a 5-year simulated period. They used two different models to perform the evaluation: one using population-based cost and transition probability parameters (Jonsson *et al.* 1999*b*), with effectiveness data based on 24-week trial results (Rogers *et al.* 1998); and the other a within-trial based model (Rogers *et al.* 1998). In their results Jonsson *et al.* compared the cost-effectiveness of 5 mg and 10 mg of donepezil with no treatment and found both to be cost-saving for both models (see Tables 8.2 and 8.3). However, an estimate of the cost-effectiveness of moving from 5 mg to 10 mg of donepezil, showed that this option is not cost-effective, with a CER of 606 750 SEK for the population-based model and 309 969 SEK for the within-trial based model (1995 Swedish Kronor (SEK)) equivalent to £UK43 862 and £UK22 407.

Neumann and colleagues (1999) used a Markov model of mild, moderate, and severe stages of AD assessed using the Clinical Dementia Rating scale to estimate the cost-effectiveness of donepezil compared to no treatment. The analysis included direct medical and non-medical costs and indirect costs associated with unpaid caregiver time, based on the costing exercise undertaken by Rice *et al.* (1993). They found that the costs of donepezil were offset by reduced costs of care arising from better cognitive functioning and delayed progression to more costly levels of care. However, they found that the size of this offsetting effect varied substantially depending on the modelling assumptions used. Their main results indicate that the cost-effectiveness of donepezil therapy depends on the duration of the therapeutic effect of the drug. If the effect lasts for 6 months, the cost-effectiveness is very poor in the initially mild and moderate groups, with cost per QALY of \$160 000 and \$440 000, respectively (1997 \$US). However, if the drug effect is sustained for 24 months, the cost-effectiveness becomes much better and in the case of patients with initially mild disease is actually cost saving (see Table 8.4). This underlines the need for reliable longer term evidence on outcomes.

Table 8.2 Cost-effectiveness of 5 and 10 mg donepezil compared with no treatment in terms of cost per patient-years in non-severe states—population-based model (1995 Swedish Kronor)

		No treatment	Donepezil 5 mg	Donepezil 10 mg
Cost	Total	760 441	744 880	757 015
	Incremental	—	–15 561	–3426
Effectiveness	Total	2.8024	3.3244	3.3448
	Incremental	—	0.522	0.5424
	ICER	—	Cost saving	Cost saving

Data taken from Jonsson *et al.* 1999*a* with permission.

Table 8.3 Cost-effectiveness of 5 and 10 mg donepezil compared with no treatment in terms of cost per patient-years in non-severe states—within trial-based model (1995 Swedish Kronor)

		No treatment	Donepezil 5 mg	Donepezil 10 mg
Cost	Total	913 399	635 768	676 368
	Incremental	—	–277 631	–237 031
Effectiveness	Total	2.0916	2.8091	2.9400
	Incremental	—	0.7175	0.8484
	ICER	—	Cost saving	Cost saving

Data taken from Jonsson *et al.* 1999*a* with permission.

Table 8.4 Cost-effectiveness in terms of cost per QALY of donepezil versus no treatment

Assumed duration of effect (months)	Cost per quality-adjusted life-year (QALY) ($US) Mild dementia	Moderate dementia
6	160 000	440 000
12	32 000	140 000
18	9 300	76 000
24	Cost saving	47 000

Data taken from Neumann *et al.* 1999 with permission.

A study retrospectively examined the claims' data of 70 AD patients in a managed-care organization before and after the introduction of donepezil treatment. The treatment resulted in a decrease in the medical costs, particularly the outpatient costs, although this was outweighed by an increase in the medication costs and hence the overall costs (Fillit *et al.* 1999).

Results of studies on rivastigmine

Fenn and Gray (1999) used clinical trial data on 1333 patients recruited internationally in two studies of rivastigmine therapy to model disease progression and associated costs. Their results indicated that health care costs (excluding drug costs) were reduced by a small amount at the end of the 26-week trial period, but that the saving increased to approximately £1100 per patient (£UK 1997) when extrapolated to a lifetime of 3 years, thus partially offsetting therapy costs and improving potential cost-effectiveness. The authors found that the largest long-term cost savings from the drug intervention are realized when treating patients with an MMSE > 20 (mild category). However, in the short run (< 2 years' life expectancy) the largest cost savings accrue to treating patients with moderate disease (MMSE 20–11).

Conclusions

Although this review has identified a substantial number of published economic studies relating to dementia, many are simple costing studies that are of little direct help to decision makers having to make resource-allocation choices concerning this patient group. Very few cost-effectiveness analyses have been undertaken in the field of dementia.

There is scope for economic evaluations of three types of intervention: programmes of patient care; caregiver support programmes; and drug and medical treatments of the disease. Economic evaluation is becoming an increasingly important part of formal regulatory requirements (e.g. in Australia), and it plays a formal part in national technology assessment agencies such as the National Institute for Clinical Excellence in the UK and CCOHTA in Canada. In view of this fact, and with the development of new drug treatments for AD and dementia, we can expect to see an increase in the number of CEAs being performed. It is therefore important for physicians to familiarize themselves with the techniques involved to help them in their critical appraisal of the published studies.

References

Alloul, K., Sauriol, L., Kennedy, W., *et al.* (1998). Alzheimer's disease: a review of the disease, its epidemiology and economic impact. *Archives of Gerontology and Geriatrics*, **27**, 189–221.

Beecham, J. (1992). *Costing services: an up-date*, PSSRU (Discussion Paper, no. 884), Canterbury: University of Kent.

Beecham, J. (1994). Collecting information: the client service receipt interview. *Mental Health Research Review*, **1**, 6–8.

Briggs, A. and Sculpher, M. (1995). Sensitivity analysis in economic evaluation: a review of published studies. *Health Economics*, **4**, 355–71.

Briggs, A. and Sculpher, M. (1998). An Introduction to Markov modeling for economic evaluation. *PharmacoEconomics*, **13**, 397–409.

Briggs, A., Sculpher, M., and Buxton, M. (1994). Uncertainty in the economic evaluation of health care technologies: the role of sensitivity analysis. *Health Economics*, **3**, 95–104.

Briggs, A. H. and Gray, A. M. (1999). *Handling uncertainty when performing economic evaluation of healthcare interventions*. Health Technology Assessment, London.

Briggs, A. H., Wonderling, D. E., and Mooney, C. Z. (1997). Pulling cost-effectiveness analysis up by its bootstraps: a non-parametric approach to confidence interval estimation. *Health Economics*, **6**, 327–40.

Brodaty, H. and Peters, K. E. (1991). Cost effectiveness of a training program for dementia carers. *International Psychogeriatrics*, **3**, 21–34.

Brouwer, W. B. F., Koopmanschap, M. A., and Rutten, F. F. H. (1997*a*). Productivity costs in cost-effectiveness analysis: Numerator or denominator: A further discussion. *Health Economics*, **6**, 511–14.

Brouwer, W. B. F., Koopmanschap, M. A., and Rutten, F. F. H. (1997*b*). Productivity costs measurement through quality of life. *Health Economics*, **6**, 253–9.

Bryan, S., Buxton, M., McKenna, M., *et al.* (1995). Private costs associated with abdominal aortic aneurysm screening: the importance of private travel and time costs. *Journal of Medical Screening*, **2**, 62–6.

Cairns, J. A. and van der Pol, M. M. (2000). *The estimation of marginal time preference in a UK-wide sample (TEMPUS) project*, Vol. 4, No. 1). Health Technology Assessment, London.

Canadian Coordinating Office for Technology Assessment (1994). *Guidelines for economic evaluation of pharmaceuticals: Canada* (1st edn). Ottawa, CCOHTA.

Cavallo, M. C. and Fattore, G. (1997). The economic and social burden of Alzheimer disease on families in the Lombardy Region of Italy. *Alzheimer Disease and Associated Disorders*, **11**, 184–90.

Clipp, E. C. and Moore, M. J. (1995). Caregiver time use: an outcome measure in clinical trial research on Alzheimer's disease. *Clinical Pharmacology and Therapeutics*, **58**, 228–36.

Coughlin, T. A. and Liu, K. (1989). Health care costs of older persons with cognitive impairments. *Gerontologist*, **29**, 173–82.

Davidoff, A. and Powe, N. R. (1996). The role of perspective in defining measures for the economic evaluation of medical technology. *International Journal of Technology Assessment in Health Care*, **12**, 9–21.

Davis, K. L., Martin, D. B., and Kane, R. A. (1997). The caregiver activity survey (CAS): development and validation of a new measure for caregivers of persons with Alzheimer's disease. *International Journal of Geriatric Psychiatry*, **1997**, 978–88.

Diener, A., O'Brien, B., and Gafni, A. (1998). Health care contingent valuation studies: a review and classification of the literature. *Health Economics*, **7**, 313–26.

Dinusson, J. and Knopman, D. (1999). Pharmacoeconomics of Alzheimer's disease. *Neurologist.*, **6**, 116–25.

Dolan, P. (1997). Modeling valuations for EuroQol health states. *Medical Care*, **35**, 1095–108.

Donaldson, C. and Bond, J. (1991). Cost of continuing-care facilities in the evaluation of experimental National Health Service nursing homes. *Age and Ageing*, **20**, 160–8.

Donaldson, C. and Gregson, B. (1989). Prolonging life at home: What is the cost? *Community Medicine*, **11**, 200–9.

Donaldson, C. and Shackley, P. (1997). Economic evaluation. In *Oxford textbook of public health* (ed. R. Detels, W. W. Holland, J. M. Ewan, *et al.*) (3rd edn), pp. 850–71. Oxford University Press, Oxford.

Drummond, M., Mohide, E., Tew, M., *et al.* (1991). Economic evaluation of a support program for caregivers of demented elderly. *International Journal of Technology Assessment in Health Care*, **7**, 209–19.

Drummond, M. F., O'Brien, B., Stoddart, G. L., *et al.* (1997). *Methods for the economic evaluation of health care programmes*. Oxford University Press, Oxford.

Drummond, M. F., O'Brien, B., Stoddart, G. L., *et al.* (2000). *Methods for the economic evaluation of health care programmes*. Oxford University Press, Oxford.

Eisenberg, J. M., Koffer, H., and Finkler, S. A. (1984). Economic analysis of a new drug: potential savings in hospital operating costs from the use of a once-daily regimen parenteral cephalosporin. *Reviews of Infectious Diseases*, **6**, S909–S923.

Ernst, R. L. and Hay, J. W. (1994). The US economic and social costs of Alzheimer's disease revisited. *American Journal of Public Health*, **84**, 1261–4.

Ernst, R. L. and Hay, J. W. (1997). Economic research on Alzheimer disease: A review of the literature. *Alzheimer Disease and Associated Disorders*, **6** (11 Suppl.), 135–45.

Ernst, R. L., Hay, J. W., Fenn, C., *et al.* (1997). Cognitive function and the costs of Alzheimer disease. An exploratory study. *Archives of Neurology*, **54**, 687–93.

EuroQol Group (1990). EuroQol: a new facility for the measurement of health-related quality of life. *Health Policy*, **16**, 199–208.

Fagnani, F., Everhard, F., Buteau, L., *et al.* (1999). Cost and repercussions of Alzheimer's disease in France: An extrapolation from the Paquid study data. *Revue de Geriatrie*, **24**, 205–11.

Feeny, D., Furlong, W., Boyle, M., *et al.* (1995). Multi-attribute health status classification systems. Health Utilities Index. *PharmacoEconomics.*, **7**, 490–502.

Feeny, D., Furlong, W., and Barr, R. D. (1998). Multiattribute approach to the assessment of health-related quality of life: Health Utilities Index. *Medical Pediatric Oncology*, **Suppl. 1**, 54–9.

Fenn, P. and Gray, A. (1999). Estimating long term cost savings from treatment of Alzheimer's disease: a modelling approach. *PharmacoEconomics.*, **16**, 165–174.

Fillit, H., Gutterman, E. M., and Lewis, B. (1999). Donepezil use in managed Medicare: Effect on health care costs and utilization. *Clinical Therapeutics*, **21**, 2173–85.

Folstein, M. F., Folstein, S. E., and McHugh, P. R. (1975). 'Mini-mental state'. A practical method for grading the cognitive state of patients for the clinician. *Journal of Psychiatric Research*, **12**, 189–98.

Fox, P. J. (1997). Service use and cost outcomes for persons with Alzheimer disease. *Alzheimer Disease and Associated Disorders*, **11** (Suppl. 6), 125–34.

Frew, E., Wolstenholme, J., and Whynes, D. (1999). Estimating time and travel costs incurred in clinic-based screening: flexible sigmoidoscopy screening for colorectal cancer. *Journal of Medical Screening*, **6**, 119–23.

Garber, A. M. and Phelps, C. E. (1997). Economic foundations of cost-effectiveness analysis. *Journal of Health Economics*, **16**, 1–31.

Gerard, K. and Mooney, G. (1993). QALY league tables: handle with care. *Health Economics*, **2**, 241–5.

Gold, M. R., Siegel, J. E., Russell, L. B., *et al.* (1996). *Cost-effectiveness in health and medicine*. Oxford University Press, Oxford.

Gray, 1995.

Gray, A. and Fenn, P. (1993). Alzheimer's disease: the burden of illness in England. *Health Trends*, **25**, 31–7.

Gutterman, E. M., Markowitz, J. S., Lewis, B., *et al.* (1999). Cost of Alzheimer's disease and related dementia in managed-medicare. *Journal of the American Geriatrics Society*, **47**, 1065–71.

Hay, J. W. and Ernst, R. L. (1987). The economic costs of Alzheimer's disease. *American Journal of Public Health*, **77**, 1169–75.

Henke, C. J. and Burchmore, M. J. (1997). The economic impact of tacrine in the treatment of Alzheimer's disease. *Clinical Therapeutics*, **19**, 330–45.

Hodgson, T. A. (1983). The state of the art of cost-of-illness estimates. *Advances in Health Economics and Health Services Research*, **4**, 129–64.

Hodgson, T. A. and Meiners, M. A. (1982). Cost-of-Illness methodology: a guide to current practices and procedures. *Milbank Memorial Fund Quarterly/ Health and Society*, **60**, 429–62.

Holmes, J., Pugner, K., Phillips, R., *et al.* (1999). Managing Alzheimer's disease: the cost of care per patient. *British Journal of Health Care Management*, **4**, 332–7.

HM Treasury (1997). *Appraisal and evaluation in central government*. HMSO, London.

Hu, T-W., Huang, L.-f., and Cartwright, W. S. (1986). Evaluation of the costs of caring for the senile demented elderly: a pilot study. *Gerontologist*, **26**, 158–63.

Huang, L-F., Cartwright, W. S., and Hu, T-W. (1988). The economic cost of senile dementia in the United States, 1985. *Public Health Reports*, **103**, 3–7.

Hux, M. J., O'Brien, B. J., Iskedjian, M., *et al.* (1998). Relation between severity of Alzheimer's disease and costs of caring. *Canadian Medical Association Journal*, **159**, 457–65.

Johannesson, M. (1995). A note on the depreciation of the societal perspective in economic evaluation. *Health Policy*, **33**, 59–66.

Johannesson, M. and Karlsson, G. (1997). The friction cost method: a comment. *Journal of Health Economics*, **16**, 249–55.

Johannesson, M., Meltzer, D., and O'Conor, R. M. (1997). Incorporating future costs in medical cost-effectiveness analysis: implications for the cost-effectiveness of the treatment of hypertension. *Medical Decision Making*, **17**, 382–9.

Johnston, K., Buxton, M. J., Jones, D. R., *et al.* (1999). *Assessing the costs of healthcare technologies in clinical trials*, Vol. 3, No. 6. NHS Health Technology Assessment, London.

Jonsson, L., Lindgren, P., Wimo, A., *et al.* (1999a). The cost-effectiveness of donepezil therapy in Swedish patients with Alzheimer's disease: a markov model. *Clinical Therapeutics*, **21**, 1230–40.

Jonsson, L., Lindgren, P., Wimo, A., *et al.* (1999*b*). Costs of mini mental state examination-related cognitive impairment. *PharmacoEconomics.*, **16**, 409–16.

Kanowski, S. (1998). Cost–benefit evaluation of drug treatment for Alzheimer's disease. *Archives of Gerontology and Geriatrics*, **6**, 275–80.

Kaplan, R. M. and Anderson, J. P. (1988). A general health policy model: update and applications. *Health Services Research*, **23**, 203–35.

Kaplan, R. M., Bush, J. W., and Berry, C. C. (1976). Health status: types of validity and the index of well-being. *Health Services Research*, **11**, 478–507.

Katz, S. and Akpom, A. (1976). Assessment of primary sociobiologic functions. *International Journal of Health Services*, **6**, 189–98.

Keen, J. (1993). Dementia: questions of cost and value. *International Journal of Geriatric Psychiatry*, **8**, 369–78.

Knapp, M. R. J., and Beecham, J. (1993). Reduced list Costings: examination of an informed short cut in mental health research. *Health Economics*, **2**, 313–22.

Knopman, D., Schneider, L., Davis, K., *et al.* (1996). Long-term tacrine (cognex) treatment: effects on nursing home placement and mortality, Tacrine Study Group. *Neurology*, **47**, 166–77.

Koopmanschap, M. A. and Rutten, F. F. H. (1993). Indirect costs in economic studies: confronting the confusion. *PharmacoEconomics*, **4**, 460–6.

Koopmanschap, M. A., and Rutten, F. F. (1996*a*). The consequence of production loss or increased costs of production. *Medical Care*, **34**(12 Suppl.), DS59–68.

Koopmanschap, M. A. and Rutten, F. F. H. (1996*b*). A practical guide forcalculating indirect costs of disease. *PharmacoEconomics*, **10**, 460–6.

Koopmanschap, M. A. and van Inveld, B. M. (1992). Towards a new approach for estimating indirect costs of disease. *Social Science and Medicine*, **34**, 1005–10.

Koopmanschap, M. A., Rutten, F. F. H., van Inveld, B. M., *et al.* (1995). The friction cost method for measuring indirect costs of disease. *Journal of Health Economics*, **14**, 171–89.

Koopmanschap, M. A., Rutten, F. F. H., van Inveld, B. M., *et al.* (1997). Reply to Johannesson and Karlsson's comment. *Journal of Health Economics*, **16**, 257–9.

Krahn, M. and Gafni, A. (1993). Discounting in the economic evaluation of health care interventions. *Medical Care*, **31**, 403–18.

Kronborg Andersen, C., Sogaard, J., Hansen, E., *et al.* (1999). The cost of dementia in Denmark: the Odense Study. *Dementia and Geriatric Cognitive Disorders*, **10**, 295–304.

Leon, J. and Neumann, P. J. (1999). The cost of Alzheimer's disease in managed care: A cross-sectional study. *American Journal of Managed Care*, **5**, 867–77.

Leon, J., Cheng, C. K., and Neumann, P. J. (1998). Alzheimer's disease care: costs and potential savings. *Health Affairs*, November/December **17**, 206–16.

Lubeck, D. P., Mazonson, P. D., and Bowe, T. (1994). Potential effect of tacrine on expenditures for Alzheimer's disease. *Medical Interface*, October, 130–8.

Luce, B. R. and Elixhauser, A. (1990). Estimating costs in the economic evaluation of medical technologies. *International Journal of Technology Assessment in Health Care*, **6**, 57–75.

Manning, W. G., Fryback, D. G., and Weinstein, M. C. (1996). Reflecting uncertainty in cost-effectiveness ratios. In *Cost-effectiveness in health care and medicine* (ed. M. Gold, J. Siegel, L. Russell, *et al.*), pp. 247–75. Oxford University Press, New York.

Max, W., Webber, P., and Fox, P. (1995). Alzheimer disease: the unpaid burden of caring. *Journal of Aging and Health*, **7**, 179–99.

Meek, P. D., McKeithan, K., and Schumock, G. T. (1998). Economic considerations in Alzheimer's disease. *Pharmacotherapy*, **18** (2, Pt 2), 68–73.

Meerding, W. J., Bonneux, L., Polder, J. J., *et al.* (1998). Demographic and epidemiological determinants of healthcare costs in Netherlands: cost of illness study. *British Medical Journal*, **317**, 111–15.

Meltzer, D. (1997). Accounting for future costs in medical cost-effectiveness analysis. *Journal of Health Economics*, **16**, 33–64.

Menzin, J., Lang, K., Friedman, M., *et al.* (1999). The economic cost of Alzheimer's disease and related dementias to the California Medicaid program ('Medi-Cal') in 1995. *American Journal of Geriatric Psychiatry*, **7**, 300–8.

Mittelman, M. S., Ferris, S. H., Shulman, E., *et al.* (1996). A family intervention to delay nursing home placement of patients with Alzheimer disease. A randomized controlled trial. *Journal of the American Medical Association*, **276**, 1725–31 [see comments].

Moore, M. J. and Clipp, E. C. (1994). Alzheimer's disease and caregiver time. *Lancet*, **343**, 239–40 [Letter].

Mushlin, A. L. and Fintor, L. (1992). Is screening for breast cancer cost-effective? *Cancer*, **69**(Suppl.), 1957–62.

Netten, A. and Dennett, J. (1999). *Unit costs of health and social care*. PSSRU University of Kent, Canterbury.

Neumann, P. J., Hermann, R. C., Berenbaum, P. A., *et al.* (1997). Methods of cost-effectiveness analysis in the assessment of new drugs for Alzheimer's disease. *Psychiatric Services*, 48, 1440–4.

Neumann, P. J., Hermann, R. C., and Weinstein, M. C. (1998). Measuring QALYs in dementia. In *Health economics of dementia* (ed. A. Wimo, B. Jonsson, G. Karlsson, *et al.*), pp. 359–70. Wiley, Chichester.

Neumann, P. J., Hermann, R. C., Kuntz, K. M., *et al.* (1999). Cost-effectiveness of donepezil in the treatment of mild or moderate Alzheimer's disease. *Neurology*, **52**, 1138–45.

Nord, E. (1995). The person-trade-off approach to valuing health care programs. *Medical Decision Making*, **15**, 201–8.

O'Brien, B., Gore, R., Hux, M., *et al.* (1999). Economic evaluation of donepezil for the treatment of Alzheimer's disease in Canada. *Journal of the American Geriatric Society*, **47**, 570–8.

O'Shea, E. and O'Reilly, S. (2000). The economic and social cost of dementia in Ireland. *International Journal of Geriatric Psychiatry*, **15**, 208–18.

Ostbye, T. and Crosse, E. (1994). Net economic costs of dementia in Canada. *Canadian Medical Association Journal*, **151**, 1457–64.

Oster, G. and Epstein, A. M. (1987). Cost-effectiveness of anti-hyperlipidemic therapy in the prevention of coronary heart disease: the case of cholestyramine. *Journal of the American Medical Association*, **258**, 2381–87.

Parsonage, M. and Neuberger, H. (1992). Discounting and Health Benefits. *Health Economics*, **1**, 71–6.

Patrick, D. L., Bush, J. W., and Chen, M. M. (1973). Methods for measuring levels of well-being for a health status index. *Health Services Research*, **8**, 228–45.

Posnett, J. and Jan, S. (1996). Indirect cost in economic evaluation: the opportunity cost of unpaid inputs. *Health Economics*, **5**, 13–23.

Rice, D. P. (1967). Estimating the cost of illness. *American Journal of Public Health*, **57**, 424–40.

Rice, D. P., Fox, P. J., Max, W., *et al.* (1993). The economic burden of Alzheimer's disease care. *Health Affairs*, **12**, 164–76.

Rocca, W. A., Hofman, A., Brayne, C., *et al.* (1991*a*). Frequency and distribution of Alzheimer's disease in Europe: a collaborative study of 1980–1990 prevalence findings. The EURODEM-Prevalence Research Group. *Annals of Neurology*, **30**, 381–90.

Rocca, W. A., Hofman, A., Brayne, C., *et al.* (1991*b*). The prevalence of vascular dementia in Europe: facts and fragments from 1980–1990 studies. EURODEM-Prevalence Research Group. *Annals of Neurology*, **30**, 817–24.

Rogers, S. L., Farlow, M. R., and Doody, R. S. (1998). A 24-week, double blind, placebo-controlled trial of donepezil in patients with Alzheimer's disease. *Neurology*, **50**, 136–45.

Rosser, R. and Kind, P. (1978). A scale of valuations of states of illness: is there a social consensus? *International Journal of Epidemiology*, **7**, 347–58.

Russell, L. B. (1986). *Is prevention better than cure?* Brookings Institution, Washington DC.

Ryan, M. (1996). *Using consumer preferences in health care decision making: the application of conjoint analysis*. Office of Health Economics, London.

Schneider, J., Kavanagh, S., Knapp, M., *et al.* (1993). Elderly people with advanced cognitive impairment in England: resource use and costs. *Ageing and Society*, **13**, 27–50.

Schumock, G. T. (1998). Economic considerations in the treatment and management of Alzheimer's disease. *American Journal of Health System Pharmacy*, **55**, S17–S21.

Sculpher, M. J. and Buxton, M. J. (1993). *The private costs incurred when patients attend screening clinics: the cases of screening for breast cancer and for diabetic retinopathy* (HERG Discussion Paper No. 10). Brunel University, Uxbridge.

Shapiro, E. and Tate, R. B. (1997). The use and cost of community care services by elders with unimpaired cognitive function, with cognitive impairment/no dementia and with dementia. *Canadian Journal on Aging*, **16**, 665–81.

Sintonen, H. (1981). An approach to measuring and valuing health states. *Social Science and Medicine*, **15**, 55–65.

Small, G. W., Donohue, J. A., and Brooks, R. L. (1998). An economic evaluation of donepezil in the treatment of Alzheimer's disease. *Clinical Therapeutics*, **20**, 838–50.

Smith, K. and Wright, K. (1994). Informal care and economic appraisal: a discussion of possible methodological approaches. *Health Economics*, **3**, 137–48.

Souetre, E. J., Qing, W., Vigoureux, I., *et al.* (1995). Economic analysis of Alzheimer's disease in outpatients: impact of symptom severity. *International Psychogeriatrics*, 7, 115–22.

Souetre, E., Thwaites, R. M. A., and Yeardley, H. L. (1999). Economic impact of Alzheimer's disease in the United Kingdom: cost of care and disease severity for non-institutionalized patients with Alzheimer's disease. *British Journal of Psychiatry*, **174**, 51–5.

Stewart, A., Philips, R., and Dempsey, G. (1998). Pharmacotherapy for people with Alzheimer's disease: a markov-cycle evaluation of five years' therapy using donepezil. *International Journal of Geriatric Psychiatry*, **13**, 445–53.

Stommel, M., Collins, C. E., and Given, B. A. (1994). The costs of family contributions to the care of persons with dementia. *Gerontologist.*, **34**, 199–205.

Torgerson, D. J., Donaldson, C., and Reid, D. M. (1994). Private versus social opportunity cost of time: valuing time in the demand for health care. *Health Economics*, **3**, 149–55.

Torrance, G. W. (1982). Preferences for health states: a review of measurement methods. *Mead Johnson Symposium for Perinatal Developmental Medicine*, **20**, 37–45.

Torrance, G. W. (1986). Measurement of health state utilities for economic appraisal. *Journal of Health Economics*, **5**, 1–30.

Torrance, G. W., Furlong, W., Feeny, D., *et al.* (1995). Multi-attribute preference functions. Health Utilities Index. *PharmacoEconomics.*, 7, 503–20.

Torrance, G. W., Feeny, D. H., Furlong, W. J., *et al.* (1996). Multiattribute utility function for a comprehensive health status classification system. Health Utilities Index Mark 2. *Medical Care*, **34**, 702–22.

Trabucchi, M. (1999). An economic perspective on Alzheimer's disease. *Journal of Geriatric Psychiatry and Neurology*, **12**, 29–38.

van Hout, B. A., Al, M. J., Gordon, G. S., *et al.* (1994). Costs, effects and C/E-ratios alongside a clinical trial. *Health Economics*, **3**, 309–19.

van Roijen, L., Essink-Bot, M. L., Koopmanschap, M. A., *et al.* (1996). Labor and health status in economic evaluation of health care: the health and labor questionnaire. *International Journal of Technology Assessment in Health Care*, **12**, 405–15.

Weinberger, M., Gold, D. T., Divine, G. W., *et al.* (1993). Expenditures in caring for patients with dementia who live at home. *American Journal of Public Health*, **83**, 338–41.

Weinstein, M. C. and Stason, W. B. (1977). Foundations of cost-effectiveness analysis for health and medical practices. *New England Journal of Medicine*, **296**, 716–21.

Weinstein, M., Fineberg, H., Elstein, A., *et al.* (1980). *Clinical decision analysis*. Saunders, Philadelphia, PA.

Weisbrod, B. A. (1961). *Economics of public health*. University of Pennysylvania Press, Philadelphia.

Welch, H., Walsh, J., and Larson, E. (1992). The cost of institutional care in Alzheimer's Disease: nursing home and hospital use in a prospective cohort. *Journal for the American Geriatric Society–Archives*, **40**, 221–4.

Whitehouse, P. J. (1997). Pharmacoeconomics of dementia. *Alzheimer Disease and Associated Disorders*, **11**(Suppl. 5), S22–32; discussion S32–3.

Whitehouse, P. J., Winblad, B., Shostak, D., *et al.* (1998). First International Pharmacoeconomic Conference on Alzheimer's Disease, Amsterdam, July 1998: Report and summary. *Alzheimer Disease and Associated Disorders*, **12**, 266–80.

Whynes, D. K. and Walker, A. R. (1995). On Approximations in Treatment Costing. *Health Economics*, **4**, 31–9.

Willan, A. R. and O'Brien, B. J. (1996). Confidence intervals for cost-effectiveness ratios: an application of Fieller's theorem. *Health Economics*, **5**, 297–305.

Wimo, A., Karlsson, G., Nordberg, A., *et al.* (1997*a*). Treatment of Alzheimer disease with tacrine: a cost–analysis model. *Alzheimer Disease and Associated Disorders*, **11**, 191–200.

Wimo, A., Karlsson, G., Sandman, P. O., *et al.* (1997*b*). Cost of illness due to dementia in Sweden. *International Journal of Geriatric Psychiatry*, **12**, 857–61.

Wimo, A., Mattson, B., Krakau, I., *et al.* (1995). Cost-utility analysis of group living in dementia care. *International Journal of Technology Assessment in Health Care*, **11**, 49–65.

Wimo, A., Wetterholm, A., Mastey, V., *et al.* (1998). Evaluation of the health care resource-utilization and caregiver time in anti-dementia drug trials—a quantitative battery. In *Health economics of dementia* (ed. A. Wimo, B. Jonsson, G. Karlsson, *et al.*), pp. 465–99. Wiley, Chichester.

Winblad, B., Hill, S., Beermann, B., *et al* (1997). Issues in the economic evaluation of treatment for dementia. Position paper from the International Working Group on Harmonization of Dementia Drug Guidelines. *Alzheimer Disease and Associated Disorders*, **11**(Suppl. 3), 39–45.

World Bank (1993). *World development report 1993: investing in health*. Oxford University Press for the World Bank edn, New York.

II | *Clinical practice*

9 Psychiatric and clinical cognitive assessment

Peter Bentham and John Hodges

Introduction

This chapter assumes the reader is familiar with the basic principles of the psychiatric interview and mental state examination, which are well covered in standard texts (Leff and Isaacs 1981). The psychiatric evaluation of an elderly patient is similar to that of a younger adult and this account focuses on areas where important differences in emphasis exist.

Aims of assessment

The psychiatric assessment interview serves several different purposes: it poses questions to obtain factual information on historical events, happenings, and activities; it acts as a stimulus to elicit emotions, feelings, and attitudes; and begins to establish a therapeutic relationship with the patient (Rutter and Cox 1981). The assessment should result in a comprehensive diagnostic formulation and, importantly, a proper assessment of need (Cm 849 1989). Risk assessment is an integral part of this process.

Preassessment information

Before attempting to see the patient, a certain amount of background information is useful. The majority of referrals come from general practitioners (GPs; i.e. primary-care physicians). Pullen and Yellowlees (1985) identified a number of key pieces of information required by psychiatrists in referral letters. It is important to establish who and what prompted the referral, in addition to having background information on the patient's psychiatric history, family history, and drug treatment. General practitioners should also be encouraged to provide medical details and clear information on how to contact informants for elderly patients. A telephone call to the GP can be useful, but may be better left until after the assessment so that questions can be better focused.

Who should assess?

The established model of specialist assessment for older people with mental health problems is via a domiciliary consultation by a hospital-based psychiatrist. An obvious advantage of this system is that the psychiatrist will be skilled at physical and mental state assessment. However, in areas where demand outstrips medical resources, community psychiatric nurses or members of community multidisciplinary teams may perform initial assessments (Coles *et al.* 1991). Claims have been made that the quality of assessment by these teams is at least as good as that obtained via a consultant domiciliary visit (Collighan *et al.* 1993), but the effectiveness of using a filter between GP and old age psychiatrist has been questioned (Jolley and Arie 1992). The case for retaining consultant home visits, versus other forms of assessment, has been reviewed by Orrell and Katona (1998) who highlight the lack of any randomized controlled trials comparing these forms of assessment.

Where and when should assessment take place?

Ideally patients should be seen within 48 hours of referral to avoid the development of both waiting lists and crises (Shah and Ames 1994). In practice, most urgent visits are made within 48 hours and non-urgent assessments within 1 week (Tullet *et al.* 1997) and this is generally found to be satisfactory.

Domiciliary assessment

Most patients referred to old age psychiatry services should be assessed initially at home, and this is particularly important when dementia is suspected. A home visit offers the advantage of assessing the patient in their natural environment. It avoids a potentially exhausting journey for those who are physically frail, reduces anxiety, and eliminates the effect of disorienting, unfamiliar hospital surroundings on the patient's mental state. Domiciliary visits enable the patient's home environment to be directly observed, they also offer the opportunity to test cognition and assess competence in daily living activities in relation to that environment. It can be informative to ask the patient to locate their medication supply or even accept their kind offer of tea and biscuits! If care is taken setting up the home visit then the problems associated with outpatient non-attendance can largely be avoided. Finally, home assessment can facilitate contact with useful informants such as neighbours and home carers when family members are unavailable.

There are some disadvantages, which can be minimized with care. The first problem may be gaining access. A normal elderly person could be forgiven for refusing access to someone presenting as a doctor who fails to carry an identity card. The patient may not answer the doctor's call because of disability, anxiety, or suspicion. If this situation is anticipated, then arrangements can be made for appropriate others to be present to reassure and facilitate access. Behaviourally disordered animals and grandchildren can threaten chaos, requiring novel adaptive responses from the interviewer! Ensuring privacy for both the patient and informant may be more difficult than in an outpatient setting. Use can, however, be made of other rooms within the home and it is usually possible to facilitate a brief one-to-one doorstep or kitchen conversation even under difficult circumstances. Finally, when visiting the elderly at home issues of personal safety must be considered; though Mrs Smith may be a nice old lady, her son or neighbour may be less endearing. Overall, domiciliary visits have no major disadvantages and may be more cost-effective than clinic-based assessments (Shah 1997).

Inpatient assessment

Approximately one-third of referrals to old age psychiatry services come from geriatric or general medicine. In many respects the alien environment of a medical ward is an unsatisfactory setting for assessment, but psychiatric input at this stage is essential if psychiatric problems are significantly impinging on the patient's medical and social management. Timing of the assessment may be important, clouded consciousness is often more evident later in the day, conversely depressive symptoms are usually worse in the morning. Assessment of psychiatric symptomatology shortly after a benzodiazepine overdose is unlikely to be reliable. It is probably best not to visit at mealtimes or during the nursing handover, because access to the patient and the informant may prove difficult.

It is common for elderly patients with acute medical problems to be treated on general medical wards. As these units are focused on providing efficient general medical care to patients of all age groups, the specialized requirements of the old age psychiatrist may not be fully appreciated. Prior to seeing the patient it is important to have read the case notes and to have interviewed someone with first-hand knowledge of the current problem. Usually this is the primary nurse, but other members of the health care team may be able to contribute.

From the medical notes it should be straightforward to identify the stated reason for admission, but it must be appreciated that often this is not the main issue. History of the onset of the problem is of great value but is often lacking in the elderly living alone; here a well-written referral letter from the general practitioner is invaluable. Past medical history should be available and it is useful to review previous admission notes. Details of medication are usually recorded but may be inaccurate, which must be borne in mind when considering the potential adverse effects of drugs. It is unlikely that a formal mental state examination will be found, although many geriatric units now record an Abbreviated Mental Test score (AMT) (Hodkinson 1972). The nursing notes are often more informative with regard to the patient's behaviour, memory, mood, sleep, appetite, and self-care. However, caution must be used when interpreting psychopathological descriptions. Disorders of thought and perception may not be what they seem, and particularly the term 'confusion' is imprecisely defined (Simpson 1984). Details of the patient's support network prior to admission can provide useful diagnostic information. It is unlikely that a patient with moderately severe dementia would have been able to survive in the community without substantial input from formal or informal carers. Perhaps the most useful information in hospital notes is the information on how to contact informants in the community, thus enabling a more complete picture to be obtained. If contact information is available prior to the hospital visit it can be extremely helpful to have a family member or friend present at the interview.

There is often the opportunity to observe the patient in the ward environment prior to the interview. This can give valuable information on the patient's conscious level and grasp of surroundings. Problem behaviours described by the nursing staff can be witnessed at first hand, enabling a better understanding of how they impact on staff, patients, and the functioning of the ward.

Having obtained the necessary background information, the visiting psychiatrist should take care in choosing an appropriate location for the interview. The nursing staff will routinely direct the doctor to the patient's bed, the most appropriate place to conduct a physical examination. Even with the curtains drawn this offers little privacy for the more verbally based psychiatric examination; moreover, the general background noise is often an impediment to communication with those who have poor hearing. Usually a private spot can be found and it is not unreasonable to ask politely if an immobile patient can be conveyed there in a wheelchair. A brief physical examination may also be required, as the medical team could have overlooked physical problems influencing the patient's mental state. Finally, it is important to remember to communicate the results of the assessment without undue delay. A clearly written name and contact telephone number are particularly useful to the medical team if further discussion is required.

Assessment in residential care homes

Psychiatrists are often asked to assess patients in residential settings. Assessment issues are similar to those discussed above. Care staff generally have limited understanding of the patient's medical state but are often more knowledgeable about their background. In taking a history it is important to ascertain when and why the patient became resident and how they initially adjusted to their new home. It is useful to enquire as to whether any changes in staff, residents, or environment preceded the onset of the presenting problem.

Outpatient assessment

Though outpatient clinic assessments are in general less satisfactory than those performed at home, there is one particular situation where a clinic assessment may offer advantages. Memory clinics have become increasingly common (Wright and Lindesay 1995). These clinics may have several functions including specialist assessment of those presenting with mild memory or other cognitive problems. Memory clinics facilitate referrals at a much earlier stage than would be expected by the traditional pathways. A common function is the early diagnosis of dementia and differential diagnosis within the dementia spectrum. This is achieved by the involvement of a multidisciplinary team including: psychiatrists, neurologists, geriatricians, neuroradiologists, psychologists, social workers, occupational therapists, nurses, and others. These clinics offer a focus of expertise particularly enabling detailed psychiatric, physical, neuroradiological, and neuropsycholgical evaluation.

The Cambridge Memory Clinic has been in existence for 10 years and has experience of assessing more than 2000 cases. Whenever possible, patients are seen by a neurologist, psychiatrist, and neuropsychologist on the same day. This avoids multiple hospital visits and allows the teams involved to hold a case conference at which the diagnosis, investigation, and management plan are formulated (Hodges *et al.* 2000). The following practice principles evolved in this clinic may help others organizing similar clinics:

- All patients referred to the clinic are asked to attend with a family member or close friend if at all possible.
- Patients are sent a 'life questionnaire' to complete in advance of the appointment, which details family history, marital history, past medical complaints, education, and current medication. They also receive the Cambridge Behavioural Questionnaire (Bozeat *et al.* 2000), which is modelled on the Neuropsychiatric Inventory (Cummings *et al.* 1994). This is completed by a carer/family member/friend and enquires about a wide range of cognitive behavioural and neuropsychiatric symptoms and activities of daily living. The information obtained from these is invaluable and saves much time in the clinic.
- Patients and their family member/friend are interviewed separately.
- All patients undergo a brief standardized cognitive evaluation, based upon theoretically motivated concepts outlined elsewhere (Hodges 1994), the Addenbrooke's Cognitive Examination (ACE) (Mathuranath *et al.* 2000).

The psychiatric interview

Assessment of the elderly patient places greater emphasis on gathering information from ancillary sources. In general psychiatry the patient can often give enough historical information to allow the formulation of an accurate diagnosis, and sometimes this is the case with the elderly. Patients with significant impairment of memory, language, or general cognitive abilities are highly unlikely to be able to give a comprehensive history. Even in early dementia, there are problems recalling information in temporal sequence, making it extremely difficult to evaluate the natural history of the illness. It must be remembered, however, that the informant history is not necessarily more accurate than the patient's. The informant may also have significant cognitive impairment or be less familiar with the patient than they would have you believe. Carers in particular will have their own agenda, which may not be overt. Indeed, different carers often have very different perspectives and various accounts may conflict with one another. Frank evasiveness is uncommon, but denial of specific problems or explanations that are clearly inconsistent with the objective evidence should raise the possibility of abuse (Rathbone-McCuan and Voyles 1982).

Establishing rapport and eliciting information

Establishing a good rapport with the patient and carer is a crucial element of the interview. First impressions are often lasting and a mishap at this point can lead to enduring difficulties. It is important to appreciate that patients may be unaware that they require assessment or that they could have forgotten the appointment. The psychiatrist should make an introduction giving their title, name, and place of work. Patients should also be addressed by their title and surname unless they express another preference. It is useful to say who requested the assessment, as the patient is often quite familiar with the referring professional, and briefly to state the reason for the visit. Make no assumptions about relationships within the home, and ascertain from the outset 'who is who'. Whilst acknowledging the patient's right to sit on their favourite chair, endeavour to arrange a suitable seating arrangement and always heed carer's warnings about 'deaf sides'. Distractions such as televisions and radios should be switched off 'so that the doctor can hear better'. A simple outline of the likely interview format should be given, including the time available. Before proceeding with the formal interview, non-verbal communication should be noted. If the patient appears angry, suspicious, or terrified, then this must be explored further. Elderly patients are often unfamiliar with the modern philosophy of community care, but they may have heard about people being 'taken away', or vaguely recall stories of the workhouse.

A failure to respond appropriately to questions could suggest a hearing impairment, indicating that a functioning aid will be required. If the patient's hearing aid can be located, check that it is switched on ('m' = microphone) and that the earpiece is clear of wax. Turn up the volume and a whistling noise should be heard. Silence may indicate flat batteries, dirty contacts, or a broken aid. Turn down the volume and insert the earpiece into the correct ear, checking that it fits snugly. Turn up the volume again to a point just before the whistling recurs and check if you can now be heard. If a hearing aid is not working it should be removed, as it simply acts as an obstruction impairing any residual hearing. When communicating with a patient whose hearing is impaired it is essential to speak slowly and clearly. Volume should be increased and it is important to check whether the patient can now hear. Shouting must be avoided as receptors for soft sounds are often more degenerated than those for loud ones, leading to the painful phenomenon of recruitment once a certain volume is reached. The elderly person who asks you to 'speak up' only to then to say 'don't shout—I'm not deaf' is not being awkward but accurately relaying the subjective experience of presbyacusis. Increasing pitch along with volume is unhelpful, as hearing loss tends to be worse for higher frequencies. Most people have some ability to lip read, therefore it is important that your face is visible, not covered by a hand, and adequately illuminated. If all else fails write questions down or try speaking through the bell of the stethoscope with the patient wearing the earpiece. Carrying a set of simple cognitive questions (e.g. the AMT) in large print is useful, as is the Brief Assessment Schedule Depression Cards (BASDEC) (Adshead *et al.* 1992) for eliciting depressive symptoms.

Generally it is better to interview at a slower pace than with younger adults to allow sufficient time for information to be processed and responses to be generated. It is probably best to start with simple non-threatening questions to set the stage for a more comprehensive assessment. Open questions should then be utilized to obtain relevant clinical information. It is important though to remain aware that older people are sometimes more cautious in their responses and may require prompting. Similarly, the current generation of elderly often attribute significant symptoms to 'old age' thereby giving false-negative answers to screening questions. Often the psychiatrist has to take a more active stance offering encouragement and utilizing more multiple-choice or forced-choice questions. Leading questions, as always, must be avoided. The complexity of questioning should be tailored to the patient's observed abilities and emotional reaction, with care being taken to avoid a catastrophic reaction (Goldstein 1942), which can lead to premature termination of the interview. The interview must be structured, but also flexible and adaptive. Information gained from the history contributes substantially to the mental state evaluation. Many aspects of the cognitive assessment can be incorporated within history-taking, without resorting to an overt formal mental test, which could be distressing to a sensitive patient. Some psychiatrists start with background history and others with the presenting complaints. Generally, formal cognitive testing is left until later but some prefer early evaluation of cognition before the patient tires (Jarvik and Wiseman 1991).

Finally, attention should be paid to the psychodynamics of the patient–doctor interaction. The patient may be old enough to be the interviewer's parent or grandparent. Transference could inhibit disclosure of distressing information to someone reminiscent of a schoolchild; similarly, countertransference (or ageism) might make one reluctant to ask sexual questions of a parent-like figure.

Setting rules

The format of the assessment and the time available should first be outlined. All things considered it is probably best to interview the patient first, even if it seems unlikely that they will be able to provide much information. This sends out a clear message that the patient is important and valued. The presence of another key person during history-taking may facilitate or inhibit the free flow of information. Patients or informants sometimes express a preference for the other person to be present or absent and it can be useful to ask what arrangement is preferred. However, it is essential to spend a brief period alone with the informant to ascertain whether there were any problems that they were unable to discuss in front of the patient. If this is the case then these problems can be discussed later over the telephone or via a clinic appointment with the carer.

Taking the history

History of present illness

The psychiatric history begins with the presenting complaints. The aim is to determine the temporal sequence of symptom development in relation to environmental events, physical health, functional ability, and treatment interventions. In patients with suspected organic disorder the history must also be supplemented by interview with an informant. It is vitally important to identify the initial symptoms and their mode of onset. Often it is difficult to obtain a clear history of the time course but this can be aided by using landmarks such as Christmas, birthdays, or holidays. Symptoms with insidious onset are usually dated imprecisely but are sometimes related to a particularly memorable situation. It is important to enquire whether any abnormality had been noticed prior to this event. If the initial problem occurred relatively suddenly a distinction should be drawn between symptoms that developed in less than 24 hours and those that developed over a few days or weeks. An acute or subacute onset of cognitive dysfunction suggests delirium or an affective illness. Next, the course of the illness must be determined. Have the presenting symptoms worsened over time and have new ones developed? Has the deterioration been smooth or irregular? If irregular has there been a stepwise deterioration with long periods of relative stability being interrupted by episodes of sudden deterioration? Is there evidence of fluctuation over shorter periods, if so is this irregular or is there a diurnal pattern with symptoms being consistently worse either in the morning or later in the day? Obtaining recent discrete examples of variations in cognitive ability or performance, possibly via a rating scale, can improve accuracy in detecting fluctuating confusion (Walker *et al.* 2000). What is the relationship between cognitive, affective, and physical symptoms?

Past psychiatric and medical illness

The information from the patient, though valuable, is likely to need supplementation by the informant or GP. It is useful to ask about periods of hospitalization and previous treatment. It must be noted, however, that treatment with electroconvulsive therapy (ECT) in the 1950s is no guarantee that the patient suffered from an affective illness. Following the interview it may necessary to ask the GP for more specific information on past illnesses.

Current prescribed medication

Good GP referral letters often contain a comprehensive computerized print-out of a patient's current medication. This should never be taken at face value and it is vital to ask what medication the patient thinks is being taken. It can be enlightening to enquire as to the purpose of the treatment and the need to adhere to the prescribed regimen. The psychiatrist should always ask to see the patient's medication supply. Containers will indicate when a drug was dispensed. By taking note of the remaining number of tablets and the frequency of administration, it is possible to estimate whether compliance has been adequate. If compliance appears to have been poor the reason should be ascertained. Possibilities to be considered are: poor motivation; lack of understanding about the medication; delusional ideas; practical problems such as huge tablets, child-proof containers and distant dispensaries; a well thought-out, adaptive, logical decision; and, importantly, impairment of prospective memory (Meacham and Singer 1977). Excessive consumption of hypnotic, anxiolytic, or analgesic medication could indicate dependence.

Non-prescribed substances

A history of alcohol consumption is an integral part of the assessment of all elderly psychiatric patients, and it should be borne in mind that elderly problem drinkers often do not volunteer this information. It is important to make an estimate of both the current level of alcohol intake (units/week) and that in the past. If the patient is or was a heavy drinker then a history of adverse physical, social, or legal consequences should be sought (see Chapter 34). Similarly for smoking, the present and past level of consumption should be asked about. Over-the-counter remedies such as St John's Wort may have important interactions with prescribed drugs, and laxative abuse can lead to a variety of problems. It is not unheard of for patients to borrow prescribed medicines from friends and relatives, and very occasionally an abuse of illegal drugs is encountered.

Family history

It is preferable to interview the patient in the presence of a relative, who has earlier been asked to allow time for questions to be answered and then to help out if information is not forthcoming. This enables the accuracy of the history to be validated and appropriate prompts to be provided. In general, the older the patient, the more difficult it is to verify the accuracy of the family history as those of their own, and particularly preceding, generations are usually unavailable. Younger people are often not well informed regarding their ancestors, however when it is particularly important to get an accurate family tree it can be useful to ask if there is a relative with a particular interest in family history. Inability to remember the names of close family members or confusion between the names of different generations is evidence of significant retrograde memory impairment. The amount of detail sought will be largely determined by the nature of the presenting problem, with particularly detailed enquiry being reserved for those with illnesses known to have a specific genetic component. As a minimum, one should attempt to ascertain the age and cause of death for parents and siblings and to ask whether anyone in the family has suffered from mental illness. Prior to the days of community care, patients with the more severe mental disorders were likely to be admitted to a psychiatric hospital. The approximate age on first admission can be a useful clue to the diagnosis as can the length of stay, treatment received, and degree of eventual recovery. To detect dementia it can be useful to ask if anyone in the family had become forgetful or confused as they got older, or had to go into a home or hospital because they were unable to look after themselves. Further clarification can be obtained by asking whether this person had ever suffered from strokes, Parkinson's disease, or other physical problems that could explain their disability. If names and dates of birth are available it may be possible to trace old medical records in hospital archives.

Personal history

Personal history is intimately interwoven with family history and much information can be gathered whilst obtaining the latter. In anxious patients, particularly those with cognitive impairment, this can be a good starting point for the interview as the questions can be more easily answered. Moderately demented patients can usually say where they were born. The narrative account of personal history offers a good opportunity to assess memory and orientation, without resorting to a formal test. Knowledge of the father's occupation may indicate something of the family's social circumstances, with unemployment in the 1920s and 1930s being particularly linked with hardship. Formal schooling was between the ages of 5 and 14 years for all but the most fortunate; however, many elderly people will tell you with pride that they could have gone to grammar school had the financial situation been more favourable. It must also be noted that between 1939 and 1945 there was considerable disruption to schooling in the cities due to bombing and evacuation, further reducing educational opportunities. Claims not to be particularly clever should be treated with caution, particularly in those with poor hearing and vision since childhood; similarly specific learning disabilities may have led to poor school performance.

Childhood abuse in its various forms may have enduring effects. Woods (1995) reports a case of frequent intrusive flashback memories still occurring nearly 70 years after the event.

Employment history can provide a very useful insight into a person's abilities, interests, and personality, although it may largely reflect limited opportunities, particularly for women. In the elderly an employment history can be very lengthy, particularly when recounted by someone with obsessional tendencies. In this situation specific questions should be used to ascertain which was the longest held job and which was the most skilled or intellectually demanding.

Marital details and information on descendants is collected in the usual way, but this may be complex when there have been several marriages. Care must be taken in interpreting information. A long marriage may not be a happy one; people remain married for reasons of security and religion as well as love. Loss events are more common in the elderly and death of a spouse is considered to be one of the highest stressors of all. Similarly, the death of a child has an enormous impact, even if that child is in his sixties. Parents at any age do not expect to outlive their children. Bereavements in early life should be asked about as they may also be important in predisposing people to psychiatric disorder in old age, particularly phobias (Lindesay 1991). Other life events that may require more detailed exploration are retirement, physical illness, exposure to criminal acts, and changes of accommodation, particularly institutionalization.

Sexual history

It is important to appreciate that elderly people may have an ongoing interest in sexual activities. Older patients are likely to have been married and if male probably still are. Psychiatrists are often reluctant to take a sexual history for a variety of reasons. However, evidence suggests that elderly people are quite willing to discuss sexual issues if given the opportunity. As a minimum, a screening question about any marital or relationship difficulties should be asked. The interviewer should be prepared to answer surprise questions of a sexual nature and remain alert to the fact that sexual problems can present in a myriad of ways (see Chapter 35).

Personality

Personality assessment can be difficult in the elderly, particularly in those with a long past history of psychiatric disorder extending back into middle age and early adult life. Stereotypical views of the elderly often portray them as being either cantankerous or stubborn, or alternatively as passive, sweet, and dependent. The psychiatrist must remain aware of the wide range of individual differences, which if anything become more marked in later life. In assessing personality, information has to be obtained from the patient and an informant who has been well acquainted, preferably for several years. However, a suitable informant may not be available for very elderly or reclusive individuals. In this situation the patient's account must be viewed with caution as the description of premorbid personality may be significantly coloured by the current mental state. It can be useful to compare the patient's perceptions with details obtained from the personal history. It is unlikely that someone who had always been anxious and lacking in self-confidence would have been able to function effectively for many years as a foreman or a barmaid. Assessment is as for younger adults, but elderly people may find it difficult to describe spontaneously their personality and more structured questioning may be required. In addition to asking about sociability, self-confidence, and relationships it is also important to ascertain how the patient coped with major life stresses in the past. Insight into changes of personality is virtually always absent and it is vital to incorporate questions about such alterations and their impact when interviewing informants.

Present social circumstances and support

Domiciliary visits facilitate direct assessment of the home environment. A keen eye can help answer several questions. Gardens can be very informative. A well-stocked, carefully planned garden may indicate a past interest and skill even if it is now untidy and overgrown. It may be possible to estimate the duration of neglect by examining the pruning state of the plants. A deliberate attempt to shade windows by bushes and trees may suggest someone of a suspicious nature. Is it easy to gain access to the property and is it secure? Is the main living area clean and tidy, if not, then is the neglect recent or longstanding? Are there any accident hazards such as loose carpets, unguarded heating appliances or steep stairs? Is there any evidence of potentially dangerous behaviour in the form of burns to furniture or pans? Are smoke alarms fitted? What are the sleeping arrangements? Has the bed been slept in? It is important to get a sight of the kitchen area and particularly the cooker to ascertain whether it is in good working order and has been safely used. A cooker in pristine condition may simply indicate that it is redundant. A peek inside the refrigerator can be very enlightening in relation to shopping abilities and food hygiene. Similarly, the bathroom and toilet should be assessed if appropriate. The presence of a large number of bottles, full or empty, may indicate alcohol abuse. Other senses should be utilized in the assessment. Incontinence can be readily detected by smell and occasionally by touch! It may really be possible to hear the neighbour shouting abuse through the wall.

A clear picture of the patient's functional ability in everyday life must be obtained. Some information may come from the patient, but particularly in those with suspected organic impairment the bulk of the information should be obtained from an informant. The patient's ability to perform basic activities of daily living such as, washing, dressing, eating, and toileting should be ascertained, along with the degree to which they are dependent on others for the performance of these functions. Similarly, instrumental activities such as, shopping, cooking, managing finances, and taking medication must be assessed. A rating instrument such as the Clifton Assessment Procedures for the Elderly (CAPE) Behaviour Rating Scale (Pattie and Gilleard 1979) can be useful to structure the informant interview. In all cases it is wise to ask whether a patient still drives a motor vehicle as some of the most unlikely people hold a licence. This is important even in functional disorders, as poor concentration or the effects of medication can impair driving ability (see Chapter 42). Other potential risky behaviour should be asked about. Has there been any behaviour indicative of intent to self-harm or aggressive behaviour towards others? Is the patient liable to fall or wander off and get lost? Are heating and cooking appliances being used safely? Are undesirable characters being invited into the home? Carers can sometimes be extremely imaginative in dealing with problem behaviours and it is useful to know what interventions have been tried and to what extent they have been successful.

It is worth trying to obtain some details of the patient's financial status. They should be in receipt of a regular income, usually a state pension, and may be eligible for other benefits such as income support or the attendance allowance. House ownership is common and may be shared with another person. It is useful to know whether savings are in joint or individual accounts, and whether the patient's affairs are being dealt with by another either on an informal or formal basis. The capacity of the patient to manage his or her own affairs should be formally assessed if there is doubt about it in this area (see Chapter 41).

The amount of informal and formal support available to the patient must be clarified, which can be neatly summarized in a social network diagram (Capildeo *et al.* 1976). The quality of this support also needs to be evaluated. It is useful to know whether home-care input is consistent and whether transport to and from the day centre is reliable. More importantly, the quality of relationships within the patient's family and circle of friends should be assessed. It is worth trying to clarify how the problem is seen from different perspectives as this may significantly affect the aims of a carer. Problems arising from differing aims can be compounded by faulty communication between different elements of the support system. Attempting to understand the way in which a support system functions helps avoid unnecessary confrontation and unwitting collusion with maladaptive relationship patterns such as scapegoating.

Carer's needs

The interview with the carer must also address their needs as well as those of the patient (see Chapter 21). It is important that the problems identified by the carer are seen to be understood and appreciated. The objective burden of care should be assessed by ascertaining exactly what the carer has to do for the patient in terms of providing assistance, supervision, and support. It can be enlightening to ask how much time is spent on these activities during a normal day. The impact of providing care on family, social, and employment life must also be taken into consideration. Subjective burden should be assessed by determining the carer's emotional and cognitive reaction to providing care. It is important to remember that clinical depression in carers is common and one should always to be vigilant for the signs. The emotional reaction to caregiving may be influenced by the quality of the past relationship between the patient and carer. Similarly, it is important to explore the carer's current perceptions of what caregiving is about, and this is clearly related to the carer's understanding of the patient's illness. Despite good intentions elderly carers are not always able to do what they feel is necessary because of problems with their own health and the psychiatrist should adopt a realistic perspective. A carer's right to have their needs assessed has now been formally recognized in the Carers Act (Department of Health 1996).

Mental state assessment

The mental state examination should follow the same format as used with a younger adult, but with an elderly patient greater emphasis should be placed on certain areas. There may also be subtle differences in symptom presentation. It is important to combine qualitative, clinically led evaluation, with quantification particularly in the cognitive domain.

Appearance and behaviour

This aspect of the examination must never be neglected. In patients with marked behavioural disturbance or where communication is difficult, careful systematic observation is likely to yield the most useful information.

The general appearance of the patient, including the state of dress and personal hygiene, must be assessed. If the patient is unkempt then an attempt should be made to estimate whether this has been a recent or more longstanding problem. Look for ingrained dirt, long fingernails, and weight loss, comparing the presentation of the patient with the state of the living environment. Incontinence should be readily apparent. Caution is indicated, however, when interpreting an immaculate appearance as this may simply reflect the excellence of care from another.

Note should be taken of the patient's level of attention and concentration prior to more formal assessment (see below). Involuntary movements of the face and/or limbs can give clues regarding long-term neuroleptic therapy or neurodegenerative disorders, particularly Huntington's disease, but these clues may be easily missed

Problem behaviours, particularly those occurring in dementia, are complex, multifaceted disturbances that are difficult to classify. Agitation is a good example. In general psychiatry, the term agitation describes a subjective mood state accompanied by objective evidence of motor restlessness. In dementia, agitation has a much broader meaning, encompassing behaviours as diverse as pacing, shouting, and sleep disturbance (Cohen-Mansfield and Billig 1986). Recent research has attempted to analyse the nature and causes of a number of the commonly encountered problems, including, wandering (Hope and Fairburn 1990), aggression (Patel and Hope 1993), eating changes (Morris *et al.* 1989), and disruptive vocalizations (Cohen-Mansfield and Werner 1997). However, it is probably best in our current state of knowledge simply to describe these abnormal behaviours objectively in their situational context.

Mood

Depression is common in the elderly, but it must be remembered that the vast majority of old people are not depressed, and it is not the norm for old people to be miserable. There is no typical presentation of depression in the elderly and there are many similarities with depression in younger adults, but perhaps there is a wider variety of presentations. Depression is easy to miss, particularly where an overt complaint of depressed mood is absent or denied. Particular problems may arise with somatic presentations and disproportionate complaints in the setting of physical illness. Similarly, marked cognitive dysfunction may be the most conspicuous feature of depression, sometimes leading to an erroneous diagnosis of dementia. The most common reason for missing depression in elderly people is simply a failure to consider it as a possible explanation for a variety of behavioural, cognitive, or emotional changes (see Chapter 27).

A negative answer to a screening question asking whether an elderly person feels sad, depressed, or miserable does not exclude depressed mood. Many older people have a tendency to minimize their feelings of sadness (Geogortas 1983) and a more detailed examination is recommended. Patients should always be asked about their usual activities, with the aim of ascertaining whether there has been any significant diminution in interest or enjoyment (anhedonia). Probably the next most productive line of enquiry is to attempt to clarify the patient's thoughts about themselves, their situation, and future prospects. Feelings of guilt, worthlessness, helplessness, and hopelessness may reflect Beck's negative cognitive triad (Beck 1967). It is also important to ask about biological symptoms such as sleep and appetite disturbance, however their significance may be difficult to interpret in the setting of physical illness. Screening questionnaires, such as the Geriatric Depression Scale (GDS) (Yesavage *et al.* 1983), have been designed specifically for the elderly, focusing on the cognitive aspects of depression and utilizing a simple 'yes/no' answering format. Many of the questions can easily be incorporated into a clinical interview and the GDS can serve as a guide to the main symptom areas that should be covered during an assessment.

As in younger adults it is vital to ask about suicidal thoughts when assessing depression in an elderly person. Suitable approaches are to enquire whether the patient has ever felt that life was not worth living or if they had ever wished for their life to come to an end. Affirmative answers should then lead on to a more detailed exploration of suicide intent, plans, and definite methods. If an elderly person has deliberately self-harmed it should be treated as an attempt to end life unless there is very good evidence to the contrary. Even if the act was in a medical sense trivial, a detailed assessment of suicidal intent must be made in every case. Old age requires people to face death and, in general, fear of death seems to become less common. Elderly people have to try and come to terms with the meaning of their existence, negotiating the 'integrity versus despair' crisis (Erikson 1965). With successful resolution many old people are content to die when their time comes. Acceptance of death is normal and must be differentiated from depressive despair and a morbid desire to terminate a miserable existence.

In dementia, the patient's ability to describe their mood state is impaired by the cognitive deficits. Language dysfunction may compromise this ability to describe thoughts and feelings and it is unlikely that the patient will be able to recall accurate details of their sleep pattern or activities. In this situation particular care needs to be taken in obtaining a detailed history from an informant. Informants may use the word 'depression' loosely to indicate a number of behavioural changes, particularly lack of interest and paucity of emotional expression. Clarification should always be sought in order to distinguish depression, which is often associated with a degree of apathy, from apathy alone, which is a common symptom in dementia and may produce a behavioural phenocopy of depression. Unlike the depressed patient, the patient with apathy is largely unaware and unconcerned about their failings. Depression must also be distinguished from emotional lability in which episodes of distress and tearfulness suddenly appear, only to resolve just as quickly.

The symptoms of mania in the elderly are similar to those in younger adults (see Chapter 29). Though not uncommon, the illness is perceived as being rare and often the diagnosis is not considered. Occasionally cognitive impairment can be marked, leading to the erroneous diagnosis of dementia or delirium. In distinguishing mania from organic personality change, it can be useful to try and differentiate the truly elated mood from euphoria, which is more of a state of contentment not justified by the circumstances.

Anxiety is a common symptom in the elderly (see Chapter 30). It may occur as a normal emotional reaction to stress such as physical illness, but it can also be the most conspicuous feature of a depressive illness. A careful search should be made for symptoms of depression or organic brain disease where anxiety presents for the first time in later life. Autonomic symptoms of anxiety such as palpitations or diarrhoea may dominate the clinical picture, resulting in referral to physicians. Some patients with disabling anxiety may appear quite relaxed at interview and deny that they have any symptoms. This can occur with phobic anxiety that has become focused on a particular situation, which is now avoided. It is therefore important to ascertain whether the patient can engage in normal daily living activities, such as venturing out alone, without experiencing excessive anxiety.

Talk and thought

In contrast to schizophrenia in younger adults, formal thought disorder is extremely rare in late-onset paranoid disorders (Chapter 32).

Mixed affective states can occur, occasionally producing a phenomenon known as 'slow flight of ideas'. Thinking has essentially the same form as in manic flight of ideas, but the flow is greatly retarded and the content is depressive. This disorder of the flow and form of thought can sometimes be mistaken as evidence of cognitive impairment.

Delusions and hallucinations

Examination of this part of the mental state is essentially the same as in younger adults, but it can prove difficult to clarify the presence of these abnormalities in more advanced dementia. True delusions should be differentiated from persecutory ideas not held with delusional intensity, which are common in dementia. The distinction between confabulation and delusions can sometimes be difficult to make but is of importance (Cummings *et al.* 1987). Visual hallucinations early in the course of dementia may suggest a diagnosis of dementia with Lewy bodies (see Chapter 24iv).

Misidentifications

The 'Capgras' and 'Fregoli' syndromes are well recognized, but three other misidentification phenomena are not infrequently encountered in patients with dementia (Förstl *et al.* 1994).

Patients exhibiting the 'phantom boarder' symptom believe, on the basis of misrecognition, that there are imaginary guests living in the house and may set extra places for dinner. The 'mirror sign' is the misidentification of the patient's own reflection in a mirror, and this may be manifest by the patient talking to their own reflection. An extreme reaction to a television programme may be indicative of the 'TV' sign, with the patient misidentifying television images and plots as real.

Cognitive examination

The following section draws heavily upon experience gained in the Cambridge Memory Disorders Clinic in which over 2000 patients have been evaluated over the past decade (Hodges *et al.* 2000). The Addenbrooke's Cognitive Examination (ACE) was developed to aid diagnosis in the clinic and enable the collection of standardized data. This has been shown to be a sensitive tool for the early diagnosis of

Alzheimer's disease and the differentiation of Alzheimer's disease from frontotemporal dementia (Mathuranath *et al.* 2000) (see the Appendix at the end of this chapter). The ACE incorporates the Mini-Mental State Examination (MMSE) (Folstein *et al.* 1975) and contains subsections that assess orientation, attention, memory, verbal fluency, spoken and written language, and visuospatial function. It requires no specialist training or equipment, and takes approximately 10 minutes to administer.

Although, brief, standardized bedside instruments, such as the MMSE and ACE, are valuable adjuncts to cognitive examination, and provide quantification, they are, however, no substitute for careful and logical evaluation by a clinician (Hodges 1994; Walsh and Darby 1999). When assessing cognition it is important to adhere to certain ground rules and follow a logical sequence, which helps avoid false-positive diagnoses. For example, tests of executive function which utilize analysis of complex verbal material would be beyond the grasp of an aphasic or amnesic patient. Likewise, a patient with an acute delirium may be unable to perform even the most basic memory tasks as a consequence of their attention deficit and ought not to be labelled amnesic.

Language deficits are relatively easy to spot on clinical evaluation, but impairment in visuospatial function is often missed.

Attention

Humans are continuously bombarded with sensory stimuli within and between sensory input modalities; loss of ability to focus and sustain attention (or alternatively: block out irrelevant 'noise') renders the individual incapable of following a specific sensory stimulus (such as a conversation) and vulnerable to random irrelevant environmental stimuli. Disorders of the frontal lobes, basal ganglia, and ascending reticular formation are particularly associated with poor attention. Breakdown in attentional processing is the most prominent deficit in delirium and occurs commonly after a closed head injury, in the middle stages of the Alzheimer's disease, in dementia with Lewy bodies, and vascular dementia (Calderon *et al.* 2001).

Assessment

Orientation depends upon both attentional processes and episodic memory, but is more vulnerable to deficits in attention. Questions of time orientation are more sensitive than those related to place. Testing personal orientation adds little; only profoundly aphasic or hysterical patients are unable to relate their own name. It should be noted that normal orientation does **not** exclude the presence of significant memory impairment: many patients with episodic memory problems (e.g. early Alzheimer's disease) remain well oriented.

Other commonly used tests of attention are serial subtraction (although some normal elderly and poorly educated subjects make errors) or reverse spelling (as in the MMSE and ACE). Another useful bedside test is asking subjects to recite the months of the year in reverse order.

Memory

Memory complaints are extremely common and it is important to apply a theoretically motivated approach to analysing symptoms according to the subcomponent of memory involved. In broad terms, memory subtypes can be considered under the following headings.

Working memory

Working memory refers to the finite amount of information that can be held by the brain 'on-line' (such as reading a phone number then holding it in mind until the number can be dialled, or solving arithmetical problems in the head). In the absence of rehearsal, such items are typically lost after a few seconds. The frontal lobes and closely associated basal ganglia structures are important for working memory. Slips of working memory are often erroneously seen by patients as the harbinger of dementia and thus they are commonly referred to memory clinics: these lapses of attention (such as forgetting why you opened the refrigerator door or went into the study, or immediately forgetting a new telephone number) are common 'normal' everyday symptoms which are increased with anxiety, but they also occur more commonly with advancing age and are a particular feature of depression.

Episodic memory

This refers to memory for events, which are specific in time and place, and unique to each individual. Difficulty with the acquisition of new event-based memories (such as the inability to recall details of a television programme or conversation with a friend despite good attention at the time) is the hallmark of early Alzheimer's disease and other causes of the amnesic syndrome. Lesions which give rise to amnesia involve the limbic system of the brain (especially the hippocampi and their connections). Retrograde memory (established prior to the insult) is typically better than anterograde (established any time after) in amnesic syndromes, and, within retrograde memory, very remote memory is classically better preserved than recent memory.

Semantic memory

Semantic memory refers to the brain's knowledge-store of word and object meanings; it includes facts such as that Paris is the capital of France, canaries are small yellow birds kept as pets, and that Ronald Reagan was a president of the United States. The inferolateral regions of the temporal lobes are particularly critical to supporting semantic knowledge. Loss of memory for words is the usual complaint in patients with semantic dementia (also known as progressive fluent aphasia) and after herpes simplex virus encephalitis. Alzheimer's sufferers show a similar phenomenon, though it is usually overshadowed by their profound episodic memory deficit (Garrard *et al.* 1997). It is important, however, to distinguish between the occasional word-finding lapse, usually for proper nouns which occurs normally (especially in later life), and the relentlessly progressive loss of vocabulary, which occurs in association with left temporal pathology.

Assessment

As mentioned above, orientation is dependent on memory and attentional processes. Working and episodic memory can be assessed using the 'name and address test' in the ACE. In this test, subjects are asked to repeat a simple 7-item name and address on three consecutive occasions (learning trials that ensure encoding) and then, without prior warning, recall is tested after 5 to 10 minutes. Patients with working memory problems show poor immediate repetition, but typically recall what they have learnt after a delay. By contrast, those with amnesia (including early Alzheimer's disease) typically repeat a name and address perfectly after each trial but show very rapid forgetting, and recall little, or nothing, after a delay of a few minutes of a distracting task. The performance of patients with subcortical pathology (Parkinson's disease, progressive supranuclear palsy, vascular dementia) improves with encouragement and a force-choice paradigm ('was it Chelmsford or Colchester?') The 3-item recall from the MMSE is too insensitive to detect anything other than severe amnesia.

Category fluency (the ability to generate exemplars from a given semantic category such as types of animals or kitchen utensils), included in the ACE, is a sensitive measure of semantic memory (see below). Semantic memory impairment also manifests as an inability to name objects and to define the meaning of words. Knowledge of famous people is tested by asking the patient to name the current and last Prime Minister, the leader of the Opposition, and the President of the USA.

Language

Numerous terms are in use to describe aphasic syndromes, though some serve more to confuse than enlighten. The terms 'expressive' and 'receptive' seem particularly to mislead: all aphasic patients have some form of difficulty 'expressing' themselves, and 'receptive' aphasia is often, erroneously, taken to mean that the patient has difficulty with incoming language only but can produce their own language perfectly well. The classic aphasia syndromes are rarely seen in the clinic and do not characterize the language deficits found in the dementias. The most important aspect of language examination is history-taking, during which the examiner should be analysing the patient's speech and language. Significant aphasia (except difficulty naming) should be readily apparent after a 5-minute conversation. In all cases, naming must be tested and patients should be asked to write a sentence; but in a busy clinic, comprehension, repetition, and examination of reading can fairly safely be omitted.

In Alzheimer's disease, impaired naming with intact conversational fluency and word comprehension (sometimes called anomic aphasia) is typically seen, and as the disease progresses comprehension and writing become impaired. Repetition and single-word reading are preserved until very late. Patients with vascular pathology show a wide range of deficits but are typically anomic. Two forms of progressive aphasia occur: non-fluent progressive aphasia, which resembles Broca's aphasia, and progressive fluent aphasia, more often referred to as semantic dementia, in which profound anomia is accompanied by impaired single-word comprehension, preserved repetition, and surface dyslexia (Hodges *et al.* 1996).

Assessment

Analysis of conversational speech is all-important with special attention to fluency, the presence of paraphasic errors, and word-finding difficulty. Speech is fluent if the patient is able to produce some well-formed sentences or phrases even if empty or anomic (e.g. 'Oh you know, the thing you put the stuff in when you're going somewhere and'). Non-fluent language, in contrast, is a consequence of a breakdown of the language production and syntactic (grammatical) aspects of language and is the hallmark of damage to Broca's area, producing laboured or 'telegraphic' speech (e.g. 'I...go...hospital'). Paraphasic errors are substitutions of a correct word for one related in sound or meaning. The former, known as phonological paraphasias, involve the substitution of related sound fragments such as 'dobble' for 'bottle'. Semantic paraphasic errors involve the substitution of words of related meaning (e.g. 'dog' for 'fox') or else of a superordinate category (e.g. 'animal' for 'fox'). In more extreme circumstances, paraphasic substitutions may not be words at all ('neologisms'). Semantic errors and word-finding pauses are very common in Alzheimer's disease and semantic dementia.

Naming

Naming is a complex task that requires the integrity of three basic processes—visuoperceptual analysis, semantic knowledge, and word access—and is, therefore, vulnerable to a wide range of pathologies. Naming should always be tested using a range of items of low frequency (not just 'pen' and 'book'). The ACE contains 12 line drawings (crown, helicopter, giraffe, camel, etc.). The type of naming error produced varies according to the locus of damage. Patients with visuoperceptive deficits produce visual errors (a 'head' for a 'mushroom', etc.), retain tactile naming, and can give correct responses when asked to put a name to a description ('What do we call the large grey African animal with a trunk?'). A breakdown in the central semantic process causes impairment in naming from all modalities and patients produce semantic errors ('dog' for 'pig'), while phonological deficits produce phonological errors regardless of the mode of input.

Comprehension

If a language disorder is suspected, comprehension should be tested starting with simple commands (such as 'point to the window, desk', etc.) and progressing to more complex two- and three-usage commands. Impaired single-word comprehension denotes pathology in the left temporal lobe, but patients with damage to more anterior structures, and those with delirium, may fail on more complex sentences.

Repetition

Lesions involving peri-Sylvian language structures are almost always associated with impaired repetition, although this may not be apparent unless multisyllabic words ('caterpillar', 'fundamental', etc.) and phrases ('no ifs ands or buts') are tested.

Reading and writing

Aphasic patients show dyslexic difficulties in keeping with their type of aphasia, thus fluent aphasics will struggle to understand the meaning of words in printed form, while non-fluent aphasics have trouble reading text. Patients with semantic deficits often show a dissociation between a retained ability to read orthographically regular (pronounced as they are spelt) words (such as mint, flint, hint, etc.) and an inability to read correctly irregular words (such as pint, cellist, island, etc.) known as surface dyslexia. Writing is a more complex ability, which draws upon central (linguistic) and more peripheral (praxic) processes and breaks down early in the dementias.

Visuospatial and perceptual disorders

Visuospatial deficits are easily overlooked unless patients are specifically examined. Therefore no cognitive evaluation is complete without asking the asking the patient to copy at least one line drawing. The ACE contains the overlapping pentagons from the MMSE, a wire cube, and the clock-drawing test.

Constructional apraxia, an inability to draw or copy line drawings is a common finding in parietal pathology, particularly with right-sided lesions. In the context of the dementias, marked deficits in visuospatial function suggest dementia with Lewy bodies (Calderon *et al.* 2001). More severe breakdown in spatial cognition causing individuals to misreach for visually guided targets, to trip on steps, or collide with furniture when walking is seen with bilateral parietal diseases and results clinically in Balint's syndrome; the features of which are simultanagnosia, optic ataxia, and ocular apraxia. Simultanagnosia is the inability to integrate and make sense of an overall visual scene in spite of preservation in the ability to identify individual elements. Ocular apraxia describes the inability to direct one's gaze to a novel visual stimulus, while optic ataxia is the inability accurately to reach for a visually guided target.

Spatial neglect is a cross-modality disorder that typically involves the neglect of all sensory information (visual, tactile, auditory) from the side contralateral to the lesion, and virtually only occurs in the context of right parietal lobe damage.

Visual neglect may be detected on clock-drawing in the ACE with omission of features to the left, but is best tested by cancellation (crossing off 'A's on a sheet of paper containing randomly arranged letters), or line-bisection tasks. Patients with severe visual neglect may even appear to be hemianopic. A milder form of neglect can be elicited by 'sensory extinction' of the neglected side during bilateral sensory stimulation.

A restricted form of impaired object recognition relates to faces. Known as prosopagnosia, the subject can no longer recognize previously familiar faces but can recognize their voices and have access to knowledge from their names. Usually bilateral (occasionally right) lesions of the inferior occipitotemporal junction are responsible.

Executive-frontal dysfunction

The term 'executive' refers to aspects of higher order brain function, such as problem-solving, reasoning, goal-setting, planning, and mental abstraction which rely upon the dorsolateral prefrontal lobes. Various methods are available to measure these phenomena though no single test offers foolproof sensitivity, so one should apply as many as possible if the index of suspicion is high.

Assessment

Letter and category-based verbal fluency are the simplest bedside tests and provide much useful information. In letter fluency, the patient is asked to generate as many words as they can think of beginning with a given letter in 1 minute. They are instructed not to use proper nouns and not just to change the endings to create new exemplars ('plant, planted, planting, etc.'). In category fluency, patients are asked to produce as many exemplars as possible from a given category in 1 minute. The ACE contains fluency for 'p' words and animals. Normal subjects usually generate 15 or more words on animal fluency and do slightly worse on the 'p' words. Patients with frontal executive deficits and basal ganglia pathology show an exaggeration of this relationship, doing poorly on category fluency and even worse on letter fluency. Patients with semantic impairments related to temporal lobe diseases, such as semantic dementia and Alzheimer's disease, typically show the reverse pattern of relatively worse performance on category fluency.

Failure to abstract meaning from proverbs ('What does, too many cooks spoil the broth mean?') is a valuable indicator, but is strongly influenced by background intellectual ability. The so-called 'cognitive estimates' test is also useful ('What is the population of Cambridge?, or 'What is the height of the Post-office Tower in London?', or 'How fast does a racehorse gallop?'), as are 'differences and similarities' ('What's the difference between a child and a dwarf?' or 'In what way are a sculpture and a piece of music similar?') (see Hodges 1994).

Orbitofrontal syndrome

The striking changes in personality and social interaction seen in patients with prefrontal lesions relate particularly to orbital (or ventral) surface damage. Though devastating in their effects on social function, such lesions are notoriously difficult to detect using neuropsychological tests. Patients lack empathy and emotional warmth: for instance, if confronted with something as serious as the hospitalization of their spouse, their primary concern may be that their mealtime routine will be disturbed. They are disinhibited and oblivious to social mores: for instance, they may be overly familiar with strangers, disregard personal space, and make inappropriate comments (often of a sexual nature) or gestures. They often make rash and irresponsible decisions such as spending money above their means. Stereotyped and ritualistic behaviours, such as insisting on always taking a particular route when shopping or repetitively closing doors in the home, are common. A useful clue is often the presence of a change in eating behaviour. Patients may become fixated on one dish; often they develop a preference for sweet foods. A lack of normal satiety means that they may overeat, often with secondary weight gain (Bozeat *et al.* 2000).

Imitation and utilization behaviour are dramatic but rare phenomena related to orbital frontal lobe damage. The patient with imitation behaviour unconsciously mimics the examiner's posture and mannerisms, regardless of how absurd they are: raising an arm in the air, placing a leg on the desk, sitting on the floor, etc. Utilization behaviour is even more striking still: the patient will use any object placed in their grasp. The classic example is the patient offered multiple pairs of spectacles who attempts to wear them all, one on top of another.

Apraxia

Motor apraxia is defined as a loss of ability to carry out skilled motor tasks that cannot be explained in terms of an elementary disorder of motor control (weakness or ataxia), primary sensory disturbance, or a global impairment of cognition. Tests of apraxia are not included in the ACE, but should be included in patients with suspected basal ganglia, frontal or parietal lobe pathology.

Ideomotor (production) apraxia

This refers to the inability to execute the motor programme for a given task (e.g. miming the use of scissors, hammer) despite adequate comprehension when done by someone else. Patients with ideomotor apraxia also have problems performing meaningless (non-symbolic) gestures. It is associated with left parietal lobe pathology.

Ideational (conceptual) apraxia

In contrast, this is a loss of knowledge of actions: there is an inability either to perform or recognize a given motor task. There is also inability to match tools correctly to these actions, thus a subject may select a screwdriver to hammer a nail. Patients with temporal lobe disease and the dementias show this form of apraxia.

Buccofacial apraxia

Buccofacial apraxia represents a specific form of apraxia, in which patients are unable to perform tasks such as licking their lips or blowing out matches to command. It is particularly associated with non-fluent aphasia, presumably as the motor programming of articulation and non-linguistic buccofacial movements share a common pathway.

Insight and judgement

The patient's understanding of their illness, its impact on function, and the perceived need for treatment should be assessed by checking what the patient thinks is wrong with them and what should be done about it. This should be interpreted in light of the wider picture derived from information obtained during the interview. Judgement is essentially the ability to act appropriately in a given situation where several options are available. It is sometimes assessed by asking about hypothetical situations, but it is probably best evaluated by assessing the patient's ability to deal effectively with everyday problems. A number of instruments have been developed for the evaluation of insight with parallel patient and carer questionnaires (Markova and Berrios 2000).

Physical examination

Psychiatric disorder in the elderly is often precipitated or complicated by physical illness (see Chapter 10). A psychiatric assessment lacking a physical examination is incomplete. A brief selective examination can be conducted in the patient's home and the psychiatrist should carry a basic selection of tools including a stethoscope and a sphygmomanometer. A more thorough assessment can usually be arranged if necessary via the outpatient clinic, but this can sometimes be difficult to facilitate because of the patient's mental state. Medical emergencies can masquerade as psychiatric disorder in the form of delirium and prompt action on the part of the psychiatrist can occasionally be life-saving.

Conclusions

This chapter has presented a practical overview of psychiatric and clinical cognitive assessment in the older person from the psychiatrist's perspective. Assessment should result in a plausible diagnostic formulation, which in turn leads to a practical management plan. It must be stressed, however, that assessment is an ongoing process and truly comprehensive assessments are best achieved systematically by utilizing the skills of a multidisciplinary team.

Appendix

ADDENBROOKE'S COGNITIVE EXAMINATION (ACE)

ADDENBROOKE'S / NORFOLK & NORWICH DEPARTMENTS OF NEUROLOGY

Name :

Date of birth :

Hospital no. :

Addressograph

Age at leaving education : _____
(school/college etc.)

Date of testing : __/__/__

Tester's name : ____________

ORIENTATION

a) What is the Year ______
Season ______
Date ±2 ______
Record errors. Day ______
Month ______

[*Score* 0 - 5]

b) Where are we Country ______
County ______
Town ______
Record errors. Hospital/building ______
Floor *Allow if almost correct.* ______

[*Score* 0 - 5]

REGISTRATION

Name three unrelated objects, taking one second to say each: eg. **lemon, key & ball**. Say them once only and ask the patient to repeat all three. *Give one point for each correct answer at first attempt. If score<3 repeat the items until the patient learns all 3.* [0 - 3]

ATTENTION/CONCENTRATION

Ask the patient to **begin with 100 and subtract 7, and keep subtracting 7**.
Stop after five subtractions (93, 86, 79, 72, 65). *Score the total number of correct subtractions.*
If score<5: Spell **WORLD backwards**. *Score is the number of letters in the correct order, eg dlorw = 4.*
Take score of better of the two tasks. Record errors: ______________ [0 - 5]

RECALL Ask for the names of the 3 objects learned in question 3. *One point for each answer.* [0 - 3]

MEMORY

a) **Anterograde Memory**:
Read the name and address and ask the patient to repeat it once you have finished. Regardless of the score after the first trial, repeat the task twice in exactly the same way. *Record errors at each trial.*

	1st trial	2nd	3rd	5 min delay
Peter Marshall	__ __	__ __	__ __	__ __
42 Market Street	__ __ __	__ __ __	__ __ __	__ __ __
Chelmsford	__	__	__	__
Essex	__	__	__	__
	/7	/7	/7	/7

Trial 1-3 [0 - 21]
5 min delay [0 - 7]

b) **Retrograde Memory:**

Record errors.

Name of PM ________
Last PM ________
Opposition Leader ________
USA President ________ [0 - 4]

VERBAL FLUENCY

a) **Letters** Ask the patient to generate as many words as possible beginning with the letter **P** in one minute; proper nouns (people and places etc) are not allowed.

b) **Animals** In the same way ask the patient to generate the names of as many **animals** as possible in one minute, beginning with **any letter of the alphabet**.

Record all responses. Error types: perseverations and intrusions.

P
(start here) *(continue)*

Animals
(start here) *(continue)*

Animal	P	Score
>21	>17	7
17-21	14-17	6
14-16	11-13	5
11-13	8-10	4
9-10	6-7	3
7-8	4-5	2
<7	<4	1

P : Total ______ No. correct ______ [0 - 7]
Animals : Total ______ No. correct ______ [0 - 7]

LANGUAGE

a) **Spontaneous speech**
Describe only
Do NOT score

- fluency (phrases>5 words)
- paraphasic errors (phonemic or semantic)
- word finding difficulties

b) **Naming** Ask the patient to name the following pictures.
Record errors.

[0 -2]

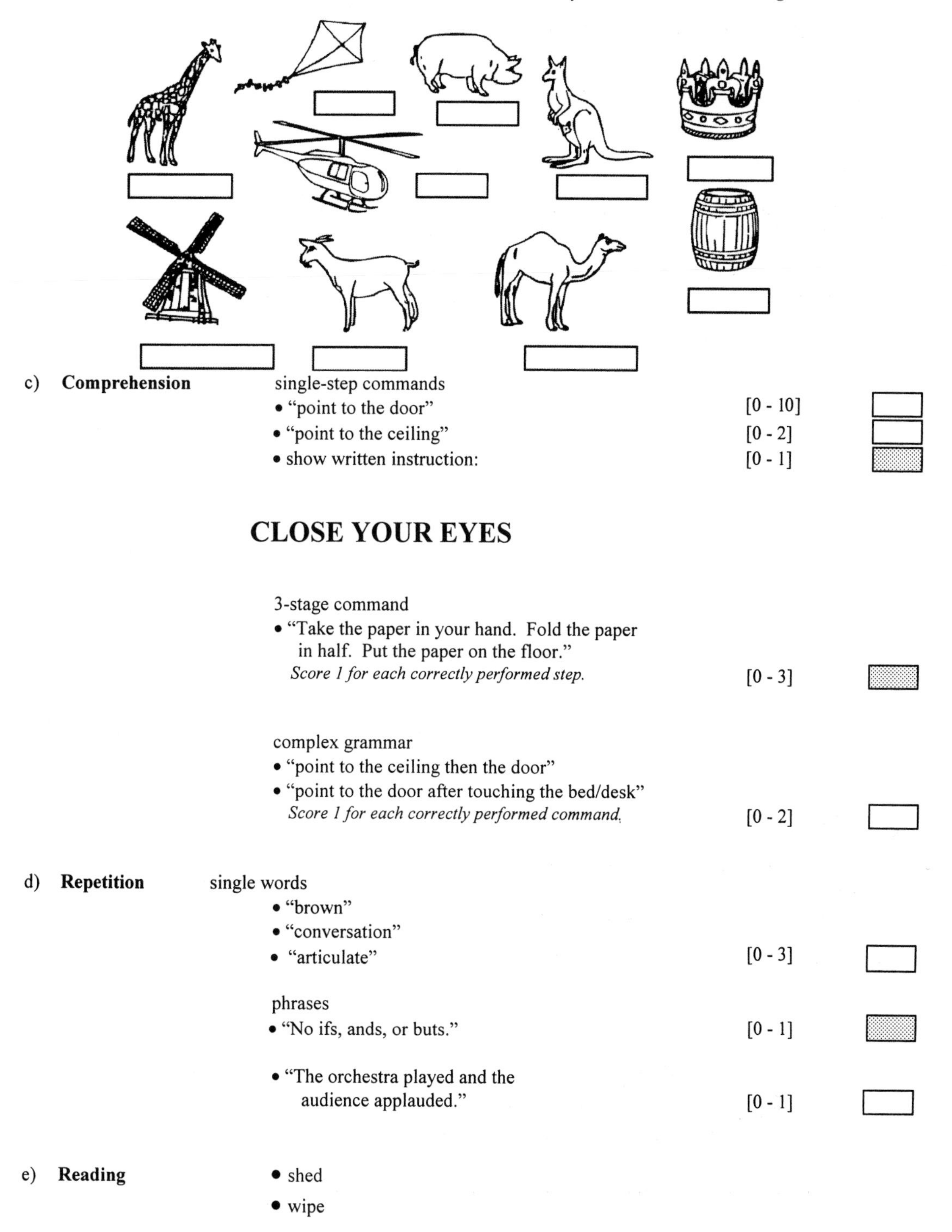

c) **Comprehension**

single-step commands

- "point to the door" [0 - 10]
- "point to the ceiling" [0 - 2]
- show written instruction: [0 - 1]

CLOSE YOUR EYES

3-stage command

- "Take the paper in your hand. Fold the paper in half. Put the paper on the floor."
  Score 1 for each correctly performed step. [0 - 3]

complex grammar

- "point to the ceiling then the door"
- "point to the door after touching the bed/desk"
  Score 1 for each correctly performed command. [0 - 2]

d) **Repetition**

single words

- "brown"
- "conversation"
- "articulate" [0 - 3]

phrases

- "No ifs, ands, or buts." [0 - 1]
- "The orchestra played and the audience applauded." [0 - 1]

e) **Reading**

- shed
- wipe

- board
- flame
- bridge *Score 1 if all regular words correct.* [0 - 1]

- sew
- pint
- soot
- dough
- height *Score 1 if all irregular words correct.* [0 - 1]

f) **Writing**

Ask the patient to **make up a sentence and write it down** in the space below.
If stuck, suggest a topic eg. weather, journey to hospital.
Score 1 for a correct subject and verb in a meaningful sentence.

____ [0 - 1]

NOW CHECK delayed recall of name and address. Record errors on page 1 and enter result into box.

VISUOSPATIAL ABILITIES

a) **Overlapping pentagons** Ask the patient to copy this diagram:

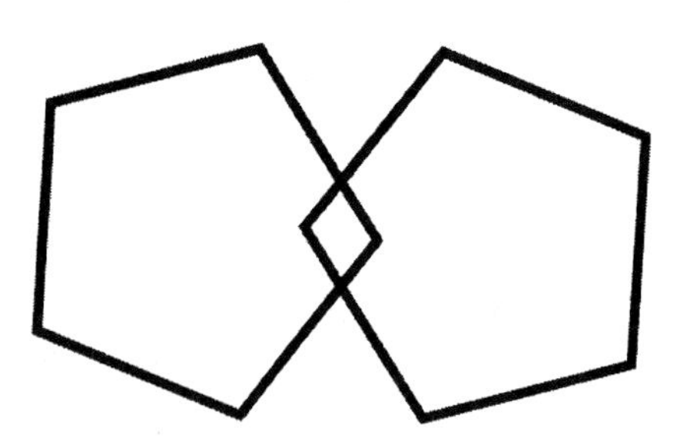

Score 1 if both figures have 5 sides and overlap. [0 - 1]

b) **Wire cube** Ask the patient to copy this drawing:

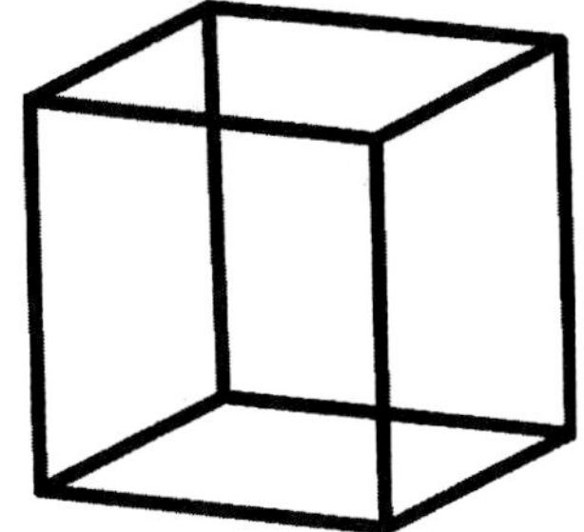

Score 1 if correct. [0 - 1] ☐

c) **Clock** Ask the patient to draw a clockface with numbers and the hands at ten past five.

Score 1 each for correct circle, numbers and hands. [0 - 3] ☐

CHECK: Have you tested and recorded the delayed recall of name and address (page 1)?

OVERALL SCORES **MMSE:** **/30** **TOTAL:** **/100**

MDP/Version 2/1999

Cut-off <88, sensitivity 0.93, specificity 0.71; cut-off <83, sensitivity 0.82, specificity 0.96 for diagnosis of dementia. Normative values based on 127 controls aged 50–80.

References

Adshead, F., Day Cody, D., and Pitt, B. (1992). BASDEC: a novel screening instrument for depression in elderly medical inpatients. *British Medical Journal*, **305**, 397.

Beck, A. T. (1967). *Depression: clinical, experimental and theoretical aspects*. Hoeber, New York.

Bozeat, S., Gregory, C. A., Lambon Ralph, M. A., and Hodges, J. R. (2000). Which neuropsychiatric and behavioural features distinguish frontal and temporal variants of frontotemporal dementia from Alzheimer's disease? *Journal of Neurology, Neurosurgery and Psychiatry*, **69**, 178–86.

Calderon, J., Perry, R., Erzinclioglu, S., Berrios, G. E., Dening, T., and Hodges, J. R. (2001) Perception, attention and working memory are disproportionately impaired in dementia with Lewy Body (LBD) compared to Alzheimer's disease (AD). *Journal of Neurology, Neurosurgery and Psychiatry*, **70**, 157–64.

Capildeo, R., Court, C., and Rose, F. C. (1976). Social network diagram. *British Medical Journal*, **1**, 143–4.

Cm 849 (1989). *Caring for people: community care in the next decade and beyond*. HMSOA, London.

Cohen-Mansfield, J. and Billig, N. (1986). Agitated behaviours in the elderly. 1. A conceptual review. *Journal of the American Geriatrics Society*, **34**, 711–21.

Cohen-Mansfield, J. and Werner, P. (1997). Typology of disruptive vocalisations in older persons suffering from dementia. *International Journal of Geriatric Psychiatry*, **12**, 1079–91.

Coles, R. J., von Abendorff, R., and Herzberg, J. L. (1991). The impact of a new community mental health team on an inner city psychogeriatric service. *International Journal of Geriatric Psychiatry*, **6**, 31–9.

Collighan, G., MacDonald, A., Herzberg, J., Philpot, M., and Lindesay, J. (1993). An evaluation of the multidisciplinary approach to diagnosis in older people. *British Medical Journal*, **306**, 821–4.

Cummings, J. L., Miller, B., Hill, M. A., and Neshkes, R. (1987). Neuropsychiatric aspects of multi-infarct dementia and dementia of the Alzheimer type. *Archives of Neurology*, **44**, 389–93.

Cummings, J. L., Mega, M., Gray, K., Rosenberg-Thompson, S., Carusi, D. A., and Gornbein, J. (1994). The Neuropsychiatric Inventory: comprehensive assessment of psychopathology in dementia. *Neurology*, **44**, 2308–14.

Department of Health (1996). *Carers (Recognition and Services) Act 1995. LAC(96)7, HSG(96)8*. Department of Health, London.

Erikson, E. H. (1965). *Childhood and society*. Norton, New York.

Folstein, M. F., Folstein, S. E., and McHugh, P. R. (1975). 'Mini-mental state'. A practical method for grading the mental state of patients for the clinician. *Journal of Psychiatric Research*, **12**, 189–98.

Förstl, H., Besthorn, C., Burns, A., Geiger-Kabisch, C., Levy, R., and Sattel, A. (1994). Delusional misidentification in Alzheimer's disease: a summary of clinical and biological aspects. *Psychopathology*, **27**, 194–9.

Garrard, P., Perry, R., and Hodges, J. R. (1997). Disorders of semantic memory. *Journal of Neurology, Neurosurgery and Psychiatry*, **62**, 431–5.

Georgotas, A. (1983). Affective disorders in the elderly: diagnostic and research considerations. *Age and Ageing*, **12**, 1–10.

Goldstein, K. (1942). *After effects of brain injuries during war*. Grune and Stratton, New York.

Hodges J. R. (1994). *Cognitive assessment for clinicians*. Oxford University Press, Oxford.

Hodges, J. R., Patterson, K. E., Graham, N., and Dawson, K. (1996). Naming and knowing in dementia of Alzheimer's type. *Brain and Language*, **54**, 302–25.

Hodges, J. R., Berrios, G. E., and Breen, K. (2000). The multidisciplinary memory clinic approach. In *Memory disorders in psychiatric practice* (ed. G. E. Berrios, and J. R. Hodges), pp. 101–21. Cambridge University Press, Cambridge.

Hodkinson, H. M. (1972). Evaluation of a mental test score for assessment of mental impairment in the elderly. *Age and Ageing*, **1**, 233–8.

Hope, R. A. and Fairburn, C. G. (1990). The nature of wandering in dementia: a community based study. *International Journal of Geriatric Psychiatry*, **5**, 239–45.

Jarvik, L. F. and Wiseman, E. J. (1991). A checklist for managing the dementia patient. *Geriatrics*, **46**, 31–40.

Jolley, D. J. and Arie, T. (1992). Developments in psychogeriatric services. In *Recent advances in psychogeriatrics* (ed. T. Arie), p. 126. Churchill Livingstone, Edinburgh.

Leff, J. P. and Isaacs, A. D. (1981). *Psychiatric examination in clinical practice* (2nd edn). Blackwell, Oxford.

Lindesay, J. (1991). Phobic disorders in the elderly. *British Journal of Psychiatry*, **159**, 531–41.

Markova, I. S. and Berrios, G. E. (2000). Insight into memory deficits. In *Memory disorders in psychiatric practice* (ed. G. E. Berrios and J. R. Hodges), pp. 204–34. Cambridge University Press, Cambridge.

Mathuranath, P. S., Nestor, P., Berrios, G. E., Rakowicz, W., and Hodges, J. R. (2000). A brief cognitive test battery to differentiate Alzheimer's disease and frontotemporal dementia. *Neurology*, **55**, 1613–20.

Meachem, J. A. and Singer, J. (1977). Incentive effects in prospective memory. *Journal of Psychology*, **97**, 191–7.

Morris, C. H., Hope, R. A., and Fairburn, C. G. (1989). Eating habits in dementia: a descriptive study. *British Journal of Psychiatry*, **154**, 801–6.

Orrell, M. and Katona, K. (1998). Do consultant home visits have a future in old age psychiatry? *International Journal of Geriatric Psychiatry*, **13**, 355–7.

Patel, V. and Hope, T. (1993). Aggressive behaviour in elderly people with dementia: a review. *International Journal of Geriatric Psychiatry*, **8**, 457–72.

Pattie, A. and Gilleard, C. J. (1979). *Manual of the Clifton Assessment Procedures for the Elderly (CAPE)*. Hodder and Stoughton, Sevenoaks, Kent.

Pullen, I. M. and Yellowlees, A. J. (1985). Is communication improving between general practitioners and psychiatrists? *British Medical Journal*, **290**, 31–3.

Rathbone-McCuan, E. and Voyles, B. (1982). Case detection of elderly abused parents. *American Journal of Psychiatry*, **139**, 189–92.

Rutter, M. and Cox, A. (1981). Psychiatric interviewing techniques: 1. Methods and measures. *British Journal of Psychiatry*, **138**, 273–82.

Shah, A. (1997). Cost comparison of outpatient and home-based geriatric psychiatry consultations in one service. *Aging and Mental Health*, **1**, 372–6.

Shah, A. and Ames, D. (1994). Planning and developing psychogeriatric services. *International Review of Psychiatry*, **6**, 15–27.

Simpson, C. J. (1984). Doctors and nurses use of the word 'confused'. *British Journal of Psychiatry*, **145**, 441–3.

Tullet, D. C., Orrell, M. W., Kalkat, G. S., and Katona, C. L. E. (1997). Domiciliary visits in old age psychiatry: Expectation and practice. *Primary Care Psychiatry*, **3**, 195–8.

Walker, M. P., Ayre, G. A., Cummings, J. L., Wesnes, K., McKeith, I. G., O'Brien, J. T., and Ballard, C. G. (2000). The clinician assessment of fluctuation and the one day fluctuation assessment scale: two methods to assess fluctuating confusion in dementia. *British Journal of Psychiatry*, **177**, 252–6.

Walsh, K. and Darby, D. (1999). *Neuropsychology. A clinical approach* (4th edn). Churchill Livingstone, Edinburgh.

Woods, R. T. (1995). Psychological treatments. 1: Behavioural and cognitive approaches. In *Neurotic disorders in the elderly* (ed. J. Lindesay), p. 11. Oxford University Press, Oxford.

Wright, N. and Lindesay, J. (1995). A survey of memory clinics in the British Isles. *International Journal of Geriatric Psychiatry*, **10**, 379–85.

Yesavage, J. A., Brink, T. L. Rose, T. L., and Lum, O. (1983). Development and validation of a geriatric depression screening scale: a preliminary report. *Journal of Psychiatric Research*, **17**, 37–49.

10 Physical assessment of older patients

Simon Winner

Introduction

In the course of comprehensive assessment of a patient who presents with psychological problems, the old age psychiatrist will wish to carry out a brief examination to detect any physical disease that might be contributing to the clinical picture. This apparently simple aim is complicated by aspects of illness in old people that can obscure the diagnosis, such as the frequent occurrence of non-specific presentations and the presence of multiple pathology. Defining a problem often requires a breadth of experience in general medicine, specific knowledge of disease in old age, and skills in setting priorities for investigations. A brief account cannot encompass all the craft and science of geriatric medicine. Instead, this chapter aims to help the old age psychiatrist to recognize those patients who might especially benefit from referral onwards to a geriatrician or other physician (internist), or back to their general practitioner for possible physical disease to be elucidated.

Some relevant characteristics of illness in old age will be illustrated, the importance of disability assessment will be discussed, and diseases which may present in disguised form to old age psychiatrists (and others) will be reviewed. The emphasis will be on common conditions and on ways that salient clinical features, including physical signs, can be picked up by the non-specialist. Reference will also be made to less common disorders that the geriatrician keeps in mind when seeing referrals. Some relevant conditions are discussed in other chapters of this book (for example, Chapter 25), while some physical signs mentioned in other chapters are described in detail here.

A successful approach to health care for old people must take the characteristic features of disease in old age into account (Evans 1981). Lack of physiological reserve means that ill old people may deteriorate rapidly if untreated, and there is a high incidence of secondary complications. Referral should therefore be made without delay, and allowance must be made for a prolonged recovery phase. In geriatric medicine, as in old age psychiatry, assessment must give due consideration to the patient's social context, housing, and income, and treatment must be augmented to include the provision of appropriate community support. Key features of disease in old age that make diagnosis more difficult include non-specific presentations, atypical manifestations, and the prevalence of multiple pathology.

Non-specific presentations of disease

Disease in old people frequently presents non-specifically and typical diagnostic features are obscured, so the physician assessing a common clinical problem must be able to recognize, in concealed form, a variety of possible causes across the spectrum of clinical medicine. Fortunately, although diagnostic features may not be obvious, they are seldom completely absent and can, in most cases, be revealed by the application of simple clinical method: taking a good history (from the patient and relatives, neighbours, and others), and carrying out a thorough physical examination, supplemented when appropriate by simple laboratory tests and radiographs. Acute confusion (delirium) is the most important example in the present context, and merits a whole chapter on its own (see Chapter 25). Much of the clinical approach described for delirium can be applied more generally, since most of the diseases listed as causes of confusion can alternatively bring about the other non-specific presentations of disease in old people that are commonly encountered, such as immobility ('off her feet'), instability (falling over), incontinence, or a general increase in dependency (see Disability below). In patients with an established psychiatric disorder, the first non-specific indication of a physical illness may be acute worsening of their mental symptoms such as agitation, confusion, or depression.

Atypical manifestations of disease

Painless myocardial infarction and 'covert' acute infection are common examples of atypical manifestations of disease in elderly patients. Truly silent myocardial infarction, that is coronary occlusion with no symptoms at all, is seen in prospective studies of young and old. Painless myocardial infarcts are commoner with increasing age (Muller *et al.* 1990) and there are persuasive explanations related to age-associated changes in autonomic function. However, many of these are not truly silent: there has often been an identifiable clinical event which may be frankly cardiac, such as left ventricular failure, or something less specific. When the assessor recognizes the significance of a relatively sudden change in general health or exercise capacity in the history, findings on examination and electrocardiography may substantiate a retrospective diagnosis of myocardial infarction as the cause. Atypical presentations have sometimes been overemphasized, and used to justify 'blind' treatments and a negative attitude to clinical assessment. Contrary to popular myth, infections in old people do not usually occur without pyrexia or other characteristic physical signs (Berman *et al.* 1987). Confusion or immobility may be the presenting symptoms, rather than specific complaints such as productive cough or dysuria, but clues as to the cause are usually present for the careful observer to find. Normal oral temperatures may be misleading, and rectal or auditory canal temperatures are more reliable (Darowski *et al.* 1991). While it is often appropriate to treat early for the possibility of infection in old people, there are few occasions when simple clinical assessment fails to provide useful confirmatory information.

Multiple pathology and multiple aetiology

The common occurrence of multiple pathology means that assessment will often reveal several disease processes in an elderly patient, and an important diagnosis may be missed among conditions irrelevant to the presenting complaint. Conversely, a single symptom may have several contributing causes, the phenomenon of multiple aetiology. Both require the assessor to keep a cool head while collecting clinical evidence. The search should not cease when a single possible cause has been found. On the other hand, patients may be harmed, more than helped, if every possible line of enquiry is investigated 'to the hilt'. Skills in setting priorities must be combined with the judicious use of accurate diagnostic techniques. Multiple aetiology contributes a layer of complexity and possible inaccuracy to the diagnostic process (Fairweather and Campbell 1991), but may also be a key to therapeutic success in geriatric medicine. In a patient who has ceased to walk, for example, several causes may be found, each making a small contribution to the problem and each giving limited scope for therapeutic intervention. The effects of several individually unimpressive interventions may aggregate to produce a major change in the patient's condition: thus, analgesics for chronic arthralgia of the hip, quadriceps exercises to help stabilize an osteoarthritic knee, withdrawing diuretics to reduce postural hypotension, and recognizing and treating mild parkinsonism can summate and lead the patient to walk again.

Disability assessment

Geriatricians supplement a traditional history and examination by assessing disability, which can usefully be defined in terms of the WHO classification of impairment, disability, and handicap (World Health Organization 1980). This classification has recently been revised, and alternative, less technical terms have been recommended ('disability' has become 'activity', and 'handicap' has become 'participation'), but these are not yet in common use (World Health Organization 1999). Disability assessment in clinical practice focuses on independence in basic activities of daily living (ADL): continence, mobility, and simple self-care activities such as washing, dressing, eating, and going to the lavatory. More complex activities such as shopping, cooking, doing the laundry, using a telephone, and handling money are sometimes called instrumental activities of daily living (IADL). Disability assessment plays several key roles. In many people, reduced performance in ADL is the first sign of failing health. A change in disability should be viewed in the same light as the onset of confusion, as a pointer to possibly remediable physical illness until proved otherwise. Disability assessment can also be the key to multiple pathology: conditions that are contributing to major or recent-onset disability usually merit priority in investigations and treatment. Its importance in rehabilitation is self-evident, and routine use of an ADL scale in the assessment and monitoring of an acute illness can help to ensure that appropriate rehabilitation goals are considered from an early stage.

Basic ADL can be summarized using a standardized assessment scale, and the Barthel index (Table 10.1) is among the most widely used and best validated (Mahoney and Barthel 1964; Collin *et al.* 1988; Wade and Collin 1988). At its simplest, the Barthel index is useful as a check-list, but summary scores are also a practical clinical tool for following progress and providing an estimate of severity. Reduced scores should always lead to scrutiny of the pattern of disability: different individuals may achieve the same score with quite different sets of problems. The Barthel index is not a substitute for detailed assessments by physiotherapists and occupational therapists, whose reports will include diagnosis of the factors contributing to current disabilities, analysis of the scope and methods for improvement, and assessment of the patient's abilities with household management tasks (IADL). The Barthel index is simply a quick snapshot of basic ADL that can be used by many different people, and has been recommended as part of a common language of assessment to enhance communication between health professionals in different disciplines (Working Group of the Royal College of Physicians and the British Geriatrics Society 1992). Regular use in the practice of old age psychiatry can be advocated. An ADL assessment used in conjunction with an assessment of cognitive function (Chapter 9) encompasses many of the important non-specific presentations of disease.

Physical assessment

The importance of recognizing a change in disability and dependency as a possible manifestation of treatable disease gives rise to the maxim in geriatric medicine that a 'social problem', such as increased demand on carers, should never receive only a 'social solution', for example admission to residential care, without taking the opportunity for a thorough medical assessment. The same principle could be applied to many patients presenting with psychological symptoms, which should not be treated as purely psychiatric illness without the physical assessment that is the subject of this chapter.

Psychiatrists vary in their confidence, training, and experience in general medicine. Some may prefer to skip the last sections of this chapter, which attempt a brief survey of conditions of particular relevance to the physical assessment of elderly psychiatric patients, with notes on physical signs and laboratory investigations. The intention is to highlight important points for the 'occasional' physician rather than give a comprehensive account, and this is especially true of the comments on physical signs. The reader is

Table 10.1 Barthel index of activities of daily living (after Collin *et al.* 1988)

Bowels	0	=	incontinent (or needs to be given enema)
	1	=	occasional accident (once per week or less)
	2	=	continent (for preceding week)
Bladder	0	=	incontinent or catheterized and unable to manage alone
	1	=	occasional accident (once per day or less)
	2	=	continent (for preceding week)
Feeding	0	=	unable
	1	=	needs help cutting, spreading butter, etc.
	2	=	independent
Grooming	0	=	needs help with personal care
	1	=	independent face/hair/teeth/shaving (implements provided)
Dressing	0	=	dependent
	1	=	needs help but can do about half unaided
	2	=	independent (including buttons, zips, laces, etc.)
Transfer: bed to chair and back			
	0	=	unable, no sitting balance
	1	=	major help (one strong/skilled or two people), can sit up
	2	=	minor help from one person (physical or verbal)
	3	=	independent
Toilet use	0	=	dependent
	1	=	needs some help, but can do something alone
	2	=	independent (on and off, dressing, wiping)
Mobility: around house or ward, indoors			
	0	=	immobile
	1	=	wheelchair independent, including corners
	2	=	walks with help of one person (physical or verbal, supervision)
	3	=	independent (but may use any aid, e.g. stick)
Stairs	0	=	unable
	1	=	needs help (physical, verbal, carrying aid)
	2	=	independent
Bathing	0	=	dependent
	1	=	independent (in and out of bath or shower)

Guidelines for the Barthel ADL Index:

1. The index should be used as a record of what a patient does, not what a patient can do.
2. The main aim is to establish the degree of independence from any help, physical or verbal, however minor and for whatever reason.
3. The need for supervision renders the patient not independent.
4. A patient's performance should be established using the best available evidence. Asking the patient, friends/relatives, and nurses are the usual sources, but direct observation and common sense are also important.
   However direct testing is not needed.
5. Usually the patient's performance over the preceding 24–48 hours is important, but occasionally longer periods will be relevant.
6. Middle categories imply that the patient supplies over 50% of the effort.
7. Use of aids to be independent is allowed.

assumed to have access to standard textbooks of general medicine (such as Weatherall *et al.* 1996) and geriatric medicine (Evans *et al.* 2000), and to a manual of clinical examination.

The emphasis is on conditions that commonly cause patients to present to psychiatrists, for example because of odd behaviour or apparent confusion, depression, or anxiety. Some less-common diseases are described that preoccupy geriatricians, usually because diagnosis opens up therapeutic opportunities. All the diseases mentioned can present in easily recognizable form, but here the focus is on disguised, atypical, or non-specific presentations. Conditions are discussed under the following headings:

(1) cardiovascular disease and related disorders;
(2) chest disease;
(3) gastrointestinal disease;
(4) malignant disease;
(5) neurological disease, dwelling on common conditions of special importance to old age psychiatrists, cerebrovascular disease, and parkinsonism, and physical signs often found in demented patients;
(6) endocrine and metabolic conditions;
(7) miscellaneous conditions.

Some overlap with Chapter 25, on delirium, is intended. As the aim is to highlight reasons for referring the patient to a geriatrician or other physician for further management, investigations and treatment are not discussed in detail, except for brief accounts of the management of stroke and Parkinson's disease.

Cardiovascular disease and related disorders

Heart failure

Perhaps surprisingly, this is one of the commonest conditions to elude detection or receive inadequate attention when old people with non-specific malaise are assessed by non-specialists. Treatment can often transform the patient. Although most old people with heart failure present with classic symptoms such as breathlessness, disguised presentations are common and may be mistaken for primary psychological illness. Tiredness and exhaustion may predominate, causing the patient to 'go off her feet', unable to exert herself enough to experience breathlessness. She may find this difficult to explain, exhibiting only apathy. Patients are sometimes sleepy, and others without overt stupor exhibit slowness of thought and action. Avoiding exhausting visits to the kitchen or lavatory may lead to self-neglect and incontinence. Similar symptoms suggestive of depression may occur without frank heart failure as a result of very fast heart rates (such as uncontrolled atrial fibrillation), with very slow rates (for example in heart block), with anaemia, and in hypothyroidism (see below).

Signs relevant to heart failure include the apex rate in atrial fibrillation (AF), which should be assessed by auscultation on the anterior chest wall since weak beats are not always palpable peripherally. AF controlled by drug therapy (digoxin and sometimes beta-blockers) should have an apex rate around 90 beats per minute. Signs of congestive cardiac failure are often misinterpreted. The jugular venous pressure can be difficult to assess, and ankle oedema is common in old people as a result of venous insufficiency in dependent limbs. A rewarding, though neglected, sign of right heart failure for the non-expert is the presence of sacral oedema, which is almost always significant. Heart failure is the commonest cause but fluid overload may be secondary to renal failure, and in a few patients the excess of tissue fluid is attributable to hypoproteinaemia, usually hepatic or renal in origin. All patients in whom sacral oedema is discovered merit further physical assessment; in those who are already known to have heart failure, this sign suggests that optimum control has not been achieved. Crackles audible in the lung bases are so common in old people that their usefulness as a sign of left ventricular failure is reduced. Breathlessness on minor exertion or at night should trigger further assessment, including a chest radiograph. General signs to be sought include clues to infective endocarditis, such as finger clubbing, splinter haemorrhages under fingernails, and retinal haemorrhages.

When heart failure is found, referral is merited so that a range of causes can be considered in the conventional manner. The specialist is always on the lookout for significant disease of the heart valves, which may present insidiously but with substantial rewards for early diagnosis: cardiac surgery can be curative and may be especially effective in old people (Working Group of the Royal College of Physicians 1991) but delay in diagnosis worsens the risks. Aortic stenosis classically causes exertional angina, breathlessness, and syncope, but some old people just feel profound exhaustion. Physical signs such as a slow-rising pulse and mid-systolic murmur are unreliable in distinguishing significant stenosis from aortic sclerosis, when a calcified valve causes turbulence without impeding blood flow (McKillop *et al.* 1991), and the physician will have a low threshold for further investigation with echocardiography. Significant and remediable mitral valve disease can also be underestimated. Referral to a physician is therefore justified for any patient in whom the old age psychiatrist detects a cardiac murmur, not least because neurological and neuropsychological presentations are common in old people with infective endocarditis, mostly due to cerebral embolism (Jones and Siekert 1989). This treatable condition is frequently unrecognized until non-specific manifestations have progressed to overt cardiac disease with irreparably damaged heart valves.

Postural hypotension

This condition should be sought in patients who are becoming immobile. Postural hypotension usually causes dizziness on rising to a standing position, leading to falls or even faints, but in some patients the relationship of light-headedness to postural change is not obvious in the presenting history, and anxiety and loss of confidence predominate. Similar symptoms may occur after meals and on exercise. The blood pressure should be measured after lying supine for 10 minutes and then 2 minutes after standing up. A fall of 20 mmHg or more in systolic pressure is usually regarded as significant. Age-associated decline in postural reflexes usually interacts with a more immediate cause, such as intercurrent infection, which may produce a temporary worsening in postural stability that lasts longer than the acute illness itself. Drugs are very frequently implicated, especially diuretics, hypotensives, antiparkinsonian drugs, and a wide variety of psychotropic medications including antidepressants, hypnotics, sedatives, and tranquillizers of all kinds. Though not always possible in psychiatric patients, stopping the causative drugs offers a simple remedy. An explanation of the phenomenon, with instructions to rise slowly, and to pause for the 'head to clear' before walking off, can alleviate symptoms and restore confidence more reliably than treatment with fluid-retaining drugs such as fludrocortisone.

Iatrogenic cardiovascular disease in old people can also take the form of pathologically slow heart rates, usually attributable to overzealous therapy with beta-blocking drugs or to digoxin toxicity, which may also cause disturbances of colour vision, confusion, anorexia, gastrointestinal upset, and cardiac arrhythmias.

Chest disease

Most chest conditions declare themselves in the clinical history and examination, or on a chest radiograph. Chronic airways disease is so common that its presence may be discounted or its severity underestimated, and mistakes are made when a new clinical development is not recognized as a complication or worsening of the underlying chest disorder. Thus, confusion may be precipitated by giving psychotropic drugs, such as 'mild' hypnotics or opiate analgesics, either via acute worsening of hypoxaemia or by causing carbon dioxide intoxication. The latter may have a subacute onset, with mental changes progressing from mild disorientation through frank delirium to stupor and coma, accompanied by warm peripheries, a bounding pulse, and the same flapping tremor that may occur in hepatic encephalopathy or uraemia ('asterixis'). Referral is appropriate, and the physician's assessment will include blood gas analysis.

Signs of chest infection should always be sought, starting with an examination of the sputum which may be purulent. Tuberculosis occasionally crops up as a cause of slowly progressive malaise in old people that may be mistaken for depression or malignancy, and a chest radiograph can be justified in most patients.

Gastrointestinal disease

Diseases of the gastrointestinal tract often declare themselves through suggestive symptoms, or are revealed by tests for causes of gastrointestinal blood loss, for example when investigating iron-deficiency anaemia. Exceptions that the physician must specifically call to mind when investigating non-specific symptoms include liver disease and alcoholism, malabsorption syndromes (which may cause weight loss in the face of a good appetite), and malignancy.

Psychiatrists will not need reminding to consider the possibility of alcohol abuse whatever the patient's declared consumption (see also Chapter 34). Intoxication can be confirmed by taking a blood sample for alcohol assay (best preserved in a fluoride oxalate/blood sugar bottle). Acute alcohol withdrawal should always be considered as a cause of anxiety, confusion, or odd behaviour, whether or not the patient has a tremor or visual hallucinations. Withdrawal is the prime suspect when a patient has an otherwise unexplained 'funny turn' or fit a couple of days after arriving in hospital, whatever the reason for admission.

Chronic liver disease sometimes progresses covertly and remains undiagnosed until intercurrent illness precipitates life-threatening hepatic encephalopathy, when confusion may progress to stupor and coma. Although most encephalopathic patients are frankly jaundiced, signs of hepatic disease may be missed unless sought, and blood tests of liver function (including prothrombin time) should be carried out in all patients. Between acute episodes of decompensation, even severe cirrhosis may have few or subtle clinical signs and biochemistry may be normal apart from a low serum albumin or a raised gamma-glutamyl transpeptidase. There should be a low threshold for referral for specialist attention. Delirium and stupor are also common in acute pancreatitis; most sufferers are clearly physically ill but the diagnosis may not be obvious until the serum amylase concentration is measured.

Severe constipation is common in old people, and faecal impaction may present non-specifically with profound malaise, or with easily remediable urinary or faecal incontinence (with spurious diarrhoea). Rectal examination should be carried out. A plain abdominal radiograph is occasionally helpful in revealing severe constipation, if the rectal examination is negative.

Malignant disease

Malignancy comes into the differential diagnosis of almost all illnesses, and may cause psychological symptoms through a variety of mechanisms including cerebral secondaries and biochemical upset. Basic clinical assessment of an elderly patient should always include a search for evidence of the commonest tumours and their possible complications. Signs meriting special attention include comparing body weight with any previous records, checking the breasts and axillary lymph nodes, the thyroid and local neck nodes, supraclavicular nodes especially on the left as a marker of intra-abdominal malignancy, any signs in the chest and abdomen including a tender irregular liver, rectal examination (for a mass, positive occult blood in the stool, and palpable prostatic malignancy), testing the spine for bony tenderness suggestive of secondaries, and checking for papilloedema. A chest radiograph may show evidence of primary or secondary tumours. Abdominal imaging by ultrasound or computed tomography (CT) may be merited, looking especially at the liver for secondaries and at the pancreas and kidneys for 'occult' primary tumours. A cranial CT scan seeking secondaries is justified in patients with neurological or psychological symptoms or signs. Blood tests should include: a full blood count and erythrocyte sedimentation rate (ESR); sodium and calcium concentrations (see below); and liver function tests, including alkaline phosphatase, which may be raised before other tests become abnormal due to liver secondaries and which is also a sensitive indicator of bony metastases. Anaemia is common, and the blood film may give clues as to the cause, for example iron deficiency or marrow infiltration.

Myelomatosis is a primary haematological malignancy with varied manifestations, including bone pain, susceptibility to infections, and renal failure. Neuropsychiatric presentations may occur via hypercalcaemia, or, more rarely, impaired cerebral perfusion from hyperviscosity due to very high blood levels of immunoglobulin. Usually the ESR is very high and immunoglobulin assay and electrophoresis contribute to the diagnosis.

Cerebrovascular disease

Cerebrovascular disease is important to the old age psychiatrist: first, when strokes present in disguised form; and, second, as a major cause of dementia. Although most strokes are obvious, covert presentations do occur, and in some patients psychological illness is suspected until neurological features are recognized which change the clinician's approach. Sudden onset of symptoms is highly suggestive of a stroke, and a history should be sought from family members and other observers with this in mind. Psychiatrists are perhaps more reliable than physicians at picking out elements of dysphasia or a visuospatial disorder from apparently confused speech or behaviour.

Dysphasia

Fluent dysphasia is occasionally difficult to recognize. The patient can seem generally confused until the observer considers word-finding difficulties and recognizes, often from irregularities in the tempo of speech, that word-substitution is taking place; perseveration and the use of neologisms are sometimes subtle. The patient usually has accompanying difficulties with understanding (receptive dysphasia), and may not be aware that her speech is difficult to interpret. The ability to name objects is often grossly abnormal, and may be revealed by the simple bedside tests of language described in Chapter 9. Dysphasia commonly results from lesions in the dominant cerebral hemisphere, and accompanying signs, usually in right-sided limbs, should be sought. Occasionally, patients respond with relief to the first person to say: 'We know you're not confused: you know what you want to say but you just can't find the words'.

Visual loss and visuospatial disorders

In addition to testing all apparently confused patients for dysphasia, the experienced geriatrician will routinely test vision, and seek evidence of visuospatial problems. The commonest visual disturbance to arise from stroke is loss of all (or part) of the field of vision to one side in both eyes, an homonymous hemianopia (or quadrantanopia). Patients may be unaware of the defect, especially when hemiparesis is mild or absent, or when there are accompanying problems with visuospatial awareness (see below). They may not be able to explain why they are walking into doorways or driving badly, and family members may object to being ignored when they are sitting in the hemianopic field. The patient's behaviour may be misinterpreted, but the alert physician should have no difficulty in eliciting relevant signs at the bedside, testing the visual fields in the conventional manner by confrontation ('I am going to test what you can see to each side: keep looking at me, and point to my finger when you first see it moving in the corner of your eye').

Visuospatial disorders attributable to cerebral damage after stroke may occur in dominant hemisphere lesions but are generally more pronounced with lesions of the non-dominant (usually right) hemisphere. They take a confusing variety of forms with a broad range of neuroanatomical correlates, often loosely summarized as 'parietal lobe dysfunction'. (For a comprehensive and highly readable account of this topic and the dysphasias see Hodges 1994.) The uncommon extremes described in textbooks serve to illustrate the kinds of problem that the astute observer will recognize frequently in milder form: some patients fail to recognize paralysed limbs (usually on the left) as their own; they may don clothes only on one side of the body (dressing apraxia); they may fail to recognize common objects despite satisfactory eyesight (visual agnosia) or intact perception of touch (astereognosis); some patients are unable to find their way around familiar places, and some cannot copy a simple drawing (constructional apraxia).

These disorders must be distinguished from simpler defects of vision and sensation which do not necessarily imply localization to the cerebral cortex. Approaches to this topic are dogged by imprecise use of language: a patient with an homonymous hemianopia (caused by a lesion anywhere along the postchiasmal visual pathways) may pay less attention to objects in her impaired field simply as a result of the blindness, and a patient with reduced sensation in her limbs will understandably fail to notice some stimuli on that side. This is often described as 'neglect' or 'inattention', but these same terms are used more precisely to describe visuospatial impairments of cortical origin. Severe inattention may cause the patient to ignore all stimuli to one side of the body. Milder degrees may be detected by bedside signs that reflect the importance of excluding hemianopia or simple sensory impairment. To demonstrate visual inattention (or extinction), the visual fields are first assessed by confrontation as above. Provided that the fields are intact when each side is tested separately, the confrontation test is completed by offering a stimulus simultaneously to both sides: if one side is consistently ignored, the patient has visual inattention. Sensory inattention is the equivalent sign using double simultaneous stimulation of light touch on the hands. In patients with demonstrable field defects or sensory impairment, no conclusions about 'parietal lobe function' can be drawn from these signs, but the observations of nurses, therapists, and family members will often draw attention to a defect. Tests involving drawing (for example a clock-face), line bisection, or star cancellation can be helpful (Hodges 1994).

Lesions of the occipital (visual) cortex can give rise to odd visual phenomena, including blindness that is denied, and, rarely, 'blind sight' when blindness is claimed but some vision is apparent from eye-movements that track moving objects which can be grasped with precision. This situation must be distinguished from hysteria and other psychological disorders, and cranial imaging can be helpful.

Signs of stroke and differential diagnosis

A systematic assessment of the physical signs of stroke begins with those discussed above: signs of cortical involvement, such as dysphasia or visuospatial impairment, and signs of a visual-field defect. The examiner should then seek vertebrobasilar signs such as ophthalmoplegia or cerebellar ataxia, and finally hemiparesis (upper motor neuron signs affecting the face, arm, and/or leg on one side of the body) and unilateral sensory impairment. These signs can give a useful bedside classification of the likely site and size of a lesion (Bamford *et al.* 1991). Signs useful for demonstrating mild hemiparesis include pyramidal drift of the outstretched arms (which should be held palm upwards, drifting towards pronation and flexion when the sign is present), and gait, because a spastic leg will tend towards extension and the toes will catch on the floor unless the limb is circumducted. When typical features of stroke and a clear history of sudden onset are absent, a cranial CT scan may help to exclude differential diagnoses such as space-occupying lesions. Here tumours are less important than the rare, but treatable, cerebral abscess, and subdural haematoma—which may follow trivial injury and may take a chronic form with impaired cognition or conscious level accompanying mild hemiparesis.

Multi-infarct disease

Patients with recurrent small strokes may present to the old age psychiatrist with multi-infarct dementia. Clinical features seldom allow certainty in distinguishing this from Alzheimer's disease and other causes of progressive dementia. However, the history of decline may have been punctuated by distinct steps, some of which may be recognizable in retrospect as discrete strokes, for example by questioning the family about accompanying transient immobility or drooping of one side of the face. Hypertension, signs of peripheral vascular disease such as bruits, and focal neurological signs increase the likelihood of cerebrovascular disease as the cause. Widespread disease causes bilateral upper motor neuron lesions in the lower cranial nerves, giving a 'pseudobulbar palsy' with dysarthria, dysphagia, and slow movements of the tongue. Upper motor neuron signs in the limbs on both sides give rise to weakness, stiffness, and clumsiness. Emotional lability and a gait with rapid small steps (*marche à petit pas*) may complete the picture. The gait disturbance in some patients with vascular dementia is frankly parkinsonian (see below), as is that associated with other forms of dementia such as Alzheimer's disease. Difficulty walking and severe urinary incontinence with relatively mild cognitive impairment suggests normal-pressure hydrocephalus, described in Chapter 24vi, p. 000.

Management of stroke

Old age psychiatrists will frequently see patients with non-acute cerebrovascular disease whose medications require review, and will occasionally diagnose acute stroke in patients under their care. The following account of their management is intended as a broad outline to enhance understanding and inform decisions about referral to a physician.

There is robust evidence from large-scale randomized trials that patients who have had a transient ischaemic attack (TIA) or stroke can be protected from further vascular events (secondary prevention) by taking aspirin at doses of 75–300 mg daily, which are as effective as higher doses with lower rates of complications such as cerebral or gastrointestinal bleeding (Antiplatelet triallists' collaboration 1994). Patients who are intolerant of aspirin can be given an alternative antiplatelet agent such as clopidogrel. Patients who continue to suffer cerebrovascular events despite aspirin may be helped by the addition of slow-release dipyridamole.

For patients in atrial fibrillation, the most effective prevention (primary and secondary) of cerebral embolism is conferred by long-term anticoagulation with warfarin, aiming for a target INR (international normalized ratio) of 2.5. While evidence suggests that this therapy is underused in eligible patients, the hazards of anticoagulation may outweigh the benefits in many elderly, frail people, and clinical judgement must be applied carefully to an individual patient's circumstances. Contraindications include a tendency to fall, and poor memory, confusion, or anything else that might worsen concordance (compliance) with daily therapy at precise but changeable doses, and with attendance for regular blood tests. Local arrangements for laboratory control must be taken into account, as should the patient's preferences following appropriate explanation. Before starting warfarin, it is advisable to investigate and treat dyspepsia or iron-deficiency anaemia, and to control hypertension. In patients under 70 years of age without hypertension, diabetes mellitus, cardiac failure or structural disease of the heart, the risks of stroke in atrial fibrillation are low enough for aspirin to be sufficient for primary prevention. There is at present no evidence to support the use of warfarin for the prevention of cerebral embolism in patients in sinus rhythm, with the exception of those with mechanical heart valves. Warfarin and aspirin should only be given together in exceptional circumstances.

Secondary prevention may be enhanced by attention to the risk factors for vascular disease, such as hypertension, obesity, smoking, and lack of physical exercise. The benefits of cholesterol-lowering drugs have not been fully elucidated in relation to cerebrovascular disease, nor for cardiovascular risk reduction in older people.

Patients with a recent TIA or a very mild, non-disabling stroke should be referred for urgent assessment (within a week) in a specialist outpatient 'neurovascular' clinic—daily aspirin can be prescribed in the meantime (150 mg is a commonly chosen dose). TIAs must be distinguished from a wide variety of other diagnoses, including migraine, and specialist clinics will select patients for rapid assessment by duplex ultrasound and cranial imaging, including magnetic resonance angiography. Carotid end-arterectomy will be considered for patients with carotid territory symptoms in association with severe carotid stenosis on the relevant side, provided that the patient is fit for surgery. To minimize the risk of recurrent events such as stroke, surgery should be carried out as soon as possible after a TIA.

The old age psychiatrist confronted with a patient with acute stroke should feel confident in making an urgent referral to a physician with a special interest, in the expectation that the patient will be admitted to hospital for organized 'stroke unit' care. There will be some exceptions, such as patients whose comorbidity makes palliative care without hospital admission appropriate, but it is difficult to predict which patients with initially severe stroke will recover, or conversely those with initially mild stroke who will deteriorate and require further care. Meanwhile, the patient's swallow should be tested, and if there is any doubt then oral intake should be restricted to prevent aspiration pneumonia. Acute stroke is primarily a clinical diagnosis, but urgent brain imaging is indicated in various circumstances, such as when trauma is suspected or if the patient is on anticoagulants (Intercollegiate Working Party for Stroke 2000). CT scanning more than 7–10 days after the stroke may no longer distinguish cerebral haemorrhage from infarction, though magnetic resonance imaging (MRI) can do so at any time. Unless treatment is considered irrelevant to the patient's circumstances, imaging should be carried out within 48 hours to allow exclusion of cerebral haemorrhage, and for the timely administration of aspirin 300 mg daily for trial-proven benefits in acute cerebral infarction. Haemorrhagic complications outweigh the benefits from any form of heparin or other anticoagulation as treatment for acute ischaemic stroke, and there is no evidence to suggest that patients with atrial fibrillation gain net benefit. Thrombolytic therapy with tissue plasminogen activator (tPA) confers benefits in terms of disability and death rates in highly selected patients, who must undergo imaging and treatment within 3–6 hours after the onset of a stroke. At present, this treatment is appropriately confined to specialist centres and randomized controlled trials.

Specialist care for acute stroke patients will include attention to hydration, pyrexia, hyperglycaemia, and blood pressure, the use of compression stockings to prevent venous thrombosis in the legs, and the implementation of early rehabilitation. Organized 'stroke unit' care has been shown convincingly in randomized controlled trials (RCTs) to improve outcomes in terms of death and disability (Stroke Unit Trialists' Collaboration 1997). Depression after stroke is so common that antidepressant therapy regardless of specific symptoms has been tested in small-scale RCTs, with variable results (Intercollegiate Working Party for Stroke 2000, p. 95)

Parkinsonism and Parkinson's disease

Parkinson's disease and related disorders of the extrapyramidal motor system are important to the old age psychiatrist for several reasons:

1. The early symptoms and signs are sometimes misinterpreted as manifestations of psychiatric disorder, particularly depression or dementia.
2. Depression commonly complicates Parkinson's disease, and dementia may accompany the later stages, especially in elderly patients.
3. Drug-induced parkinsonism is frequently attributable to medications used in psychiatry.
4. Anti-parkinsonian drugs frequently cause confusion or hallucinations.
5. Features of parkinsonism may supervene in several of the organic dementias, including Alzheimer's disease and vascular dementia (see Chapters 24ii and iii, respectively).

Idiopathic Parkinson's disease is common in old people, having a steep rise in prevalence with age to approximately 2% of people over 80 years (Mutch *et al.* 1986). Diagnosis and management can be complex. The disease is variable in onset and in its rate of progression. Effective drug treatment is available, but the powerful actions of these drugs in modulating neurotransmission are reflected in their potent side-effects. The suspicion of Parkinson's disease in a patient presenting to the psychiatrist should prompt specialist referral to a geriatrician or neurologist. This brief account will concentrate on helping the old age psychiatrist to recognize the diagnosis when the presentation is disguised, and includes an outline of current treatment.

Clinical features of Parkinson's disease

Parkinson's disease (PD) has an insidious onset. The commonest presenting feature is tremor, often unilateral at first, sometimes mild and intermittent, and therefore overlooked. The other classical features—hypokinesia, rigidity, and postural instability—occasionally raise questions about the patient's mental health before their true significance is realized. Facial hypokinesia may cause relatives to report that the patient always seems miserable and never smiles, with a perpetual blank stare. Inability to initiate movements, such as getting out of a chair, may be misinterpreted as apathy: 'She just sits there doing nothing all day long'. Characteristic difficulties with walking may give an impression of bizarre behaviour: inability to start walking contrasts with a tendency once on the move for the pace to increase, sometimes uncontrollably (festinant gait). 'Freezing' into immobility in the middle of a walk or other activity can be spectacular and inexplicable to the victim and witness alike. Patients have difficulty explaining why they cannot move their limbs to prevent falls, or why they dress so slowly. Slowness when writing or handling money may be mistaken for cognitive impairment. Fear of falling and feelings of terror when unable to turn over in bed at night may add understandable anxiety to the clinical picture.

Once the diagnosis is suspected, specific aspects of the history should be clarified. Asking patients to describe in detail what happens when they try to walk may be revealing: parkinsonian patients simply describe the inability to move and do not give elaborate explanations, and they have often discovered 'tricks' that help them to start, such as imagining they are stepping over something on the ground, or trying to step on particular parts of a patterned floor. Mobility often varies with the time of day, and patients should always be asked about an inability to turn in bed at night. Problems with swallowing and constipation are commonly under-reported and should be sought.

Facial hypokinesia is sometimes subtle, and the observations of family members, carefully elicited, can help to confirm a suspicion. Parkinsonian patients classically blink less than normal, though normal rates are hard to define. The positive glabellar tap has traditional status but lacks specificity (see below). Even a few brief beats of the characteristic coarse tremor, usually seen in the hands at rest, offer support for the diagnosis, as does frank cogwheel rigidity, but many old people exhibit small degrees of increased tone without other features. The patient should be watched getting out of a chair, and the gait should be examined. The characteristic stooped posture may not be present in the early stages, but arm-swinging may be reduced, festinant (hurrying) walking may be observed, and watching a patient turn may demonstrate instability. The specialist will assess disability by observing activities of daily living, and will carry out timed tests, such as a 10-metre walk and the time taken to dress the upper half of the body. Handwriting may be characteristically cramped (micrographia), and its appearance and the time taken to copy out a paragraph can be useful for later comparisons.

Specialist referral is advocated, partly to protect patients who do not have Parkinson's disease from the hazards of inappropriate therapy. Benign essential tremor is the commonest movement disorder of old age and is frequently misdiagnosed. This tremor is usually absent at rest and worse with actions such as raising a cup to the lips, moreover there is no accompanying bradykinesia or rigidity. In syndromes of multiple system atrophy, parkinsonism characteristically unresponsive to levodopa therapy accompanies a failure of upward gaze in progressive supranuclear palsy and postural hypotension in the Shy–Drager syndrome.

Drug-induced parkinsonism

In elderly patients, iatrogenic parkinsonism may be as common as idiopathic PD, can produce identical symptoms and signs, and often goes unrecognized by general practitioners (Wilson and MacLennan 1989). Its lack of recognition has also been reported among psychiatric residents (Hansen *et al.* 1992). Drugs vary in their potency for causing parkinsonism and other extrapyramidal effects such as dyskinesias. The main culprits are the phenothiazines, thioxanthenes, butyrophenones (haloperidol), and metoclopramide. Other drugs implicated include alpha-methyldopa, reserpine, tetrabenazine, cinnarizine, and some 'atypical' antipsychotics. Most cases are attributable to drugs that are among the least potent but are in widespread use. The use of prochlorperazine and metoclopramide as antiemetics in old people should be decreased, using domperidone as an alternative when necessary; it should be borne in mind that many prescriptions for dizziness (such as prochlorperazine and cinnarizine) carry risks that outweigh the benefits. In old age psychiatry, thioridazine has been supplanted by risperidone which has fewer extrapyramidal effects, but these may be significant and long-term use should be minimized. Parkinsonism may persist for many months following withdrawal of the causative drugs. Treatment with anticholinergic antiparkinsonian drugs (see below) or larger than usual doses of levodopa may be successful but is often limited by confusion. The follow-up of survivors has shown that a high proportion subsequently develop idiopathic PD, suggesting that drug-susceptibility may be identifying latent disease (Wilson and MacLennan 1989).

Treatment of Parkinson's disease

Options for the treatment of PD and the management of complications have become more complex in recent years (Drug and Therapeutics Bulletin 1999), and, along with the difficulties with diagnosis described above, justify referral to a geriatrician or neurologist.

Levodopa preparations are the most effective antiparkinsonian drugs for the relief of motor deficits (hypokinesia, gait disturbance, instability on turning), but this is at the expense of the eventual onset of motor complications, such as on–off fluctuations and dyskinesias—choreoathetoid, lurching, and jerking hyperkinetic movements which can be disfiguring, disabling, exhausting, and painful. These often coincide with peak blood levels of levodopa, and may be helped by the use of frequent small doses and controlled-release preparations. Levodopa is given as a combined-preparation with a peripheral decarboxylase inhibitor (PDI, as co-beneldopa or co-careldopa) to increase delivery to the brain and decrease peripheral side-effects such as postural hypotension and gastrointestinal upset. The precise combination will depend on the desired daily dose of levodopa, ensuring that even when this is low, sufficient PDI is delivered. Details of preparations and dosing regimes are well described in the British National Formulary (BNF). The many side-effects of levodopa include nausea (for which phenothiazine derivatives should be avoided, and domperidone may be prescribed), confusion, and hallucinations. Patients usually prefer to administer their own medications for optimal effect, and as the disease progresses they often choose doses which induce dyskinesias, rather than accept immobility with reduced doses. Problems can occur in patients who develop impairment of memory or cognition while retaining control of their drugs: surges of confusion, hyperactivity, and dystonia attributable to levodopa toxicity may be recognized by accompanying extremes of sweating and tachycardia.

To postpone the onset of motor complications from sustained levodopa therapy, it is usual to delay starting treatment until disability from PD has significantly affected the patient's quality of life. There is increasing concern that even the small levodopa doses traditionally used to confirm the diagnosis may prime the early PD patient to the onset of dyskinesias. Alternative antiparkinsonian agents are increasingly used for early stages of the disease.

Selegilene, a monoamine-oxidase-B inhibitor, has a modest beneficial effect on PD symptoms, and may have a place in early disease to delay the need for levodopa. Its widespread use as an adjunct to levodopa to reduce 'end-of-dose' deterioration has been clouded by the suspicion of an increased death rate.

Trials of dopamine receptor agonists, such as bromocriptine, lisuride, pergolide, and apomorphine, versus levodopa in early PD have been disappointing, but three newer drugs, cabergoline, pramipexole, and ropinirole, are beginning to show promise. In a trial with a 5-year follow-up, motor deficits were somewhat greater in patients initially treated with ropinirole rather than levodopa, but functional abilities were similar in the two groups. Supplementary levodopa was given as required for the control of motor symptoms, but ropinirole significantly postponed the onset of dyskinesias and reduced their severity

(Rascol 2000). Unwanted effects include nausea and hallucinations.

Anticholinergic drugs, such as trihexyphenidyl (benzhexol) and orphenadrine, are particularly effective for tremor, and are also used in drug-induced parkinsonism, but their use in elderly patients is limited by their tendency to cause confusion, as well as blurred vision, urinary problems, and a dry mouth (though this can be useful when excessive salivation is a problem in late PD). Amantidine has a mild antiparkinsonian effect, but can cause confusion and hallucinations in old people. Entacapone is a catechol-O-methyl transferase (COMT) inhibitor, a new class of drug which aims to increase the clinical response to levodopa by increasing the amount that reaches the brain. Unwanted effects include worsening of dyskinesias, and nausea, and liver function tests should be monitored. Surgical techniques for treating drug-resistant tremor and disabling dyskinesias are under evaluation in specialized centres, and include the creation of lesions in or near the basal ganglia (thalamotomy, pallidotomy, and subthalamotomy) and the implantation of electrical stimulators.

Problems in distinguishing Parkinson's disease from depression have been mentioned above. Depression is also a frequent accompaniment of the disease, affecting up to 50% of patients. Drug treatment must take account of interactions with the disease and with antiparkinsonian drugs. Selective serotonin-reuptake inhibitors (SSRIs) have been recommended as the drugs of first choice (Allain 2000), although there have been case-reports implicating some preparations as inducers of parkinsonism. By contrast, tricyclic antidepressants can improve motor symptoms, but can cause troublesome delusions, confusion, and postural hypotension in parkinsonian patients. SSRIs in combination with selegilene can cause the rare, but dangerous, serotonin syndrome.

The old age psychiatrist may be asked to advise on the neuropsychiatric complications of drug therapy in the late stages of PD, when a balance must be struck between mobility and confusion, hallucinations, delusions, paranoia, and sleep disturbance. Atypical neuroleptic drugs, such as clozapine and olanzapine, have been reported as being useful in selected patients for the control of psychotic symptoms, allowing levodopa therapy to continue (Wolters *et al.* 1996).

Neurological signs, ageing, and dementia

A wide variety of age-associated changes in neurological function have been described, including deterioration in the senses of smell, vision, and hearing, and in somatic sensation, especially of vibration. The common textbook assertion that ankle jerks are frequently absent in old people has been called into question by a survey showing intact reflexes in 94% of 200 consecutive elderly admissions, tested by a plantar-strike method (Impallomeni *et al.* 1984). A large-scale, cross-sectional survey of the prevalence of abnormal neurological signs in apparently healthy old people has shown age-associated increases in the prevalence of paratonia (a mild increase in resting tone sometimes called Gegenhalten), in failure of vertical gaze both upwards and downwards, in abnormalities of visual tracking movements, and also in the prevalence of two so-called primitive reflexes: a positive glabellar tap and an abnormal snout reflex (Jenkyn *et al.* 1985).

Primitive reflexes are present in human infants but disappear with maturation of the central nervous system. Their reappearance later in life is generally attributed to the release of brainstem activity from the regulatory activity of higher centres. These signs are often recorded in demented patients, and may be elicited as follows:

1. *Glabellar tap*: the centre of the forehead is tapped regularly and repeatedly by the examiner's finger, positioned to avoid causing a visual threat. Normally, only the first two or three taps produce a blink. Continued reflex blinking constitutes an abnormal response.
2. *Palmomental reflex*: the thenar eminence of a hand is stroked. An abnormal response consists of reflex contraction of the mentalis muscle on the same side, producing wrinkling of the chin and sometimes curling of the lower lip.
3. *Snout reflex*: the examiner gently, but firmly, applies an index finger to the philtrum and lips. An abnormal response consists of

pouting, pursing, or puckering the lips, with contraction of the orbicularis oris muscle. Normally there is no response.

4. *Suck reflex*: stroking the perioral region on one side elicits abnormal pursing and sucking movements, with turning of the head towards the stimulus.
5. *Grasp reflex*: introducing the examiner's fingers into the subject's hand between the thumb and forefinger evokes abnormal reflex grasping by flexion of the subject's fingers.
6. *Traction sign*: the subject's flexed fingers are gently extended by the examiner's fingers. An abnormal response consists of hooking the fingers.

Primitive reflexes have been found to be associated with Alzheimer's disease (Huff *et al.* 1987), along with diminished olfaction and astereognosis. A large-scale survey found them to be significantly more common in patients with dementia of various types (Alzheimer's, vascular, and associated with Parkinson's disease) than in non-demented subjects (Hogan and Ebly 1995). Despite a strong association, however, primitive reflexes were found to lack sufficient sensitivity to be useful in the diagnosis of dementia.

Endocrine and metabolic diseases

Endocrine and metabolic diseases feature prominently in accounts of the psychiatric manifestations of organic disease (Lishman 1997).

Thyroid disorders

Diseases of the thyroid gland are common, presentations are varied and often non-specific, and apart from aggressive or late-presenting malignancy they are usually curable. The thyroid should be palpated, local lymph nodes should be sought, and an enlarged gland should be auscultated, seeking a bruit. Hypothyroidism should be considered in all apparently depressed patients, looking for accompanying features such as cold intolerance, alopecia, a puffy face, slow-relaxing reflexes, cerebellar ataxia, or the rare sign of pretibial myxoedema. Occasional hypothyroid patients present with bizarre psychiatric symptoms: myxoedematous madness (Asher 1949). Thyrotoxicosis may lie behind anxiety states, hyperactivity, or odd behaviour, and may cause heat-intolerance. Eye signs (lid retraction, lid lag, and exopthalmos) should be sought, along with warm peripheries, a fine tremor, tachycardia which persists during sleep, or atrial fibrillation. The rare phenomenon of lethargic thyrotoxicosis, when very high levels of thyroid hormones are found in an apparently depressed patient, is said to carry special risks.

The laboratory test of choice is a measurement of serum thyroid-stimulating hormone concentration (TSH), using a modern highly sensitive assay. A normal TSH concentration excludes hypothyroidism and hyperthyroidism, apart from a few rare exceptions (Rae *et al.* 1993). However, an abnormal TSH result requires cautious appraisal since both high and low levels may be the result of non-thyroidal illness in a euthyroid patient. This is due to the complex interaction of many factors which include: the timing and severity of the illness; the possible effects of drugs (including steroids, oestrogens, and amiodarone); and resultant effects on the binding and metabolism of thyroid hormones, especially the conversion of thyroxine (T4) to tri-iodothyronine (T3). When the TSH level is abnormal, the interpretation of assays of T4 and T3 depends, to some extent, on whether it is hypo- or hyperthyroidism that is suspected on clinical grounds. A high TSH with a low T4 indicates hypothyroidism, but other combinations are more problematic and referral to a specialist is strongly advised.

Disorders of blood glucose

Hypoglycaemia should be suspected as a contributor to psychological disturbance in any patient taking antidiabetic medications, and where the timing of symptoms may relate to meals. Blood glucose measurements can often be carried out at home by a carer taught to use test sticks. Long-acting oral hypoglycaemics, such as glibenclamide, are often implicated, whereas short-acting drugs, such as tolbutamide or gliclazide, are safer. When a failure by the patient to take medication is not considered by the physician, persistently high sugars may lead to increases in prescribed doses, so that admission to hospital or the arrival of a caring relative may precipitate catastrophic hypoglycaemia simply by ensuring compliance.

Hyperglycaemia in elderly patients may lead to ketoacidosis, but non-ketotic hyperosmolar states are also common. Both are life-threatening medical emergencies, and confused patients with high blood glucose levels should be referred for urgent inpatient management before coma ensues.

Renal failure

Psychiatric features are common in the presentation of patients with renal failure, varying from drowsiness to behavioural changes, memory impairment, mood fluctuations, frank delirium, and occasionally psychosis (Lishman 1997, pp. 555–63). Most patients are obviously physically ill, but some remain undiagnosed until blood tests reveal very high urea and creatinine levels (over 400 μmol/l). In men, a common cause is obstruction to urine flow by prostatic hypertrophy or carcinoma, revealed by palpation of the bladder and rectal examination.

Hyponatraemia

A reduction in the plasma concentration of sodium is a frequent cause of confusion in elderly patients, and can result in stupor and coma. The effects depend partly on the speed with which it has developed—so that sometimes delirium occurs with only modest reductions in sodium level, whilst, occasionally, patients remain alert and lucid with plasma sodium concentrations of 119 mmol/l and below. In surveys of general hospital patients, chest infections and diuretic drugs are common causes; antidepressants and carbamazepine feature prominently in patients shared by old age psychiatrists and physicians. Hyponatraemia is often dilutional even without frank signs of fluid overload, and responds to oral fluid restriction after treatment or removal of the cause. Referral is frequently indicated, since it can be difficult to identify those patients who are water-depleted and because other possible causes of hyponatraemia range widely through renal, hepatic, cardiac, and pituitary disease to the production of an antidiuretic hormone analogue by a carcinoma of the bronchus. Recovery speeds vary, and symptoms may not resolve until a week or so after the serum sodium level returns to normal.

Hyper- and hypocalcaemia

Hypercalcaemia may cause a variety of mental disturbances, ranging from mild behavioural changes through depression to psychosis and dementia. Other symptoms include tiredness, constipation, thirst, urinary frequency, and muscular weakness. Once a raised level has been confirmed, in a fasting blood specimen corrected for serum albumin concentration, the patient should be referred to a physician for investigation of possible causes, including malignancy (metastatic and non-metastatic), hyperparathyroidism, and drugs.

Significant hypocalcaemia is less common, may also cause a variety of psychological symptoms including irritability and lethargy, and may be accompanied by muscular spasm. Causes include malabsorption syndromes, vitamin D deficiency, and hypoparathyroidism which may emerge years after damage to the glands during thyroid surgery.

Adrenal disorders

Addison's disease (hypoadrenalism) is a rare cause of insidiously worsening malaise that may be mistaken for depression, and weight loss is usual. Cushing's syndrome (cortisol excess) is uncommon. However, many sufferers have psychiatric complications, such as depression or psychosis, which also occur with chronic corticosteroid therapy for disorders such as asthma.

Miscellaneous conditions

Urinary tract infections

Urinary infections are common, and often present non-specifically with confusion, anorexia, or fatigue. Asymptomatic bacteriuria is also frequent in old people, and a positive culture on a midstream urine specimen (MSU) can contribute to the diagnostic problems posed by multiple pathology (see above). However, early antibiotic treatment is often justified while awaiting the results of MSU and blood cultures, especially in patients with known renal tract abnormalities, an indwelling or recent urinary catheter, pyrexia, or a raised white cell count or C-reactive protein (CRP). Urinalysis using reagent strips which test for the presence of nitrite and leucocytes can be useful: infection is unlikely if both are absent and there are no urinary symptoms. Positive results should be confirmed with an MSU.

Anaemia

The non-specific malaise often caused by anaemia may be extreme, with immobility, apathy, and self-neglect. Falls and confusion may also occur and a blood count and film can be justified in all patients presenting to psychiatrists and physicians, with further investigations on conventional lines according to the results. Mild macrocytosis on the film may reflect alcohol excess or hypothyroidism, and more severe degrees are found in folate or vitamin B_{12} deficiencies, possible contributors to dementia (Lishman 1997, pp. 587–93).

Hip fractures

Proximal femoral fractures are common, and are missed surprisingly often in old people who may be able to walk for a few days on an impacted fracture, especially if cognitive impairment or drugs are masking pain. Careful examination and appropriate radiographs may be rewarding.

Giant-cell arteritis

This interesting condition usually causes headaches or visual disturbance, sometimes associated with pain around the shoulder girdle or pelvis (polymyalgia rheumatica). Patients occasionally present non-specifically with malaise, weight loss, or pyrexia, a few have strokes or fits, and a variety of neuropsychiatric syndromes have been described, including fluctuating delirium with memory impairment (Pascuzzi *et al.* 1989). Treatment with corticosteroids usually relieves the symptoms and may prevent sudden blindness. Hence the alert geriatrician actively considers giant-cell arteritis in a wide variety of patients, assessing the temporal arteries (for overlying erythema, absence of pulsation, tenderness, and induration), checking the blood for a raised ESR and CRP, and proceeding to temporal artery biopsy. Urgent steroid therapy pending biopsy may be justified (Drug and Therapeutics Bulletin 1993).

Hazards in the home

Assessing a confused patient in her own home is of particular value to an old age psychiatrist, and two conditions that may arise from a hazardous home environment merit special consideration: hypothermia and carbon monoxide poisoning.

Life-threatening hypothermia in old people may progress gradually, with slowness of thought and action manifest for days before the onset of frank confusion, stupor, and eventually coma. This is an example of multiple aetiology: age-associated impairments of thermal sensation and thermoregulatory reflexes are prevalent amongst apparently well, old people (Exton-Smith 1981). Chronic diseases such as hypothyroidism may contribute, and acute illnesses such as a chest infection or myocardial infarction can produce a sudden worsening of body temperature control. Psychotropic drugs are often implicated, and phenothiazines can have a specific effect on hypothalamic thermoregulatory function. Social and cultural factors complete the mixture, since many old people live in badly insulated houses, are unwilling to spend scarce resources on heating (especially because they do not feel the cold, see above), and believe that it is healthy to sleep by an open window whatever the weather. Clues include cold central body parts such as axillae and groins, and signs that mimic hypothyroidism such as slow movements, a hoarse voice, and a puffy face.

Standard mercury thermometers are generally inaccurate below 36.5 °C, therefore core temperatures, rectal or tympanic, should be measured with a low-reading device. Urgent referral to hospital is indicated for treatment by slow warming, and for attention to potentially lethal complications such as cardiac arrhythmias.

Carbon monoxide poisoning may result from faulty heating and ventilation systems, and deaths are sometimes preceded by several days of morning confusion, sleepiness or agitation, headache, and nausea that improve on leaving the house. Thinking of the possibility can be life-saving.

Conclusions

In summary, a basic assessment for physical disease in elderly psychiatric patients should begin with a detailed history from the patient and anyone else who can be contacted, including a full drug history. The patient's disabilities should be recorded, and use of the Barthel index of ADL is recommended. If not already fully assessed, cognitive function should be surveyed with a brief test. On physical examination, special attention should be paid to signs relevant to heart failure (especially the apex rate and sacral oedema), cardiac murmurs, supine and erect blood pressure, the temporal arteries, abnormalities in the chest and abdomen including rectal examination and stigmata of liver disease, and evidence of malignancy (including lymphadenopathy in the neck), and thyroid disease. Neurological assessment should include a search for Parkinson's disease and signs compatible with stroke, especially dysphasia, visuospatial disorders, and visual-field defects. The gait should be assessed, and the optic fundi checked for papilloedema. Physical examination should include measuring rectal (or auditory meatus) temperature (see also Chapter 25, Table 25.6).

The investigations to be carried out will vary according to the clinical findings and will depend on local facilities and the location of the patient. Ideally, even patients seen at home should have a blood test, with samples sent for haemoglobin measurement, white cell count, blood film examination, and ESR as well as tests for CRP, blood sugar, creatinine and urea, sodium, potassium, liver function, calcium, and thyroid function (beginning with an assay of TSH). In addition, patients with delirium and others in whom infection must be excluded should have a chest radiograph, a midstream urine sample tested for leucocytes and nitrites and sent for culture, and blood cultures (see also Chapter 25, Table 25.6). Referral to a physician is justified whenever doubts remain, or results are unexpected.

This chapter has mainly been concerned with the question of when a patient should be suspected of having a physical disease. It is often more difficult to decide when such disease has been satisfactorily excluded. Once again, precise criteria will vary between patients depending on the reasons for the original suspicion. When seeking evidence of infection, if the history, expert physical examination, and the tests listed above neither reveal cause for concern nor suggest further lines of investigation, detailed surveillance over a few days should be undertaken. If symptoms, signs, body temperature, and repeat tests of white cell count and CRP remain satisfactory, acute infections may generally be considered to have been excluded, at least to the point where surveillance can be relaxed pending further clinical events. For other forms of physical disease in psychiatric patients, thorough clinical assessment should be followed by surveillance over a longer period. When initial evaluation has not yielded a physical diagnosis and psychiatric management has begun, follow-up assessment after an appropriate interval should be offered. Indeed, continuity and follow-up are the hallmarks of appropriately careful medical practice.

References

Allain, H., Schuck, S., and Mauduit, N. (2000). Depression in Parkinson's disease. *British Medical Journal*, **320**, 1287–8. [editorial]

Antiplatelet triallists' collaboration (1994). Collaborative overview of randomised trials of antiplatelet therapy – I: Prevention of death, myocardial infarction, and stroke by prolonged antiplatelet therapy in various categories of patients. *British Medical Journal*, 308, 81–106.

Asher, R. (1949). Myxoedematous madness. *British Medical Journal*, **ii**, 555–62.

Bamford, J., Sandercock, P., Dennis, M., Burn, J., and Warlow, C. (1991). Classification and natural history of clinically identifiable subtypes of cerebral infarction. *Lancet*, **337**, 1521–6.

Berman, P., Hogan, D. B., and Fox R. A. (1987). The atypical presentation of infection in old age. *Age and Ageing*, **16**, 201–7.

Collin, C., Wade, D. T., Davis, S., and Horne, V. (1988). The Barthel ADL index: a reliability study. *International Disability Studies*, **10**, 61–3.

Darowski, A., Najim, Z., Weinberg, J., and Guz, A. (1991). The febrile response to mild infections in elderly hospital inpatients. *Age and Ageing*, **20**, 193–8.

Drug and Therapeutics Bulletin (1993). The management of polymyalgia rheumatica and giant cell arteritis. *Drug and Therapeutics Bulletin*, **17**, 65–8.

Drug and Therapeutics Bulletin (1999). Developments in the treatment of Parkinson's disease. *Drug and Therapeutics Bulletin*, **37**, 36–40.

Evans, J. G. (1981). Institutional care. In *Health care of the elderly* (ed. T. Arie), pp. 176–93. Croom Helm, London.

Evans, J. G., Williams, T. F., Michel, J. and Beattie, L. (2000). *Oxford Textbook of Geriatric Medicine* (second edition). Oxford University Press, Oxford.

Evans *et al.* (2000).

Exton-Smith, A. N. (1981). The elderly in a cold environment. In *Health care of the elderly* (ed. T. Arie), pp. 42–56. Croom Helm, London.

Fairweather, D. S. and Campbell, A. J. (1991). Diagnostic accuracy. The effects of multiple aetiology and the degradation of information in old age. *Journal of the Royal College of Physicians of London*, **25**, 105–10.

Hansen, T. E., Brown, W. L., Weigel, R. M., and Casey, D. E. (1992). Underrecognition of tardive dyskinesia and drug-induced parkinsonism by psychiatric residents. *General Hospital Psychiatry*, **14**, 340–4.

Hodges, J. R. (1994). *Cognitive assessment for clinicians*. Oxford University Press, Oxford.

Hogan, D. B. and Ebly, E. M. (1995). Primitive reflexes and dementia: results from the Canadian Study of Health and Aging. *Age and Ageing*, **24**, 375–81.

Huff, F. J., Boller, F., Lucchelli, F., Querriera, R., Beyer, J., and Belle, S. (1987). The neurologic examination in patients with probable Alzheimer's disease. *Archives of Neurology*, **44**, 929–32.

Impallomeni, M., Kenny, R. A., Flynn, M. D., and Pallis, C. A. (1984). The elderly and their ankle jerks. *Lancet*, **i**, 670–2.

Intercollegiate Working Party for Stroke (2000). *National clinical guidelines for stroke*. Royal College of Physicians, London.

Jenkyn, L. R., Reeves, A. G., Warren, T., Whiting, R. K., Clayton, R. J., Moore, W. W., *et al.* (1985). Neurologic signs in senescence. *Archives of Neurology*, **42**, 1154–7.

Jones, H. R. and Siekert, R. G. (1989). Neurological manifestations of infective endocarditis. Review of clinical and therapeutic challenges. *Brain*, **112**, 1295–315.

Lishman, W. A. (1997). *Organic psychiatry*. Blackwell Scientific, Oxford.

McKillop, G. M., Stewart, D. A., Burns, J. M. A., and Ballantyne, D. (1991). Doppler echocardiography in elderly patients with ejection systolic murmurs. *Postgraduate Medical Journal*, **67**, 1059–61.

Mahoney, F. I. and Barthel, D. W. (1964). Functional evaluation: the Barthel index. *Maryland State Medical Journal*, **14**, 61–5.

Muller, R. T., Gould, L. A., Betzu, R., Vaceck, T., and Pradeep, V. (1990). Painless myocardial infarction in the elderly. *American Heart Journal*, **119**, 202–4.

Mutch, W. J., Dingwall-Fordyce, I., Downie, A. W., Paterson, J. G., and Roy, S. K. (1986). Parkinson's disease in a Scottish city. *British Medical Journal*, **292**, 534–6.

Pascuzzi, R. M., Roos, K. L., and Davis, T. E. (1989). Mental status abnormalities in temporal arteritis: a treatable cause of dementia in the elderly. *Arthritis and Rheumatism*, **32**, 1308–11.

Rae, P., Farrar, J., Beckett, G., and Toft, A. (1993). Assessment of thyroid status in elderly people. *British Medical Journal*, **307**, 177–80.

Rascol, O., Brooks, D., Korczyn, A., *et al.* for the 056 Study Group. (2000). A five-year study of the incidence of dyskinesia in patients with early Parkinson's disease who were treated with Ropinirole or levodopa. *New England Medical Journal*, **342**, 1484–91.

Stroke Unit Trialists' Collaboration (1997). Collaborative systematic review of the randomised trials of organised inpatient (stroke unit) care after stroke. *British Medical Journal*, **314**, 1151.

Wade, D. T. and Collin, C. (1988). The Barthel ADL index: a standard measure of physical disability? *International Disability Studies*, **10**, 64–7.

Weatherall, D. J., Ledingham, J. G. G., and Warrell, D. A. (1996). *Oxford textbook of medicine*. Oxford University Press, Oxford.

Wilson, J. A. and MacLennan, W. J. (1989). Review: drug-induced parkinsonism in elderly patients. *Age and Ageing*, **18**, 208–10.

Wolters, E. C., Jansen, E. N. H., Tuynman-Qua, H. G., *et al.* (1996). Olanzapine in the treatment of dopaminometic psychosis in patients with Parkinson's Disease. *Neurology*, **47**, 1085–7.

Working Group of the Royal College of Physicians (1991). Cardiological intervention in elderly patients. *Journal of the Royal College of Physicians of London*, **25**, 197–205.

Working Group of the Royal College of Physicians and the British Geriatrics Society (1992). *Standardised assessment scales for elderly people*. Royal College of Physicians, London.

World Health Organization (1980). *The international classification of impairments, disabilities and handicaps*. World Health Organization, Geneva.

World Health Organization (1999). ICIDH-2: international classification of functioning and disability. (Beta-2 draft). *www.who.int/icdh/* (accessed 17 November 2000).

11 Psychological assessment and treatment

Bob Woods and Georgina Charlesworth

Introduction

The last 20 years have seen major growth in the application of psychological theories and principles to the problems faced by older people and their families. In the UK, clinical psychology is seen as a core component of a mental health service for older people, but, just as important, there is increasing recognition of the need for psychological perspectives and approaches across all disciplines in old age psychiatry.

Our approach is holistic; we consider mental health problems in late life to be best understood as an interaction between biological, social, environmental and psychological factors. The contribution of each of these to the presenting problems varies from case to case, from time to time. We take a lifespan developmental approach, recognizing that the person presenting *now* has a lifetime of experiences and relationships, which contribute to their current situation and their attempts to cope with and adapt to changes now being experienced. Psychological treatment must be based on thorough assessment, and tailored carefully to the individual circumstances of the case.

This chapter outlines the contribution of psychological perspectives to old age psychiatry, before considering in detail psychological assessment of cognitive abilities and other important areas of function. Psychological therapies, and the adaptations required in applying them to older people, are discussed, with a detailed consideration of psychological approaches for use with older people with cognitive impairment. Finally, we review the evidence-base for the efficacy of these approaches. Readers wishing to pursue these topics in more detail are recommended to consult relevant chapters in the *Handbook of the clinical psychology of ageing* (Woods 1996*a*). An updated selection of these chapters is also available (Woods 1999*a*).

What psychological approaches are applicable?

There are four branches of psychology of particular value in work with older people. They can be used either within or outside the psychiatric diagnostic system across the wide range of presenting problems seen in old age psychiatry:

1. *Clinical*—application of psychological models to understand and reduce emotional distress (e.g. depression, anxiety, anger, shame), and address behaviours experienced as unhelpful by the patient, families, or staff. As examples: interpersonal or communication models can be used to modify difficult patterns of staff–patient interaction; behavioural analysis can provide detailed data on the triggers and reinforcers for a specific behaviour (e.g. wandering).
2. *Health*—application of psychological models to understand and, if appropriate, adapt unhelpful health-related behaviours (e.g. non-compliance with medication, frequent complaints about somatic symptoms) and responses to physical illness.
3. *Cognitive*—investigation of thinking processes and the impact of thoughts upon emotions and behaviour, and vice versa (used within both

clinical and health psychology). For example, the concept of cognitive appraisal is useful in understanding people's responses to both external events (e.g. changes in social networks) and internal processes (e.g. their own thoughts, feelings, and behaviours).

4. *Neuropsychology*—identification and measurement of perceptual abilities and cognitive functions, such as memory, language, information processing, and planning. For example, neuropsychological assessment data can be used to aid the diagnostic process in memory clinics.

Using psychological approaches in mental health services for older people

Some psychological approaches can be used by all members of a psychiatric team, and are an integral part of good practice. For example, an awareness of one's own and others' 'cognitive appraisals' is central to achieving good communication. Cognitive appraisal refers to the meaning of an event or situation from the point of view of the appraiser, together with the associated emotion. As appraisal is heavily influenced by expectations and prior experiences, two people can come away from the same situation with very different views on what took place. To minimize the differences in view between clinician and patient, it is necessary to adhere to good principles of communication, which demand not simply consideration of the delivery of information. For example, this will not only involve adapting vocabulary, style, and content to match the knowledge and abilities of the listener, and providing written or taped information to support the spoken consultation, but also checking out the other's understanding of what has been said.

Considering the patient's response to diagnostic disclosure

Being given a psychiatric diagnosis is a potentially traumatic life-event. The response to receiving a diagnosis is highly individual, and, will depend upon an individual's appraisal of the meaning of the diagnosis and prognosis, and of their own ability to deal with it (i.e. their 'self-efficacy'). For example, responses to being told a diagnosis of an anxiety disorder may include: relief ('Oh, it's an "anxious stomach"—I thought that I had cancer'); disbelief and anger ('I am not anxious, I have heart problems. I knew that they hadn't investigated thoroughly'); fear ('What will happen to me?', 'What will people think?'); hopelessness ('So, I'm just a worried old woman. I might as well book my place in that Home'); helplessness ('I've been a worrier all my life—I can't do anything about it now'). Checking out the individual's appraisal of the diagnosis and prognosis increases the likelihood that misunderstandings will be identified and corrected early on. Similarly, knowing something of the patient's perceived self-efficacy in being able to cope with the illness will influence the intervention plan.

Amongst the most difficult diagnoses both to give and to receive are those of the chronic, degenerative, and debilitating conditions such as Alzheimer's disease and vascular dementia. In the past, clinicians have tried to 'protect' patients by not 'breaking the bad news' (Rice and Warner 1994). However, there is increasing awareness of the importance of the process of sharing diagnostic information with both the patient and family to facilitate accommodation and adjustment to the condition, and to allow for preparation for the future. 'Breaking bad news' well, requires good communication skills, sensitivity to the individual, and a considerable investment of time before, during, and after the assessment process. Prediagnostic counselling is the time to explain the assessment procedures clearly in a manner that the person can understand, and at the level of detail that matches the person's need for knowledge. The patient should be informed of the uses to which the information will be put, and their perception of the possible outcomes explored. For example, a neuropsychological assessment may result in advice about competence to drive. Providing feedback from assessments is an important part of the diagnostic process and should not simply be fitted into a 5-minute slot at the end of a session; time must be allowed, and further sessions scheduled as necessary, for the client to talk through the implications of the results and diagnosis they have received (Husband 1999).

When a person is referred, they may have already been told their physical and mental health diagnoses, or they may have been prescribed treatments without diagnostic disclosure. Either way, it is important to clarify their understanding of previously received information and treatments. The person's distress is sometimes attributable to misunderstandings and subsequent catastrophic thinking. For example, being told that a test result is negative can be interpreted in two ways—either as 'all clear' or 'bad news'.

Psychological assessment and formulation

Psychologists use a variety of techniques to collect historical and current information, including different questioning styles within an interview, psychometric questionnaires, observational or self-monitoring data, and existing case notes. The aim of an assessment will determine its nature, but, for the most part, psychologists will aim to draw up individual 'formulations' or 'case conceptualizations' which draw on psychological theory and provide a framework for understanding the cause and maintenance of presenting problems. From the formulation, an individual action plan for interventions can be devised.

A range of tools is available for assessing attributes of personality, emotional states, social environment, self-efficacy, coping, perceptions of illness, cognitive abilities and processes, and behavioural reactions. These are used to inform the individual formulation, in the context of other information, and are not intended to be viewed in isolation. Given the particular salience of cognitive function in mental health problems in late life, we will first consider neuropsychological assessment before outlining other areas of assessment.

Assessment of cognitive function

Numerous purposes may underlie an assessment of cognitive function (Woods 1999*b*). In addition to the common use of neuropsychological assessment in contributing to the diagnostic evaluation of dementia, it may also be used to monitor change over time, or for assisting with assessment of competence, or for evaluating treatments and services, for example. A distinction needs to be made between diagnostic (or categorical) and descriptive assessment strategies. In the past, cognitive tests were often devised to maximize their efficiency, in terms of specificity and sensitivity, by placing the person assessed into one category or another. This approach did not necessarily lead to the development of useful measures of psychological functions, and, by encouraging diagnostic allocations on the basis of only one type of evidence, could lead to significant diagnostic errors.

A moment's consideration of the nature of dementing disorders will illustrate the folly of relying on a cut-off score below which patients are said to have dementia, where the assessment is simply of current cognitive function. Dementia involves, by definition, a reduction from some previous level of function. Those who previously functioned at a higher level will inevitably take longer to reach a fixed cut-off threshold than those with a lifelong lower level of function, and their dementia will not be detected at such an early stage. Conversely, a person functioning at a low level may, through normal variation (perhaps mediated by mild health problems, sensory difficulties, or simply an 'off' day!), score on some occasions below the threshold, and appear to have dementia when they in fact do not. The consistent finding that the most widely used screening test for dementia, the Mini-Mental State Examination (Folstein *et al.* 1975), is strongly educationally biased, illustrates this problem (e.g. Orrell *et al.* 1992).

Descriptive assessment, on the other hand, aims to provide a profile of the person's function, their strengths and weaknesses. Comparisons are made both within the person's profile, and with estimates of the person's previous level of performance. It may inform the diagnostic process, but failure in any area will lead to a consideration of the possible reasons for difficulty, rather than an automatic assignment to a diagnostic category. Interpreting the results of a cognitive assessment is far from straightforward. If the person's cognitive function has changed, it is necessary to consider whether these changes are consistent with those associated with normal ageing. An extensive literature documents that, on average, most cognitive functions show some age-related decline by the seventh decade, even when cohort effects are controlled for. However, there is also a consistent finding of increased individual variation, i.e. individual patterns of change vary widely (Schaie 1990). The main contributory factors to this increased variation are considered to be health problems such as hypertension and diabetes, but many other factors may apply in the individual case. Amongst these should be noted sensory deficits, fatigue, the unfamiliarity of the tests and testing situation, language and cultural differences, and the adverse effect on performance that comes from the individual's propensity to evaluate their own performance negatively (e.g. 'I was never any good with figures').

These factors emphasize the skill and care that is required to obtain a valid cognitive profile. Having taken these factors into account, perhaps the best indicator of the extent to which the changes exceed those that could be accounted for by other processes is whether the person's relative position in their age group has reduced greatly, so that someone who was performing well above average is now performing at an average level, or someone who was previously at the average level is now well below. Such comparisons require the test to have good norms for the relevant age groups (which are unfortunately not available for all tests).

How can the person's previous level of ability be estimated? It is rare for an actual test score to be available. Most commonly, premorbid levels of intellectual ability are estimated from word reading tests, such as the National Adult Reading Test (Nelson and Willison 1991), as this is an ability which appears to be relatively spared by ageing and dementia. However, its use can be problematic where the person's first language is not English, where the person has major visual problems, or a dysphasia. Then it may be necessary to rely on demographic data, such as level of education attainment and occupational history; regression equations have been described to assist with this (Crawford *et al.* 1989). However in the individual case, little weight should be given, without supporting evidence, to an absence of attainment (e.g. leaving school at 14 years of age, employment in a manual job), in view of the limited educational and occupational opportunities that were available in youth for some of today's older people. An alternative way of estimating change is to interview others who have known the person over a period of time, using questions targeted on specific changes in ability and performance. The Informant Questionnaire on Cognitive Decline in the Elderly (IQCODE; see Jorm *et al.* 1989) provides a useful framework for achieving this.

There are a number of areas to assess in carrying out a full cognitive assessment. Indeed the fact that the diagnostic criteria for dementia require 'global' change indicates the need for avoiding a narrow focus in assessment. Woods (1999*b*) and Crawford *et al.* (1998) give examples of tests commonly used. However, new tests are being published rapidly, but clinicians will often have their own older 'favourites', drawn, appropriately, from experience in assessing a large number of older people. The areas that would typically be covered are listed below. They are assessed in widely used brief batteries such as the Cambridge Cognitive Capacity Scale (CAMCOG; Roth *et al.* 1988) and the Middlesex Elderly Assessment of Mental State (MEAMS; Golding 1989):

- intellectual function;
- memory and learning—a range of aspects including verbal and non-verbal memory; free recall and recognition memory; immediate and delayed memory;
- attention and concentration;
- speed;
- language;
- executive functioning—planning, problem-solving, flexible thinking;
- perceptual abilities;
- constructional abilities.

In selecting a cognitive test, the following points should be considered:

- Are adequate norms available, appropriate for this person's age and educational level and cultural background?
- How difficult is the test? Will the patient find it too easy and be bored, or will it expose them to repeated overt failure, and risk losing their cooperation and motivation?
- Are the test materials appropriate for older adults? Is the person's vision good enough to cope with any written materials or drawings? Do the materials appear childish, and risk offending the person's dignity?
- Are parallel forms of the test available, if it is likely that follow-up assessment will be required? If repeat testing is envisaged, the person's initial score needs to be in the middle of the range possible on that test, to give scope for change in either direction.
- Does the test relate clearly to a specific cognitive function and/or real-life abilities—what does performance on this test indicate?
- How long will it take to administer this test? Will the person be tired and less able to concentrate towards the end of it?

A good strategy is to begin with one of the briefer batteries mentioned above, and select further tests, if required, based on the person's profile of performance and response.

Assessment of non-cognitive aspects

This section describes the assessment of mood, well-being, behaviour, and need. There is a variety of assessment tools, which include self-report and 'other', or proxy, report options. They can be used in assessment as a way of comparing an individual to the 'norm', or to assess the degree of severity of symptomatology, and can be used to track change during treatment. Questionnaires listing symptoms with which a client identifies may provide a useful demonstration that they are not alone in their situation. Questionnaires should be selected carefully, taking into account the content of the questions, the complexity of the response format, and their psychometric properties, particularly their reliability and validity. Respondents should be given a rationale for the use of the questionnaire, and it should be emphasized that there are no 'right' or 'wrong' answers.

Self-report measures may be useful even where the patient has a marked cognitive impairment. Mozley *et al.* (1999) have shown that people with a moderate degree of dementia are able to give a reasonable account of their circumstances, and that such accounts can be a rich source of information. To supplement the person's own views, the usual approach is to ask an informant to complete an appropriate scale, based on their observations of the person over a given period. This has the advantage of being naturalistic and tapping into real-life function, but is dependent on the availability of a reliable relative, friend, or member of staff who has enough contact with the person to provide detailed and accurate information. There is increasing evidence that such ratings may be influenced by the informant's own mood and strain levels (Teri and Truax 1994).

A compendium of assessment scales and psychometric questionnaires for use with older adults is now available (Burns *et al.* 1999). Along with descriptions and reviews, the original scales are reproduced wherever permission has been given. NFER-Nelson produce portfolios of measures for mental health and health psychology, including measures of coping and self-efficacy, some of which are appropriate for older adults.

Depression

A widely recommended psychometric instrument used specifically to measure depression in older adults is the Geriatric Depression Scale (GDS; Yesavage *et al.* 1983). The GDS uses a 'forced-choice' yes–no response format, with 30-, 15-, 10-, and 4-item versions available (see Burns *et al.* 1999). The 15-item version has gained popularity given its brevity combined with good correlation with the full 30-items. The 30-item version includes questions on memory, concentration, decision-making, and clarity of mind, which therefore affects its validity as a depression measure for people with cognitive impairments. Perhaps the most well-known psychometric measure for depression is the Beck Depression

Inventory (BDI). The reliability of the full 21-item version has been demonstrated with older adults (Gallagher *et al.* 1982), and a 13-item short form has been devised (Foelker *et al.* 1987). However, use of the BDI with older adults has been criticized as it includes somatic elements and has a complex response format (choosing between four different statements for each item). Its use for measuring depression in people with dementia is not recommended (Wagle *et al.* 2000). The BDI has been substantially revised to form the BDI-II, which has yet to be fully validated in elderly populations. The Center for Epidemiological Studies depression scale (CES-D) is used widely in Europe, and it formed the basis of the measure used in the EURODEP studies. It has high sensitivity and specificity for depression screening in older adults (Beekman *et al.* 1997), but its properties as a measure of change are less well established. In a comparative investigation of psychometric measures for screening and detecting change, Boddington and colleagues (2000) concluded that the SelfCARE-D (Bird *et al.* 1987) and GDS-15 performed better than the BDI and visual analogue scales when compared to independent psychiatric screening using the ICD-10 diagnosis and rating of severity and the Montgomery Asberg Depression Rating Scale (MADRS). Informant rating scales for depression in people with dementia include the Cornell Scale (Alexopoulos *et al.* 1988) and the Depressive Signs Scale (Katona and Aldridge 1985).

Anxiety

Psychometric measures of anxiety have been developed more recently than those for depression. A brief measure devised specifically for use with physically ill people is the anxiety scale from the Hospital Anxiety and Depression Scale (HADS—Kenn *et al.* 1987; Flint and Rifat 1996). However, the psychometric properties of the seven anxiety items have not received as much attention as those for depression. Recently, the FEAR questionnaire has been developed as a rapid screening instrument for generalized anxiety in elders (Krasucki *et al.* 1999). A large number of specific measures have been developed for the key aspects of each anxiety diagnosis, but these have rarely been validated on older populations. The RAID is an example of an informant rating scale for anxiety symptoms in dementia (Shankar *et al.* 1999).

Well-being and quality of life

Although depression and anxiety reflect important aspects of (lack of) well-being, measures are being developed to evaluate aspects not confined to clinical disorders. For older people, 'life satisfaction' (e.g. Bigot 1974; Gilleard *et al.* 1981*a*) has traditionally been evaluated to assess adaptation and happiness with life. For people with moderate to severe dementia, well-being may be evaluated using direct observation methods such as Dementia Care Mapping (Kitwood and Bredin 1992) or the Positive Response Schedule (Perrin 1997), where this is appropriate (see below).

There is much activity in developing quality-of-life measures for people with dementia (Lawton 1997), with debate concerning definitions and methods (Rabins and Kasper 1997; Selai and Trimble 1999), and a number of scales appearing (Brod *et al.* 1999).

Caregiver well-being is often assessed using the General Health Questionnaire (GHQ) (Goldberg 1978), which has versions of different lengths including 60-, 30-, 28-, and 12-item questionnaires. Where the concern is to assess the specific impact of the caregiving, scales such as the Relatives Stress Scale (Agar *et al.* 1997; Greene *et al.* 1982) which address caregiving issues directly, may be preferred. Ramsay *et al.* (1995) provide a review of this area.

Behaviour

Two main approaches are commonly used for assessing behaviour and self-care. The first is to ask someone who knows the person well—a relative or careworker—to complete a rating scale according to that person's behaviour over a specified period. Numerous rating scales are available, varying greatly in scope, focus, and depth. Little and Doherty (1996) provide a detailed review of such scales. The second method is to observe the person directly, either in a structured situation or in his/her natural environment. The Structured Assessment of Independent Living Skills (SAILS) (Mahurin *et al.* 1991) is an example of the former approach; the Patient Behaviour Observation Instrument (Bowie and Mountain 1993), where observations are recorded on a hand-held computer, exemplifies the latter.

The choice of method and scale should be determined by the purpose of the assessment. Direct observation is most easily carried out in a residential home, ward environment, or a structured standardized setting, and is useful for commonly occurring behaviour, but it would be little use in assessing, say, aggressive behaviour occurring only two or three times a week (Brooker 1995). Rating scales may focus on the person's abilities and competence, or on behavioural problems, or may mix the two areas. Generally, it is more difficult to obtain reliable ratings from staff of problem behaviours than of the person's self-care ability, and it is good practice to ask staff to complete the scale in a small group, and to chart challenging behaviour which occurs infrequently.

Some scales have been devised especially for family members providing care at home to complete; these include the Problem Check List (Agar *et al.* 1997; Gilleard 1984) and the Behaviour and Mood Disturbance Scale (Greene *et al.* 1982).

Needs assessment

The identification of the person's unmet needs is an important aspect of devising an intervention plan. Several schedules are available to assist with this process, for example the Camberwell Assessment of Need for the Elderly (CANE—Reynolds *et al.* 2000) and the Care Needs Assessment Pack for Dementia (CARENAP-D—McWalter *et al.* 1998). The former is not dementia-specific. Both schedules allow assessment of the needs of carer alongside those of the patient.

Psychological therapies

Readers familiar with psychotherapeutic approaches used with younger adults will find that most of these have also been used with older adults. There are some psychological approaches devised specifically for older people, such as reminiscence and life review (Woods and McKiernan 1995; Schweitzer 1998), which exist as 'stand alone' therapies, as well as being used within integrative approaches such as cognitive behaviour therapy (CBT) and cognitive analytic therapy (CAT). Psychotherapeutic work may be individual- or group-based, with the latter offering an enjoyable and engaging opportunity to communicate and share experiences. Psychodynamic and family therapies will not be discussed in this chapter, as they are covered elsewhere in the volume.

Techniques vs. relationship

Psychological therapies often have clearly defined techniques and 'technologies'. To name but a few, CBT uses daily thought records, activity schedules, and behavioural experiments, and in CAT there are sequential diagrammatic formulations and 'goodbye' letters. There has been considerable debate about the relative benefits of different schools of psychotherapy for people of all ages, with a general recognition of the importance in all therapies of a good therapeutic relationship. Indeed, with the current generation of older adults 'being psychotherapeutic' may well be more important than 'doing psychotherapy', particularly with people with dementia (Cheston 1998). Good psychotherapeutic listening skills, being open to hearing the emotional significance of what the person says, having the ability to tune in to symbolic and metaphoric communication, and possessing the ability to be reflective with the person, will be invaluable in understanding more fully the emotional world of the person and their responses to events. Again, these skills are useful for treating people with dementia (Mills 1997) as well as for those who are cognitively intact.

Are adaptations necessary?

Adaptations to therapies are often suggested for use with older adults, but the adaptations are not made for age *per se*. Indeed, given the heterogeneity of the older adult population, it is possible for therapy to progress more smoothly and with greater success in some older adults than with some people of younger years. Adaptations are most likely to be necessary for individuals (irrespective of age) with one or more of the following: adverse life circumstances; cognitive impairment; sensory impairments; chronic illness or physical disabilities; dependency upon others or poor social networks; 'anti-therapy' beliefs; and, finally, chronic psychological difficulties or a poor coping history. Given that the majority of older adults referred to psychiatric services will have one or more of the above, common therapy adaptations are considered in more detail below.

Adversity

Changes in health (e.g. chronic physical or cognitive disabilities), in close relationships (e.g. bereavement, enforced shift from spouse to caregiver), and in wider social networks (e.g. relocation to a new community) are adverse life circumstances that often trigger referral to therapy services (Thompson 1996). Additional contributors to adverse circumstances include poverty and ageism in society.

Strategies for therapy in adverse life circumstances have been developed by clinicians working in the field of life-threatening illness. In cognitive therapy, for example, different strategies are used for realistic negative automatic thoughts (NATs) compared to NATs that contain biases and do not reflect the objective evidence. Realistic NATs are addressed either through the use of pragmatic strategies and/or more 'radical' strategies that follow from the identification of the underlying meaning of NATs (Liese and Larson 1995; Moorey 1997). Pragmatic strategies are those that help clients to accept thoughts and to develop appropriate coping skills. They may be either problem-focused (intended to make an impact upon the situation) or emotion-focused (intended to modulate a person's emotional response to the situation).

Patients' life circumstances can trigger a sense of helplessness and hopelessness in clinicians too, along with the belief that 'nothing can be done'. In an attempt to do something, clinicians may try to spot areas where change is possible and try to offer hope by giving advice and suggestions. However, unsolicited advice can exacerbate a sense in the client of being isolated and misunderstood. False hope, similar to false reassurance, offers short-lived relief, but in the longer term it damages the bond of trust between the clinician and patient. Therapy in adversity must therefore be compassionate towards the patient's circumstances, and achieve the difficult balance between hope and realism.

Cognitive impairment

To participate in any talking therapy where 'cognitive shifts' are the mechanism of change, the patient needs certain cognitive abilities. These include the ability to: attend, concentrate, encode and remember the spoken word; identify, differentiate and label emotions; access and verbally describe thoughts and images; integrate new learning and generalize from the specific to the general; take a 'meta-perspective' (i.e. think about the process of thinking) and think 'flexibly'. The greater the cognitive impairments of patients, the more flexible therapists must be in their approach to play to the patients' strengths or compensate for their disabilities. For example: demands on memory may need to be reduced; the patient may need to learn 'pretherapy' skills such as identifying and labelling emotions and thoughts, or 'decentering' so that different perspectives can be taken. Development of such adaptations is becoming increasingly important, given the increasing interest in offering psychological therapies for anxiety, depression, and adjustment to loss to people with dementia. Again, as an alternative to adaptation a clinician may choose to use behavioural strategies, such as relaxation, with the aim of bringing about physiological and behavioural change without cognitive mediation.

Physical health status

Sensory impairments and mobility problems must be taken into account as an individual enters therapy, but the presence of a disability does not necessarily make therapy less effective (Kemp *et al.* 1991/2). Rybarczyk and colleagues (1992) list six important elements in therapy for people with disability-related mood disorders, namely: resolve practical barriers to participation; accept depression as a separate and reversible problem; limit excess disability; counteract the loss of important social roles and autonomy; and challenge the perspective of being a 'burden'. Psychological approaches in medicine and surgery (Salmon 2000) are relevant to work with older people. For example, many older people experience painful arthritis; a psychological approach to coping and management has been shown to reduce depression and pain in people with this condition (Barlow *et al.* 1997). Psychological approaches can be used in addition to physical treatments, or at times when pharmacotherapy is limited due to potential adverse effects.

'Anti-therapy' beliefs

It has often been assumed that older adults prefer passively receiving medication to engaging in therapies involving active participation. Naturally, some people are rightly wary about becoming involved in an approach unfamiliar to them and their generation, but this does not equate to 'anti-therapy' beliefs. Reservations about psychological therapy may be due to: belief that the mind and body are wholly separate entities, and certainty that their condition is 'of the body'; the sense of hopelessness about the future commonly seen in depression; internalized ageist beliefs such as 'you can't teach an old dog new tricks'; a low sense of self-efficacy, combined with excessive trust in the power of the medical profession. On some occasions, choosing not to engage in therapy has been seen as a self-protective stance against re-exposure to regrets from the past. Hopelessness and ageist beliefs are barriers to therapy, and must be identified early on if therapy is to have any chance of success. Education about the interconnectedness of the mind and the body may be necessary, using for example the explanations for psychological involvement that are often used in pain clinics. (The explanation given is that seeing a psychologist does not mean that a person's physical symptomatology is considered to be 'all in the mind'. Rather, the reason for seeing the psychologist is that physical symptoms lead to psychological consequences such as worry, fear, depression, and anger and these emotions can trigger off further body sensations thus making the situation even more difficult. The psychological approach will take into account both the initial symptoms and the psychological reaction to them.)

Dependency upon others

Often it is not the older person who has made the request for referral to psychiatric services, but others who have prompted it. People who prompt their own referral are more likely to show preparedness to engage with services than those referred at others' request, where the referred individual has taken a passive role, accepting their dependency upon others, or where they are actively fighting against the other's control. It is important to bear in mind the role of family members and friends in both the support of the referred person, but also in the unwitting exacerbation of problems. When carrying out therapy with a 'disempowered' individual, it is not reasonable to expect them to have great influence upon more powerful others around them. In such cases, it may be appropriate to involve others in interventions, or indeed for others to become the 'target' of the intervention.

Chronicity of problems

The duration of presenting problems influences the goals of therapy for two reasons. First, the individual may have accepted the problems as part of their identity, e.g. 'I'm a depressive', and second, they may have a long history of previous interventions, many with poor outcome. The history of interventions, and the individual's view of these, becomes an important part of the assessment, as does identifying previously used ways of coping (successful or unsuccessful).

Conversely, an individual may have an identity as independent and able, following a life of success in both work and home life, and be struggling to adapt to disabilities and dependence. The loss of positive beliefs may be as instrumental in depression as the triggering of negative ones (James *et al.* 1999).

Stages of therapy

Various authors have identified stages of therapy, most typically including 'preparation', 'intervention', and 'termination' phases. The typical length of brief therapies with older adults is 16 to 20 one-hour sessions (Dick *et al.* 1996; Yost *et al.* 1986). The initial preparation or 'socialization' phase includes the establishment of trust and rapport between the client and therapist, sharing their expectations of the therapy, and determination of desired outcomes or goals. Developing collaboration between the therapist and client takes time and effort, especially in settings where the client expects and/or prefers the medical model of the professional as the 'expert' who prescribes interventions. This initial phase is important, and cannot be rushed. Premature attempts to move into the intervention phase (for example, offering an 'adaptive alternative' to a negative automatic thought during the assessment for cognitive therapy) are at best futile and at worst damaging to the relationship. The intervention phase is where the client and therapist work together to attain the goals. The content will depend upon the individual conceptualization and the therapeutic approach being used. The termination phase encompasses the preparation for ending therapy, and may include the use of relapse-prevention techniques.

Goals

Psychological therapies do not offer a 'cure' for physical illness, nor do they promise to change life situations since goals must be realistic for an individual's circumstances. However, appraisals of self-efficacy (perceived ability to cope) and control (perceived ability to influence one's current and future internal and external environment) have been shown to be important predictors of good outcome in both physical and mental health. Increasing an individual's sense of self-efficacy and control may become tasks of therapy (Krantz 1995). In addition, the concept of 'excess disability' offers a hopeful view on the potential for psychosocial interventions. By aiming to reduce excess disability while accepting a degree of 'unalterable disability', we can hope to improve quality of life for the older person, including people with dementia and their caregivers.

The goals of psychotherapy are less clear when individuals do not seem to have 'insight' into their difficulties, including people with dementia. The lack of insight might be seen as arising from defence mechanisms of denial and repression, and therefore an appropriate goal for psychotherapeutic intervention, or alternatively they may be taken to be an exclusion factor for psychological therapy. With those who have awareness and insight, the goal may be to assist the person come to terms with and adjust to the losses of ability and function.

Psychological treatment in dementia care

In a social psychological, person-centred approach, Kitwood (1997) argued that the clinical presentation of dementia is not simply a manifestation of neuropathological impairment, but the complex interaction for each individual of the social environment, personality and life experiences, physical health status, and even medication side-effects. Kitwood (1993) expressed this understanding of the variety of influences on the presentation of dementia in a simple equation:

$$D = P + B + H + NI + SP;$$

where: D = dementia; P = personality; B = biography; H = physical health; NI = neurological impairment; SP = social psychology.

In effect, the suggestion is that the person with dementia may well appear more impaired, or to have a more severe level of dementia than is necessitated by the actual neuropathological damage that has been sustained (i.e. they have excess disability). Kitwood's approach emphasizes the need for holistic assessment; in addition to assessing a person's cognitive function, there is a need for an understanding of his/her life story, preferences, interests, values, relationships, achievements, and disappointments. Furthermore, Kitwood draws our attention to the social environment surrounding the person, suggesting that often it can constitute a 'malignant social psychology', devaluing, diminishing, dehumanizing, and depersonalizing the person, leading to greater disability and dysfunction. Examples of a malignant social psychology would include infantilization, disempowerment, and objectification (Kitwood 1990). Kitwood showed how these features were everyday occurrences in most care settings, emphasizing that these were not generally the product of malicious abusive carers, but a flawed response arising from the limited skills and sensitivity that most of us exhibit in the presence of cognitive impairment.

Three broad areas of psychological approaches may be identified, emphasizing cognitive, emotional, or behavioural goals, and these will be considered in turn. In each case, current good practice is based on understanding and valuing the personhood of the person with dementia, and it aims to reduce the person's apparent excess disability.

Cognitive-based

There is a growth of interest in applying cognitive rehabilitation techniques to people with dementia (Camp *et al.* 1996; Arkin 1997; Clare *et al.* 1999). These approaches, using principles and methods derived from cognitive psychology, are proving helpful with people who have experienced other forms of brain trauma (Wilson 1989). These approaches may be seen as the successors to earlier, perhaps rather simplistic, cognitive retraining programmes, such as reality orientation (Holden and Woods 1995). Two major strategies may be considered (see also Woods 1996*b*) and are described below.

Reducing cognitive load

If cognitive demands can be reduced, retained abilities may be maximized. This may be achieved through environmental adaptations, such as careful and clear signposting, reducing the number of irrelevant and distracting sources of stimuli, and making use of familiar, well-learned associations wherever possible. A small homely unit, with a few, consistent staff, and many familiar items and possessions in the person's own room, will pose less cognitive demands than a large institution, with long corridors, many other residents, and a frequently changing staff group.

External memory aids also assist by reducing the need for effortful, self-initiated cognitive processes. Memory aids shown to be helpful in single-case studies include watches, diaries, and specially made booklets or wallets containing relevant pictures and information (Hanley and Lusty 1984; Bourgeois 1990, 1992). If such aids are to act as retrieval cues, they need to be placed so that the person will encounter the cue at the relevant time. Specific training is usually needed to ensure that cues will be regularly used by the person with dementia. In several studies where people with dementia have been trained to find locations in a hospital ward or nursing home, signposting alone had less impact than training to use the signposts and other landmarks in the environment (Hanley 1981; Gilleard *et al.* 1981*b*; Lam and Woods 1986).

Enhancing learning

Whilst learning is of course almost always impaired in dementia, some learning remains possible (see Miller and Morris 1993, pp. 113–15, for a summary of the relevant research). Indeed, rates of forgetting are relatively unimpaired after the first 10 minutes or so; if material can be adequately registered, retention is feasible. Several methods for assisting acquisition have been described:

- Spaced retrieval involves the learning of one item at a time, with the retrieval period being increased gradually each time the person correctly retrieves the item (Camp and Schaller 1989; McKitrick *et al.* 1992). The active process of retrieval is thought to be important in consolidating the memory for the item. If the person is unable to retrieve the item, they are prompted, and the retrieval interval is then reduced, before being built up once again. Camp *et al.* (1996) report the successful use of the spaced retrieval procedure in order to teach the person with dementia to make use of a memory aid (a calendar).

- Recently, attention has been drawn to the benefits of ensuring, as far as possible, that the learning proceeds without the person making errors; such errors often serve to interfere with effective learning, in that the person is likely to remember the error in competition with the correct response. Clare *et al.* (1999) describe the errorless learning procedure, where prompts are used to guide the person into giving the correct response, and guessing is discouraged.
- Procedural learning, where encoding proceeds through a motor act, or practice of a sequence of movements, has also been shown to be relatively intact in dementia (Bird and Kinsella 1996), and has been applied to enhancing the performance of everyday skills in several studies (e.g. Zanetti *et al.* 1997).

Emotion-based

Validation therapy (Feil 1993) has attracted wide use in dementia care. It is focused on the emotional communication of the person with dementia, in contrast to the cognitive emphasis of other approaches. The preliminary evidence for its effectiveness as a therapy 'package', is mixed (Toseland *et al.* 1997). However, as a communication approach it has much to commend it, as it enables care-staff to listen respectfully and sensitively to the feelings expressed. Confrontations regarding dates and times and chronology are avoided by responding to feelings rather than facts, and the importance of tailoring responses to the individual's characteristics is recognized. Feil draws attention to unresolved conflicts and trauma emerging in the midst of the dementia, surfacing in ways that are at first difficult to interpret and understand. Sometimes knowledge of the person's life story helps to piece together the drama being re-enacted. For example, it helps to know that the patient who becomes angry and aggressive when he encounters a locked door was once a prisoner-of-war. The importance of providing a safe, containing environment where strong emotions can be expressed and validated cannot be overemphasized if such individuals are to be helped.

Feil suggests that in the context of dementia, universal needs and longings emerge: the need for safety, to feel loved, to have purposeful activity, to have others to love and care for. Miesen (1992, 1993) describes the pattern of behaviour in which the person is frequently searching for a parent, talking about them as if alive, as 'parent fixation'. He explains this in terms of the person's need for a safe, secure attachment figure, in the midst of the puzzling, perplexing world of dementia. Bender and Cheston (1997) identify four 'discrete states' of emotional response in dementia: anxiety; depression; grief; and despair/terror. Solomon and Szwarbo (1992) have similarly drawn attention to issues of loss, anxiety, fear, and even terror, but they also highlight the high prevalence of anger and suspiciousness in the 86 patients they interviewed (58% and 35%, respectively). The range of powerful emotions present, and the lessened availability of socially acceptable means of expressing them, may be an important factor in the challenging behaviour seen in dementia.

Behavioural

It is the non-cognitive features of dementia that are experienced as most taxing and stressful by families and careworkers (Donaldson *et al.* 1998). Some of these features are clearly related to the person's emotional state, mood, and anxiety. Hope *et al.* (1997) suggest there are three distinct behavioural syndromes in dementia: overactivity (including aimless walking); aggressive behaviour; and psychosis (hallucinations, persecutory ideas, and extreme anxiety). However, the elaboration of typologies of, say, wandering (Hope and Fairburn 1990), aggression (Stokes 1989; Ware *et al.* 1990), and sexual problems (Haddad and Benbow 1993) support the need for a multifactorial understanding of such difficulties. For instance, two people may both be said to 'wander', but the actual behaviour and its function may be quite different.

Challenging behaviour is seen psychologically as an expression of an unmet or poorly communicated need (Stokes 1996). The person's learned, sophisticated means of meeting basic needs are damaged by the dementia, exposing a 'dysfunctional and at times grotesque distortion of goal-directed communication and conduct' (Stokes 1996, pp. 616). Thus aggression occurs most often during intimate care, when plausibly the person feels most vulnerable and threatened; shouting out may reflect a physical pain that cannot be adequately communicated, or a need for contact by the person who feels abandoned and desolate when familiar others are not in view; wandering may, for some, reflect a search for something or someone familiar and safe, in a place that appears strange and frightening. Magai and Cohen (1998) have shown an association between behavioural disturbance and the person with dementia having been rated (by a family carer) as having had a longstanding insecure attachment style. This provides further support for the notion that in dementia we see the person's raw attempts to remain safe and secure, stripped of the layers of socialization that normally surrounds all our attempts at 'attention seeking'.

There remains a tendency for difficult behaviour to be seen as a property of the person with dementia, rather than as arising in interaction with the care environment. Thus, difficult behaviour is seen as leading to increased carer strain (e.g. Donaldson *et al.* 1997). The inter-relationship between carer strain and challenging behaviour might better be seen as a dynamic process; a carer under strain may be much more critical of the person with dementia (Bledin *et al.* 1990) and have less adaptive coping mechanisms; the person with dementia may respond to negative interactions with greater anxiety or agitation; this may lead to further strain in the caregiver; so the cycle continues. Carer strain changes the emotional climate for the person with dementia too, and they may well respond to a negative atmosphere with behaviour that is viewed as challenging.

In the residential context, interventions for challenging behaviour may be viewed as successful where staff perceive the behaviour as less difficult to manage, even if its frequency does not change (Moniz-Cook *et al.* 1998). The factors which cause staff to find behaviour more challenging include their own anxiety, as well as features of the home environment (Moniz-Cook *et al.* 2000). Again, challenging behaviour is, in part, related to the perception, appraisal, and approach of the caregiver. The detailed observational approach developed by Kitwood, Dementia Care Mapping (Kitwood and Bredin 1992), is useful in helping staff to see more clearly the perspective of the individual person with dementia, and to recognize that what at first seems a behaviour problem is actually a response to the strange, puzzling, and sometimes frightening situation in which the person finds him/herself.

The psychological approach to challenging behaviour in dementia (see Woods and Bird 1999) is based on careful, individualized assessment of the person's cognitive function, style of coping, life story, and social network, together with these key questions:

- What areas are presenting difficulty or distress to the patient or caregivers?
- Is the person's behaviour causing distress? (If not, leave well alone.)
- What is the patient actually doing, when, and under what circumstances?
- Why might the patient be behaving in this way? What aspects of the person's physical condition or the environment may be contributing?
- What can realistically be changed? If the distress arising from the behaviour is not to the patient but to others, then their reactions might be the target for change, rather than the behaviour *per se*.

An individualized intervention plan may be devised from such an assessment, using, where appropriate, cues to prompt more appropriate and adaptive behaviour (Bird *et al.* 1995).

The evidence-base for psychological interventions in late life

Psychological treatments for older adults are gradually being empirically tested (Woods and Roth 1996). Using the criteria developed by the American Psychological Association Division of Clinical Psychology (APA DCP), Gatz and colleagues (1998) concluded that:

- behavioural and environmental treatments for behaviour problems in dementia patients are 'well-established', and that:
- cognitive, behavioural, and brief psychodynamic therapies for depression are 'probably efficacious', as are:
- life review for individuals with symptoms of depression or living in settings that restrict independence; and
- CBT for sleep disorders; support for carers based upon a psychoeducational model; and, memory and cognitive retraining for dementia patients.

Reviews of psychosocial treatments for depression have identified benefits (Scogin and McElreath 1994; Koder *et al.* 1996; O'Rourke and Hadjistavropoulous 1997; McCusker *et al.* 1998), even with the physically ill (Draper 2000). Cognitive behavioural approaches are particularly suited to research trials. For example, in a review of the literature up to 1994, Koder *et al.* (1996) identified 18 papers about cognitive therapy for depression in older adults, seven of which contained outcome data; and Gatz and colleagues (1998) identified 11 studies that met the APA DCP criteria. Dolores Gallagher-Thompson's and Larry Thompson's team have produced a substantial body of work using pleasant-activity scheduling and thought challenging with depressed older adults and depressed caregivers (see Thompson 1996 for a review). Maintenance interpersonal psychotherapy has recently been shown to be effective in reducing the risk of relapse in older people who have recovered from depression, especially when used in combination with medication (Reynolds *et al.* 1999). Problems of anxiety have been targeted in far fewer trials, but clinical reports suggest cognitive–behavioural therapy (CBT) is just as effective as with younger people (e.g. King and Barrowclough 1991).

The body of literature on psychotherapeutic work with people with dementia is growing (see Cheston 1998 for a review), and outcome measures are now being included in treatment trials (Kipling *et al.* 1999). Techniques include progressive muscle relaxation (which can be learned through procedural learning) (Suhr *et al.* 1999) and increasing pleasurable life events (Thompson *et al.* 1990; Teri and Uomoto 1991; Teri *et al.* 1997). Indeed, Teri and colleagues (1997) demonstrated that their approach of training family caregivers to manage depression in the person with dementia resulted in improvements in mood for both the people with dementia and their caregivers.

There has been some controversy regarding the use of cognitive retraining approaches in dementia. Efforts to reduce the cognitive load, to target the person's resources on areas of importance to him/her, to provide an environment where intact memory function is less important, will be of benefit to most people with dementia. Questions are raised regarding the more intensive memory programmes described, for example by Arkin (1997) or Clare *et al.* (1999). These programmes inevitably draw attention to the memory deficit, and require a shared understanding that such a problem exists, and that the person wishes to work to improve their memory function. Even in the early stages of dementia, it is not yet clear what proportion of patients would be able and willing to focus on their memory difficulties in this way. Anxiety regarding the difficulties may in fact interfere with the learning process—in the study reported by Josephsson *et al.* (1993), the failure of one of the four people with dementia to show learning was attributed to high levels of anxiety. Even where the person is keen to proceed with memory exercises, this may serve as a way of coping with intense fears and anxieties, which, in the authors' clinical experience, may surface in frustration with the cognitive exercises. The American Psychiatric Association's Practice Guideline (1997) for the treatment of patients with dementia draws attention to case reports of anger, frustration, and depression, and concludes: 'Cognition-oriented treatments...are unlikely to be beneficial...and do not appear to warrant the risk of adverse events'. Some of the concerns arise from the well-documented misuse of reality orientation (RO) (Dietch *et al.* 1989), and do serve to reinforce the importance of a sensitive, individualized, person-centred approach to cognitive rehabilitation (Holden and Woods 1995). In fact, the evidence for the effectiveness of reality orientation, in achieving improvements in verbal orientation and in behavioural function, is relatively well established (Spector *et al.* 2000). The fall from favour of RO related more to the attempts to apply it in a standardized (and too often patronizing) way to all patients, without individualizing its application so that the goals of intervention would be relevant and important to the person receiving it.

The evidence-base for other dementia-care approaches is less well established, with very few good trials available of reminiscence or validation approaches, despite their wide use in dementia care. The success of behavioural approaches, noted by Gatz *et al.* (1998) is mainly in series of single- cases, and more substantial work is also required in demonstrating how these approaches may be applied to a wider range of patients and difficulties. Thus, while there is considerable scope for evidence-based practice in this area, there is a need for further development of approaches and evaluations that reflect, as far as possible, the realities of clinical practice, where interventions must be devised that meet complex individual needs, and where the context of care often exerts a significant influence on outcome.

References

Agar, S., Moniz-Cook, E., Orbell, S., Elston, C., and Wang, M. (1997). Measuring the outcome of psychosocial intervention for family caregivers of dementia sufferers: a factor analytic study. *Aging and Mental Health*, **1**, 166–75.

Alexopoulos, G. S., Abrams, R. C., Young, R. C., and Shamoian, C. A. (1988). Cornell Scale for Depression in Dementia. *Biological Psychiatry*, **23**, 271–84.

American Psychiatric Association (1997). Practice guideline for the treatment of patients with Alzheimer's disease and other dementias of late life. *American Journal of Psychiatry*, **154**(5 Suppl.), 1–39.

Arkin, S. M. (1997). Alzheimer memory training: quizzes beat repetition, especially with more impaired. *American Journal of Alzheimer's Disease*, **12**, 147–58.

Barlow, J. H., Williams, B., and Wright, C. C. (1997). Improving arthritis self-management among older adults: 'Just what the doctor didn't order'. *British Journal of Health Psychology*, **2**, 175–86.

Beekman, A. T., Deeg, D. J., van Limbeek, J., *et al.* (1997). Criterion validity of the Center for Epidemiologic Studies Depression Scale (CES-D): results from a community-based sample of older subjects in the Netherlands. *Psychological Medicine*, **27**, 231–5.

Bender, M. P. and Cheston, R. (1997). Inhabitants of a lost kingdom: a model for the subjective experiences of dementia. *Ageing and Society*, **17**, 513–32.

Bigot, A. (1974). The relevance of American life satisfaction indices for research on British subjects before and after retirement. *Age and Ageing*, **3**, 113–21.

Bird, M. and Kinsella, G. (1996). Long-term cued recall of tasks in senile dementia. *Psychology and Aging*, **11**, 45–56.

Bird, A. S., Macdonald, A. J. D., Mann, A. H., and Philpot, M. P. (1987). Preliminary experience with the SELFCARE (D): a self-rating depression questionnaire for use in elderly, non-institutionalized subjects. *International Journal of Geriatric Psychiatry*, **2**, 31–8.

Bird, M., Alexopoulos, P., and Adamowicz, J. (1995). Success and failure in five case studies: use of cued recall to ameliorate behaviour problems in senile dementia. *International Journal of Geriatric Psychiatry*, **10**, 305–11.

Bledin, K., MacCarthy, B., Kuipers, L., and Woods, R. T. (1990). Daughters of people with dementia: expressed emotion, strain and coping. *British Journal of Psychiatry*, **157**, 221–7.

Boddington, S., Krasuki, C., and Cook, J. (2000). To BDI or GDS: which depression rating scale to use with older people? Paper presented at the *PSIGE Annual conference*, Birmingham July 2000.

Bourgeois, M. S. (1990). Enhancing conversation skills in patients with Alzheimer's disease using a prosthetic memory aid. *Journal of Applied Behavior Analysis*, **23**, 29–42.

Bourgeois, M. S. (1992). *Conversing with memory impaired individuals using memory aids: a memory aid workbook*. Winslow Press, Bicester, Oxford.

Bowie, P. and Mountain, G. (1993). Using direct observation to record the behaviour of long-stay patients with dementia. *International Journal of Geriatric Psychiatry*, **8**, 857–64.

Brod, M., Stewart, A. L., Sands, L., and Walton, P. (1999). Conceptualization and measurement of quality of life in dementia: the dementia quality of life instrument (DQoL). *Gerontologist*, **39**, 25–35.

Brooker, D. J. R. (1995). Looking at them, looking at me; a review of observational studies into the quality of institutional care for elderly people with dementia. *Journal of Mental Health*, **4**, 145–56.

Burns, A., Lawlor, B., and Craig, S. (1999). *Assessment scales in old age psychiatry*. Martin Dunitz, London.

Camp, C. J. and Schaller, J. R. (1989). Epilogue: spaced-retrieval memory training in an adult day-care center. *Educational Gerontology*, **15**, 641–8.

Camp, C. J., Foss, J. W., O'Hanlon, A. M., and Stevens, A. B. (1996). Memory interventions for persons with dementia. *Applied Cognitive Psychology*, **10**, 193–210.

Cheston, R. (1998). Psychotherapeutic work with people with dementia: a review of the literature. *British Journal of Medical Psychology*, **71**, 211–31.

Clare, L., Wilson, B. A., Breen, K., and Hodges, J. R. (1999). Errorless learning of face–name associations in early Alzheimer's disease. *Neurocase*, **5**, 37–46.

Crawford, J. R., Stewart, L. E., Cochrane, R. H. B., Foulds, J. A., Besson, J. A. O., and Parker, D. M. (1989). Estimating premorbid IQ from demographic variables: regression equations derived from a UK sample. *British Journal of Clinical Psychology*, **28**, 275–8.

Crawford, J. R., Venneri, A., and O'Carroll, R. E. (1998). Neuropsychological assessment of the elderly. In *Comprehensive clinical psychology: geropsychology* (ed. B. Edelstein), pp. 133–69. Elsevier, New York.

Dick, L. P., Gallagher-Thompson, D., and Thompson, L. W. (1996). Cognitive-behavioral therapy. In *Handbook of the clinical psychology of aging* (ed. R. T. Woods), pp. 509–44. Wiley, Chichester.

Dietch, J. T., Hewett, L. J., and Jones, S. (1989). Adverse effects of reality orientation. *Journal of the American Geriatrics Society*, **37**, 974–6.

Donaldson, C., Tarrier, N., and Burns, A. (1997). The impact of the symptoms of dementia on caregivers. *British Journal of Psychiatry*, **170**, 62–8.

Donaldson, C., Tarrier, N., and Burns, A. (1998). Determinants of carer stress in Alzheimer's disease. *International Journal of Geriatric Psychiatry*, **13**, 248–56.

Draper, B. M. (2000). The effectiveness of the treatment of depression in the physically ill elderly. *Aging and Mental Health*, **4**, 9–20.

Feil, N. (1993). *The Validation breakthrough: simple techniques for communicating with people with 'Alzheimer's type dementia'*. Health Professions Press, Baltimore, MD.

Flint, A. J. and Rifat, S. L. (1996). Validation of the Hospital Anxiety and Depression Scale as a measure of severity of geriatric depression. *International Journal of Geriatric Psychiatry*, **11**, 991–4.

Foelker, G. A., Shewchuk, R. M., and Niederehe, G. (1987). Confirmatory factor analysis of the short form Beck Depression Inventory in elderly community samples. *Journal of Clinical Psychology*, **43**, 111–18.

Folstein, M. F., Folstein, S. E., and McHugh, P. R. (1975). 'Mini Mental State': a practical method for grading the cognitive state of patients for the clinician. *Journal of Psychiatric Research*, **12**, 189–98.

Gallagher, D., Nies, G., and Thompson, L. W. (1982). Reliability of the Beck Depression Inventory with older adults. *Journal of Consulting and Clinical Psychology*, **50**, 152–3.

Gatz, M., Fiske, A., Fox, L. S., Kaskie, B., Kasl-Godley, J. E., McCallum, T. J., *et al.* (1998). Empirically validated psychological treatments for older adults. *Journal of Mental Health and Aging*, **4**, 1–45.

Gilleard, C. J. (1984). *Living with dementia*. Croom Helm, Beckenham.

Gilleard, C. J., Willmott, M., and Vaddadik, S. (1981*a*). Self report measures of mood and morale in elderly depressives. *British Journal of Psychiatry*, **138**, 230–5.

Gilleard, C., Mitchell, R. G., and Riordan, J. (1981*b*). Ward orientation training with psychogeriatric patients. *Journal of Advanced Nursing*, **6**, 95–8.

Goldberg, D. (1978). *Manual of the General Health Questionnaire*. NFER-Nelson, Windsor.

Golding, E. (1989). *Middlesex Elderly Assessment of Mental State*. Thames Valley Test Company, Titchfield, Hampshire.

Greene, J. G., Smith, R., Gardiner, M., and Timbury, G. C. (1982). Measuring behavioural disturbance of elderly demented patients in the community and its effect on relatives: a factor analytic study. *Age and Ageing*, **11**, 121–6.

Haddad, P. M. and Benbow, S. M. (1993). Sexual problems associated with dementia: Part 1: problems and their consequences. *International Journal of Geriatric Psychiatry*, **8**, 547–51.

Hanley, I. G. (1981). The use of signposts and active training to modify ward disorientation in elderly patients. *Journal of Behaviour Therapy and Experimental Psychiatry*, **12**, 241–7.

Hanley, I. G. and Lusty, K. (1984). Memory aids in reality orientation: a single-case study. *Behaviour Research and Therapy*, **22**, 709–12.

Holden, U. P. and Woods, R. T. (1995). Positive approaches to dementia care (3rd edn). Churchill Livingstone, Edinburgh.

Hope, R. A. and Fairburn, C. G. (1990). The nature of wandering in dementia: a community-based study. *International Journal of Geriatric Psychiatry*, **5**, 239–45.

Hope, T., Keene, J., Fairburn, C., McShane, R., and Jacoby, R. (1997). Behaviour changes in dementia—2: are there behavioural syndromes? *International Journal of Geriatric Psychiatry*, **12**, 1074–8.

Husband, H. J. (1999). The psychological consequences of learning a diagnosis of dementia: three case examples. *Aging and Mental Health*, **3**, 179–83.

James, I. A., Kendell, K., and Reichelt, F. K. (1999). Conceptualizations of depression in older people: the interaction of positive and negative beliefs. *Behavioural and Cognitive Psychotherapy*, **27**, 285–90.

Jorm, A. F., Scott, R., and Jacomb, P. (1989). Assessment of cognitive decline in dementia by informant questionnaire. *International Journal of Geriatric Psychiatry*, **4**, 35–9.

Josephsson, S., Backman, L., Borell, L., Bernspang, B., Nygard, L., and Ronnberg, L. (1993). Supporting everyday activities in dementia: an intervention study. *International Journal of Geriatric Psychiatry*, **8**, 395–400.

Katona, C. L. E. and Aldridge, C. R. (1985). The dexamethasone suppression test and depressive signs in dementia. *Journal of Affective Disorders*, **8**, 83–9.

Kemp, B. J., Corgiat, M., and Gill, C. (1991/2). Effects of brief cognitive-behavioral group psychotherapy on older persons with and without disabling illness. *Behavior, Health and Aging*, **2**, 21–8.

Kenn, C., Wood, H., Kucyj, M., Wattis, J. P., and Cunane, J. (1987). Validation of the Hospital Anxiety and Depression Rating Scale (HADS) in an elderly psychiatric population. *International Journal of Geriatric Psychiatry*, **2**, 189–93.

King, P. and Barrowclough, C. (1991). A clinical pilot study of cognitive-behavioural therapy for anxiety disorders in the elderly. *Behavioural Psychotherapy*, **19**, 337–45.

Kipling, T., Bailey, M., and Charlesworth, G. (1999). The feasibility of a cognitive behavioral therapy group for men with mild/moderate cognitive impairment. *Behavioural and Cognitive Psychotherapy*, **27**, 189–93.

Kitwood, T. (1990). The dialectics of dementia: with particular reference to Alzheimer's disease. *Ageing and Society*, **10**, 177–6.

Kitwood, T. (1993). Towards a theory of dementia care: the interpersonal process. *Ageing and Society*, **13**, 51–67.

Kitwood, T. (1997). *Dementia reconsidered: the person comes first.* Open University Press, Bucks.

Kitwood, T. and Bredin, K. (1992). A new approach to the evaluation of dementia care. *Journal of Advances in Health and Nursing Care*, **1**, 41–60.

Koder, D. A., Brodaty, H., and Anstey, K. J. (1996). Cognitive therapy for depression in the elderly. *International Journal of Geriatric Psychiatry*, **11**, 97–107.

Krantz, S. E. (1995). Chronic physical disability and secondary control: appraisals of an undesirable situation. *Journal of Cognitive Psychotherapy*, **9**, 229–48.

Krasucki, C., Ryan, P., Ertan, T., Howard, R., Lindesay, J., and Mann, A. (1999). The FEAR: a rapid screening instrument for generalised anxiety in elderly primary care attenders. *International Journal of Geriatric Psychiatry*, **14**, 60–8.

Lam, D. H. and Woods, R. T. (1986). Ward orientation training in dementia: a single-case study. *International Journal of Geriatric Psychiatry*, **1**, 145–7.

Lawton, M. P. (1997). Assessing quality of life in Alzheimer disease research. *Alzheimer Disease and Associated Disorders*, **11**(Suppl. 3), 91–9.

Liese, B. S. and Larson, M. W. (1995) Coping with life-threatening illness: a cognitive therapy perspective. *Journal of Cognitive Psychotherapy*, **9**, 19–34.

Little, A. and Doherty, B. (1996). Going beyond cognitive assessment: assessment of adjustment, behaviour and the environment. In *Handbook of the clinical psychology of ageing* (ed. R. T. Woods), pp. 475–506. Wiley, Chichester.

McCusker, J., Cole, M., Keller, E., Bellavance, F., and Berard, A. (1998). Effectiveness of treatments of depression in older ambulatory patients. *Archives of Internal Medicine*, **158**, 705–12.

McKitrick, L. A., Camp, C. J., and Black, F. W. (1992). Prospective memory intervention in Alzheimer's disease. *Journal of Gerontology*, **47**, P337–P343.

McWalter, G., Toner, H., McWalter, A., Eastwood, J., Marshall, M., and Turvey, T. (1998). A community needs assessment: the Care Needs Assessment Pack for Dementia (Carenap-D)—its development, reliability and validity. *International Journal of Geriatric Psychiatry*, **13**, 16–22.

Magai, C. and Cohen, C. I. (1998). Attachment style and emotion regulation in dementia patients and their relation to caregiver burden. *Journal of Gerontology*, **53B**, P147–P154.

Mahurin, R. K., DeBettignies, B. H., and Pirozzolo, F. J. (1991). Structured assessment of independent living skills: preliminary report of a performance measure of functional abilities in dementia. *Journal of Gerontology*, **46**, P58–66.

Miesen, B. M. L. (1992). Attachment theory and dementia. In *Care-giving in dementia* (ed. G. Jones and B. M. L. Miesen), pp. 38–56. Routledge, London.

Miesen, B. M. L. (1993). Alzheimer's disease, the phenomenon of parent fixation and Bowlby's attachment theory. *International Journal of Geriatric Psychiatry*, **8**, 147–53.

Miller, E. and Morris, R. (1993). *The psychology of dementia.* Wiley, Chichester.

Mills, M. A. (1997). Narrative identity and dementia: a study of emotion and narrative in older people with dementia. *Ageing and Society*, **17**, 673–98.

Moniz-Cook, E., Agar, S., Silver, M., Woods, R., Wang, M., Elston, C., *et al.* (1998). Can staff training reduce behavioural problems in residential care for the elderly mentally ill? *International Journal of Geriatric Psychiatry*, **13**, 149–58.

Moniz-Cook, E., Woods, R., and Gardiner, E. (2000). Staff factors associated with perception of behaviour as 'challenging' in residential and nursing homes. *Aging and Mental Health*, 4, 48–55.

Moorey, S. (1997). When bad things happen to rational people: cognitive therapy in adverse life circumstances. In *Frontiers of cognitive therapy* (ed. P. Salkovskis), pp. 450–69. Guilford Press, New York.

Mozley, C. G., Huxley, P., Sutcliffe, C., Bagley, H., Burns, A., Challis, D., *et al.* (1999). 'Not knowing where I am doesn't mean I don't know what I like': cognitive impairment and quality of life responses in elderly people. *International Journal of Geriatric Psychiatry*, **14**, 776–83.

Nelson, H. E. and Willison, J. (1991). *National Adult Reading Test: test manual.* NFER-Nelson, Windsor.

O'Rourke, N. and Hadjistavropoulos, T. (1997). The relative efficacy of psychotherapy in treatment of geriatric depression. *Aging and Mental Health*, **1**, 305–10.

Orrell, M., Howard, R., Payne, A., Bergmann, K., Woods, R., Everitt, B. S., *et al.* (1992). Differentiation between organic and functional psychiatric illness in the elderly: an evaluation of four cognitive tests. *International Journal of Geriatric Psychiatry*, 7, 263–75.

Perrin, T. (1997). The positive response schedule for severe dementia. *Aging and Mental Health*, **1**, 184–91.

Rabins, P. V. and Kasper, J. D. (1997). Measuring quality of life in dementia: conceptual and practical issues. *Alzheimer Disease and Associated Disorders*, **11**(Suppl. 3), 100–4.

Ramsay, M., Winget, C., and Higginson, I. (1995). Review: measures to determine the outcome of community services for people with dementia. *Age and Ageing*, **24**, 73–83.

Reynolds, C., Frank, E., Perel, J. M., Imber, S. D., Cornes, C. and Miller, M. D. (1999). Nortriptyline and interpersonal psychotherapy as maintenance therapies for recurrent major depression: a randomized controlled trial in patients older than 59 years. *Journal of the American Medical Association*, **281**, 39–45.

Reynolds, T., Thornicroft, G., Abas, M., Woods, B., Hoe, J., Leese, M., *et al.* (2000). Camberwell Assessment of Need for the Elderly (CANE)—development, validity and reliability. *British Journal of Psychiatry*, **176**, 444–52.

Rice, K. and Warner, N. (1994). Breaking the bad news: what do psychiatrists tell patients with dementia about their illness? *International Journal of Geriatric Psychiatry*, **9**, 467–71.

Roth, M., Huppert, F. A., Tym, E., and Mountjoy, C. Q. (1988). *CAMDEX—Cambridge examination for mental disorders of the elderly*. Cambridge University Press, Cambridge.

Rybarczyk, B., Gallagher-Thompson, D., Rodman, J., Zeiss, A., Gantz, F. E., and Yesavage, J. (1992). Applying cognitive-behavioral psychotherapy to the chronically-ill elderly: treatment issues and case illustration. *International Psychogeriatrics*, **4**, 127–40.

Salmon, P. (2000). *Psychology of medicine and surgery—a guide for psychologists, counselors, nurses and doctors*. Wiley, Chichester.

Schaie, K. W. (1990). Intellectual development in adulthood. In *Handbook of the psychology of aging* (3rd edn) (ed. J. E. Birren and K. W. Schaie), pp. 291–309. Academic Press, San Diego.

Scogin, F. and McElreath, L. (1994). Efficacy of psychosocial treatments for geriatric depression: a quantitative review. *Journal of Consulting and Clinical Psychology*, **62**, 69–74.

Schweitzer, P. (ed.) (1998). *Reminiscence in dementia care*. Age Exchange, London.

Selai, C. and Trimble, M. R. (1999). Assessing quality of life in dementia. *Aging and Mental Health*, **3**, 101–11.

Shankar, K. K., Walker, M., Frost, D., and Orrell, M. W. (1999). The development of a valid and reliable scale for rating anxiety in dementia (RAID). *Aging and Mental Health*, **3**, 39–49.

Solomon, K. and Szwarbo, P. (1992). Psychotherapy for patients with dementia. In *Memory function and aging-related disorders* (ed. J. E. Morley, R. M. Coe, R. Strong, and G. T. Grossberg), pp. 295–319. Springer, New York.

Spector, A., Davies, S., Woods, B., and Orrell, M. (2000). Reality orientation for dementia: a systematic review of the evidence for its effectiveness. *Gerontologist*, **40**, 206–12.

Stokes, G. (1989). Managing aggression in dementia: the do's and don'ts. *Geriatric Medicine* (April), 35–40.

Stokes, G. (1996). Challenging behaviour in dementia: a psychological approach. In *Handbook of the clinical psychology of ageing* (ed. R. T. Woods), pp. 601–28. Wiley, Chichester.

Suhr, J., Anderson, S., and Tranel, D. (1999). Progressive muscle relaxation in the management of behavioural disturbance in Alzheimer's disease. *Neuropsychological Rehabilitation*, **9**, 31–44.

Teri, L. and Truax, P. (1994). Assessment of depression in dementia patients: association of caregiver mood with depression ratings. *Gerontologist*, **34**, 231–4.

Teri, L. and Uomoto, J. M. (1991). Reducing excess disability in dementia patients: training caregivers to manage patient depression. *Clinical Gerontologist*, **10**, 49–63.

Teri, L., Logsdon, R. G., Uomoto, J., and McCurry, S. M. (1997). Behavioral treatment of depression in dementia patients: a controlled clinical trial. *Journal of Gerontology*, **52B**, P159–P166.

Thompson, L. W. (1996). Cognitive-behavioral therapy and treatment for late-life depression. *Journal of Clinical Psychiatry*, **57**(Suppl. 5), 29–37.

Thompson, L. W., Wagner, B., Zeiss, A., and Gallagher, D. (1990). Cognitive/behavioural therapy with early stage Alzheimer's patients: an exploratory view of the utility of this approach. In *Alzheimer's disease: treatment and family stress* (ed. E. Light and B. D. Lebowitz), pp. 383–97. Hemisphere, New York.

Toseland, R. W., Diehl, M., Freeman, K., Manzanares, T., and McCallion, P. (1997). The impact of validation group therapy on nursing home residents with dementia. *Journal of Applied Gerontology*, **16**, 31–50.

Wagle, A. C., Ho, L. W., Wagle, S. A., and Berrios, G. E. (2000). Psychometric behaviour of the BDI in Alzheimer's disease patients with depression. *International Journal of Geriatric Psychiatry*, **15**, 63–9.

Ware, C. J. G., Fairburn, C. G., and Hope, R. A. (1990). A community based study of aggressive behaviour in dementia. *International Journal of Geriatric Psychiatry*, **5**, 337–42.

Wilson, B. A. (1989). Designing memory-therapy programmes. In *Everyday cognition in adulthood and late life* (ed. L. W. Poon, D. C. Rubin, and B. A. Wilson), pp. 615–38. Cambridge University Press, Cambridge.

Woods, R. T. (ed.) (1996*a*). *Handbook of the clinical psychology of ageing*. Wiley, Chichester.

Woods, R. T. (1996*b*). Cognitive approaches to the management of dementia. In *The cognitive neuropsychology of Alzheimer-type dementia* (ed. R. G. Morris), pp. 310–26. Oxford University Press, Oxford.

Woods, R. T. (ed.) (1999*a*). *Psychological problems of ageing: assessment, treatment and care*. Wiley, Chichester.

Woods, R. T. (1999*b*). Psychological assessment of older people. In *Psychological problems of ageing: assessment, treatment and care* (ed. R. T. Woods), pp. 219–52. Wiley, Chichester.

Woods, R. T. and Bird, M. (1999). Non-pharmacological approaches to treatment. In *Diagnosis and management of dementia: a manual for memory disorders teams* (ed.

G. Wilcock, K. Rockwood, and R. Bucks), pp. 311–331. Oxford University Press, Oxford.

Woods, R. T. and McKiernan, F. (1995). Evaluating the impact of reminiscence on older people with dementia. In *The art and science of reminiscing: theory, research, methods and applications* (ed. B. K. Haight and J. Webster), pp. 233–42. Taylor and Francis, Washington DC.

Woods, R. T. and Roth, A. (1996). Effectiveness of psychological interventions with older people. In *What works for whom? A critical review of psychotherapy research* (ed. A. Roth and P. Fonagy), pp. 321–40. Guilford Press, New York.

Yesavage, J. A., Brink, T. L., and Rose, T. L. (1983). Development and validation of a geriatric depression scale: a preliminary report. *Journal of Psychiatric Research*, **17**, 37–49.

Yost, E. B., Beutler L. E., Corbishley, M. A., and Allender J. R. (1986). *Group cognitive therapy: a treatment approach for depressed older adults*. Pergamon Press, New York.

Zanetti, O., Binetti, G., Magni, E., Rozzini, L., Bianchetti, A., and Trabucchi, M. (1997). Procedural memory stimulation in Alzheimer's disease: impact of a training programme. *Acta Neurologica Scandinavica*, **95**, 152–7.

12 Neuroimaging in the elderly: radiological and electrophysiological tools and findings

Hans Förstl and Frank Hentschel

Age-related changes

Brain morphology changes during the normal ageing process. Morphological imaging with computed tomography (CT) and magnetic resonance imaging (MRI) shows an increase of the intracranial cerebrospinal fluid (CSF) space, which is accentuated after the age of 50. In contrast to clearly disease-related alterations, these age-related changes are not focally accentuated. Ventricular volume increases by 0.3 ml/year, subarachnoidal volumes by 0.6 ml/year. Cortical grey matter density declines after 60 years of age (polioaraiosis), and the grey to white matter volume ratio increases. White matter changes (leucoaraiosis or white matter lesions, WML) are associated not only with cortical atrophy and age, but also with stroke, myocardial infarction, fibrinogen, factor VIIIa activity, hypertension, and blood cholesterol concentration. Mild impairment of cognitive performance in non-demented individuals is correlated with white matter lesions and cortical atrophy including hippocampal atrophy. Coronal or transversal MRI sections offer an excellent view of the hippocampus (Figs 12.1(a)–(d)). The best results are obtained when the gantry is tilted according to the course of the optic nerves at an angle of 20° negative to the canthomeatal line along the hippocampal axial lane.

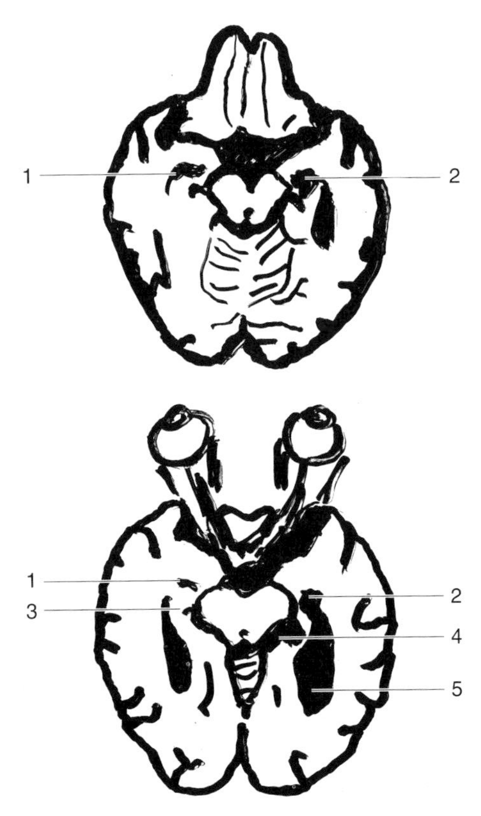

Fig. 12a Transverse.

Sketches of radiological anatomy seen on CT and MRI scans.

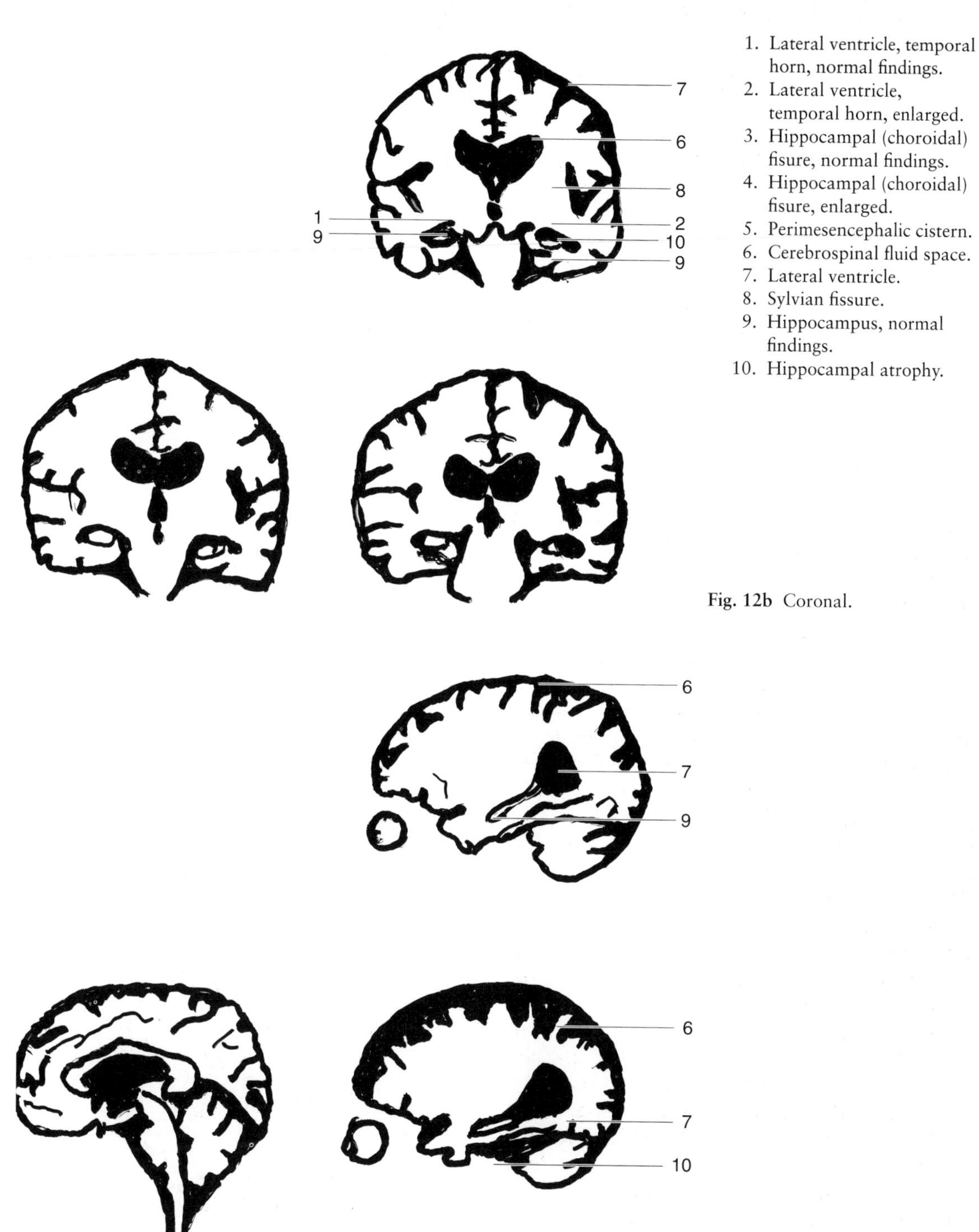

1. Lateral ventricle, temporal horn, normal findings.
2. Lateral ventricle, temporal horn, enlarged.
3. Hippocampal (choroidal) fisure, normal findings.
4. Hippocampal (choroidal) fisure, enlarged.
5. Perimesencephalic cistern.
6. Cerebrospinal fluid space.
7. Lateral ventricle.
8. Sylvian fissure.
9. Hippocampus, normal findings.
10. Hippocampal atrophy.

Fig. 12b Coronal.

Fig. 12c Sagittal.

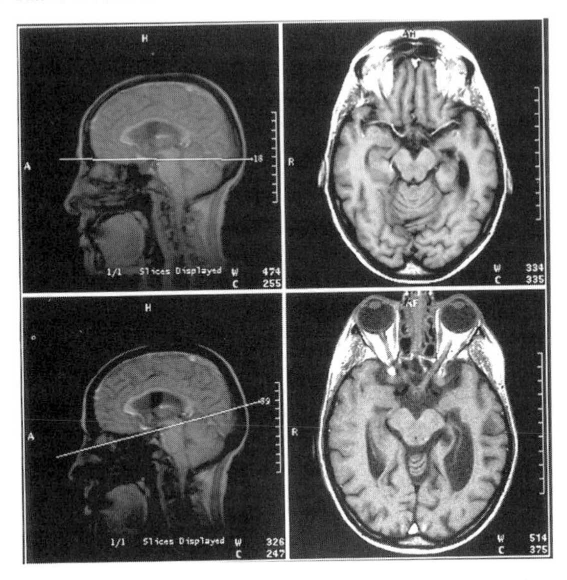

Fig. 12.1.1 MRI, T1w; study of the hippocampal formation using different techniques. Patient, 68 years, female; clinically diagnosed Alzheimer's disease. Hippocampal atrophy with enlargement of both temporal horn and parahippocampal fissure on the left. Transverse imaging with standard orientation and scout view (*top right*), angulated imaging (*bottom right*; see text), and scout view (*left*).

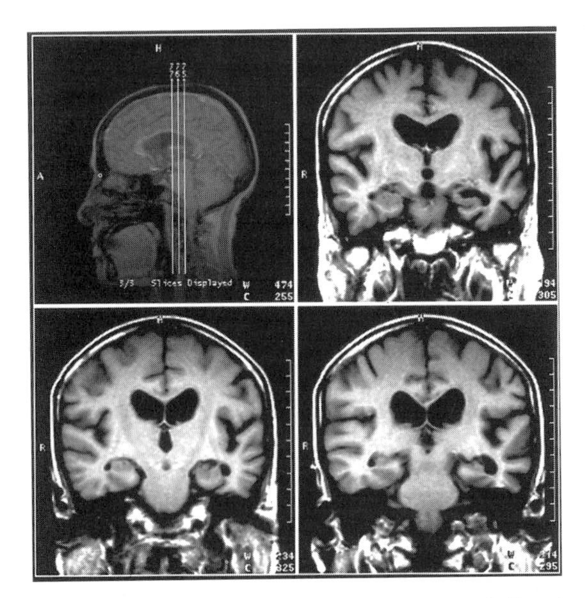

Fig. 12.1.2 Coronal orientation; scout view (*top left*) and consecutive images (6 mm, gap 20%).

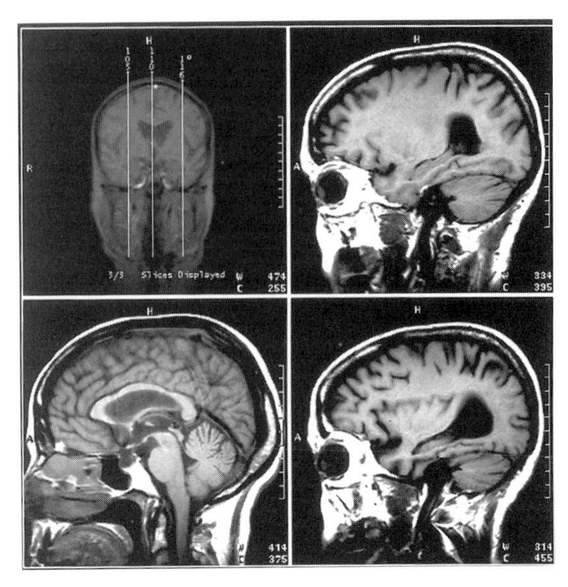

Fig. 12.1.3 Saggital orientation; scout view (*top left*); the left hippocampus (*bottom*) is smaller than the opposite hippocampus. Note the decreased diameter of dorsal corpus callosum (*bottom left*).

The prevalence of *white matter changes* is 11% in the fourth and 83% in the seventh and later decades. Neuropsychological testing reveals a reduction in attention, speed, and abstract reasoning, but there is no obvious relationship to so-called neurological soft signs (Baum *et al.* 1996). Periventricular frontal caps are histopathologically associated with changes in the ependymal cell wall, subependymal gliosis, and age-associated myelin loss. Lacunar lesions in the deeper or subcortical white matter are a consequence of perivascular myelin reduction (Virchow–Robin spaces), whereas larger patchy and confluent white matter changes are due to microangiopathy-related ischaemia (Fazekas *et al.* 1998*a*, 1998*b*). Patients with white matter lesions are at an increased risk of developing cerebral infarcts and manifest dementia, and they are subject to increased mortality.

The *hippocampus*, part of the limbic system, is of great importance for declarative—primarily episodic (biographical)—memory. In cognitively intact individuals, their future cognitive function in old age can be predicted from the size of the hippocampus. Hippocampal atrophy can be demonstrated in one-third of all healthy elderly (Golomb *et al.* 1996).

In normal controls the right hippocampus is larger than the left; decreased asymmetry and hippocampal atrophy can predict the development of dementia, representing a very early preclinical stage of Alzheimer's disease (AD).

EEG (electroencephalography) changes

Normal ageing is typically accompanied by decreasing posterior dominant power and frequency after the fifth decade, reduced alpha-blocking after eye opening, and a mild and intermittent increase of theta activity which may be accentuated over the left temporal lobe. These changes may be less marked in strictly selected elderly normals. Until the seventh decade, beta-activity may increase, particularly during emotional stress; fast frontal beta-power is correlated with cognitive performance. The photic driving response, the synchronization of the occipital EEG signal with rhythmical light stimuli, is impaired. After the age of 70, these alterations usually become more accentuated, but even then delta-power is not increased in normal people. There are complex gender differences in the pattern of age-related changes, and, therefore, gender-based norms are necessary for quantitative comparisons between normal and subtle pathology.

Mild cognitive impairment

Hippocampal atrophy can be found in two-thirds of patients with mild cognitive impairment (Jack *et al.* 1998, 1999).

Since the hippocampus is a vulnerable structure affected in a large number of disease processes, hippocampal atrophy is therefore diagnostically non-specific (DeLeon *et al.* 1997). Pure hippocampal sclerosis may even imitate early AD (Ala *et al.* 2000). A large hippocampal volume predicts better cognitive performance in old age, whereas hippocampal atrophy in patients with mild cognitive impairment predicts the manifestation of dementia. Medial temporal lobe measurements increase the predictive accuracy, even though the absence of medial temporal lobe atrophy does not preclude the development of dementia (Jack *et al.* 1999; Visser *et al.* 1999). It is still unclear whether hippocampal atrophy or measurement of the entorhinal cortex is the best marker for the future development of dementia (Juottonen *et al.* 1998, 1999; see Table 12.1).

One study showed that positron emission tomography (PET) measurements of cerebral glucose metabolism begin to decrease before the

Table 12.1 Contribution of morphological investigations to the diagnosis and differential diagnosis of dementias (%)

Population	Region	Sensitivity	Specificity	% Correct classification
Early AD vs. C	Entorhinal cortex	80	94	87
	Perirhinal cortex	73	81	77
	Temporopolar cortex	73	78	76
	Total perirhinal cortex	83	84	84
	EC both + gender	94	90	92
AD vs. C	Hippocampus	80	91	86
	Entorhinal cortex	80	94	87
	Hippocampus + age	87	94	90
	EC + age	90	94	92

AD, Alzheimer's disease; C, matched controls, EC, entorhinal cortex. After Juottonen *et al.* 1998, 1999, modified with permission.

onset of observable memory decline, whereas hippocampal volume only declines in conjunction with memory deficits (Reiman *et al.* 1998). A number of groups found that atrophic brain changes accelerate the clinical manifestation of cognitive deficits (Förstl *et al.* 1996*b*, *c*; Fox 1998, 1999), but it must be emphasized that significant, however less dynamic, brain changes occur in the long preclinical phase of AD. Entorhinal and hippocampal atrophy can be expected in the preclinical stages of AD, whereas other forms of dementia may be heralded by different structural and functional brain changes.

As brain atrophy and early functional changes can be regarded as risk factors for an imminent development of dementia, evidence for a large cognitive reserve can be considered as a protective factor. There is evidence from a number of studies that a larger head size is associated with a lower probability of poor cognitive performance in old age (e.g. Reynolds *et al.* 1999)—a view not supported by every author (Jenkins *et al.* 2000). However, better educated individuals can tolerate more severe brain atrophy before developing equivalent cognitive disturbances (Kidron *et al.* 1997; Coffey *et al.* 1999). The main difficulty in interpreting such findings is due to the inter-relationship between genetic and social background, brain size, education, and the eventual manifestation of a dementia, which is usually established by the cross-sectional evaluation of cognitive impairment using standard neuropsychological tests.

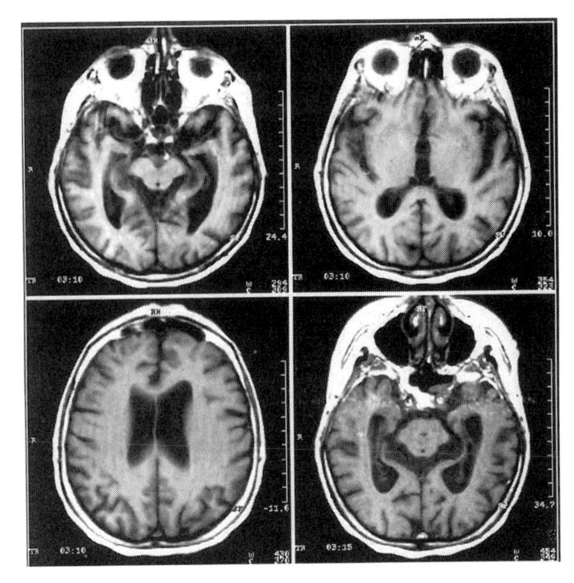

Fig. 12. 2 Patient, 78 years, female, clinically diagnosed Alzheimer's disease. MRI transversal T1w (T_R 600 ms, T_E 17 ms, 2 acqu). Marked dilatation of cerebrovascular spaces with emphasis of both Sylvian and parahippocampal fissures. Note different information on transverse imaging (*top left*) and angulated imaging (*bottom right*) with regard to median temporal lobe.

Alzheimer's disease

The normal CT or MRI scan in a demented patient is compatible with a diagnosis of Alzheimer's disease (AD). However, the majority of patients with manifest AD show a loss of grey and white matter volume (Salat *et al.* 1999), significant hippocampal atrophy (Jack *et al.* 1998), and temporoparietal hypoperfusion. A significant correlation between hippocampal atrophy and declarative memory deficits has been consistently verified (Fama *et al.* 1997; Mori *et al.* 1997; Pantel *et al.* 1997; Mauri *et al.* 1998; Peterson *et al.* 2000). In contrast, it has been impossible to show consistent associations between non-declarative functions and hippocampal volume; or performance on declarative memory tests and the volumes of other brain areas. A study of demented patients affected by the Kobe earthquake in Japan in 1995 demonstrated a relationship between amygdala atrophy and emotional event memory (Mori *et al.* 1999). Unspecific vascular changes in the white matter are often detected, most frequently in patients with familial AD (Coffman *et al.* 1990) (Fig. 12.3).

Hippocampal measurements can be used to statistically discriminate between groups of patients with AD and non-demented controls. Coronal or transverse MRI sections offer an excellent view of the hippocampus, whereas the best CT results are obtained when the gantry is tilted at an angle of 20° negative to the canthomeatal line along the hippocampal axial plane (see above). Hippocampal atrophy is correlated with temporoparietal hypoperfusion

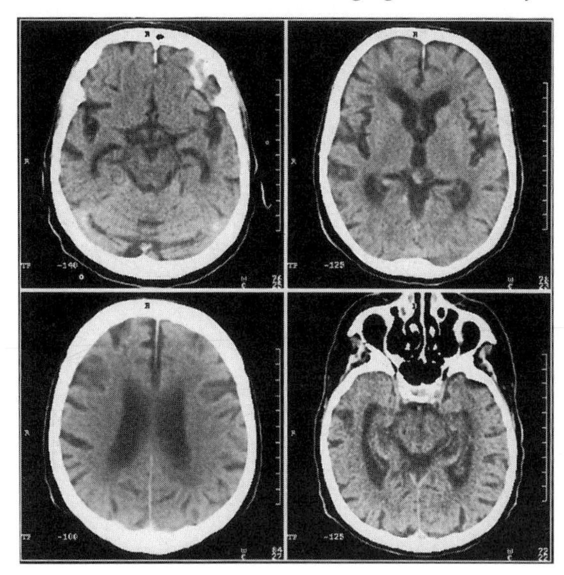

Fig. 12.3 Patient, 74 years, female; clinically diagnosed Alzheimer's disease and a positive family history (dementia in father, mother, and aunt). CT transverse (70 mA, 130 kV). Unexpected findings with discrete dilatation of cerebrospinal fluid spaces and discrete dilatation around the ventricles accentuated around the parahippocampal fissure (*bottom right*). Note periventricular hypodensity ('leucoaraiosis'), often seen in familial AD.

and hypometabolism as demonstrated with single-photon emission computed tomography (SPECT) and PET (Lavenu *et al.* 1997; Yamaguchi *et al.* 1997). Patients with AD activate large distributed neuronal networks in widespread brain areas, which are not activated by normal elderly subjects during the same task (Desgranges *et al.* 1998; Bäckman *et al.* 1999).

Several methods can be used to improve the identification of patients with very early AD, for example high-resolution measurement of the entorhinal cortex, where the neurofibrillary degeneration begins in the majority of patients (Bobinski *et al.* 1999), functional neuroimaging during neuropsychological tasks testing the individual patient's limits (Buck *et al.* 1997; Desgranges *et al.* 1998; Bäckman *et al.* 1999; Pietrini *et al.* 1999), and PET imaging of acetylcholinesterase activity (Kuhl *et al.* 1999; Reed *et al.* 1999). Arterial, spin-label magnetic resonance imaging yields high-resolution morphological and functional imaging without the use of ionizing radiation (Alsop *et al.* 2000). All these methods are expected to provide further insight on the brain, but we must accept that the brain changes have different (low) levels of specificity and sensitivity. It is insufficient to define one simple distance or planimetric measurement, but it is necessary to consider clusters of changes to distinguish between the various degenerative dementias (Table 12.2).

Morphological brain changes are not only significantly correlated with alterations of perfusion and metabolism as examined with SPECT and PET, but also with functional brain changes observed with EEG. Conventional EEG

Table 12.2 Clusters of atrophy to distinguish between the degenerative dementias

Diagnosis	Cortex	Hippocampus	Corpus callosum
AD	temporal	early and pronounced	posterior
Dementia with Lewy bodies	temporal	late and mild	none
Frontotemporal degeneration	frontotemporal (Gyr.temp.ant.)	late and mild	anterior
Corticobasal degeneration	unilateral frontotemporal pre-Rolandic region	late and mild	intermediate

in patient's with AD demonstrates an accentuation of age-related changes: a nearly symmetrical decrease of the occipital dominant rhythm and power, with an increase of theta- and, more specifically, delta-power in the later stages of illness. None of these findings are obligatory or diagnostic, and a normal conventional EEG recording can be considered compatible with the diagnosis. In contrast, statistically, a normal *quantitative* EEG has a high negative predicting power for AD. The usual findings in early AD are mild decreases in the mean EEG frequency, dominant occipital activity, decreased alpha/theta ratio, lower beta-power, and increases of the relative and absolute theta-power together with disorganization of EEG topography and impairment of the photic driving response. Significant decreases of normal alpha-power (8–12 Hz) and increases of slow-wave power in the delta and theta bands have been confirmed (Förstl *et al.* 1996*a–c*; Pucci *et al.* 1999). These changes are particularly severe in patient's with early-onset AD. The decreases of alpha- and the increases of delta- and theta-power are correlated with the severity of cognitive deficits, e.g. memory, attention, and verbal tests (Förstl *et al.* 1996*a,c*). Both visually examined and quantitative EEG are widely underestimated in comparison to other much more expensive and fancy neuroimaging tools (Besthorn *et al.* 1997; Claus *et al.* 1999). A successful diagnostic discrimination between AD and normal ageing in more than 85% of patients can be achieved, provided the synchronicity and complexity of the EEG signals are taken into consideration. Coherence or synchronicity may reflect neuronal coupling or connectivity, whereas complexity may reflect the subtlety of neuronal tuning (Besthorn *et al.* 1997, Wada *et al.* 1998, Jelles *et al.* 1999*a & b*). Relative theta-power is a sensitive discriminator between ageing and dementia, whereas the occipital/frontal alpha ratio allows an efficient statistical distinction to be made between groups of patients with AD and vascular dementia. Figure 12.4 shows a comparison of band-power spectra between matched samples of normal

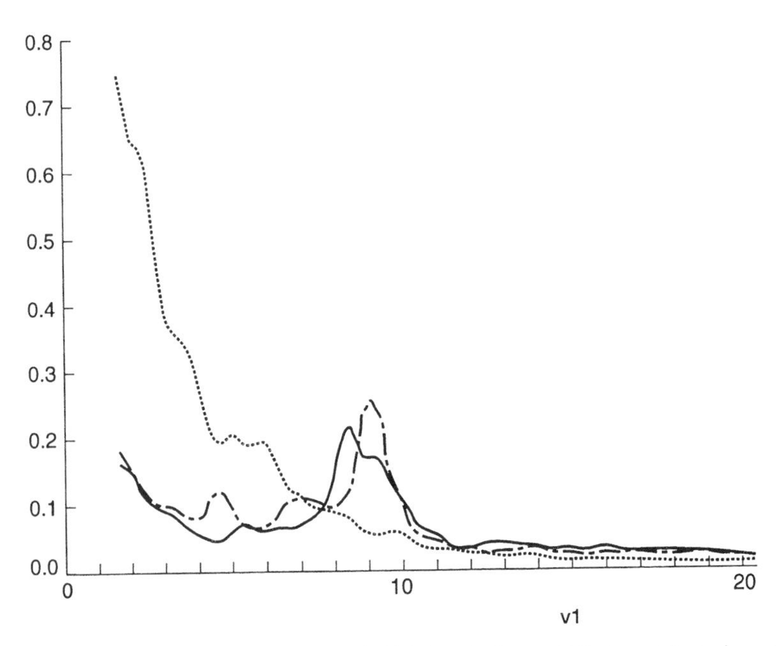

Fig. 12.4 Averaged power-spectra from 10 patients with Alzheimer's disease (AD; dotted line), frontal lobe degeneration (dashed line), and normal elderly controls (continuous line). Delta- and theta-power are increased in AD, but closely similar in frontal lobe degeneration and normal ageing (x axis, log transformed power at Fz).

elderly controls, patients with AD, and those with frontal lobe degeneration.

Both morphological and functional abnormalities increase during the course of AD; for instance, an annual increase in the intracranial cerebrospinal fluid volume of almost 2% and an annual decrease of the alpha/theta-power ratio of 0.1 has been observed (Förstl *et al.* 1996*b*, *c*; Fox *et al.* 2000). Moreover, decreases of alpha- and beta-activity were found to be independent predictors of mortality (Claus *et al.* 1998).

Dementia with Lewy bodies

A new variant of dementia has attracted great interest over the last decade, the Lewy-body variant of AD or dementia with Lewy bodies (McKeith *et al.* 1996). The consensus criteria for a clinical diagnosis of this variant require the exclusion of ischaemic brain disease, and mention a generalized cortical atrophy with prominent frontal lobe changes (McKeith *et al.* 1996). Recent studies have confirmed that the mediotemporal lobe atrophy is comparably less severe in the Lewy-body variant than the pure form of AD (Hashimoto *et al.* 1998; Lippa *et al.* 1998; Barber *et al.* 1999, 2000*a*). Functional neuroimaging studies have demonstrated a decreased occipital perfusion with relatively well-preserved temporoparietal perfusion in the Lewy-body variant (Donnemiller *et al.* 1997; Ishii *et al.* 1999). Tracer studies have revealed a more severe impairment of dopamine transport and function in the Lewy-body variant compared to AD (Donnemiller *et al.* 1997; Walker *et al.* 1999). A severe loss of choline-acetyltransferase in the Lewy-body variant due to a double pathology, with Lewy bodies plus neurofibrillary tangles and Alzheimer plaques in the basal nucleus of Meynert, may explain the greater slowing of the EEG in the Lewy-body variant compared to AD; temporal slow-wave transients have been observed as a correlate of more frequent confusional states in the Lewy-body variant (Briel *et al.* 1999; Barber *et al.* 2000*b*). An REM-sleep behaviour disorder with bursts of vigorous movement of the arms and legs accompanied by vocalization during sleep is a not infrequent manifestation of the Lewy-body variant, and can be confirmed polysomnographically (Boeve *et al.* 1998).

Lobar atrophies (e.g. Pick's disease)

Patients with the frontotemporal variant of these lobar disorders show the expected frontally accentuated brain atrophy (Fig 12.5) and normal EEG activity (Förstl *et al.* 1996*a*). The comparably severe frontal lobe atrophy with nearly normal mediotemporal lobe structures has now been demonstrated by a number of groups (Kaufer *et al.* 1997; Lavenu *et al.* 1998; Lieberman *et al.* 1998; Frisoni *et al.* 1999). Other studies have attempted to distinguish patients with frontotemporal degeneration from patients with typical AD on the basis of quantitative EEG (Yener *et al.* 1996; Neary *et al.* 1998). In their study, Elfgren and colleagues (1996) showed that the decrease in frontal blood flow is associated with impaired clinical performance. Slowly progressive aphasia and semantic dementia with left prefrontal or left temporal brain atrophy are rare variants of these diseases. A direct relationship between temporal lobe atrophy and semantic memory has been demonstrated by Mummery *et al.* (2000). Posterior or progressive biparietal atrophies can be atypical early presentations of AD (Mackenzie Ross *et al.* 1996).

Other degenerative dementias with motor symptoms

Modern diagnostic criteria for Parkinson's disease (Gelb *et al.* 1999) mention a narrowing of the substantia nigra pars compacta which can be shown on heavily T2-weighted MRI scans. Tracer studies show a decreased striatal uptake. Clear lines cannot be drawn between pure AD at one extreme, pure Parkinson's disease at the other, and the Lewy-body variant of AD in the middle. It is both realistic and advantageous to assume a spectrum of neurodegenerative diseases with a

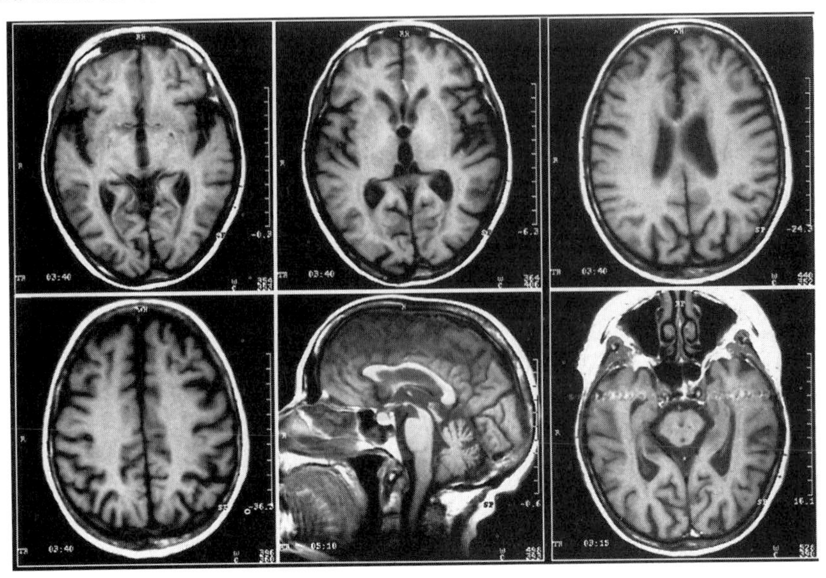

Fig. 12.5 Patient, 76 years, female; clinically diagnosed frontotemporal lobar atrophy. MRI T1w. Enlargement of the Sylvian fissure (*top, left and middle*); asymmetrical enlargement of the lateral ventricle (*top right*) and frontal cortical atrophy (*top right* and *bottom left*); in sagittal direction (*bottom middle*) circumscribed atrophy of the frontal corpus callosum; no significant enlargement of the parahippocampal fissures (*bottom right*).

mixture of plaques, neurofibrillary tangles plus Lewy bodies, and usually superimposed vascular changes. Between 10 and 20% of all patients with Parkinson's disease will develop severe dementia. Occasionally, patients without significant Alzheimer-type changes can be observed, and dementia in those is correlated with the density of Lewy neurites in the area CA2 hippocampal field (Churchyard and Lees 1997). The disconnection between the dentate gyrus, entorhinal cortex, septal nuclei, hypothalamus, and the CA1 field may contribute to dementia in patient's with Parkinson's disease. Demented patients with Parkinson's disease cannot be reliably distinguished from patients with AD on the basis of functional neuroimaging studies (Turjanski and Brooks 1997) as both groups show temporoparietal and, occasionally, frontal perfusion and metabolic changes. A decreased fluorodopa uptake in the caudate nucleus and frontal cortex is associated with impaired verbal fluency, working memory, and attentional functioning (Rinne *et al.* 2000). An association has been observed between dopamine transport, density of the putamen and caudate nucleus, and prefrontal functioning in non-demented Parkinson patients (Müller *et al.* 2000). Striatal, cerebellar, and brainstem volumes are often normal in patients with pure idiopathic Parkinson's disease.

Structural neuroimaging makes a significant contribution to the identification of patients with vascular parkinsonism (Winnikates and Jankovic 1999). Patients with atypical parkinsonian syndromes demonstrate a number of morphological brain changes. For instance, significant reductions in mean striatal and brainstem volumes can be seen in patients with multiple system atrophy and progressive supranuclear palsy (Schulz *et al.* 1999; Soliveri *et al.* 1999). Furthermore, while patients with pure Parkinson's disease exhibited a loss of cholinergic innervation to the cerebral cortex, the PET study of acetylcholinesterase activity indicated a preferential loss of cholinergic innervation of the thalamus in progressive supranuclear palsy. Corticobasal degeneration is characterized morphologically by an asymmetrical frontoparietal atrophy including basal ganglia and the substantia nigra (Hentschel

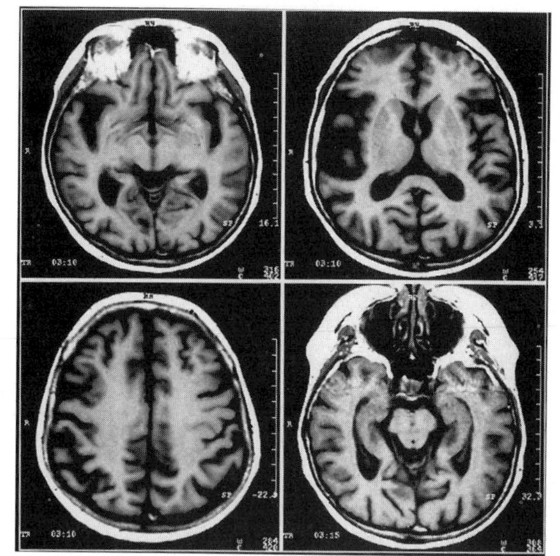

Fig. 12.6(a) Patient, 71 years, female; clinically diagnosed corticobasal degeneration. MRI transverse, T1w (T_R 600 ms, T_E 17 ms, 2 acqu.) different enlargement of Sylvian fissure (*top*); right-hand side enlargement of the subarachnoidal cerebrospinal fluid space with emphasis of the pre-Rolandic region (*bottom left*); no significant enlargement of the parahippocampal fissures (*bottom right*).

et al. 1998; Soliveri *et al.* 1999; see Fig. 12.6(a)). An atrophy of the corpus callosum has been described by Yamauchi *et al.* (1998). Both corticobasal degeneration and progressive supranuclear palsy show mediofrontal hypoperfusion, but the alterations are more widespread and asymmetrical in corticobasal degeneration (Okuda *et al.* 2000). A systematic comparison of these three atypical parkinsonian syndromes revealed the indicative features listed in Table 12.3 (Schrag *et al.* 2000). Subcortical gliosis is sometimes observed by neuroradiologists or neuropathologists (Fig. 12.6(b)).

Vascular dementia

Detailed diagnostic criteria and pathophysiological considerations of this second leading cause of dementia in the elderly is presented elsewhere in this book (Chapter 24iii). Neuroimaging is obligatory for a diagnosis (according to the NINDS–AIREN) and helps to distinguish between the following forms of vascular dementia:

Table 12.3 Criteria for the differentiation of progressive supranuclear palsy (PSP), multiple system atrophy-pontine (MSA-P), and multiple system atrophy with predominant cerebellar parkinsonism (MSA-C)

PSP	MSA-P	MSA-C
Midbrain diameter on axial scans	Hyperintense putaminal rim	Dilatation of the fourth ventricle
Signal increase of the midbrain	Putaminal hyperintensity*	Atrophy of the medullar dentate nucleus, middle cerebellar peduncles, pons inferior olives
Dilatation of the third ventricle	Atrophy of the dentate nucleus	Signal increase of the cerebellum, middle cerebellar peduncles, pons (hot-cross bun sign), inferior olives
Frontal or temporal lobe atrophy	Dilatation of the fourth ventricle	
Signal increase in the globus pallidus	Signal increase in the cerebellum middle cerebellar peduncles, pons (hot-cross bun sign)	
Atrophy or signal increase of the red nucleus		

*On 0.5-T-scan. After Schrag *et al.* 2000, modified with permission.

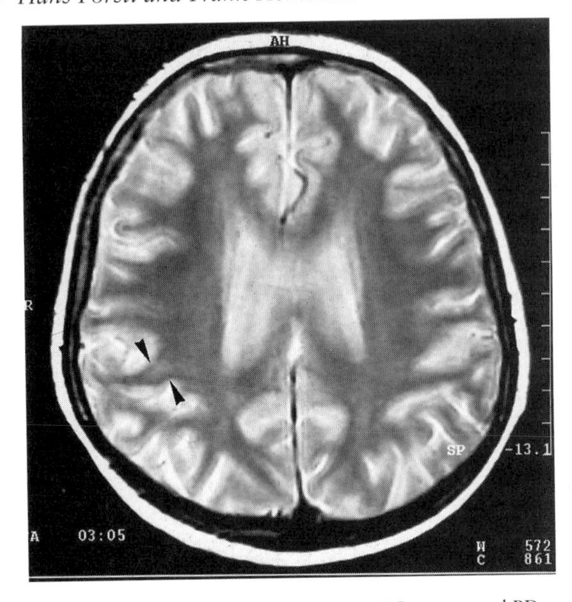

Fig. 12.6(b) Same patient as in (a). MRI transversal PDw (T_R 3400 ms, T_E 15 ms, 2 acqu.). Hyperintense subcortical gliosis on the right (arrows; see text).

- large-vessel infarcts localized in the anterior, medial, posterior cerebral arteries and watershed territories or association areas (so-called multi-infarct dementia, MID);
- small-vessel disease affecting the basal ganglia and white matter with multiple lesions (Fig. 12.7) or diffuse and extensive lesions (Fig. 12.8) (extensive subcortical white matter lesions are frequently referred to as Binswanger's disease or subcortical arterio-sclerotic encephalopathy, SAE);
- bilateral paramedian thalamic or fornix infarcts, which lead to severe memory deficits (so-called strategic infarcts).

There is not just one vascular dementia, but a multitude of causes and vascular pathologies that can cause extensive cognitive impairment. The identification of vascular factors in demented patients, which has been improved by advanced MRI techniques (e.g. FLAIR-sequences, Fig 12.9), is of great importance, as potential interventions go beyond simply symptomatic measures. Neurodegenerative changes of the Alzheimer and

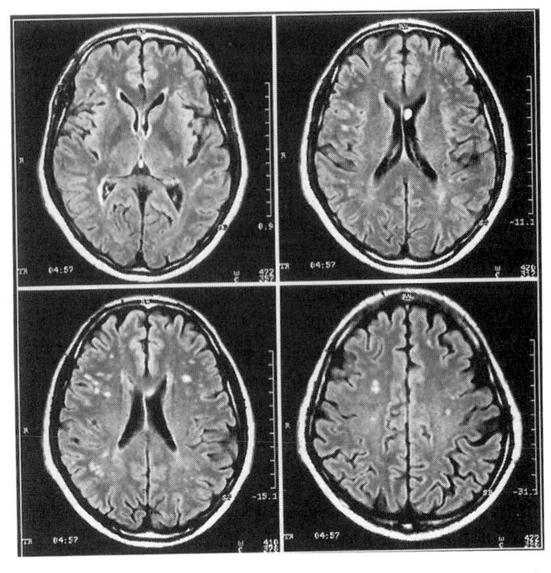

Fig. 12.7 Patient, 46 years, male; microangiopathy with multiple subcortical white matter hyperintensities and frontal predominance (multiple risk factors,, E.g. hypertension, hypercholesteraemia, ...). MRI transversal, FLAIR (T_R 9000 ms, T_I 2500 ms, T_E 110 ms, 2 acqu.).

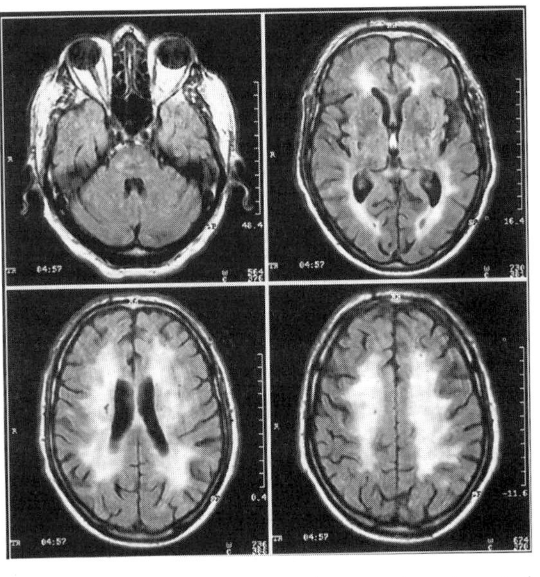

Fig. 12.8 Patient, 67 years, male; extensive subcortical vascular pathology with hyperintense confluent lesions (subcortical arteriosclerotic encephalopathy, SAE; Binswanger's disease) MRI transverse, FLAIR (T_R 9000 ms, T_I 2500 ms, T_E 110 ms, 2 acqu.). Note hyperintense lesions within the pons (*top left*).

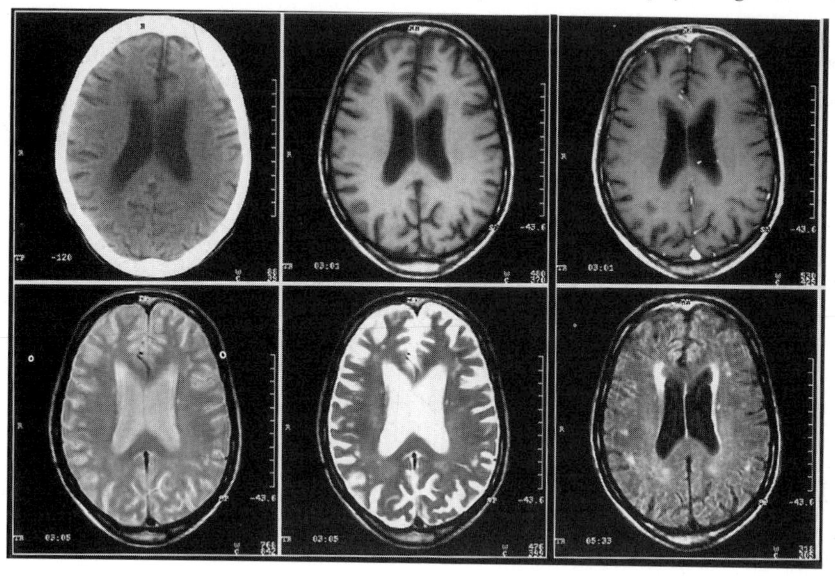

Fig. 12.9 Comparison of different imaging techniques to detect vascular changes (all slices on the level of cella media of lateral ventricles). Patient, 79 years, male; microangiopathy. CT (*top left*) (70 mA, 139 kV) clearly showing leucoaraiosis; MRI T1w without (*top middle*) and with contrast media (*top right*) no detection of relevant changes in the white matter (T_R 570 ms, T_E 17 ms, 2 acqu.); MRI PDw (T_R 3400 ms, T_E 15 ms, 2 acqu.) with discrete hyperintense changes (*bottom left*); MRI T2w (T_R 3400 ms, T_E 105 ms, 2 acqu.) with markedly white matter lesions (*bottom middle*); MRI FLAIR (T_R 9000 ms, T_I 2500 ms, T_E 110 ms, 2 acqu.) with the best detection of white matter changes (*bottom right*).

other types of dementia can co-occur with vascular brain changes (Snowdon *et al.* 1997). This has been supported by recent studies which documented that one-sixth of the patients suffering ischaemic stroke suffered from pre-existent dementia (Hénon *et al.* 1997), and that preferentially those patients who display a pre-existent mediotemporally accentuated brain atrophy develop poststroke dementia (Hénon *et al.* 1998). Both the localization and extent of brain damage determine the profile and severity of cognitive deterioration. Functional changes caused by vascular lesion are of decisive importance, and it appears that subcortical lacunar infarctions in the white matter, the basal ganglia, and the thalamus are most critical (Longstreth *et al.* 1998; Kwan *et al.* 1999). Diffusion-weighted MRI allows the identification of fresh infarcts and demonstrates that vascular brain changes are ongoing processes (Choi *et al.* 2000).

EEG power spectra are linked to metabolic changes in vascular dementia (Szelies *et al.* 1999) and to clinical deficits. Event-related potentials (ERP) demonstrate a prolonged central processing time for novel stimuli (Yamaguchi 2000). Focal EEG abnormalities—usually intermittent, lateralized slow waves, or spike and sharp waves—are found in 75% of patients with multi-infarct dementia. There are no significant differences between multi-infarct dementia, other forms of vascular dementia, and AD regarding the mean background parameters of qEEG, but the occipital/frontal power ratio is higher in any form of vascular dementia than in AD. Coherence is decreased between disconnected areas usually linked by short corticocortical and corticosubcortical fibres. However, the differential diagnostic validity of EEG for vascular dementias appears to be clearly inferior to neuroradiological methods.

Cerebral autosomal dominant arteriopathy with subcortical infarcts and leucoencephalopathy (CADASIL) is a rare but important variant of vascular dementia. A significant inverse correlation between cognitive performance and lesion volume has been described in this disease (Dichgans *et al.* 1999).

Creutzfeldt–Jakob disease

Creutzfeldt–Jakob disease, a rapidly progressive form of dementia, is caused by proteinaceous infectious agents (prions). Conspicuous sharp waves in the EEG which couple with myoclonic jerks can be observed in the advanced stages of illness. Sometimes a rapidly progressive unspecific brain atrophy with occasional frontal accentuation and subcortical changes can be seen, but the absence of significant brain changes is much more characteristic in the early stage. The caudate nucleus and putamen show an increased signal in T2w-imaging. Recently, so-called diffusion-weighted MRI has been recommended to reveal hyperintensities in the basal ganglia or thalamus. These can be symmetrical or asymmetrical, and reflect a patient's clinical deficits (Bahn and Piero 1999; Na *et al.* 1999; Yee *et al.* 1999). The 'pulvinar sign', bilateral thalamic hyperintensity in T2-proton weighted-images due to a thalamic gliosis, is currently considered most distinctive (Zeidler *et al.* 2000).

AIDS–dementia complex

Global brain atrophy due to progressive white matter lesions and almost unaffected grey matter can often be observed in this complex (Kim *et al.* 1996; Thurnher *et al.* 1997). Focal perfusion changes are detected earlier than morphological changes and can be reversible (Smirniotopoulos *et al.* 1997).

The subacute encephalitis caused by HIV infection leads to periventricular circumscribed or confluent white matter lesions which need to be distinguished from a papovaviridae infection (progressive multifocal leucoencephalopathy, PML) (Kim *et al.* 1996, Thurnher *et al.* 1997). Opportunistic infections of the central nervous system are frequent in patients with AIDS. Two of the most common cerebral complications—the *Toxoplasma gondii* abscess and lymphoma—are virtually indistinguishable by CT or MRI.

Normal-pressure hydrocephalus (NPH)

NPH is characterized clinically by the triad of fluctuating cognitive impairment, incontinence, and gait disturbance. Neuromorphologically, large lateral and small, fourth ventricle, periventricular hypodensities are found together with small superior interhemispheric fissures and sulci. These morphological changes can be seen with cranial CT, whereas MRI is necessary to observe the typical 'fluid void sign' (Figs 12.10(a), (b)). The hyperdynamic cerebrospinal fluid movement can sometimes cause a reversible signal extinction ('fluid void') at the aqueduct, but more often this occurs at the cerebrospinal junction. Volumetric measurements can distinguish NPH from AD in typical cases (Kitagaki *et al.* 1998), but, again, the two diseases can coincide. If severe mediotemporal lobe atrophy is observed—a sign of

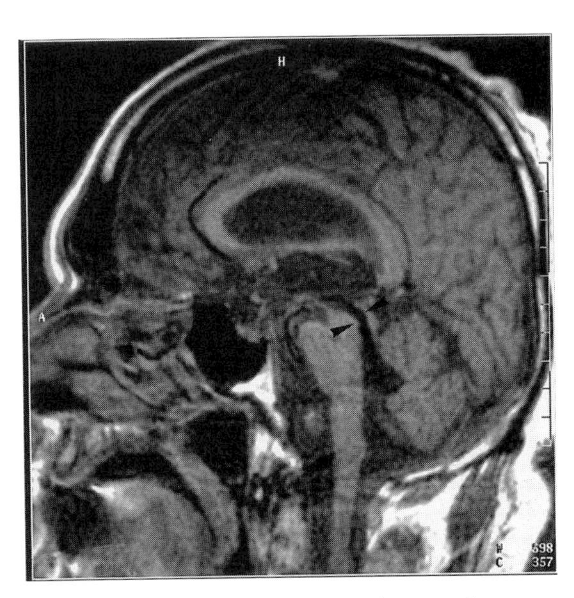

Fig. 12.10(a) Patient, 59 years, male; normal-pressure hydrocephalus with gait disturbance and urinary incontinence. MRI sagittal, T1w (T_R 450 ms, T_E 14 ms, 2 acqu.).

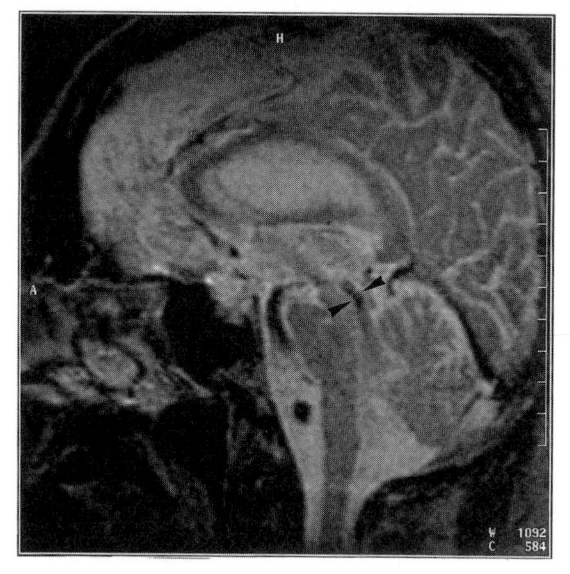

Fig. 12.10(b) Same patient as in (a). MRI sagittal, T2w (T_R 2200 ms, T_E 80 ms, 2 acqu.). Note specific 'fluid void sign' in the enlarged cerebral aqueduct with 'whirling' of cerebrospinal fluid in the fourth ventricle (arrows in both figures). Note fluid void in both, Basilar artery and the deep veins in the midsagittal slices.

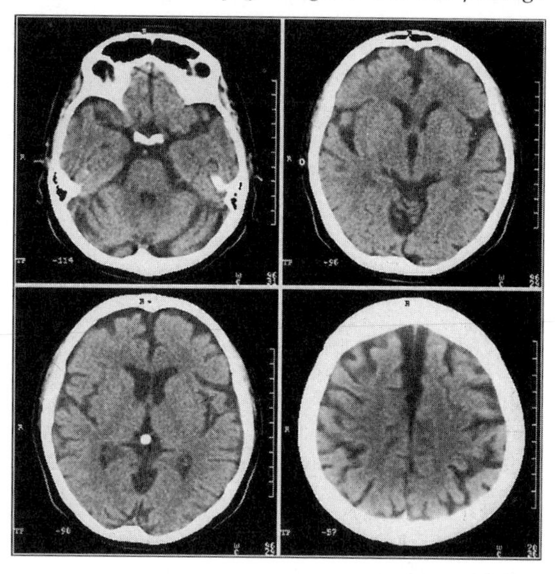

Fig. 12.11 Patient, 37 years, female; with chronic alcohol addiction; first delirium tremens. CT transversal (70 mA, 139 kV). Atrophy of cerebellum (*top left*), vermis cerebelli (*top right*), and frontal cortex (*bottom*) with marked dilatation of the anterior fissure (*bottom right*).

AD—shunting will be of questionable benefit. No single morphological parameter can identify those patients with NPH who will benefit from ventriculoperitoneal shunting. Reductions of glucose metabolism and perfusion, frontally and periventricularly, are potentially reversible after operation (Talbot and Testa 1995). A prevalent problem is not only the comorbidity with AD, but also with other systemic and brain diseases (e.g. Formiga *et al.* 2000). Tumours and inflammatory conditions have to be ruled out before a diagnosis of NPH is made.

Alcohol-induced brain changes

A number of such changes can be visualized neuroradiologically, and may occur in isolated or combined form:

- commonly, frontal cortical atrophy with fissure widening of the rostral interhemispheric fissure and cerebellar atrophy, usually most pronounced around the vermis (Fig 12.11);
- chronic subdural haematoma, often after minor head injuries,
- Wernicke–Korsakoff encephalopathy, sometimes with identifiable haemorrhagic changes in the mamillary bodies and tissue alterations in the dorsomedial thalamic nuclei;
- focal callosal atrophy and hemispheric white matter changes (Marchiafava–Bignami syndrome); and
- central pontine or extrapontine myelinolysis, a frequent, but unspecific, sequel of chronic alcohol abuse following the rapid normalization of hyponatraemia with intravenous fluids.

MRI is clearly superior to CT in demonstrating the last three alterations. Functional neuroimaging reveals a decrease in cerebral blood flow and metabolism, being most accentuated in the prefrontal lobe and cerebellum. In alcohol-related dementia, infra- and supratentorial atrophy, third and lateral ventricular enlargement (Oslin *et al.*

1998), improvements in the white matter volume loss and the hippocampal, hemispheric, and cerebellar volumes have been demonstrated in abstinent alcoholics (Shear *et al.* 1994; Liu 2000). Electroencephalographically, increased slow-wave activity persists during abstinence (Oslin *et al.* 1998). The high prevalence of extensive cerebrovascular changes satisfying the diagnostic criteria for vascular dementia in elderly male alcoholics represents an unexpected finding (Fisman *et al.* 1996). Vascular changes can also play a major role in the mamillary pathology of the alcohol-related Wernicke–Korsakoff syndrome (Fisman *et al.* 1996), in the white matter and corpus callosum lesions of the Marchiafava–Bignami disease (Ferracci *et al.* 1999), and in central pontine or extrapontine myelinolysis, demonstrated particularly well in MRI-FLAIR sequences.

Confusional states (delirium)

Little work has been done on the structural causes and functional changes in confusional states. Alcohol intoxication and alcohol withdrawal are well-known causes of confusional states. The Lewy-body variant of AD (McKeith *et al.* 1996) is a form of dementia in which superimposed confusional states are of diagnostic significance. All forms of severe somatic or brain diseases leading to cerebral hypoperfusion, hypoxia, or a significant cholinergic/aminergic imbalance may cause confusional states. Therefore, the expected neuroimaging findings are highly variable and reflect the underlying illness (Förstl 1998).

A systematic investigation revealed that confusional states are more common in late-onset (mixed) AD and forms of vascular dementia with widespread cerebral damage, and much less frequent in the predominantly cortical forms of dementia (Robertson *et al.* 1998).

Old studies, now almost forgotten, have repeatedly demonstrated the superior diagnostic validity of a simple EEG for the differential diagnosis of confusional states associated with severe EEG alterations. Likewise in other more chronic and irreversible forms of cognitive impairment (for example AD), quantitative EEG often needs to be employed to detect the much more subtle alterations in the mild and moderate stages.

Schizophrenia-like illness

The co-occurrence between late-onset schizophrenia and neuroimaging evidence of organic brain changes exceeds expectation. White matter abnormalities indicating increased vascular risk, unsuspected vascular lesions, and ventricular enlargement have been described. Recent work has confirmed subcortical changes, e.g. increased periventricular and thalamic signal intensity in proton-weighted MRI sequences (Sachdev *et al.* 1999), with inconspicuous findings at the corpus callosum, cerebellum (Sachdev and Brodaty 1999*a* and *b*), and largely intact mediotemporal lobe structures (Denihan *et al.* 2000).

Depression

Somatic and brain diseases, often with a chronic course and pain syndromes, are frequently associated with depression in the elderly. Cerebrovascular abnormalities are often found. A diagnosis of 'vascular depression' does not require a causal or temporal relationship between the development of psychopathology and a stroke, which is an important conceptual difference compared to poststroke depression (Alexopoulos *et al.* 1997*a,b*; Krishnan *et al.* 1997). An onset of depression after age 65 and evidence of cerebrovascular disease or a vascular risk factor are sufficient for the diagnosis to be made. The diagnosis of vascular depression is supported by: cognitive deficits, with impaired planning and sequencing of 'purposeful' action; psychomotor slowing, and mildly depressive symptoms, e.g. feelings of guilt; impaired judgement; mildly impaired activities of daily living; and no evidence of a positive family history of depression.

Several authors have demonstrated increased white matter hyperintensity in patients with late-onset depression (e.g. Simpson *et al.* 1997). Mild volume reductions in grey matter of the prefrontal, mediotemporal, caudate, hippocampal, and amygdala have also observed (Kumar *et al.* 1997; Greenwald *et al.* 1997; Shah *et al.* 1998; Ashtari *et al.* 1999). The severity of these alterations may be correlated with cognitive impairment (Ashtari *et al.* 1999; Kramer-Ginsberg *et al.* 1999). However, it has been stressed in several studies that these morphological changes and differences compared with elderly controls are not very large (Greenwald *et al.* 1997; Ashtari *et al.* 1999; Palsson *et al.* 1999). The observation of a poor treatment response in patients with subcortical and also with grey matter changes is of great clinical importance (Shah *et al.* 1998; Simpson *et al.* 1998). SPECT and PET studies have consistently demonstrated cerebral hypoperfusion in depressed elderly in the prefrontal (Klemm *et al.* 1996; Iidaka *et al.* 1997) and paralimbic areas (Klemm *et al.* 1996). The degree of hypoperfusion is correlated with age and with the severity of depression (Iidaka *et al.* 1997), but normalization of cerebral perfusion leads to an improvement in the affective state (Jaracz *et al.* 1996). As there is such ample evidence for a relationship between vascular changes and depression in the elderly, it appears debatable whether vascular factors should be considered relevant in just one subgroup of elderly depressed patients.

Summary and recommendations

In elderly patients with psychiatric problems, morphological investigations with CT and MRI, sometimes even functional neuroimaging with SPECT or PET, are strongly recommended if there is a suspicion of:

- degenerative dementia (e.g. AD, lobar atrophy, Huntington's chorea, etc.);
- vascular changes (multiple cortical infarcts, subcortical vascular encephalopathy, thalamic infarction, etc.); or
- tumour, inflammation, post-traumatic brain lesions, hypoxia, and normal-pressure hydrocephalus as causes of secondary psychosis.

Little additional information can be gained by morphological or functional brain imaging if:

- recent brain scans are available;
- no remarkable morphological and functional alterations can be expected (e.g. in long-lasting illnesses with presenile onset and no conceivable clinical change); or
- if the patient's condition does not allow a technically satisfactory examination.

EEG is a widely available, inexpensive, and non-invasive tool, with excellent time-, but limited spatial resolution. Its validity is probably underestimated in the English speaking countries and possibly overestimated elsewhere. Advanced and cheap methods of EEG analysis are widely available and their clinical importance is likely to increase in all parts of the world.

Paroxysmal discharges (spikes or sharp waves) and focal and generalized changes of the EEG background activity in organic brain disease can often be detected by the visual inspection of conventional analogue paper-and-ink recordings. The new quantitative analysis of digitized EEG data (qEEG) offers improved reliability and comparability between individuals or groups of patients and allows the investigation of subtle changes in the course of an illness. Various statistical approaches and parameters have been employed in the investigation of elderly psychiatric patients, for example:

- spectral analysis or Fourier transformation of the EEG signal in a defined frequency band (delta-, theta-, alpha-, beta-power);
- correlations between different electrode locations yielding the coherence or synchronicity of the EEG signal;
- transformations derived from chaos-theory yielding the dimensionality or complexity of the signals.

Conventional EEG will probably retain its importance for the diagnosis of acute and severe organic psychosis, even though it may be surpassed by qEEG in the early diagnosis of chronic degenerative brain disease.

Recent technical advances

We are guilty of not having mentioned the latest developments in MRI technology and nuclear medicine until this point, because it appears unlikely that the ordinary elderly patient will benefit from these advances before the next edition of this book.

Diagnostic neuroimaging has traditionally attempted to distinguish structural findings in neurodegenerative, vascular, and other forms of dementia from one another and from normal ageing. The contribution of novel MRI sequences and functional investigations to these tasks is currently being evaluated.

The development of spiral (helical-, volume-) CT allows a 3-dimensional reconstruction of large-volume organs. The availability of MRI machines has increased worldwide, and the time needed for investigation has been reduced with the help of new MRI sequences. FLAIR- and magnetization-transfer techniques, as well as perfusion- and diffusion-weighted investigations are gaining increasing scientific and clinical importance (Ulug and Zijl 1999; Chun *et al.* 2000; Hentschel 2000). Identical MRI machines yield high morphological resolution together with functional investigations of blood flow and

Table 12.4 Pros and cons of different neuroimaging methods

	CT	MRI	PET/SPECT
Measurement	density	relaxation time	radioactivity
Resolution	1–2 mm	<1 mm	7 to 8 mm (ring system) 14 to 17 mm (head-camera)
Result	morphology (limited functional findings)	morphology (functional including metabolism (MRS))	functional (perfusion, metabolism, receptors, and neurotransmitters)
Duration	seconds (single layer)	seconds (single layer) up to 30 min (several complete sequences)	seconds (perfusion) to minutes (glucose metabolism)
Radiation exposure	low (mSV)	none	MBq to GBq depending on ligand (which can be injected or inhaled)
Noise level	low	up to 100 dB	none
Contraindications	claustrophobia	bioelectrical instruments (i.e. pacemakers), metals (artefacts, warming), claustrophobia	claustrophobia
Advantages	cheap, wide availability	morphological and functional studies with one machine and without radiation exposure ('one-stop-shop')	diagnostics of receptors, neurotransmission, etc.
Disadvantage	radiation; low sensitivity	relatively expensive, increasing availability	low availability, high radiation exposure, poor spatial resolution compared to CT and MRI

metabolites. Magnetic resonance spectroscopy (MRS) of protons or phosphorus permit the intravital measurement of cerebral metabolism (Ernst *et al.* 1997; Pfefferbaum *et al.* 1999; Stoppe *et al.* 2000). Although these techniques and functional MRI are already established in neuroscience laboratories, their transfer into relevant clinical psychiatric studies is fraught with difficulties. Some of the morphological and functional alterations associated with diseases in old age psychiatry are not as clearly defined as experimental paradigms used in basic sciences' studies. Individual premorbid variance is large and is further enhanced by the type and severity of superimposed illness. Motivation and compliance is a major issue in some of the functional studies. The pros and cons of CT, MRI, and PET or SPECT are summarized in Table 12.4.

Our position is critical regarding the clinical—not the scientific—importance for the next decade of the impressive methodological advances we have seen over the last 5 years (Förstl and Hentschel 2000).

References

Ala, T., Beh, G. O., and Frey, W. H. (2000). Pure hippocampal sclerosis, a rare cause of dementia mimicking Alzheimer's disease. *Neurology*, **54**, 843–8.

Alexopoulos, G. S., Meyers, B. S., Young, R. C., Campbell, S., Silbersweig, D., and Charlson, M. (1997*a*). 'Vascular depression' hypothesis. *Archives of General Psychiatry*, **54**, 915–22.

Alexopoulos, G. S., Meyers, B. S., Young, R. C., Kakuma, T., Silbersweig, D., and Charlson, M. (1997*b*). Clinically defined vascular depression. *American Journal of Psychiatry*, **154**, 562–5.

Alsop, D. C., Detre, J. A., and Grossmann, M. (2000). Assessment of cerebral blood flow in Alzheimer's disease by spin-labeled magnetic resonance imaging. *Annals of Neurology*, **47**, 93–100.

Ashtari, M., Greenwald, B. S., Kramer-Ginsberg, E., *et al.* (1999). Hippocampal/amygdala volumes in geriatric depression. *Psychological Medicine*, **29**, 629–38.

Bäckman, L., Andersson, J. L. R., Nyberg, L., Winblad, B., Nordberg, A., and Almkvist, O. (1999). Brain regions associated with episodic retrieval in normal aging and Alzheimer's disease. *Neurology*, **52**, 1861–70.

Bahn, M. M. and Piero, P. (1999). Abnormal diffusion-weighted magnetic resonance images in Creutzfeldt–Jakob disease. *Archives of Neurology*, **56**, 577–83.

Barber, R., Cholkar, A., Scheltens, P., Ballard, C., McKeith, I. G., and O'Brien, J. T. (1999). Medial temporal lobe atrophy on MRI in dementia with Lewy bodies. *Neurology*, **52**, 1153–8.

Barber, R., Ballard, C., McKeith, I. G., Gholkar, A., and O'Brien, J. T. (2000*a*). MRI volumetric study of dementia with Lewy bodies, a comparison with AD and vascular dementia. *Neurology*, **54**, 1304–9.

Barber, R., Varma, A. R., Lloyd, J. J., *et al.* (2000*b*). The electroencephalogram in dementia with Lewy bodies. *Acta Neurologica Scandinavica*, **101**, 53–6.

Baum, K. A., Schulte, C., Girke, W., *et al.* (1996). Incidental white-matter foci on MRI in 'healthy' subjects: evidence of subtle cognitive dysfunction. *Neuroradiology*, **38**, 755–60.

Besthorn, C., Zerfass, R., Geiger-Kabisch, C., *et al.* (1997). Discrimination of Alzheimer's disease and normal ageing by EEG data. *Electroencephalography and Clinical Neurophysiology*, **103**, 241–8.

Bobinski, M., DeLeon, M. J., Convit, A., *et al.* (1999). MRI of entorhinal cortex in mild Alzheimer's disease. *Lancet*, **353**, 38–40.

Boeve, B. F., Silber, M. H., Ferman, T. J., *et al.* (1998). REM sleep behavior disorder and degenerative dementia. An association likely reflecting Lewy body disease. *Neurology*, **51**, 363–70.

Briel, R. C. G., McKeith, I. G., Barker, W. A., *et al.* (1999). EEG findings in dementia with Lewy bodies and Alzheimer's disease. *Journal of Neurology, Neurosurgery and Psychiatry*, **66**, 401–3.

Buck, B. H., Black, S. E., Behrmann, M., Caldwell, C., and Bronskill, M. J. (1997). Spatial- and object-based attentional deficits in Alzheimer's disease. Relationship to HMPAO-SPECT measures of parietal perfusion. *Brain*, **120**, 1229–44.

Choi, S. H., Na, D. L., Chung, C. S. *et al.* (2000). Diffusion-weighted MRI in vascular dementia. *Neurology*, **54**, 83–9.

Chun, T., Filippi, C. G., Zimmermann, R. D., and Ulug, A. M. (2000). Diffusion changes in the human brain. Am J Neuroradiology, **21**, 1078–1083.

Churchyard, A. and Lees, A. J. (1997). The relationship between dementia and direct involvement of the hippocampus and amygdala in Parkinson's disease. *Neurology*, **49**, 1571–6.

Claus, J. J., DeVisser, B. W. O., Walstra, G. J. M., *et al.* (1998). Quantitative spectral electroencephalography in predicting survival in patients with early Alzheimer disease. *Archives of Neurology*, **55**, 1105–11.

Claus, J. J., Strijers, R. L. M., Jonkman, E. J., *et al.* (1999). The diagnostic value of electroencephalography in mild senile Alzheimer's disease. *Clinical Neurology*, **110**, 825–32.

Coffey, C. E., Saxton, J. A., Ratcliff, G., Bryan, R. N., and Lucke, J. F. (1999). Relation of education to brain size in normal aging—implications for the reserve hypothesis. *Neurology*, **53**, 189–96.

Coffman, J. A., Torello, M. W., Bornstein, R. A. *et al.* (1990). Leukoaraiosis in asymptomatic adult offspring of individuals with Alzheimer's disease. *Biological Psychiatry,* **27**, 1244–48.

DeLeon, M. J., George, A. E., Golomb, J., *et al.* (1997). Frequency of hippocampal formation atrophy in normal aging and Alzheimer's disease. *Neurobiology of Aging*, **18**, 1–11.

Denihan, A., Wilson, G., Cunningham, C., *et al.* (2000). CT measurement of medial temporal lobe atrophy in Alzheimer's disease, vascular dementia, depression and paraphrenia. *International Journal of Geriatric Psychiatry*, **15**, 306–12.

Desgranges, B., Baron, J.-C., de la Sayette, V., *et al.* (1998). The neural substrates of memory systems impairment in Alzheimer's disease. A PET study of resting brain glucose utilization. *Brain*, **121**, 611–31.

Dichgans, M., Filippi, M., Brüning, R., *et al.* (1999). Quantitative MRI and CADASIL. Correlation with disability and cognitive performance. *Neurology*, **52**, 1361–7.

Donnemiller, E., Heilmann, J., Wenning, G. K., *et al.* (1997) Brain perfusion scintigraphy with 99mTc-HMPAO or 99mTc-ECD and 123I-β-CIT single-photon emission tomography in dementia of the Alzheimer-type and diffuse Lewy body disease. *European Journal of Nuclear Medicine* 1997, **24**, 319–25.

Elfgren, C. I., Ryding, E., and Passant, U. (1996). Performance on neuropsychological tests related to single photon emission computerised tomography findings in frontotemporal dementia. *British Journal of Psychiatry*, **169**, 416–22.

Ernst, T., Chang, L., Melchior, R., and Mehringer, C. M. (1997). Frontotemporal dementia and early Alzheimer disease: differentiation with frontal lobe H-1-MR spectroscopy. *Radiology*, **203**, 829–36.

Fama, R., Sullivan, E. V., Shear, P. K., *et al.* (1997). Selective cortical and hippocampal volume correlates of Mattis dementia rating scale in Alzheimer disease. *Archives of Neurology*, **54**, 719–28.

Fazekas, F., Schmidt, R., Kleinert, R., *et al.* (1998*a*). The spectrum of age-associated brain abnormalities: their measurement and histopathological correlates. *Journal of Neural Transmission*, **53**(Suppl.), 31–9.

Fazekas, F., Schmidt, R., and Scheltens, P. (1998*b*). Pathophysiologic mechanisms in the development of age-related white matter changes of the brain. Dement Geriatr Cogn Disord, **9**(Suppl.), 2–5.

Ferracci, F., Conte, F., Gentile, M., *et al.* (1999). Marchiafava-Bignami disease. *Archives of Neurology*, **56**, 107–10.

Fisman, M., Ramsay, D., and Weiser, M. (1996). Dementia in the elderly male alcoholic—a retrospective clinico-pathological study. *International Journal of Geriatric Psychiatry*, **11**, 209–18.

Formiga, F., Mascaro, J., Chivite, D., *et al.* (2000). Reversible dementia due to two coexistent diseases. *Lancet*, **355**, 1154.

Förstl, H. (1998). Organic psychiatry. In *Textbook of psychiatry and psychotherapy* (ed. M. Berger), pp. 261–344. Urban and Schwarzenberg, Munich.

Förstl, H. and Hentschel, F. (2000). Contribution of neuroimaging to the differential diagnosis of dementias and other late life psychiatric disorders. *Reviews in Clinical Gerontology*, **10**, 55–68.

Förstl, H., Besthorn, C., Hentschel, F., Geiger-Kabisch, C., Sattel H., and Schreiter-Gasser, U. (1996*a*). Frontal lobe degeneration and Alzheimer's disease: a controlled study on clinical findings, volumetric brain changes and quantitative electroencephalography data. *Dementia*; **7**, 27–34.

Förstl, H., Besthorn, C., Sattel H., *et al.* (1996*b*). Volumetric brain changes and quantitative EEG in normal ageing and Alzheimer's disease. *Nervenarzt*, **67**, 53–61.

Förstl, H., Sattel, H., Besthorn, C., *et al.* (1996*c*). Longitudinal cognitive, electroencephalographic and morphological brain changes in ageing and Alzheimer's disease. *British Journal of Psychiatry*; **168**, 280–6.

Fox, N. C., Warrington, E. K., Seiffer, A. L., Agnew, S. K., and Rossor, M. N. (1998). Presymptomatic cognitive deficits in individuals at risk of familial Alzheimer's disease. A longitudinal prospective study. *Brain*, **121**, 1631–9.

Fox, N. C., Warrington, E. K., and Rossor, M. N. (1999). Serial magnetic resonance imaging of cerebral atrophy in preclinical Alzheimer's disease. *Lancet*, **353**, 2125.

Fox, N. C., Cousens, S., Scahill, R., *et al.* (2000). Using serial registered brain magnetic resonance imaging to measure disease progression in Alzheimer's disease. *Archives of Neurology*, **57**, 339–44.

Frisoni, G. B., Laakso, M. P., Beltramello, A., *et al.* (1999). Hippocampal and entorhinal cortex atrophy in frontotemporal dementia and Alzheimer's disease. *Neurology*, **52**, 91–100.

Gaup (1906).

Gelb, D. J., Oliver, E., and Gilman, S. (1999). Diagnostic criteria for Parkinson disease. *Archives of Neurology*, **56**, 33–9.

Golomb, J., Kluger, A., DeLeon, M. J., *et al.* (1996). Hippocampal formation size predicts declining memory performance in normal aging. *Neurology*, **47**, 810–13.

Greenwald, B. S., Kramer-Ginsberg, E., Bogerts, B., *et al.* (1997). Qualitative magnetic resonance imaging findings in geriatric depression. Possible link between later-onset depression and Alzheimer's disease? *Psychological Medicine*, **27**, 421–31.

Hashimoto, M., Kitagaki H., Imamura, T., *et al.* (1998). Medial temporal and whole-brain atrophy in dementia with Lewy bodies. *Neurology*, **51**, 357–62.

Hénon H., Pasquier, F., Durieu, I., *et al.* (1997). Preexisting dementia in stroke patients. Baseline frequency, associated factors, and outcome. Stroke, **28**, 2429–36.

Hénon H., Pasquier, F., Durieu, I., *et al.* (1998). Medial temporal lobe atrophy in stroke patients: relation to pre-existing dementia. *Journal of Neurology, Neurosurgery and Psychiatry*, **65**, 641–7.

Hentschel, F., Zerfaß, R., Becker, G., Beyreuther, K., and Förstl, H. (1998). Neuroradiological findings in

Alzheimer's disease due to a presenilin mutation. *Fortschr Röntgenstr*; **168**, 97–100.

Hentschel, F. (2000). Verfahren radiologischer Bildgebung in der Psychiatrie. In *Bildgebende Verfahren in der Psychiatrie* (ed. G. Stoppe, F. Hentschel, and D. L. Munz), pp. 2–37. Thieme, Stuttgart.

Iidaka, T., Nakajima, T., Suzuki, Y., Okazaki, A., Maehara, T., and Shiraishi, H. (1997). Quantitative regional cerebral flow measured by Tc-99M HMPAO SPECT in mood disorder. *Psychiatry Research*, **68**, 143–54.

Ishii, K., Yamaji, S., Kitagaki H., Imamura, T., Hirono, N., and Mori, E. (1999). Regional cerebral blood flow difference between dementia with Lewy bodies and AD. *Neurology*, **53**, 413–16.

Jack, C. R., Peterson, R. C., Xu, Y. C., *et al.* (1998). Hippocampal atrophy and apolipoprotein E genotype are independently associated with Alzheimer's disease. *Annals of Neurology*, **43**, 303–10.

Jack, C. R., Petersen, R. C., Xu, Y. C., *et al.* (1999). Prediction of AD with MRI-based hippocampal volume in mild cognitive impairment. *Neurology*, **52**, 1397–403.

Jaracz, J., Rajewski, A., Junik, R., Sowinski, J., and Gembicki, M. (1996). The assessment of regional cerebral blood flow using HMPAO-SPECT during depressive episode and in remission. *Psychiatria Polska*, **30**, 757–69.

Jelles, B., Strijiers, R. L. M., Hoojier, Ch., *et al.* (1999*a*). Non-linear EEG analysis in early Alzheimer's disease. *Acta Neurologica Scandinavica*, **100**, 360–8.

Jelles, B., van Birgelen, J. H., Slaets, J. P. J., *et al.* (1999*b*). Decrease of non-linear structure in the EEG of Alzheimer patients compared to healthy controls. *Clinical Neurology*, **110**, 1159–67.

Jenkins, R., Fox, N. C., Rossor, A. M., *et al.* (2000). Intracranial volume and Alzheimer disease, evidence against the cerebral reserve hypothesis. *Archives of Neurology*, **57**, 220–4.

Juottonen, K., Laakso, M. P., Insausti, R., *et al.* (1998). Volumes of the entorhinal and perirhinal cortices in Alzheimer's disease. *Neurobiology of Aging* 19, 15–22.

Juottonen, K., Laakso, M. P., Partanen, K., *et al.* (1999). Comparative MR analysis of the entorhinal cortex and hippocampus in diagnosing Alzheimer's disease. *American Journal of Neuroradiology*, **20**, 139–44.

Kaufer, D. I., Miller, B. L., Itti, L., *et al.* (1997). Midline cerebral morphometry distinguishes frontotemporal dementia and Alzheimer's disease. *Neurology*, **48**, 978–85.

Kidron, D., Black, S. E., Stanchev, P., *et al.* (1997). Quantitative MR volumetry in Alzheimer's disease. Topographic markers and the effects of sex and education. *Neurology*, **49**, 1504–12.

Kim, D. M., Tien, R., Byrum, C., and Krishnan, K. R. (1996). Imaging in acquired immune deficiency syndrome dementia complex (AIDS dementia complex): a review. *Progress in Neuropsychopharmacology and Biological Psychiatry*, **20**, 349–70.

Kitagaki H., Mori, E., Ishii, K., *et al.* (1998). CSF spaces in idiopathic normal pressure hydrocephalus: morphology and volumetry. *American Journal of Neuroradiology* 19, 1277–84.

Klemm, E., Danos, P., Grünwald, F., Kasper, S., Möller H. J., and Biersack H. J. (1996). Temporal lobe dysfunction and correlation of regional cerebral blood flow abnormalities with psychopathology in schizophrenia and major depression—a study with single photon emission computed tomography. *Psychiatry Research*, **68**, 1–10.

Kramer-Ginsberg, E., Greenwald, B. S., Krishnan, R. R., *et al.* (1999). Neuropsychological functioning and MRI signal hyperintensities in geriatric depression. *American Journal of Psychiatry*, **156**, 438–44.

Krishnan, K. R., Hays, J. C., and Blazer, D. G. (1997). MRI-defined vascular depression. *American Journal of Psychiatry*, **154**, 497–501.

Kuhl, D. E., Koeppe, R. A., Minoshima, S., *et al.* (1999). *In vivo* mapping of cerebral acetylcholinesterase activity in aging and Alzheimer's disease. *Neurology*, **52**, 691–9.

Kumar, A., Schweizer, E., Zhisong, J., *et al.* (1997). Neuroanatomical substrates of late-life minor depression. A quantitative magnetic resonance imaging study. *Archives of Neurology*, **54**, 613–17.

Kwan, L. T., Reed, B. R., Eberling, J. L., *et al.* (1999). Effects of subcortical cerebral infarction on cortical glucose metabolism and cognitive function. *Archives of Neurology*, **56**, 809–14.

Lavenu, I., Pasquier, F., Lebert, F., *et al.* (1997). Association between medial temporal lobe atrophy on CT and parietotemporal uptake decrease on SPECT in Alzheimer's disease. *Journal of Neurology, Neurosurgery and Psychiatry*, **63**, 441–5.

Lavenu, I., Pasquier, F., Lebert, F., *et al.* (1998). Explicit memory in frontotemporal dementia: the role of medial temporal atrophy. Dement Geriatr Cogn Disord, **9**, 99–102.

Lieberman, A. P., Trojanowski, J. Q., Lee, V. M. Y., *et al.* (1998). Cognitive, neuroimaging, and pathological studies in a patient with Pick's disease. *Annals of Neurology*, **43**, 259–65.

Lippa, C. F., Johnson, R., and Smith, T. W. (1998).The medial temporal lobe in dementia with Lewy bodies: a comparative study with Alzheimer's disease. *Annals of Neurology*, **43**, 102–6.

Liu, R. S. N., Lemiuex, L., Shorvon, S. D., *et al.* (2000). Association between brain size and abstinence from alcohol. *Lancet*, **355**, 1969.

Longstreth, W. T., Bernick, C., Manolio, T. A., *et al.* (1998). Lacunar infarcts defined by magnetic resonance imaging of 3660 elderly people. The cardiovascular health study. *Archives of Neurology*, **55**, 1217–25.

McKeith, I., Galasko, D., Kosaka, K., *et al.* (1996). Consensus guidelines for the clinical and pathologic diagnosis of dementia with Lewy bodies (DLB). *Neurology*, **47**, 1113–24.

Mackenzie Ross, S. J., Graham, N., Stuart-Green, L., *et al.* (1996). Progressive biparietal atrophy: an atypical presentation of Alzheimer's disease. *Journal of Neurology, Neurosurgery and Psychiatry*, **61**, 388–95.

Mauri, M., Sibilla, L., Bono, G., Carlesimo, G. A., Sinforiani, E., and Martelli, A. (1998). The role of morph-volumetric and memory correlations in the diagnosis of early Alzheimer dementia. *Journal of Neurology*, **245**, 525–30.

Mori, E., Yoneda, Y., Ymamshita H., Hirono, N., Ikeda, M., and Yamadori, A. (1997). Medial temporal structures relate to memory impairment in Alzheimer's disease: an MRI volumetric study. *Journal of Neurology, Neurosurgery and Psychiatry*, **63**, 214–21.

Mori, E., Ikeda, M., Hirono, N., Kitagaki H., Imamura, T., and Shimomura, T. (1999). Amygdalar volume and emotional memory in Alzheimer's disease. *American Journal of Psychiatry*, **156**, 216–22.

Müller, U., Wächter, T., Barthel, H., *et al.* (2000). Striatal $[^{123}I]\beta$-CIT SPECT and prefrontal cognitive functions in Parkinson's disease. *Journal of Neural Transmission*, **107**, 303–19.

Mummery, C. J., Patterson, K., Price, C. J., *et al.* (2000). A voxel-based morphometry study of semantic dementia: relationship between temporal lobe atrophy and semantic memory. *Annals of Neurology*, **47**, 37–44.

Na, D. L, Suh, C. K., Choi, S. H., *et al.* (1999). Diffusion-weighted magnetic resonance imaging in probable Creutzfeldt–Jakob disease. *Archives of Neurology*, **56**, 951–7.

Neary, D., Snowden, J. S., Gustafson, L., *et al.* (1998). Frontotemporal lobar degeneration—a consensus on clinical diagnostic criteria. *Neurology*, **51**, 1546–54.

Okuda, B., Tachibana H., Kawabata, K., *et al.* (2000). Cerebral blood flow in corticobasal degeneration and progressive palsy. *Alzheimer Disease and Associated Disorders*, **14**, 46–52.

Oslin, D., Atkinson, R. M., Smith, D. M., and Hendrie H. (1998). Alcohol-related dementia: proposed clinical criteria. *International Journal of Geriatric Psychiatry*, **13**, 203–12.

Palsson, S., Aevarsson, O., and Skoog, I. (1999). Depression, cerebral atrophy, cognitive performance and incidence of dementia. *British Journal of Psychiatry*, **174**, 249–53.

Petersen, R. C., Jack, C. R., Xu, Y. C., *et al.* (2000). Memory and MRI-based hippocampal volumes in aging and AD. *Neurology*, **54**, 581–7.

Pfefferbaum, A., Adalsteinsson, E., Spielman, D., Sullivan, E. V., and Lim, K. O. (1999). *In vivo* brain concentrations of *N*-acetyl compounds. Creatine and choline in Alzheimer disease. *Archives of General Psychiatry*, **56**, 185–92.

Pietrini, P., Furey, M. L., Alexander, G. E., *et al.* (1999). Association between brain functional failure an dementia severity in Alzheimer's disease: resting versus stimulation PET study. *American Journal of Psychiatry*, **156**, 470–3.

Pucci, E., Belardinelli, G., Cacchio, G., *et al.* (1999). EEG power spectrum differences in early and late onset forms of Alzheimer's disease. *Clinical Neurophysiology*, **110**, 621–31.

Reed, B. R. and Jagust, W. J. (1999). Opening a window on cerebral cholinergic function—PET imaging of acetylcholinesterase. *Neurology*, **52**, 680–2.

Reiman, E. M., Uecker, A., Caselli, R. J., *et al.* (1998). Hippocampal volumes in cognitively normal persons at genetic risk for Alzheimer's disease. *Annals of Neurology*, **44**, 288–91.

Reynolds, M. D., Johnston, J. M., Dodge H. H., DeKosky, S. T., and Ganguli, M. (1999). Small head size is related to low Mini-mental State Examination scores in a community sample non demented older adults. *Neurology*, **53**, 228–9.

Rinne, J. O., Portin, R., Ruottinen, H., *et al.* (2000). Cognitive impairment and the brain dopaminergic system in Parkinson disease. *Archives of Neurology*, **57**, 470–5.

Robertson, B., Blennow, K., Gottfries, C. G., and Wallin, A. (1998). Delirium in dementia. *International Journal of Geriatric Psychiatry*, **13**, 49–56.

Sachdev, P. and Brodaty, H. (1999*a*). Mid-sagittal anatomy in late-onset schizophrenia. *Psychological Medicine*, **29**, 963–70.

Sachdev, P. and Brodaty, H. (1999*b*). Quantitative study of signal hyperintensities on T2-weighted magnetic resonance imaging in late-onset schizophrenia. *American Journal of Psychiatry*, **156, 12** 1958–67.

Sachdev, P., Brodaty H., and Rose, N. (1999). Schizophrenia with onset after 50 years. *British Journal of Psychiatry*, **175**, 416–21.

Salat, D. H., Kaye, J. A., and Janosky, J. S. (1999). Prefrontal grey and white matter volumes in healthy aging and Alzheimer disease. *Archives of Neurology*, **56**, 338–44.

Schrag, A., Good, C. D., Miszkiel, K., *et al.* (2000). Differentiation of atypical parkinsonian syndromes with routine MRI. *Neurology*, **54**, 697–702.

Schulz, J. B., Skalej, M., Wedekind, D., *et al.* (1999). Magnetic resonance imaging-based volumetry differentiates idiopathic Parkinson's syndrome from multiple system atrophy and progressive supranuclear palsy. *Annals of Neurology*, **45**, 65–74.

Shah, P. J., Ebmeier, K. P., Glabus, M. F., and Goodwin, G. M. (1998). Cortical grey matter reductions associated with treatment-resistant chronic unipolar depression. *British Journal of Psychiatry*, **172**, 527–32.

Shear, P. K., Jerrigan, T. L., and Butters, N. (1994). Volumetric magnetic resonance imaging quantification of longitudinal brain changes in abstinent alcoholics. *Alcoholism, Clinical and Experimental Research*, **18**, 172–6.

Simpson, S., Talbot, P. R., Snowden, J. S., and Neary, D. (1997). Subcortical vascular disease in elderly patients with treatment resistant depression. *Journal of Neurology, Neurosurgery and Psychiatry*, **62**, 196–7.

Simpson, S., Baldwin, R. C., Jackson, A., and Burns, A. S. (1998). Is subcortical disease associated with a poor response to antidepressants? Neurological, neuropsychological and neuroradiological findings in late-life depression. *Psychological Medicine*, **28**, 1015–26.

Smirniotopoulos, J. G., Koeller, K. K., Nelson, A. M., and Murphy, F. M. (1997). Neuroimaging—autopsy correlations in AIDS. *Neuroimaging Clinics of North America*, **7**, 615–37.

Snowdon, D. A., Greiner, L. H., Mortimer, J. A., *et al.* (1997). Brain infarction and the clinical expression of Alzheimer disease. The nun study. *Journal of the American Medical Association*, **277**, 813–17.

Soliveri, P., Monza, D., Paridi, D., *et al.* (1999). Cognitive and magnetic resonance imaging aspects of corticobasal degeneration and progressive supranuclear palsy. *Neurology*, **53**, 502–7.

Stoppe, G., Bruhn, H., Pouwels, P. J. W., *et al.* (2000). Alzheimer disease: absolute quantification of cerebral metabolites in vivo using localized proton magnetic resonance spectroscopy. *Alzheimer's Disease and Associated Disorders*, **14**, 112–19.

Szelies, B., Mielke, R., Kessler, J., and Heiss, W. D. (1999). EEG power changes are related to regional cerebral glucose metabolism in vascular dementia. *Clinical Neurophysiology*, **110**, 615–20.

Talbot, P. R. and Testa, J. (1995). The value of SPECT in dementia. *Nuclear Medicine Communications*, **16**, 425–37.

Thurnher, M. M., Thurnher, S. A., Muhlbauer, B., *et al.* (1997). Progressive multifocal leucoencephalopathy in AIDS, initial and follow-up CT and MRI. *Neuroradiology*, **39**, 611–18.

Turjanski, N. and Brooks, D. J. (1997). PET and the investigation of dementia in the parkinsonian patient. *Journal of Neural Transmission*, **51** (Suppl.), 37–48.

Ulug, A. M. and Zijl, P. C. M. (1999). Orientation-interdependent diffusion imaging without tensor diagnonalization, anisotropy definitions based on physical attributes of the diffusion elipsoid. *Journal of Magnetic Resonance Imaging*, **9**, 804–13.

Visser, P. J., Scheltens, P., Verhey, F. R. J., *et al.* (1999). Medial temporal lobe atrophy and memory dysfunction as predictors for dementia in subjects with mild cognitive impairment. *Journal of Neurology*, **246**, 477–85.

Wada, Y., Nanbu, Y., Jiang, Z. Y., Koshino, Y. and Hashimoto, T. (1998). Interhemispheric EEG coherence in never-medicated patients with paranoid schizophrenia: analysis at rest and during photic stimulation. *Clinical Electroencephalography*, **29**, 170–6.

Walker, Z., Costa, D. C., Ince, P., McKeith, I. G., and Katona, C. L. E. (1999). In-vivo demonstration of dopaminergic degeneration in dementia with Lewy bodies. *Lancet*, **354**, 646–7.

Winnikates, J. and Jankovic, J. (1999). Clinical correlates of vascular Parkinsonism. *Archives of Neurology*, **56**, 98–102.

Yamaguchi, S., Meguro, K., Itoh, M., *et al.* (1997). Decreased cortical glucose metabolism correlates with hippocampal atrophy in Alzheimer's disease as shown by MRI and PET. *Journal of Neurology, Neurosurgery and Psychiatry*, **62**, 596–600.

Yamaguchi, S., Tsuchiya H., Yamagata, S., *et al.* (2000). Event-related brain potentials in response to novel sounds in dementia. *Clinical Neurophysiology*, **111**, 195–203.

Yamauchi, H., Fukuyama, H., Nagahama, Y., *et al.* (1998). Atrophy of the corpus callosum, cortical hypometabolism, and cognitive impairment in corticobasal degeneration. *Archives of Neurology*, **55**, 609–14.

Yee, A. S., Simon, J. H., Anderson, C. A., Sze, C. I., and Filley, C. M. (1999). Diffusion-weighted MRI of right-hemisphere dysfunction in Creutzfeldt–Jakob disease. *Neurology*, **52**, 1514–15.

Yener, G. G., Leuchter, A. F., Jenden, D., *et al.* (1996). Quantitative EEG in frontotemporal dementia. *Clinical Electroencephalography*, **27**, 61–8.

Zeidler, M., Sellar, R. J., Collie, D. A., *et al.* (2000). The pulvinar sign on magnetic resonance imaging in variant Creutzfeldt–Jakob disease. *Lancet*, **355**, 1412–18.

13 Psychopharmacology in the elderly

Philip Wood

Introduction

Physicians caring for elderly patients need to concern themselves with how an ageing physiology, biochemistry, and intellect interact with drug treatments. Only in recent times have new drugs been subjected to concerted efforts to measure these effects, and thus the most explicit data are largely restricted to these new drugs. For most, it is necessary to apply the general principles of changes in pharmacokinetics and dynamics associated with ageing. Clearly it is difficult to disentangle changes due to ageing *per se* from those due to disease, and it is often unnecessary as the former are usually swamped by the latter. It is not always possible to provide set rules about dosage adjustments for the elderly, simply because patients differ so much. On occasions where research is either lacking or divergent, an overly dogmatic statement may be made in the interests of simplicity. Unless otherwise stated the term 'elderly' is taken to mean those patients over the age of 65 years. Drugs used or encountered by psychiatrists are used as examples wherever possible, even though more thoroughly researched alternatives exist.

Age-related changes in physiology relevant to drug handling (Table 13.1)

A schematic outline of drug handling is given in Fig. 13.1.

The reader is reminded that, put simply, pharmacokinetics are how the body affects drugs, and pharmacodynamics are how drugs affect the body.

Table 13.1 Age-related changes relevant to drug handling

Elevation of gastric pH
Reduction of gastric emptying rate
Reduction of splanchnic blood flow
Thinning and reduction of absorptive surface
Decline in total body size in advanced age
Relative increase in total body fat until advanced age
Decline in metabolically active tissue
Decline in total body water
Reduction in plasma albumin
Slight and variable increase in Al acid glycoprotein
Reduction in liver mass
Redistribution of regional blood flow away from liver and kidney
Reduction in hepatic microsomal enzyme activity
Reduction in glomerular filtration
Reduction in renal tubular function

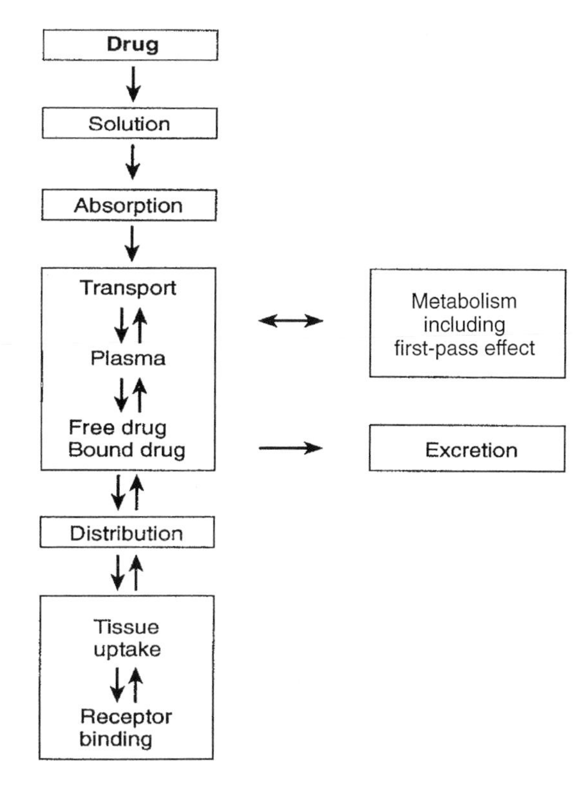

Fig. 13.1 Schematic outline of drug handling.

Pharmacokinetics

There is still some doubt whether certain age-related physiological changes are due to ageing or debility (Swift and Triggs 1987). What is more certain is that the elderly as a population are more often sick, and are more likely to suffer chronic disease states. However, certain age-associated changes do occur and will be briefly reviewed.

Absorption and transport

Whilst the rate and extent of drug absorption from the gastrointestinal tract is largely unaltered in the elderly, there are still some changes in gastric pH and gut-wall metabolism that affect the bioavailability of some compounds, for example L-dopa and the benzodiazepine clorazepate. In the elderly, the reduced steady-state concentrations of clorazepate are partly a result of reduced gastric acid concentration (Stevenson *et al.* 1980). A threefold increase in the bioavailability of L-dopa is seen because the level of dopa decarboxylase is reduced in the stomach wall of the elderly (Evans *et al.* 1980), and as a result the elderly require lower starting dosages. Conversely, those patients with delayed gastric emptying have lower levels due to loss through metabolism (Bianchine *et al.* 1971). After oral dosing of diazepam, elderly patients exhibit a slower rise in blood levels and minor prolongation of the drug's half-life (Klotz *et al.* 1975). Slow-release preparations, for example nifedipine, have a much longer half-life in the elderly, which reflects absorption rather than elimination kinetics.

Studies of drug–protein binding in the elderly have been inconsistent, perhaps reflecting mixed patient selection, variations in the techniques used to assay drugs, and the temporary changes in acute-phase proteins, e.g. α-acid glycoprotein which rises and falls with inflammation. Furthermore, plasma protein represents only part of the total available protein for binding throughout the whole body. However, a number of reports note a decrease in bound fractions of diazepam, lorazepam, and clobazam, but an increase in the bound fraction of chlorpromazine (Swift and Triggs 1987). The pharmacokinetics of chlorpromazine is further complicated by avid hepatic elimination (high-clearance). Clinical significance is seen only in those drugs which have a narrow therapeutic window, or a small volume of distribution. Changes in serum albumin in the well elderly are modest and have little influence on the carriage of drugs, apart from those agents which are highly plasma bound (Bender *et al.* 1975). Furthermore, decreased binding may offset decreased clearance, leaving no net effect since less drug is delivered to the liver. Underlying pathological states that influence the serum protein concentrations must also be taken into account. Elevations of α-acid glycoprotein, an acute-phase reactant known to increase non-specifically in response to infection, inflammation, cancer, trauma, and, to a lesser extent, age (Abernethy and Kerzner 1984), can lead to increased cationic drug binding and thus a reduced free-drug fraction, for example imipramine and chlorpromazine (Piafsky *et al.* 1978). In general, the influence of protein binding is not clinically significant, and any effect tends to be overshadowed by the more important changes in elimination (Grandison and Boudinot 2000).

Body composition

Body composition can be expected to have an important effect on the distribution and the handling of drugs. Due to the relative increase in body fat in the elderly, lipophilic drugs can be expected to have an increased apparent volume of distribution and thus clearance, for example trazodone (Miller *et al.* 1987) and diazepam. In contrast, hydrophilic drugs (and alcohol is a good example) will have a decreased volume of distribution, and potentially high plasma concentrations.

Elimination

Liver metabolism

Research has shown that certain drug metabolic pathways are influenced by ageing. The bioavailability of orally administered drugs depends on their absorption and metabolism. Since absorption is relatively unaffected by ageing, whereas metabolism by the gut wall and the liver may be markedly reduced, an increase in bioavailability is most apparent with drugs that are highly metabolized. This is demonstrated in a measured reduction in the first-pass effect, that is to say less drug is removed after absorption into the portal vein as the drug passes through the liver to the systemic circulation (Castleden and George 1979), since:

(1) there is a reduction in liver mass, blood flow, and perfusion with age;
(2) the prevalence of slow acetylator status is increased in the elderly (Gachalyi *et al.* 1984);
(3) there is a modest decline in oxidative metabolism in the elderly.

Drugs undergoing hepatic phase-I metabolism (oxidation/reduction/hydrolysis), for example phenothiazines, are likely to be more slowly metabolized. Microsomal oxidative enzyme activities and affinities are reduced by about 6% for every 10 years of age (Sotaniemi *et al.* 1997), and possibly more so in the frail elderly. Drugs undergoing conjugation (phase II), which increases water solubility, are much less likely to be influenced. Overall, one can expect to see drugs that are oxidized in the liver to have a prolonged half-life as their clearance is reduced.

Renal excretion

One of the most important and consistent effects on drug handling in the elderly results from a decline in renal function, on average a reduction of 35% in those over 65 years of age compared to the young. Numerous examples of these changes exist (Turnheim, 1998). It is important to realize that this change is not uniform across the elderly, and in the 'healthy' elderly few clinically significant changes are noted (Fliser *et al.* 1999). The diminution of renal clearance is accentuated in those elderly with other medical problems, such as renal and heart disease, diabetes, hypertension, and atherosclerosis. Not only is this important for any water-soluble drug excreted unchanged in the urine, but also for any water-soluble active metabolites produced by the liver. An example of this effect is 2-OH-desipramine, the major metabolite of desipramine (Kitanaka *et al.* 1982).

Pharmacodynamics

Little is known about receptor status and age, and it is unclear whether a change in receptor affinity or density explains the apparent increase in sensitivity of the elderly to, for example, benzodiazepines (Castleden *et al.* 1977; Greenblatt *et al.* 1991; Albrecht *et al.* 1999) and isoprenaline, and the reduced sensitivity to propranolol. The increased sensitivity of the elderly to some drugs is far more likely to reflect disease rather than ageing *per se* (Davies and Castleden 1988). Small single-dose studies in otherwise healthy individuals have demonstrated that older subjects are more likely to develop orthostatic hypotension whilst taking thioridazine and, to a lesser extent, remoxipride. In this study, sedation differed little, although it could be more of a problem in those with deficient cholinergic function (Swift *et al.*

1999). Studies of tardive dyskinesia using ageing rats have shown enhanced receptor sensitivity, increased numbers of dopamine receptors (Burr *et al.* 1977), and substantially increased adrenergic receptor binding, compared to younger animals, in the cerebral cortex after pretreatment with neuroleptics (Misra *et al.* 1981).

Adverse drug reactions (ADRS)

Incidence

It is estimated that approximately 30% of all medical admissions to hospital are related to adverse drug events. Up to 16% of patients admitted to psychogeriatric wards have side-effects persisting from psychotropic medication. The incidence rises with age (Frisk *et al.* 1977), with the number of drug reactions per hospital admission reaching 5.6% in patients over 60 years of age (Smidt and McQueen 1972).

Although epidemiological data on drug toxicity have many confounding variables, for those drugs with a strong anticholinergic effect (for example, imipramine, amitriptyline, clomipramine, doxepin, maprotiline), the incidence of ADRs is 1.2%. For other antidepressants the incidence is significantly lower (0.6% $p < 0.05$). For the lower potency neuroleptics (for example, thioridazine) the risk is nearer 0.8%. When used in combination with 'anticholinergic' antidepressants the risk rises to 1.5% in those over 45 years of age (Schmidt *et al.* 1987).

Causes

Several factors contribute to the increased propensity for ADRs in the elderly:

1. There is a higher incidence of coexistent illnesses, which not only increase the likelihood of other potentially interacting drugs being prescribed but also expose the patient to problems with the complicated and frequently altering drug regimens. For example, the increased treatment complexity translates to increased difficulties in communication: the physician may wrongly believe that the patient has stopped taking a previously prescribed medication. There is an increased likelihood of many doctors being involved at multiple locations, and each may lack accurate information regarding the patient's drug history, let alone appreciate interactions with less than familiar drugs. Coexistent illness often precipitates organ failure, leading to alterations in bioavailability and, eventually, to changes in plasma drug levels.
2. Not only do more women take medications than men but they also live longer, leading to a cohort effect in the latter years of life.
3. The number of prescriptions increases directly with age, so that over 75% of the elderly population receive prescribed drugs. Multiple drug prescriptions are also more common and, associated with this complexity, is a reduction in compliance, including irregular drug-taking habits. Psychotropic drug use follows similar patterns, with institutionalized patients being prescribed psychotropic drugs more frequently than their community-based controls (Zawadski *et al.* 1978). In one American community study, 70% of patients with non-psychiatric health problems were receiving sedatives and hypnotics in addition to their other prescriptions (Lech *et al.* 1975).
4. Altered drug kinetics expose the body to higher levels of drugs, and thus increased side-effects. Stopping drugs can also lead to altered kinetics through a reduced effect on enzyme induction (for example, the antiepileptics and barbiturates), lowered competition during renal secretion, and possibly through alterations in renal blood flow. Altered gastric emptying can increase the bioavailability of some drugs, for example L-dopa.
5. Altered pharmacodynamics may mean enhanced drug action, even if there is no significant change in kinetics.
6. There is a consistent association between the current use of long half-life hypnotics, anxiolytics, tricyclic antidepressants, or antipsychotics and an increased risk of hip fracture in the elderly, as well as an increase in

risk associated with increased drug dose (Ray *et al.* 1987).
7. The risk for toxic delirium increases steadily with age, being sixfold greater in those over 60 than those under 60 years of age (Schmidt *et al.* 1987).

Clinical presentation

The typical patient at high risk from adverse drug reactions is a small, elderly female, with a previous history of adverse drug reactions and allergies, who has multiple chronic illnesses, and in whom both renal and mental function is failing. In all instances, the doctor is wise to be highly suspicious that medications are at least partly responsible when changes in a patient's condition are noted. Since not all adverse drug reactions fit into the clear-cut 'rash and eosinophilia' pattern, the possibility that a patient with a non-specific presentation might have an adverse drug reaction needs to be kept in mind. Aspects of the history and clinical findings which increase the likelihood of ADR include: a temporal relationship between a drug prescription and the illness, usually 2–3 weeks; the patient noting that they are 'not so well' since starting the new drug; mild fever; rash; eosinophilia; and deranged liver function tests (LFTs—usually elevations in gamma-glutamyl transferase (GGT) or alanine transaminase (ALT). In those drugs with known adverse side-effects such as tricyclic antidepressants, it is worth enquiring for symptoms of postural hypotension, constipation, urinary retention, and confusion, and looking for appropriate signs. In any case of doubt it is recommended that all non-essential drugs be withdrawn and close monitoring of the patient be maintained. If the drugs are later deemed necessary and no suitable alternative is available, then a rechallenge is warranted if the earlier ADR produced no cardiovascular effects. Rechallenge is likely to produce positive results within 2 weeks. All ADRs should be reported, even if it is a known effect, as this is the only way that continually revised ADR figures for all drugs can be maintained. The patient's notes and medication chart should be clearly labelled, the patient's general practitioner (GP) notified, and the yellow ADR card sent off to the appropriate authority.

Individual drug groups

Antipsychotics

There is a range of widely differing drugs in this class. Each has an individual profile and, as a result, individual clinicians tend to get to know a few of the group and use these in preference to others. The major classes and subclasses are:

(1) phenothiazines:
  (a) aliphatic, for example chlorpromazine (Largactil),
  (b) piperidenes, for example thioridazine (Melleril),
  (c) piperazines, for example trifluperazine (Stelazine);
(2) butyrophenones, for example haloperidol;
(3) thioxanthenes, for example piperazine, thiothixene;
(4) diphenylbutylpiperidines, for example pimozide;
(5) azepines, for example clozapine;
(6) benzisoxazoles, for example risperidone;
(7) thienobenzodiazepine/dibenzodiazepine, e.g. olanzapine, quetiapine;
(8) benzamides, e.g. amisulpride.

As the pharmacological effects of the phenothiazines are very broad, these expose the patient to a large number of common side-effects (see Table 13.2).

The atypical antipsychotics have a wider range of receptor blocking activity, ranging from relatively pure D_2 receptor antagonism (e.g. amisulpride) through to D_2/serotonin-$5HT_2$ antagonists (e.g. risperidone and ziprasidone) to multireceptor antagonists (e.g. olanzapine and quetiapine).

Pharmacokinetics

In general, the antipsychotics, including the 'atypical antipsychotics' are well absorbed, have substantial first-pass metabolism in the liver, and are widely distributed throughout the body. They

Table 13.2 Profiles of the major antipsychotic drugs

Drug	Potency Eq. dose (mg)*	Sedative effects	Extra-pyramidal effects dose (mg)	Usual** starting (mg)
Chlorpromazine	100	High	Moderate	10–25 b.d./t.d.s.
Thioridazine	100	Moderate	Low	10–25 b.d./t.d.s.
Haloperidol	4	Low	High	2–3
Trifluoperazine	5	Moderate	High	2–3
Thiothixine	5	Moderate	High	2–3
Pimozide	4	Moderate	High	1–2
Flupenthixol decanoate		Low	Moderate	≈20
Fluphenazine decanoate		Low/mod	High	≈12.5
Clozapine	50–100	High	Low	12.5 daily
Risperidone	2	Low	Low	0.5 b.d.
Olanzapine	2	Low	Low	1–2
Sertindole	1	Low	Low	0.5–1

*Chlorpromazine has been arbitrarily assigned a value of 100 for the sake of comparison, but cannot be reliably related to the extremely long-acting preparations.
**For the elderly.
b.d. twice per day
t.d.s. three times per day

have high tissue-binding and are slowly eliminated, and therefore have a relatively long duration of action. There is only mild enzyme induction. It is generally advisable to reduce the dose, at least initially, in elderly patients (especially in the physically ill) by about one-half to two-thirds of that used in the young. The various potencies and side-effect profiles of the phenothiazines make it possible for the clinician to make an informed choice to suit the circumstances (see the section on physical illness, p. 302).

Side-effects

All antipsychotics block D_{1-4} receptors to varying degrees, although the D_2 receptor appears to be more important in terms of psychosis. Unfortunately this receptor also mediates the extrapyramidal system pathways, block of which produces varying degrees of extrapyramidal side-effects (EPSE) (see Table 13.3). This is less of a problem with the atypical antipsychotics (Sweet and Pollock 1998) as the effects are offset by the additional affinity to the serotoninergic receptors. In general, the higher the S_2/D_2 ratio, the less EPSE. The α-adrenergic-1 blockade causes orthostatic hypotension and, coupled with blockade of histamine-1 receptors, some sedation. Table 13.4 compares the newer agents with haloperidol by way of illustration.

Table 13.3 Effects of antipsychotics

Block D_1 and D_2, D_3 dopamine receptors (in varying ratios)
Block α receptors
Anticholinergic
Antihistamine
Serotonin antagonism
Antiemetic

Anticholinergic activity may lead to dry mouth, urinary hesitancy, and possible overflow incontinence, constipation, and (to a lesser extent) blurred vision in the elderly. Paradoxically, the anticholinergic effects can be protective against extrapyramidal side-effects (see below). A quinidine-like effect has been ascribed to phenothiazines, along with some direct myocardial depression which can, at high levels, precipitate cardiac failure. The cardiographic changes such as QT prolongation and inverted T and U waves are

Table 13.4 Relative effect of antipsychotics on various receptors

Receptor blockade	Chlorpromazine	Haloperidol	Clozapine	Respiridone	Olanzapine
D_1	+++	+++	+++	+++	+++
D_2	+++	++++	+++	++++	+++
D_3	++++	++++	+.	++++	+++
D_4	++++	+++++	++++	+++++	++++
H_1	+++	+.	++++	++++	++++
ACh	+++	+.	+++	±	++++
a_1	++++	+.	+++	+++++	+++
a_2	0	+.	+++	++++	0
5-HT_1	0	+.	0	0	++++
5-HT_2	++++	+++	++++	+++++	++++
DA uptake	+.	+.	±	+.	?

Note: abbreviated list below, (best seen in pharmacology texts)
D_1: dopamine type 1, possibly mediates antipsychotic effects;
D_2: dopamine type 2, depending on the areas of the brain as to the effect on +ve or –ve symptoms in schizophrenia;
D_3: dopamine type 3, possible effects negative psychotic symptoms;
D_4: dopamine type 4, possible effects positive symptoms;
H_1: histamine type, leads to sedation;
ACh: acetylcholine, leads to dry mouth, etc., and mitigates EPSE;
a_1: alpha type 1, leads to postural hypotension;
a_2: alpha type 2, leads to sexual dysfunction;
5-HT_1: 5-hydroxytryptamine type 1, has an antidepressant/antiaggressive effect;
5-HT_2: 5-hydroxytryptamine type 2, mitigates EPSE of D_2 etc

probably benign, but in patients with myocardial disease and conduction defects, high doses should be avoided, especially with thioridazine (Ballenger 1987). With the doses usually employed in the elderly, there are generally few toxic effects on the eye (for example, corneal or lenticular opacities) and retinal pigmentation is rarely seen. The skin in the elderly is seemingly more sensitive to the effects of neuroleptics, with an apparent increased incidence of slate-coloured pigmentation (Hader 1965); however, no evidence has been presented to show an increase in hypersensitivity or photosensitivity reactions. Clozapine can cause a serious granulocytopenia or agranulocytosis.

Extrapyramidal side-effects

Extrapyramidal side-effects do not seem to be related to antipsychotic activity. Thioridazine has fewer extrapyramidal side-effects, especially compared with the butyrophenones and those drugs with an aliphatic side chain. The 'atypical antipsychotics' increase the ratio between antipsychotic activity and extrapyramidal side-effects, and may be of benefit in a minority of elderly people in whom parkinsonism or tardive dyskinesia is a significant problem (Geddes *et al.* 2000).

Pseudo-Parkinson's disease

This is typically a triad of bradykinesia, rigidity, and (to a lesser extent) tremor. Although termed pseudo-Parkinson's the condition is virtually indistinguishable from idiopathic Parkinson's disease. The likelihood of precipitating the condition rises with dose and remits with reduction of dose. There may be a delay in expression of the condition for up to several years, but 70% occur within 1 month and 90% within 3 months of initiation of treatment. (Marsden *et al.* 1975). The elderly, women, and those with organic brain disease are at greatest risk. Spontaneous improvement on stopping treatment is usually seen within a few weeks, although an unfortunate few remain symptomatic for years, and some exhibit signs again later in life. However, one must remember that there is a 1–2% incidence of dyskinesias in those elderly people who have never had antipsychotic medication.

The condition is helped by anticholinergic drugs such as orphenadrine, procyclidine, etc.

There is no advantage in using these drugs prophylactically, which cause additional anticholinergic side-effects and may increase the risk of a later development of tardive dyskinesia (American Psychiatric Association 1980). Downward adjustment of the dose or a change to thioridazine may be of benefit if the problem occurs. Anticholinergic treatment withdrawal may be attempted after 4–6 months. Amantadine can ameliorate the condition, but L-dopa is not generally indicated for the treatment of pseudo-Parkinson's disease because dopaminergic drugs tend to exacerbate the psychiatric condition.

Tardive dyskinesia (TD)

TD is a repetitive, involuntary movement of the tongue, lips, mouth, trunk, and limbs secondary to drug use. It differs only in aetiology from idiopathic orofacial dyskinesia. Paradoxically, it not only appears whilst the patient is taking the neuroleptic, but more commonly appears following withdrawal, even up to years later. It relates to the gradual loss of dopamine receptor blockade in the striatum, and the possible emergence of receptor supersensitivity. The prevalence increases with age, and it is more common in women. The repetitive chewing movements seen in otherwise normal elderly people may be a subset of the condition. It is wise to exclude other coincidental causes such as the stereotyped movements seen in schizophrenia, focal dystonia, Huntington's disease, Wilson's disease, and rheumatic chorea. The emergence of the problem is more strongly related to the duration of treatment than to absolute dose. Approximately 10–20% of patients taking a neuroleptic for a year or more develop appreciable symptoms. Plasma levels are not related. TD lasts for years, even after stopping the offending drug. Mehta *et al.* (1977) showed that 11/13 elderly patients with TD had symptoms for over 5 years.

Again, paradoxically, the treatment consists of cautiously reducing (by approximately 10% weekly) the offending drug, which unfortunately may worsen the psychiatric condition. Usually a month or two, but occasionally up to 2 years, may elapse before the symptoms abate. An attempt at control using another neuroleptic, such as pimozide, or by augmenting acetylcholine release with physostigmine can be tried. Clonazepam and lithium, along with many other medications, have been tried in this rather difficult condition. The best advice remains that prevention is better than cure—that is to say, restricting the use of antipsychotics to those clearly in need and using the minimum effective dose. There may be some advantage in using the atypical antipsychotics, in particular, clozapine. Fortunately, the condition does not seem to be uniformly or relentlessly progressive, so the clinician faced with a patient requiring a neuroleptic can be comforted by this fact; fortunately, the patient is rarely as concerned as the doctor or relatives.

In summary, increasing age increases the likelihood of developing tardive dyskinesia whilst on psychotropic medication, and decreases the likelihood of recovery.

Akathisia

Because this causes restlessness with hand, finger, and foot movement it can be mistaken for agitation, but it is seen without autonomic disturbance or distress in the patient. The lack of response to anticholinergics, and the reduction in symptoms associated with a reduction of a neuroleptic, suggest postsynaptic receptor blockade is the problem, possibly in the mesolimbic area.

Dyskinesia and dystonia

The classical oculogyric exaggerated posturing frequently seen in the young is rare in the elderly. It occurs soon after initiation of treatment and responds to anticholinergics. The atypical antipsychotics may have advantages (the incidence of these symptoms is lower), but published experience in the elderly is lacking.

Antidepressants

Tricyclic antidepressants (TCA)

Pharmacokinetics

Absorption is complete for most agents in this group and, similarly, there is substantial first-pass metabolism. The TCAs are highly protein bound (90%) and have a wide distribution with a predilection for the heart, lungs, kidneys, and adrenals. TCAs are subject to substantial oxidative degradation in the liver, although demethylation occurs in the case of amitriptyline and imipramine. The decreased metabolic capacity in the elderly reduces first-pass metabolism, contributes to the prolongation of plasma half-lives, and increases the steady-state levels on repeated standard dosage. Since some metabolic byproducts have both antidepressant and other side-effects, the net effect is complicated and difficult to predict.

In general, for a given dose, amitriptyline plasma levels show a weak correlation with age. In a study by Schultz *et al.* (1983), mean systemic clearance did not appear to change with age (in those older than 65 years), although the half-life was longer in elderly patients (21 against 16 hours). They also had an increased volume of distribution (17 against 14 l/kg). Bioavailability remained essentially unaltered with ageing. There is a weak correlation between the half-life of nortriptyline and age, and for both drugs there is much individual patient variation (Braithwaite *et al.* 1979). Despite this wide variation in plasma levels between individuals, some authors have shown that steady-state levels can be predicted from single-dose kinetics, for example nortriptyline (Dawling *et al.* 1980) and amitriptyline (Dawling *et al.* 1984). Pharmacodynamic data suggest a narrow therapeutic window and little relationship between plasma levels and side-effects (Swift and Hewick 1987).

Side-effects

Effects on the heart

Cardiotropic side-effects limit TCA use in patients with unstable heart disease. This may not necessarily be due to the effect on left ventricular performance (Glassman *et al.* 1983), but on conduction and through postural blood-pressure control (Rodstein and Som Oei 1979). Described effects include:

1. An accentuation of postural blood-pressure drop, probably through blocking norepinephrine (noradrenaline) reuptake centrally, leading to increased receptor stimulation and hence inhibition of peripheral sympathetic activity. The best predictor of this is a pretreatment postural fall in blood pressure. Thus, extreme care is required in those elderly with postural hypotension, autonomic impairment, and heart disease.
2. A possible negative inotropic effect, although this is generally unimportant unless the patient has severe heart failure.
3. A quinine-like effect which leads, in toxic states, to bundle-branch patterns, QRS widening, and occasionally heart block. This quinine (Class 1)-like effect may have some theoretical uses in ventricular arrhythmias, but, in general, the drugs are not used in patients with heart disease, including those with conduction disturbance (PR prolongation and bundle-branch block).
4. Like all Class 1 drugs, toxic doses cause arrhythmias, but there is conflicting evidence concerning an increased risk of sudden death in association with TCAs.

Lofepramine is favoured in many geriatrics units in the United Kingdom. It is more lipophilic than most TCAs and thus is likely to have good penetration into the brain. It is metabolized into desipramine, but cardiotoxicity is low and safety in overdose is reported as high.

Anticholinergic side-effects

The TCAs are noted for their anticholinergic side-effects. Clinical experience suggests that the elderly are particularly prone to toxic confusional states, dry mouth, constipation, retention of urine (especially in the male), and occasionally precipitation of glaucoma. Nevertheless, many elderly patients take their TCAs successfully and without adverse effects, provided there is close attention to dosage. TCAs differ in their frequency and severity of side-effects (see Table 13.5).

Potential interactions

Interactions with antihypertensives such as guanethidine, debrisoquine, bretylium, and

Table 13.5 Relative severity of side-effects of some commonly used antidepressants

Drug	Relative anticholinergic action	Relative sedative action	Postural hypotension
Amitriptyline	+++	+++	++
Imipramine	+++	+++	++
Doxepin	+++	+++	++
Nortriptyline	++	++	±
Protriptyline	++	+	++
Desipramine	+	+	+/++
Lofepramine	+	±	+
Maprotiline	++	++	+
Trazodone	+	+	+
Mianserin	±	++	+
Serotonin agonists	0	–	±
Moclobemide (RIMA)	0	–	0

bethanidine are more often described than seen, especially as these drugs are obsolete as antihypertensives. It should not be forgotten that methyl-dopa and clonidine can have their effect antagonized by TCAs. Administration of TCAs with adrenergic agents such as anaesthetics and cough and cold remedies can accentuate the adrenergic action. Co-administration of barbiturates tends to lower TCA levels through enzymatic induction, as does smoking, whereas neuroleptics increase them. Smokers tend to experience fewer side-effects than non-smokers.

Tetracyclic antidepressants

Reduced anticholinergic and cardiotropic profiles favour this group, which includes mianserin. Daytime sedation can limit the usefulness of some compounds. Mianserin has been associated with aplastic anaemia, and thus a blood count after the fourth week of starting the drug is advisable.

Serotonin agonists (SSRIs)

These agents may have some advantages due to the lack of sedation, cardiotoxicity, and anticholinergic side-effects. They have proved to be almost as effective and safer than the TCAs. The main side-effects are gastrointestinal upset (nausea and vomiting), headache, sleep disturbances, and weight loss as well as hyponatraemia, but there is some minor variation between the members of this group.

Fluvoxamine, fluoxetine, and paroxetine are inhibitors of the neuronal presynaptic reuptake of serotonin. Paradoxically, although trazodone and mianserin have effects on serotonin, they act more like antagonists than agonists and thus are excluded from this brief description of effects in the elderly. A summary of pharmacokinetic data for the elderly is shown in Table 13.6 (Freeman 1988; Dechant and Clissold 1991; Murdock and McTavish 1992; Palmer and Benfield 1994).

Bioavailability is generally high and maximal plasma levels are reached at 2–8 hours. Serotonin agonists are metabolized in the liver and their metabolites excreted in urine. Their mean half-life (terminal phase) is not consistently increased in the elderly, although, in the case of paroxetine, initial dosages should be at the low end of the suggested adult dosage. Interference with other oxidized drugs can occur, increasing the half-life by reducing clearance. Fluoxetine, norfluoxetine (the major metabolite of fluoxetine), and paroxetine are potent inhibitors of the hepatic isoenzyme P450IID6, whereas sertraline has much

Table 13.6 Serotonin agonists and reversible monoamine oxidase inhibitors

Drug	Absorption	Elimination	V_d l/kg	Plasma binding (%)	Active metabolite	Half-life (half-life active metabolite)	Interactions
Fluoxetine	High	Demethylation	26	95	Yes	1–3 days (7-15 days)	Low
Fluvoxamine	High	Demethylation	5	77	No	13–19 hrs	Warfarin Digoxin
Sertraline	High, slow	Demethylation, Oxidation	≈20	97	Weak	25–26	Minimal
Paroxetine	High	Conjugation	>10	95	Weak	>24 h, variable	Minimal
Moclobemide	High	Oxidation	≈80	50	Weak	1–2 hrs	Cimetidine Pethidine dextromethorphan

weaker inhibitory effects on its activity. Inhibition of P450 isoenzymes can cause potentially dangerous increases in the plasma levels of a number of drugs, including TCAs, neuroleptics, and mood stabilizers, such as carbamazepine. However, in general, these selective serotonin reuptake inhibitors (SSRIs) are reported not to interfere in a significant way with other drugs, and nor do they potentiate the deleterious effects of alcohol. An exception is fluvoxamine's interference with warfarin metabolism, which leads to an increase in prothrombin time and an increase in digoxin excretion (Murdock and McTavish 1992). The onset of action of serotonin agonists appears to be no quicker than with the TCAs. There are few demonstrable effects on cardiovascular indices, and, although the effect on ECG and other cardiac indices are apparently less than with the TCAs, clinical data are lacking. EEG effects are more akin to those seen with desipramine; attention span and reaction times were improved in volunteer studies. In general, reported data show that SSRI dosage adjustments appear to be unnecessary in elderly depressed patients.

Monoamine oxidase inhibitors (MAOI)

With care, these drugs are useful in the treatment of depression in the elderly. Although phenelzine metabolism is possibly affected by acetylator status, it appears that the actual dose is more important than the acetylator status of the patient (Tyrer *et al.* 1980). Out of five studies reviewed by Pare, three suggested that response is better in slow acetylators (Pare 1985), and that, in general, doses used by physicians are too low. Few data exist on their use in the elderly, but early workers reported a high incidence of hepatotoxicity. Obviously extreme caution needs to be exercised in patients with hypertension, cardiovascular disease, and those in whom compliance with dietary restrictions cannot be expected. In some studies, deprenyl, a specific MAO-B inhibitor which has a more favourable side-effect profile, has been shown to have an antidepressant effect if given in adequate doses (30–50 mg). At these doses, it is possible that MAO-A is also inhibited (resulting in postural hypotension and reactions with cheese).

Theoretically, depression associated with dementia in the elderly should be responsive to treatment with MAOIs due to the elevated MAO levels in the brain. However, evidence in support of this is limited (Ashford and Ford 1979). TCAs can interact adversely with MAOIs, the most potent interactions being with clomipramine and the least with trimipramine. Tranylcypromine is the most interactive of the MAOIs and isocarboxazid the least. A washout period before starting or changing from a MAOI should be considered (see Table 13.7).

Table 13.7 Interchange and co-administration of various antidepressants

From	to TCAs	to SSRIs	to RIMAs	to MAOIs
TCAs	NA	Potential increase in plasma concentrations of both drugs	No washout	2 week washout. Probably contraindicated together.
SSRIs	Potential increase in plasma concentrations of both drugs	NA	No washout	2–4 week washout
RIMAs	Well tolerated, avoid clomipramine. Suggest start TCA first	no washout	NA	Few data
MAOIs	3 week washout	2 week washout	? washout	NA

Reversible inhibitors of monoamine oxidase subtype A (RIMA)

The best described agent in this class is moclobemide, which has a broad spectrum of antidepressant activity. An advantage over the irreversible MAO inhibitors is that it causes only minimal potentiation of the pressor response to dietary tyramine (the so-called 'cheese effect'). Consequently, the risk of a potentially fatal hypertensive crisis, a major deterrent to the wider acceptance of the irreversible MAOIs, is substantially reduced, and the need for dietary precautions is minimized. Moclobemide is largely devoid of the anticholinergic adverse effects, symptomatic postural hypotension, and weight gain variously associated with the tricyclic antidepressants and irreversible MAO inhibitors, and appears considerably safer on overdosage than the tricyclic and second generation antidepressants. Due to virtually complete metabolism in the liver, doses should be reduced by approximately one-half in those patients continuing to take cimetidine. Because of the potential for severe central nervous system adverse drug reactions, concomitant administration with clomipramine should be avoided, as should be co-administration with selegiline. Potentiation of opiates is possible. There are no data to suggest that the dose needs to be altered in the elderly *per se*, but doses may need to be reduced to one-third to one-half in those with hepatic impairment. Renal-impaired patients do not require a dose adjustment (Fitton *et al.* 1993).

Lithium

Pharmacokinetics

The low therapeutic index of lithium and the changes in lithium handling in the elderly lead to the need for careful monitoring of this drug and for heightened awareness of toxicity in the elderly. Lithium levels are heavily dependent on the renal excretion of the drug. The plasma half-life is normally approximately 20 hours, but is between 36 and 49 hours in the elderly since clearance drops from 25 ml/min to 10 ml/min in the over 75-year-old group. The volume of distribution is also likely to be reduced (Sproule *et al.* 2000). Thus, on average, lithium doses necessary to maintain therapeutic levels are approximately 50% lower in the elderly than in the young. However, there is much interpatient variation, and age contributes only 14% of the variation seen between individuals (Hewick *et al.* 1977). Therefore, the dose should be carefully titrated for each patient. Those patients on diuretics (who are more likely to have a sodium deficiency) are more prone to a reduced clearance of lithium, hence putting them at a greater risk of toxicity. When giving a diuretic to a patient established on lithium, doctors should check serum lithium levels one week later. The dose may have to be reduced by approximately 30%. Levels must be measured in the steady state, 12 hours after the last dose. Levels above 1 mM, or even less in the elderly, carry a serious risk of toxicity (Foster *et al.* 1977), and most psychogeriatricians aim for 0.4–0.6

mEq in the very old. If mood control, side-effects, and previous measurements are stable, then a maximum 3 monthly interval of measurement is reasonable.

Toxicity

Toxicity is reflected in patient apathy, sluggishness, coarse irregular hand tremor and muscle twitches, muscular weakness, ataxia, difficulty with speech, as well as nausea, vomiting, and diarrhoea. In those with bipolar disorders there may be an increase in the severity of tremor. Most of these symptoms are non-specific enough not to be easily appreciated in the elderly. They are relatively insidious in onset and slow to resolve, often lagging behind blood levels when the drug is withheld. The problem is not commonly seen as monitoring is widely practized, but intercurrent illness, worsening renal failure, and failing compliance or confusion put the elderly at greater risk. A lithium level in the 'therapeutic range' does not preclude a diagnosis of toxicity. In the case of severe illnesses associated with a drop in urine output, such as severe bouts of vomiting and diarrhoea, the patient should be instructed to stop taking the lithium for the duration of the problem and to seek medical advice if the symptoms last for more than 36 hours. Whilst this advice in most cases is sufficient to avoid toxicity, there is such variability among patients that each case must be judged on its merits. Where there is doubt, lithium levels should be measured: at weekly intervals during periods of illness. Lithium should be restarted as soon as possible, as a relapse in symptoms can be seen as early as 7–10 days after stopping the drug if renal function has returned to previous levels.

Acute changes after initiation of therapy include: gastrointestinal irritation (nausea and loose bowel motions), fine hand tremor, a nephrogenic diabetes insipidus with polyuria and polydipsia. In many patients, these subside, but they can be quite persistent. Chronic effects include weight gain, oedema, hypothyroidism, goitre, and leucocytosis. Thyroid function tests (TFTs), especially TSH, help to differentiate those drug features from that of myxoedema. Before treatment, patients should have TFTs, ECG, urea and electrolytes (U + E), and creatinine clearance calculated, to assess pre-existing renal, cardiac, and thyroid function. It is recommended that U + Es be repeated within 4 weeks, and the TFTs within 3 months, of initiation of lithium therapy in the elderly. If all is stable, 6-monthly TFT checks should be sufficient.

Antiepileptics

Carbamazepine

The psychotropic effects, as opposed to the antiepileptic effects, of carbamazepine are utilized to help in the management of bipolar affective disorders. Its mode of action is unclear, but the depressant effect on catecholamine turnover and on glutamate release may be important. Carbamazepine autoinduces its own metabolism via the hepatic mono-oxygenase system, and quite commonly the hepatic transaminases are elevated. For this reason, and because of the possible exacerbation of liver failure, liver transaminases should be assayed before carbamazepine commencement, within the first month of treatment, and periodically thereafter. Similar advice is given for obtaining a leucocyte count, in view of the rare, but important, persistent agranulocytosis and aplastic anaemia. Transient drops in the leucocyte count are more common. Forewarning may be seen in the form of a persistent sore throat, easy bruising or bleeding, and fever.

Through enzyme induction, carbamazepine can reduce the plasma concentrations of drugs metabolized in the liver, including imipramine and certain benzodiazepines. Conversely, other drugs, such as fluoxetine, can increase carbamazepine levels. Assaying plasma levels will help the clinician minimize the risk of toxicity. Just as with lithium, signs of mild toxicity may be subtle, especially in the elderly. The clinician should avoid being lulled into a false sense of security by levels within the 'normal range'. An increase in confusion, unsteadiness and falls, hypotension, constipation, urinary retention, and an ADH-like effect causing hyponatraemia are worthy of mention as possible signs of toxicity.

Sodium valproate

Sodium valproate is rapidly absorbed and almost completed metabolized in the liver, and has a variable half-life of about 8–20 hours. Although the pharmacokinetics differ between the young and the old, the clinical significance of this is debatable. Serum levels are poorly correlated with beneficial effects.

Amphetamines

These agents have extremely restricted use in the elderly since they have the potential to induce addictive and psychotic states, but *occasional* use under strict supervision has been advocated to activate and enhance mood (Clark 1978). Contraindications include the presence of cerebrovascular disease, hyperthyroidism, hypertension, glaucoma, movement disorder, and epilepsy. MAOIs interact with amphetamines and thus a 2-week washout period is necessary between changing therapies.

Potential interactions when changing or adding to other antidepressant groups

Not uncommonly, side-effects and questionable efficacy lead to a need to change from one antidepressant to another. However, the prescriber needs to be aware of potential interactions between the different classes (Table 13.7). While MAOIs and TCAs both increase norepinephrine (noradrenaline) levels in the synaptic cleft, the clinical significance of this remains unclear, with the exceptions of those mentioned in Table 13.7 Some TCAs and SSRIs inhibit each other's metabolism which, in turn, increases their respective plasma concentrations.

Sedatives, anxiolytics, and hypnotics

Benzodiazepines

Pharmacokinetics (see Table 13.8)

Both the long- and the short-acting benzodiazepines are quickly and completely absorbed from the gastrointestinal tract, although alcohol seems to enhance absorption. The longer half-life benzodiazepines, for example diazepam, tend to have good lipid solubility. The initial short action is due to the drug's distribution into fat and muscle. Once the uptake sites are saturated, drug clearance depends on hepatic metabolism. With the decline in lean body mass (relative increase in total body fat) in the elderly, there is an increased apparent volume of distribution giving a plasma half-life in an 80-year-old about four times that of a person in their twenties. However, there is no change in the plasma clearance of the benzodiazepines, and therefore not much change in the plasma concentrations achieved with the regular use of, for example, diazepam. Accumulation in the elderly is no more likely than in the young (Ives and Castleden 1983). In the shorter acting, more water-soluble group, evidence of pharmacokinetic changes in the elderly is lacking.

Table 13.8 Summary of pharmacokinetic data of the benzodiazepines

Type and examples	Metabolism/ elimination	Lipid solubility	Change, old vs. young	
			Half-life	V_d
Long-acting, e.g. Diazepam	Oxidation to active metabolites	High	Increased 70–200%	Increased
Medium-acting, e.g. Temazepam	Conjugation	Medium	No change	No change
Short-acting, e.g. Triazolam Midazolam	Oxidation, No active metabolites	Medium	No change	No change

Metabolism
Benzodiazepines are metabolized in the liver, and some metabolically active products may have β-elimination half-lives as long as or even longer than the parent compound. Where the products are glucuronides (conjugates), then renal impairment may become significant (for example, lorazepam and oxazepam). Because glucuronidation is relatively well preserved even in cirrhosis, these drugs become the benzodiazepines of choice in those with poor liver function. Cigarette smokers tend to exhibit less CNS depression with diazepam, probably through induction of hepatic microsomal enzymes. This may also be true for those patients accustomed to alcohol and those taking other inducing agents such as phenytoin.

Pharmacodynamics
All benzodiazepines cross the blood-brain barrier and bind to specific benzodiazepine receptors. The receptor concentration is highest in the central cortex, hippocampus, and the cerebellum. The effect of ageing on these receptors is, as yet, unknown, but it is thought that the ageing brain is more sensitive to the effects of benzodiazepines (Castleden *et al.* 1977; Swift *et al.* 1985; Klotz 1998).

Withdrawal from benzodiazepines
The dependency potential of benzodiazepines means that occasionally there is a need to withdraw these drugs from patients. Inadvertent withdrawal in the elderly is often the first indication of dependence, but only if it is recognized for what it is. The presentation can be non-specific, with agitation, confusion, and hallucinosis heading the list. The association with an intercurrent illness allows the condition to masquerade as a toxic confusional state, prevents the patient from taking their regular prescription, and may lead medical staff to believe that benzodiazepines are contraindicated. Treatment is represcription of the offending drug, or immediately placing the patient on a long-acting agent such as diazepam, in equivalent dose (see Table 13.9). It should be noted that it is impossible to give precise equivalent dosages as the different drugs have widely varying half-lives (Higgitt *et al.* 1985; Taylor 1989). A long-acting benzodiazepine evens out the peaks and troughs in plasma levels and sets the stage for managed withdrawal. Unless the patient has specific psychiatric problems, a history of seizures, or other medical problems such as heart disease, admission to hospital should be unnecessary. Admission is advised for the frail elderly or those who have poor supervision. The general rule is, first, to substitute a long-acting drug, and then to withdraw it slowly. Substitution of an equivalent dose may take up to 10 days (longer if the patient cannot be closely supervised). It is advisable to warn the patient of possible increased daytime somnolence. Increased anxiety, tremor, and insomnia indicate that the substituted dose is inadequate, but can also represent the underlying psychological disturbance, especially when low levels are reached. Following successful substitution, withdrawal can be in 2-mg decrements per

Table 13.9 Benzodiazepine dosage equivalents

Drug	Dose equivalent to 10 mg diazepam	Half-life (hours)	Half-life active metabolite
Chlordiazepoxide	20 mg	5–30	36–200
Diazepam	10 mg	20–100	36–200
Lorazepam	1–2 mg	10–20	
Nitrazepam	10–15 mg	15–38	
Oxazepam	20 mg	4–15	
Temazepam	20 mg	8–22	
Triazolam	0.5 mg	2–5	

week, where the daily dose is over 15 mg; 1-mg decrements where it is between 10 and 15 mg; and 0.5-mg decrements where the dose is less than 5 mg per day. Individual tailoring of dosages may prove necessary. Alternative drug therapy with sedative and anxiolytic antidepressants may be useful in some more difficult cases but, clearly, one problem may be substituted for another! Once again, prevention is better than cure, and dependence can be markedly reduced by clear explanations at the time of initial prescription. Explanations include warning of insomnia and possible nightmares (even after short courses), explicit reasons for usage, and giving short courses for all except those with psychotic states. Finally, repeat prescriptions should not be given without clinical review.

Non-benzodiazepine hypnotics

These are a new group of hypnotics which are central gamma-aminobutyric acid (GABA) chloride receptor agonsits and, therefore, have a sedative effect; examples are zopiclone, zolpidem, and zaleplon. In the elderly, there is no appreciable decline in the bioavailability of these drugs, but there is a slight prolongation of the half-life of zopiclone from 5 hours to approximately 6 hours at age 65 years, and 8 hours in those over 74 years. This is probably due to the effect of a reduction in liver mass, as the metabolic degradation is via the oxidative, decarboxylation, and demethylation pathways. Zaleplon has a high first-pass metabolism. Dosing over 7 days does not lead to accumulation in the elderly. In those with severe hepatic insufficiency, half-lives can increase by over 60%, but only mild prolongation is seen with renal impairment (creatinine clearance at 30 ml/min) (Galliot *et al.* 1987; Noble *et al.* 1998; Holm and Goa 2000). Although none of these effects has been clearly demonstrated to be of clinical significance, the recommendation for use in both the elderly and those with hepatic insufficiency is to reduce the initial doses of these agents to about 50% of that used in the young.

There are reported to be fewer residual and adverse effects on psychomotor performance, and also fewer effects on memory in the elderly than with comparable doses of benzodiazepines. When co-prescribed with TCAs, it is recommended that the therapeutic effect of the TCA is monitored, as metabolism of the TCA may be enhanced (Caille *et al.* 1984).

Barbiturates

There are no good indications for barbiturates to be newly prescribed in the elderly. However, attempts to withdraw patients from these drugs when given in low dose are often difficult and of questionable benefit. The risk of altered vitamin D metabolism, which can lead to osteomalacia and reduced serum calcium levels, should be borne in mind for patients on long-term barbiturate treatment. Due to the induction of liver enzymes, other drugs, such as phenytoin, warfarin, and some TCAs, may be metabolized more rapidly.

Chloral hydrate

This hypnotic is still used, despite there being safer and more effective alternatives. Chloral hydrate is a prodrug, needing to be metabolized to trichloroethanol (TCE) to exert any hypnotic effect. There is no evidence that this is altered in the elderly. TCE has an elimination half-life of 8 hours. Like most hypnotics, chloral hydrate is subject to tachyphylaxis. Because trichloroacetic acid binds to plasma proteins, it may displace other bound drugs. Chloral hydrate also potentiates the effect of alcohol and has a narrow therapeutic window, with lethal depression of respiration occurring at only 10 g. Its addictive potential is high and withdrawal is quite unpleasant.

Clomethiazole

Clomethiazole is rapidly absorbed but undergoes substantial first-pass hepatic metabolism. In the elderly, there is wider variation in bioavailability and peak concentrations, but there is no change in the elimination half-life (Briggs *et al.* 1980). After intravenous delivery its half-life is prolonged in the elderly, presumably due to the reduction in hepatic blood flow (Castleden and George 1979). No accumulation seems to occur after repeated dosing in the elderly, but, irrespective of this, there does seem to be some residual sedation after single doses of 384 mg (Castleden *et al.* 1979). It is recommended that this drug is reserved as an alternative to benzodiazepines in those patients undergoing alcohol withdrawal or nocturnal confusion, which may be due to the excessive use of alcohol.

Drugs in the treatment of the dementias

There is a vast literature relating to these conditions, but it is difficult to make much sense of it due to the variation in patient selection and assessment, lack of control groups, and variable study design. In recent years, large multicentre trials of a wide variety of drugs have been in progress. The first drug to receive any acceptance at all was tacrine (THA), and more recently donezepil and rivastigmine. While there is continuing debate as to their merits, there is no doubt about their toxicity, as may be expected from cholinergic agents. These agents are covered in more detail in Chapter 24vii.

Physical illnesses

Introduction

The vast majority of pharmacokinetic work has been performed in healthy populations, some of whom were aged patients. Few, if any, pharmacodynamic studies have taken place in the sick elderly. In an effort to provide practical examples of how disease states may affect drug handling, each major system will be briefly outlined.

Cardiovascular disease

Significant heart disease leads to a decline in renal clearance. In severe congestive heart failure, liver congestion reduces liver perfusion. Thus, the TCAs and phenothiazine may have reduced first-pass metabolism, decreased clearance, and increased plasma concentrations. Orthostatic hypotension is also increasingly significant (Glassman *et al.* 1983). Conversely, TCAs tend to antagonize the adrenergic-blocking antihypertensives, thus potentially worsening the control of hypertension. Serotonin reuptake inhibitors, mianserin, and to a lesser extent lofepramine, are probably the best choice of antidepressant in patients with cardiovascular disease, although most TCAs are only a major danger at high dosages. Diuretics enhance sodium loss and reduce the excretion of lithium, although loop diuretics are generally safer than thiazides.

An agitated patient in heart failure, who has no other obviously treatable toxic delirium, places an additional burden on the heart, and thus an antipsychotic agent may be of clear benefit. Thioridazine[1] has a reasonable balance in terms of sedation, lack of side-effects, and a lesser degree of blockade (see Table 13.3). Any α-adrenergic receptor blockade may lead to reduced blood pressure and can increase the likelihood of falls; however, there are drugs marketed for the treatment of heart failure which do block α-adrenergic receptors. Angiotensin-converting enzyme inhibitor drugs can potentiate the postural hypotensive effect of chlorpromazine and possibly other phenothiazines

Respiratory disease

Respiratory disease, especially chronic and progressive conditions, clearly engenders anxiety. Where there is considerable and reasonable distress (namely, where other medical therapy has been maximized) anxiolytics are indicated, but the clinician needs to be aware of the risks of respiratory depression, dysphoric, and habituation effects. Modest doses of a reasonably long-acting benzodiazepine, such as diazepam, are often used. In higher doses, all benzodiazepines have the potential for depressing the respiratory centre. If sedation rather than an anxiolytic effect is wanted, then zopiclone is probably safer (Muir *et al.* 1983). The dose of TCAs does not usually need to be altered outside the general guidelines for aged and frail patients unless the patient is on high doses of steroids, where the effect of the latter is potentiated. Agents with high anticholinergic activity may dry secretions, which may be to the detriment of some patients with tenacious sputum. Due regard should be given to the variable sedative activity of the various tricyclics. Treatment of psychotic states and toxic delirium in patients with chronic airways disease may be life-saving. In these instances, where respiratory failure and drugs are seemingly in a vicious circle, the elderly (and often not so frail) patient is best treated with haloperidol. Chlorpromazine is also useful for its sedative effects, but has the disadvantage of its greater effect on postural hypotension. Low doses, such as 0.5–1 mg haloperidol twice daily or chlorpromazine 25 mg twice daily, can also be effective when used as anxiolytics. The long-term use of these drugs is not recommended, due to the risk of precipitating a tardive dyskinesia, which can be particularly disabling by further impairing respiratory movements. Haloperidol has seemingly few complications except in significant overdose, where respiration needs to be artificially supported. Occasionally, hyperthermia may result, but is rarely serious and often ascribed to the previous agitation, the work of breathing, or an intercurrent infection. The mild vasodilatory effects of chlorpromazine, 5–10 mg, may be sufficient to dissipate heat if continued antipsychotic medication is warranted. Dantrolene is rarely indicated. Some physicians have reached for the atypical antipsychotics, but few data exist on their relative merits in such circumstances. Intercurrent illness, including pneumonia, can push steady-state concentrations of TCAs up into the toxic range (Dawling *et al.* 1980, 1984).

Central nervous system disease

Epilepsy

The phenothiazines infrequently cause convulsions, especially at high doses. They may lower the threshold for fits in known epileptics, alcohol and barbiturate withdrawal, or Alzheimer's disease and vascular dementia where fits have complicated the primary condition. Temporal lobe epilepsy itself is associated with psychiatric manifestations. Antidepressants can lower the fit threshold and destabilize epileptic patients receiving medication. Depression may coexist with epilepsy, but there are no clear reports of improvement in either state upon successful treatment of the other. The enzyme inductive effect of some antiepileptic medications can enhance the urinary excretion of chlorpromazine (by 18%) (Forrest *et al.* 1970), and also lead to a decline in the plasma levels of tricyclic antidepressants.

Glaucoma

All drugs with anticholinergic side-effects can, in rare cases, precipitate glaucoma, but there are few problems with patients already established on treatment for glaucoma.

Stroke

Poststroke depression is a defined and not uncommon entity. Treatment with tranquillizers and antidepressants may impair cognitive skill, and therefore should not be used unless other strategies have failed (Allen *et al.* 1988). Small studies suggest that TCAs are effective (Lipsey *et al.* 1983) and may improve function (Reding *et al.* 1986). There are no data on what happens to antidepressant penetration of the blood-brain barrier after stroke.

Parkinson's disease

Anticholinergic side-effects of drugs tend to summate, leading in extreme cases to the central cholinergic syndrome which is very hazardous to the elderly. There is also a tendency to worsen constipation and urinary hesitancy. Psychotic symptoms, as a result of antiparkinsonian medications, are not uncommon and are particularly disturbing; however, antipsychotics such as clozapine and risperidone may be effective in controlling these symptoms. In general, complete control of parkinsonian features proves very difficult while the patient remains on any antipsychotic medication.

Dementia

Dementia as a syndrome is so common in the community that it is bound to be found in association with other pathologies. Rarely are there problems with using non-psychoactive pharmaceuticals in such patients. Extra vigilance is required when drugs are needed to control some behavioural or psychological problem. Psychotropics are reputed to be more likely to induce greater confusion in a dementing patient, but clear evidence for this is lacking. This issue warrants further research. There is greater sensitivity to the parkinsonian effects of antipsychotics in those patients with Lewy-body variant dementia (McKeith *et al.* 1992). Timing of dosing should be such that any daytime effect is minimized. Too often, benzodiazepines and major tranquillizers are used too late in the evening, the patient sleeps well into the morning, and is greatly confused late in the afternoon—thus contributing to the 'sundown syndrome'.

Renal disease

Renal impairment is not uncommon in the elderly, and the rate of creatinine clearance reduces with age. Where the primary drug or its metabolite is active and dependent on excretion, drug-level monitoring and dose reductions warrant consideration. For example, nortriptyline levels remain much the same, but metabolite levels rise substantially: 10–20 times higher than in patients with normal renal function, especially in those patients on haemodialysis. It remains unclear if this influences the clinical outcome, in that the metabolites are of uncertain clinical activity (Young *et al.* 1984). Risperidone doses need to be halved in patients with renal (and hepatic) impairment.

Urinary incontinence

If urinary incontinence in the male is due to prostatic obstruction, then it would be ill-advised to use a TCA with potent anticholinergic activity, and it is important to be aware that antipsychotics, especially chlorpromazine and thioridazine, do possess anticholinergic activity. Conversely, in the case of a patient with an unstable bladder, the TCA of choice would be imipramine.

Endocrine disease

Diabetes

The clinician needs to be aware of the state of the renal, cardiac, and peripheral vascular function (see above). Many older diabetics have a degree of autonomic dysfunction, which this predisposes them to the hypotensive effects of many drugs. MAOIs enhance the hypoglycaemic effect of hypoglycaemic agents.

Thyroid disease

In hyperthyroid states, phenothiazines may exacerbate the tachycardia; so it is ill-advised to use tricyclics or MAO inhibitors, as their toxic properties are accentuated (Shader *et al.* 1970). Where clearly indicated in hypothyroid states, tricyclics have been used successfully. However, phenothiazines have been reported to precipitate hypothermic coma, and minor tranquillizers obscure thyroid function tests (Shader *et al.* 1970). Lithium should be avoided until the thyroid state has been stabilized for approximately 2–3 months.

Adrenal disease

Psychiatric disturbance may be seen in patients on high doses of adrenocorticoids. Psychosis is reported to respond well to phenothiazines (Hall *et al.* 1979), but to be exacerbated by the use of tricyclic antidepressants (Hall *et al.* 1978). In the case of hypocortisolism, psychotropic drugs have been reported to accentuate the existing hypotension and clearly should be avoided.

Gastrointestinal disease

Hepatic disease

In patients with hepatic impairment, the use of those drugs which are eliminated by hepatic metabolism needs to be modified by a reduction in

Table 13.10 Drugs used in patients with hepatic disease

Class of drug	Safer drugs	Less safe
Benzodiazepines/ Sedatives	Temazepam Oxazepam	Diazepam Clomethiazole
Antipsychotics	Cautious use of all, reduce dose to approximately $\frac{1}{4}$–$\frac{1}{3}$, especially if oral doses given	All can precipitate coma, avoid all, especially chlorpromazin in cholestasis

dose and occasionally frequency—for example, antipsychotics used for a sedative effect. There are few data that specifically address the use of the more established drugs in patients with hepatic impairment (see Table 13.10), with the possible exception of olanzapine (Caccia 2000).

Peptic ulcer disease

Both cimetidine and disulfiram decrease the clearance of chlordiazepoxide and diazepam, but not oxazepam, and plasma concentrations of the TCAs are increased by cimetidine through a reduction in liver metabolism. Antacids tend to reduce the absorption of phenothiazines by up to 45% (Forrest *et al.* 1970).

Drug prescribing and compliance

All too often, those prescribing medications forget to identify the hoped-for endpoint. To avoid this, an increased emphasis needs to be placed on diagnosis and communication with patient and their carers. Drug dosages need to be tailored to the patient, after assessing the impact of both the primary disorder and coincident organic conditions. A good general rule is to 'start low, go slow'. Due thought, explanation, and simple advice should be given regarding the side-effects. For example, a fall secondary to postural hypotension may be avoided by simply suggesting that the patient rises slowly, takes adequate fluids, and is especially careful in the morning, etc. Alteration in bowel and bladder habit may be alleviated by maintaining dietary bulk and the judicious use of bulk laxatives. Carers can be an important source of information and observation, and thus it is worth the small investment of time in educating them to look for signs of primary and side-effects. These observations may then be used as a prearranged indication either for dose adjustment or for a return for advice. Specific advice with regard to the method of initiation, follow-up, and dose alteration cannot be given here, but general principles can be followed (see Table 13.11). (Table 13.12 provides a summary of the major psychopharmaceuticals and their actions.) The trial of therapy should be long enough to achieve the anticipated endpoint. If there is no satisfactory result and the dose appears to be adequate, then alternative diagnosis and treatment should be considered. Generally, one benzodiazepine can be substituted for another within its 'length of action class', but rarely does it help much to do so. TCAs can be substituted for one another, but substitution to or from serotonin agonists and MAOI warrants review of the product data (see above). One phenothiazine can be substituted for another at an equivalent dose.

The clinician should clarify the reasons for dose and drug alterations in the notes, to avoid a therapeutic impasse and to allow informed review in the future. Drug plasma-level monitoring, especially for TCAs, goes some way to assuring the clinician that satisfactory levels have been achieved, and thus can increase confidence that any lack of response is not due to an inadequate dose. Drug dosage adjustment without the benefit of plasma-level monitoring is reasonable for

Table 13.11 Psychopharmaceutical drug prescribing in the elderly

Drug group	Initiation of therapy	Initial monitoring	Dose adjustment	Monitoring	Trial period
Benzodiazepines,					
– long acting	Diazepam, half dose dose	Next day, then alternate days	Weekly to monthly	1–3 monthly	2–3 weeks
– short acting	Temazepam, low normal dose	Next day then alternate days	For short-term use only	Not applicable	1–2 weeks
Phenothiazines					
– oral preparations	Low normal adult dose	Inpatient alternate Outpatient weekly	2-weekly	1–3 monthly	4–6 weeks
– depot preparations	Low normal adult dose oral)	2-weekly (usually in combination with	1–2 monthly	3 monthly	6 months
Anti-depressants – TCAs	Low normal adult dose. Single dose kinetic data may be of use in dose finding	1–2 weekly	2–4 weekly	3 monthly	6–8 weeks
– Serotonin agonists	Normal ?lower dose, see data sheets	1–2 weekly	2–4 weekly	3 monthly	6–8 weeks
Lithium	75–100 mg daily increasing to 6–800 mg daily over 2 weeks	Weekly, or twice weekly if higher starting dose. are used	2–3 weekly	1–3 monthly	6–8 weeks

TCAs after 3 weeks, despite their half-life being in the order of 24–30 hours. If no effect is seen by 6–8 weeks, alternatives need to be considered. MAOI have similar constraints. Psychotropics are usually effective to some degree within the half-life of the drug, and dose adjustments can be made even from day to day for the shorter acting drugs. Depot preparations should only be adjusted from month to month.

One may expect that the elderly are at special risk for problems with poor compliance due to their tendency to have multiple pathologies, complicated drug regimes, and a concomitant high incidence of memory impairment and confusion. Despite the difficulties in comparing the various studies on compliance, these expectations largely hold true (Schwartz *et al.* 1962; Davis 1968; Crooks and Parkin 1977). Problems associated with poor compliance and possible solutions are outlined in Table 13.13.

Emphasis needs to be given to education and counselling (McDonald *et al.* 1977). Any misconceptions and ambivalence with regard to the illness should be explored and corrected using simple and concise instructions. Important points should be stated twice, at the beginning and at the end of the interview. Childproof bottles are often difficult for some elderly people to open, as are many blister packs. Dosette-type containers can be used in selected patients. Up-to-date drug-dosing cards with drug prescriptions identical to those on the bottle help everyone. Reducing and simplifying drug regimens should always be attempted. Ideally, there should be no more than two or three drugs administered once or possibly twice a day, preferably timed to meals. Where supervision is required, once-daily regimens have obvious advantages. The practitioner should encourage the patient to bring all medications to the clinic.

Drug Group name	Absorption— onset of action	Binding	Metabolism	Excretion	Half-life	Clearance	Comment
Benzodiazepines –*Group 'A'*: diazepam clobazam chlordiazepoxide flurazepam	Well absorbed,some increase in volume of distribution—0.5–1.5 h	High, possibly some reduction in the elderly	Liver oxidation, probably reduced in the elderly	Metabolites via the kidney	Prolonged	Slightly reduced	Lipophilic, reduction of dose of younger adults is advised, especially in the frail
–*Group 'B'*: lorazepam oxazepam temazepam lormetazepam	Well absorbed onset may be slowed in the elderly, for example oxazepam 0.7–5.8 h	High or oxidised	Liver, conjugated via the kidney	Metabolites effect	Minimal	Minimal effect	More polar (water soluble) normal dose tolerance higher.
Barbiturates	Well		Liver	Metabolites via the kidney (some active)	Prolonged in the elder	Reduced	Induce liver enzymes
Phenothiazines	Well	High	Liver, substantial first-pass metabolism	Metabolites via the kidney	Possibly prolonged poorly understood	Reduced, but poorly understood	Dose reduction warranted in the elderly
Antidepressants –*Tricyclics*	Complete	High	Liver, substantial first-pass metabolism, oxidative, some active metabolites	Metabolites via the kidney	Prolonged but wide scatter in the data Dependent on the primary drug	Moderately reduced, but wide scatter in the data	Dose reduction warranted especially in the frail elderly
–*Serotonin-reuptake inhibitors*	Well	High	Liver	Metabolites via the kidney	Somewhat prolonged but variable clinical significance	Midly reduced, but overlaps with data from the young	Dose reduction generally not warranted, except perhaps in the frail elderly
–*MAOI* pheneizine, isocarboxid	Well	Moderate–high	Liver, acetylation[a]	Metabolites via the kidney	Lack of data ?2–4 h ?prolonged in the elderly	Lack of data	Acetylator status is less important than dose in determining effect[b]
–*Lithium*	Complete	Minimal	None	Via kidney, reduced in sodium depletion	Prolonged over and above that due to reduction in renal function[c]	Reduced	Reduced dose strongly advised, monitor levels

[a]From Pare (1985); [b]From Tyrer *et al.* (1980); [c]from Hewick *et al.* (1977).

Table 13.13 Helping the elderly with compliance with drug administration

Relevant questions	Possible solutions
Does the patient and carer understand and accept the diagnosisand the need for medication?	Spend time in clarifying the problem, potential solutions, and drug effects. Identify action to be taken if side-effects are seen.
Does the patient and/or the carer have good enough mentation to remember to take the drug?Are there ways to improve the patient's memory to take the drug such as strategic placement of the drug near other patterned activities?	Tactfully explore this problem and provide a drug-dosage card, drug dispensing container, e.g. dosette, or request nursing staff to help. Occasionally other attendants are willing to assist in providing reminders either by phone or calling in.
Is the bottle clearly visible, labelled with the dose, the reason for taking it, and is it able to be opened by the patient? Is the drug dispensed in childproof (and often elderly, proof) bottles or blister packs?	Drug containers should be accessible (simple screw-topped clear bottles are best), and the pharmacist should be warned of any difficulties the patient may experience, e.g. poor co-ordination or vision. A bold printed instruction such as 'For depression, take two tablets at night', 'For the heart' will enhance patient understanding.
Are there more than four drugs and do they have to be taken more than twice during the day?	Simplify drug regimes in both number of drugs and timing of administration. Ideally there should be a once or twice daily regimen.

Drug studies and research techniques

Reading and interpreting the literature on drugs

The clinician is constantly reading reports of drug studies, approached by representatives of drug companies, and subject to the claims of advertising. Thus clinicians need to be able to assess the pertinent facts for themselves, and be able to come to a reasoned judgement. Features of drug studies will be listed below and guidance given on how to assess such studies. It is also worthwhile remembering that there is a publication bias against 'negative' studies. The Cochrane Library and collaborative groups offer considerable information in selected areas, especially with regard to the review of randomized clinical trials. Local and international sites are readily accessible via the Internet.

Was the hypothesis for the study clearly stated? Too complicated a hypothesis will prove all the more difficult to analyse. A clear diagnostic protocol needs to be identified in the 'Methods' section, and evidence needs to be given in the 'Results' that the study population conformed to the stated diagnosis and progressed much as one would expect. This can be amply demonstrated by looking at the control group (either placebo or 'conventional' drug). Many papers are made more difficult to interpret by having new or modified diagnostic and assessment criteria, with no presented or published evidence for the reliability (between-raters or test-retest), sensitivity, or specificity of the tests used. It is apparent that even proven psychometric instruments are imperfect, but at least published data in their utility are available. A drug-evaluation trial is not the best proving ground for a new psychometric or diagnostic instrument.

Drug-evaluation trials need to have clear predetermined relevant endpoints. The time course of the trial needs to be clinically relevant; as some trials are too short and leave the reader wondering if benefit or deleterious effects would have been seen after a longer period. Follow-up of patients after withdrawal or termination is often pertinent, as some drugs have persistent effects. Crossover trials need to be carefully analysed to avoid both contamination from a lack of washout time, and an order effect (where one group, having been on a persistently active drug, maintains that effect through the second part of the trial even though no drug can be found in the plasma).

How would the hypothesis have normally been tested? Most drug-intervention trials are conducted in a double-blind fashion, with either a placebo or a currently accepted standard for comparison. There is a tendency to avoid head-to-head trials between two newer (and, as is often claimed, more effective and less toxic) drugs. This leaves a lingering doubt about how such drugs compare. A review of relevant authoritative papers will also help to reassure the reader that the study has followed accepted practices, and, where different methods have been used, these need to be clearly reasoned.

Was the trial powerful enough? This is an essential part of trial design and the reader should know whether the trial had the statistical power to achieve a result or not. Unfortunately, it is likely that if the figures are not stated then the calculations were not done. Thus, reports should state the probability that the investigator would like to have of achieving statistical significance at, say, the 4% level. This is not simple and forces investigators to clarify the differences that they would like to achieve, and relies, to a degree, on prior knowledge. Whilst these calculations are somewhat complicated, it is possible to use nomograms (Gore and Altman 1982).

Did the trial choose a relevant subject group? Populations vary between inpatients and outpatients, rural and urban, old and young, social class, etc. Thus, the patients whom the reader normally sees may not have similar demographic characteristics to those in published studies. For example, a tertiary referral centre may pick up highly selective populations, and extrapolation of the data to differing populations is hazardous. Finally, any drug study stating that it is concerned with the 'elderly' needs to give a definition of 'elderly' or 'aged', and to present descriptive statistics such as mean, range, and (if the population is large enough) a standard deviation from the mean. One must appreciate that a patient of 65 years of age is hardly into the elderly age group, whereas an 80-year-old clearly is.

If the reader is finally persuaded that the trial has enough merit to warrant a change in clinical practice, then it is usually worth discussing with colleagues and looking out for commentary in authoritative journals. Timely summaries and reviews of a more consensus type appear in the *Drug and Therapeutics Bulletin*, the *Drugs and Prescriber's Journal*, or may be found on the Internet in the Cochrane Library, and others. These journals tend to follow the trends rather than lead them. The *British Medical Journal*, in its advice to authors (Style matters 1990), presents more detailed guidelines for writing papers. This is a good checklist to go through for both critical reading and the design of drug trials. Other research-orientated journals are too numerous to mention.

Considering the relative lack of good information upon which much of this chapter has been based, the reader may well be correctly persuaded that there is a need for more work to be done for the elderly. Should the reader be persuaded that they wish to redress the imbalance, the following section may be of benefit.

Research into pharmacology in the elderly

Designing a psychopharmacological research project in old age psychiatry should reflect an intelligent reading of research papers. Needless to say, design, let alone implementation, looks a lot easier than it is, and the benefit of gaining experience from association with an active research group cannot be overstated. Such an opportunity will quickly disabuse the researcher of the mistaken idea that time for research will be easy to find, and that research is cheap to run. This section is biased toward pharmaceutical research.

The most important issue in research is to define the question in as precise a manner as possible. This forms the basis of a hypothesis, and then leads to a clearer idea of research aims. It immediately becomes apparent that clear definitions of terms are necessary. For example, even the word 'old' needs to be defined. Is 'old' more than 65 years of age, or is it more than 80 years of age? Clarity of definitions and description of the population base is needed. Are 'normals' to be included, and in the case of intervention research, how are the controls to be chosen?

The choice of measurement tools is important, and ideally the instrument should be chosen from those already tried, tested, and well respected. If no suitable instrument exists, a protocol should be designed to establish the utility of the instrument. Perhaps the researcher should be encouraged by noting that a paper describing the new instrument and another using it, means that two papers can go on a CV rather than one!

An early discussion with the statistician is time well spent. It often offers a forum for clarification of the hypothesis and the tools with which proof is to be collected. The statistical techniques to be used need to be discussed and settled on as early as possible, as this will determine the number of subjects and the power of the study. If the study is truly breaking new ground, making power calculations impossible, a pilot study may be the best route to take. As a result, the researcher should be amply rewarded by a clearer hypothesis, a better use of instruments, and an adequate sample size. It will also help determine the frequency and power of assessment, and patient tolerance. In some cases, a pilot study will prove to the workers that more measures may not be more instructive, but rather merely fatigue the assessor and patient alike. Non-treatment factors affecting outcomes may also become apparent. Overlooked problems with pilot studies are that the researcher has often tired of the subject by the time the pilot is complete, and that 'negative' results tends to militate against conducting a full study. By rights, a pilot study is never really able to prove the hypothesis, just alter a likelihood. Before shelving a small study it is worth remembering that a good 'negative' study should be published just as much as a 'positive' one.

Defining the population (subjects) will lead to inclusion and exclusion criteria. Remember, the elderly are quite likely to have concomitant medical problems and to be taking medications. What conditions are likely to make the study unsafe or unreliable? Too stringent criteria will make recruitment difficult. Actual recruitment procedures and case-finding will need to be thought about. Allow generous time for case-finding, as patients seem to melt away when it comes to actual recruiting. Too slow a recruitment will lead to workers drifting away and suitable cases being missed. Therefore, diplomatic approaches to other workers in the field may be necessary. Descriptive studies can have a more variable source of subjects, so there is all the more need to define the population. Are the subjects to be out and about and independent (recruit from service, interest, and church groups), in care (residential and nursing homes), or clinical patients? Geographical population-based studies are the most difficult to establish as they are truly labour-intensive, and require a strong relationship with general practitioners who use up-to-date, computerized age–sex registers.

The ethical consequences of using various controls needs to be considered. Is any group of patients going to be clearly disadvantaged, such as receiving no treatment, when there may be a clear treatment option? What is the ratio between the various groups to be? Are there going to be various doses of the drug tested in parallel? Is there to be an enrichment phase (taking the responders only and then randomly testing them) or a dose-finding phase when the best tolerated dose is to be ascertained? All these aspects alter the power and therefore the number of recruits necessary. They also alter how the trial will be later seen and probably criticized.

Randomization into groups usually presents no major problem with the wide use of computer-generated lists. If a multicentre trial is envisaged, smaller blocks of patients will need to be randomized to avoid unbalanced groups within any one centre. Checks will need to be kept to prove that the groups are matched, and that there is some method of breaking the code in the event of a crisis, without unblinding the researchers.

Documentation and data recording is best not left to the medical staff on the team as they are notoriously poor at this! Pharmaceutical research especially requires a degree of obsessional behaviour. The tediousness of this aspect is minimized by clear forms with easy data-entry techniques. Designing the form to be 'computer friendly' is also a boon for the data-entry process. This usually means having the data on one margin, and in clearly defined 'boxes'.

For drug research the form, packaging, and labelling will benefit from the attention of a pharmacist. Compliance will need to be assessed. An aspect that exercises ethics committees is the detection and handling of side-effects. Clear lines of communication and 'good clinical practice' must be clearly apparent. This includes patient consent, confidentiality, data handling, monitoring, and audit. Other matters to establish are developing a standard operating procedure (manuals for workers), indemnity, funding, archives, and final publication of results.

Under what circumstances can the patient 'exit' the trial, and how is that coped with? Are drop-outs to be replaced? If so, how will this affect any intention-to-treat analysis? Longer trials can be severely compromised by this phenomenon, as intercurrent illness, subject fatigue, and even random deaths can severely detract from the final power of the sample. In research into older adults these factors can be significant in the sample-size calculation. What are the endpoints? These need to be decided before starting. What are the primary variables (clear data which can be taken for evidence of benefit or detriment), and are there to be any secondary variables (supportive data that will help, but are not to be taken for 'stand alone' evidence of change)? Is there to be an interim analysis to avoid proceeding with a clearly dangerous process?

Much help in the above aspects is given by funding bodies, who tend towards standardized formats for grant applications. However, some research may not go through such rigours, but this should not result in a sloppy approach. As a rule of thumb, approximately one-third of the time and energy spent in conducting research goes into the project planning, one-third into the study itself, and one-third on the analysis and write-up. There are a number of useful texts on the subject, two of which are listed in order of increasing detail of coverage (Pocock 1983; Munro 1988).

Note

1. A warning was issued on 11 December 2000 to British doctors by the chairman of the Committee on Safety of Medicines (CEM/CMO/2000/18) about the cardiotoxicity of thioridazine, in particular prolongation of the QTc interval and life-threatening ventricular arrhythmias. In fact, this advice related to the 'second-line treatment of schizophrenia in adults' and the elderly were not specified. However, it is likely that thioridazine will be prescribed less and less by old age psychiatrists in the coming years. (http://www.doh.gov.uk/cmo/cemcmo200018.pdf and http://www.fda.gov/medwatch/safety/2000/mellar.htm).

Appendix

Definitions and formulae

Pharmacology: The process of absorption, distribution, localization, transport, biotransformation, and excretion of a drug.

Pharmacodynamics: The study of the biochemical, physiological, and psychological effects of drugs and their mechanism of action, including the correlation of actions with the structure and chemical nature of drugs.

Half-life: Plasma drug half-life, the time taken for half of the drug to be lost from the blood plasma. Thus:

$$t_{1/2} = \frac{0.0693 \times Vd}{\text{Clearance}}$$

Vd: Apparent volume of distribution. This describes the amount of drug in the whole body relative to that in plasma. This factor is independent of clearance.

Clearance: This is the best index of the body's ability to eliminate a drug, and is the sole determinant of the tendency for the body to accumulate a drug to a given steady state:

$$C_{ss} = \frac{\text{Dose}}{\text{Dosing interval}} \times \frac{1}{\text{Clearance}}$$

(C_{ss} = the plasma drug concentration at steady state).

Creatinine clearance: A measure of renal function. Best simply estimated in the elderly by the Cockcroft and Gault (1976) formula:

Creatinine clearance =

$$\frac{(140\text{–age (years)} \times \text{weight (kg)}}{815 \times \text{plasma creatinine (mmol/L)}} \times 0.85 \text{ (females))}$$

References

Abernethy, D. R. and Kerzner, L. (1984). Age effects on alpha-acid glycoprotein concentration and imipramine plasma protein binding. *Journal of the American Geriatrics Society*, **32**, 705–8.

Albrecht, S. Ihmsen, H., Hering, W., Geisslinger, G., Dingemanse, J., Schwilden, H., *et. al.* (1999). The effect of age on the pharmacokinetics and pharmacodynamics of midazolam. *Clinical Pharmacology and Therapeutics*, **65**, 630–9.

Allen, C. M. C., Harrison, M. J. G., and Wade, D. T. (1988). Management of cognitive and emotional problems. In *The management of acute stroke*, pp. 185–91. Castle House Publications, Tunbridge Wells.

American Psychiatric Association (1980). Tardive dyskinesia: summary of a task force on the late neurological effects of antipsychotic drugs. *American Journal of Psychiatry*, **137**, 1163–72.

Ashford, J. W. and Ford, C. V. (1979). Use of MAO inhibitors in elderly patients. *American Journal of Psychiatry*, **136**, 1466–7.

Ballenger, B. R. (1987). Antipsychotic agents. In *Clinical pharmacology in the elderly* (ed. C. G. Swift), pp. 343–64. Marcel Dekker, New York.

Bender, A. D., Post, A., Meier, J. P., Higson, J. E., and Reichard, G. (1975). Plasma protein binding of drugs as a function of age in adult human subjects. *Journal of Pharmacological Science*, **64**, 1711.

Bianchine, J. R., Calmlin, L. R., Morgan, J. P., Dujunvne, C. A. and Lassagna, L. (1971). Metabolism and absorption of L-3,4 dyhydroxyphenylalanine in patients with Parkinson's disease. *Annals of the New York Academy of Sciences*, **179**, 126–39.

Braithwaite, R. A., Montgomery, S., and Dawling, S. (1979). Age, depression and tricyclic antidepressant levels. In *Drugs and the elderly* (ed. J. Crooks and H. Stevenson), pp. 133–44. MacMillan, London.

Briggs, R. S., Castleden, C. M., and Craft, C.A. (1980). Improved hypnotic treatment using chlormethiazole and remazepam. *British Medical Journal*, **280**, 601–4.

Burr, D. R., Creese, I., and Snyder, S. H. (1977). Antischizophrenic drugs: chronic treatment elevates dopamine receptor binding in brain. *Science*, **196**, 326–8.

Caccia, S. (2000). Biotransformation of post-clozapine antipsychotics: pharmacological implications. *Clinical Pharmacokinetics* **38**, 393–414.

Caille, G., Du Souich, P., Spenard, J., Lacasse, Y., and Vezina, M. (1984). Pharmacokinetic and clinical parameters of zopiclone and trimipramine when administered simultaneously to volunteers. *Biopharmaceuticals of Drug Disposition*, **5**, 117–25.

Castleden, C. M. and George, C. F. (1979). The effect of ageing in the hepatic clearance of propranolol. *British Journal of Clinical Pharmacology*, **7**, 49–54.

Castleden, C. M., George, C. F., Marcer, D., and Hallet, C. (1977). Increased sensitivity to nitrazepam in old age. *British Medical Journal*, **1**, 10–12.

Castleden, C. M., George, C. F., and Sedgwich, E. M. (1979). Chlomethiazole—no hangover effect but not an ideal hypnotic for the young. *Postgraduate Medical Journal*, **55**, 15960.

Clark, A. N. G. (1978). Morale and motivation. *Practitioner*, Committee on Safety of Medicines 2000 **220**, 735–7.

Cockcroft, D. W. and Gault, M. H. (1976) Prediction of creatinine clearance from serum creatinine. *Nephron*, **16**, 31–41.

Crooks, J. and Parkin, D. M. (1977). The problem of compliance in drug therapy. In *Advanced medicine* (series): Vol. 3 *Topics in therapeutics* (ed. R. G. Shanks), pp. 11631. Pitman Medical, London.

Davies, K. N. and Castleden, C. M. (1988). Ageing and receptors. In *Advanced geriatric medicine* (ed. J. G. Evans and F. I. Caird), pp. 161–70. John Wright, Bristol.

Davis, M. S. (1968). Physiologic, psychological and demographic factors in patient compliance with doctor's orders. *Medical Care*, **6**, 115.

Dawling, S., Crome, P., Braithwaite, R. A. and Lewis, R. R. (1980). Nortriptyline therapy in elderly patients: dosage prediction after single dose pharmacokinetic study. *European Journal of Clinical Pharmacology*, **18**, 147–50.

Dawling, S., Ford, S., Rangedara, D. C., and Lewis, R. R. (1984). Amitriptyline dosage prediction in elderly patients from plasma concentrations at 24 hr after a single 100 mg dose. *Clinical Pharmacokinetics*, **9**, 261–6.

Dechant, K. L., and Clissold, S. P. (1991). Paroxetine. A review of its pharmacodynamic and pharmacokinetic properties, and therapeutic potential in depressive illness. *Drugs*, **41**, 225–53.

Evans, M. A., Triggs, E. J., Broe, G. A., and Saines, N. (1980). Systemic availability of orally administered L-dopa in the elderly parkinsonian patient. *European Journal of Clinical Pharmacology*, **17**, 215–21.

Fitton, A., Faulds, D., and Goa, K. L. (1993). Moclobemide. A review of its pharmacological properties and therapeutic use in depressive illness. *Drugs*, **43**, 561–96.

Fliser, D., Bischoff, I., Hanses, A., Blocks, S., Joest, M., Ritz, E., *et al.* (1999). Renal handling of drugs in the healthy elderly. Creatinine clearance underestimates renal function and pharmacokinetics remain virtually unchanged. *European Journal of Clinical Pharmacology*, **55**, 205–11.

Forrest, F. M., Forrest, I. S., and Serra, M. T. (1970). Modification of chlorpromazine metabolism by some other drugs frequently administered to psychiatric patients. *Biological Psychiatry*, **2**, 53–8.

Foster, J. R., Gershell, W. K., and Goldfarb, A. (1977). Lithium treatment in the elderly. 1. Clinical Usage. *Journal of Gerontology*, **32**, 299–302.

Freeman, H. (1988). Progress in antidepressant therapy. Fluoxetine: a comprehensive overview. *British Journal of Psychiatry*, **153**, Supplement 3.

Frisk, P. A., Cooper, J. W., and Campbell, N. A. (1977). Cornmunity-hospital pharmacist detection of drug-related problems upon patient admission to small hospitals. *American Journal of Hospital Pharmacy*, **34**, 738–42.

Gachalyi, B., Vas, A., Hajós, P., and Kádor, A. (1984). Acetylator phenotypes: effect of age. *European Journal of Clinical Pharmacology*, **26**, 43–5.

Galliot, J., LeRoux, Y., Houghton, G. W., and Dreyfus, J. F. (1987). Critical factors for pharmacokinetics of zopiclone in the elderly and in patients with liver and renal insufficiency. *Sleep*, **10**, 7–21.

Geddes, J., Freemantle, N., Harrison, P., and Bebbington P (2000). Atypical antipsychotics in the treatment of schizophrenia: systematic overview and meta-regression analysis. *British Medical Journal*, **321**, 1371–6.

Glassman, A. H., Johnson, L. L., Giadina, E. V., Walsh, T., Roose, S. P., Cooper, T. B. *et al.* (1983). The use of imipramine in depressed patients with congestive heart failure. *Journal of the American Medical Association*, **250**, 1997–2001.

Gore, S. M. and Altman, D. C. (1982). *Statistics in practice*. British Medical Association, London.

Grandison, M. K. and Boudinot, F. D. (2000). Age-related changes in protein binding of drugs: implications for therapy. *Clinical Pharmacokinetics*, **38**, 271–90.

Greenblatt, D. J., Harmatz, J. S., Shapiro, L., Engelhardt, N., Gouthro, T. A. and Shader, R. I. T. I. (1991). Sensitivity to triazolam in the elderly. *New England Journal of Medicine*, **324**, 1691–8.

Hader, M. (1965). The use of selected phenothiazines in elderly patients. *Mount Sinai Journal of Medicine*, **32**, 622–33.

Hall, R. C. W., Popkin, M. D., and Kirkpatrick, B. (1978). Tricyclic exacerbation of steroid psychosis. *Journal of Nervous and Mental Disorders*, **166**, 738–42.

Hall, R. C. W., Popkin, M. K., Stickney, S. K., and Gardner, E. (1979). Presentation of the 'steroid psychosis'. *Journal of Nervous and Mental Disorders*, **167**, 229–36.

Hewick, D. S., Newbury, P., Hopwood, S., Naylor, G., and Moody, J. (1977). Age as a factor affecting lithium therapy. *British Journal of Clinical Pharmacology*, **4**, 201–5.

Higgit, A. C., Lader, M. H., and Fonagy, P. (1985). Clinical management of benzodiazepine dependence. *British Medical Journal*, **291**, 688–90.

Holm, K. J. and Goa, K. L. (2000). Zolpidem: an update of its pharmacology, therapeutic efficacy and tolerability in the treatment of insomnia. *Drugs*, **59**, 865–89.

Ives, D. R. and Castleden, C. M. (1983). Clinical and pharmacological considerations in the use of diazepam in the elderly. *Geriatric Medicine Today*, **2**, 36–9.

Kitanaka, I., Ross, R. J., Cutler, N. R., Zavadil, A. P., and Potter, W. Z. (1982). Altered hydroxydesipramine concentrations in elderly depressed patients. *Clinical Pharmacology and Therapeutics*, **31**, 51–5.

Klotz, U. (1998) Effect of age on pharmacokinetics and pharmacodynamics in man. *International Journal of Clinical Pharmacology and Therapeutics*, **36**, 581–5.

Klotz, U., Avant, G. R., Hoyumpa, A., Schenker, S., and Wilkinson, G. R. (1975). The effects of age and liver disease on the disposition and elimination of diazepam in adult man. *Journal of Clinical Investigation*, **55**, 347.

Lech, S. V., Friedman, G.D., and Ury, H. K. (1975). Characteristics of heavy users of outpatient prescription drugs. *Clinical Toxicology*, **8**, 599–610.

Lipsey, J. R., Robinson, R. G., Pearlson, G. D., Rao, K., and Price, T. R. (1983). Nortriptyline treatment of post-stroke depression. *Lancet*, **i**, 297–300.

McDonald, E. T., McDonald, J. B., and Phoenix, M. (1977). Improving drug compliance after hospital discharge. *British Medical Journal*, **2**, 618.

McKeith, I., Fairbairn, A., Perry, R., Thompson, P., and Perry, E. (1992). Neuroleptic sensitivity in patients with senile dementia of Lewy body type. *British Medical Journal*, **305**, 673–8.

Marsden, C. D., Tarsy, D., and Baldessarini, R. J. (1975). Spontaneous and drug induced movement disorders. In *Psychiatric aspects of neurological disease* (ed. F. Benson and D. Blumer), pp. 219–66. Grune and Stratton, New York.

Mehta, D., Mehta, S., and Mathews, P. (1977). Tardive dyskinesias in psychogeriatric patients. *Journal of the American Geriatrics Society*, **25**, 545–7.

Miller, L. G., Greenblatt, D. J., Friedman, H., Burstein, E., Scavone, J. M., and Harmatz, J. S. (1987). Trazodone kinetics in old age. *Clinical Pharmacology and Therapeutics*, **41**, 210.

Misra, C. H., Shelat, H., and Smith, R. C. (1981). Influence of age on the effects of chronic fluphenazine on receptor binding in rat brain. *European Journal of Pharmacology*, **76**, 317.

Muir, J., Defouilley, C., Arlati, S., Locquet, R., and Aubrey, P. (1983). Sleep-disordered breathing in COPD patients: incidence of zopiclone vs placebo. *American Review of Respiratory Diseases*, **4**, 137.

Munro, A. J. (1988). *Clinical trials procedure: notes for doctors*. Association for Clinical Research, London.

Murdock, D. and McTavish, D. (1992). Sertraline: a review. *Drugs*, **44**, 604–24.

Noble, S., Langtry, H. D., and Lamb, H. M. (1998). Zopiclone. An update of its pharmacology, clinical efficacy and tolerability in the treatment of insomnia. *Drugs*, **55**, 277–302.

Palmer, K. J. and Benfield, P. (1994). Fluvoxamine. A review of its pharmacodynamic and pharmacokinctic properties, and therapeutic potential in non-depressive illness. *CNS Drugs*, **1**, 57–87.

Pare, C. M. B. (1985). The present status of monoamine oxidase inhibitors. *British Journal of Psychiatry*, **146**, 576–84.

Piafsky, K. M., Borgaå, O., Odar Cederöf, I., Johansson, C., and Sjöqvist, F. (1978). Increased plasma protein binding of propranolol and chlorpromazine mediated by disease induced elevations of plasma α acid glycoprotein. *New England Journal of Medicine*, **299**, 1435–9.

Pocock, S. J. (1983). *Clinical trials—a practical approach*. Wiley, Chichester.

Ray, W. A., Griffin, M. R., Schaffner, W., Baugh, D. K., and Melton, J. (1987). Psychotropic drug use and the risk of hip fracture. *New England Journal of Medicine*, **316**, 363–9.

Reding, M. J., Orto, L. A., Winter, S. W., Fortuna, I. M., Ponte, P. D., and McDowell, F. H. (1986). Antidepressant therapy after stroke. A double blind trial. *Archives of Neurology*, **43**, 763–5.

Richelson, E. (1999). Receptor pharmacology of neuroleptics: relation to clinical effects. *Journal of Clinical Psychiatry*, **60** (Suppl. 10), 5–14.

Rodstein, M. and Som Oei, L. (1979). Cardiovascular side-effects of longterm therapy with tricyclic antidepressants in the aged. *Journal of the American Geriatrics Society*, **27**, 231–3.

Schmidt, G., Grohmann, R., Strauss, A., Spiess Kiefer, D., Lindmeier, D., and Miller Oerlinghausen, B. (1987). Epidemiology of toxic delirium due to psychotropic drugs in psychiatric hospitals. *Comprehensive Psychiatry*, **28**, 242–9.

Schultz, P., Turner-Tamiyasu, K., Smith, G., Giacomini, K. M., and Blaschke, T. F. (1983). Amitriptyline disposition in young and elderly normal men. *Clinical Pharmacology and Therapeutics*, **33**, 360–6.

Schwartz, D., Wang, M., Zeitz, L., and Goss, M. E. (1962). Medication errors made by elderly chronically ill patients. *American Journal of Public Health*, **52**, 2018.

Shader, R. I., Belfer, M. L., and di Mascio, A. (1970). Thyroid dysfunction. In *Psychotropic drug side effects: clinical and theoretical perspectives* (ed. R. I. Shader and A. DiMascio), pp. 25–45. Williams and Wilkins, Baltimore, MD.

Smidt, N. A. and McQueen, E. G. (1972). Adverse reactions to drugs: a comprehensive hospital inpatient survey. *New Zealand Medical Journal*, **76**, 397–401.

Sotaniemi, E. A., Arranto, A. J., Pelkonen, O., and Pasanen, M. (1997). Age and cytochrome P450-linked drug metabolism in humans: an analysis of 226 subjects with equal histopathologic conditions. *Clinical Pharmacology and Therapeutics*, **61**, 331–9.

Sproule, B. A., Hardy, B. G., and Shulman, K. I. (2000). Differential pharmacokinetics of lithium in elderly patients. *Drugs and Aging*, **16**, 165–77.

Stevenson, I. H., Salem, S., O'Malley, K., Cusak, B., and Kelly, J. G. (1980). *Age and drug absorption. In Drug absorption* (ed. L. F. Prescott and W. S. Nimmo), pp. 235–61. Adis Press, Sydney.

Style Matters. (1990). Guidelines for writing papers. *British Medical Journal*, **300**, 38.

Sweet, R. A. and Pollock, B. G. (1998). New atypical antipsychotics. Experience and utility in the elderly. *Drugs and Aging*, **12**, 115–27.

Swift, C. G. and Hewick, D. S. (1987). Drug treatment of depressive illness. In *Clinical pharmacology in the elderly* (ed. C. G. Swift), pp. 443–71. Marcel Dekker, New York.

Swift, C. G., Swift, M. R., Ankier, S. I., Pidgen, A., and Robinson, J. (1985). Single dose pharmacokinetics and pharmacodynamics of oral loprazolam in the elderly. *British Journal of Clinical Pharmacology*, **20**, 119–28.

Swift, C. G. and Triggs, E. J. (1987). Clinical pharmacokinetics in the elderly. In *Clinical pharmacology in the elderly* (ed. C. G. Swift), pp. 31–82. Marcel Dekker, New York.

Swift, C. G., Lee, D. R., Maskrey, V. L. Yisak, W. Jackson, S. H., and Tiplady, B. (1999). Single dose pharmacodynamics of thioridazine and remoxipride in healthy younger and older volunteers. *Journal of Psychopharmacology*, **13**, 159–65.

Taylor, D. (1989). Guidelines for withdrawing benzodiazepines. *British Journal of Pharmaceutical Practice*, Marc, 106–10.

Turnheim, K. (1998). Drug dosage in the elderly. Is it rational? *Drugs and Aging*, **13**, 357–79.

Tyrer, P., Gardener, M., Lambourn, J., and Whitford, M. (1980). Clinical and pharmacokinetic factors affecting response to phenelzine. *British Journal of Psychiatry*, **136**, 359–65.

Young, R. C., Alexopolous, G. S., Shamolan, C. A., Manley, M. W., Amiya, A. K., and Kutt, H. (1984). Plasma 10-hydroxynortriptyline in elderly depressed patients. *Clinical Pharmacology and Therapeutics*, **35**, 540–4.

Zawadski, R. T., Glazer, G. B., and Lurie, E. (1978). Psychotropic drug use among institutionalised and noninstitutionalised Medicaid-aged in California. *Journal of Gerontology*, **33**, 825–34.

14 *Clinical practice: social work with older persons*

Martin Bradshaw

Introduction

The role of social workers in relation to older people changed substantially during the period 1990–1995. Until that time, a considerable proportion of social services resources were directed towards child care, with local authorities providing a significant level of residential care places and some help in the home as their main contribution to meeting the needs of dependent elders. The full implementation of the Community Care Act in 1993 resulted in a radical review of social care, and of the functions of various professional and manual staff. Further developments have been promoted by the 'modernization' agenda of a new Labour government that seeks to enhance social inclusion of older citizens. This chapter sets out to explain the current contribution of social care staff to the assessment, treatment, and care of older people with mental health problems. It is divided into three main areas:

1. *The socioeconomic context*—contains a brief summary of issues leading to the introduction of 'community care', with a review of key factors confronting health and social services authorities in the new millennium.
2. *Legal issues*—summarizes the main legal remedies available for the protection of vulnerable adults, which usually involve social workers in the assessment and implementation of statutory orders.
3. *Care management of individual clients*—provides an explanation of the direct contribution of 'Care Managers' to the assessment and ongoing care of older people, with case examples of multidisciplinary working.

Socioeconomic background

The progressive increase in the numbers and dependency of older people throughout the 1980s presented central and local government with a range of policy and resource problems, which involved both health and social service agencies. Social security funding mechanisms encouraged the trend for elderly patients to be discharged from NHS hospitals into residential and nursing homes. This exodus of frail and mentally ill people resulted in a massive expansion of private care establishments. Many thousands of patients were enabled to live nearer to their relatives, in accommodation that was generally superior to the large wards of centralized hospitals. There was not, however, an equivalent transfer of staff and skills to the independent sector, and the quality of care varied considerably across the country. Transfers from hospital were largely funded through state benefits, available on demand after a simple means test. Although health authorities were able to reduce the numbers of long-stay beds, the cost of social security benefits to central government increased rapidly, with no direct control over placement levels. A solution was urgently required that would limit central costs and introduce an assessment of need before state funding was authorized.

As financial costs rose, there was a parallel growth in the 'consumer' movement, which began to permeate the health and social care sectors. Patients and clients expected a more personal service, based on their individual needs. They were no longer prepared to accept a system whereby individuals could be assessed many times for a range of different services, with little choice or coordination between service providers. While patients could choose residential or nursing-home care without a professional assessment (subject only to the means test), there was no equivalent right to choose care at home. Thus a 'perverse incentive' towards expensive institutional care had been created, at the central government's expense.

The Community Care Act, 1990

Following a report by Sir Roy Griffiths, the Community Care Act, 1990 was finally implemented in 1993, after a series of delays due to the financial and technical problems associated with such a radical shift in welfare service provision. Local authorities were given substantial grants to develop community care services, using revenue that would otherwise have been committed to new residential and nursing-home placements. Around 85% of this funding had to be spent in the independent sector, in order to protect the stability of existing providers for an interim period. The Act had six key objectives for service improvement and delivery (Department of Health 1989):

(1) to promote the development of domiciliary, day, and respite services to enable people to live in their own homes wherever feasible and sensible;
(2) to ensure that the service providers make practical support for carers a high priority;
(3) to make proper assessment of need, and good case management the cornerstone of high-quality care;
(4) to promote the development of a flourishing independent sector alongside good-quality public provision;
(5) to clarify the responsibilities of agencies and so make it easier to hold them accountable for their performance;
(6) to secure better value for the taxpayers' money by introducing a new funding structure for social care.

The reforms introduced by the Community Care Act were expected to take at least a decade to settle down, since they involved major developments in organizational culture and professional practice. Many services became more flexible and responsive to individual needs within months of implementation, particularly out of normal working hours. In one shire county for example, the number of independent agencies providing care at home rose from 12 to over 40 in 2 years from 1993. This dramatic expansion enables carers to receive support at night and at weekends, whereas personal care was previously available mainly during office hours, Monday to Friday. Individual clients who are fortunate enough to obtain these services now have a real alternative to institutional care. However, the development in services has not been matched by sufficient financial resources. Local authorities have been faced with rising expectations, higher dependency levels, and reduced admissions to long-stay NHS care. The average length of stay of older people in acute hospitals has fallen progressively, increasing the pressure on local authorities to care for highly dependent clients at home. At the same time, grants from central government towards their base budgets have been reduced so that the perceived effect of 'Community care' for many people is a worse service. The social care system does not generally use waiting lists to manage excessive demand. Instead, 'eligibility criteria' are devised as a method of controlling the number of people deemed to qualify for a particular service. A central feature of the 1990s was the progressive tightening of these criteria, to the point where a relatively small number of highly dependent people receive substantial 'packages' of care, while many less-dependent older people have no access to help such as shopping or cleaning. This excessive allocation of resources to relatively few individuals has been recognized by health and social care planners, since it tends to create a 'dependency culture'. Central government grants at the beginning of the new century are now weighted towards preventing dependence, and 'intermediate care' services that aim to rehabilitate and maximize independence.

Responsibility for continuing care

Although one of the key objectives for the new Act was to clarify responsibility for care provision, this has not unfortunately been the case in practice. Prior to 1993, legislation was relatively clear about the provision and funding of health care for older people. The NHS provided long-term care in hospital for geriatric patients, or private individuals could choose to place themselves into nursing homes with financial assistance from social security funds. Social services departments were expressly forbidden to purchase or provide health care. Under the Community Care Act, local authorities were given powers to purchase nursing-home care, and encouraged to facilitate the discharge of highly dependent patients from hospital. At a time when NHS budgets were under increasing pressure it was perhaps inevitable that confusion should arise, since social services apparently had significant amounts of new money to purchase care for highly dependent patients with some health care needs. The term 'cost-shunting' accurately describes professional practice in some areas. Both health and social services' authorities had a direct incentive to encourage individual patients to remain under the care of the 'other' authority for as long as possible. While joint commissioning of services has helped to reduce the tension between statutory authorities, such initiatives often founder because of the financial pressures on respective authorities.

The trend towards increased social services' purchasing of 'health' care involves a fundamental shift away from services that are free at the point of delivery. Local authorities apply a means test for most care provision, but there is growing public resistance to charging for long-term care. A series of test cases in the late 1990s confirmed the right of individuals to free health care, and the 'NHS Plan' (2000) includes a decision that the nursing element of long-term care shall be funded by the state. However, most of the costs remain the responsibility of the individual apart from Scotland, where long-term personal care is free. This is likely to remain a turbulent area of public and professional debate for years to come; the costs of subsidizing care for dependent older people are very high, and government policies continue to seek reduced taxation as a primary goal.

The cost of 'community care'

While increased choice of services has been a key policy objective of both central and local government, there has been significant confusion about the relationship between cost and choice under the community care legislation. Local authorities have to manage finite budgets within a framework that lacks clarity about limits to the amount and type of service that can be expected following an assessment. A particular example of this financial uncertainty is the question of a 'ceiling' to the cost of care at home. In many urban areas, services can now be provided as required, 7 days a week, by a combination of local authority and independent agencies. The net cost of even a modest home-care package can rapidly exceed the cost of an independent residential placement, and some authorities have attempted to introduce limits to the amount of care at home they are prepared to fund. Any policy change in this area will have a major impact on elderly mentally ill patients, as they tend to require above average levels of support at home by nature of their unpredictable care demands.

In structural terms, the Community Care Act can be interpreted as having broadly achieved the key objectives of integrated assessment and flexible services that enable older people to stay in their own homes for as long as possible. However, these dramatic changes to professional practice will fall far short of achieving their potential benefit unless adequate funding is made available through central government grant mechanisms. One of the strong ironies of the new 'mixed economy of welfare' is that services can be cut back to reach budget targets much more easily by non-renewal of external contracts. Thus flexible care support provided by private and voluntary agencies is extremely vulnerable to funding cuts by local politicians seeking to balance a difficult budget. Conversely, residential homes directly run by the local authority are notoriously hard to close, with the net result that a disproportionate amount of available resources remains committed to institutional rather than domiciliary-care services.

Funding changes introduced in the NHS Plan will reduce the financial incentives for local authorities to place older people in private residential or nursing homes. A major review of the housing benefit regulations undertaken in the late 1990s will result in substantial new revenue transfers to local authorities by 2003 under the

'Supporting people' legislation. This funding will enable higher levels of support to be provided at home, reducing still further the incentive to placement in long-term care.

Statutory legal protection for vulnerable adults

There are two principal statutes available to protect vulnerable adults when their judgement is impaired through mental disorder, or they are thought to be seriously at risk due to environmental or other factors: The Mental Health Act, 1983 and Section 47 of The National Assistance Act, 1948.

The Mental Health Act, 1983

This Act gives social workers a central function in the care and protection of mentally disordered people. It provides a series of checks and balances that empower doctors to recommend compulsory admission to hospital, but give the social worker or 'nearest relative' the right to make the formal application for admission and discharge. A fundamental review of this Act is underway, and is likely to result in a series of changes to the process of assessment and compulsory admission.

Approved social workers

In order to carry out many of the specific duties under the Act, local authorities have to appoint an appropriate number of 'approved social workers' (ASWs). Individual patients can be detained in hospital for long periods under this legislation, and staff who are empowered to make such applications have to be specially trained, and undergo periodic refresher courses. The role of the ASW is unique in local authority terms, since they act as independent practitioners when using the Mental Health Act, and then are not subject to the usual management controls. The decision to admit a patient to hospital against their will cannot be overturned by a more senior officer of the authority. If a detained patient wishes to appeal against the decision, there is recourse to an independent tribunal that is completely separate from the social services department.

The Act assigns three principal duties to the ASW:

(1) to safeguard the civil liberties of the patient, and ensure that all proper procedures have been followed;
(2) to ensure that admission to hospital or guardianship is the appropriate course of action 'in all the circumstances of the case', and that reasonable alternatives to admission have been explored;
(3) to arrange for the least restrictive method of securing the necessary treatment recommended by appropriately qualified doctors.

The process of assessment

It is not intended to give a detailed breakdown of all the main provisions of the Mental Health Act in this chapter. The following paragraphs indicate essential elements of the most commonly used sections, to explain the approach taken by ASWs in fulfilling their statutory duties.

When a referral is received, the ASW is responsible for coordinating the assessment and following the patient right through the process until admission or alternative care is arranged. The ASW will arrange for the patient to be interviewed by her/himself and two doctors, one of whom should ideally have previous knowledge of the patient. Unless the case is of extreme urgency (when a single recommendation by one doctor can be used for up to 72 hours), one of the doctors must be approved under Section 12 of the Act as having special experience in the diagnosis and treatment of mental disorder. If the patient is not known to either of the doctors, then two 'Section 12 approved' practitioners should be asked to conduct the interview. This particular requirement is designed to protect the civil liberty of vulnerable patients, who can become subject to a 6-month detention order after an emergency assessment by three professionals with no previous knowledge of the circumstances.

The ASW gathers information about the patient from relatives, carers, and other appropriate sources such as the GP or hospital notes. When interviews have been completed the ASW must discuss the case with at least one of the two doctors, and decide if admission to hospital is appropriate. There are two principal options available: 'Section Two' involves admission for assessment followed by treatment (for up to 28 days), while 'Section Three' permits compulsory admission for treatment for up to 6 months.

Guardianship

Some patients may not require admission to hospital for treatment, yet still need a measure of compulsion to ensure their safety and general welfare. The Mental Health Act makes specific provision for this group of vulnerable adults through the guardianship procedures. The criteria are similar to those of Section Three, in that patients must be suffering from mental illness or severe mental impairment of a degree that warrants reception into guardianship, and action has to be necessary in the interests of the welfare of the patient or others. The 'guardian' is often the local social services authority, but can also be any other person accepted by the local authority (usually a relative). Guardianship orders last for 6 months, and can then be renewed for a further 6 months with annual reviews thereafter.

When an order has been made in respect of an older person, the guardian has three potential areas of control:

(1) to require the patient to reside in a specified place;
(2) to require the patient to attend at specified places and times for the purpose of medical treatment, occupation, education, or training—however, the patient cannot be compelled to receive treatment under this Section;
(3) to require access to the patient to be given, at any place where the patient is residing, to any registered medical practitioner, ASW, or other specified person (for example, a community psychiatric nurse or domiciliary-careworker).

The combination of these three powers can give the guardian a significant degree of influence over the life of an elderly person who needs additional protection. However, the use of guardianship procedures has been relatively limited since the introduction of the Mental Health Act in 1983. While the intention of this part of the Act is clear, there is a lack of direct powers to enforce the guardianship order. Although the patient can be 'required' to live in a particular place, there is no specific authority for that patient to be removed from one place to another. A frequent difficulty facing medical and social work practitioners is that of the demented older person who refuses to leave their home to live in nursing-home care. An ASW can legitimately apply for a guardianship order under these circumstances, but has no authority to actually remove the patient to the nursing home. This effectively means that the patient has to be admitted to hospital under Section Two or Three, then transferred, or removed from their home, to the nursing home using strong persuasion and the rather vague protection of the guardianship order. Most ASWs are reluctant to take the latter course, since they are extremely vulnerable to accusations of ageist practice and abuse of civil liberties.

The fundamental weakness of current guardianship procedures is that to work effectively they depend on a significant degree of cooperation from the patient. If the mentally disordered individual does not have sufficient insight or comprehension of the implications of the order, it will be relatively ineffective. Paradoxically, if the patient does understand the need to accept control or supervision, the order may be unnecessary.

The use of Mental Health Act procedures presents particular ethical and professional issues in protecting elderly patients. Dementing illnesses are increasingly common as the number of very elderly people increases, and 'community care' policies encourage medical and social work professionals to maintain patients at home whenever possible. Relatives are not always persuaded that elderly people should be allowed to remain at home, where they are perceived to be 'at risk'. Families can exert considerable pressure on social services staff to place vulnerable older people in residential or nursing homes, even where this may not be in the long-term interest of the individual concerned. The Human Rights Act (which came into force in 2000) will strengthen the rights of individual patients still further, and is likely to result in a reduction in compulsory admissions.

Section 47, The National Assistance Act, 1948

The second legal option available to safeguard the welfare of older people is found in the National Assistance Act. Section 47 differs fundamentally from the Mental Health Act in that it can be used where there is no diagnosis of mental disorder. A person can be removed from their home to a 'place of safety' (usually a hospital or residential home), if they are living in excessively squalid conditions and refusing appropriate support. A typical case would involve an elderly person with a fractured leg, refusing to go to hospital for treatment. Living conditions can deteriorate rapidly when there is a sudden loss of mobility, since use of a toilet can be difficult. The patient effectively becomes incontinent, but may refuse help or treatment. In this situation, there is enormous pressure for the authorities to 'do something', yet the elderly person has a right to determine how they wish to live.

Section 47 differs fundamentally from the Mental Health Act powers available to social workers, because the patient has very limited right of appeal. Only one doctor is involved, and relatives do not have a power of veto. However, in some situations there may be no apparent alternative to the temporary removal of an elderly person with an abnormal personality to a place of safety, in order to prevent them suffering serious harm as a result of self-neglect.

This order is rarely used, because there are many ethical concerns about the right of medical practitioners to intervene where an elderly person has decided that they do not wish to receive treatment for a potentially life-threatening condition. The right to refuse treatment is well established for younger people who are not suffering from mental illness, and accusations of 'ageism' can be hard to refute when similar principles are not applied to older patients.

Informal protection of vulnerable adults

The proportion and overall numbers of mentally disordered people in residential and nursing homes continue to rise as NHS long-stay care is increasingly transferred to the independent sector. Many of these patients are incapable of making informed choices about where they wish to live, and frequently express the desire to leave the establishment. This presents health and social care professionals with a considerable dilemma. The formal legal position is that all residents of independent and local authority homes must be free to leave at any time, unless (exceptionally) they are formally detained under Mental Health Act powers in a registered mental nursing home. Staff who restrain informal residents in any way, or repeatedly persuade them to remain in the home, could be open to charges of assault or illegal imprisonment. However, if they fail to prevent patients from coming to harm, care staff can be accused of negligence. When relatives have undertaken the painful experience of admitting a mentally disordered father or mother to a residential home, they expect a 'duty of care' from medical and social care staff. This includes (not unreasonably) ensuring that the elderly person is under appropriate supervision to prevent injury to themselves or others. In order to protect the civil liberties of vulnerable residents, the guardianship powers available under the Mental Health Act can certainly be used, although some doctors are reluctant to describe dementia as a mental illness under the terms of the Act. However, the sheer numbers of mentally disordered elderly people in institutional care make guardianship an impossibility for most of them given the current resources, even if this was appropriate. Many social services departments are hardly able to maintain sufficient ASWs to provide assessments for acutely ill patients needing compulsory admission to hospital. Guardianship procedures involve a minimum of several days work, and require senior management approval if the local authority is to act as the guardian. Each case has then to be properly reviewed, with formal reports given at appropriate intervals. While this level of intervention may be desirable to protect civil liberty, it is clearly not always achievable.

Some social services authorities are establishing a form of 'interim' civil liberty protection for residents. While accepting the impossibility of managing several hundred guardianship orders, they are not prepared to sanction the 'common sense' detention of elderly people without some measure of authority. As an absolute minimum, these interim procedures should contain an official medical report confirming that the resident is mentally disordered. Without such a statement, no elderly person should be prevented from leaving a residential or nursing home if they so wish. In addition to the medical report, there needs to be a summary of the problem behaviour (e.g. leaving the home and wandering into traffic), and a list of recommended methods of dealing with the behaviour. This will include an estimate of the risks involved, and a consensus about how much freedom the resident should be allowed in all the circumstances of the case. Thus it may be agreed that an elderly person should be permitted to walk unescorted outside the home, even though there is a significant chance that they may on occasions become lost. The alternative for that individual might be an excessive degree of restriction, which would lead to an unacceptably low quality of life.

General guidance issued to staff must include statements about any prohibited action, such as tying patients to chairs or the use of fixed trays and tilt-back chairs to prevent free movement. There will frequently be strong disagreement between professional staff from different disciplines about the use of particular equipment (for example cot sides), but these disputes must be resolved at the drafting stage if the guidance is to be effective. The final part of the form should include a statement from relatives or an independent advocate to the effect that they agree to the measures proposed for the protection of the 'vulnerable adult'. Where there is any significant disagreement between professional staff and relatives/advocates, consideration should be given to an assessment under the Mental Health Act. No informal procedures should ever deny access to review by an ASW or 'approved' doctors.

While these procedures have no formal legal authority, they offer considerable reassurance to staff, relatives, and residents. The constraints on an individual are clearly stated; and if an unfortunate incident occurs, it can be clearly demonstrated that all concerned acted in the best interests of the patient. There is obviously a workload implication for residential and medical staff, but the additional protection of 'vulnerable adult' procedures are a significant improvement to practice standards in the care of older people.

Similar principles apply to mentally disordered older people living in their own homes, although the legal and ethical issues are more complex. For example, a dementing patient may repeatedly turn on the cooker, but forget to light the gas. It has been common practice for social workers to arrange safer forms of heating and cooking to prevent injury to their client and others, yet where the individual resists intervention there is no statutory authority for action. Some relatives lock the door behind them when they leave, to prevent the disordered person from wandering into traffic. Paid care staff are then expected to continue the routine, but the risk of the individual being unable to escape in case of fire is deemed to be excessive by many practitioners. The elderly person would, in these circumstances, be virtually imprisoned in their own home. Again, procedures for the protection of vulnerable adults who live at home should specify measures that are acceptable, such as the use of alternative fuels. They should also prohibit excessive restriction of liberty, particularly because of the risks associated with fire.

Decision-making by mentally incapacitated adults is a complex area of ethics, involving a range of statutes. A consultation paper 'Who decides' (Lord Chancellor's Department 1997) reviewed existing legislation, and a series of changes to the law is expected by 2003.

Care management of individual clients

Social work with older people has undergone a radical transformation over the last 25 years. As recently as the 1970s, most qualified social workers were deployed in statutory child care and child protection tasks. A relatively small number were based in hospitals, providing advice and support to inpatients and preparing arrangements for their discharge. The level of domiciliary care available was extremely limited, often restricted to a 'home help' service of cleaning and housework in school hours from Monday to Friday. Casework would typically involve unqualified welfare assistants arranging basic support, or persuading older people to accept admission to residential care because there were no reasonable alternatives available.

During the 1980s, social work with adult clients was given higher priority and professional status as the numbers of disabled older people continued to rise. Complex multidisciplinary assessments began to be accepted as necessary to maintain this type of client at home. This trend has created a separate set of problems, since the volume of assessment work threatens to overwhelm the number of qualified practitioners available. Many authorities are now introducing a form of triage, where only the most complex and high-risk cases receive input from care managers, while less-qualified staff undertake routine reviews and basic case work.

Social care for older persons is now provided by a wide spectrum of paid and informal carers, whose individual skills range from basic personal care, to highly qualified ASWs and care managers with many years of practice experience. While the model of care provision will differ according to the type of team and local professional preference, there are fundamental similarities in approach across the country. This final section sets out the broad principles of 'care management', then demonstrates how they are applied in practice through a number of case examples.

In order for any individual to receive a service appropriate to their needs, the following steps are usually required:

1. *Case-finding*—While most elderly clients are referred directly to social services by GPs, hospitals, or relatives, the local authority has a duty to ensure that potential service users are identified, through a range of media. The Community Care Act gives high priority to the provision of straightforward information that helps users and carers find their way through the complex pattern of services provided by statutory and independent agencies. It is no longer deemed sufficient to wait for appropriate clients to refer themselves to social services, and liaison arrangements with GP practices are increasingly common. The 'over-75' checks conducted by primary health care teams are a useful way of identifying unmet social and health care needs.
2. *Referral*—Once a potential service user has been identified from any source, they have to be referred to the local social services office. While detailed arrangements vary, basic information on needs and circumstances is required. Referrals can be accepted from professional staff, older people themselves, their carer, or any other interested person.
3. *Screening*—Requests for assistance range from simple services such as walking sticks, through to admission to residential or nursing homes. The screening process ensures that urgent cases receive high priority, while cases that fall below certain 'eligibility criteria' may have to wait for a substantial time before assessment.
4. *Assessment*—A central aim of the Community Care Act is to reduce the number of assessments for each client. In the past, older people underwent a series of assessments for different services, often with different criteria at each stage. The individual was being evaluated against the rules for the service, rather than the service being tailored for the particular needs of the person. Social work, medical, and nursing assessments were frequently not accepted by other disciplines, and patients were asked similar questions about their disability by each successive practitioner. The trend under 'community care ' is towards holistic assessment, with the care manager drawing on a range of expertise to produce a rounded view of the client's needs. There is of course a requirement for specialist medical assessment in complex cases, but the hospital-based care manager will endeavour to integrate the treatment regime into the social care assessment where appropriate. Unfortunately, thorough holistic assessments are often impossible because of the pressure to discharge patients rapidly from acute settings.

The results of the assessment will normally be made available to the older person (and their relatives if necessary), so that details can be verified, and the views of all concerned can be recorded. A welcome feature of modern practice is the status given to the needs of the carer. This is an essential component of any holistic assessment, since the capacity and willingness of carers to continue their support for the patient is central to the decision about levels of paid-care input required. Informal or 'family' carers now have the right to a separate assessment of their social and health needs, which may of course conflict with the wishes of the older person. In extreme cases, the carer may have a different care manager to ensure fair representation of the rights of each member of the household or family.

5. *Notification of assessed charge*—While the assessment of need does not take any account of an ability or willingness to pay, most services arranged or provided by the local authority are means-tested. This is an increasingly contentious area of social care, but it is important to inform potential users of their likely financial contribution at an early stage in the process. Regrettably, many individuals with substantial disabilities refuse to consider any help when faced with paying the full cost of their care. In some cases, it may even be cheaper for them to pay private agencies directly rather than use the local authority as an intermediary. This option may appear superficially attractive, in that it reduces the bureaucracy involved and gives direct control to the older person. However, the service user is then completely dependent on the care provider for monitoring any change in needs, and for summoning additional support. There is much less security, and no access to the professional skills of the care manager or associated disciplines in a coordinated manner.

   Test cases in the late 1990s have confirmed that patients discharged from compulsory treatment orders under the Mental Health Act do not have to pay for their after-care.

6. Care planning—When agreement has been reached in principle to the provision of care support, detailed planning then takes place to identify the type of care required at different times of the day and night. The 'care plan' will specify which tasks have to be undertaken, by which type of staff, in what time frame. The plan is drafted by the care manager, then usually checked with the user or their relative/carer to ensure that it will meet the identified needs. This document is then used as a 'shopping list' to secure appropriate care from local providers.

7. *Purchasing and arranging of care*—Care managers have more or less choice about the range of services depending on the local political climate and the state of the 'mixed economy of care'. The Community Care Act explicitly encourages the use of independent sector providers, and gives financial incentives for local authorities to purchase services externally. If care is arranged from 'internal providers', this is a relatively straightforward process using residential homes or home care services run directly by the authority. The care is provided by staff who work for the social services department, to standards set down by their own management.

   Where care is arranged from an independent provider, more complex mechanisms are employed, involving the use of contracts and purchasing budgets. Each team or care manager will have access to a set budget, which they use to assemble a 'care package' fitting the requirements set out in the care plan. Most authorities operate a system of 'accreditation' for independent residential/ nursing homes and domiciliary-care agencies, which allows local purchasers to buy care from providers who have demonstrated that they meet certain quality and price standards. These care costs are then invoiced to the local authority on a regular basis.

8. *Monitoring and review*—One of the reasons for introducing the improved assessment and monitoring procedures in 1993 was that clients were often allocated services that subsequently became inappropriate for their changing needs. However, the volume and complexity of care packages have prevented care managers from reviewing them as frequently as was intended by the community care reforms. Regular reassessment is an essential element of good care arrangements, and some authorities have introduced reviewing officers at a lower level of qualification to ensure that at least a minimum number of reviews are carried out.

The principles of care management are integrated into the 'care programme approach', which operates in multidisciplinary teams caring for older people with mental health problems. Each individual patient has a specified care plan, and a named 'key worker' who is responsible for coordinating action to fulfil the care plan. This structured method of meeting need is particularly important when patients are discharged from hospital, since complex care arrangements have to be initiated across a number of professional disciplines within a short time.

Summary of social care provision

A principal objective of care management procedures is to make appropriate help available to the client and their carers, in order to maximize their independence and improve their quality of life. The range of services that was actually in place up to 1993 depended largely on local preference and historical accident. The number of day-care or residential places per head of population varied substantially across the country, and services are still predominantly concentrated in urban areas. As 'purchaser/provider' divisions of responsibility become established in social services' departments, the analysis of unmet need and service deficits has assumed a much higher priority. Local authorities are now required to produce 3-year plans, identifying how services are to be developed, and inviting comment on the use of public funding for welfare provision. Targets are set for improvement in key areas. This approach should gradually lead to a more even distribution of essential social care facilities across each local authority area.

The precise mix of provision will depend on available funding and local political and professional preference. Local authorities have to demonstrate 'best value' in the way they procure care for their population. However, most of the services described below should be available to clients who meet the relevant eligibility criteria. Cost will vary according to local charging policies.

Sheltered housing

The provision of supported housing is primarily a function of housing authorities rather than social service departments, although recent reforms in local government structure have brought the two responsibilities much closer together. Schemes are either managed directly by the local authority or, increasingly, by independent housing associations. The accommodation is usually purpose-built, with some form of support from a resident or visiting warden. Each tenant will have an alarm call system, so that in an emergency they can summon help via a central switchboard

There has been a substantial expansion in sheltered housing in the past decade, and many older people have benefited from an improvement in their accommodation. It is, however, important to be aware of the limitations of this type of environment, particularly for people with mental health needs. Personal care is not generally available from wardens, and the allocation of staff time for individual tenants is extremely limited. Wardens are primarily responsible for alerting other agencies to problems, rather than providing a direct care service themselves. Housing associations tend to rely increasingly on peripatetic staff who may visit several schemes from a central base.

Older people and their relatives often have an unrealistic expectation of the support available, and believe that a move to sheltered housing is justified because there will always be someone to look after them. In reality, most personal care will actually come from domiciliary-care staff who are based outside the housing complex. This level of support can often be supplied in the existing household without the inevitable distress caused by a change of accommodation.

The relatively low staffing levels mean that supervision of dementing or depressed patients will be minimal, and it is not generally advisable for people with significant mental health needs to be moved into sheltered housing unless sufficient support is available from external statutory or informal sources. Sheltered housing is also not necessarily the answer to loneliness, since tenants live in separate flats and may only have occasional opportunities to mix with other people. New funding arrangements from 2003 will result in the responsibility for 'support' in sheltered housing schemes being transferred to social services departments.

Residential care

Residential homes are either run directly by the local authority, or by private and voluntary organizations. Care managers can purchase places in independent homes, albeit within a limited budget, and a formal contract is then signed by the resident or their representative. Private individuals can also place themselves directly into independent residential homes without the assistance of a care manager, if they do not require financial support from the state. All residential homes are registered and inspected by the local authority.

Older people living in residential care should not require the 24-hour availability of qualified nursing staff. If they need this level of care at the point of admission, they should be directed towards a nursing home or a 'dual-registered' home that can provide residential and nursing care within the same establishment. Staffing levels in residential homes are generally lower than in nursing homes. The willingness of proprietors to accept residents with significant mental health problems varies according to skill levels, building design, and operational philosophy. The dividing line between residential and nursing-home care is difficult to define, but some highly effective specialist residential homes do provide excellent care for older people with dementing illnesses. These establishments tend to have enhanced staffing levels, and will often segregate their physically frail residents from those suffering from severe mental illness. Care managers and local authority inspectors will be able to advise carers and medical colleagues on the appropriate choice of a home to suit particular needs.

Nursing homes

Nursing homes are run by private or voluntary organizations, since local authorities are prohibited from the direct provision of nursing care. Places can be purchased in the same way as in residential homes, except that a certificate is required from an officer of the health authority confirming that the patient is suitable for admission to a nursing home. There is a shortage of specialist nursing-home places for mentally ill patients in many areas, resulting in delays in hospital discharge and relatives having to travel long distances. Private nursing homes now provide the majority of long-stay care for high-dependency patients who are unable to live at home, with NHS hospitals primarily offering an assessment and respite service, and residual long-stay care for patients who are extremely difficult to place in the independent sector. Nursing and residential homes are registered and inspected by the same authority from 2003.

Older people who are funded by the local authority in residential and nursing homes have to make a means-tested contribution to the cost of their care, and will pay the full cost if the capital they own exceeds a prescribed limit. They should receive regular reviews of their needs by a care manager or reviewing officer, at least every 6 months. As with most services provided under contract from external organizations, there is a limited budget available. Placement rates are directly linked to the length of stay of existing patients; as older people suffering from dementing illnesses tend to live longer than physically frail residents, many authorities are now facing a demand for institutional care that far exceeds their funding capacity. The 'nursing' element of this type of care will be funded by the state from 2001.

Day care

Day services cover a wide range of provision, where older people retain their own homes but go out to purpose-built centres or residential and nursing homes for part of the time. Transport is usually arranged by the local authority, and can include the use of taxis or specialist vehicles. Day centres use a combination of volunteers and paid staff to provide meals, activities, and personal care. While traditionally these services operated from mid-morning to mid-afternoon, there is now a trend for centres to be open longer hours, including weekends in some areas. Specialist units designed for supporting carers of mentally ill clients can offer care through the evening or at night, to alleviate the exhaustion experienced by carers when sleep patterns are continually disrupted. These facilities are often used as the base for multidisciplinary teams which provide assessment and therapeutic service to mentally ill patients and their carers.

While comprehensive day services can offer essential respite to carers, there may be difficulties in their use by patients who experience significant levels of confusion. The process of getting a confused person ready for transport at a particular time can be extremely stressful for carers, and patients often experience increased levels of agitation for some time after their return home. Careful assessment and planning can reduce these effects, but the change in environment may prove too disruptive in some cases. Care managers have to weigh up the benefits to the carer of a break for a few hours against the extra pressure of preparing for the journey and settling the patient afterwards.

Lunch clubs

While day centres provide direct personal care, lunch clubs offer a midday meal and companionship to older people. They are usually run by the voluntary sector in church halls and community centres, and can accept referrals directly from individuals or their carers. This type of support is invaluable to elderly people who live alone, and helps to alleviate loneliness and associated depression. As traditional family networks become more dispersed through changed working patterns and marital breakdown, the role of these local support networks is central to maintaining older people at home with a reasonable quality of life. As with many day centres, the potential benefits extend far beyond the short period actually spent in the club. Volunteers can befriend elderly people and offer additional help and friendship at other times, complementing the support available from relatives and neighbours.

Domiciliary meals service

The traditional 'meals-on-wheels' service consists of hot meals prepared centrally and then distributed in vans or private cars to clients who are unable to prepare hot food for themselves. This approach has been reviewed by many authorities as a result of concern about the nutritional value and temperature of meals by the time they reach the consumer. In rural areas, a wide range of alternatives can now be made available, including frozen meals for reheating in the home, deliveries from local schools, pubs, or residential homes, and the use of domiciliary care staff to prepare food for high-risk clients. The element of supervision is critically important for people with dementing illnesses, because they may need a lot of encouragement to eat regular meals. Although it is relatively expensive to provide a carer for the period of a meal, this is an essential part of good community support for mentally impaired clients, and a direct consequence of maintaining such individuals outside institutional settings.

Domiciliary care services

Help in the home for older persons has developed substantially in recent years. Following assessment by the care manager, a 'package' of support can be provided either directly by staff employed by the local authority, or from independent agencies under contract. Care in the home is increasingly targeted at the more dependent clients; in some areas it is now possible to provide assistance 7 days a week to older people who are completely bedfast or wheelchair-bound. Care staff receive training in the care and management of severely disabled people, and are expected to perform some quite sophisticated tasks that were previously the responsibility of district nurses. Night-care services are also becoming established, and are of particular benefit in monitoring older people who have disturbed sleep patterns.

Out-of-hours services

As community care policies take effect, the number of highly dependent people being maintained at home is rising, and there will inevitably be unpredictable breakdowns in care provision. All social service departments have arrangements to respond to crises that occur out of normal working hours. These consist of access to advice by telephone, backed up by social workers who can be called out in an emergency to assess referrals that cannot wait until the next working day. At the extreme, ASWs are available to coordinate formal assessments under the Mental Health Act, leading to compulsory admission to hospital if necessary. Emergency admissions to residential care can also be undertaken, although it is more usual for substantial care packages to be set up to hold the situation until a full assessment can be made by the local staff. Emergency duty teams will attempt to liaise with relevant practitioners as part of their assessment, but will make short-term care arrangements on the information available at the time, and then report to day-service colleagues as soon as possible to ensure continuity.

As the trend towards multidisciplinary working continues, crisis intervention teams are becoming established across the country. These services typically include psychiatric nurses, social workers, and 'support workers' who can offer assistance with a wide spectrum of care in the home. Crisis teams usually work extended days, and the aim in many areas is for them to operate 24 hours a day to prevent unnecessary hospital admission. Rapid response by skilled staff within hours to deteriorating mental health in older persons can often support family carers to the point where they no longer request compulsory admission.

Incontinence laundry service

Studies of unplanned admissions to residential and nursing homes have repeatedly demonstrated that carers can be pushed to breaking point by episodes of incontinence which are beyond their capacity to manage. While the increased availability of washing machines and tumble driers has reduced the impact of this problem, chronic incontinence remains difficult for many elderly carers to cope with unless they have additional help. Most local authorities provide or arrange for the collection and laundry of soiled clothing and bed-linen on a regular basis. This is an essential service which is highly valued by carers.

Aids and adaptations

Relatively minor disabilities can cause major disruption to the life of an elderly person, causing a loss of independence out of proportion to the medical problem. Local authorities have a duty under the Chronically Sick and Disabled Persons Act to assess disability and provide appropriate aids and adaptations to alleviate the effects of disability. Assessments are usually carried out by qualified occupational therapists, who then arrange for equipment to be delivered and installed. This can range from, for example, bath seats, small items to help with operating taps, electric hoists, through to major adaptations to improve access to buildings, and wheelchair or stair lifts.

Counselling

The process of care management includes an element of counselling as part of assessment, in order to help clients and carers decide what sort of help they need, and what plans they wish to make for the future. Unfortunately the pressures of new assessments and administration involved in setting up care packages prevent care managers from spending as much time as they would like in counselling clients and carers. This change from previous practice in adult care is regretted by many practitioners, particularly when working with carers of dementing older people. While practical assistance with personal care is clearly of fundamental importance, the emotional response of a spouse to their partner's changed personality is an equally important area for social work intervention. In the area of respite care, it may take several months for a spouse to build up sufficient trust in the care manager to agree to let their partner attend day or residential care for even a short period. There are frequently some initial problems in settling into a new routine, which may be used as an excuse for an ambivalent carer to cancel the arrangement prematurely. Without this relationship, the service is less likely to be successful, and the carer will be at greater risk of complete breakdown in their capacity to support the older person.

Staff in specialist multidisciplinary teams will usually have a greater opportunity to work in more detail with their clients, but general caseloads will restrict most care managers to limited counselling time.

Limitations of community care services

While high levels of support can be of tremendous value in maintaining highly dependent people in their own homes, there are three important factors which must be considered when care managers are contemplating a complex care package. First, the development of more flexible and comprehensive care provision at home means that it can be technically possible to dress, feed, and monitor severely demented patients in the community. This may appear to be a direct and appropriate response to demands from relatives or a carer living in the home. However, it is essential for professional staff to stand back from the situation and review the overall effect on quality of life for both patient and carer. An 'intensive' care package may consist of four or more hours of care every day, but this still leaves the client or carer unsupported for long periods. Day care may help to alleviate the stress or risk, but there may come a point where the complexity of arrangements actually increases the difficulties experienced by the service users. An important question for care managers at reviews is therefore to ask how the client (where appropriate) and carer feel about the arrangements that have been made. Even when all reasonable support has been provided, there may still not be enough security and reassurance, particularly where clients suffer from severe memory deficits. In these circumstances, admission to residential or nursing-home care may well be preferable. This option should certainly be considered if the mental state of the client has deteriorated to the point where she no longer recognizes her surroundings. The notion of 'remaining at home' takes on a different dimension when the individual cannot identify members of her family, or is unable to derive any feelings of security from previously cherished possessions.

The second issue which must be addressed is the cost of the care arrangements weighed against the benefits, and the cost of alternative provision. Community care reforms have forced both health and social care staff to become much more conscious of financial constraints. As control of resources is devolved to team and even care manager level, it is clear that any expenditure on one client will prevent another from receiving a service, assuming a fixed budget. For many physically disabled older people who cooperate fully with paid carers, it is possible to demonstrate that most of their basic needs can be met by about four home-care visits a day. However, some severely demented clients could receive twice this level of service and still be at considerable risk because of the varied and unpredictable nature of their needs for supervision. The combination of 'quality of life' and cost factors could therefore indicate that this group of patients may be more appropriately supported by institutional care in the long term. Where there is a clear diagnosis of a progressive deterioration in a dementing illness, there is a strong argument for admitting such patients to institutional care before they or their carers reach crisis point. This view runs counter to a simplistic interpretation of the community care ideology, but may actually lead to a significant improvement in the quality of life of both patients and carers. At present, resource constraints and a perception that residential/nursing-home admission is somehow evidence of 'failure', have resulted in practitioners often waiting for care arrangements to break down before they arrange admission. However, the reforms were designed to ensure that people who could appropriately be diverted from institutional care should remain at home. It is quite consistent with the spirit of the Act to recommend earlier admission to institutional care for severely demented patients, so that they can receive appropriate supervision, care, and support at all times of the day and night.

The third factor to consider is the availability of careworkers. Complex packages of care require high volumes of labour-intensive support, often delivered during unsocial hours. In the south of England, unemployment has fallen to extremely low levels and most social care providers experience great difficulty in recruiting and retaining staff. Community care policies have assumed that the supply of labour will always be adequate, but this is not the case in more prosperous regions. The problem is exacerbated by competition from the retail and light industrial sectors, to the extent that some providers have to recruit staff from abroad and offer subsidized accommodation and enhanced wage rates. Unless the supply of labour can be improved, further extension of community care services will be severely restricted.

The following examples demonstrate how care management principles can be applied in practice for the benefit of older people with mental health needs.

Case 1

Mrs A. was an 84-year-old widow who lived alone in an owner-occupied house in a large town. She had raised two of her own children and two from a second marriage, all now retired themselves. Following the death of her husband some 10 years previously she had continued to live in the family home with minimal support and occasional visits from her step-children who lived locally. Her own children had moved away, but kept in touch by telephone.

For the past 2 years, Mrs A. had employed a private home carer for 2 hours a week, who did the shopping, collected her pension, and paid bills. Although Mrs A. suffered from mild arthritis in her hips and knees, she was relatively independent, and could wash, dress, and feed herself with no difficulty. She was always pleased to see visitors, although there were longstanding tensions with her step-children which dated back to her treatment of them as children 50 years ago. There was no involvement with social services, and the GP had not seen Mrs A. for 2 years.

Early one morning, neighbours found Mrs A. lying in her garden, having fallen sometime during the night. No reason could be identified for her being in the garden after dark. She was admitted to hospital and found to have broken her left wrist. No plaster was necessary, but the arm was in a sling and could not be used. After an overnight stay she was discharged to live with her stepson for a few days while she got over the shock of her fall.

A week later, social services received a referral from the GP requesting admission to residential care for his patient, who apparently could not return home. Relatives were apparently refusing to provide further care, and a crisis was imminent.

The duty care manager visited the next day to assess the situation. Mrs A. was most cooperative on interview, and assured him that she was well able to cope at home. Although the broken wrist was an inconvenience, she would arrange extra help and did not want further assistance. Throughout the conversation, the stepson was shaking his head and clearly disagreeing with her view of events. As the interview progressed, it became evident that Mrs A. had a completely unrealistic estimation of her ability to care for herself. She was unable to get out of a chair unaided, and could not use the stairs to get to the only toilet. During the past week, there had been several episodes of urinary incontinence while relatives had been out shopping, because Mrs A. had been unable to summon assistance. Under more detailed questioning, it was clear that Mrs A. had substantial short-term memory deficits, and was disoriented in time and place. While presenting as confident and self-assured, she confabulated whenever she was asked detailed questions about her home situation. She firmly rejected the option of a temporary admission to residential care.

When interviewed separately, the stepson confirmed that he and his wife were unable and unwilling to accommodate Mrs A. for more than another couple of days. Both had full-time jobs, and had taken their full leave entitlement. It was clear that relations with Mrs A. had always been strained, and that care was provided more from a sense of duty than from a strong concern for her welfare. The stepson reported that Mrs A. had been sleeping a lot during the day, and was awake intermittently throughout the night, seemingly unaware of the time.

Following discussion with the GP and various other members of the family by telephone, the care manager arranged for Mrs A. to return home with four visits a day from domiciliary care staff, with a monitoring visit during the night by a peripatetic care team. A referral for full assessment was made to the multidisciplinary team specializing in support for elderly mentally ill clients, as it was anticipated that the situation could deteriorate quite rapidly.

Discussion

This example demonstrates how a relatively small change in disability (a broken wrist) can reveal a catalogue of other problems which had been concealed by the client's lifestyle. The care manager hypothesized that there had been a progressive deterioration in Mrs A.'s mental state, which had been masked because her private carer had been taking on more responsibility for day-to-day decisions. The 'safest' option would have been for the client to be admitted to residential care on a temporary basis, with the intention of a return home when the wrist had healed. However, given the firm refusal of Mrs A. to consider this outcome, the best that could be offered was additional support at home. It was essential for relatives to be involved in this decision, and to have all the risks explained to them in advance. While Mrs A. did not have sufficient insight into her situation to make an informed decision about her future, it was not considered appropriate to use powers available under the Mental Heath Act to force her to leave her home at this stage. The risk of falling was relatively low while Mrs A. was confined to a chair, but would increase if she was subsequently able to get up without assistance.

The case would require frequent review by the multidisciplinary team, to ensure that risks were monitored at regular intervals. The care manager would seek to encourage links with a local residential or nursing home through day-care arrangements, to begin to prepare the ground for a possible admission. This would reduce the transitional stress on Mrs A. if the home situation breaks down as seems likely at some point in the future.

Case 2

Mr B. was an 88-year-old widower, who had lived alone in a small village since the death of his wife some 5 years previously. His son and daughter visited every month, but Mr B. was relatively independent and did not need any assistance with housework or personal care. Over a period of about a year, his behaviour began to change, and relatives noticed that he was becoming extremely forgetful. Rubbish began to accumulate throughout the house, and Mr B. stopped going out. On two occasions, neighbours had noticed a strong smell of gas, and had found the sitting-room gas fire switched on, but unlit. Mr B. smoked around 10 cigarettes a day, and there was evidence of several recent burns to furniture where cigarettes had been left on the fabric. His daughter contacted social services for advice after the fire brigade was called to a small fire in the kitchen caused by a frying pan being left on the stove, then setting light to towels. She had repeatedly found her father to be very cold, having failed to switch on any heating during severe winter weather.

Following a detailed assessment, the care manager recommended a series of measures to reduce the chances of a major fire occurring, and to ensure that adequate heating was provided. These included installation of electric night-storage heaters with hidden switches, changing the gas stove for an electric version, and replacing the gas fire with a modern automatic ignition fire. It was also suggested that the armchair used by Mr B. was replaced by a new chair filled with fire-retardant padding. Several weeks of patient negotiation with the client were then needed to secure his agreement to the changes, since he did not consider they were necessary.

Discussion

The risk of fire is understandably one of the most serious concerns associated with progressive memory impairment. Pressure from relatives and members of the public for GPs and social workers to 'do something' is frequently intense, yet there are no formal legal powers to modify domestic equipment without the agreement of the householder. This type of case is often reviewed in a multidisciplinary case conference, in order to protect the civil liberties of the individual, and afford some sharing of the risk between the professional staff and relatives involved. If the degree of dementia suffered by the patient is extreme, it may be considered appropriate to override their objections to improved safety measures. It is essential for decisions taken to be recorded formally, particularly where the client is left in a high-risk situation. Where it is impossible to reduce the risk to an acceptable level (for example, where small fires are repeatedly caused as a result of smoking), the only option may be compulsory removal of the patient to a more secure environment such as a nursing home. This course of action is only taken after considerable debate, since the stress and reduced quality of life resulting from the decision may have a serious or even fatal effect on the individual. A strong justification for removal is the protection of other people, where the patient lives in some form of multi-occupied housing, and there is a high risk of fire or gas explosion resulting from their behaviour.

Case 3

Mrs C. lived with her husband in council accommodation. They were both over 80, and had been married for 54 years. Mrs C. suffered from multi-infarct dementia, and was receiving regular support from the community psychiatric nurse. Medication was reviewed monthly during domiciliary visits by the psychogeriatric consultant from the sector team.

A referral was made to the social services department when Mrs C. became more agitated, and started to reject the help of her husband. She would verbally abuse him, and attempt to strike him if he tried to prevent her leaving the house late at night. On several occasions she had become disoriented while returning from the shops, and had to be brought home by the police. Mr C. was becoming exhausted by the strain of caring for his wife, but insisted that it was his duty to keep her at home for as long as possible. Several members of the family lived locally, but had been discouraged from calling at the house because of Mrs C.'s hostile attitude towards visitors.

The care manager spent several hours interviewing the couple, both together and separately. It was agreed that a carer would initially call three times a week, to get to know Mr and Mrs C., and assist with personal care tasks. When confidence had been established, the level of visits was increased, so that Mr C. could go out and visit his daughter. At a later stage, day care was arranged in a nearby residential home, with the carer acting as escort to reduce the stress for Mrs C. On two nights a week, a sitter was provided to allow Mr C. to have a proper rest. This combination of domiciliary and day services was sufficient to allow Mr C. to continue in his caring role for a further 18 months. His wife's mental health then deteriorated rapidly, and she was admitted to a specialist unit within the residential home. The community psychiatric nurse and psychogeriatrician continued their support in the residential home. Mr C. visited his wife daily until she died 9 months later.

Discussion

Relatives can experience powerful feelings of guilt when caring for someone they have known and loved for many years. The fear of institutional care (still referred to as the 'workhouse' in some areas) remains very strong, and these two factors combined can lead to prolonged resistance to support from statutory agencies. The design of care plans appropriate to individual circumstances is central to the success of any services that are offered. Some people respond extremely well to day care, and this can build up to 5 or even 7 days a week if necessary. For others, relief care in the home is more acceptable. The skill of care management involves offering available services at the right time, in the right amount, so that clients and carers can choose what they need, having had some experience of the available options. Where severe dementia is involved, it will usually be advisable to develop links with a residential or nursing-home setting, since the client is likely to need some form of institutional care in the long term. While the spouse or other carer may be adamant that they wish to continue to look after the client at home, there is always the possibility of sudden disability or even death of the carer. This is a relatively common occurrence, since dementing patients are often in better physical health than their carer. If relationships have been established with a residential or nursing home, it is much easier for all concerned to make the transition if necessary.

Where carers live with the mentally disordered client, there can be a direct conflict between their respective interests, and in these situations both parties have to be treated as clients in their own right. Separate assessments can be arranged, from different care managers if necessary. Although the mentally infirm partner may refuse admission to institutional care, this should not necessarily force their spouse to continue to provide full-time supervision. The carer must be allowed to meet her reasonable needs for the benefit of her own health and well-being, even if this results in a breakdown of care arrangements for the partner. Care managers may have to defend the interests of the carer against strong and sustained pressure from other family members, who can resort to moral blackmail to prevent what they see as the stigma of admission to a nursing home. While case conferences are not necessarily the best way of seeking the views of all concerned, they can be very useful as a way of clarifying the different perspectives and assuring relatives that their opinions are being considered. Unless there is formal evidence of mental disorder, the social services' department has no legal authority to implement decisions, but considerable influence can be exerted over apparently intractable situations, especially if the GP is prepared to endorse the proposed plan of action.

The importance of multidisciplinary working cannot be overemphasized. While detailed operational arrangements differ widely across the country, professional staff must coordinate their input to complex situations. In particular, care managers should seek to arrange full psycho-geriatric assessment to ensure that everything possible has been done to diagnose and treat psychiatric disorders in their elderly clients.

Use of technology in social care for older persons

The use of alarm pendants by older persons living alone is now widespread. These simple devices offer a means of summoning assistance, providing security in the case of falls or sudden illness. There is, however, little systematic use of technology to support people with dementia. A pan-European project 'Astrid' (A social and technological response to meeting the needs of individuals with dementia and their carers) (Marshall 2000) has shown how technology can benefit people with dementia. Examples include calendar clocks that help to maintain orientation in time, sensors to warn carers when their relative is trying to leave the house, and gas, flood, or fall detectors. Sophisticated surveillance devices can now detect when the normal routine of a dementing person changes, alerting family or professional carers that a check visit may be required. This level of intrusion into individual homes raises ethical issues for care managers, but if the alternative is some form of institutional care then many families will prefer to accept the loss of privacy. Two-way video communication is also being tested in a number of pilot sites as a way of supplementing check visits by careworkers.

References

Department of Health (1989). *Caring for people: community care in the next decade and beyond.* HMSO, London.

Lord Chancellor's Department (1997). *Who decides?* The Stationery Office, London.

Marshall, M. (2000). *Astrid: a guide to using technology within dementia care.* Hawker Publications, London.

Secretary of State for Health (2000). *The NHS plan—a plan for investment. A plan for reform.* HMSO, Norwich.

15 Psychometric assessment in the elderly

Karen Ritchie

Introduction

Psychometric assessment implies the quantification of observations of behaviour, cognition, and affect, and as such is an important adjunct to psychogeriatric assessment in both the clinical and research setting. The step from observation to measurement is also important in the contribution it frequently makes to furthering our understanding of a given health problem at a conceptual level. As Blalock (1968 and 1970) has pointed out, 'measurement considerations often enable us to clarify our theoretical thinking and to suggest new variables that should be considered...careful attention to measurement may force a clarification of one's basic concepts and theories.'

This chapter will first consider some of the theoretical issues specific to the psychometric evaluation of elderly populations, and, second, will review the use which has been made of psychometric techniques in the evaluation of senescent cognitive disorder.

Conceptual considerations

Assessment models

Two principal models have governed our conceptualization of mental disorder. On the one hand the dichotomic medical model clearly distinguishes normal fluctuations in mental functioning (e.g. transient feelings of sadness, or ageing-associated memory impairment) from psychiatric pathology (e.g. severe depression, dementia). This model construes psychiatric disorder as a disease process whose aetiology is separate from that of 'normal' ageing. Measures based on this model refer to pathological behaviours which are not seen in normal populations (for example, aphasia, apraxia, insomnia, hallucinations) and thus clearly differentiate healthy and unhealthy cohorts.

The psychological model, on the other hand, conceptualizes mental functioning in terms of a normal distribution. This model assumes that affective and cognitive problems are to some degree present in all elderly persons; poor mental health being defined in terms of degree of discomfort, or a statistically significant deviation from an established norm. Measures based on this model are therefore dimensional rather than categorical and present the problem of determining a suitable cut-off point for 'abnormality'. The determination of an appropriate cut-off point for this type of measure is partly a statistical problem, but it also depends on changing social conceptualizations of dysfunction. Increasing emphasis on the quality of life of the elderly, and an increasingly optimistic view of what should constitute the normal health status of the elderly person, have undoubtedly led to a lowering of the threshold for what is considered 'acceptable' discomfort.

Given that the biological mechanisms underlying mental disorder are generally only partially understood (Michels and Marzuk 1993), diagnosis commonly relies on observations of the non-specific behavioural consequences of mental disorder, which are dimensional rather than categorical variables. The situation thus frequently arises that mental disorders now commonly considered to be discontinuous with normal ageing (for example Alzheimer's disease, depressive illness) are commonly diagnosed by reference to non-specific dimensional variables such as sadness, motor speed, memory performance. As a result, measures of mental health status in the elderly are often based on both the psychological and medical models. For example, neuropsychological measures of cognitive functioning commonly take the form of dimensional behavioural measures (based on the psychological model) such as word fluency and verbal recall. However, such tests also permit the investigator to observe the existence of dichotomous signs (indicative of pathology according to the medical model) such as perseveration, dyskinesia, aphasia, and visual field neglect. More recently the development of functional neuroimaging techniques has served to draw together the two approaches, by the visualization of the functional anatomical correlates of performance on laboratory tests of cognition in both normal and pathological states. The reader is referred to Cabeza and Nyberg (1997) for an overview of advances in functional imaging using positron-emission tomography, and to Nyberg (1998) for magnetic resonance imaging.

When developing a measuring instrument for the diagnosis or screening of mental disorder in the elderly, some consideration should be given to its underlying conceptual assumptions as these will play an important part in the scoring of items and in assessing validity. In the case of the medical model, discriminability may be improved by increasing the number of items relating to disease-specific symptoms and reducing those relating to non-specific symptoms. In the case of measures based on the psychological paradigm, adjustment is more commonly required at the cut-off point according to symptom prevalence and severity in the target population. This point is discussed below in relation to screening instruments.

The definition of 'normality' in elderly populations

An important consideration in the development of measures of mental functioning in the elderly, irrespective of whether the medical or psychological model is adhered to, is the question of what is 'normal' at a given age. All too often 'normal' performance is taken to be the average performance of an age cohort from which elderly persons with mental disorder have been excluded. This practice has undoubtedly underestimated true normal performance, due to the inclusion of persons in the so-called normal group who have subclinical pathologies and other conditions likely to mask true ability (notably sensory impairments and coexisting physical illness). Advances in medical technology have also permitted the identification of previously unrecognized pathology in so-called 'normal' elderly brains. A notable example in large-scale general population studies has been the observation through magnetic resonance imaging of white matter lesions, which are related to non-progressive attentional and memory deficits and depressive symptomatology (Breteler *et al.* 1994; Skoog *et al.* 1996)

Over the last century, rapid changes in environmental factors likely to have an important influence on mental functioning (education, medical care, nutrition, protection from adverse environmental exposure) have given rise to important age-cohort effects. That is, younger elderly are likely to have benefited from more favourable conditions than the oldest old—including greater familiarity with questionnaires and psychometric tests. It is thus not surprising that the marked differences seen between age groups in test performance in cross-sectional studies often disappear when the same behaviours are studied longitudinally. This point is particularly important in the context of cognitive assessment, and it has been nicely illustrated by Schaie (1983) who studied cognitive functioning in elderly persons over a 21-year period. Although cross-sectional age comparisons showed a significant drop in mean performance with age, over the 21 years of the study individual age cohorts in fact showed very little deterioration—apart from the over 80-year-old group. Drawing on the example of cardiovascular disease, Manton and Stallard (1988) raised the point that disorders once thought to be an inevitable feature of the ageing process are now being redefined as pathologies: '...age criteria are tending to disappear and what is considered to be the normal state for an elderly person is not very different from that of younger adults'.

Measurement issues in geriatric assessment

In developing tests for elderly populations a number of specific problems arise. Perhaps the most important, and yet most neglected, is that of the heterogeneity observed within age cohorts. The performance of children is so highly predictable at a given age that it has been possible to construct normative developmental scales, which rapidly detect social and cognitive delays and abnormalities. With age, however, standard errors on almost all behavioural measures fan out to such an extent that the 'normal' performance of elderly age cohorts is extremely difficult to characterize. This is partly due to interindividual differences in inherent ability, and partly due to interactions with extrinsic factors such as varying general health profiles. This implies that, with age, normal levels of functioning should be established on increasingly large samples. In most cases the opposite has been the case, so that normative data at high ages are usually unreliable.

A second issue, as touched on above, is the problem of the high prevalence of sensory impairment and multiple pathologies in elderly populations, and the difficulties inherent in developing measures that are independent of these factors. It is known, for example, that respiratory disorders, which show an increasing prevalence with age, may have an important impact on test performance (Grant *et al.* 1982), as may also medications commonly taken by the elderly such as digitalis. Elderly populations have a high prevalence of sensory impairment. Very few tests have been developed specifically for elderly persons who have visual or auditory problems. The inventive clinician may consider, however, making use of the tactile tests included in child assessment batteries. Unfortunately many of the psychometric measures available for use with the elderly have been validated on 'selected' populations free of impairment and disease (and their validity for the majority of elderly persons who do not fall into this category remains unknown).

A further problem is the high level of illiteracy and low levels of education often found in elderly populations. Education differentials raise two major problems. The first is the difficulty inherent in the development of 'education fair' measures, which do not produce, for example, high false-positive rates in the assessment of cognitive deficit in the poorly educated or false-negative rates in elderly persons with high levels of education. A number of statistical techniques have been developed that may assist in the evaluation of item bias, such as the use of statistical weighting using either a non-parametric or stratified regression method (Kittner *et al.* 1986) and item-response theory (IRT), a derivative of latent structure analysis (Teresi and Golden 1994). The second problem is the question of whether in adjusting for education effects in psychometric tests the researcher is not in fact removing the effects of a true risk factor. This point is discussed at length in relation to cognitive testing in the elderly by Berkman (1986).

High rates of institutionalization in elderly populations, particularly amongst the oldest old and the socially isolated, raises further difficulties in psychometric assessment. For example, the imposition of institutional regimes makes the differentiation of aptitude (what the elderly person is actually able to do) from performance (that which he habitually does in everyday life) at times rather difficult. This factor is particularly likely to affect measures of the consequences of mental illness such as activities of daily living (ADL) scales and informant measures of performance. The stress associated with the move to long-term care and the isolated nature of institutional life together may have a significant effect on the performance on both affective and cognitive measures. Performance on cognitive tests has been shown to drop significantly immediately after entry into an institution (Wells and Jorm 1987; Ward *et al.* 1990; Ritchie and Fuhrer 1992) with only partial restitution after a three month period (Wells and Jorm 1987). Ward *et al.* (1990) report a mean drop of four points on the Mini-Mental State Examination (Folstein *et al.* 1975), and Ritchie and Fuhrer (1992) observed that elderly persons with mild senile dementia living in the community performed better on this test than normal elderly people living in institutions. The principal difficulty lies in differentiating true changes in mental status, which may be due to institutionalization (or may have been the cause of institutionalization), from transient adjustment effects.

A general problem has been that tests used with the elderly are commonly tests developed for use with younger adults. The problem is not only one of content (adapting test materials to older populations) but also of one at a more fundamental level, where little thought has been given to the ways in which information processing might evolve at higher ages. Theories of cognitive development are primarily concerned with childhood changes, and it is assumed that cognitive processes once mature in early adolescence do not evolve further. Research in this area is clearly needed to determine whether differences between younger and older adults are due to deterioration or adaptive evolution of cognitive processes. For example, small children rely heavily on rote memory, which requires no analysis of information content. With age there is an increasing ability to learn by association and condensation; new information is linked with existing information and retained in a summarized form. This permits the retention of larger amounts of information. Interestingly enough, assumptions that elderly people have poorer memories than younger persons is often based on performance on tests of rote recall (for example, list learning), rather than précis recall (requesting the subject to retain a summary of a text) on which older persons perform better.

Psychometric measures of cognitive functioning in the elderly

Interest in the assessment of cognitive functioning in the elderly has undoubtedly been further stimulated by concern, on the part of both health planners and clinicians, that ageing of the population may be giving rise to what Kramer (1980) has termed a 'rising pandemic of mental disorders and associated chronic diseases and disabilities'. At a population level it has been estimated (for example, in the United Kingdom, France, and Australia) that one year of senile dementia per capita may be expected in the over 60-year-old population (Ritchie *et al.* 1993*b*, 1994*a*,*b*). For mental health service providers cognitive disorder is costly—not only does the elderly person with cognitive impairment require assistance with activities of daily living, but also his judgement is impaired so that assistance may be required for decision-making. Additionally, it has been demonstrated that the caregivers of elderly persons with cognitive disorders have a significantly increased risk of both physical and mental illness (Gilleard *et al.* 1984; Kiecolt-Glaser *et al.* 1987).

A large number of tests have appeared in the literature that not only aim to identify cognitive dysfunction in the elderly, but also to assess its functional consequences for the purposes of planning care and evaluating the impact of therapeutic intervention. These instruments principally involve the direct examination of the elderly person through questions assessing his memory, orientation, language, and visuospatial performance. Given the inherent difficulties involved in requesting self-report from persons with cognitive difficulties, increasing interest has been given in recent years to informant measures, which provide information on premorbid ability, degree of change over time, and ability to perform activities of daily living.

Within the field of geriatric psychiatry, psychometric evaluation of cognitive functioning has served three main purposes: screening for cognitive impairment; differential diagnosis of disorders affecting intellectual performance; and evaluation of the consequences of cognitive impairment. Each of these will be considered in turn. Table 15.1 provides summary information on most of the validated psychometric measures of cognitive performance that have been used with elderly subjects. The table indicates the name of the test, its more commonly known acronym, the country and the language in which it has been

Table 15.1 Psychometric tests developed for the assessment of cognitive performance in the elderly[a]

Test name	Author[b]	Country	Function
Alzheimer Disease Assessment Scale (ADAS)	Rosen (1984)	US	T
Amsterdam Dementia Screening Test (ADS)	De Jonghe (1994)	Holland	S
Alters Konzentrations Test (AKT)	Geiger-Kabisch (1993)	Germany	SC
Behaviour Dyscontrol Scale (BDS)	Grigsby (1992)	UK	SC
Behavioral Pathology in AD (Behave-AD)	Harwood *et al.* (1998)	US	C
Batterie d'Evaluation de la Démence (BED)	Signoret (1982)	France	D
Behavioral and Emotional Activities in Dementia	Sinha (1992)	US	T, C
Cognitive Abilities Screening Instrument (CASI)	Liu (1994)	China	S
Canberra Interview for the Elderly (CIE)	Henderson (1994)	Australia	D
Clinical Check List	Hare (1978)	US	S
Clock Drawing Test (CDT)	Ainslie (1993)	US	S
Cambridge Contextual Reading Test (CCRT)	Beardsall (1994)	UK	P
Cognitive Performance Test (CPT)	Burns (1994)	US	C
CERAD Neuropsychological Battery	Welsh (1994)	US	D
Cognitive Screening Test (CST)	Ponds (1992)	Holland	S
Computerized Neuropsychol. Test Battery (CNTB)	Veroff (1991)	US	C
Clifton Assessment Scale (CAPE)	Clarke (1991)	US	C
Cambridge Exam. for Mental Disorders (CAMDEX)	Roth (1988)	US	C, D
CAMDEX-N (Dutch Version)	Neri (1994)	US	C, D
Dementia Rating Scale (DRS)	Rosser (1994)	US	C, D
Structural Interview for the Diagnosis of Alzheimer's type and multi-infarct dementias (ENEDAM)	Morinigo (1990)	Spain	D
Détérioration Cognitive Observéé (DECO)	Ritchie (1992)	France	S
East Boston Memory (EBMT)	Albert (1991)	US	S, C
Echelle Comportement et Adaptation (ECA)	Ritchie (1991)	France	C, T
Evaluation Cognitive par ordinateur (ECO)	Ritchie (1992)	France	SC, D
Extended Scale for Dementia (ESD	Helmes (1992)	Canada	C, D
Functional Assessment Staging (FAST)	Sclan (1992)	US	SC
Gedragsobservatieschool-geriatrie (GOS-G)	Gorissen (1994)	Holland	D
Guy Advanced Dementia Schedule (Guy-ADS)	Ward (1993)	US	D, S
Hierarchic Dementia Scale (HDS)	Ronnberg (1994)	Sweden	D, C
Hasegawa Dementia Scale (HDS)	Gao (1991)	China	S
Hierarchic Dementia Scale	Cole and Dastoor (1996)	Canada	SC
Hodkinson Test	Gomez de Caso (1994)	Spain	D, C
Hodkinson Abbreviated Mental test	Rocca (1992)	Italy	C, S
Informant questionnaire on cognitive decline in the elderly (IQCODE)	Jorm (1991)	Australia	D, S
Iowa Screening Test	Eslinger (1985)	US	S, SC
Kew Cognitive Map	McDonald (1969)	US	S
London Psychogeriatric rating Scale (LPRS)	Reid (1991)	US	SC
Mattis Dementia Rating Scale	Coblentz (1973)	UK	S
Mental Status Questionnaire (MSQ)	Kahn (1960)	US	S
Mini-Mental State Examination (MMSE)	Folstein (1975)	US	S
Mini-Object Test	Still (1983)	US	S
Mémoire de Prose	Capitani (1994)	Italy	C
Memory Impairment Screen (MIS)	Buschke *et al.* (1999)	US	S
Modified Ordinal Scales for Psychological Development (M-OSPD)	Auer and Reisberg (1996)	US	C
N-ADL	Nishimura (1993)	Japan	C
NM Scale	Nishimura (1993)	Japan	C
National Adult Reading Test (NART)	Nelson (1982)	UK	P, C
Nurse's Observation Scale for Geriatric patients (NOSGER)	Tremmel (1993)	UK	D, C
Nunberg Alters Inventar (NAI)	Pek (1992)	Hungary	C, T

Table 15.1 *contd*

Test name	Author[b]	Country	Function
Neuropsychiatric Inventory (NPI)	Cummings (1994)	US	D
Observation Psycho Geriatrics (OPG)	Duine (1991)	Holland	C
Qualitative Evaluation of Dementia (QED)	Royall (1993)	US	C
Refined ADL Assessment Scale (R-ADL)	Tappen (1994)	US	C, D
Short portable Mental Status Questionnaire (SPMSQ)	Albert (1991)	US	S, C
Syndrom Kurztest (SKT)	Kim (1993)	Germany	C, T
Severe Impairment Battery (SIB)	Panisset (1992)	France	C
Structured Interview for the diagnosis of dementia of Alzheimer Type, Multi-Infarct Dementia and dementias of other etiology (SIDAM)	Zaudig (1992)	Germany	D
Structured Assessment of Independent Living Skills (SAILS)	Mahurin (1991)	US	C
Telephone Assessed Mental State (TAMS)	Lanska (1993)	US	D, S
Troublesome Behaviour Scale (TBS)	Asada (1994)	Japan	D

[a]The tests are classified according to function: screening of cognitive disorder (S), assessment of a specific cognitive function (SC), differential diagnosis (D), assessment of the impact of therapeutic intervention (T), estimation of premorbid intelligence level (P), or for the evaluation of the consequences of cognitive disorder (C).
[b]Only the first author is given.

developed, and the purpose for which it has been developed. The three main uses of cognitive measures (screening, diagnosis, and assessment of consequences) are discussed below.

Screening tests

In mediaeval Britain, the *Prerogativa Regis* (a Crown document later adopted as common law) established tribunals in 1392 for the screening of cognitive impairment to ensure protection of the afflicted individual and to provide assistance in the management of his financial affairs (Tomlins 1822). It is interesting to note that this examination consisted of questions to the individual relating to temporal and spatial orientation, memory, calculation, and reasoning. The content is in fact strikingly similar to the many screening tests for dementia in current use. Table 15.1 describes many of these tests, but more extensive reviews may be found in Israel *et al.* (1986) and Ritchie (1988).

Screening tests for cognitive impairment in the elderly may generally be divided into three categories:

(1) brief mental status examinations consisting of single-item assessments of orientation, memory, and reasoning such as the Mini-Mental State Examination (Folstein *et al.* 1975), the Mental Status Questionnaire (Kahn *et al.* 1960), the Kew Cognitive Map (McDonald 1969), and the Abbreviated Mental Test (Qureshi and Hodkinson 1974);
(2) abbreviated neuropsychological batteries designed to target specific cognitive functions known to be affected by dementing disease, such as the Iowa battery (Eslinger 1985) and the Memory Impairment Screen (Buschke *et al.* 1999); and
(3) informant tests designed to estimate the degree of cognitive decline from premorbid levels of functioning, such as the proxy questionnaire from the Blessed Scale (Blessed *et al.* 1968), DECO (Ritchie and Fuhrer 1992, 1996), the IQCODE (Jorm and Korten 1988), and the CAMDEX family interview (Roth *et al.* 1988).

Preference has generally been given to the first type of test, undoubtedly because of its high face validity, although the other two methods have been found to be equally discriminative. While formerly considered an adjunct to the clinical examination, informant report has now been demonstrated by a number of researchers to be as highly discriminant in screening for cognitive disorder as direct examination of the elderly person himself, and less subject to education effects (Jorm and Korten 1988; Ritchie and Fuhrer 1992, 1996). Informant methods also appear to be unaffected by institutionalization (Ritchie and Fuhrer 1992). A combination of informant and cognitive screening tests has been shown to have better discriminability than either method alone (Mackinnon and Mulligan 1998).

Most screening tests show quite high levels of discriminability in case-control studies typically designed with an equal case to non-case ratio—using relatively clear-cut cases of cognitive impairment, and normal subjects free of likely confounding characteristics, respectively. Not surprisingly, the performance of these same tests is seen to drop dramatically when used in the community setting. This is partly due to the fact that prevalence rates of cognitive disorder in the community are much lower than in case-control studies, and the level of cognitive impairment is often much milder, giving rise to poorer positive and negative predictive values. Brayne and Calloway (1991) have demonstrated, for example, that the positive predictive value of the Mini-Mental Status examination falls from 89% when the case:non-case ratio is 1:10, to only 59% when it is 1:50. Similarly, Ritchie and Fuhrer (1996) observed that the discriminability of an informant questionnaire fell from 90% in a case-control study to 79% in a community study. Weinstein and Fineberg (1980) have pointed out that this problem can, to a large extent, be overcome by adjusting the cut-off point of a screening test according to the predicted prevalence of the disease within the target population. For example, a downward adjustment of the cut-off point on an informant questionnaire was found by Ritchie and Fuhrer (1996) to improve discriminability in the community setting by 10%.

Diagnostic instruments

Psychometric tests may also be used to assist the differential diagnosis of disorders responsible for cognitive impairment in the elderly. These tests derive from experimental studies in cognitive psychology applied in clinical practice in the field of neuropsychology. Quantifiable tasks have thus been developed which are capable of isolating the specific cognitive subsystems affected by diseases and clinical syndromes, such as implicit and semantic memory (Huff *et al.* 1986; Ritchie *et al.* 1993*a*; Beardsall and Huppert 1994), perception, localization, and analysis of visual stimuli (Salthouse 1982; Rosen 1983; Ska and Nespoulous 1987), and syntax and phoneme comprehension (Bayles 1982). Despite the proliferation of focalized testing methods in the field of cognitive processing research in normal adults, and their demonstrated utility in differential diagnosis, surprisingly few of these tests are being carried over into everyday clinical practice. A recent survey across developed countries suggests that reliance is still predominantly placed on older tests such as the Wechsler Memory and Intelligence scales (Sullivan and Bowden 1997).

Neuropsychometric tests targeting specific cognitive processes have now been used in the differential diagnosis of senile dementia of the Alzheimer type (Almkvist *et al.* 1993; Kertesz and Clydesdale 1994; Rosser and Hodges 1994), and subtypes of Alzheimer's disease (Mann *et al.* 1992; Richards *et al.* 1993; Stern *et al.* 1993; Lundervold *et al.* 1994), vascular dementia (Almkvist *et al.* 1993; Kertesz and Clydesdale 1994), frontotemporal degeneration and Lewy-body disease (Filley *et al.* 1994; Grossman *et al.* 1998), depression (Masserman *et al.* 1992), Huntington's disease (Masserman *et al.* 1992; Lundervold *et al.* 1994; Rosser and Hodges 1994; Rich *et al.* 1997), progressive supranuclear palsy (Rosser and Hodges 1994), and Parkinson's disease (Stern *et al.* 1993; Lundervold *et al.* 1994; Westwater *et al.* 1997). Cognitive testing has also been used to monitor the effects of adverse environmental exposure in the elderly such as surgery and anaesthesia (Moller *et al.* 1998; Ancelin *et al.* 2000).

The psychometric tests used in the diagnosis of pathologies in elderly subjects have varied widely between studies, thus making comparisons between clinical centres very difficult. In response to this problem, psychometric tests targeting specific cognitive functions have been incorporated into standardized comprehensive diagnostic batteries designed for the differential diagnosis of psychogeriatric illness, such as the CAMCOG which forms part of CAMDEX (Roth *et al.* 1988), the mental status examination of the Canberra Interview for the Elderly (Henderson *et al.* 1994), and the cognitive assessment component of the SIDAM (Zaudig *et al.* 1991). The National Institute on Aging has also established a series of collaborative studies to standardize cognitive measurement in the elderly (Buckholtz and Radebaugh 1994).

Measurement of the consequences of psychiatric disorder

Increasing interest in the impact of psychiatric illness on the quality of life, on caregiving services, and on the caregivers themselves has led to the more recent development of psychometric tests designed to assess the *consequences* of cognitive disorder. In this context, terms such as 'disability' and 'dependency' are often used, but with little precision. The International Classification of Impairments, Disabilities, and Handicaps (ICIDH) provides a useful conceptual framework for considering the consequences of disease by differentiating three levels: impairment (the consequences of disease at the level of body organs and systems); disability (interference with the activities performed by the individual); and handicap (the social consequences of disease). At the impairment level psychometric tests measure changes in cognitive processes (memory, language, attention) as discussed above. However, it is at the level of disability that most work has been done in this area, with numerous scales having been developed to describe the impact of cognitive dysfunction on behaviour and social adaptation. Examples of this type of scale are the Neuropsychiatric Inventory, assessing behavioural and emotional changes in dementia (Cummings *et al.* 1994), the Troublesome Behaviour Scale (Asada *et al.* 1994), and the Refined ADL Assessment Scale (Tappen 1994). Other scales assess deterioration in daily activities corresponding to specific changes in cognitive processing, for example the Functional Assessment Staging Scale (Sclan and Reisberg 1992), the BEHAVE-AD (Harwood *et al.* 1998), and the Cognitive Performance Test (Burns *et al.* 1994). Tests have also been developed to monitor residual functioning in severely impaired subjects based on the Piagetian model such as the M-OSPD (Auer and Reisberg 1996) and the Hierarchic Dementia Scale (Cole and Dastoor 1996).

Computerized cognitive assessment

Although automated cognitive testing has been reported in the literature since the late 1960s, it has only become popular as a routine clinical procedure in the past few years. This is mainly due to three important developments: the ability to simulate complex imagery; the microcomputer; and the touch screen. The most important of these has undoubtedly been the development of the microprocessor, which has not only dramatically decreased the cost of automated testing, but also greatly increased its flexibility such that users can design their own testing programmes with little expense and can transfer results to other software for analysis.

The most obvious advantage of computerized cognitive testing is the possibility of standardizing stimulus presentation; an advantage which has led to the recent computerization of existing manual tests such as the Progressive Matrices and Mill Hill Vocabulary Test (Watts *et al.* 1982). By the end of the 1960s a review of cognitive tests adapted for computer administration had already appeared in the literature (Gedye and Miller 1969). A further advantage of computer administration is the significant reduction in administration time. Computerization also permits the use of extremely complex administration procedures, which may be tailored to suit individual needs. This possibility has led to the development of 'adaptive' or 'tailored' testing, in which the test content is determined for each individual as a function of each response made in the course of the testing period. In this way difficulty levels can be adjusted according to the ability of the subject.

Item selection algorithms generally follow one of three branching models: item to item via predetermined structures; subtest to subtest; or as a function of a complex rule specified by a mathematical testing model. Item to item branching strategies are the simplest form of adaptive testing, having a triangular or pyramidal structure when drawn graphically. Inter-subtest branching strategies are similar, except that each node in the diagram now consists of several items rather than one. This gives fewer nodes, but allows for re-entrant nodes in which only a portion of the items in a subtest need to be administered before branching to another. Model-based branching is based on item response, or latent trait theory, assuming that item responses are probabilistically related by a specified function to a continuous underlying trait or ability. Theoretical models of branching systems and scoring methods for adaptive testing are described in greater detail by Vale (1981) and Dewitt and Weiss (1976). These articles also provide practical guidelines for the construction of branching strategies.

Reliable data recording has been a persistent problem in both research and clinical investigations, as it is at this point that both conscious and unconscious interviewer bias may exert a strong influence. This problem has been repeatedly reported in the literature relating to behavioural evaluation since the 1940s (Guest 1947). Most of us are familiar with this issue and no matter how well interviewers are trained, the investigator can never be sure if the coded response is truly an accurate representation of the subject's behaviour. Computer testing has greatly alleviated this difficulty. Computerized testing provides an interactive environment in which the subject can respond directly to the stimulus via a keyboard or tactile screen, and where the response is registered immediately by the program without the intermediary of an interviewer or response coder. In this way the investigator may incorporate a control system into the program, through which he may check at the end of a session that all items have been presented by the interviewer.

While earlier tests generally only recorded simple information such as 'right' or 'wrong', computer technology has permitted the development of complex automated decision-making. For example, the program may automatically record persistent perseveration between tasks (where subjects continue to attend to stimuli relevant to a previous task), or visual-field neglect (where the subject responds only to items in one part of the screen). Direct interaction between the respondent and the testing apparatus permits the accurate recording of reaction times and response latencies. The latter is of particular interest in follow-up studies, as an increased response time in subsequent administrations of a test is often a more sensitive indicator of early cognitive deficit than is error rate. In this way complex observations may be recorded even where the examination is carried out by lay interviewers. For example, Fagot *et al.* (1993) describe a haptic recognition task in which the computer records the number and duration of hand contacts with each stimulus, and the ECO cognitive battery for the elderly (Ritchie *et al.* 1993*a*) automatically records visual-field neglect and rotation errors in a matching-to-sample task.

In the early years of computerized test development, investigators (and in particular clinicians) expressed doubts as to the feasibility of presenting elderly subjects with computer hardware, and they frequently rejected computerized testing as being detrimental to the clinician–patient relationship. On the other hand, the growing number of reports of the use of computerized testing with the elderly suggest that in practice there is very little difficulty (Morris 1985; Carr *et al.* 1986). In the first place, many elderly persons now own their own microcomputers and many others have had some experience with them. Additionally, elderly people generally find computer-generated tests far more interesting and less threatening than paper and pencil tests administered by an interviewer—the latter situation is often negatively associated with school experiences, and the elderly person often feels he is being judged by the younger interviewer.

For readers interested in the use of computerized cognitive assessment some points are perhaps worth noting. Development of a computerized test or battery of tests first involves the selection of both hardware and software. The options available are presently so numerous that it is impossible to cover them all within the scope of this chapter. An early review of the question is provided by Underwood (1978) and Dewitt and Weiss (1976), who describe software systems for implementing adaptive testing on a generalized timesharing computer and a real-time mini-computer. Researchers are generally guided by practical limitations. In computerized testing for the laboratory research of a specific cognitive function, the user generally seeks out the hardware and software that is best able to demonstrate and manipulate the cognitive function under investigation.

On the other hand, if the tests are designed for multicentre use, then standardization becomes an important consideration. Preference may then be given to widely used systems, such as IBM or MacIntosh which have user-friendly software packages well suited to the development and rapid modification of adaptive cognitive tests. If the test is to be used in general population studies, lightweight portable hardware should be considered. A limitation of this technology has been the poor quality of the screens, which has subsequently limited their use to the scoring of responses. However, with the development of monochrome LCD displays, the quality is now greatly improved. A separate monitor will be required if response latencies are to be recorded, although the manufacturers of MacIntosh and IBM PC are in the process of developing laptop models which may incorporate a touch screen.

If response latencies are to be recorded in different research sites, then care should be exercised to ensure standardization of hardware. The evolution of computer technology has been accompanied by a rapid increase in the speed of microprocessor operation. Variations are therefore likely to exist between computers in the accuracy of reaction time or response latency measures, especially if the program controls timing by 'delay loops', as is the case with older computers such as the Apple II series. Alternatively, timing may be controlled by the software using the computer's time-of-day clock. Even so, with IBM-compatible computers absolute timing can still only reach 0.1 of a second, which, while generally adequate for the estimation of response time in clinical studies, may not be adequate for experimental examination of reaction time. For MacIntosh computers the 'tic' rate permits a timing accuracy of 34 ms using software commands to the system clock. Timing accuracy can be increased for IBM-compatible computers through BIOS modifying software (see Graves and Bradley (1991) for a description of this procedure), and for MacIntosh using special public-domain software, timing routines as described by Westall *et al.* (1986, 1989).

Display clarity depends upon the graphic standard used by the software. The relative advantages of different standards should be taken into consideration when selecting test software. Earlier standards, such as CGA (Color Graphics Adapter), give figures with relatively poor resolution. Therefore, stimuli requiring finer detail or portraying dimensionality are best programmed by more advanced graphics standards, such as EGA (Enhanced Graphics Adapter) or VGA (Visual Graphics Array). On the other hand, with lower resolution, graphics can be drawn more quickly on the screen and the display and response timing of the test is easier to coordinate.

When adapting existing paper and pencil cognitive tests for computer administration, reliability and validity should be established, even where this has previously been done for the manually administered form. Watts *et al.* (1982) have shown, for example, that the computerized version of the Ravens Progressive Matrices gave absolute levels approximately 5 points lower than obtained by the paper and pencil version of the test. Furthermore, normative data collected using one type of visual display unit may not apply if the display type and quality are altered—especially when changing from a cathode ray tube to the liquid crystal displays used in laptop machines. It may also be necessary to test alternative administration methods to reduce error due to the test presentation method. Banderet *et al.* (1988) compared two versions of a computerized addition task with the original paper and pencil version. The first version required subjects to enter answers from a keyboard, and despite pretest typing practice, subjects were 35% slower with the keyboard than with the paper and pencil version. Furthermore, scores obtained from the computer version were less stable over time. An alternative computerized multiple-choice version was found to be not only more stable than either the paper and pencil or original computer task, but also more sensitive to the experimental condition.

Persons wishing to develop their own tests may do so economically by using ready-made software systems for test development. These systems provide the necessary formats and paradigms for the user to construct his own cognitive tests for both research and clinical use. Examples of this type of software are the Psylab system for MacIntosh (which may be obtained from Dr Y. Joanette, Hôpital Côte-des-Neiges, Montréal) and the Micro Experimental Laboratory (MEL) for IBM PC compatibles (Schneider 1988). A specialist program for the construction of language comprehension tests has also been developed by Walczyk (1993).

Finally, while as noted above, subject acceptance is generally not a problem, Kane and Kay (1992) stress that previous experience with computers may constitute an important source of variance in test performance in the elderly, especially when the subject is required to manipulate a number of keys on a keyboard. Variation between subjects is likely to be even greater with cross-cultural data collection and in groups with a wide age range. It is thus important to standardize as far as possible for subject familiarity. This should not be left to the interviewer, who may introduce significant error variance at this point. The test program should incorporate standardized practice trials, to bring all subjects up to an equivalent pretest level of competency in manipulating response devices before commencing the testing procedures.

Table 15.2 provides a list of currently available computerized cognitive tests suitable for use with elderly persons and the hardware required for their administration.

Conclusions

A large number of psychometric tests have been developed for the evaluation of the mental health status of the elderly person. In this chapter we have considered developments specifically in the field of cognitive dysfunction and its behavioural consequences. Computerized testing methods have greatly expanded the functions which may be measured, and have also increased efficiency and reliability. Perhaps the greatest shortcoming

Table 15.2 Computerized cognitive tests suitable for use with elderly populations

Test	Author	Hardware
Abbo Cognitive Performance Test (ACPT)	unpublished*	MacIntosh
Adaptive Rate Continuous Performance Test (ARCPT)	Buschbaum and Sosteck (1980)	Apple II/IBM PC
Automated Portable Test System (APTS)	Bittner *et al.* 1986	IBM compatible
Automated Psychological Screening (B-MAPS)	Acker and Acker (1982)	IBM/MacIntosh
Cambridge Neuropsychological Test (CANTAB)	Sahakian and Owen (1992)	IBM PC
Cambridge Mental Disorders of the Elderly (CAMDEX)	Roth *et al.* (1988)	IBM PC
Computergestützte Neuropsychologische Testanordnung (CNAT)	unpublished**	Atari
Evaluation Cognitive par Ordinateur (ECO)	Ritchie *et al.* (1993*a*)	MacIntosh
Geriatric Mental State (GMS-AGECAT)	Copeland *et al.* (1986)	PDP 11/34
Memory Assessment Clinics Battery (MAC)	Larrabee *et al.* (1991)	AT&T 6300
Psychomotor and Visuospatial Tasks	Hofman *et al.* (2000)	IBM PC
Selective Reminding Tests (SRTs)	Kane and Perrine (1988)	IBM PC
Walter Reed Performance Assessment Battery (WRPAB)	Thorne *et al.* (1985)	IBM PC

*Abbo Enterprises, 7334 Girard Ave, La Jolla CA 92037.
**Reischies and Wilms, Psychiatrische Klinik und Poliklinik der Freie Universität Berlin, 1987.

at the moment is the assumption that information processing in normal elderly persons is the same as that for young adults. Little consideration has been given to the possibility that an upper extension to existing theories of cognitive and emotional development may be required (that is beyond childhood and adolescence to different phases of adult life) if psychometric testing is to be adequately adapted to elderly populations.

References

Acker, W. and Acker, C. (1982). *Bexley Maudsley Automated Psychological Screening and Bexley Maudsley Category Sorting Test: manual*. NFER-Nelson, Windsor.

Ainslie, N. K. and Murden, R. A. (1993). Effect of education on the clock-drawing dementia screen in non-demented elderly persons. *Journal of the American Geriatrics Society*, **41**, 249–52.

Albert, M., Smith, L. A., Scherr, P. A., Taylor, J. O., Evans, D. A., and Funkenstein, H. H. (1991). Use of brief cognitive tests to identify individuals in the community with clinically diagnosed Alzheimer's disease. *International Journal of Neuroscience*, **57**, 167–78.

Almkvist, O., Backman, L., Basun., H., and Wahlund, L. O. (1993). Patterns of neuropsychological performance in Alzheimer's disease and vascular dementia. *Cortex*, **29**, 661–73.

Ancelin, M. L., de Roquefeuil, G., and Ritchie K. (2000). Anesthesia and postoperative cognitive dysfunction in the elderly: a review of clinical and epidemiological observations. *Revue d'Epidémiologie et de Santé Publique* **48**, 459–72.

Asada, T., Yoshioka, M., Morikawa, S., Koyama, H., Kitajima, E., Kawasaki, K., *et al.* (1994). Development of a troublesome behaviour scale (TBS) for elderly patients with dementia. *Japanese Journal of Public Health*, **41**, 518–27.

Auer, S. R. and Reisberg, B. (1996). Reliability of the Modified Ordinal Scales of Psychological Development: a cognitive assessment battery for severe dementia. *International Psychogeriatrics*, **8**, 225–31.

Banderet, L. E., Shukitt, B. L., Walthers, M. A., Kennedy, R. S., Bittner, A. C., and Kay, G. G. (1988). Psychometric properties of three addition tasks with different response requirements. *Proceedings of the 30th Annual Meeting of the Military Testing Association*. Veteran's Administration, Arlington, VA.

Bayles, K. A. (1982). Language function in senile dementia. *Brain and Language*, **16**, 265–80.

Beardsall, L. and Huppert, F. A. (1994). Improvement in NART word reading in demented and normal older persons using the Cambridge Contextual Reading Test. *Journal of Clinical and Experimental Neuropsychology*, **16**, 232–42.

Berkman, L. F. (1986). The association between educational attainment and mental status examinations: of etiologic significance for senile dementias or not? *Journal of Chronic Disease*, **39**, 171–4.

Bittner, A. C., Carter, R. C., Kennedy, R. S., Harbeson, M. M., and Krause, M. (1986). Performance evaluation tests for environmental research (PETER): evaluation of 114 measures. *Perceptual and Motor Skills*, **63**, 683–708.

Blalock, H. M. (1968). The measurement problem. In *Methodology in social research* (ed. H. M. Blalock and A. Blalock), pp. 3–18. McGraw-Hill, New York.

Blalock, H. M. (1970). Estimation measurement error using multiple indicators and several points in time. *American Sociological Review*, **35**, 101–10.

Blessed, G., Tomlinson, B. E., and Roth, M. (1968). The association between quantitative measures of dementia and of senile change in the cerebral gray matter of elderly subjects *British Journal of Psychiatry*, **114**, 797–811.

Brayne, C. and Calloway, P. (1991). The case identification of dementia in the community: a comparison of methods. *International Journal of Geriatric Psychiatry*, **5**, 309–16.

Breteler, M. M. B., van Amerongen, N. M., van Swieten, J. C., Claus, J. J., Grobbee, D. E., van Gijn, J., *et al.* (1994). Cognitive correlates of ventricular enlargement and cerebral white matter lesions on magnetic resonance imaging. *The Rotterdam Study*; *Stroke*, **25**, 1109–15.

Buckholtz, N. S. and Radebaugh, T. S. (1994). National Institute on Aging collaborative studies in the standardization of cognitive measures. *Alzheimer Disease and Associated Disorders*, **8** (Suppl.), 214–16.

Burns, T., Mortimer, J. A., and Merchak, P. (1994). Cognitive Performance Test: a new approach to functional assessment in Alzheimer's disease. *Journal of Geriatric Assessment and Neurology*, **7**, 46–54.

Buschbaum, M. S. and Sostek, A. J. (1980). An adaptive rate continuous performance test: vigilance and reliability for 400 male students. *Perceptual and Motor Skills*, **51**, 707–13.

Buschke, H., Kusianski, G., Katz, M., Stewart, W. F., Sliwinski, M. J., Eckholdt, H. M., *et al.* (1999). Screening for dementia with the memory impairment screen. *Neurology*, **15**, 231–8.

Cabeza, R. and Nyberg, L. (1997). Imaging cognition: an empirical view of PET studies with normal subjects *Journal of Cognitive Neuroscience*, **9**, 1–26.

Capitani, E., Della-Sala, S., Laiacona, M., and Marchetti, C. (1994). Standardization and use of a test of memory of prose. *Bollettino di Psicologia Applicata*, **209**, 47–63.

Carr, A. C., Woods, R. T., and Moore, B. J. (1986). Automated cognitive assessment of elderly patients: a comparison of two types of response device. *British Journal of Clinical Psychology*, **25**, 305–6.

Clarke, M., Jagger, C., Anderson, J., Battcock, T., Kelly, F., and Stern, M. C. (1991). The prevalence of dementia in a total population: a comparison of two screening instruments. *Age and Ageing*, **20**, 396–403.

Coblentz, J. M., Mattis, S., Zingesser, L. H., Kasoff, S. S., Wisniewski, H. M., and Katzman, R. (1973). Presenile dementia: clinical aspects and evaluation of cerebrospinal fluid dynamics. *Archives of Neurology*, **29**, 299–308.

Cole, M. G. and Dastoor, D. P. (1996). The Hierarchic Dementia Scale: conceptualization. *International Psychogeriatrics*, **8**, 205–12.

Copeland, J. R. M., Dewey, M. E., and Griffiths-Jones, H. M. (1986). A computerized diagnostic system and case nomenclature for elderly subjects: GMS and AGECAT. *Psychological Medicine*, **16**, 89–99.

Cummings, J. L., Mega, M., Gray, K., Rosenberg-Thompson, S., Carusi, D. A., and Gornbein, J. (1994). The Neuropsychiatric Inventory: comprehensive assessment of psychopathology in dementia. *Neurology*, **44**, 2308–14.

De Jonghe, J. F., Krijgsveld, S., Staverman, K., Lindeboom, J., and Kat, M. G. (1994). Differentiation between dementia and functional psychiatric disorders in a geriatric ward of a general psychiatric hospital using the Amsterdam dementia screening test. *Nederlands Tijdschrift voor Geneeskunde*, **138**, 1668–73.

Dewitt, L. J. and Weiss, D. J. (1976). Hardware and software evolution of an adaptive ability measurement system. *Behavior Research Methods and Instrumentation*, **8**, 104–7.

Duine, T. J. (1991). Validity of a new psychogeriatric behavior observation scale for application in nursing homes and homes for the aged. *Tijdschrift voor Gerontologie en Geriatrie*, **22**, 228–33.

Eisdorfer, C., Cohen, D., Paveza, G. J., Ashford, J. W., Luchins, D. J., Gorelick, P. B., *et al.* (1992). An empirical evaluation of the Global Deterioration Scale for staging Alzheimer's disease. *American Journal of Psychiatry*, **149**, 190–4.

Eslinger, P. J., Damasio, A. R., Benton, A. L., and Van Allen, M. (1985). Neuropsychologic detection of abnormal mental decline in older persons. *Journal of the American Medical Association*, **253**, 670–4.

Fagot, J., Lacreuse, A., and Vauclair, J. (1993). Haptic discrimination of nonsense shapes: hand exploratory strategies but not accuracy reveal laterality effects. *Brain and Cognition*, **21**, 212–25.

Filley, C. M., Kleinschmidt-DeMasters, B. K., and Gross, K. F. (1994). Non-Alzheimer fronto-temporal degenerative dementia. A neurobehavioural and pathologic study. *Clinical Neuropathology*, **13**, 109–16.

Folstein, M. F., Folstein, S. E., and McHugh, P. R. (1975). 'Mini Mental State' a practical method for grading the cognitive state of patients for the clinician. *Journal of Psychiatric Research*, **12**, 189–98.

Gao, Z. (1991). Assessment of Hasegawa's Dementia Scale for screening and diagnosis of dementia in the elderly. *Chinese Journal of Neurology and Psychiatry*, **24**, 258–261.

Gedye, J. L. and Miller, E. (1969). The automation of psychological assessment. *International Journal of Man–Machine Studies*, **2**, 237–62.

Geiger-Kabisch, C. and Weyerer, S. (1993). The Geriatric Concentration Test. Results of a study of patients over 65 years of age in Mannheim. *Zeitschrift für Gerontologie*, **26**, 81–5.

Gilleard, C. J., Belford, H., Gilleard, E., Whittick, J. E., and Gledhill, K. (1984). Emotional distress among the supporters of the elderly mentally infirm. *British Journal of Psychiatry*, **145**, 172–7.

Gomez de Caso, J. A., Rodriguez-Artalejo, F., Claveria, L. E., and Coria, F. (1994). Value of Hodkinson's test for detecting dementia and mild cognitive impairment in epidemiological surveys. *Neuroepidemiology*, **13**, 64–8.

Gorissen, J. P. (1994). Structure of the Behavior Observation Scale—Geriatrics. *Tijdschrift voor Gerontologie en Geriatrie*, **25**, 58–62.

Grant, I., Heaton, R., McSweeney, A., Adams, K., and Timms, R. (1982). Neuropsychological findings in chronic obstructive pulmonary disease. *Archives of Internal Medicine*, **142**, 1470–6.

Graves, R. E. and Bradley, R. (1991). Millisecond timing on the IBM PC/XT and PS/2: a review of the options and corrections for the Graves and Bradley algorithm. *Behavior Research Methods Instruments and Computers*, **23**, 377–9.

Grigsby, J., Kaye, K., and Robbins, L. J. (1992). Reliabilities, norms and factor structure of the Behavioral Dyscontrol Scale. *Perceptual and Motor Skills*, **74**, 883–92.

Grossman, M., Payer, F., and Onishi, K. (1998). Language comprehension and regional cerebral defects in frontotemporal degeneration and Alzheimer's disease. *Neurology*, **50**, 157–63.

Guest, L. (1947). A study of interviewer competence. *International Journal of Opinion and Attitude Research*, **1**, 17–19.

Hare, M. (1978). Clinical checklist for the diagnosis of dementia. *British Journal of Medicine*, **2**, 266–7.

Harwood, D. G., Ownby, R. L., Barker, W. W., and Duara, R. (1998). The behavioral pathology in Alzheimer's Disease Scale (BEHAVE-AD): factor structure among community-dwelling Alzheimer's disease patients. *International Journal of Geriatric Psychiatry*, **13**, 793–800.

Helmes, E., Merskey, H., Hachinski, V. C., and Wands, K. (1992). An examination of psychometric properties of the extended scale for dementia in three different populations. *Alzheimer Disease and Associated Disorders*, **6**, 236–46.

Henderson, A. S., Jorm, A. F., Mackinnon, A., Christensen, H., Scott, L. R., Korten, A. E., *et al.* (1994). A survey of dementia in the Canberra population: experience with ICD-10 and DSM-III criteria. *Psychological Medicine*, **24**, 473–82.

Hofman, M., Seifritz, E., Krauchi, K., Hock, C., Hampel, H., Neugebauer, A., *et al.* (2000). Alzheimer's disease, depression and normal ageing: merit of simple psychomotor and visuospatial tasks. *International Journal of Geriatric Psychiatry*, **15**, 31–9.

Huff, F. J., Corkin, S., and Growdon, J. H. (1986). Semantic impairment and anomia in Alzheimer's disease. *Brain and Language*, **28**, 235–49.

Israel, L., Waintraub, L., and Fillenbaum, G. G. (1986). Assessing the dementias in clinical practice and population surveys: review of the literature since 1965. In *Senile dementias: early detection* (ed. A. Bes), pp. 117–25. John Libbey Eurotext, Paris.

Jorm, A. F., Scott, R., Cullen, J. S., and Mackinnon, A. J. (1991). Performance of the informant questionnaire on cognitive decline in the elderly (IQCODE) as a screening test for dementia. *Psychological Medicine*, **21**, 785–90.

Jorm, A. F. and Korten, A. (1988). Assessment of cognitive decline in the elderly by informant interview. *British Journal of Psychiatry*, **152**, 209–13.

Kahn, R. L., Godfarb, A. I., and Pellack, M. (1960). Brief objective measures for the determination of mental status in the aged. *British Journal of Psychiatry*, **117**, 326–8.

Kane, R. L. and Kay, G. G. (1992). Computerized assessment in neuropsychology: a review of tests and test batteries. *Neuropsychology Review*, **3**, 1–17.

Kane, R. L. and Perrine, K. R. (1988). Construct validity of a nonverbal analogue to the selective reminding verbal learning test. *Paper presented at the meeting of the International Neuropsychological Society*, New Orleans, LA, INS.

Kertesz, A. and Clydesdale, S. (1994). Neuropsychological deficits in vascular dementia vs Alzheimer's disease. *Archives of Neurology*, **51**, 1226–31.

Kiecolt-Glaser, J. K., Glaser, R., Shuttleworth, E. C., Dyer, C. S., Ogrocki, P., and Speicher, C. E. (1987). Chronic stress and immunity in family care-givers of Alzheimer's disease victims. *Psychosomatic Medicine*, **49**, 523–35.

Kim, Y. S., Nibbelink, D. W., and Overall, J. E. (1993). Factor structure and scoring of the SKT test battery. *Journal of Clinical Psychology*, **49**, 61–71.

Kittner, S. J., White, L. R., Farmer, M. E., Wolz, M., Kaplan, E., and Moes, E. (1986). Methodological issues in screening for dementia: the problem of education adjustment. *Journal of Chronic Disease*, **39**, 163–70.

Kramer, M. (1980). The rising pandemic of mental disorders and associated chronic diseases and disabilities. *Acta Psychiatrica Scandinavica*, **62**, 282–97.

Lanska, D. J., Schmitt, F. A., Stewart, J. M., and Howe, J. N. (1993). Telephone-Assessed Mental State. *Dementia*, **4**, 117–19.

Larrabee, G. J., West, R. L., and Crook, T. H. (1991). The association of memory complaint with computer-simulated everyday memory performance *Journal of Clinical and Experimental Neuropsychology*, **13**, 466–78.

Liu, H. C., Chou, P., Lin, K. N., Wang, S. J., Fuh, J. L., and Lin, H. C. (1994). Assessing cognitive abilities and dementia in a predominantly illiterate population of older individuals in Kinmen. *Psychological Medicine*, **24**, 763–70.

Lundervold, A. J., Karlsen, N. R., and Reinvang, I. (1994). Assessment of sub-cortical dementia in patients with Huntington's disease, Parkinson's disease, multiple sclerosis and AIDS by a neuropsychological screening battery. *Scandinavian Journal of Psychology*, **35**, 48–55.

McDonald, C. (1969). Clinical heterogeneity in senile dementia. *British Journal of Psychiatry*, **115**, 267–71.

Mackinnon, A. and Mulligan, R. (1998). Combining cognitive testing and informant report to increase accuracy in screening for dementia. *American Journal of Psychiatry*, **155**, 529–35.

Mahurin, R. K., DeBettignies, B. H., and Pirozzolo, F. J. (1991). Structured assessment of independent living skills: preliminary report of a performance measure of functional abilities in dementia. *Journal of Gerontology*, **46**, 58–66.

Mann, U. M., Mohr, E., Gearing, M., and Chase, T. N. (1992). Heterogeneity in Alzheimer's disease: progression rate segregated by distinct neuropsychological and cerebral metabolic profiles. *Journal of Neurology, Neurosurgery and Psychiatry*, **55**, 956–9.

Manton, K. G. and Stallard, E. (1988). *Chronic disease modeling: measurement and evaluation of the risks of chronic disease processes*. Charles Griffin, London.

Masserman, P. J., Delis, D. C., Butters, N., Dupont, R. M., and Gillin, J. C. (1992). The subcortical dysfunction hypothesis of memory deficits in depression: neuropsychological validation in a sub-group of patients. *Journal of Clinical and Experimental Neuropsychology*, **14**, 687–706.

Michels, R. and Marzuk, P. M. (1993). Progress in psychiatry. *New England Journal of Medicine*, **329**, 552–60.

Moller, J. Y., Cluitmans, P., and Rasmussen, L. S. (1998). Long-term postoperative cognitive dysfunction in the elderly: ISPOCD1 Study. *Lancet*, **351**, 857–61.

Morinigo, A., Zaudig, M., Mittelhammer, J., and Hiller, W. (1990). Description y validez ' Test-Retest ' de le ENEDAM. *Actas Luso Espanolas de Neurologia Psiquitria y Ciencias Afines*, **18**, 396–402.

Morris, R. G. (1985). Automated clinical assessment. In *New directions in clinical psychology* (ed. F. Watts), pp. 121–38. Wiley, Chichester.

Nelson, H. E. (1982). *National Adult Reading Test*. NFER-Nelson, London.

Neri, M., Roth, M., Mountjoy, C. Q., and Andermacher, E. (1994). Validation of the full and short forms of the CAMDEX interview for diagnosing dementia. *Dementia*, **5**, 257–65.

Nishimura, T., Kobayashi, T., Hariguri, S., Takeda, M., Fukunaga, T., Inoue, O., *et al.* (1993). Scales for mental state and daily living activities for the elderly: clinical behavioral scales for assessing demented patients. *International Psychogeriatrics*, **5**, 117–34.

Nyberg, L. (1998). Mapping episodic memory. *Behavioral Brain Research*, **90**, 107–14.

Panisset, M., Roudier, M., Saxton, J., and Boller, F. (1992). A battery of neuropsychological tests for severe dementia; an evaluation study. *Presse Médicale*, **21**, 1271–4.

Pek, G. and Fulop, T. (1992). The Hungarian version of the Nuremberg Geronto-psychological inventory. *Orvosi Hetilap*, **132**, 2319–22.

Ponds, R. W., Verhey, F. R., Rozendaal, N., Jolles, J., and Deelman, B. G. (1992). Screening for dementia: validity of the cognitive screening test and the Mini-Mental State Examination. *Tijdschrift voor Gerontologie en Geriatrie*, **23**, 94–9.

Qureshi, K. N. and Hodkinson, H. M. (1974). Evaluation of a ten-question mental test in the institutionalized elderly. *Age and Ageing*, **3**, 152–7.

Reid, D. W., Tierney, M. C., Zorzitto, M. L., Snow, W. G., and Fisher, R. H. (1991). On the clinical value of the

London Psychogeriatric rating Scale. *Journal of the American Geriatrics Society*, **39**, 368–71.

Rich, J. B., Campodonico, J. R., Rothlind, J., Bylsma, F. W., and Brandt, J. (1997). Perseverations during paired-associate learning in Huntington's disease. *Journal of Clinical Experimental Neuropsychology*, **19**, 191–203.

Richards, M., Bell, K., Dooneief, G., Marder, K., Sano, M., Mayeux, R., *et al.* (1993). Patterns of neuropsychological performance in Alzheimer's disease patients with and without extrapyramidal signs. *Neurology*, **43**, 1708–11.

Ritchie, K. (1988). The screening of cognitive impairment in the elderly: a critical review of current methods. *Journal of Clinical Epidemiology*, **41**, 635–43.

Ritchie, K. and Fuhrer, R. (1992). A comparative study of the performance of screening tests for senile dementia using receiver operating characteristics analysis. *Journal of Clinical Epidemiology*, **45**, 627–37.

Ritchie, K. and Fuhrer, R. (1996). The validation of an informant screening test for irreversible cognitive decline in the elderly: performance characteristics within a general population sample. *International Journal of Geriatric Psychiatry*, **11**, 149–56.

Ritchie, K. and Ledésert, B. (1991). The measurement of incapacity in the severely demented elderly: the validation of a behavioural assessment scale. *International Journal of Geriatric Psychiatry*, **6**, 217–26.

Ritchie, K., Allard, M., Huppert, F. A., Nargeot, C., Pinek, B., and Ledésert, B. (1993*a*). Computerized cognitive examination of the elderly (ECO): the development of a neuropsychological examination for clinic and population use. *International Journal of Geriatric Psychiatry*, **8**, 700.

Ritchie, K., Jagger, C., Brayne, C., and Letenneur, L. (1993*b*). Dementia-free life expectancy: preliminary calculations for France and the United Kingdom. In *Calculation of health expectancies* (ed. J. M. Robine, C. D. Mathers, M. R. Bone, and I. Romieu), pp. 233–40. John Libbey Eurotext, Paris.

Ritchie, K., Mathers, C., and Jorm, A. F. (1994*a*). Dementia-free life expectancy in Australia. *Australian Journal of Public Health*, **18**, 149–52.

Ritchie, K., Robine, J. M., Letenneur, L., and Dartigues, J. F. (1994*b*). Dementia-free life expectancy in France. *American Journal of Public Health*, **84**, 232–6.

Rocca, W. A., Bonaiuto, S., Lippi, A., Luciani, P., Pistarelli, T., Grandinetti, A., *et al.* (1992). Validation of the Hodkinson abbreviated mental test as a screening instrument for dementia in an Italian population. *Neuroepidemiology*, **11**, 288–95.

Ronnberg, L. and Ericsson, K. (1994). Reliability and validity of the Hierarchic Dementia Scale. *International Psychogeriatrics*, **6**, 87–94.

Rosen, W. G. (1983). Neuropsychological investigation of memory, visuoconstructional, visuoperceptual and language abilities in senile dementia of the Alzheimer type. In *The dementias* (ed. R. Mayeux and W. G. Rosen), pp. 51–63. Raven Press, New York.

Rosen, W. G., Mohs, R. C., and Davis K. L. (1984). A new rating scale for Alzheimer's disease. *American Journal of Psychiatry*, **4**, 1356–64.

Rosser, A. E. and Hodges, J. R. (1994). The Dementia Rating Scale in Alzheimer's disease, Huntington's disease and progressive supranuclear palsy. *Journal of Neurology*, **241**, 531–6.

Roth, M., Huppert, F. A., Tym, E., and Mountjoy, C. Q. (1988). *CAMDEX: The Cambridge Examination for Mental Disorders of the Elderly.* Cambridge University Press, Cambridge.

Royall, D. R., Mahurin, R. K., Cornell, J., and Gray, K. F. (1993). Bedside assessment of dementia type using the qualitative evaluation of dementia. *Neuropsychiatry, Neuropsychology and Behavioral Neurology*, **6**, 235–44.

Sahakian, B. J. and Owen, A. M. (1992). Computerized assessment in neuropsychiatry using CANTAB: discussion paper. *Journal of the Royal Society of Medicine*, **85**, 399–402.

Salthouse, T. A. (1982). *Adult cognition: an experimental psychology of human aging.* Springer-Verlag, New York.

Schaie, K. W. (1983). The Seattle Longitudinal Study: a twenty-one year exploration of psychometric intelligence in adulthood. In *Longitudinal studies of adult psychological development* (ed. K. W. Schaie), pp. 64–135. Guilford Press, New York.

Schneider, W. (1988). Micro experimental laboratory: an integrated system for IBM PC computers. *Behavior Research Methods Instruments and Computers*, **20**, 206–17.

Sclan, S. G. and Reisberg, B. (1992). Functional assessment staging in Alzheimer's disease: reliability, validity, and ordinality. *International Psychogeriatrics*, **4**(Suppl. 1), 55–69.

Signoret, J. L. (1982). *Batterie d'Estimation de la Démence.* Service de Neurologie, Hôpital de la Salpêtrière, Paris, Unpublished Manuscript.

Sinha, D., Zemlan, F. P., Nelson, S., Bienenfeld, D., Thienhaus, O., Ramaswamy, G., *et al.* (1992). A new scale for assessing behavioral agitation in dementia. *Psychiatry Research*, **41**, 73–8.

Ska, B. and Nespoulous, J. L. (1987). Pantomimes and aging. *Journal of Clinical Experimental Neuropsychology*, **9**, 754–66.

Skoog, I., Berg, S., Johansson, B., Palmertz, B., and Andreasson, L. A. (1996). The influence of white matter lesions on neuropsychological functioning in demented and non-demented 85-year olds. *Acta Neurologica Scandinavica*, **93**, 142–8.

Stern, Y., Richards, M., Sano, M., and Mayeux, R. (1993). Comparison of cognitive changes in patients with Alzheimer's and Parkinson's disease. *Archives of Neurology*, **50**, 1040–5.

Still, C., Goldsmith, T., and Mallin, R. (1983). Mini-object test: a new brief clinical assessment for aphasia-apraxia-agnosia. *Southern Medical Journal*, **76**, 52–4.

Sullivan, K. and Bowden, S. (1997). Which tests do neuropsychologists use? *Journal of Clinical Psychology*, **53**, 657–61.

Tappen, R. M. (1994). Development of the refined ADL Assessment Scale for patients with Alzheimer's and related disorders. *Journal of Gerontological Nursing*, **20**, 36–42.

Teresi, J. A. and Golden, R. R. (1994). Latent structure methods for estimating bias, item validity and prevalence using cognitive and other geriatric screening measures. *Alzheimer Disease and Associated Disorders*, **8**(Suppl.), S291–8.

Thorne, D., Genser, S., Sing, H., and Hegge, F. (1985). The Walter Reed Performance Assessment Battery. *Neurobehavioral Toxicology and Teratology*, **7**, 415–18.

Tomlins, T. E. (1822). *Statutes of the Realm*. Eyre and Strahan, London.

Tremmel, L. and Spiegel, R. (1993). Clinical experience with the NOSGER: tentative normative data and sensitivity to change. *International Journal of Geriatric Psychiatry*, **8**, 311–17.

Underwood, M. A. (1978). Computerized adaptive testing and personnel accessioning system design. In *Computerized Adaptive Testing Conference, Minneapolis, University of Minnesota, Department of Psychology, Psychometric Methods Program* (ed. D. J. Weiss). University of Minnesota, Minneapolis.

Vale, CD. (1981). Design and implementation of a microcomputer-based adaptive testing system. *Behaviour Research and Instrumentation*, **13**, 399–406.

Veroff, A. E., Cutler, N. R., Sramek, J. J., Prior, P. L., Mickelson, W., and Hartman, J. K. (1991). A new assessment tool for neuropsychopharmacologic research: the computerized Neuropsychological Test Battery. *Journal of Geriatric Psychiatry and Neurology*, **4**, 211–17.

Walczyk, J. (1993). A computer program for constructing language comprehension tests. *Computers in Human Behavior*, **9**, 113–16.

Ward, H. W., Ramsdell, J. W., Jackson, J. E., Renvall, M., Swart, J. A., and Rockwell, E. (1990). Cognitive function testing in comprehensive geriatric assessment: a comparison of cognitive test performance in residential and clinical settings. *Journal of the American Geriatrics Society*, **38**, 1088–92.

Ward, T., Dawe, B., Procter, A., Murphy, E., and Weinman, J. (1993). Assessment in severe dementia: the Guy's Advanced Dementia Schedule. *Age and Ageing*, **22**, 183–9.

Watts, K., Baddeley, A. D., and Williams, M. (1982). Automated tailored testing using Raven's Matrices and Mill Hill Vocabulary Tests: a comparison with manual administration. *International Journal of Man-Machine Studies*, **17**, 331–44.

Weinstein, M. C. and Fineberg, H. V. (1980). *Clinical decision analysis*. W. B. Saunders, Philadelphia.

Wells, Y. and Jorm, A. F. (1987). Evaluation of a special nursing home unit for dementia sufferers: a randomized controlled comparison with community care. *Australian and New Zealand Journal of Psychiatry*, **21**, 524–31.

Welsh, K. A., Butters, N., Mohs, R. C., Beekly, D., Edland, S., Fillenbaum, G., *et al.* (1994). The Consortium to Establish a Registry for Alzheimer's Disease (CERAD). Part V. A normative study of the neuropsychological battery. *Neurology*, **44**, 609–14.

Westall, R., Perkey, M. N., and Chute, D. L. (1986). Accurate millisecond timing on Apple's MacIntosh using Drexel's millitimer. *Behavior Research Methods Instruments and Computers*, **18**, 307–11.

Westall, R., Perkey, M. N., and Chute, D. L. (1989). Millisecond timing on the Apple MacIntosh: updating Drexel's millitimer. *Behavior Research Methods Instruments and Computers*, **21**, 540–7.

Westwater, H., McDowall, J., Siegert, R., Mossman, S., and Abenethy, D. (1997). Implicit learning in Parkinson's disease: evidence from a verbal version of the serial reaction time task. *Journal of Clinical Experimental Neuropsychology*, **20**, 413–18.

Zaudig, M. (1992). A new systematic method of measurement and diagnosis of 'mild cognitive impairment' and dementia according to ICD-10 and DSM-III-R criteria. *International Psychogeriatrics*, **4**(Suppl. 2), 203–19.

Zaudig, M., Mittelhammer, J., Hiller, W., Pauls, A., Thora, C., Morinigo, A., *et al.* (1991). SIDAM: a structured interview for the diagnosis of dementia of the Alzheimer type, multi-infarct dementia and dementias of other aetiology according to ICD-10 and DSM III-R. *Psychological Medicine*, **21**, 225–36.

16 Dynamic psychotherapy with older persons

Mark Ardern

Introduction

A recent survey of 100 psychotherapy departments in the UK has indicated that older people still appear to be being short-changed (Murphy 2000). The belief persists that this age group are either not worthy of, or do not benefit from, dynamic psychotherapy. We can speculate on the reasons for this: older people may be seen as too psychologically rigid to waste valuable NHS time. At the same time, psychotherapy has, in an increasingly evidence-based world, had to justify its place as an effective and worthwhile treatment (Corvin and Fitzgerald 2000; Margison *et al.* 2000). It is not surprising then that dynamic psychotherapy with older persons is a relatively novel option, at least in this country.

Nevertheless a healthy interest is growing in the idea that this form of treatment may provide an alternative, or additional help, for some older people who are in difficulty (see, for example, Nemiroff and Colarusso 1985; Martindale 1995; Wheelock 1997).

There are some general principles that writers in the field have emphasized. First, dynamic psychotherapy is likely to require modification in this age group (Porter 1997). It is possible to combine therapy with other forms of management, such as social manipulation or medication (Gabbard 2000). Time constraints are not necessarily a drawback and may actually aid in the motivation for psychological work (Hildebrand 1986). Finally, a new, more informed and assertive, generation of old people are likely to request psychotherapy by way of 'consumer choice'. Sadly, as with family therapy and schizophrenia (Lam 1991), not all treatments of proven value are wholeheartedly embraced by services.

This chapter concentrates on the practice of dynamic psychotherapy with patients who might be referred to old age psychiatrists. More intensive and detailed accounts of psychoanalysis with the elderly have been published elsewhere (for example, Sandler 1978; Hubback 1996; Wharton; 1996).

The emotional challenges of later life

Before considering the pathological derailments that can occur in later life, it is appropriate to dwell on normal adaptations. A parallel would be that we cannot make sense of abnormal grief reactions until we are familiar with the healthy manifestations of mourning.

Despite debate as to when it begins, old age is a fact. The state of 'being old' is less obvious. Some people are viewed as old well before their time. Others appear to remain young in spirit until a ripe old age. Although genetic factors and the inexorable biology of ageing will influence agedness, the experience of 'feeling old' remains an individual one (Thompson 1993). Even when we are truly old we tend to view old age as 'someplace else' (Wheelock 1997). To grow old gracefully implies a pleasing harmony between subjective experience and chronological age. Western culture, where youth is idealized and old age denigrated, does little to foster this harmony. Older people's views of themselves will be distorted by what they perceive around them in the media and society (Midwinter 1991). So we can end up feeling and behaving as is expected of us, a process that has been described as 'malignant mirroring' (Zinkin 1983; Evans 1998). Given the power of these influences, elderly people's fears of being a burden or nuisance are not therefore necessarily signs of personal neurosis, but are perhaps evidence of a collective neurosis.

That said, a successful adaptation to ageing is principally centred on personality make up. Personality derives from genes and early life experiences; they are the bricks which supply the architecture of character. As there are no imminent prospects of replacing these bricks, we are left only with the possibility of their rearrangement. Dynamic psychotherapy is aimed at helping elderly people do some of this rearranging themselves.

We know that deficient parenting or some other early trauma will sensitize the individual to reacting in particular ways to later stressors. This is the justification for considering infant observation to be an essential component of an analytical training. From a dynamic viewpoint, psychiatric breakdown in later life can be traced back to the source of these vulnerabilities. This form of psychotherapy makes the connection between today's distress and yesterday's experience. In short, it tries to uncover meaning. Using Winnicott's terminology, a 'good enough' early life will provide the foundations for a robust personality structure better equipped to face the phase of life we call 'old age'.

What should we expect from old age?

Unlike in young adulthood, where opportunities and hopes seem limitless, middle age brings with it the realization that our time is finite (Jaques 1965). Ambitions have to be modified and some relinquished altogether. The events that happen to force this reappraisal have been extensively described (see, for example, King 1980; Gutmann 1987). To summarize, as old age approaches we are confronted with losses, some concrete and others more conceptual. Even if we are fortunate enough to encounter few of these, the *threats* of losing what we already have are real enough. Friends die, and others are forced to move home. A daunting prospect is that of retirement, which usually heralds a downturn of income, status, and worth. Ill health and social isolation further threaten to undermine our autonomy.

It is normal therefore to view old age with some apprehension. Losses as they occur will be accompanied by emotional pain. Mourning involves a painful transition, in which we let go of that we have loved. If negotiated successfully, mourning has its rewards. It gives courage in facing future uncertainties, and opens up the possibility of new attachments.

Fundamentally dynamic psychotherapy helps patients move through their difficulties in giving up old hopes and wishes. It also enables energy to be released from regrets towards a new found creativity (Limentani 1995). As Jung pointed out: 'we cannot live the afternoon of life according to the programme of life's morning' (Jung 1931; and quoted by Porter 1997). An ideal old age is an unattainable goal, and yet we can hold on to a notion that old age is a disease which might be curable. A few years ago we heard of the elderly French lady who lived to the fantastic age of 122 (Ritchie 1997). Reports of longevity make vivid reading; but they also carry the fear that such states of old age are in themselves desirable.

Gender, partners, and society

There has been some suggestion that men have more problems in adjusting to ageing than women. Studies of bereavement in later life have shown that the death of a wife has a more serious impact on the physical and mental well-being of the partner than the death of a husband (Parkes 1992). Generally speaking, men and women tend to become more androgynous with age (Martin 1992). Some of this is due to endocrine changes, but social factors are important. Women normally expect to outlive their husbands, and in the contemporary elderly British couple the woman assumes a more dominant role. A husband may have to learn how to adapt to domesticity for the first time. With retirement, and adult children having left home, partners will find themselves spending more time with each other (Brok 1992). Sexual relationships can become strained. For example, a decline in sexual potency, or a fear of this, may undermine the man's sense of identity. The woman may be inhibited from voicing her sexual needs, a matter made worse by societal myths surrounding an asexual old age. In extreme old age, men will increasingly find themselves living in a world of women and, by contrast, less at ease with sharing confidences. For some men this will increase their experience of isolation, perhaps especially for those who end up in institutional care.

The practitioner of dynamic psychotherapy will require not just a knowledge of his individual patient's life history, personality, and defence mechanisms. He will have to acknowledge a range of biological and sociocultural matters of relevance to old people and the real world in which they live.

Old age that goes wrong

For a minority of people old age is approached not with trepidation but with dread. The old lady who barricades her home (and by inference her mind) to unwelcome intruders; the sociable entertainer who once charmed his audience, now finds that frailty and incontinence are met with disgust. With advancing years flirtatiousness can easily be interpreted as lechery. As a consequence we may witness a rigid reinforcing of defence mechanisms, or, eventually, their manifest fracturing.

It is not possible to describe all the means by which old people succumb psychologically to the vicissitudes of late life. The final common pathway is often clinical depression. But the routes to psychiatric illness, or at least the psychodynamic ones, can be considered by attention to latent flaws in personality structure. Buildings that collapse do not do so just because of earthquakes or hurricanes. Their downfall is usually ascribed to vulnerabilities in design or construction. The most durable structures are designed to move in the face of adversity. When psychic upheavals happen, so it is with people.

Narcissism

The term 'narcissism', like depression, is a perplexing one since it is rooted in different theoretical concepts (see, for example, Sandler *et al.* 1991). Often in psychiatry the word carries pejorative overtones of a childish self-centredness. And yet a healthy narcissism, roughly synonymous with pride, exists in all of us. It enables us to preserve our self-esteem and identity. With narcissism the healthy adult values and even loves himself a little. By contrast, those lacking narcissism have no self-worth and do not care for themselves.

Some psychoanalysts refer to 'narcissistic injuries' (Kohut 1971). By this is meant the result of external assaults on the ego. If narcissism is used excessively as a defence then the inevitable attacks, which come about in old age, cause profound psychic damage.

Case 1

Dr A. was a competent and conscientious general practitioner whose self-esteem was closely invested in his success in his work. Academic prowess had been a goal which served to appease his father's disdain. At 65 he was reluctantly forced to retire early following a serious heart attack. He had never anticipated giving up work, since unconsciously his self-worth had been entirely based on his role as a doctor. Dr A. craved, and until now had received, admiration from his patients. Shortly after he gave up work he became severely depressed. Now that the source of his nourishment had dried up, life lost its purpose.

A more overt demonstration of narcissistic hunger was articulated by an elderly man who had been fussed over as a child. In a long-term group the patient complained that, although he enjoyed receiving Christmas cards, the effort of sending them was too much trouble. His arresting comment to the group leaders, 'We just want to be loved without having to love back', encapsulated his life's experience (previously quoted by Martindale 1995 and Ardern 1999).

Obsessionality

As with narcissism, obsessional traits can be assets. An internalized sense of right and wrong and a degree of order enables us to live in society. Without a super-ego we have no capacity to experience guilt or shame. People who are excessively obsessional are, however, prone to problems if the harsh demands they set themselves begin to fuel guilty preoccupations about potential failure. The workaholic is driven to manic activity, redoubling efforts to succeed in his career. (Dr A. above was not only a casualty of his narcissism but also of his obsessionality.) Furthermore, the obsessional character is inherently inflexible in the face of adversity, and this rigidity, once a benefit, now becomes a hindrance to change.

Obsessional people can find psychotherapy problematic since they easily feel humiliated. They may consciously enter therapy in a dutiful manner, but find themselves undermining the therapist's expertise with rational and intellectual challenges. In this way the unconscious defences strive to keep emotions out of the treatment. Emotions, with their unpredictable nature, are alien to obsessional people. Dynamic psychotherapy will involve these patients' struggle with mastery. In time it may be possible for the patient to modify his aspirations and come to realize that real strength involves some plasticity.

The dependent personality

All of us need people. But for some individuals this need dominates their way of life. People with dependent personalities find the experience of being alone intolerable. They do not feel whole in the absence of 'the other'.

Old age is a time of loss and renegotiation of relationships. This can bring about jealousies and escalating demands for attention. Demands are often perceived by the recipient as overwhelming. As quickly as the dependent person moves towards the object of his desire, the faster the object retreats. The gulf is filled with something else; often alcohol, pleas for more medication, or an excessive interest in doctors.

Dependent people have usually experienced childhood insecurities in attachment and spend their lives searching for substitutes. Sometimes these substitutes, in the form of health professionals, are at first only too happy to oblige. In time, though, a dawning realization may occur that relief of the patient's distress is only temporary.

The dependent personality may give the appearance of a stoical (pseudo) independence; a condition which the author has termed 'counterdependence' (Ardern 1997). This is a reaction formation, due to faulty ' basic trust'. For people with this variant of the dependent personality, who hover in a no-man's land between being smothered or abandoned, intimacy is shunned. The void may not be apparent to the outsider since such people have become expert at accumulating a wide circle of acquaintances. The caring professions are attractive careers to 'counterdependent' people because their own unconscious needs for attachment become projected into even more needy patients. Retirement is a watershed, and the dependence associated with old age rekindles anxiety. A lifetime's phobic avoidance of dependence now has to be faced.

Frustrating as it is for the scientist in us, human beings do not lend themselves to be classified so neatly. Terms such as 'narcissism' and 'counterdependence' will be regarded by some theorists as representing the same fundamental pathology. The dynamic psychotherapist helps to formulate the dominant characteristics (and their origins) which block the road to a happier old age.

Death

Young people seem not to consider death as a possibility, readily taking dangerous risks even in play. It is important to remember that death's almost exclusive relegation to old age is quite new in our history. The young may, in today's society, have even more reason to consider themselves immortal. The older person's view of death is likely to be governed by previous experience, particularly in relation to the age and mode of parental death (Martindale 1998). For some, death hangs overhead like a persecuting cloud; for others it offers a sanctuary from worries. Death may signify an abandonment for individuals with poorly formed 'internal objects'. The approach of death and attacks on the Self by pain or disfigurement are frequently voiced concerns of older people. Few people want to die alone or in a humiliated state of disintegration; most want to be confident of remaining alive in other's minds once gone.

The unique meaning of death to the individual older person will determine its importance (or not) in dynamic psychotherapy.

Transference and countertransference

Central to all dynamic psychotherapies are the phenomena of transference and countertransference. As has been said, 'countertransference is dangerous only when it is forgotten about' (Menninger, quoted by Newton and Jacobowitz 1999). Since both span the generations, even a young therapist can be perceived by his patient as a parental figure. It is difficult when a patient old enough to be our parent behaves more like our child; this provokes confusing feelings in the therapist. The therapist is tempted into instructing the patient, but this protective urge is often mixed with contempt, typified by unwelcome thoughts in the therapist that the patient should 'act her age' (Ardern 1999, p. 265).

The older patient is likely to be envious of his younger therapist, but defends himself from conscious awareness of this feeling by a more acceptable idealization of his therapist. This may initially gratify the therapist's own narcissistic concerns about his therapeutic skills, and the younger the therapist the more likely these anxieties are to be troubling.

As the relationship deepens the therapist should anticipate the emergence of the transference of the patient's negative feelings (Nemiroff and Colarusso 1985). One of the pervading concerns, which does not sit comfortably in the minds of young therapists, is the patient's unconscious preoccupation with impending dependence. The dependability of the therapist is therefore especially crucial for the elderly (Martindale 1989). Absences, and the eventual termination of therapy, provide a useful symbolic focus for work with this phenomenon. Abrupt endings, initiated by an inexperienced therapist, often reflect anxieties in the therapist about dealing with this topic.

Since brain disease is most prevalent in the elderly, therapists may mistakenly attribute psychological symptoms to organic deterioration, rather than psychic conflict (Settlage 1996). A therapist feeling 'stuck' may experience his 'discovery' of organic illness as reconfirmation of his diagnostic prowess. This zeal is an understandable reaction in a therapist keen to be reassured on his competence, and wishing to fend off thoughts of his own therapeutic impotence.

Apart from these general themes which occur in the therapeutic relationship, particular ones will emerge that more specifically belong to the individual patient or individual therapist.

For example, where the patient has a sensitivity about being judged harshly, even the most tentative interpretation from the therapist may be received by the patient, and felt by the therapist, as persecutory. Where a patient reminds the therapist of one of his own parents, with whom he still has unresolved Oedipal issues, his reaction to the patient will be problematic (Rechtshaffen 1959).

Finally, we see in our older patients that which may come our way in time. A relatively objective view of old age may become obscured in old age psychiatry by an impression of old age as inevitably associated with degeneration and illness. Prejudices such as these may reinforce pessimism that dynamic psychotherapy offers little.

Therapeutic alternatives

In contrast to Freud's (over quoted) dictat about mental life ceasing in middle age (Freud 1905), most contemporary writers emphasize that psychological development continues throughout life (Erikson 1966; Porter 1997), and that the unconscious remains 'timelessly intact' (Crusey 1985). The therapeutic process is therefore the same in the elderly as in the younger patient (Settlage 1996).

Dynamic psychotherapy with older people can likewise be brief or long term, insight-orientated or supportive. Patients can be seen either individually or in groups. In addition, these approaches are now being supplemented with creative therapies, such as art and music therapy.

Brief therapy

A patient's motivation to seek help may be enhanced in a crisis. Powerful precipitants to psychological disturbance such as physical illness, as with Dr A. (Case 1, above), bring to the fore unconscious frailties. A person's defensive structures which are adaptive at age 30 may be ineffective at age 65 (Wheelock 1997). As this developmental adaptation breaks down, a therapeutic opportunity arises.

Brief therapy seizes upon the crisis and aims to get the patient 'back on the road' somewhat wiser (Quick 1996). Although not specifically researched in the elderly, various brief therapies have been described with younger adults (for example, Bauer and Kobos 1987; Sifneos 1987).

Case 2

Mrs B. was the unloved sibling of a sister who died in childhood. Mrs B. later married a man who was abusive to her. Subsequently, their own daughter committed suicide, and a year before being referred to the old age psychiatry service, Mrs B.'s husband died. Mrs B. started to binge-drink alcohol, partially aware that this was an attempt to blot out her grief for her dead husband. This awareness did not prevent a series of 'revolving-door' admissions for detoxification. The focus of brief therapy was to explore the meaning of her drinking, not only in relation to her husband, but in her more unconscious belief that she was *responsible* for her sister's death and her daughter's suicide; all of which were reinforced by malicious comments from other family members. This matter of responsibility had led to Mrs B. feeling she was a person inherently dangerous to others. The drinking was not just an anaesthetic but self-destructive. It became clearer that her reasons for pushing away medical and social help were because she felt she *deserved* to be dead herself.

In this example, though the crises were managed in a conventional way, the immediate aftermath offered a 'window of opportunity' to foster the patient's insight into the reasons for her self-destructiveness. The patient was helped to make a connection between her compulsive drinking and the dangerousness she was attempting to erase.

Long-term psychotherapy

Case 3

A 65-year-old talented cartoonist, Mr C. was referred by his GP who was worried about the patient's disclosure of vague longstanding suicidal feelings. Mr C.'s wife had died several years ago from a wasting disease. Mr C. had taken antidepressants, but complained they only made him 'artificially brighter' with no effect on more deep-seated despair.

Mr C. was referred for long-term psychotherapy. He described how his parents were 'remote' and admitted that he was in the habit of avoiding too much display of feelings.

As expected, Mr C. punctually attended his appointments with the therapist. He tended to agree with whatever the therapist said and for months never showed irritation. In spite of gentle encouragement, he made excuses as to why his artwork could not be brought in to the sessions.

The therapist liked the patient, but in supervision she discussed her increasing frustration about wanting to shake the patient out of his deadness. A breakthrough came when Mr C. reported an outburst of fury towards his female partner. The partner had switched off the radio when Mr C. was engrossed in listening to his favourite composer. The therapist found herself identifying with this 'switching off' by the patient's partner. The therapist ventured an interpretation about Mr C.'s rage towards others (parents, dead wife, and the therapist herself) and how eagerness to please concealed his shame about 'causing so much trouble'.

Here the focus of therapy was more intangible. The first task was to engage Mr C. in a meaningful relationship with the therapist. A major obstacle to this was the patient's core dilemma of both fearing abandonment and of wanting to preserve his remoteness. In supervision, the therapist's exasperated countertransference reaction to the patient's overcompliance was examined. The 'switching off' incident allowed feelings to be brought into the room. Following the therapist's interpretation, the patient began to trust the therapist enough to bring his artwork without fear of criticism. The therapist's holiday break stimulated the patient's jealousy, which he now voiced openly. Over time the patient found it possible to express a range of feelings towards the therapist. In parallel his creativity improved. Despite continued anxieties about ending up like his wife in a disintegrated state, Mr C. had become emotionally alive. It became possible for him to face old age and its uncertainties.

Supportive psychotherapy

Dynamic psychotherapy in the setting of the old age psychiatry department is most likely to take the supportive form. A review of supportive psychotherapy is provided by Holmes (1995). A basic premise is that the patient's resources are insufficient to allow personality change. The prospect of insight is limited. One aim of supportive psychotherapy is to locate breaches in the patient's defensive structure. These are then bolstered by the therapist's active encouragement.

A difference between simple counselling and this form of supportive psychotherapy is that with the latter the therapist constructs a psychodynamic formulation. Partly this helps the therapist to avoid stepping on 'land mines', which might alienate the patient, or, worse still, precipitate psychiatric illness. The therapist observes the transference and countertransference, but by and large keeps these ideas to himself. Although some writers advocate the use of interpretation, it has to be assumed that major factors in the success of supportive psychotherapy are the therapist's reliability and empathy. Patients may not need to be seen frequently but, in order to allow their internalization of a good object, they will have to be sure that the therapist is psychically available.

For some patients the therapist may conclude that weaning away is not possible. In these cases the patient's dependence is actively cultivated. The notion of encouraging dependence can seem alien in a society that increasingly talks of 'empowerment' (Bell 1996). The boundaries of supportive psychotherapy overlap with other psychological therapies which incorporate modelling and reinforcement.

Case 4

Mr D., an 80-year-old man, has been seen in the psychiatric outpatient clinic for 30 min every 2 months for 10 years by the same doctor. He is on lithium therapy for previous manic and depressive episodes following a myocardial infarct. The doctor has decided that Mr D. will need to be seen indefinitely. The patient goes from doctor to doctor for various bodily symptoms, part of a lifelong hypochondriacal concern. Although married to a woman young enough to be his daughter, he has become infatuated with an even younger woman living abroad. This infatuation has the quality of an adolescent 'crush' that threatens to destabilize his mental health. The doctor is aware that Mr D.'s relationships arise from a narcissistic vulnerability, also demonstrated by the patient's attempted invasion into the doctor's personal life. Mr D. insists on calling the doctor by his Christian name, asking about his hobbies and holidays, and, being a 'special case', relishing the attention of the occasional medical student.

The doctor deals with the immediate threat of an unrequited affair by forcefully discouraging the patient's unrealistic aspirations.

By combining limit-setting (for example, maintaining the 2-month boundary) with some personal disclosures from the doctor, a compromise is achieved. This partially gratifies the patient's needs. In parallel, the young woman with whom Mr D. is infatuated agrees to offer companionship. Her evident relief is stated over the telephone to the patient: 'Please give your doctor my good wishes'.

Although Mr D. remains fragile, he has recently survived a coronary artery by-pass graft without psychiatric breakdown.

Group therapy

Dynamic group psychotherapy is an alternative (and ostensibly cheaper) option to individual therapy. Although it is not appropriate to describe the theory and practice of group therapy here (see Yalom 1985), there are some important differences between group therapy with older adults and that undertaken with younger patients. Several authors have written up their experiences of psychodynamic groups with older members (Finkel *et al.* 1994; Evans 1998), including child survivors of the Holocaust (Tauber and Van der Hal 1998). The main potential advantage of group therapy is obvious; groups provide possibilities for patients to use each other as well as the therapist to observe themselves in relationships. In their transferences, members are free to make all sorts of misattributions among themselves (Marrone 1984). Leszcz (1990) suggests that for older people the process of pairing might not be a destructive 'subgrouping' but be of self-restorative value. In a similar way the author acknowledges the potential benefits of extra-group socialization, which is often unavoidable in treatment settings such as day hospitals (Ardern 1997).

Therefore group psychotherapy with older people is likely to require a greater tolerance of behaviours by members than the rarefied experience of those running groups for younger (and implicitly more independent) patients.

To the elderly the experience of sitting in a room together to talk about feelings is likely to be an unusual one. Many help-seeking elderly people participate in social groups in day centres. These groups, while no doubt helpful to some, usually go out of their way to *avoid* uncomfortable feelings, especially if these involve anger directed towards the organizers. A predetermined focus to the meeting, although superficially cohesive, often acts to ensure that 'hot potatoes' are avoided.

Dynamic group psychotherapy aims to provide a safe setting in which no subject is taboo. The disclosure of hitherto well-guarded concerns will only occur if therapists foster a climate of trust and are non-judgmental. Choosing a setting where such a group can flourish away from extraneous intrusions is not always easy.

Patient selection should ensure that the risk of scapegoating is lessened. Usually applied exclusion criteria, such as cognitive impairment, may not necessarily be desirable (Hunter 1989), but an equivalent degree of psychological mindedness among members should be sought. Martindale (1995) warns against mixing patients with too great a heterogeneity in psychological functioning.

The early functions of the therapists include a shepherding role: deciding when and how to contact unreliable attenders. Patients will be vigilant as to how the therapist(s) navigate this without being seen to be bullying, nannying, or neglectful. In elderly groups, absences are more sinister to members, perhaps denoting serious ill health or even death. With two therapists there is a better chance of continuity should either be away. Two therapists can usefully reflect and write up sessions in mutual supervision, though the use of an outside supervisor is advisable. Closed groups offer some advantages in cohesiveness and deeper work. However, over a long period, patients' absences or death can provide a sense of erosion along the lines of 'ten green bottles'. Open groups, which allow new members, have obvious merits, but they may convey ideas of substitutes in a soccer team. An initial duration of a group is likely to be a year, with the possibility of extension. Planned breaks are important as opportunities for discussion around loss.

Elderly members are less likely than younger ones to express openly their negative feelings towards therapists. Younger therapists may mistakenly assume that no such feelings exist, or may avoid enquiry, being tempted to 'let sleeping dogs lie'. Complaints against therapists may then be directed at a safer target, for example towards other doctors or the NHS in general. Therapists should be alert to these displacements.

Somatization often emerges in an elderly group. Older patients will be less used to, and less ready to accept, a psychological interpretation of their physical symptoms. Therapists are wise to be cautious in this area, and any treatments which patients receive from other sources should be acknowledged as important. Members may come to realize that their symptoms have other meanings too.

Group psychotherapy gives space to therapists to observe and reflect more easily than in individual therapy. In a mature group some patients will act as co-therapists, which is not necessarily a defensive manoeuvre. Working with an experienced group therapist provides a valuable learning opportunity for an inexperienced trainee, where as co-therapist he has the privilege of hearing the anxieties and frustrations of older people. Both patients and therapists can thereby enhance their psychodynamic skills.

Insight—Case 5

In a group for elderly patients, all with a previous history of depression, one member who had problems in acknowledging her neediness described returning to her home as a child to find it bombed. One wall remained, supporting a fireplace on which, surrounded by rubble, was a glass vase still intact. Being a mature group, one of the members quickly spotted the patient's identification with the vase, commenting that she perhaps felt like the vase that had survived but remained fragile. In this group, members had become more expert in making interpretations to each other, bringing insight to their bewilderment.

Envy—Case 6

In the same group, a forthcoming break was announced by the therapists. There was speculation among members that therapists needed a break as they were so exhausted. It was also assumed that the therapists were going on holiday together—something extravagant, like a cruise. The envy that the therapists could afford this and were physically fit enough to enjoy it was evident. Later on the patients wondered if they would be remembered (at the time the group sessions ran). This possibility contrasted with an earlier assumption that the therapists, once on holiday, would be rid of all thoughts of work.

Trust—Case 7

A particularly anxious woman had spent her childhood in care. In the group she commented that she had 'never known love'. She became panicky when disclosing longstanding suicidal ideas, fearing that the therapist's reaction to this might be to place her in 'care' in a mindless way. One of the other members broke in, demanding an assurance from the therapist that confidentiality in the group was sacrosant. The therapist hurriedly agreed, but in supervision she became aware that her compulsive reassurance might require consideration. It was decided that the therapist would raise the subject again in the next group, pointing out that there *may* be occasions when it would be right to breach confidentiality. This might, for example, involve reporting serious suicidal intent to the patient's own psychiatrist. The group was able to realize that this could be reasonable and indeed caring. Subsequently, this patient has become less panicky. Having experienced a new kind of parenting, she is now more able to trust that her disclosures will not undermine the therapist's composure.

Assertiveness—Case 8

Several patients attended a group run in a day hospital. The timing of the group meant that those attending the group missed afternoon tea at the end of the working day. The members had discussed this outside and then requested that the therapists might consider adjusting the time. The therapists recognized that the social function of the day hospital for these isolated people was an important matter. Even more important, this was the first time that the patients had challenged the therapists' arrangements. The therapists agreed to hold the group earlier. The patients' assertiveness in daring to ask had not resulted in a refusal but in a change for the better. The patients began to speculate that being assertive in other ways might make it possible for them to improve their lives. They toyed with the concept of negotiation rather than passively accepting what was on offer without question.

Creative therapies

As with the interpretation of dreamwork, creative therapies provide another road by which the unconscious becomes accessible. Art and music are two media which are increasingly considered in psychodynamic therapy with older people (Waller and Gilroy 1992; Hanser and Thompson 1994). These alternatives may be less threatening for the elderly and more enjoyable. Even where creative therapists do not embark on interpretation with patients, the work produced (on paper or audiotape) can be informative for the multidisciplinary team. These representations of patients' preoccupations can also give a powerful display of change over time.

Mistakes

It might be assumed that dynamic psychotherapy, even if not of benefit to patients, can do no harm.

However, as with medication, any treatment with the power to change may do so with adverse consequences (see, for example, Casement 1985; Strupp 1994). There are some generally accepted views on predictors of poor outcome for different types of patient (Mace 1995). It is a reality that many old people with psychological problems also have concurrent physical illness, are socially isolated, and poor. Since the therapist has to accept these facts he will have to be flexible in his approach. Patients with reduced mobility may require special attention, so that arranging transport to sessions, or an alternative setting, may be necessary. Physical contact between the therapist and the patient, if not undertaken to gratify the therapist, can be helpful. The therapist may need to make extra efforts to communicate with people who have sensory deprivation (see below). Even so, things can go wrong. Here are two examples:

Example 1

An experienced non-medical psychotherapist had been seeing an 85-year-old lady on a private basis each week for about a year. The patient had become worried about going outdoors and this was compounded by dizziness and palpitations. Fearing for her future, she made escalating demands on her family which left them exhausted and resentful. (Cohler and Galatzer-Levy (1990) have pointed out that adult children's response to ageing parents will be partly determined by the responses they received from them.) As a consequence, there were discussions between the patient and her family about how it might be time to go into an old people's home. The psychotherapist was drawn into these discussions with the family. The patient was less and less able to listen to the psychotherapist's interpretations about her bodily symptoms. Eventually the psychotherapist asked for the opinion of a psychiatrist who concluded that the patient had an agitated depression. The patient agreed to take paroxetine and one month later was back to her normal self. The patient broke off therapy, refusing to see the psychotherapist again.

Fortunately the psychotherapist had been able to spot that both she and her patient were floundering. The psychotherapist's perceived allegiances to the family increased the patient's distress, as did the continued interpretations. The patient was angry at not being heard, and felt guilty that she could not 'pull herself together'. Even though the psychotherapist eventually secured the treatment for the patient that she needed, any chance of post-treatment reflection was lost.

In a survey of psychoanalysts training in New York, attitudes towards the concurrent prescribing of antidepressant medication with analysis were surprisingly positive. Of 43 patients with a mood disorder, 36 were judged by their analyst not only to have improved in mood, but to have an enhanced analytic process (Donovan and Roose 1995).

Example 2

A 75-year-old single lady with a long history of hospitalization for depression was accepted into a group run by two psychiatrists, one of whom was also a psychoanalyst. The patient was hard of hearing but initially enthusiastic. As the weeks in the group passed she frequently misheard other members who became irritated with her apparent lack of sensitivity. In turn she became argumentative and began to accuse the therapists of trying to provoke her. This then extended into delusional ideas that the therapists had planted agents in her Church congregation to 'do therapy' to her. She was perplexed that the therapists would institute such a regime. Eventually one of the therapists saw her alone and, recognizing she had developed a paranoid psychosis, prescribed an antipsychotic. The patient improved but remained suspicious of the group and never returned. The group itself was terrified by witnessing the emergence of mental illness in its midst, and wondered if it was usual for patients to be driven mad by group therapy.

In this instance the therapists were so eager to find group members that they turned a blind eye to warning signs in the patient's extensive case notes. With hindsight it should have been apparent that this was a recipe for uncontainable projections.

Dynamic psychotherapy and the NHS institution

Since many elderly patients will be unsuitable for dynamic therapy, is there a role for the psychotherapist in the old age team?

Several authors have emphasized the stress induced in staff caring for older people, and the unwitting damage that can be inflicted on patients (Zagier Roberts 1994; Terry 1996; Ardern *et al.* 1998; Ardern 1999; Garner 1999).

A team with high morale and a clear sense of purpose is inherently of benefit to patients. One which is split and at war with itself will lead to patients being caught in the crossfire. Thus the psychotherapist can help psychiatric teams to work together, as well as supervising those team members who wish to practise psychotherapy (Holmes and Mitchison 1995; Adshead 1998).This may be the most cost-effective way of employing the skills of a consultant psychotherapist.

Conclusions

Not before time is dynamic psychotherapy being considered as a potentially valuable aspect of psychiatry in the elderly. In the United States there is already a wealth of literature on the subject (in addition to references throughout this text see Duffy (1999)). In relieving older people's distress we may need to place ourselves in their shoes. The psychodynamic model strives to ensure that we do not enact our own frustrations on patients who remind us of parents or grandparents. The theoretical framework is no less rigorous than with younger patients. At present in the UK, limits to the practice of dynamic psychotherapy in this age group are apparently set by the lack of opportunities for training and supervision. Since old age psychiatry departments are eclectic in their function, psychodynamic expertise should reduce competitive splits between biological, social, and psychological approaches to treatment.

The Tavistock Centre in London has recently introduced a yearly part-time course for professionals working with the elderly. Readers may wish to access the website of the Association for Psychoanalytic Psychotherapy in the NHS (APP), within which is the Older Adults Section. (*www.app-nhs.org.uk*).

Acknowledgement

The author would like to thank anonymous patients and professionals referred to in this chapter. Special thanks are given to Gina Elie, secretary.

References

Adshead, G. (1998). Psychiatric staff as attachment figures. Understanding management problems in psychiatric services in the light of attachment theory. *British Journal of Psychiatry*, **172**, 64–9.

Ardern, M. (1997). Psychotherapy and the elderly. In *Advances in old age psychiatry: chromosomes to community care* (ed. C. Holmes and R. Howard), pp. 265–76. Wrightson Biomedical, Petersfield.

Ardern, M. (1999). Psychodynamic aspects of old age psychiatry. In *Everything you need to know about old age psychiatry* (ed. R. Howard), pp. 253–66. Wrightson Biomedical, Petersfield.

Ardern, M., Garner, J., and Porter, R. (1998). Curious bedfellows: psychoanalytic understanding and old age psychiatry. *Psychoanalytic Psychotherapy*, **12**, 47–56.

Bauer, G. and Kobos, J. (1987). *Brief therapy: short-term psychodynamic intervention.* Aronson, New Jersey.

Bell, D. (1996). Primitive mind of state. *Psychoanalytic psychotherapy*, **10**, 45–57.

Brok, A. J. (1992). Crises and transitions: gender and life stage issues in individual, group and couples treatment. *Psychoanalysis and psychotherapy*, **10**, 3–16.

Casement, P. J. (1985). *On learning from the patient.* Routledge, London.

Cohler, B. J. and Galatzer-Levy, R. M. (1990). Self meaning and morale across the second half of life. In *New dimensions in adult development* (ed. R. A. Nemiroff and C. A. Colarusso), pp. 214–63. Basic Books, New York.

Corvin, A. and Fitzgerald, M. (2000). Evidence-based medicine: psychoanalysis and psychotherapy. *Psychoanalytic psychotherapy*, **14**, 143—51.

Crusey, J. E. (1985). Short-term psychodynamic psychotherapy with a sixty-two-year-old man. In *The race against time: psychotherapy and psychoanalysis in the second half of life.* (ed. R. A. Nemiroff and C. A. Colarusso), pp. 147–66. Plenum Press, New York.

Donovan, S. J. and Roose, S. P. (1995). Medication use during psychoanalysis: a survey. *Journal of Clinical Psychiatry*, **56**, 177–8.

Duffy, M. (ed.) (1999). *Handbook of counselling and psychotherapy with older adults.* Wiley, New York.

Erikson, E. (1966). Eight ages of man. *International Journal of Psycho-analysis*, **2**, 281–300.

Evans, S. (1998). Beyond the mirror: a group analytic exploration of late life depression. *Aging and mental health*, **2**, 94–9.

Finkel, S., Metler, P., Wasson, W., Berte, K., Bailey, N., Brauer, D. *et al.* (1994). Group therapy in the elderly. In *Functional psychiatric disorders of the elderly* (ed. E. Chiu and D. Ames), pp. 478–98. Cambridge University Press, Cambridge.

Freud, S. (1905). On psychotherapy. *Standard edition* (1964), Vol. 7, pp. 257–68. Hogarth, London.

Gabbard, G. O. (2000). A neurobiologically informed perspective on psychotherapy. *British Journal of Psychiatry*, **177**, 117–22.

Garner, J. (1999).Psychotherapy and old age psychiatry. *Psychiatric Bulletin*, **23**, 149–53.

Gutmann, D. L. (1987). *Reclaimed powers: towards a new psychology of men and women in later life*. Basic Books, New York.

Hanser, S. B. and Thompson, L. W. (1994). Effects of a music therapy strategy on depressed older adults. *Journal of Gerontology*, **49**, 265–9.

Hildebrand, P. (1986). Dynamic psychotherapy with the elderly. In *Psychological therapies for the elderly* (ed. I. Hanley and M. Gilhooly), pp. 22–40. Croom Helm, Beckenham.

Holmes, J. (1995). Supportive psychotherapy. The search for positive meanings. *British Journal of Psychiatry*, **167**, 439–45.

Holmes, J. and Mitchison, S. (1995). A model for an integrated psychotherapy service. *Psychiatric Bulletin*, **19**, 209–13.

Hubback, J. (1996). The archetypal senex: an exploration of old age. *Journal of Analytical Psychology*, **41**, 3–18.

Hunter, A. J. G. (1989). Reflections on psychotherapy with ageing people, individually and in groups. *British Journal of Psychiatry*, **154**, 250–2.

Jaques, E. (1965). Death and the mid-life crisis. *International Journal of Psycho-analysis*, **46**, 502–14.

Jung, C. G. (1931). The stages of life. In *Collected works, 1960*, Vol. 8 (ed. H. Read, M. Fordham, and G. Adler), pp. 387–403. Routledge, London.

King, P. (1980). The life cycle as indicated by the nature of the transference in the psychoanalysis of the middle aged and elderly. *International Journal of Psycho-analysis*, **61**, 153–60.

Kohut, H. (1971). *The analysis of self*. Hogarth, London.

Lam, D. (1991). Psycho-social family interventions in schizophrenia: a review of empirical studies. *Psychological Medicine*, **21**, 423–41.

Leszcz, M. (1990). Towards an integrated model of group psychotherapy with the elderly. *International Journal of Group Psychotherapy*, **40**, 379–99.

Limentani, A. (1995). Creativity and the third age. *International Journal of Psycho-analysis*, **76**, 825–33.

Mace, C. (1995). *The art and science of assessment in psychotherapy*. Routledge, London.

Margison, F. R., Barkham, M., Evans, C., McGrath, G., Mellor-Clark, J., Audin, K. *et al.* (2000). Measurement and psychotherapy: evidence-based practice and practice-based evidence. *British Journal of Psychiatry*, **177**, 123–30.

Marrone, M. (1984). Aspects of transference in group analysis. *Group Analysis*, **XVII**, 179–94.

Martin, C. (1992). The elder and the other. *Free Associations*, **3**, 341–54.

Martindale, B. (1989). Becoming dependent again: the fears of some elderly patients and their younger therapists. *Psychoanalytic Psychotherapy*, **4**, 67–75.

Martindale, B. (1995). Psychological treatments II: psychodynamic approaches. In *Neurotic disorders in the elderly* (ed. J. Lindesay), pp. 114–37. Oxford University Press, Oxford.

Martindale, B. (1998). On ageing, dying, death and eternal life. *Psychoanalytic psychotherapy*, **12**, 259–70.

Midwinter, E. (1991). *Out of focus: old age, the press and broadcasting*. Centre for Policy on Ageing, London.

Murphy, S. (2000). Provision of psychotherapy services for older people. *Psychiatric Bulletin*, **24**, 181–4.

Nemiroff, R. A. and Colarusso, C. A. (1985). *The race against time: psychotherapy and psychoanalysis in the second half of life*. Plenum Press, New York.

Newton, N. A. and Jacobowitz, J. (1999). Transferential and countertransferential processes in therapy with older adults. In *Handbook of counseling and psychotherapy with older adults* (ed. M. Duffy), pp. 21–40. Wiley, New York.

Parkes, C. M. (1992). Bereavement and mental health in the elderly. *Reviews in Clinical Gerontology*, **2**, 45–51.

Porter, R. (1997). The psychoanalytic psychotherapist and the old age psychiatry team. In *Psychiatry in the elderly* (2nd edn) (ed. R. Jacoby and C. Oppenheimer), pp. 257–68, Oxford University Press, Oxford.

Quick, E. K. (1996). *Doing what works in brief therapy: a strategic solution focused approach*. Academic Press, London.

Rechtshaffen, A. (1959). Psychotherapy with geriatric patients: a review of the literature. *Journal of Gerontology*, **14**, 73–84.

Ritchie, K. (1997). Eugeria, longevity and normal ageing. *British Journal of Psychiatry*, **171**, 501.

Sandler, A. M. (1978). Problems in the psychoanalysis of an ageing narcissistic patient. *Journal of Geriatric Psychiatry*, **11**, 5–16.

Sandler J., Person, E. S., and Fonagy, P. (ed.) for the International Psychoanalytical Association (1991). *Freud's 'on narcissism: an introduction'*. Yale University Press, New Haven, CT.

Settlage, C. F. (1996). Transcending old age: creativity, development and psychoanalysis in the life of a centenarian. *International Journal of Psycho-analysis*, **77**, 549–64.

Sifneos, P. (1987). *Short-term dynamic psychotherapy: evaluation and technique*. Plenum Press, New York.

Strupp, H. (1994). *When things get worse. The problem of negative effects in psychotherapy*. Aronson, London.

Tauber, Y. and Van der Hal, E. (1998). Countertransference and life-and-death issues in group psychotherapy with child Holocaust survivors. *American Journal of Psychotherapy*, **52**, 301–12.

Terry, P. (1996). *Counselling the elderly and their carers*. Macmillan, London.

Thompson, P. (1993). I don't feel old: the significance of the search for meaning in later life. *International Journal of Geriatric Psychiatry*, **8**, 685–92.

Waller, D. and Gilroy, A. (ed.) (1992). *Art therapy: a handbook*. Open University Press, Buckingham.
Wharton, B. (1996). In the last analysis: archetypal themes in the analysis of an elderly patient with early disintegrative trauma. *Journal of Analytical Psychology*, **41**, 19–36.
Wheelock, I. (1997). Psychodynamic psychotherapy with the older adult: challenges facing the patient and the therapist. *American Journal of Psychotherapy*, **51**, 431–44.
Yalom, I. D. (1985). *The theory and practice of group psychotherapy* (3rd edn). Basic Books, New York.
Zagier Roberts, V. (1994). Caring and uncaring in work with the elderly. In *The unconscious at work: individual and organisational stress in the human services* (ed. A. Obholzer and V. Zagier Roberts), pp. 75–83. Routledge, London.
Zinkin, L. (1983). Malignant mirroring. *Group Analysis*, **XVI**, 113–26.

17 Family therapy with ageing families

Eia K. Asen

Introduction

The clinical awareness of the enormous significance of families for the psychological and physical well-being of older people has been slow to make an impact upon family therapists (Gilleard *et al.* 1992). There are only a few family therapy services for older adults and their relatives in existence. In a review article, Flori (1989) found that age was negatively correlated with the likelihood of patients receiving family therapy. Ageism may be partially responsible for this, with the emphasis on 'saving the young', perhaps because the elderly are perceived as having lived their lives (Ivey *et al.* 2000). The marital and family therapy literature on working with ageing families is relatively modest (Van Amburg *et al.* 1996), with few papers and books (Keller and Bromley 1989; Neidhardt and Allen 1993; Richardson *et al.* 1994). This chapter describes the development of family systems therapy, outlines guidelines for family assessments, and details specific family therapy techniques that can be used when dealing with adult patients and their families who present with psychological problems or illness in later life.

The evolution of systemic family therapy

The term 'family therapy' is something of a misnomer for two reasons: first because the notion of 'family' is open to many interpretations if not attacks; and, second, because the term 'therapy' may be quite unacceptable to a family. The term 'family' is frequently read as implying an intact, two-parent, heterosexual couple with two children and two pets, with the man the breadwinner, the woman the homemaker, and possibly some doting grandparents providing the occasional relief. Clearly such a picture can unjustifiably ascribe a pathological nature to other family forms, such as gay or lesbian couples, single parents with children, childless couples, and unattached elderly persons. However, as we now have in our cultures many different forms of committed relationships it is not necessary to have a traditional family in order to be at the receiving end of family therapy: any relationship lends itself to a systemic or family therapy approach. As to the term 'therapy', this can imply the presence of an illness or dysfunction that requires a cure and it may therefore be perceived as inappropriate by some clients.

Despite these limitations the term 'family therapy' continues to be used. In the field of psychological approaches it applies both to a conceptual framework and to a treatment modality. It is important to make the distinction between family therapy as a specific psychological treatment method, and family therapy as a way of conceptualizing psychological and psychosocial disturbance. The latter, namely 'thinking families'—or even 'thinking systems'—is an important framework for any clinician involved in the assessment of a patient, the family, and the social context.

Gregory Bateson is usually credited with being the father of the family therapy movement. An anthropologist himself, he led a group of researchers in Palo Alto in the 1950s studying the patterns of schizophrenic transaction and communication. He and his team postulated that the schizophrenic's family was shaping his thought processes through the often bizarre communication requirements imposed on him (Bateson *et al.* 1956; Bateson 1978). Bateson and his co-workers also observed that the family seemed to require a symptomatic person for its functioning: if the 'identified patient' got better then the family was destabilized, with the result that someone else in the family appeared to get worse. Moreover, the group also observed that at times the whole family resisted or blocked the clinical improvement of the patient—as if they 'needed' the patient to remain unwell. Jackson (1957) named this phenomenon 'family homeostasis' and described the family as a 'system' which has a variety of properties, such as hierarchies, boundaries, overt and covert conflicts between specific members, coalitions, and so on. The idea that the family was an 'open system' (von Bertalanffy 1968) implied that it was part of a number of different social contexts: the extended family, the neighbourhood, the cultural setting, etc. In the systemic model individuals and families are seen as being part of a larger suprasystem, behaving according to a set of explicit or implicit rules, and it is these rules which are thought to govern interpersonal behaviours and communications (Watzlawick *et al.* 1967). Sometimes problem behaviours are so interlinked that it is impossible to distinguish between cause and effect—or what came first:

He: 'I only nag because you are so forgetful.'
She: 'But I can't remember anything if you always have a go at me.'
He: 'If you weren't upsetting me all the time I would stop nagging...'
She: 'If you stopped nagging I wouldn't be upset and I could concentrate more and remember things.'

Such recursive processes are termed 'circular', with certain communications leading to certain responses, which in turn trigger further communications and responses. These repetitive loops form an 'interaction pattern' in which both partners, as in the above example, can become trapped. Characteristically each person views his or her actions merely as a response to the other's responses or behaviours. It is often only possible for an outside observer to see the almost absurd circularity of some such interactions. Family systems therapy (or systemic family therapy, as it is often referred to) aims to challenge and disrupt such stuck interactions and dysfunctional patterns, so that new forms of communication and interaction can emerge. Family therapy with older adults and their families aims to foster better relationships between family members of different generations and, more specifically, to achieve more appropriate support or independence for older family members (Richardson *et al.* 1994). As a result there are now a whole range of family therapy approaches on which clinicians working with elderly patients and their families can draw.

The major family therapy approaches

Over the past four decades quite a number of systemic approaches have emerged in a variety of different contexts, both private and public. In practice, most therapists draw on a whole range of ideas and techniques. This section summarizes the leading systemic practices.

Structural family therapy

Many of the concepts of this form of therapy (Minuchin *et al.* 1967; Minuchin 1974) are based on a normative model of family functioning. It postulates that families function particularly well when certain structures prevail, such as intrafamilial hierarchies, clear boundaries, and appropriate communication patterns. Family structure becomes visible through the interactions of the various subsystems—the children, parents, or grandparents. Each family negotiates boundaries between the different generations. Grandparents, for example, are regarded as intrusive if the parents find them interfering with the care of their offspring who get caught up between the two parties, each demanding that the children side with the one against the other: a situation known as *triangulation*. Here the relative absence of boundaries between the parental and grandparental generation can contribute to family conflicts. The therapist's task is to intervene in such a way as to make the family structure approximate to the normative model of family life, with an emphasis on clearly defined boundaries and hierarchies. Techniques employed include the direct challenging of absent or rigid boundaries, 'unbalancing' the family equilibrium by temporarily joining with one member of the family against others, or setting 'homework' tasks designed to restore hierarchies (Minuchin and Fishman 1981). The structural approach is very active, with the therapist encouraging family members to 'enact' problems in the consulting room so that the ways in which communications become blocked or interactions get stuck can be studied '*in vivo*'. The therapist's job is then to keep the problem on the boil long enough for the family to find a new solution.

Strategic family therapy

In this approach (Haley 1963) the clinician designs interventions or 'strategies' to fit the problem (Hoffman 1981). Therapy initially does not appear to focus on the family as a whole, but rather narrowly on the nature of the presenting symptom and the 'identified' patient. The underlying assumption is that the symptom is being maintained by the apparent 'solution'—the very behaviours that seek to suppress it. For example, the 'anxious' elderly woman may elicit her son's overprotectiveness, a solution which may well perpetuate the problem. A structural therapist would tend to view overprotectiveness as a dysfunctional aspect of family organization, and therefore challenge those communication patterns linked to the presenting problem. Strategic therapists, however, would not concern themselves with the more general dysfunctional behaviours unless these are presented as problems. Instead, they focus on the problem brought by the client or family in an attempt to solve it (Watzlawick *et al.* 1974; Haley 1977; Herr and Weakland 1979). Theory has it that if the presenting problem changes, then a domino effect can be observed in other interactions and behaviours. Strategic therapists use 'reframing' as a major technique. The family's or client's perceived problem(s) are put into a different meaning-frame which provides new perspectives. This new way of viewing things can bring about changes in communication and behaviours. For example, reframing forgetfulness as the older adult's wish to give someone else a role, may be a useful challenge to an ingrained belief that this older adult is incompetent or hopeless. The strategic therapies are primarily symptomatic approaches and therapy is usually not a long-term enterprise.

Milan systemic approach

This form of therapy focuses on multigenerational family patterns, looking at the struggles of different family members over several generations (Boscolo *et al.* 1987). It involves making elaborate hypotheses about how, for example, longstanding rivalries within a sibling group become reactivated around the time of their elderly parent's illness, and how this, in turn, affects the older person's mental state. Such hypotheses lead to the design of interventions that take into account the anticipated attempts of the family to disqualify the therapy. The resulting 'counter-paradoxes' prescribed by the Milan team (Selvini Palazzoli *et al.* 1978) are aimed at recommending 'no change' in the hope that the family would resist this command and do the opposite, namely change—if only to defeat the therapist(s)! To confirm or refute hypotheses about family process and to arrive at these interventions, the Milan team perfected a particular interviewing technique: circular questioning (Selvini Palazzoli *et al.* 1980). The therapist conducts the family session mostly by asking questions, seeking information about people, their differences, and the various relationships and their specific characteristics. Such questions might, for instance, be triadic in that they ask person A, the grandfather for example, about his perception of aspects of the relationship between person B, grandmother, and C, grand-daughter. Talking about this in the presence of everyone inevitably produces plenty of feedback on which therapists base their next questions. Families and their individual members cannot help but get involved in thinking about the intricacies of their relationships with one another. A process is triggered whereby family members question each others' assumptions and behaviours and this can lead to new ways of communicating and relating.

Social constructionist and narrative approaches

Recently, the prescriptive style of the Milan systemic approach has given way to a critique of scientific objectivity, namely the traditional view that the observer (or clinician) stands outside the process observed. Inspired by the writings of physicists, neuroscientists, and philosophers (Capra 1975; Maturana and Varela 1972; von Foerster 1981, respectively), the 'post-Milan' therapists (Boscolo *et al.* 1987) focus on how the observer actually constructs what is being observed. The so-called 'reality' therapists believe that what they perceive should no longer be seen as something objectively 'out there': instead, reality is seen as 'invented', reflecting the therapists' own cultures and inherent belief systems. As each culture has its own dominant discourses and narratives (Foucault 1975), therapists need to examine how their language and cultural assumptions shape problem definitions. Interactions between patients, families, and clinicians reflect deeply embedded assumptions inherent in the traditional clinical discourses of experiences and relationships. In this sense, dominant professional discourses create a 'problem-determined system' (Anderson *et al.* 1986). If in therapeutic encounters the patients' experiences are treated as evidence of illness or pathology, then these experiences can only be explored within a pathology-oriented framework. This is very limiting, particularly if the narratives in which patients and their families 'story' their experiences—or have these 'storied' by others (psychiatrists, for example)—do not fit these experiences. Therefore significant aspects of their lived experience will not fit, or will even contradict, the dominant narrative (White and Epston 1990). Systemic narrative therapy attempts to help patients and their families find new ways of making sense of their experiences and to evolve new 'stories', with therapy being seen as a mutually validating conversation out of which change can occur. New interviewing techniques, often referred to as therapeutic conversations, have been developed in which both family and therapist 'co-evolve' or 'co-construct' their very own ways of describing the family system, so that it no longer needs to be viewed or experienced as problematic (Jones 1993). Such therapeutic conversations can actively challenge the contextual influences of cultural assumptions, stereotypes, or beliefs, such as ageism. Roper-Hall (1993) describes how this was done when a 71-year-old widow stated that she was too old to learn to drive. The therapist curiously enquired how the patient thought her age made a difference, and got an explanation regarding her lack of confidence. The therapist replied: 'So if you could find a way to increase your confidence, learning to drive might seem more possible?' This was followed by exploring some of the implications: 'If you did that, who would be more surprised, your older or your younger friends?' The patient seemed puzzled at first, but then started challenging her own thinking: 'Why should I be too old to drive?!' The characteristics of a post-Milan therapist are said to be those of a clinician who is 'democratic' and realistic about the possibility of change, taking non-judgemental and multipositional stances.

Contextual family therapy

This approach (Boszormenyi-Nagy 1988) emphasizes the healing relationships brought about through a growth in family commitment and trust, with the development of loyalty, fairness, and reciprocity, and with great emphasis on intergenerational interventions (Anderson and Hargrave 1990). Techniques used include life-review, using props such as family photo albums, family trees, and scrapbooks to reconsider the past and make peace with certain aspects of life to date. Involving other family members in this task brings in new perspectives and facilitates discussion. Video life reviews with older adults and their families are an effective tool in helping them to 're-story' past events with new meanings (Hargrave 1994). These reviews have a historical and evaluative dimension and promote stronger relational ties. They also deal with transition issues such as easing everyone through difficult developmental challenges and dealing with emotional pain.

Behavioural and psychoeducational approaches

Behavioural systemic work is generally based on the principles of social learning theory (Jacobson and Margolin 1979). A behavioural analysis is made at the outset, targeting specific family problems that need to be addressed. For each of these problems, well-defined goals are set out, with therapeutic interventions designed to achieve these. Communication training, contingency contracting, problem-solving training, limit setting, and operant-conditioning strategies are some of the techniques employed (Falloon 1988). Much emphasis is placed on searching for creative solutions from within the family, with the therapist in the role of facilitator rather than expert problem-solver. The psychoeducational approach (Leff *et al.* 1982) has strong behavioural elements, though it also draws on techniques from other family therapy models. Psychoeducational therapy aims to reduce expressed emotion (EE; critical comments and overinvolvement). Three separate therapeutic strategies are employed to achieve this goal in working with seriously mentally ill patients and their families: (1) educational sessions for the family—about the illness and the part the family can play in keeping the patient well; (2) a fortnightly relatives' group—to share experiences and solutions; and (c) family sessions (Kuipers *et al.* 1992). Such combined multilevel work is rare when it comes to treating older adults and their families. Psychoeducation more often takes the form of designing interventions to alleviate carer stress, reflecting the bias towards the needs of carers and the presumed passivity of the 'objects' of care (Richardson *et al.* 1994).

Solution-focused therapies

De Shazer (1985) used the observation that most symptoms and problems have a tendency to fluctuate. A depressed older person, for example, is sometimes more and at other times less depressed. The use of rating scales and a deliberate focus on those times when the depressive symptoms are absent leads to the identification of 'exceptions', which then form the basis of the solution. Patients and their families are encouraged to amplify the solution patterns of behaviours, with the aim of driving the problem patterns into the background (George *et al.* 1990, Iveson 1990).

Integrated approaches

It will be apparent from the above that there a number of different schools of family therapy with fairly diverse concepts, techniques, and theories of change. Whilst there are those purist family therapists who adhere to one particular dogma with missionary zeal, the majority of clinicians working in the field tend to find their own integrated approach, drawing on a whole range of different ideas and practices. Clearly, family therapy interventions need to be sensitive to the setting in which they are carried out: different approaches may be needed, for example, if one works in a GP surgery as opposed to working in an old people's home. The practice of family therapy is no longer confined to special rooms equipped with one-way mirrors, cameras, microphones, and teams of four. Family therapy has moved from its elitist stance and is becoming user-friendly (Treacher and Carpenter 1993). Home-based work or outreach family therapy (Clark *et al.* 1982) is now no longer uncommon in working with the elderly and their families.

Family assessment

Before prescribing family therapy it is wise to undertake a family assessment. This is a complex process. It looks at the elderly person in relation to the wider family and the social context, evaluating how family and helpers affect the older adult and his/her illness or problem. The family assessment also requires an appraisal of how the older person's illness affects the family and helpers. Family assessments are the basis for determining whether and how much the family can be a resource for containing or changing the presenting problems—and whether therapy is indicated or not.

The order in which a family assessment is carried out may vary, but the major ingredients are the same: problem identification, assessment of family relationships and communication patterns, assessment of the professional and agency network, and assessment of the wider social and cultural setting.

Assessing the family's coping mechanisms in practice

The mnemonic PRACTICE (Christie-Seely 1984) is a family assessment tool which helps the clinician to look at problems in context:

P Presenting problem
R Roles and rules
A Affect
C Communication
T Time in family life-cycle
I Illness
C Community
E Environmental

P—Assessing the presenting problem

The problem can be the illness itself, its result (e.g. the need for hospitalization), or the effect it has on other family members (e.g. a spouse's depression or a grandchild's behavioural problem). In practice, a family assessment starts with a description of the problem(s) by each family member, who can be asked in turn to give an opinion. To elicit the relevant information the clinician asks each person about the problem and how it affects everyone:

1. How does each person see the problem?
2. Is there agreement or disagreement about what constitutes a problem? When (and by whom) was it first noticed?
3. What is the effect of the illness on each family member?
4. Who is most/least affected?
5. What is each person's explanation and expectation?

In listening to each family member's account, the clinician can highlight the effects of the problem on everyone and get family members to talk to one another directly, encouraging them to use their own problem-solving skills.

R—Assessing family roles and rules

Acute or chronic illness in the family can change and even reverse roles. In cases of serious acute illness, the medical care system may take over major family roles, at times conflicting with parental roles. Hospitalized older adults may find it particularly difficult having to cope with a new system of rules imposed on them which do not tally with those at home. Many families find it difficult to compete with the round-the-clock nursing care that hospitals can provide, resulting in the family being tempted to leave an elderly person in hospital or a nursing home for much longer than needed. The following questions can help to clarify traditional and new family roles and rules:

1. How is the family (re-)allocating roles and functions?
2. Who anticipates/experiences role strains?
3. What is the power structure in the family?
4. How do family members agree about doing things differently?
5. Is the patient denying/overusing the sickness role?
6. What is the role of the helping system? How does it aid and/or block the family?

The clinician's task is to get the family members to talk openly about the ill person's change of role and help them consider drawing up new rules for short- and long-term survival.

At times it may be necessary to convene a professional network meeting with the family to discuss and allocate appropriate roles to the various helpers and family members.

A—Assessing affect

It is widely known that there are considerable personal and cultural differences as regards when and how much emotion people show. In many families the acute or chronic illness of an older adult is frequently accompanied by an initial phase of dazed denial, followed by anxiety, hope, and fear, and not infrequently considerable resentment towards the ill member. In assessing the affective status of family members, a number of issues need to be addressed:

1. What is the predominant emotional tone in the family?
2. Is anyone controlling the family mood?
3. Who is most/least able to talk about feelings?
4. Are all family members able to express both positive and negative emotions? How appropriate is that?
5. What is the non- and paraverbal family language?
6. How has the family dealt with illness in the past?

The clinician's task is to assess, as well as to facilitate, the open expression of grief and encourage the sharing of other feelings.

C—Assessing communication

Clarity of communication is not only an important issue for the family but also for the medical care team. The clinician often has the task of helping his colleagues give clear information to the family, as well as helping the family to ask important questions and get them answered:

1. Who talks *to* whom? Who talks *for* whom?
2. Who, if anybody, is the 'family switchboard'?
3. How direct is communication between family members?
4. Who blocks whom at what points?
5. What are the covert messages (para- and non-verbal)?
6. How critical/supportive are communications?
7. When does communication become confused or confusing?

The clinician can challenge a seeming conspiracy of silence regarding diagnosis. Given their age and the seriousness of their illness, the elderly patient may need help in dealing with 'unfinished business' and in getting the family to consider how to make the best of the time left.

T—Assessing the time in the family life-cycle

The family life-cycle provides a framework for understanding the predicament of elderly family members and for giving it a historical perspective (Carter and McGoldrick 1989; Sanbourn and Bould 1991). Retirement, widowhood, grandparenthood, illness, and dependency are the predictable stages at this point. When a young adult leaves home this can create space for the care of an older person. How the family copes with transitions in later life depends very much on the system they themselves have created over the years, and how that system adjusts to losses and new demands. Successful family functioning requires flexibility in structures, roles, and responses to new challenges (Walsh 1989). In the family assessment, data about past and present family functioning can be elicited by asking:

1. Which major family transitions are imminent or have taken place?
2. What effects is illness having on the anticipated changes of the family structure?
3. How is family life going to change if the illness gets better or worse?

I—Assessing the illness history

How families view illness varies a great deal, reflecting social and cultural values. The meanings that families attach to symptoms need to be explored by the clinician in relation to the family's personal, educational, and cultural background:

1. What are the family's beliefs and fears about ageing and illness?

2. Who (if anyone) feels responsible for illness?
3. What are the beliefs about how illness is spread?
4. How have previous generations coped with old age and carer issues?
5. What are the patterns of health and illness in previous generations?
6. What is the family's experience of past and present relationships with health professionals?

Systemic work has to focus on interventions with the social networks of older adults: often a single interview can be sufficient to mobilize or reassure the existing support system (Pottle 1984).

C—Assessing community resources

Illness in the elderly often requires intensive care at home or hospitalization. The family's support network will determine to what extent the patient can be managed in the home environment. Here the extended family plays an important role, and the clinician needs to evaluate the family's coping mechanisms; social ties and support have a major influence on health:

1. Does the family want to accept the outside world or would it prefer to close ranks and cope by itself?
2. Who is perceived by whom as being potentially helpful?
3. What role could the extended family and friends play?
4. What other social support structures are available?
5. What are the family strengths? Which familiar coping strategies can be relied on? Which can't?
6. Which alternative coping strategies could be explored?

Here the clinician may wish to encourage the family to consider the pros and cons of accepting appropriate amounts of help from the extended family or other sources.

E—Assessing environmental factors

The environment within which the patient and family live is an important factor for their health: this includes housing, financial and employment situation, medical and educational facilities, religious links with the community—and, last but not least, ethnicity. Family structures and family relations are very culture-dependent and extremely relevant to the place of the elderly. These include very diverse concepts about: authority relations; sex-role and generational differences; different emphases on lineal versus collateral kin; on the interdependence of nuclear families; and visiting and mutual aid relationships (Markides and Mindel 1987). (Lineal kin are direct ascendants or descendants, e.g. grandparents, parents, and children. Collateral kin are of the same generation, e.g. siblings and first cousins.) Families differ a great deal in how they relate to external, non-family support systems and to what extent they expect care to be provided entirely from within the family (Boyd-Franklin 1989). What seems to make sense in one cultural context may be a sign of failure in another. Here are some questions that address the social and cultural contexts within which families live:

1. What is culturally acceptable, given this family's particular ethnicity?
2. How much is the family linked with the local community?
3. Where are strong links—where does the family feel isolated?
4. What is the financial/work situation?
5. What is the housing/neighbourhood like?
6. Does the family experience racism?
7. Which community resources are available (e.g. self-help groups, church, or other culturally relevant settings)?

'Thinking families' also means 'thinking systems', and a good family clinician will see the larger social, cultural, and political context as affecting the health of the family. Not taking this into account means somehow confirming the pathology of the individual without looking at the pathological contributions society makes.

It is possible to conceptualize systemic family assessment as a set of different layers which all need to be examined in turn, but not necessarily in any specific order. Using a family systems approach means seeing the older adult in

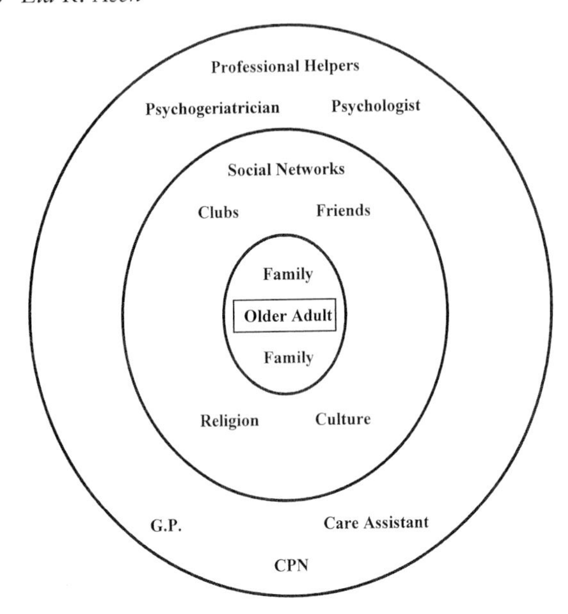

Fig. 17.1 The older adult in context.

context—and this is graphically represented in Fig. 17.1.

Not uncommonly the first point of contact for the clinician may be the elderly person alone. Chapter 9 in this volume outlines the principles and practice of the psychiatric examination of the older adult. Older adults frequently claim they have 'no family' or that the family is 'not important'. If clinicians unquestioningly accept this, they are likely to miss important information and the opportunity to use the family as a central resource. In the (often only temporary) absence of family members it is possible to undertake a 'family assessment by proxy'. This means interviewing in such a way that the views of important others are represented. Working systemically with an individual involves asking the older adult a number of questions that focus deliberately on his or her relationship with members of the family (Jenkins and Asen 1992). This gives valuable information on how certain family issues may maintain or contribute to the present problems. Examples of such questions are:

1. When you are very down, who among your family or friends is most affected?
2. Who, if anyone, do you feel isn't really bothered?
3. How does X respond when you are very low?
4. Who gets most irritated about you being so forgetful?
5. Of all the people who worry about you, who is the most/who the least helpful?

This way of questioning induces thought, reflection, self-questioning and can often itself be 'therapeutic' in that it reveals potentially new ways of viewing one's own predicament in relation to others. This can open up new channels, particularly if such reflections are shared with other family members.

From family assessment to family therapy

Where assessment ends and therapy begins is often quite difficult to determine. In the field of family work this dividing line would often seem artificial: all family assessments have a potentially therapeutic function—and there is an assessment function to every therapeutic session. It could be argued that bringing the family together in front of a neutral clinician is itself a major intervention. The assessment format itself is not only designed to provide answers for the examining clinician, but it also aims to generate new information for the patient and family members. For example, hearing other family members speculate about certain aspects of relationships that involve the listener can evoke powerful thoughts and feelings, such as being misunderstood or found out, and can lead to intensive discussion and interaction. This in itself can be therapeutic, because it challenges long-held beliefs and facilitates communication around issues that usually cannot be talked about openly. The sensitive clinician will know when the family resists discussing certain issues, and will then make a decision as to how wise it is to probe further at that point or whether to leave this for another time.

Many family therapists ask 'the family' to attend for the first session, but in practice will see whoever turns up. It is not uncommon for the number of clients attending the actual therapy sessions to increase over time—from one person to as many as six or ten, including members of the extended family or relevant others. For example, a woman in her eighties may well turn up with a neighbour who is more involved in her well-being than members of her family. However, what also can be elicited and explored is why her own children did not come. It may be important to invite the older person and her relevant others for what could be called family *work* rather than family *therapy*—a notion that may carry connotations of blame. Other family members can be invited by letter or by a phone call explaining how and why it might be useful for them to attend.

Whilst it is difficult to produce a satisfactory manual detailing any form of psychotherapy (Jones and Asen 2000), a brief attempt will be made here to give a broad outline of the shifting focus and processes of family therapy with the elderly. The first stages of therapy are often problem-focused, with the emphasis on getting the various members to come to some agreement as to what is most urgent and needs to be tackled first. This can take some time since not infrequently each family member has quite a different agenda. In fact, the failure to reach a consensus may well be the most urgent problem that the family as a whole has: one son may want to make peace and just ensure that the next year is as stress-free as possible; his sister feels the need to settle old scores and use therapy as an opportunity to tell her mother all she had not been able to tell her for the past 53 years. The elderly parents may see the purpose of family meetings as sorting out their relationship with their grandchildren and ensuring they can see them more regularly, whereas yet another family member may be of the opinion that the elderly couple should use the sessions to tackle, once and for all, their longstanding marital problems. The therapist can feel tempted to intervene and try to rescue the situation by setting the goals himself or providing a focus, particularly if everyone turns to him for advice. Giving such advice may defuse conflicts in the short-term, but is unlikely to result in the family developing its own problem-solving strategies.

It is only once the immediate presenting problems have been tackled that the family can look at the more long-term issues with which they have to cope. Consequently, the first few sessions may be dominated by Milan systemic circular questions (Selvini Palazzoli *et al.* 1980), spiced with structural (Minuchin 1974), strategic (Herr and Weakland 1979), and solution-focused (de Shazer 1985) techniques. During later phases of therapy contextual (Boszmorenyi-Nagy 1988), re-storying (Pocock 1995), or relapse-prevention work (Asen and Tomson 1992) may be more central.

Common issues in treating the elderly and their families

Iveson (1990) makes the point that three assumptions tend to inform the work of family therapists: older people's 'belongingness' (e.g. being full members of society); their responsibility for their actions; and their capacity to make choices. Believing in these until proved otherwise, rather than assuming the opposite, may empower older adults rather than overprotect them. Getting the balance right is rarely easy. If we protect older people from themselves we end up making key decisions for them. If we protect them from their families or from their neighbours, we can be in danger of undermining them. Yet, if we don't, we may put them at risk. One way or another, this remains a constant dilemma for any clinician. The next section illustrates specific issues and scenarios that can benefit from family therapy intervention.

Illness and the ageing family

Serious illness and impending death have major effects on the family. Carer stress and exhaustion, another family member developing related symptoms, collective denial and neglect of the older person all are symptoms of the family failing to adjust appropriately to this family crisis. Research shows that both the psychological and physical health of spouses and children of chronically ill elderly people are negatively affected, and that it is especially the female spouses of elderly male patients who are at risk (Kriegsman *et al.* 1994). The question as to which offspring should be responsible for the elderly relatives can stir up considerable feelings all round. Which family member chooses—or is designated—to do the caregiving is not only related to the caregiving demands, geographical proximity, or gender, but is also influenced by family legacy (Glaberman 1995). Children who have been exempted or excused from family responsibilities in childhood, appear to be unencumbered as adults when faced with caregiving responsibilities for a relative with Alzheimer's disease. Since family legacy influences who is the primary caregiver, family interventions need to address these long-term issues. It is not enough merely to focus on enabling caregivers to ask for help from relatives or on teaching them how to set limits. To help such 'unencumbered children' (Glaberman 1995) escape from their chronic uninvolved roles may require a transgenerational, re-storying approach.

Old business revived

Most families create, over time, their own stories or myths, and the past is painted in certain ways so that points about the present can be made. Sometimes myths exist to hide shameful events or secrets. Not infrequently, when people reach the end of their lives, the time has come for them and their relatives to question some of the myths and let out certain carefully guarded secrets. Reviving and dealing with old business in the present to improve things for more than one generation is one of the major tasks of family therapy.

Case 1

Both Mr and Mrs Brown were in their mid-80s when his depression and dementia suddenly became more serious. Mrs Brown developed cancer and their three children, all in their forties and fifties and with their own families, became involved in their care. The oldest son Peter, a doctor, tried to handle the medical side of it. The other son John, a lawyer, managed the legal side, and their sister Imogen, a nurse, was dispatched to deal with the practical day-to-day issues. For a few weeks this arrangement worked adequately, but gradually many old conflicts surfaced. A referral for family therapy was made by the old age psychiatrist, after a physical fight had broken out between the two brothers—in front of their parents. The first few family meetings involved only the siblings who were barely on speaking terms. Peter was accused of interfering with the treatment of both parents by constantly changing doctors, hospitals, and medication. John was charged with not handling the money matters honestly, and making arrangements that benefited, above all, his own family. Imogen was blamed for siding with her mother against her father. She, in turn, accused her brothers of sticking only to their professional roles rather than getting their 'hands dirty'—and so on. Soon old unfinished business had surfaced: resentment of the two younger siblings towards their older brother who they believed had always enjoyed the privileged position of the older son and was now likely to inherit the major part of the family fortune. He pointed out that it had not been an easy position, as he had been made his mother's confidant from a very young age. In this role he had learned that she had had three major affairs which had to be kept top secret. However, somehow this so-called secret had become common knowledge, though everyone seemed to subscribe to the myth that father had never found out about it. Imogen explained how she had felt totally neglected by her father and how angry she was about being asked to help out whenever it suited her parents.

The initial family work consisted of six family sessions, with only the siblings present. This helped to put past and present issues into perspective and resulted in the siblings cooperating with one another—for the benefit of their parents—rather than continuing to re-enact the fights of their childhood. It was only then that two meetings in the parents' home with the whole family were convened. It turned out that father had known all along about the affairs but had been too angry to confront his wife. Many other issues were brought up, with the siblings now balanced enough not to let their own agenda interfere with the short-term management of their parents. Family work helped to develop a care plan to which all members of the family could subscribe with the minimum of conflict between the adult children. A few months later the elderly parents asked for some marital therapy 'to settle some old issues once and for all'.

Married to the sick role

Chronic disease in the elderly has clearly wide-ranging effects on the family (Griegsman *et al.* 1994). But illness can also become a weapon to get at others. Repetitive self-harm, for example, contains elements of an attack on one's family. Illness can also act as 'superglue', holding together relationships that might otherwise fall apart. Such illness bonds are not uncommon and often characterized by scenarios where one person is the 'patient' and the other the 'nurse'. Physical or psychological illness then becomes the *raison d'être* for the relationship, and all parties seem to have a lot invested in keeping 'it', the real or imaginary illness, going. For example, a woman in her late seventies was treated as an invalid by her husband years after she had made a complete recovery from a brain haemorrhage. Referring constantly to her 'illness', he succeeded in making her feel so helpless and dependent that she thoroughly 'learned' to doubt her own judgement. In family therapy sessions her strengths were identified and the couple were set tasks for her to increase her competence step-by-step. In the event, it emerged that the major obstacle to her recovery was her husband's resistance to letting go of the power position he had obtained as a result of her illness years ago. Given that elderly people are more likely to be physically frail, there is plenty of scope for using illness in their daily battles.

Case 2

Mr Smith, in his eighties, was seriously diabetic and suffered frequent hypoglycaemic attacks. During these he would call for his wife and ask her to prepare a meal urgently. Mrs Smith, in her late seventies, suffered from what she herself called intractable back pain. She claimed that her pain was too severe to get out of bed. Mr Smith would prick his finger and take a quick blood sugar to verify his hypoglycaemic status and show the alarming results to his wife. Mrs Smith would then point to her 'pain-thermometer', kindly, though probably unwisely, fitted by one of the leading neurological hospitals in the country, which by means of a red flashing light, prominently displayed on her chest, signalled that she was 'objectively' in severe pain. Arguments between both partners would break out, each claiming to be more ill than the other and 'proving' it by referring to objective blood sugar and pain levels. At the point of referral the situation had become hopelessly stuck. Couple therapy initially focused on how each of them could survive their attacks and make themselves safe. A little later some work was done to help them understand how they had arrived at such an absurd impasse. Mrs Smith revealed that it all started some 50 years ago on the night of their wedding when Mr Smith had danced all night with his ex-girlfriend. It was soon after the honeymoon that she developed back pain ('this made me sick') and her husband patiently looked after her for years until he himself became a 'patient'. Therapy sessions helped them to talk about how much and little they cared for one another. Some progress was made in that they changed their expectations about how much each could and should rely on the other.

Marital therapy for octogenarians

It is never too late for couple-work and a few sessions can sometimes bring about significant shifts (Carni 1989). This may be particularly indicated when a depressed older adult lives with a high EE spouse. Such work can be framed as 'partner-assisted therapy', otherwise the spouse may feel blamed for the partner's depression (Jones and Asen 2000). The major issues that emerge as triggering or maintaining depression are: past affairs (often half a century ago!); retirement after a very busy life involving a lot of travel; and overinvolvement of a parent with a grown-up son or daughter, which fuels rivalries or produces battles over the family inheritance. Some partners never give up hope of changing the other—even if this has not proved a realistic proposition over the preceding decades. Helping people to accept the other for what he or she is may prove impossible. Family therapists can challenge the couple and ask them how many years they might wish to continue to waste, trying to achieve the seemingly impossible. In many respects, couple therapy for this age group is not much different from the approach one would choose with younger clients. Change is possible at any age, although the goals with the elderly might be fairly modest and centre on some improvements in decision-making or certain aspects of communication. For example, the eternal complaint that 'she never listens to me' can be addressed by asking how he could be better heard or how he would have to talk so that she might find it bearable or possible to listen to him. Simple tasks, such as '4 minutes each' or 'slow motion replay' (Asen 1995), are designed to rehearse new communication patterns and facilitate better interaction between hopelessly stuck partners.

Grandparenthood as an antidepressant

Old age is often thought of as a time of loss—loss of friends, health, job, status, etc. The elderly, semirebelliously hovering in their 'third adolescence' between dependence and independence, do not fit easily into society, frequently breaking rules and antagonizing others. Their unpredictable behaviour is randomly attributed to senility or wisdom, much to the annoyance of their offspring and the continuous amusement of their grandchildren. It is often overlooked how much mutual benefit can be derived for grandparents and grandchildren alike, from connecting the two generations. Family therapists will wish to concentrate their efforts on promoting intergenerational work, encouraging this natural alliance. However, this is not always unproblematic since the generation in between, namely the parents, may disapprove of the grandparental input.

Case 3

Jackie, a woman in her forties, felt that her own mother (Mary, aged 75) had neglected her when she was a child. However, she realized that Mary, in her role as grandmother, seemed to have a much closer relationship with her 7-year-old daughter Jodie. This brought back painful memories. Jackie increasingly saw her mother as a rival for Jodie's love, and felt that Jodie was being thoroughly spoilt by her grandmother. Consciously or unconsciously, Jackie started to block her mother seeing Jodie, and eventually she stopped her own mother from having access to Jodie altogether. Since Mary had quite distinct views of how inadequate Jackie was as a mother, this further reinforced old powerful dynamics. The casualty in this conflict was Jodie who very much missed seeing her grandmother. Family work involving the three generations proved useful, with benefits not only for Jackie and her mother, but three, if not four, generations (Whitaker 1982).

The elderly as a lifetime job

The part the family plays in influencing illness is frequently underestimated: even when organic brain disease is present, the family's responses can affect the course and outcome of the condition (Davis 1997). For example, if the grown-up children, because of their own anxieties, behave in overly responsible ways, they may soon find themselves involved in a cycle where the more they do for their parents, the more helpless the parents become, with ever-increasing demands, burden, guilt, and resentment. The vicious cycle of family overfunctioning/elderly underfunctioning can maintain or hasten symptoms labelled as senility (Walsh 1989). After careful assessment, an over-responsible adult daughter, for example, can be assisted through family therapy to consider whether it might be more helpful to her father if she challenges him to do certain things by himself, rather than having them done for him. Similarly, an underinvolved sibling may in therapy be questioned about his reluctance or inability to share the burden with the overcaring dutiful daughter.

Underestimating the skills and assets of an elderly patient is very common, but blind acceptance of such views or beliefs makes them come true. Sometimes it may suit adult children to become (over-) involved in their elderly parents' lives: perhaps to avoid issues in their own marriages, perhaps because their own children have left home and there is now a void in their lives that can be filled by fussing over someone else. Hanson (1991) has pointed out that the 'patienting process' isolates dementia sufferers, whose behaviours are constantly defined as wrong or inappropriate. Being invalidated leads the sufferers to isolate themselves further, with the result that they are increasingly ignored and lose touch. Helping the family to identify the dementia sufferer's strengths and looking for exceptions to behaviours symptomatic of dementia, can result in the older adult gaining confidence and feeling useful in some domains of life.

Conclusions—indications for family therapy

Carpenter (1994) carried out a project in a primary health care setting and found that almost a third of referrals of older adults mentioned marital or family problems. Grief counselling and current family and marital relationship conflicts were most often the focus for subsequent work. However, in only 9% were formal conjoint family therapy sessions conducted. Clearly, there is a need for family interventions, but the 'when' and 'what' requires some discussion. Earlier in this chapter a distinction was made between 'thinking families' and 'family systems' therapy as a form of treatment. The former is a framework that helps the clinician to view the older adult in context, thus informing and contributing to overall treatment and management plans. In other words, the combination of 'thinking families' and 'thinking systems' is an indispensable infrastructure for any modern clinician. Family therapy as a treatment modality has some very specific applications, some of them described above. In addition, this form of therapy may be considered in cases of: elder abuse; resistance to an elder's independence; elderly parents struggling as caregivers for dependent adult children; postretirement issues; having to make decisions to institutionalize an elderly person.

Family therapy is a useful intervention in the hands of experienced clinicians who have undertaken a recognized systemic training over a number of years. Its application needs to be based on clients' needs and research findings, rather than being guided by dogmatic unsubstantiated claims. Much damage can be caused by insensitive clinicians who, for example, think it absolutely necessary to confront all painful issues immediately, whatever the risk of such an approach to the older person's health. Family therapy cannot be prescribed against the wishes of those meant to receive it. Meeting with the family from time to time, framed as 'discussing issues', is a low-key family therapy intervention that can be more helpful than formal, ritualized family therapy. Change is almost always a slow process and its pace needs to be dictated by the family rather than be forced upon it. Montalvo (1993) points out that clinical errors occur when clinicians have too narrow or too wide a focus and persist in a course of action that is not of help to the patient. His suggested remedies for lessening the possibility of error are an excellent illustration of good systemic practice and include the following:

- be alert to coexisting problems;
- make preliminary assessments before intervening in the patient's interpersonal world;
- establish the 'when' and 'how' of symptom display—to search for contemporary forces that maintain symptoms;
- understand changes in decisions of the patient, the caregivers, or the providers—to protect the independence of the clinician's assessment (Montalvo 1993).

Family therapy is often only thought of as a last resort, rather than being an approach which, in most cases, could and should be part of the overall management plan comprising diagnostic, preventive, and therapeutic aspects. Teams which include a family therapist as a permanent member of staff are able to utilize different perspectives and to provide specialized inputs from different individuals and disciplines (Ross *et al.* 1992). Moreover, professionals working with the elderly can re-examine who their clients or patients are: is it 'just' the elderly patient or could it be the family? Surely there is little argument that if the family can cope better, then this must be better for the elderly—not to mention the mental health of future generations of the very same family. And this is where family work with the elderly can also have a useful preventive function.

References

Anderson, H., Goolishian, H. A., and Windermand (1986). Problem determined systems: toward transformation in family therapy. *Journal of Strategic and Family Therapy*, **4**, 1–13.

Anderson, W. T. and Hargrave, T. D. (1990). Contextual family therapy and older people: building trust in the intergeneration family. *Journal of Family Therapy*, **12**, 311–20.

Asen, K. E. and Tomson, P. (1992). *Family solutions in family practice*. Quay Publications, Lancaster.

Asen, K. E. (1995). *Family therapy for everyone: how to get the best out of living together*. BBC Books, London.

Bateson, G., Jackson, D., Haley, J., and Weakland, J. (1956). Toward a theory of schizophrenia. *Behavioural Science*, **1**, 251–64.

Bateson, G. (1978). The birth of a matrix or double bind and epistemology. In *Beyond the double bind* (ed. M. Berger), pp. 39–64. Brunner/Mazel, New York.

Boscolo, L., Cecchin, G., Hoffman, L., and Penn, P. (1987). *Milan systemic family therapy*. Basic Books, New York.

Boszormenyi-Nagy, I. (1988). *Foundations of contextual therapy*. Brunner/Mazel, New York.

Boyd-Franklin, N. (1989). *Black families in therapy: a multisystems approach*. Guilford Press, New York.

Capra, F. (1975). *The Tao of physics*. Fontana/Collins, London.

Carni, E. (1989). *To deal or not to deal with death: family therapy with three enmeshed older couples. Family Therapy*, **16**, 60–8.

Carter, B. and McGoldrick, M. (ed.) (1989). *The changing family life-cycle: a framework for family therapy* (2nd edn). Allyn and Bacon, Boston.

Carpenter, J. (1994). Older adults in primary health care in the United Kingdom: an exploration of the relevance of family therapy. *Family Systems Medicine*, **12**, 133–48.

Christie-Seely, J. (ed.) (1984). *Working with families in primary care*. Preager, New York.

Clark, T., Zalis, T., and Sacco, F. (1982). *Outreach family therapy*. Aronson, New York.

Davis, L. L. (1997). Family conflicts around dementia home-care. *Families, Systems and Health*, **15**, 85–98.

de Shazer, S. (1985). *Keys to solutions in brief therapy*. W. W. Norton, New York.

Falloon, I. R. H. (1988). Behavioural systems therapy: systems, structures and strategies. In *Family therapy in Britain* (ed. E. Street and W. Dryden), pp. 101–26. Open University Press, Milton Keynes.

Flori, D. E. (1989). The prevalence of later life family concerns in the marriage and family therapy journal literature (1976–1985): a content analysis. *Journal of Marital and Family Therapy*, **15**, 289–97.

Foucault, M. (1975). *The archaeology of knowledge*. Tavistock, London.

George, E., Iveson, C., and Ratner, H. (1990). *Problem to solution*. Brief Therapy Press, London.

Gilleard, C., Lieberman, S., and Peeler, R. (1992). Family therapy for older adults: a survey of professionals' attitudes. *Journal of Family Therapy*, **14**, 413–22.

Glaberman, J. (1995). The unencumbered child: family reputation and responsibilities in the care of relatives with Alzheimer's disease. *Family Process*, **34**, 87–99.

Griegsman, D., Penninx, B., and van Eijk, J. (1994). Chronic disease in the elderly and its impact on the family: a review of the literature. *Family Systems Medicine*, **12**, 249–67.

Haley, J. (1963). *Strategies of psychotherapy*. Grune and Stratton, New York.

Haley, J. (1977). *Problem-solving therapy*. Jossey- Bass, San Francisco.

Hanson, B. G. (1991). Parts, players, and 'patienting': the social construction of senile dementia. *Family Systems Medicine*, **9**, 267–74.

Hargrave, T. D. (1994). Using video life reviews with older adults. *Journal of Family Therapy*, **16**, 259–68.

Herr, J. J. and Weakland, J. H. (1979). *Counseling elders and their families: practical techniques for applied gerontology*. Springer, New York.

Hoffmann, L. (1981). *Foundations of family therapy*. Basic Books, New York.

Iveson, C. (1990). *Whose life? Community care of older people and their families*. BT Press, London.

Ivey, D. C., Wieling, E., and Harris, S. M. (2000). Save the young—the elderly have lived their lives; ageism in marriage and family therapy. *Family Process*, **39**, 163–75.

Jackson, D. (1957). The question of family homeostasis. *Psychiatric Quarterly* (Suppl.), **31**, 79–90.

Jacobson, N. S. and Margolin, G. (1979). *Marital therapy: strategies based on social learning and behavior exchanges principles*. Brunner/Mazel, New York.

Jenkins, H. and Asen, K. (1992). Family therapy without the family: a framework for systemic practice. *Journal of Family Therapy*, **14**, 1–14.

Jones, E. (1993). *Family systems therapy*. Wiley, Chichester.

Jones, E. and Asen, E. (2000). *Systemic couple therapy and depression*. Karnac, London.

Keller, J. and Bromley, M. (1989). Psychotherapy with the elderly: a systemic model. *Journal of Psychotherapy and the Family*, **5**, 291–46.

Kriegsman, D. M. W., Penninx, B., and van Eijk, J. (1994). Chronic disease in the elderly and its impact on the family: a review of the literature. *Family Systems Medicine*, **12**, 249–67.

Kuipers, L., Leff, J., and Lam, D. (1992). *Family work for schizophrenia: a practical guide*. Gaskell, London.

Leff, J., Kuipers, L., Berkowitz, R., Eberlein-Vries, R., and Sturgeon, D. (1982). A controlled trial of social intervention in the families of schizophrenic patients. *British Journal of Psychiatry*, **141**, 121–34.

Markides, K. S. and Mindel, C. H. (1987). *Ageing and ethnicity*. Sage, London.

Maturana, H. R. and Varela, F. J. (1972). *Autopoiesis and cognition: the realization of living*. Reidel, Dordrecht.

Minuchin, S., Montalvo, B., Guerney, B. G., Rosman, B. L., and Schumer, F. (1967). *Families of the slums*. Basic Books, New York.

Minuchin, S. (1974). *Families and family therapy*. Tavistock, London.

Minuchin, S. and Fishman, C. (1981). *Family therapy techniques*. Harvard University Press, Cambridge, MA.

Montalvo, B. (1993). Cautionary tales from geriatrics: eight ideas for the health provider. *Family Systems Medicine*, **11**, 89–99.

Neidhardt, E. R. and Allen, J. A. (1993). *Family therapy with the elderly*. Sage Publications, London.

Pocock, D. (1995). Searching for a better story: harnessing modern and post-modern positions in family therapy. *Journal of Family Therapy*, **17**, 149–73.

Pottle, S. (1984). Developing a network-orientated service for elderly people and their carers. In *Using family therapy*. (ed. J. Carpenter and A. Treacher), pp. 149–65. Blackwell, Oxford.

Richardson, C. A., Gilleard, C., Lieberman, S., and Peeler, R. (1994). Working with older adults and their families—a review. *Journal of Family Therapy*, **16**, 225–40.

Ross, J. L., Yudin, J., and Galluzzi, K. (1992). The geriatric assessment team: a case report. *Family Systems Medicine*, **10**, 213–18.

Roper-Hall, A. (1993). Developing family therapy services with older adults. In *Using family therapy in the 90s* (ed. J. Carpenter and A. Treacher), pp. 185–203. Blackwell, Oxford.

Sanborn, B. and Bould, S. (1991). Intergenerational caregivers of the oldest old. In *Families: intergenerational and generational connections* (ed. S. K. Pfeifer and M. Sussan), pp. 000–00. Haworth Press, New York.

Selvini Palazzoli, M., Boscolo, L., Cecchin, L., and Prata, G. (1978). *Paradox and counterparadox*. Aronson, New York.

Selvini Palazzoli, M., Boscolo, L., Cecchin, G., and Prata, G. (1980). Hypothesizing, circularity, neutrality: three guidelines for the conductor of the session. *Family Process*, **19**, 3–12.

Treacher, A. and Carpenter, J. (1993). User-friendly family therapy. In *Using family therapy in the 90s* (ed. J. Carpenter and A. Treacher), pp. 8–31. Blackwell, Oxford.

van Amburg, S. M., Barber, C. E., and Zimmerman, T. S. (1996). Ageing and family therapy: prevalence of ageing issues and later life concerns in marital and family therapy literature. *Journal of Marital and Family Therapy*, **22**, 195–203.

von Bertalanffy, L. (1968). *General Systems Theory: foundations, development, applications*. Penguin Books, Harmondsworth.

von Foerster, H. (1981). *Observing systems*. Intersystems, Seaside, CA.

Walsh, F. (1989). The family in later life. In *The changing family life-cycle: a framework for family therapy* (2nd edn) (ed. B. Carter and M. McGoldrick), pp. 312–32. Allyn and Bacon, Boston.

Watzlawick, P., Jackson, D., and Beavin, J. (1967). *Pragmatics of human communication*. W. W. Norton, New York.

Watzlawick, P., Weakland, J., and Fish, R. (1974). *Change: principles of problem formation and problem resolution*. W. W. Norton, New York.

Whitaker, C. (1982). *From psyche to system*. Guilford Press, New York.

White, M. and Epston, D. (1990). *Narrative means to therapeutic ends*. W. W. Norton, New York.

18 Clinical practice: primary care with the elderly mentally ill

Helen J. Graham

The general practitioner (GP) gives personal, primary, and continuing care to individuals, families, and a practice population, irrespective of age, sex, and illness. His aim is to make early diagnoses; include and integrate physical, psychological, and social factors in considerations about health and illness; and will undertake the continuing management of patients with chronic, recurrent, or terminal illnesses; will know how and when to intervene, through treatment, prevention, and education.

This concept of care (Leewenhorst Statement 1974, quoted in Taylor and Taylor 1988) gives GPs a unique involvement with the full range of health problems of elderly people in the context of their families and the community. General practitioners are familiar with most aspects of mental illness in elderly patients, much of which is ill-defined and interwoven with the complexities of the many personal, social, and medical problems of this age group. Good primary care also involves the rational use of hospital-based resources, which is achieved through the general practitioner's role as a 'gate-keeper' to specialist services. Conversely, effective specialist care involves the cooperation of the GP.

The delivery of primary health care and general practitioner services

In the United Kingdom, GP services are an integral part of the National Health Service (NHS). Each GP has responsibility for a defined population, each patient being required to register and remain with a personal general practitioner unless application is formally made to change doctor. The GP is responsible for the provision of care for all registered patients, 24 hours a day and for 365 days a year. This situation has encouraged group practice through the sharing of clinical responsibilities. From 1st April 1999, primary care groups have been introduced nationally, each serving a local population of between 60 000 and 150 000 patients. Each group consists of elected general practitioners and local health and social care professionals who work together with patients and health authorities. Primary care groups will bring together primary and community services, and will be charged with the responsibility of improving the health of their local community, developing locality services, commissioning secondary care, and implementing clinical governance. Many plan to become primary care trusts and will be financially responsible for providing community services (Shapiro 2000). Individual practices have the option of negotiating separate NHS practice-funding under the personal medical services pilot scheme. This allows practice-based contracts for a full range of patient services in a health authority, the employment of salaried GPs, or, of continuing with direct health authority funding within their primary care group. Following the Primary Care Act of 1997, a framework for delivering services was established through a national scheme of general medical services administered by local health authorities: an administrative section of the National Health Service responsible for primary care, pharmacy, and optician services. Recent health strategies aim to implement health improvement programmes in priority areas of health, including mental illness and older people (Department of Health 1999*a* and 2001).

Increasing patient demand for out-of-hours care and a national commitment to explicit standards of care defined in a set of National Service Frameworks (Department of Health 1999*b*) has led to the development of a range of innovative primary care services. In addition to registering with a local GP, patients may use primary care walk-in centres which are located in public places such as supermarkets and railway stations. The subcontracting of emergency services has brought about radical changes in the provision of out-of-hours primary care. Patients have access to first-level health advice through a nationwide, direct-access telephone service, called NHS Direct, which is staffed by nurses who advise on self-care, GP or specialist referral, or the use of local services. Most general practitioners belong to out-of-hours 'cooperatives', which are based in emergency centres and provide care for populations of up to one million. Patients who request out-of-hours care are initially advised by a doctor or nurse by telephone, accounting for half of all calls. If a medical consultation is advised, patients attend a primary care centre, accounting for one-third, or are managed by home visit, accounting for one-quarter. About half of all out-of-hours calls from patients aged over 65 result in a home visit, and of these, patients aged over 75 have a hospital admission rate seven times that of infants (Salisbury *et al.* 2000). The integration of social workers into the cooperatives facilitates urgent 'sectioning' of patients and emergency admission to residential care.

Epidemiology of general practice care of the elderly

The average list size for a general practitioner is 1845 patients, based on the total numbers of full- and part-time doctors (Department of Health 2000). The national average percentage of elderly patients aged 65–74 is 8.3% and aged over 75 it is 7.4%. A full-time GP with a list size of 2000 patients can expect to care for approximately 165 patients aged between 65 and 74 (8.3%) and 146 patients aged over 75 (7.3%), about 40 (2%) of whom will be over 85 years of age. The list may be 'personal', as in a single-handed practice or in a group practice where doctors consult only with their own registered patients, or the list may be 'combined' where patients are free to consult any doctor in a group practice.

Average annual consultation rates for adults increase with age, with 3.0 contacts for patients aged 16–65, 4.3 for patients aged 65–74, and 5.1 for those aged over 75. Contact rates are 17% higher in elderly people living in communal establishments and 8% higher in elderly people living alone than those living in standard accommodation (McNeice and Majeed 1999). Women consult more frequently than men. For patients aged 65–74 years the annual consultation rates are 4.8 for men, and 5.3 for women; and for those over 75 years, 6.4 for men and 7.1 for women (RCGP 1995). Older people have fewer patient-initiated visits, and are more likely to attend for follow-up of established disease. Because of their reduced mobility, they require more home visits than younger patients—about one-third and two-thirds of total consultations, respectively, in those aged 75–84 and 85 and over being at home. For all age groups, 25% of home visits are to patients aged 75–84 and 15% to people aged over 85 years. Of patients aged 65 years and over living in communal establishments, 66% of doctor contacts are in the home compared to 18% of those living in standard accommodation. To compensate for this additional workload, GPs receive weighted capitation fees for patients aged over 65 years. Additional payments are made for newly registered patients who have a simple health screening, and for patients who reside in an area of deprivation. In England, deprivation is determined by the use of the 'Jarman Index', this identifies areas or Enumeration Districts which can be expected to generate a high workload for a practitioner. The index has four levels of deprivation derived from a scoring system based on eight factors. In relation to an older population this includes the number of elderly living alone, the number of residents in ethnic households, the degree of household overcrowding, and numbers who have moved house (Department of Health 2000).

Screening and monitoring disease in the elderly

The reservoir of unreported illness in elderly patients assessed at home (Williamson *et al.* 1964) has been demonstrated in many general practice-based studies, and has led to the opinion that opportunistic case finding or screening is more appropriate to the needs of older patients. Evidence for the benefits of screening in studies using controlled trials is equivocal (Tulloch and Moore 1979; Hendricksen *et al.* 1984; Vetter *et al.* 1984). Changes in general practice in the NHS (Health Departments of Great Britain 1989) require GPs to offer all patients aged 75 years and over an annual health assessment. This may be delegated to other members of the primary health care team such as the practice nurse or health visitor. The assessment should include: the offer of a visit, to see the home environment and to find out whether carers and relatives are available; social, mobility, and mental assessments; assessment of continence, and general function; and a review of medication. It has been reported that only half of the elderly population offered checks accepted and that there is no standardized approach or use of screening instruments for the detection of psychological morbidity (Nocon 1993). Of patients who accepted checks, 98% considered them to be useful, although some who were at high health risk were falsely reassured (McIntosh and Power 1993). Over half of GPs reported that they rarely detected new mental health problems (Chew *et al.* 1994). An increased rate of detection of dementia and depression occurred if screening instruments were inserted into patient notes and used opportunistically, although this was not found to alter clinical practice (Iliffe *et al.* 1994).

The use of computerized patient lists for screening, audit, and research

The use of computers for patient registration and practice management is almost universal in primary care. Increasing numbers of practices hold electronic patient records that contain computerized medical histories and consultations, and have switched to computer-generated prescribing (Fig. 18.1). Screening and monitoring disease and disability can be undertaken using the computerized registration details of patients, although these are limited by the input of clinical details (Fig. 18.2).

The electronic patient list has superseded the previously used Age–Sex Register, in which patients were listed by year of birth, with names ordered alphabetically in a card index. The increasing use of the electronic patient record in surgery consultations and the electronic transfer of patient information between general practice and hospitals and laboratories are bringing about a process of seamless care and paperless clinical practice. Most software programs include clinical activity measures such as appointments, diagnostic indices based on clinical diagnosis or problem presentation, prescribing information, hospital links for the transfer of laboratory results and appointment bookings, and links with the local health authority to effect a rapid transfer of registration data. Most systems have a prevention display, adjusted for patients' age and sex, using 'headers' which appear on the screen during the consultation to alert the user to important information, such as eligibility for screening for the over-75 age group or drug allergies. This encourages proactive care and health promotion.

When patient diagnoses are entered using the READ system based on the international classification of diseases (Department of Health 1993), the health and therapeutic indices of patients can be closely monitored. A systematic search of the patient database using a READ code or defined sociodemographic characteristics can identify patients within a defined group and can be used as a disease register. The widespread use of computers for prescribing enables drug names to be used as key search words to identify patients with specific diagnoses. For example, a search using the names of commonly prescribed antidepressant drugs is more likely to identify patients treated for depression than using 'depression' as the key search word.

Full Report

Mrs. Marjorie Robertson	**02/11/1915**	**Female**	**NHS13456**	**Applied**

Address
12 View Hill London Se22 SE22 0RG

Communication numbers
Telephone - home 0171 567 1234

Problems

Atrial Fibrillation	Started: 14/07/2000	Ended:
Depression - management of	Started: 14/04/2000	Ended:
Heart failure	Started: 15/12/1999	Ended:
Currently Relevant	Started: 03/01/1996	Ended:

Allergy and Intolerance

27/04/1995	Allergy	Moderate	PENICILLIN V tabs 250mg

Medical History

26/06/2000	[V]Fitting or adjustment of cardiac pacemaker
14/05/2000	Atrial fibrillation and flutter
04/05/2000	Palpitations
14/04/2000	O/E - depressed
06/12/1999	Home visit elderly assessment

Repeat Masters

DIGOXIN tabs 125micrograms	Until: 15/11/2000	Last issued: 15/08/2000	Number of issues:	1 of 12
ONCE DAILY				
SERTRALINE tabs 50mg	Until: 15/11/2000	Last issued: 15/08/2000	Number of issues:	1 of 6
ONCE DAILY				
WARFARIN SODIUM tabs 3mg	Until: 03/10/2000	Last issued: 15/08/2000	Number of issues:	1 of 6
EVERY DAY				

Acute and Repeat Issue Therapy

17/02/2000	issued	CO-AMILOFRUSE tabs 2.5mg+20mg	Supply: (30) tablet(s)	IN THE MORNING

Consultation

26/06/2000	Discharge details	
25/05/2000	Letter from Outpatients	
14/05/2000	Surgery consultation	Dr. Jack Kerrush
04/05/2000	Surgery consultation	Dr. Jack Kerrush
14/04/2000	Out of hours, Practice	Dr. William Preston
15/12/1999	Acute visit	Miss Ellie Nabule
06/12/1999	Clinic	Miss Ellie Nabule

Blood pressure

04/05/2000	BP 190/110	recall due:
06/12/1999	BP 180/105	recall due:

Referrals and Requests
11/05/2000 Refer for Palpitations at Cardiology department of with
by: Dr. Jack Kerrush

Fig. 18.1 Computer display in GP surgery: sample medical history and therapy history. (Reproduced from the ViSion program by kind permission of VAMP Health.)

Problems of age–sex registers

Despite advances in information technology, problems occur with the maintenance of accurate age–sex registers—which are initially provided by the local health authority. Through direct computer links with primary care, the health authority centralizes patient registration data and forwards medical records when patients change doctors. Inaccuracies increase with the age of the population, due partly to increased mortality (Bowling and Jacobson 1989) and partly to errors in, or omission of, address notifications associated with population movement and new patient registrations. This leads to list inflation, in which patients are wrongly included when they have died or moved away. Such patients are untraceable and are referred to as 'ghosts'. Less of a problem

Full Report

Mrs. Marjorie Robertson **22/07/1921** **Female** **4628081042**

Address

Communication numbers
Telephone - home

Problems

Osteoarthritis	Started: 12/09/2001	Ended:
Chest Infections	Started: 05/10/2000	Ended:
Chronic Obstructive Pulmonary Disease	Started: 11/01/2000	Ended:
Currently Relevant	Started: 30/10/1995	Ended:

Advice Given
14/08/1996 Advice to patient - subject Advice GENERAL

Agencies
14/08/1996 Domiciliary services Dr. Jim Kelly

Diet
14/08/1996 Diet - patient initiated Eating habits: Good Type of diet:

Exercise
14/08/1996 Exercise grading Moderate X2 WEEKLY KCH OSTEOPOROSIS CLASS Dr. Jim Kelly

Hearing (over 75 years)
14/08/1996 O/E - hearing tested-8th nerve Treatment being received WEARS AID Dr. Jim Kelly

Mental cognitive
14/08/1996 O/E - state of mind Referral

Mental emotional state
14/08/1996 O/E - state of mind Referral Dr. Jim Kelly

Mobility level
14/08/1996 Mobile outside with aid Mobile outside with aid

Physical health
14/08/1996 Geriatric health exam. Treatment being received OSTEOPOROSIS C/O KCH Dr. Jim Kelly

Sleep pattern
14/08/1996 [D]Sleep disturbances Satisfactory Dr. Jim Kelly

Vision in the elderly
14/08/1996 Ophthalmological monitoring Satisfactory C/O OPTICIAN Dr. Jim Kelly

New Registration Consultation
17/01/2000 New patient screen Seen by: Dr. G Adam Clinician: Dr. S Woods

Over 75 years check
14/08/1996 Geriatric screening Seen by: Dr. Jim Kelly Clinician: Dr. H Tegner

Urinalysis - Glucose
14/08/1996 Urine test for glucose Nil

Urinalysis - Protein
14/08/1996 Urine protein test Nil

Allowances received - Elderly
14/08/1996 OAP PENSION

Carers - elderly
14/08/1996 Domiciliary services MANAGES ALL OWN DOMESTIC CHORES & GARDEN

Foot care
14/08/1996 Feet examination ATTENDS THE SURGERY

Next of kin - elderly
14/08/1996 Relation: Other relative MRS VERONICA CASE - DAUGHTER IN LAW

Optician last seen
14/08/1996 Seen by optician 1994

Risk factors - elderly
14/08/1996 Risk factors: Yes HYPERTENSION (TREATED) - OSTEOPOROSIS

Hygiene - elderly
14/08/1996 Geriatric health exam. Hygeine Home: Good Personal: Good

Fig. 18.2 Computer display in GP surgery: sample prevention history. (Reproduced from the ViSion program by kind permission of VAMP.)

is list deflation, where care is provided for patients but names have been omitted from the register due to administrative errors. Some patients may have moved within the practice area but have failed to notify their change of address. Patient turnover is variable and is higher in inner-city areas. A study of patients aged 75 years and over observed a turnover of 13% in one year, in addition to a 10% death rate (Graham and Livesley 1986). Bowling and Jacobson (1989) using the Health Authority list of a deprived inner city area found that addresses were inaccurate for half the patients aged 65–74 years, two-fifths of those aged 75–84 years, and two-thirds of those aged 85 years and over. The implications of such errors in health screening programmes, population surveys, and research is considerable in terms of time expenditure, and the accuracy of denominator values used in epidemiological studies.

'At-risk' groups

A universal approach to screening and monitoring has tended to distract attention from the usefulness of focusing care on 'at risk' groups of elderly people. Patients who are non-consulters have been studied in detail to discover whether they are an at-risk population. Of patients aged 75 years and over who had not consulted their GP in the previous year, just over 50% who were visited needed action for simple and remediable conditions (Williams 1998). Other studies (Ebrahim *et al.* 1984) found few unreported problems and concluded that non-consulters constituted a health elite. Selected screening of elderly patients to identify those most 'at-risk' was pioneered by Barber *et al.* (1980), using a postal questionnaire to patients aged 70 years and over which focused on medicosocial problems. This eliminated 20% of patients who had no at-risk factors. The remainder were seen by their GPs, of whom 91% were found to have problems requiring attention. Freer (1987) recommended opportunistic consultation-based screening of elderly patients using a modification of Barber's questionnaire: with the use of this instrument they found that less than 30% of screened patients required follow-up.

The detection of mental illness in elderly patients

The possibility of early detection of psychiatric disorder was explored in studies of general practice patients aged 65 years and over in Newcastle-upon-Tyne (Bergmann 1981). The research team encouraged the early referral of patients by their GPs. This produced a referral rate of 2.8% in the practice population aged 65 years and over. An epidemiological approach using a screening questionnaire with the same population found a total prevalence of 21.9% estimated psychiatric morbidity. The conclusion drawn was that GPs referred only those patients who were very ill, and that, generally, the proportion of known cases was very low. Most surveys suggest that about 80% of elderly people who live in the community do not suffer from a disabling psychiatric disorder. It is possible to define the vulnerable groups from epidemiological and other research to include: older people aged 75 years and over; those who live alone; older people recently bereaved; those recently discharged from hospital; those requiring home help and community services; those asking for residential care; those planning to give up their homes for any other reason (Bergmann and Jacoby 1983); those who have moved home within the last two years; and those who are divorced or separated (Taylor *et al.* 1983).

The epidemiology of mental illness in general practice

The prevalence of mental illness in the community is difficult to establish because of variations in screening criteria and the populations screened. Over 7% of people of all age groups consulted their GP about mental illness, with consulting rates increasing with age (RCGP 1995). Medical services deal only with the visible tip of the 'iceberg' of mental illness and handicap. Using the prevalence rates found in the Newcastle-upon-Tyne study of patients aged 65 years and over who lived at home (Kay *et al.* 1964), a GP with a list of 2000 patients of whom 300 are aged 65 years and over could expect: 30 (10%) with an organic brain syndrome; 93 (31%) with a functional disorder, of whom 78 (26%) would suffer an affective disorder; 6 (2.0%) with schizophrenia, paraphrenia, and paranoid states; and a further 8 (2.6%) with other disorders such as mental subnormality, marked personality deviations, or hypochondriasis. Clarke *et al.* (1984) showed that organic brain disorders may be less common, with a prevalence of 1.6% in a large general practice survey. National morbidity statistics from general practice show that dementia is associated with an annual incidence of 1.6 new patients per GP, an annual prevalence of 3.6 patients consulting per GP per year, and an annual workload of 7.4 consultations per GP (RCGP 1995).

The presentation of mental illness in general practice

Despite the substantial psychiatric morbidity found on screening, most psychiatric illness appears to be 'invisible ' to GPs (Williamson *et al.* 1964, Goldberg and Bridges 1987). Williamson found that of people aged 65 years and over, 87% of those who suffered from dementia, 71% of those with depression, 61% of those with neurosis, and 25% of those with paranoid states did not have the diagnosis recorded in the general practice notes. Yet a study of patients aged over 65 attending a surgery found that less than 12% of patients aged 65 years and over were undiagnosed for depression by their GPs, although this excluded non-consulters and the housebound (Macdonald 1986).

Patients with psychiatric illness, therefore, tend not to present to care, and when they do, the GP does not always suspect, or record, the diagnosis. The significance of undetected depression has recently been questioned, and research into the outcome of depression has yielded conflicting results. Non-recognition of depression has failed to show serious measurable effects on outcome (Goldberg *et al.* 1998). A diagnosis of depression should be seen as a marker of the severity of the depression (Dowrick and Buchan 1995). General practitioner problems relating to the diagnostic omission of depression include the lack of clear diagnostic criteria, and the time constraints of an average doctor–patient consultation of 8 minutes in which a complex mix of medical, psychological, and social problems have to be addressed. Despite the difficulties in the detection of mental illness, psychiatric problems in elderly patients commonly present to the GP in a variety of ways.

Affective disorders

Patients who suffer from affective disorders may present with mood change, anxiety, poor appetite, sleep disturbance, and the expression of negative statements. Frequent surgery attendances for multiple symptoms suggest hypochondriasis and anxiety states. Older patients are more likely than younger patients to present with somatic symptoms when they are psychologically unwell. The multiple pathology of advancing age encourages somatization, especially when associated with underlying mood disturbance. Patients' problems may be presented by relatives who express anxiety over changed behaviour, observed mood swings, or reduced social responsiveness. Sometimes it is the GP who detects depression through a patient's apparent mood changes over successive consultations, or through casual requests for treatment.

Examples of common presentations include:

(1) A depressed 87-year-old feels 'out-of-sorts' and wants a 'tonic'.
(2) 'Stronger sleeping tablets' are requested through the receptionist by an elderly housebound patient who lives alone and who insists that the previous medication no longer works. On visiting, the patient is found to be lonely and depressed.
(3) Repeated requests by an ambulant patient 'to do away with me because I'm a burden to everyone' suggests an underlying depression.

The clustering of mental illness episodes around major life events (Murphy 1982) in which there is a sense of loss: notably bereavement, but also moving home, and loss of function and independence (for example, through strokes (House 1987), myocardial infarction, or amputation), makes elderly patients particularly likely to present at such times. Grief, stress, and emotional pain associated with these events, or their anniversaries, may lead to obvious sadness and depression, exacerbation of coexistent disease, or an increase in psychosomatic symptoms, particularly those which reflect illness in the ' lost' relative. The following history is illustrative:

Case 1

An 80-year-old widow consulted with exacerbation of longstanding tinnitus and a feeling of being 'drained'. She added that the following day was the anniversary of her husband's death and she would visit the cemetery. She left without treatment, commenting that she felt better for talking as she always felt so alone.

Major personal illness, physical deterioration (Murphy 1982), and an inability to perform activities of daily living (Iliffe *et al.* 1993) are associated with concomitant depression, as are viral infections (especially influenza) and frequent falls (Vetter and Ford 1989). Excessive alcohol intake can mask depression, although Dewar and Jones (1990) demonstrated in their community survey that heavy consumption tended to be in those with least physical, mental, and social disability. Social problems may signify underlying mental illness through requests for rehousing, for help with marital or family relationships, or through failure to cope with day-to-day activities.

Acute confusional states

Emergency visits to elderly patients with acute delirium are generally made at the request of alarmed relatives or neighbours. They are usually associated with acute physical illness and nearly always require emergency admission of the patient for investigation. Common acute causes in general practice are pneumonia, urinary tract infections, severe congestive cardiac failure, dehydration, drug toxicity, and metabolic causes such as diabetic ketoacidosis. Subacute presentation can occur with a subdural haematoma following a recent fall—which may not be mentioned by the patient.

Case 2

An 84-year-old sufferer from Parkinson's disease, which was well controlled on levodopa, suddenly became confused with visual hallucinations. Careful inspection of his medication found that he had been prescribed a double dose of levodopa in error. Omission of the tablets for three days before resuming the lower dose resulted in remission.

Psychotic illness

Elderly patients with delusions, hallucinations, and persecutory ideas are more likely to suffer from depressive illness, although a minority will have schizophrenia or paraphrenia. The GP may detect ideas of reference, or paranoia, often involving neighbours, when conversing with the patient. Sometimes, inconsistencies in the history will alert the GP to a delusional state, as illustrated in the following histories:

Case 3

A 68-year-old patient who lived alone and was independent in self-care requested repeated home visits for recurrent ill-defined abdominal pains which had been diagnosed as irritable bowel syndrome. She attributed each episode of pain to her noisy next-door neighbours whose voices, heard through the adjoining wall, accused her of various misdemeanours. The story seemed convincing until it was observed that she lived in an end-of-terrace house and had no neighbours. She was subsequently diagnosed as suffering from paraphrenia, and responded to treatment with thioridazine.

Case 4

An 87-year-old woman who lived alone as a lodger in a family house developed persecutory ideas about her landlady who, she thought, wanted to get rid of her. She imagined people in her living room who sometimes tried to take her away. She also confused day with night. The landlady asked her GP to visit because she was wandering around the house at night. She had lost 13 kg in weight, and had a haemoglobin of 8 g per 100 ml. Further investigation found no active physical disease. She was diagnosed as having a paranoid psychotic illness which subsequently improved on trifluoperazine.

Behaviour disorders and personality changes

General practice contains a small number of elderly patients who are eccentric, or who have difficult or aggressive personalities. Sometimes reclusive patients pose problems of non-compliance, particularly if they are ill and refusing help from neighbours and the primary health care team. Unravelling the ethical implications of these situations is challenging, particularly when patients with no demonstrable cognitive impairment fully accept the consequences of their decisions to refuse care, or to live in unhygienic or unheated homes. A psychiatric opinion lends support to the GP, particularly if use of statutory procedures such as Section 47 of the National Assistance Act 1948 is being considered.

Dementia

The diagnosis of dementia is obscured by its insidiousness, and by the lack of insight in the sufferer. Familiarity with patients in general practice encourages a less-critical appraisal of the clinical situation in routine consultations, which can lead to a missed diagnosis. Population screening for dementia in the over-65s is not recommended—a case-finding approach being preferred (Eccles *et al.* 1998). A high index of suspicion and a proactive approach using diagnostic guidelines increases the diagnostic yield and facilitates appropriate selection for referral (Van Hout *et al.* 2000).

A history of loss of functioning in daily activities is a better indicator than complaints of memory loss (Eccles *et al.* 1998). Unreliable histories, a dishevelled appearance, failure to recognize the doctor after years of interactive personal care, non-compliance with treatment in a previously compliant patient, hoarding of medication, and a poor coping ability at home evident on visiting all suggest dementia. Suspicions recorded in patients' notes help prompt further evaluation at subsequent contacts, and aid earlier diagnosis.

Indirect presentation of a demented patient is common and is the cue for the GP to take constructive action. Relatives or neighbours may consult, expressing concern about a patient's increasing memory loss, reduced social responsiveness, unaccounted financial expenditure, or vulnerability to fraud. A deteriorating home situation may be described in which forgetfulness leads to domestic disasters such as flooding, gas leaks, kitchen fires from burnt-out cooking utensils, or security problems with unlocked doors and windows. Key workers, such as receptionists or community pharmacists, may report difficulties in patients' management of repeat prescribing. The district nurse may observe disorientation of a patient visited for other needs, or a health visitor may report a family crisis precipitated by failure to cope with a person suffering from undiagnosed dementia, as illustrated in the following history:

Case 5

A young mother with a 5-month-old baby was visited at home by her health visitor who noted postnatal depression. Before the birth, the mother had been so concerned about her father's memory loss that without seeking advice she had taken him in to live in their two-bedroom, local-authority rented flat. The strain of caring for her baby and her confused father in overcrowded conditions proved too difficult. Referral of her father to the department of old age psychiatry confirmed the diagnosis of Alzheimer's dementia. Attendance by the father at a day centre and rehousing of the family led to remission of the mother's depression.

Management of the patient with dementia

The GP as diagnostician

As the diagnosis of dementia is often based on guess-work, non-demented patients may be given a diagnosis of cognitive impairment in error. General practitioners are often reluctant to use brief cognitive tests and to question relatives of patients who appear to be demented for fear of causing distress (O'Connor *et al.* 1993). The initial assessment includes a careful history from the patient, the carer, and information from the patient's notes. It is usually possible to differentiate the slow progression of Alzheimer's dementia from the sudden deterioration in memory or coping ability of multi-infarct dementia, which is often associated with a history of stroke or transient ischaemic episodes. A search for a reversible cause of dementia at the initial assessment is important. A history of a recent fall suggests the possibility of a subdural haematoma and, if suspected, immediate referral to a geriatrician or neurologist should be made. A review of medication, to include drugs prescribed within the practice and by emergency medical or specialist services, may identify an incorrect dosage which is causing intellectual impairment. Sedatives, tranquillizers, anti-parkinsonian agents, and hypotensives are among offending drugs. Adjustment or withdrawal of these will clarify the diagnosis. Depression masquerading as dementia ('pseudo-dementia') should be considered and, if suspected, a trial of antidepressants is indicated. Normal-pressure hydrocephalus, hypothyroidism presenting as dementia, syphilis, hypercalcaemia, and vitamin deficiencies as the cause of, rather than the result of, dementia are rarities in practice. A physical examination of the patient, particularly to detect anaemia, cardiac disorders, neurological evidence of previous stroke, and undiagnosed malignancy, is essential. Baseline investigations to include a full blood count, erythrocyte sedimentation rate, biochemistry, thyroid function tests, and syphilis serology provide a good medical evaluation prior to further assessment, although the results are more likely to detect coexistent medical pathology than aid the differential diagnosis of dementia. The correction of iron- or vitamin-deficient anaemias, the control of cardiac arrhythmias, and treatment of hypothyroidism is good medical practice, but there is a risk of the GP diverting clinical interest into 'medicalization of the patient' rather than confronting the management of the underlying dementia.

The main decision to be taken at this stage is whether to refer the patient for further assessment and management. This depends on local service provision, and whether the patient lives alone or with a family or carers who are available, able, and willing to provide care. Exploring the feelings of patients and carers, and consideration of the available options, supplemented by an assessment of the patient's needs by the district or community nurse, provides a sound preparation before taking decisions. The advantages of early referral to an old age psychiatry service include: early confirmation of the diagnosis without duplication of investigations in general practice; ease of planning appropriate support services, including day care; greater carer satisfaction through reassurance that the problem has been thoroughly addressed; and the early familiarity with the home situation by professional staff, to facilitate management of future crises. If the patient can be accompanied by a carer who can confirm the history, referral to an old age psychiatry outpatient department, multidisciplinary assessment clinic, or memory clinic is the preferred approach of some clinicians. Others recommend an initial domiciliary visit to the patient in the presence of relatives and the GP to supplement the presentation of the problem, and allow discussion of a suitable care plan. As a consequence of increased emphasis on community services, specialist 'outreach' clinics in old age psychiatry have been established in some general practices. These are more convenient than hospital outpatient visits and less distressing for both patient and carer.

Case 6

The warden of a sheltered housing unit requested a GP to visit an 81-year-old female resident who had been 'going down-hill' mentally for the past few weeks with memory loss, intermittent confusion, incontinence, and difficulty with self-care. The patient had a past history of atrial fibrillation and transient ischaemic episodes from cerebral emboli, and had been commenced on warfarin. The warden recalled a fall six weeks earlier, after which the patient had been examined at hospital and reassured that no injury had occurred. Re-referral for further investigation resulted in the detection of chronic bilateral subdural haematomas on CT scan, with no cerebral atrophy. Following surgery, her confusion cleared. Despite only a partial recovery of her memory, she was again able to cope alone.

Long-term management of patients with dementia

The GP, as the leader of the primary health care team, is responsible for coordinating and directing the long-term clinical management of patients with dementia. Social services departments are responsible for the social care and support of the patient. Care should be tailored to the needs and circumstances of individual patients and carers, and should be multifactorial in approach. The aims of care are to: manage the patient at home for as long as possible; treat underlying medical conditions or disability; support the carers (both formal and informal); and manage behaviour and relationship problems.

General practitioner knowledge of the availability and the limitations of community care in the patient's locality are important. Whether the patient lives alone or with relatives, and the extent to which relatives can cope with the stress of caring, influences outcome. Apart from home care assistants, statutory and voluntary services play minor roles in supporting patients in the home (Jones *et al.* 1983) as most community care is undertaken by lay workers (Luker and Perkins 1987).

The success of maintaining the patient at home depends on the quality of the relationship with the carer. Of the supporters of elderly people living alone, 42% were prepared to accept permanent residential care for them compared with 5% of supporters who had been living with the old person for 50 years or more. The likelihood of being supported when one is demented is increased if one has been living with a person for a very long time—an average of 36 years (Bergmann and Jacoby 1983).

Involvement of the community nurse at the outset, regardless of whether the patient lives alone or with carers, provides a multidisciplinary approach to identifying the needs of both patient and carers. Respecting the limitations of carers, identifying how each person can contribute, and knowing which services can supplement care are important. Support services include: social services for home care assistants, meals-on-wheels, clubs and carer support groups, advice on financial benefits, and respite care; physiotherapy or occupational therapy for aids and adaptations; voluntary-sector sitting services and contact with self-help groups such as the Alzheimer's Disease Society. Dependence on services will be greater where a patient lives alone. The aim should be to provide daily contact with the home. If a patient living alone suffers from severe dementia, it may be necessary to abandon community care after a short trial and arrange for admission to residential care.

Regular visits by the GP, community nurse, or health visitor will enable continuing review of the patient, support the carers, and monitor the need for further intervention. Distressing problems arising with the progression of dementia include sleep disturbance, nocturnal wandering and shouting, incontinence, and immobility. The prescription of a night tranquillizer such as clomethiazole, 1–2 capsules, helps to reduce nocturnal disturbance or, at lower doses, to control daytime agitation. Advice on regular toileting to encourage continence and, if incontinence is a problem, the provision of aids such as pads, pants, and protective mattress sheets are available through the community nursing services. Referral to the community physiotherapist and occupational therapist for assessment, including provision of aids and appliances, will assist with problems of mobility.

The 1993 community care reforms placed increased emphasis on care at home, with social services assuming responsibility for assessing patients' care and social needs in contrast with the previous service-led provision. This enables elderly people to live in their own home through the provision of day care, domiciliary care, and respite care. Welfare benefits are intended to help defray the costs of caring for a person with a disability. They include: Disability Living Allowance with care and mobility components for those aged under 65 years; Attendance Allowance if aged over 65 with special rules if terminally ill; Housing Benefit; Invalid Care Allowance for carers aged between 16–65 who are spending at least 35 hours weekly caring for a severely disabled person; Income Support; and Council Tax benefits (Department of Social Security 2000). The Orange Badge Scheme of parking concessions allows people with severe mobility to park close to shops and will help the carer to retain greater freedom.

The treatment of underlying coexisting medical conditions in addition to dementia should be continued if supervision is available. The continuation of drugs for treating hypertension in patients with vascular dementia is controversial, with some clinicians claiming it is difficult to justify (Whalley 1989). Others maintain a contrary view. General practitioners are sometimes swayed by pharmaceutical companies to prescribe new drugs which have been used for the prevention or relief of dementia, but it is recommended that GPs do not initiate therapy in dementing patients (Eccles *et al.* 1998). There is no convincing evidence that these are effective.

The demented patient who lives alone

Caring for elderly demented patients who live alone poses special problems, and is usually only possible through the goodwill of neighbours. Because access to the home is unreliable, arrangements should be made with neighbours for them to hold emergency keys. Neighbours are reassured by contact with the GP and by discussion about when to request help. Unless carers or the community nurse can supervise drugs it is injudicious to continue prescribing. Single, demented patients may cause concern over security, and personal road and home safety. The local police welcome information about these vulnerable residents and this is particularly encouraged if there is a local neighbourhood security scheme. When eventually these patients require admission to a protected environment, a residential care or nursing home is more appropriate than a sheltered housing unit in which the need to familiarize with new surrounding and still live independently will accentuate confusion.

Case 7

A demented 84-year-old woman who had no relatives lived alone with difficulty. The social services arranged admission to a nearby sheltered housing unit. Within a short time she appeared more confused, her room became squalid, she roamed the streets, and was frequently returned by the police. She developed paranoid behaviour, attacked several residents, and was formally admitted to hospital under Section 2 of the Mental Health Act. She was subsequently transferred to a nursing home for the elderly mentally infirm. It would have been more appropriate to have admitted her there directly from her own home after careful assessment, rather than into sheltered housing.

Caring for the carers—the role of the GP

General practitioners have a vital role in supporting carers. The majority of carers perceive that of all health service employees, GPs have the greatest power to improve their lives (Carers Association 1998). While most GPs are aware of this, they frequently fail to confront the difficulties carers face. A survey of elderly dependants living in the community found the following effects on carers: one-quarter felt their health to be adversely affected; one-quarter felt their social life was impaired; one-sixth felt their family life had suffered; and almost one-fifth, especially daughters, reported unbearable stress (Kings Fund Carers Unit 1989; Jones and Peters 1992). Carers need information about services and benefits, despite the limited availability of financial support (Department of Health 1999*c*). Receptionists and health-promotion nurses may be approached for information and they should have access to a regularly updated directory of local services, which should include National Health Service, local authority, and voluntary and private sector provision. Most areas have carer support groups but, although they are generally perceived as beneficial and helpful, they do not reduce the burden or alter the stress of looking after someone with a dementing illness (Eccles *et al.* 1998).

At a personal level, carers expect realistic information about dementia, the implications of the diagnosis and its prognosis, and how to make best use of the available facilities. Services should be adapted to individual circumstances and the needs of the carer and the patient, with regard to differing racial, cultural, and religious backgrounds. The carer should be accepted as a contributing member of the care team, and effective communication encouraged through discussion and the keeping of clear, concise records. For housebound patients, a shared-care record retained in the home to which all involved in care are invited to contribute regularly, will maintain continuity and improve communication.

The mental and physical health of carers is paramount if community care is to be a realistic, long-term possibility. Usually the carer and the carer's family are registered with the practice and, as it is the family who bear the major burden of caring for elderly people, the GP is the pivotal support for the family unit. This role should include advice to carers on their personal health, acknowledging the carers' crucial contributions and problems, and emotional support by counselling the carer on their attitudes and expectations. The stress experienced by carers who look after demented elderly patients has been shown to lead to psychiatric morbidity (Argyle *et al.* 1985), in addition to common physical problems such as tiredness, musculoskeletal strains, and insomnia caused by heavy physical demands. Carers of people with psychiatric disorders, particularly women carers, have an increased risk of depression (Livingston *et al.* 1996). Referral to the community nurse to teach the practical skills needed for home nursing and to reassure carers that correct procedures have been adopted will minimize physical strain. Vigilance by the GP to detect early signs of strain or poor coping will help avert crises.

How well a carer copes depends on her personality, health, and the quality of the premorbid relationship with the dependent person (Anderson 1987). Carers experience a 'living bereavement'. Recognition of the importance to the carer of clinging to memories, and of maintaining the appearance of the patient as an expression of success in the carer's role, will improve morale and self-esteem.

Respite care

Carers are at risk of increasing isolation and exhaustion through the intensity of their 24-hour responsibility. To prevent this and to delay institutionalization, the GP should emphasize the value of relief care on a daily basis provided by day centres or sitting services, and in the long term by the rotation of care with other family members or through planned regular admissions to respite beds in residential care or hospital. Since the introduction of the Community Care Act statutory service providers are required to assist and support carers, and health authorities are required to finance respite care (Department of Health 1995). Respite care is arranged by referral to social services by the patient's carer or GP, and should be planned in advance to enable relatives to book holidays. Although respite admission provides an opportunity for multidisciplinary assessment of the patient, and may delay institutionalization of the patient, it does not seem to reduce the overall burden of the carer (Eccles *et al.* 1998). Heavily dependent patients may need regular admissions, for example, for two out of every six weeks, to ease the strain. Relatives appreciate the opportunity of visiting the home or hospital beforehand to gain confidence in the staff and the surroundings. Otherwise, the family may have reservations about delegating care to staff who are less familiar with the patient's condition than themselves. However, although many carers perceived relief admission to be beneficial to many aspects of their lives (Pearson 1988), and expressed a wish for more respite care, there has been no observable improvement in their emotional well-being (Homer and Gilleard 1994).

Disadvantages for the carer include difficulties of visiting patients in hospital, and feelings of sadness, loneliness, or even guilt. The possible risk of increased mortality from bronchopneumonia (Rae *et al.* 1986) should be discussed with the carer, although Howarth *et al.* (1990) found that this was not significant. However, some carers refuse offers of help or, indeed, any support. Others may stoically underplay the strain of caring, and deny the seriousness of the illness in their relative. The outlook in such situations is poor. The GP, however, should be aware of possible underlying depression in the carer as an explanation of this behaviour. The following history illustrates this:

Case 8

A 68-year-old married woman who had refused help in the care of her demented husband was admitted to hospital after taking an overdose of sleeping tablets. On recovery, she was found to be depressed. She commented that she could think of no other solution to coping with her sick husband. Her depression responded well to antidepressants, and she eventually agreed to her husband attending a day centre.

Situations which require hospital admission

A point may be reached when the carer is no longer willing, or able, to cope. Increasing debility of the patient outstrips the tolerance of the carer and is particularly likely to occur when sleep disturbance, incontinence, and general immobility are problems (Sanford 1975). The patient then requires long-term care. Awareness of elder abuse is important as a symptom of strain in the carer. If suspected, the GP should refer to social services for an assessment for transfer to a place of safety in hospital or residential care.

Acute admissions occur when the carer unexpectedly becomes ill, or when a mildly demented patient who lives alone suffers a self-limiting illness which, under normal circumstances, would not require admission. In some areas 'Hospital at home' schemes are available and may be more appropriate. They provide comprehensive nursing at home for people who would traditionally have been cared for in hospital. Out-of-hours emergency calls by relatives who infrequently visit a mildly demented patient living alone and insist that 'something must be done' before their return home, is not an uncommon crisis, and can be an expression of their own guilt.

General practitioners and specialist services

General practice acts as a filter to specialist medical services. Although factors such as the clinical skills and interests of doctors, the availability of specialist services, and patients' expectations influence referral rates, there is substantial variation in the referral rates of individual GPs, with rates varying up to 20-fold (Moore and Roland 1989). Much of the variation in mental health services has been shown to be associated with population demographics, morbidity, and the effect of provider differences within secondary care (Melzer *et al.* 1999). The restructuring of the NHS has brought about a shift of resources from hospital to community, with community-based mental health teams now widespread in the UK. Locality commissioning of specialist services by the recently established primary care groups and trusts has powers and responsibilities to develop health care strategies for local populations. The range of services include primary care-based specialist clinics, community mental health centres, community 'shifted' outpatient or 'outreach' clinics, and domiciliary visiting by a psychiatrist or community psychiatric nurse (Goldberg and Jackson 1992; RCGP 1993). Community care is popular with patients and should allow the GP to be involved with patient management. However, in a study of specialist outreach clinics there was no increased interaction between specialists and GPs (Bailey *et al.* 1994). Community psychiatric nurses in general practice have been identified as providing primarily patient support and patient assessment in 46% and 13% of referrals, respectively (Briscoe and Wilkinson 1989). Domiciliary visiting may be arranged directly at the request of the GP and a hospital- or community-based specialist, or it may be incorporated into a practice-based outreach clinic for patients who cannot attend hospital or the surgery on medical grounds and who need a diagnosis or treatment. They are costly in time and resources, and it is questionable whether the same management outcome could be achieved by telephone consultation between the GP and the specialist. Domiciliary consultations can be helpful in the following situations: the assessment of patients in difficult home circumstances; where there is unwillingness of patients or carers to take up care recommendations; the initial evaluation of a patient recently presenting with significant memory impairment; an assessment under the Mental Health Act; or, clarification of the appropriateness of care by an old age psychiatrist or geriatrician where symptom overlap occurs. Referral to a geriatrician is indicated, if, in addition to psychiatric symptoms, the patient is acutely ill, especially if the patient is confused or if a life-threatening physical illness is present.

Case 9

A woman of 83 years who has lost contact with her family lives alone in a bed-sit. flat. Another lodger, a 48-year-old unemployed man who drinks excessively, repeatedly requests visits from the GP because of his concern over her deteriorating health and the need for rehousing. She suffers from maturity-onset diabetes (apparently controlled by diet), iron-deficiency anaemia, and episodes of congestive cardiac failure with fluctuating levels of confusion. Her accommodation is filthy and her appearance neglected, yet she shops regularly for her pension and food for herself and the other lodger. She has refused a home-care assistant and meals-on-wheels. Social services report that she is capable of making her own decisions, but are concerned about possible physical abuse by the lodger. Admissions to the geriatric unit for acute illness have resulted in self-discharge before a psychiatric assessment has been arranged. At a routine visit, her GP notes her poor performance on a mental test and arranges a domiciliary visit by a psychiatrist, who considers that she has only minimal mental impairment. She agrees to visits by the community psychiatric nurse and to attend the psychiatric day unit for further assessment.

Hospital communication

The success of a patient's rehabilitation following hospital discharge depends on the adequacy and timing of information provided to the GP at the time of discharge. Initial notification by telephone or facsimile (fax) in advance is more likely to encourage an early home visit by the GP than if only a letter is sent. Prompt discharge letters should include information on the patient's care needs, particularly in relation to community services and carer support, medication, general condition, and follow-up requirements. Sending discharge letters with patients to be handed to the GP is unreliable, especially when patients have poor mobility, live alone, or suffer memory loss. Williams and Fitton (1990) in a study of the causes of re-admission of elderly patients, found that lack of discharge information to the GP was three times more common than failure of the GP to visit a recently discharged patient after notification.

Good specialist communication from outpatient departments and day-hospitals is essential for continuity of care (RCP 1994). First attendances, discharges, a change in the treatment or condition of a patient should be reported, as should the annual progress of patients attending for long-term care. Letters should summarize the findings at consultation, should contain an assessment and management plan, and have educational value for the GP (Westerman *et al.* 1990).

When patients are discharged or managed in outpatient departments, effective liaison between hospital staff and GPs is essential when patient medication is initiated or changed. For patients under consultant supervision, medication should normally be prescribed in hospital and dispensed in the hospital pharmacy for not less than 14 days at discharge, or after referral to and treatment in outpatient units. In situations where the consultant requests that the GP should continue treating, the consultant should give the GP prior notification, in adequate time, of the patient's diagnosis and details of drug therapy. The doctor who signs the prescription has the legal responsibility for the consequences of drug treatment, and must not prescribe without adequate clinical information. It is therefore unacceptable for hospital staff to expect GPs to do so (Department of Health 1991).

Intermediate care

The development of care schemes that are intermediate between acute hospital care and long-term institutional care has led to a range of alternative provision. Further expansion of these are planned (Pollock 2000). Many schemes involve specialists in the medicine and psychiatry of old age in the direct provision of care, or in advising on care protocols or planning. This involves cooperative working with other agencies, including primary care groups, social services, and the voluntary and private sectors. For acute care, recent developments aim to bridge the hospital trusts and the local authorities and may include innovative services such as 'hospital at home' or 'supported discharge' schemes in which the patient is discharged early from hospital and supported by intensive home nursing. 'Rapid response' services may be available to support acutely ill patients at home and prevent admission. There is evidence that hospital-at-home care is an effective complementary form of health care that is acceptable to both patients and carers. However, its cost-effectiveness is uncertain and the provision of hospital-at-home schemes is variable (Corrado 2000). An alternative to acute hospital admission is the use of small community hospitals or nursing homes in which inpatient care is provided by GPs and multidisciplinary teams who usually have recourse to specialist advice. This is a useful option when insufficient home care or community support makes continuing home care untenable, particularly when mentally impaired patients require acute generalist care or rehabilitation. Although community hospitals are more a feature of rural practice, innovative projects in urban areas have led to the establishment of community care centres (Higgs 1985) which offer inpatient and rehabilitation facilities. Many of these offer day-hospital provision under the supervision of the patient's own GP.

Rehabilitation, continuing-care schemes, and palliative care may be provided by community outreach teams, or domiciliary and outpatient therapy services as alternatives to day-hospital or inpatient care. Respite care is nowadays more likely to be provided in the patient's own home, by care staff from social or voluntary services, or in a local nursing home as alternatives to hospital admission.

Residential care

Residential care includes nursing homes and residential care homes. Of the total places, 48% are provided by the independent sector, 29% by independent nursing homes, and 22% by local authority homes. In homes for elderly people, it was reported that 31% were for residents with learning difficulties and 13% were for elderly mentally infirm people or those with mental illness (Department of Health 1999*d*). The independent sector provides 91% of all places in residential homes. Of the population aged over 65 years, 9% live in residential care outside hospital, although this varies across the country (OPCS 1993). Since the introduction in 1993 of the NHS and Community Care Act 1990 there is a statutory requirement for social services to undertake a preadmission assessment. Patients or their relatives seeking admission to a home apply for a 'needs assessment' using a standard referral form from their local health authority. Residential homes arrange for local GPs to register residents as patients for the provision of general medical services, which include acute and long-term care and the implementation of preventive health measures such as annual immunization against influenza. A policy statement by the British Geriatric Society (1990) recommended that patients should have their personal choice of doctor and, where possible, maintenance of the relationship with their previous GP. Large numbers of elderly people in residential care suffer high levels of physical dependency and depression, which result in increased consultation, prescribing, and referral rates for the GP (Andrew 1988). A doubling of workload for patients in nursing homes compared to other patients over the age of 74 years has been recorded (Carlisle 1999). A study on elderly people in residential care found a prevalence of 28% for depression and 87% for dementia in local authority homes, and 35% for depression and 74% for dementia in private and voluntary sector accommodation (Harrison *et al.* 1990). Few depressed patients in residential care receive appropriate management. The outcome of depression in residents can be improved by enhancing the clinical skills of GPs and care staff, and by providing depression-related health education and activity programmes (Llewellyn-Jones *et al.* 1999).

Terminal illness at home

A GP can expect an average of 20 deaths from the list each year, of which about one-quarter will be at home (OPCS 1994). Most of these will be older patients, some of whom will suffer from mental illness. In the last year of life patients develop most of their symptoms at home. It is the GP who coordinates their care, both for those who die at home, and, in the time preceding admission, for those who die in hospital. About 70% of demented elderly people die from bronchopneumonia, a finding confirmed on postmortem (Burns *et al.* 1990), while sudden death (for example, from cardiovascular disease, pulmonary embolus, septicaemia) accounts for 30%. When a patient with dementia becomes ill with a respiratory infection, the GP should discuss the poor prognosis with relatives and discover their preference for home or hospital care. Of increasing interest to the public is the making of an advance directive about future health, in which a patient declares that life-saving measures should not be instituted should he or she develop irreversible cognitive impairment or other advanced disease (Doyal 1995). However, only a minority of GPs were aware of the recommended code of practice for making living wills (Collins 1999). The organization EXIT advises that patients inform their GP of their decision to make an advanced directive, and a copy of the statement should be filed with their health records. As competence to complete an advance directive involves understanding possible future clinical situations, the GP may be asked to assess a patient before he/she writes their directive (Fazel 1999).

Whatever the mental status of a patient, the principles of good terminal care apply. These include: mouth care, the control of distressing symptoms such as pain, or retained upper respiratory tract secretions; the involvement of community nurses; and the need for emotional support. Despite the long-term opportunity of adjusting to dementia as a fatally progressive disease, the intensity and intimacy of caring leaves the main carer bereft of a role after a patient's death. An expected sense of relief may be dominated by a bereavement requiring much consolation and counselling, yet such support from primary care is not always forthcoming. Although recently advocated as an area of prevention in primary care, practices are divided over whether bereavement support should be proactive or reactive (Harris and Kendrick 1998).

Prescribing in general practice

NHS expenditure on drugs, dressings, and appliances prescribed by GPs is rising annually, although the main increases have been in lipid-lowering drugs and antipsychotic agents. To offset these increases, GPs are urged to increase their generic rather than proprietary prescribing rates. In 1997 generic prescribing accounted for an average of 60% of drugs (Department of Health 1997). Nurse prescribing schemes are also being piloted in general practice. Longitudinal trends in prescribing for non-institutionalized elderly patients aged 65 years and over have shown an increase in the number of drugs prescribed (Rumble and Morgan 1994), This study demonstrated a positive association between age and the number of drugs taken. While the use of anxiolytics declined, the taking of hypnotics increased over the 4 years of the study. Sleep disorders in elderly patients are the most common reason for prescribing central nervous system-acting drugs in general practice. Cartwright and Smith (1988) showed that 15% of people aged over 65 years were taking sedatives and hypnotics, 90% of whom had been started on their medication outside hospital. The side-effects of hypnotic drugs include accentuated acute sedation through enhanced central nervous system sensitivity, and unwanted residual sedation with postural instability and impaired cognitive and psychomotor performance. The need for these drugs, particularly the benzodiazepines, should be questioned before prescribing because of their potential for physical and psychological dependence, and tolerance.

Medication should be considered only when insomnia is severe, disabling, or causing extreme distress and should be prescribed in short courses of 2–4 weeks only (*British National Formulary* 2000). Hypnotics should be prescribed in short courses and small doses using drugs with short half-lives such as clomethiazole and temazepam (Swift 1993).

When prescribing for depression, the tricyclic group and related drugs should be the first choice (*British National Formulary* 2000), although there has been a major increase in use of selective serotonin reuptake inhibitor drugs (PACT 1994), with paroxetine having been shown to be more effective than fluoxetine (Geretsegger *et al.* 1994). General practitioners, however, tend not only to prescribe subtherapeutic doses of antidepressants (Orrell *et al.* 1995), but also seem reluctant to treat for the recommended minimum of at least one year and to continue for two years to minimize the risk of relapse or recurrence (Old Age Depression Interest Group 1993).

General practitioners manage drug therapy for patients with long-term illness through repeat prescribing systems. The administration of these systems is variable, with many practices having inadequate control of the process which is wasteful and potentially dangerous for patients (Zermansky 1996). Good GP care in the prescribing of drugs for elderly patients involves:

(1) review of the appropriateness of medication and dosage at initial prescription and in continuing therapy;
(2) ensuring that the patient and carer understand the purpose and nature of the medication;
(3) the prescribing of lower drug doses, generally starting on 50% of the dose prescribed to younger adults;
(4) prescribing simple regimes with full and clear instructions of how and when to take medication—statements such as 'take as required', 'PRN', and 'as instructed by the physician' should be avoided for regular medication;
(5) checking the labelling of medicine containers for legibility with regard for the patient's vision;
(6) the maintenance of clear documentation of prescribed drugs: for the patient, with a repeat prescription card, computer printout, or 'tablet timetable'; for the practice, on the patient's records including the computer; and with the hospital if the patient has shared care;
(7) an efficient repeat prescribing system with a clear practice policy on the frequent review of prescriptions.

Repeat prescribing should be avoided for certain groups of elderly patients:

(1) the acutely ill;
(2) those who are depressed—clinical review should be undertaken at the renewal of each monthly prescription;
(3) those with impaired renal, hepatic, or cardiac function, who should be monitored for systems' deterioration and adjustment of drug dosage;
(4) those with a history of heavy alcohol intake;
(5) those with dementia who should not be prescribed drugs unless they can be supervised by a carer or community nurse;
(6) those who are withdrawing from antidepressants or long-term anxiolytics. This should be done slowly over 2–3 months to detect an early relapse for depression. Patients taking benzodiazepines or clomethiazole require stepwise dose reduction over several weeks or sometimes months before stopping (*British National Formulary* 2000) to prevent withdrawal symptoms.

The use of computers as an aid to efficient prescribing

Computer-based, decision-support systems and learning-support tools for general practice have been developed through a system known as PRODIGY (Prescribing RatiOnally with Decision support In General practice studY). When GPs enter a diagnosis into their clinical computer, this system suggests a range of treatment options including medicines to prescribe and non-drug advice (Purves 1998; SCHIN 2000). The Prescription Pricing Authority issues quarterly statements on personal prescribing to each GP. These are known as PACT analyses (prescribing analyses and costs) or an electronic format known as e-PACT. This has stimulated greater interest in prescribing policies, use of practice formularies, and generic formulations and has resulted in more rational and economic prescribing while proving acceptable to patients (Dowell *et al.* 1995).

The use of computers for repeat prescribing offers the potential for safer prescribing, although opportunities for quality assurance are often missed (McGavock 1999). The initial prescription is typed in by the doctor (Fig. 18.3) and can be used to set the repeat prescribing programme. Limits may be entered to control the number of repeats allowed by administrative staff before the doctor requires a review of the patient. For example, a patient on hypotensives may be allowed repeat prescriptions at monthly intervals

```
Repeat Masters
DIGOXIN TAB 125mcg             Until: 05/03/1996          Number of issues of 6
CO-DANTHRAMER SUS              Until: 05/03/1996          Number of issues of 6
FRUMIL TAB                     Until: 05/03/1996          Number of issues of 6
PREDNISOLONE TAB 2.5mg         Until: 05/03/1996          Number of issues of 6
WARFARIN TAB 1mg               Until: 05/03/1996          Number of issues of 6
PARACETAMOL CAP 500mg          Until: 05/03/1996          Number of issues of 4

Acute and Repeat Issue Therapy
18/09/1995  issued  SERTRALINE TAB 100mg          Quantity  28  1 op of 28             1 A DAY
20/06/1995  issued  PREDNISOLONE E/C TAB 2.5mg    Quantity  1   1 op of 50             3 DAILY
20/06/1995  issued  WARFARIN TAB 1mg              Quantity  28                         1 A DAY
20/06/1995  issued  FRUMIL TAB                    Quantity    1 op of 28 (2 X 14)      1  A DAY
```

Fig. 18.3 Computer display in GP surgery: sample therapy history. (Reproduced from the ViSion program by kind permission of VAMP Health.)

for 3 months without consulting, but, in the fourth month, will be required to visit the GP for a blood pressure measurement before receiving further prescriptions. All prescriptions obtained by repeat prescribing, however, must be signed by a doctor before being dispensed. Dictionaries held within the computer check the spelling and dosage, and thereby minimize errors.

Research opportunities—methodological issues

General practice provides a wealth of opportunities for research. To achieve a whole-population approach in epidemiological surveys or in studies of community care it is worth considering the potential of general practice. Advantages include: the possibility of a more accurate database compared to the electoral register; a personal approach to the patient through the GP which results in higher response rates; access to patients' medical records; and the GPs' personal knowledge and contact with patients which facilitates data collection and interpretation of results. Criteria for the selection of suitable practices include: efficient practice organization; a computerized age–sex register with health authority links; good liaison with hospital services, and, if possible, the use of training practices where there is a commitment to high standards of care, audit, and research. The question of whether to involve multiple small practices or one large group practice should be considered along with the demographic balance of the practice populations. This avoids the use of skewed population samples and ensures the recruitment of a sufficient patient numbers.

Having enlisted the cooperation of an interested practitioner, it is essential to gain consent from partners and, at the outset, to visit the practice to explain the project to all the staff. The acceptability of protocols, letters, questionnaires, and pilot studies should be confirmed with GPs, before seeking approval from local research ethical committees, the Local Medical Committee of the Health Authority, and before submitting grant applications.

Establishing a link with a key practice administrator and a GP from each practice facilitates effective organization. In communicating with patients it is essential to provide information on the research project and its potential benefits. The identity of the research clinician and the relationship with the practice should be explained. Patients appreciate a choice of venue for an interview, usually from home, the surgery, or the hospital. An identity card, a letter of introduction from the link GP, and a contact telephone number is advisable for security reasons to reassure patients, relatives, and neighbours. It is essential with door-to-door surveys to inform the local police because of the high index of suspicion aroused in neighbours. Because of the lead-in time in setting up the research and interviewing, a check on a patient's health status prior to visiting will avoid the distress of including an acutely ill or recently deceased subject. A common problem when interviewing in the community is how to respond to patients' requests for medical advice. As the interviewer is not providing general medical care, any difficulties should be referred to the patient's doctor. Patients may alert practices when surveys involve questions of a medical nature. The success of research in general practice depends on respect for the relationship between the patient, the neighbourhood, and the GP.

Research may involve the use of general practice records without the knowledge of or consent of the subjects. Most GPs or research ethical committees do not object, as health authorities use general practice lists for screening purposes. However, the researcher has an obligation of confidentiality. It is unacceptable to contact a patient from such a list without prior permission from the patient's GP.

On completion of the research, feedback to the general practices involved helps to integrate the results with the clinical needs of patients, and to foster a sense of purpose and satisfaction. It is courteous to acknowledge the contributions of GPs in papers submitted for publication. Indeed, if a GP has personally collected research data, joint authorship should be considered. This will provide a sense of goodwill that may lead to further fruitful collaboration with general practice.

References

Anderson, R. (1987). The unremitting burden on carers. *British Medical Journal*, **294**, 73–4.

Andrew, R. A. (1988). Analysis of a GP's work in a private nursing home for the elderly. *Journal of the Royal College of General Practitioners*, **38**, 546–8.

Argyle, N., Jestice, S., and Brook, C. P. (1985). Psychogeriatric patients: their supporters problems. *Age and Ageing*, **14**, 355–60.

Bailey, J. J., Black, M. E., and Wilkin, D. (1994). Specialist outreach clinics in general practice. *British Medical Journal*, **308**, 1083–6.

Barber, J. H., Wallis, J. B., and McKeating, E. (1980). A postal screening questionnaire in preventive geriatric care. *Journal of the Royal College of General Practitioners*, **30**, 49–51.

Bergmann, K. (1981). Geronto-psychiatric prevention. In *Epidemiology and prevention of mental illness in old age*. (ed. G. Magnusson, J. Neilson, and J. Buch), pp. 87–92. Proceedings of the Nordic Geronto-Psychiatric Symposium, Silkeborg.

Bergmann, K. and Jacoby, R. (1983). The limitation and possibilities of community care for the elderly demented. In *Elderly people in the community: their service needs*, pp. 141–67. HMSO, London.

Bowling, A. and Jacobson, B. (1989). Screening: the inadequacy of population registers. *British Medical Journal*, **298**, 545–6.

Briscoe, M. and Wilkinson, G. (1989). General practitioners' use of community psychiatric nursing services: a preliminary survey. *Journal of the Royal College of General Practitioners*, **39**, 412–14.

British Geriatrics Society. (1990). Private and Voluntary Homes. In *Policy Statement No 4*. British Geriatrics Society, London.

British National Formulary, No. 39. (2000). Chapter 4—Central nervous system, pp. 163–7, 184–95. British Medical Association and Royal Pharmaceutical Society of Great Britain, London.

Burns A., Jacoby, R., Luthert, P., and Levy, R. (1990). Cause of death in Alzheimer's disease. *Age and Ageing*, **19**, 341–4.

Carers Association. (1998). *Ignored and invisible? Carers experience of the NHS*. Carers National Association, London.

Carlisle, R. (1999). Do nursing home residents use high levels of general practice services? *British Journal of General Practice*, **49**, 645–6.

Cartwright, A. and Smith, C. (1988). *Elderly people: their medicines and their doctors*. Routledge and Kegan Paul, London.

Chew, C., Wilkin, D., and Glendinning, C. (1994). Annual assessment of patients aged 75 years and over: GP and practice nurses views and experiences. *British Journal of General Practice*, **44**, 263–7.

Clarke, M., Clarke, S., Odell, A., and Jagger, C. (1984). The elderly at home: health and social status. *Health Trends*, **16**, 3–7.

Collins, K., Lightbody, P., and Gilhooly, M. (1999). Living wills: a survey of the attitudes of GPs in Scotland. *British Journal of General Practice*, **49**, 641–2.

Corrado, O. J. (2000) Caring for older hospital-at-home patients. *Age and Ageing*, **29**, 97–8

Department of Health. (1991). *Responsibilities of prescribing between hospital and general practice*. Department of Health Publications, London.

Department of Health. (1993). *A national thesaurus of clinical terms in Read Codes*. NHS Executive, HMSO, London.

Department of Health. (1995). *NHS responsibilities for meeting continuing health care needs*. HSG (95) 8. BAPS, Health Publications Unit, Heywood, Lancashire.

Department of Health. (1997). *On the state of the public health: annual report of the Chief Medical Officer of the Department of Health for the year 1996*. The Stationery Office, London.

Department of Health. (1999*a*). *National Service Framework for Mental Health: modern standards and service models*. Department of Health Publications, London.

Department of Health. (1999*b*). *Saving lives: our healthier nation*. The Stationery Office, London.

Department of Health. (1999*c*). *Caring about carers: a national strategy for carers*. Department of Health Publications, London.

Department of Health. (1999*d*). *Local authority personal social services, community care statistics: 1998*. Department of Health, Wetherby, Leeds.

Department of Health. (2000). *Statistical bulletin (2000/8). Statistics for General Medical Practitioners in England and Wales: 1989–99*. Department of Health Publications, London.

Department of Health (2001). *National Service Framework for Older People*. Department of Health Publications, London.

Department of Health and the Welsh Office (1989). *General Practice in the National Health Service: a New Contract*. Department of Health, London.

Department of Social Security. (2000). *A catalogue of leaflets, posters and information*. Benefits Agency, Manchester.

Dewar, R. and Jones, D. (1990). *Determinants of alcohol consumption in the elderly: a community survey*. British Geriatrics Society, Autumn Meeting Abstracts, London.

Dowell, J. S., Snadden, D., and Dunbar, J. A. (1995). Changing to generic formulary: how one fundholding practice reduced prescribing costs. *British Medical Journal*, **310**, 505–8.

Dowrick, C. and Buchan, I. (1995). Twelve month outcome of depression in general practice: does detection make a difference? *British Medical Journal*, **311**, 1274–6.

Doyal, L. (1995). Advance directives. *British Medical Journal*, **310**, 612–13

Ebrahim, S., Hedley, R., and Sheldon, M. (1984). Low levels of ill health among elderly non-consulters in general practice. *British Medical Journal*, **289**, 1273–5.

Eccles, M., Clarke, J., Livingston, M., Freemantle, N., and Mason, J. (1998). North of England evidence based guidelines development project: guideline for the primary care management of dementia. *British Medical Journal*, **317**, 802–8.

Fazel, S., Hope, T., and Jacoby, R. (1999). Assessment of competence to complete advance directives: validation of a patient centred approach. *British Medical Journal*, **318**, 493–7.

Freer, C. B. (1987). Consultation-based screening of the elderly in general practice: a pilot study. *Journal of the Royal College of General Practitioners*, **37**, 455–6.

Geretsegger, C., Bohmer, F., and Ludwig, M. (1994). Paroxetine in the elderly depressed patient: randomised comparison with fluoxetine of efficacy, cognitive and behavioural effects. *International Clinical Psychopharmacology*, **9**, 25–9.

Goldberg, D. and Bridges, K. (1987). Screening for psychiatric illness in general practice: the GP versus the screening questionnaire. *Journal of the Royal College of General Practitioners*, **37**, 15–18.

Goldberg, D. and Jackson, G. (1992). Interface between primary care and specialist mental health care. *British Journal of General Practice*, **42**, 267–8.

Goldberg, D., Privett, M., Utson, B., *et al.* (1998). The effects of detection and treatment on the outcome of major depression in primary care: a naturalistic study in 15 cities. *British Journal of General Practice*, **49**, 1840–4.

Graham, H. and Livesley, B. (1986). Changes in the population aged over 75 of an urban general practice: implications for screening. *British Medical Journal*, **292**, 453–4.

Harris, T. and Kendrick, T. (1998). Bereavement care in general practice: a survey in South Thames region. *British Journal of General Practice*, **48**, 1560–4.

Harrison, R., Savla, N., and Kafetz, K. (1990). Dementia, depression and physical disability in a London borough: a survey of elderly people in and out of residential care and implications for future developments. *Age and Ageing*, **19**, 97–103.

Health Departments of Great Britain. (1989). *General practice in the National Health Service: the 1990 contract*. Appendix A, pp. 19–20. Health Departments of Great Britain.

Hendricksen, C., Lund, E., and Stromgard, E. (1984). Consequences of assessment and intervention among elderly people; a three year randomised controlled trial. *British Medical Journal*, **289**, 1522–4.

Higgs, R. (1985). Example of intermediate care: the new Lambeth Community Care Centre. *British Medical Journal*, **291**, 1395–7.

Homer, A. C. and Gilleard, C. J. (1994). The effect of inpatient respite care on elderly patients and their carers. *Age and Ageing*, **23**, 274–6.

House, A. (1987). Depression after stroke. *British Medical Journal*, **294**, 76–8.

Howarth, S., Clarke, C., Bayliss, R., Whitfield, A. G., Semmence, J., and Healy, M. J. (1990). Mortality in elderly patients admitted for respite care. *British Medical Journal*, **300**, 844–7.

Iliffe, S., Tai, S. S., Haines, A., Booroff, A., Goldenberg, E., Morgan, P., *et al.* (1993). Assessment of elderly people in general practice. 4. Depression, functional ability and contact with services. *British Journal of General Practice*, **43**, 371–4.

Iliffe, S., Mitchley, S., Gould, M., and Haines, A. (1994). Evaluation of the use of brief screening instruments for dementia, depression and problem drinking among elderly people in general practice. *British Journal of General Practice*, **44**, 503–7.

Jones, D. A. and Peters, T. J. (1992). Caring for elderly dependants: effects on the carers' quality of life. *Age and Ageing*, **21**, 421–8.

Jones, D. A., Victor, C. R., and Vetter, N. J. (1983). Carers of the elderly in the community. *Journal of the Royal College of General Practitioners*, **33**, 707–10.

Kay, D. W., Beamish, P., and Roth, M. (1964). Old age mental disorders in Newcastle upon Tyne. *British Journal of Psychiatry*, **110**, 146–58.

Kings Fund Carers Unit. (1989). *Doctors, carers and general practice*. MSD Foundation, London.

Llewellyn-Jones, R. H., Baikie, K. A., Smithers, H., *et al.* (1999). Multifaceted shared care intervention for late life depression in residential care: randomised controlled trial. *British Medical Journal*, **319**, 676–82.

Livingston, G., Manela, M., and Katona, C. (1996). Depression and other psychiatric morbidity in carers of elderly people living at home. *British Medical Journal*, **312**, 153–6.

Luker, K. A. and Perkins, E. S. (1987). The elderly at home: service needs and provision. *Journal of the Royal College of General Practitioners*, **37**, 248–50.

MacDonald, A. J. (1986). Do GPs 'miss' depression in elderly patients? *British Medical Journal*, **292**, 1365–7.

McGavock, H. (1999). Repeat prescribing management—a cause for concern? *British Journal of General Practice*, **49**, 343–7.

McIntosh, I. B. and Power, K. G. (1993). Elderly people's views of an annual screening assessment. *British Journal of General Practice*, **43**, 189–92.

McNeice, R. and Majeed, A. (1999). Socio-economic differences in general practice consultation rates in patients aged 65 and over: prospective cohort study. *British Medical Journal*, **319**, 26–8.

Melzer, D., Watters, L., Paykel, E., Singh, K., and Gormley, N. (1999). Factors explaining the use of psychiatric services by general practices. *British Journal of General Practice*, **49**, 887–91.

Moore, A. T. and Roland, M. O. (1989). How much variation in referral rates among GPs is due to chance? *British Medical Journal*, **298**, 500–2.

Murphy, E. (1982). Social origins of depression in old age. *British Journal of Psychiatry*, **141**, 135–42.

Nocon, A. (1993). GPs assessments of people aged 75 and over: identifying the need for occupational therapy services. *British Journal of Occupational Therapy*, **56**, 123–7.

O'Connor, D. W., Fertig, A., Grande, M. J., Hyde, J. B., Perry, J. R., Roland, M. O., *et al.* (1993). Dementia in general practice: the practical consequences of a more positive approach to diagnosis. *British Journal of General Practice*, **43**, 185–8.

Old Age Depression Interest Group. (1993). How long should the elderly take anti-depressants? A double-blind placebo controlled study of continuation/prophylaxis therapy with dothiepin. *British Journal of Psychiatry* **162**, 175–82.

OPCS (Office of Population, Censuses and Surveys). (1993). *Census: communal establishments, 1991*, Great Britain. HMSO, London.

OPCS (Office of Population, Censuses and Surveys). (1994). *Mortality statistics general for England and Wales, 1992*. Series DH127. HMSO, London.

Orrell, M., Collins, C., Shergill, S., and Katona, C. (1995). The management of depression in the elderly by GPs. Part (i)—The use of anti-depressants. *Family Practice*, **12**, 5–11.

PACT Standard Report. (1994). *PPA 3rd quarter 1994/5*. Prescription Pricing Authority, Jesmond, Newcastle-upon-Tyne.

Pearson, N. D. (1988). An assessment of relief hospital admissions for elderly patients with dementia. *Health Trends*, **20**, 120–1.

Pollock, A. M. (2000). Will intermediate care be the undoing of the NHS? *British Medical Journal*, **321**, 393–4.

Purves, I. N. (1998). PRODIGY: implementing clinical guidance using computers. *British Journal of General Practice*, **48**, 1552–3.

Rae, G. S., Bielawska, C., Murphy, P. J., and Wright, G. (1986). Hazards for elderly people admitted for respite and social care. *British Medical Journal*, **292**, 240.

RCGP (Royal College of General Practitioners), Office of Population Censuses and Surveys, Department of Health and Social Security (1995). *Morbidity statistics from general practice: fourth national study 1991–1992*. Her Majesty's Stationery Office, London.

RCGP (Royal College of General Practitioners). (1993). *Shared care of patients with mental health problems*. Report of a Joint Royal College Working Group. Royal College of Psychiatrists and Royal College of General Practitioners. Occasional paper 60. Royal College of General Practitioners, London.

RCP (Royal College of Physicians) (1994). *Geriatric day hospitals. Their role and guidelines for good practice*. Royal College of Physicians of London.

Rumble, R. H. and Morgan, K. (1994). Longitudinal trends in prescribing for elderly patients: two surveys four years apart. *British Journal of General Practice*, **44**, 571–5.

Salisbury, C., Trivella, M., and Bruster, S. (2000). Demand for and supply of out of hours care from GPs in England and Scotland: observational study based on routinely collected data. *British Medical Journal*, **320**, 618–21.

Sanford, J. R. (1975). Tolerance of debility in elderly dependants by supporters at home: its significance for hospital practice. *British Medical Journal*, **3**, 471–3.

SCHIN (Sowerby Centre for Health Informatics at Newcastle). (2000). Prodigy: practical support for clinical governance. Newcastle. *www.prodigy.nhs.uk*.

Shapiro, J. (2000). The new primary care organisations: one year on. *British Medical Journal*, **320**, 887–8.

Swift, C. G. (1993). *Sleep and sleep problems in elderly people. ABC of sleep disorders*, pp. 37–40. *BMJ* Publishing group, London.

Taylor, J. and Taylor, D. (1988). *The Assessment of General Medical Training in General Medical Practice*, pp. 10–11. University of York, York.

Taylor, R., Ford, G., and Barber, H. (1983). *The elderly at risk: a critical review of problems and progress in screening and case finding*. Age Concern Research Unit, London.

Tulloch, A. J. and Moore, V. L. (1979). A randomized controlled trial of geriatric screening and surveillance in general practice. *Journal of the Royal College of General Practitioners*, **29**, 733–42.

Van Hout, H., Vernooij-Dassen, M., Poels, P., Hoefnagels, W., and Grol, R. (2000). Are GPs able to accurately diagnose dementia and identify Alzheimer's disease? A comparison with an outpatient memory clinic. *British Journal of General Practice*, **50**, 311–12.

Vetter, N. J. and Ford, D. (1989). Anxiety and depression scores in elderly fallers. *International Journal of Geriatric Psychiatry*, **4**, 159–63.

Vetter, N. J., Jones, D. E., and Victor, C. R. (1984). Effect of health visitors working with elderly patients in general practice: a randomised controlled trial. *British Medical Journal*, **288**, 369–72.

Westerman, R. F., Hull, F. M., Bezemar, P. D., and Gort, G. (1990). A study of communication between GPs and specialists. *British Journal of General Practice*, **40**, 445–9.
Whalley, L. J. (1989). Drug treatments of dementia. *British Journal of Psychiatry*, **155**, 595–611.
Williams, E. I. (1984). Characteristics of patients aged over 75 not seen during one year in general practice. *British Medical Journal*, **288**, 119–21.
Williams, E. I. and Fitton, F. (1990). General practitioner response to elderly patients discharged from hospital. *British Medical Journal*, **300**, 159–61.
Williamson, J., Stokoe, I. H., Gray, S., Fisher, M., Smith, A., McGhee, A., *et al.* (1964). Old people at home: their unreported needs. *Lancet*, **1**, 1117–20.
Zermansky, A. G. (1996). Who controls repeats? *British Journal of General Practice*, **46**, 643–7.

19 Liaison old age psychiatry in the general hospital

Michael Philpot, Declan Lyons, and Tom Reynolds

Introduction

During the second half of the twentieth century two factors led to the emergence of liaison psychiatry: the gradual move of mental health inpatient units out of the asylums and into general hospitals, and the growing interest in the complex interaction between physical and mental disorder. This chapter reviews: the basic principles of service provision; surveys of the scope of mental disorder in general hospitals and the activities of liaison services; and the evidence for the effectiveness of interventions made.

The principles of liaison service provision

The terminology of liaison psychiatry has been developed within general psychiatry, but is equally apt for old age psychiatry. The consultation-only model involves the psychiatric assessment of patients on general hospital wards at the request of a referring doctor. Advice is given, but no further contact or responsibility is necessarily taken. Responsibility for identifying those patients with psychiatric problems lies with the medical or surgical team, as does the responsibility of carrying out the advised management. 'True' liaison involves a more integrated approach, in which the psychiatrist seeks to influence clinical management more pervasively by increased contact with general hospital staff, perhaps by becoming a member of the medical team (White 1990). Consultation–liaison, as it is practised in most hospitals, is a compromise between these two models and depends largely on the resources of the service and the priorities of the psychiatrists involved. Old age psychiatry services are increasingly based in the community with a primary care focus, and in many services referrals of patients from general hospital wards may have to take second place (Benbow and Dawson 1994). The principles briefly listed here could be applied to any aspect of service provision within old age psychiatry. Solutions to each will depend largely on local factors.

- *Accessibility.* Access to the service should be well advertised and easy to follow. Referrals might be made by phone or fax. There should be one entry point for referrals: referrers should not be 'bounced' around different departments until they find the right one. The service should set a standard response time and be able to advise the referrer when the assessment will be made. Ideally, emergency consultation should be available.
- *Effective communication.* The service should encourage clearly made referrals in which the background details and the reasons for the request are plainly stated. Specific forms are best designed and distributed for this purpose. Ideally the results of the consultation should be fed-back to the referring doctor in person or by phone. Succinct handwritten notes should be made in the medical records, avoiding a lengthy psychiatric clerking and theoretical specu-

lation. Advice should be problem-orientated and straightforward. A typewritten letter may follow to embellish the permanent record but, as this will probably arrive in the patient's notes some days later, it should not replace direct communication.

- *Clear limits of responsibility*. In most cases, the consulting doctor does not become responsible for the patient's subsequent management. The old age psychiatry service should not be seen as a 'dumping ground' for difficult patients whose discharge has been delayed for social care reasons.
- *Activity monitoring*. There should be an effective means of counting the overall workload. It is an unwritten principle of health care management that activity that is not counted did not occur.
- *Special links*. It is desirable to develop proactive links with, for instance, the geriatric, orthopaedic, and stroke units. The reasons for this are developed in subsequent sections of this chapter. These links might be reciprocal so that, for example, a geriatrician might carry out a visiting clinic on the acute old age psychiatry wards.
- *Resources*. The service may be provided by doctors, nurses, or psychologists with adequate training, experience, and supervision. Staff sessions should be 'ring fenced' and sufficient for new and follow-up visits.

Historically, liaison has been provided from generic old age psychiatry services. In the United Kingdom there are still very few dedicated and separately funded liaison teams. Lipowski (1983) argued that 'geropsychiatry' should be part of general liaison, on the grounds that the skills associated with the concept of liaison take priority over the specialist skills of old age psychiatry. In our experience, this is not the case and there is a positive advantage for the patient in being assessed by a member of the team responsible for the postdischarge management of the psychiatric problem. However, as stated above (under *Clear limits of responsibility*) this does not usually happen.

The prevalence of psychiatric disorder in the elderly in general hospitals

Older people occupy approximately 50% of all general hospital beds at any one time. For the report year 1996/97 people over 65 years of age comprised 50.5% of all Finished Consultant Episodes (that is, discharges from hospital) in England and Wales (Office of National Statistics 1999). This proportion has remained virtually the same for nearly 30 years (Bergmann and Eastham 1974). Studies of this patient group have generally shown a higher prevalence of psychiatric disorder than that found in community surveys. Prevalence rates for the major disorders are summarized in Table 19.1. This is based on a selected series of prevalence studies carried out in medical and surgical inpatients over the last 20 years (Kitchell *et al.* 1982; Cooper 1987; Feldman *et al.* 1987; Johnston *et al.* 1987; Koenig *et al.* 1988*a*, 1991, 1997; O'Riordan *et al.* 1989; Ramsey *et al.* 1991; Burn *et al.* 1992; Ardern *et al.* 1993; Jackson and Baldwin 1993; Kok *et al.* 1995; Luttrell *et al.* 1997; Clément *et al.* 1999; Sinoff *et al.* 1999; Holmes and House 2000; Uwakwe 2000). It will be seen that a rather large range of values is given for each disorder. The reasons for this variation are numerous. They include the setting in which patients were assessed, the age of the patients studied, the recruitment methods used, whether inclusion and exclusion criteria were applied (or even stated), whether valid and reliable

Table 19.1 The prevalence of psychiatric disorders in elderly physically ill inpatients (see text for references)

Diagnosis	Prevalence range (%)
Depression	5–58
Delirium	5–15
Dementia	3–40
Cognitive impairment (non-specific)	3–88
Schizophrenia	1–8
Alcoholism	1–16
Anxiety disorders	1–9

assessment tools were used, whether comorbidity was accepted or a hierarchical approach (that is, a single diagnosis) was given, and the diagnostic scheme used. In addition, the timing of the assessment and its frequency also play a part, particularly in disorders whose features may fluctuate over hours or days. Despite disagreement over the precise prevalence figures, the majority of studies determining the presence of the whole range of disorders rank depression as the most prevalent, with organic disorders (dementia and delirium) usually a close second. Some physical disorders have attracted more research attention than others. Patients admitted to hospital for the repair of hip fractures have been particularly well studied (reviewed by Holmes and House 2000). The subject of psychiatric disorders following stroke, myocardial infarction, or during the course of cancer is dealt with later in this chapter.

Clearly many patients are suffering from psychiatric disorder before they enter hospital and may already be known to specialist services: the dementias, chronic functional illnesses, and substance abuse are particularly relevant here. Concurrent medical and surgical illness may exacerbate symptoms in these disorders. Other patients develop psychiatric problems as a result of their physical disorder, its treatment, or simply by being in hospital. Between one-third and one-half of elderly patients develop delirium during their hospital admission (Levkoff *et al.* 1992; Brauer *et al.* 2000) and this is often associated with pre-existing cognitive impairment. However, delirium following cataract surgery is surprisingly infrequent and associated with the use of benzodiazepines as a premedication (Milstein *et al.* 2000).

There are some intriguing omissions from the liaison literature relating to older patients. There has been little systematic collection of data concerning somatization disorder or hypochondriasis. However, with a community prevalence rate of between 0.1 and 36% (Sheehan and Banerjee 1999), depending on the age of the sample and the criteria used, rates are likely to be high in hospital inpatients. These estimates largely exclude patients with depression, in whom hypochondriacal symptoms are relatively common (Wood *et al.* 1987). Similarly, systematic information concerning patients admitted following deliberate self-harm is surprisingly limited, given the serious clinical implications of this behaviour occurring for the first time in older people.

Liaison referrals to old age psychiatry services

Referrals of older patients comprise a substantial proportion of all referrals to liaison services (Lipowski 1983; Mainprize and Rodin 1987). In contrast to the actual prevalence of disorders in the patient group, referrals to liaison services are most commonly for dementia and delirium (perhaps because of behaviour and placement issues) and then depression. Table 19.2 gives an indication of the case-mix of referrals made from general hospital units (Benbow 1987; Mainprize and Rodin 1987; Pauser *et al.* 1987; Poynton 1988; Scott *et al.* 1988; Anderson and Philpott 1991; Wrigley and Loane 1991; Burn *et al.* 1992; Clément *et al.* 1999).

Reasons for referral vary and may depend on the local responsibilities of the liaison service as well as on the perceived skills of the service itself and the benefit to the referring team. Requests for advice on the management of psychiatric illness should clearly be the primary reason for referral. Benbow and Dawson (1994) have provided a typology of liaison problems, which is shown in Table 19.3. To this list can be added the often vexing request to 'assess for

Table 19.2 Case-mix of referrals to liaison old age psychiatry services (see text for references)

Diagnosis	Proportion of total Referrals to service (%)
Dementia	3–46
Delirium	5–25
Alcoholism	0–16
Schizophrenia	0–4
Depression	11–32
Anxiety disorders	3–5
Other disorders	2–26
No psychiatric disorder	3–19

Table 19.3 Classification of liaison problems in old age psychiatry (after Benbow and Dawson 1994)

Somatic presentation of psychological disorder
Psychological reaction to physical illness
Physical illness complicating psychiatric disorder
Psychosocial factors complicating physical illness
Psychiatric disorder delaying discharge
Anticipated failure to cope after discharge
Assessment of mental capacity

placement'. Some liaison services may be swamped by such requests (Wrigley and Loane 1991). Good practice demands that patients receive an appropriate set of assessments prior to discharge from hospital, particularly if the patient is to be transferred to a residential or nursing home (British Geriatrics Society 1995). This report emphasized the need to plan hospital discharge for elderly people with great care so as to avoid failure of service provision, which might in turn provoke an early relapse of the medical condition and subsequent readmission. In this context, delays in discharge ought not to be considered a mismanagement of beds. Whether old age psychiatrists need to be involved in the care-planning of every patient with mental disorder is debatable. However, a long wait for placement adds to the dissatisfaction of general hospital staff who see many mentally ill patients as 'bed-blockers' and may develop a low tolerance of any behavioural or emotional disturbance (Health Advisory Service 2000).

In parts of the UK, geriatricians and old age psychiatrists have the additional responsibility of identifying those patients eligible for National Health Service (NHS) continuing care (Department of Health 1995). Health and local authorities were instructed to draw up criteria defining those most in need of NHS care, but left the details to be decided at a local level. Thus, different criteria apply in each area of the country. The process is intended to ensure that the most disabled patients, those requiring intensive nursing care and speedy access to medical supervision, can obtain this care without charge. Referrals for this purpose often involve an assessment of the patient's competence (see Chapter 40). Patients who are deemed to require institutionalization to cater for their care needs but who refuse, in favour of returning home, present special problems. Lengthy negotiation may be necessary in such cases, perhaps with an intervening psychiatric admission to assist the process.

Preadmission psychiatric assessment is also recommended in the United States before patients are admitted to nursing homes under the auspices of the Omnibus Budget Reconciliation Act of 1987 (OBRA-87; Borson *et al.* 1997). However, this provision is not always used where appropriate. Borson *et al.* (1997) found that only 10% of new nursing-home residents were referred for assessment and that 55% had unmet mental health needs.

The very low rate of patient referral based on the actual or expected numbers of mentally ill elderly patients admitted to general hospitals is well documented. Where actual referral rates have been estimated these have rarely exceeded 3% (Poynton 1988; Burn *et al.* 1992). This rate was also found in a study carried out in a Nigerian hospital (Uwakwe 2000). Crisp (1968) stated that the availability and inclination of the psychiatrist was the main factor that determined the referral rate, but White (1990) eloquently summarized the possible reasons for non-referral and these are listed in Table 19.4. (The reasons have been reordered.)

There is a good deal of evidence that general hospital personnel are poor at identifying psychiatric illness (Feldman *et al.* 1987; Koenig *et al.* 1988*b*; Ardern *et al.* 1993; Jackson and Baldwin 1993). In one study, junior medical staff failed to identify one-third of patients with definite cognitive impairment, despite the fact that many of the patients had been described as confused or demented by the referring general practitioner (Ardern *et al.* 1993). Recognition of depression may be poorer in older patients who are often referred for other reasons, such as a lack of coping (Clarke *et al.* 1995). Feldman *et al.* (1987) found that junior medical staff identified only half of the patients with depression and anxiety, but were no more likely to identify severe depression than mild depression. Similarly, Ames and Tuckwell (1994) reported that 80% of depressed patients were discharged without documented plans for the management of their

Table 19.4 Reasons cited for non-referral of medical inpatients to psychiatrists (after White 1990)

Physician unaware of need for psychiatric intervention
Physician unaware of possibility of psychiatric intervention
Physician unaware of benefits of psychiatric intervention
Physician believes psychiatric disorder incurable
Poor working relationship between physician and psychiatrist
Psychiatric service dissatisfies physician
Physician feels he does not know patient well enough
Physician fears patient's emotions
Physician unable or unwilling to spare time for psychological issues
Denial of significance of psychological issues
Psychiatric language useless to physician
Physician believes patient is disadvantaged by being labelled as a psychiatric case
Physician believes patient too physically ill
Physician believes every doctor should be able to treat psychiatric illness
Patient refuses psychiatric referral

depression. In another study, nurses identified only 38% of patients previously identified as depressed using a structured interview (Jackson and Baldwin 1993). Koenig *et al.* (1988*b*) found that only 20% of depressed patients had depressive symptoms recorded in their medical notes. Even after being informed of the diagnosis, medical staff only started treatment in 13% of the patients. The remainder had relative or absolute contraindications to tricyclic antidepressants. The situation had not improved 10 years later, when the same group found that only 13% of depressed patients had been treated at any time during their admission or follow-up with an antidepressant, predominantly amitriptyline in small doses (Koenig *et al.* 1997). Farrell and Ganzini (1995) reported that 42% of patients referred for assessment of depression actually had delirium, although the patients endorsed depressive symptoms like low mood, feelings of worthlessness, and thoughts of death.

Referring doctors may be dissatisfied with the liaison service provided. Kaufman and Bates (1990) found that dissatisfaction among geriatricians in the UK was largely related to a deficiency of beds for patients with dementia. No published study has yet documented the 'user' satisfaction of a liaison service: such matters may be subject to local audit. However Loane and Jeffreys (1998) determined that 90% of the recommendations they had given had been acted upon, although they do not describe the 10% in which advice was not followed.

Of the reasons for non-referral cited in Table 19.3, some may be amenable to intervention. The use of simple screening tools, the education of general hospital staff, and the introduction of more proactive working arrangements have all been examined and will be reviewed in the following sections.

Screening tools for psychiatric disorder in the medically ill

It has been argued that the use of simple screening tests might improve the detection of psychiatric illness by general hospital medical or nursing staff, and thus increase the referral rate and appropriateness. Screening tests for cognitive impairment are described in more detail in Chapter 15, but brief tests such as the Mini-Mental State Examination (MMSE; Folstein *et al.* 1975) and the Abbreviated Mental Test (AMT; Qureshi and Hodkinson, 1974) are widely used. Whether their use has led to better management of patients has not been systematically examined. A similar case applies to tests for delirium or reversible cognitive disorder (e.g. Inouye *et al.* 1990; Treloar and Macdonald, 1997).

Screening tests for depression have been the subject of many validity and reliability studies in medically ill older people. For screening purposes, prior to more detailed assessment, tests with a high sensitivity and low false-negative rate are to be preferred. Tests may be more 'easily' administered if they can be completed in questionnaire form by the patient. However, severely depressed patients may not care to complete questionnaires and serious disorders may be overlooked. Of the self-rating scales currently in use, the Geriatric Depression Scale (Yesavage *et al.* 1983) has received the most attention. Originally in a 30-item form, the 15-item and 4-item versions have been derived and tested in a variety of settings. Both shorter versions perform well (Jackson and Baldwin, 1993; Shah *et al.* 1997; Clément *et al.* 1999), but a high false-positive rate has been reported with the longer version (Koenig *et al.* 1992; Kok *et al.* 1995), although Ramsey *et al.* (1991) found 100% sensitivity. Similar problems bedevil rating scales originally developed for use in young adults. The Zung Depression Rating Scale and the Popoff Index of Depression (Kitchell *et al.* 1982), the General Health Questionnaire (Johnston *et al.* 1987), the Hospital Anxiety and Depression Scale (Davies *et al.* 1993), and the Center for Epidemiological Studies Depression Scale (CES-D; Clément *et al.* 1999) have all performed indifferently in this patient group. Scales incorporating 'physical' or somatic symptoms of depression, which may be confounded by concurrent physical illness, tend to perform less well. Schein and Koenig (1997) reported that the use of a two-stage scoring process increased the validity of the CES-D, and suggested that the cut-points of screening tests developed for other patient groups needed adjustment for use in medically ill elderly people.

Interviewer-rated scales are more time-consuming but gain in being applicable to more severely depressed and withdrawn patients. The Brief Assessment Scale for Depression (BAS-DEP; Shah *et al.* 1997) and the Even Briefer Assessment Scale for Depression (EBAS-DEP; Allen *et al.* 1994) both perform acceptably and require little training in their use. The Brief Assessment Scale Depression Cards (BASDEC; Adshead *et al.* 1992) is a novel method that involves the patient simply endorsing statements about depression which are printed on cards. Evans (1993) has developed a 15-item combined interview and observation scale specifically for use in medically ill elderly, in response to some of the problems identified with other scales. In the United Kingdom, a consensus conference (Royal College of Physicians 1992) recommended the use of the full GDS for depression and the AMT for cognitive impairment, as well as the Philadelphia Geriatric Center Morale Scale to assess subjective well-being (Lawton 1975). However, it is not known whether this guidance has been widely implemented.

The Short Anxiety Screening Test (Sinoff *et al.* 1999) has been developed to identify anxiety symptoms and their severity rather than the disorder *per se*, but its performance is compromised in the presence of depression. The CAGE questionnaire (Ewing 1984) for the identification of alcoholism is a popular tool, although it has been found to perform poorly in older people (Luttrell *et al.* 1997). In this study, low sensitivity was also found with the Michigan Alcoholism Screening Test—Geriatric version (Blow *et al.* 1992). The authors devised a new two-stage screening test known as the UCL Screen (Luttrell *et al.* 1997). The very simple stage one item is 'Do you drink alcohol in a typical week?'

The outcome of psychiatric disorder in medically ill older patients

Studies of outcome have focused on two particular variables of interest: length of hospital stay and time to death. Patients with delirium spend longer in hospital than those without (Francis *et al.* 1990; Levkoff *et al.* 1992; Stevens *et al.* 1998; Holmes and House 2000), are more likely to be institutionalized following discharge (Francis *et al.* 1990; Levkoff *et al.* 1992), and die sooner (Caraceni *et al.* 2000; Holmes and House 2000). Increased mortality may be associated with the severity of the medical condition involved rather than the resultant delirium (Francis *et al.* 1990). Full resolution of delirium is relatively rare by the time the patient is discharged: Levkoff *et al.* (1992) reported that only 21% patients had experienced full resolution of their symptoms 3 months after discharge. Holmes and House (2000) reported that pre-existing dementia had similar effects on the outcome of patients admitted for the treatment of hip fractures. The presence of cognitive impairment (all causes) increased the length of hospital stay owing to a shortage of suitable nursing-home beds.

There is less agreement between studies concerning the effects of depression on these outcome measures. Some studies have found no effect on the length of stay or time to death (Finch *et al.* 1992; Shah 1998). Others have demonstrated that depression significantly reduces survival, independent of age, medical illness, or disability (Arfken *et al.* 1999), and is associated with reduced quality of life (Unutzer *et al.* 2000). Ganzini *et al.* (1997) found that survival was improved in depressed patients who responded to antidepressant treatment. Koenig *et al.* (1989*a*) reported that short-term survival (at 5 months) was reduced for depressed patients who were still in hospital. No effect was found in those who were discharged, suggesting that death was a function of chronic disability necessitating hospitalization rather than depression *per se*. Shah *et al.* (2000*b*) found that suicidal ideation and the degree of handicap predicted mortality in depressed patients during a 6-month, follow-up period.

Intervention studies in liaison old age psychiatry

Organizational changes

A number of studies (particularly from the UK) have documented changes in referral rates and quality before and after the introduction of specialist old age psychiatry liaison. An increase in total referrals was found in some surveys (Poynton 1988; Scott *et al.* 1988; Anderson and Philpott 1991). The latter survey carried out over an 8-year period showed an increase in depression cases and a decrease in delirium cases, suggesting more appropriate use of the service. In studies by Scott *et al.* (1988) and Baheerathan and Shah (1999) the introduction of a consultation–liaison approach involving a senior trainee psychiatrist led to a reduction in inappropriate referrals, particularly requests for social care. The impact of the service change reported by Baheerathan and Shah (1999) seems to have been in reducing overall liaison working time, bringing consequent financial savings. Collinson and Benbow (1998) described the introduction of a nurse to perform liaison assessments. The main benefit appears to have been to reduce the waiting time to assessment and thereby improve the reputation of the service. A similar nursing-based service has been described in long-term care (Pajarillo *et al.* 1997). Some services include liaison psychologists, offering short-term cognitive–behavioural treatments or family work, but no reports have yet been published on the effectiveness of this approach. Lastly, Strain *et al.* (1991) introduced screening for psychiatric disorder in patients admitted with hip fractures. The average time in hospital was shortened by about 2 days and this translated into a substantial financial saving.

Although not strictly an intervention study, Swanwick *et al.* (1994) compared the liaison service in one hospital, by an on-site psychiatric team providing a consultation-only approach, with the service in another hospital, in which a dedicated visiting senior psychiatrist practised an active liaison approach. The 'active' model led to greater diagnostic accuracy by referring teams, but no overall increase in referral numbers.

There have been only two randomized-controlled trials (RCT) of organizational interventions—both from the same research group. The introduction of a geriatric psychiatry consultant providing detailed assessment, treatment advice, and weekly follow-up for 8 weeks was compared to 'usual' care (Cole *et al.* 1991). Although there were trends showing some improvement in psychiatric symptom measures and functional status, these did not reach statistical significance. Control patients left hospital sooner on average but more of the experimental group were discharged home. A later study employed the same management but was limited to patients with delirium assessed within 24 hours of admission (Cole *et al.* 1994). This time, significant improvements in cognition and behaviour were noted in the experimental group.

The development of joint facilities between old age psychiatry and geriatrics has been advocated. Jointly managed wards have been described (Arie and Dunn 1973; Pitt and Silver 1980; Farragher and Walsh 1998), but generally this concept has not been widely taken up. In the UK such wards may now be impossible to set up as psychiatry and general hospital services are often run by financially independent organizations, even though they may share a hospital site. Benbow and Dawson (1994) describe the success of joint outpatient clinics where the specialist consultants assess and review patients alongside each other. Lastly, some academic and clinical departments are shared between the geriatrics and old age psychiatry. Arie (1994) describes the prototype of this arrangement in Nottingham. A Masters degree in Clinical Gerontology, intended for trainees in old age psychiatry and geriatrics, has been popular at our teaching hospital. Fourth-year medical students now experience old age psychiatry within a teaching block incorporating paediatrics, geriatric medicine, and palliative care and thereby acquire a developmental perspective. Joint training of junior medical staff, shared case conferences and journal clubs, and joint continuing medical education have all been advocated as ways of improving the relationship between services for the elderly (Royal Colleges of Psychiatrists and Physicians 1999). However, Waller and Hillam (2000) have highlighted the dispiriting results of attempting to educate non-psychiatric medical staff with the aim of improving identification and documentation of depression in older patients. Staff were given a training session and advised to use a screening rating scale. Patients' notes were examined before and after the intervention. No patients' notes contained even a basic mental state examination either before or after the training. Although pre-existing depression and medication was usually noted, the medical staff were generally unwilling to be involved in the treatment of depression—which they felt was 'best left to the psychiatrists'.

Treatment trials in depression

Physical illness, particularly chronic physical illness, and disability are known to be associated with poor outcome in depressed elderly patients (Cole and Bellevance 1997). Gill and Hatcher (1999) published a meta-analysis of 19 antidepressant trials in medically ill adults of all ages. Tricyclic antidepressants appeared marginally more effective than selective serotonin reuptake inhibitors. Active drugs were more effective than placebo. Drop-outs were more likely with tricyclic antidepressants. Draper (2000) has pointed out that this analysis failed to take account of acute or chronic illness status, and this appears to have an effect on the response to treatment. Altogether six RCTs have been carried out of the effects of drugs in medically ill depressed older people; these are summarized in Table 19.5. (Trials in stroke patients are described later in this chapter.) The results suggest that antidepressants may be useful in stable medical conditions, as part of general rehabilitation, but may be of less benefit in acute medical illness. However, the treatment period and the dose may have been insufficient in the study by Tan *et al.* (1994). Evans *et al.* (1997) found that patients with severe medical illnesses responded well if they tolerated at least 5 weeks of treatment. The study by Wallace *et al.* (1995) is the only RCT to date involving methylphenidate, but did not record response in any systematic way. The crossover design also presents problems in a condition like depression. However, the rapid

Table 19.5 Randomised placebo controlled trials in the drug treatment of depression in medically ill elderly patients (mixed diagnoses)

Name	Year	Sample size	Mean age (years)	Trial duration (weeks)	Acute or chronic medical condition	Active drug and daily dose	Comparison with placebo
Lakshmanan et al.	1986	24	76	3	Acute	Doxepin 10–20 mg	Active drug better
Katz et al.	1990	30	84	7	Acute	Nortriptyline means 65 mg	Active drug better
Borson et al.	1992	36	61	12	Acute	Nortriptyline mean 67 mg	Active drug better
Tan et al.	1994	63	80	4	Chronic	Lofepramine 70 mg	No difference
Wallace et al.	1995	16	72	8 days	Chronic	Methylphenidate 10–20 mg	Active drug better
Evans et al.	1997	82	80	8	Chronic	Fluoxetine 20 mg	No difference

action of methylphenidate may suggest an advantage over conventional treatments for depression.

Two further drug trials are worth mentioning, if only to emphasize the poor response to the treatment of depression in acute medical illness. Schifano *et al.* (1990) compared mianserin and maprotiline. The overall patient response was disappointing, although mianserin appeared marginally to be more effective. Lastly, Koenig *et al.* (1989*b*) managed to recruit 41 patients from nearly 700 screened medical patients for a planned RCT of nortriptyline versus placebo. The trial was abandoned as the drug was contraindicated in 80% of the potential patients.

There have been no RCTs of electroconvulsive therapy (ECT) in the elderly medically ill, although a number of case series suggest that it is safe and effective for the treatment of severe depression in patients with cardiac disease (Zielinski *et al.* 1993) or following stroke (Currier *et al.* 1992). The (usually) short-term nature of acute general hospitalization militates against the use of lengthy psychological therapies. However, a trial of interpersonal counselling in elderly hospitalized patients with subsyndromal depression reported modest improvements in depressive symptom severity at 6-month follow-up (Mossey *et al.* 1996).

Management of depression in special conditions and settings

Heart disease

Myocardial infarction is a serious condition with a high, early mortality. Those who survive are likely to face a future of disability and reduced activity. Schleifer *et al.* (1989) found that 45% of patients admitted to hospital met criteria for depression 10 days after the myocardial infarction and 33% remained depressed at 3 months. Frasure-Smith *et al.* (2000) reported that 31% of older patients developed mild to moderate depression (as identified by a screening rating scale). At follow-up one year later, health care costs—for outpatient or emergency room visits—were 40% higher in the depressed compared to the non-depressed survivors. Kaufmann *et al.* (1999) found that depression was an independent predictor of death at 12 months following the index event. They suggested the need for prospective studies to assess the impact of the aggressive treatment of depression on survival in this patient group.

Depression also has a negative influence on the outcome of more chronic cardiovascular disorders. Koenig (1998) reported that 37% of older patients with congestive heart failure had major depression compared to a prevalence of 17% in cardiac patients without heart failure. Minor depression was found in 22%. The depressed patients often remained symptomatic for a long time, used more health resources, and had a more severe medical condition. Most were not treated with antidepressants or received psychotherapy. Mortality is also increased in this group, depressed patients being twice as likely to die within 2 years (Murberg *et al.* 1999; Herrmann *et al.* 2000). Personality type may play a role in outcome. Denollet *et al.* (2000) reported an association between type-D personality (that is, high negative affectivity and social inhibition) and the poor prognosis of depressed patients with heart failure.

The management of heart disease may itself provoke a depressive illness, either as a psychological reaction to a treatment such as cardiac surgery (Oxman *et al.* 1994) or as a pharmacological effect of treatment with drugs such as beta-blockers or calcium-channel blockers (Lindberg *et al.* 1998; Dunn *et al.* 1999). There is also evidence that older people with mental disorders are far less likely to be offered treatments such as revascularization (Druss *et al.* 2000).

Inadequate drug treatment of depression has, in the past, been attributed to the fear that tricyclic antidepressants might exacerbate cardiac rhythm disturbances in older patients. Postural hypotension, atrial and ventricular arrhythmias, and heart block may arise and lead to sudden death in cardiac patients (*British National Formulary* 2000). Selective serotonin reuptake inhibitors offer a safer alternative. Roose *et al.* (1998) directly compared the efficacy of paroxetine with nortriptyline in older outpatients with ischaemic heart disease. The drugs were equally effective and approximately 60% of patients responded. However, there were many more serious adverse cardiac events in the group taking nortriptyline. The tricyclic significantly reduced the heart rate variability, a factor believed to be associated with sudden death. Poor social network support and social disability is also a risk factor for depression and adverse cardiac outcome (Murberg *et al.* 1998). Management of the depressed cardiac patient will therefore involve the withdrawal, if possible, of drugs that may promote depression, the careful choice of an antidepressant, and counselling and social support. However, the effectiveness of such a package of care in older patients has yet to be evaluated.

Cancer

Cancer is a major cause of death and morbidity in older people, with more than half of new cases occurring in those aged 65 or older (Gosney 1998). Turner *et al.* (1999) have pointed out that older patients get less-aggressive treatment and, perhaps as a consequence, have a worse prognosis. They blame ageism in health care for this state of affairs. They also underline the fact that 75-year-olds have a further life expectancy of about 10 years. Prevalence rates for major depression depend partly on the site of the cancer, but on average the overall rate in older people is approximately 25% (Massie and Holland 1990). This rate is not particularly different from other chronic medical conditions (Hosaka and Aoki 1996; Given *et al.* 2000). Kurtz *et al.* (1997) found that lung cancer was especially debilitating and that a poor level of physical function was associated with comorbid conditions like depression. The 'young-old' were particularly at risk in this respect (Kurtz *et al.* 2000). The same research group also reported that survival was not associated with depressive disorder but with the loss of mobility and severity of pain (Kurtz *et al.* 1994; Given *et al.* 2000). However, caregiver depression was related prospectively to the patient's survival and this was, in turn, related to the degree of the patient's incapacity (Kurtz *et al.* 1994).

Clearly the prevalence of a comorbid depression depends partly on the symptom threshold used in the diagnosis. Criteria emphasizing the presence of somatic symptoms and concerns tend to underestimate the prevalence (Chochinov *et al.* 1994; Newport and Nemeroff 1998). It may be difficult to distinguish between the categories of adjustment reaction and depressive episode owing to symptom overlap. Somatization disorder can also confound the diagnosis. Anxiety is a common symptom that may interfere with both investigation and treatment. The common-sense clinical approach is to adopt a low diagnostic threshold, so as to avoid missing a treatable depression (Newport and Nemeroff 1998).

As with heart disease, cancer treatments themselves may be depressogenic. Biological stressors such as chemotherapy and radiotherapy, the paraneoplastic syndromes, as well as certain drugs like vincristine, procarbazine, tamoxifen, and ondansetron have all been implicated in provoking depression (Massie and Holland 1990).

It is known, mainly from work in young and middle-aged women with breast cancer, that survival may be determined by the psychological response to the disease (Watson *et al.* 1999). Counselling methods that instil 'fighting' spirit, improve day-to-day coping, and reduce anxiety may have some benefit, reduce the incidence of depression, and improve survival (Hellbom *et al.* 1998). Adaptations of cognitive–behavioural therapy can also be useful and may be more effective than simple counselling (Moorey *et al.* 1998). However, little formal study has yet been made of these techniques in elderly patients.

Antidepressants should have a role in the treatment of depressed cancer patients, even when anxiety predominates, but there are surprisingly few studies in this area. Ravazi *et al.* (1999) found that trazodone, in an open trial, effectively relieved anxiety in patients with breast cancer. Kugaya *et al.* (1999) described a small open trial of tricyclic antidepressants in terminally ill patients. Symptomatic improvement occurred after only one week of treatment.

There has been a widely held belief that people get less anxious about death as they get older. The evidence for this is limited, but some studies have found older people to be 'philosophical' about death (Kastenbaum 1992). Older people are often not afraid to talk about death and adjustment may be enhanced by open communication with the family. The open expression of a wish to die may alert medical staff to the presence of depression. Macdonald and Dunn (1982) found this sentiment to be common in a mixed sample of community- and nursing-home residents. It predicted subsequent mortality but was not necessarily associated with depressive illness. However, Shah *et al.* (2000*a*) could not replicate this finding. Forsell (2000) found that whilst 12% of an elderly sample expressed a wish to die, the majority of them did have a mental disorder. Similarly, fear of death and the dying process is found more frequently in mentally ill older people (Sullivan *et al.* 1998).

Some patients, their families, and their doctors collude to avoid mentioning death, even when suffering is severe and the prognosis obviously poor (Quill 2000). The liaison team may have a role here in helping those involved discuss the inevitable. Initiating end-of-life discussions earlier and more systematically might allow patients to make more informed choices, achieve better palliation of symptoms, and work on issues of life closure (Quill 2000). It is also important to elicit what the patient sees as important at this stage of life. Steinhauser *et al.* (2000) found that pain and symptom management, the ability to communicate with one's physician, preparation for death, and the opportunity to achieve a sense of completion were important to most patients.

Stroke

Stroke is the third most common cause of death in the developed world. Each year in Europe 1 million people out of a population of 500 million suffer a stroke, the majority occurring in the elderly (Brainin *et al.* 2000). The association between depression and cerebrovascular disease has been investigated for more than 50 years (Rao 2000). Poststroke depression has received much attention in the last two decades. Initial reports of the high prevalence of major depression following stroke, up to 50% in some inpatient studies (Robinson and Starkstein 1990), have been tempered by the lower rates found in rehabilitation units and the community (Burvill *et al.* 1995). However, Andersen *et al.* (1994*a*) reported an incidence of depression of 41% during the first year after a stroke, most cases developing during the first few months. It has been argued that studies of this problem have used inadequate control groups. Lieberman *et al.* (1999) found no difference in the incidence of depression following stroke or hip fracture.

The diagnosis of depression in patients following stroke is problematic. House *et al.* (1989) suggested that what most patients actually experienced was emotionalism (or emotional lability) rather than depression. Other symptoms, such as anxiety and agoraphobia, apathy, and pathological crying may complicate the clinical picture (Burvill *et al.* 1995). Changes in appetite, sleep, or interest may indicate depression or be a normal adjustment response to physical disability (Fedoroff *et al.* 1991). Gainotti *et al.* (1999) found that reactive symptoms predominated in the early phase after stroke and endogenous symptoms came to the fore in the later stages. Sembi *et al.* (1998) reported that 10% of patients developed a syndrome akin to classical post-traumatic stress disorder.

Early studies suggested that poststroke major depression was a function of lesion location rather than of disability (Robinson *et al.* 1983; Starkstein *et al.* 1987). As if to strengthen this view, the same group found that only minor depression was related to physical disability (Morris *et al.* 1994). Recovery is often delayed in depressed patients who may also be more severely disabled by the stroke itself (Mayo *et al.* 1991; Van de Weg *et al.* 1999).

The early identification and treatment of poststroke depression would therefore appear to be a critical function for the liaison old age psychiatrist. Table 19.6 summarizes a number of drug trials in patients with poststroke depression, treatment beginning either in the early phase of recovery after stroke (acute) or when the patient's medical condition had stabilized (chronic). The evidence suggests that antidepressants and methylphenidate have a beneficial effect, not only on mood, but also on physical function. Positive effects may be more pronounced in the later phase of recovery. Andersen *et al.* (1994*b*) found that

Table 19.6 Randomised placebo controlled trials in the drug treatment of post-stroke depression

Name	Year	Sample size	Mean age (years)	Trial duration (weeks)	Acute or chronic medical condition	Active drug and daily dose	Comparison with placebo
Lipsey et al.	1984	34	61	4–6	Chronic	Nortriptyline 50–100 mg	Active drug better
Reding et al.	1986	27	64	4 (mean)	Acute	Trazodone mean 200 mg	Active drug improved activities of daily living
Andersen et al.	1994b	28 38	67 67	6 Chronic	Acute chronic group only	Citalopram 10–40 mg	Active drug better in
Dam et al.	1996	52[1]	62	12	Chronic	Maprotiline 150 mg Fluoxetine 20 mg	Fluoxetine improved physical recovery
Grade et al.	1998	21[1]	68	3	Chronic	Methylphenidate 30 mg	Active drug improved physical recovery
Palomaki et al.	1999	100[1]	56	52	Chronic	Mianserin 60 mg	No difference in incidence of depression
Robinson et al.	2000	104[1]	61	12	Chronic	Nortriptyline 100 mg Fluoxetine 40 mg	Nortriptyline better than fluoxetine at treating depression, anxiety and activities of daily living
Wiart et al.	2000	31	64	6	Acute	Fluoxetine 20 mg mood only	Active drug improved

Note: [1], sample included depressed and non-depressed patients citalopram was only better than placebo in depressed patients treated later than 6 weeks after their stroke. They suggested that depressive illnesses occurring early tended to recover spontaneously. Some trials have included non-depressed patients on the grounds that antidepressants may have a preventive effect (Dam *et al.* 1996; Grade *et al.* 1998; Palomaki *et al.* 1999; Robinson *et al.* 2000). In the first two of these studies, the active drug had little effect on the mean depression scores, but improvement was seen mainly in measures of physical function. The incidence of poststroke depression in the placebo group of the Finnish study (Palomaki *et al.* 1999) was unusually low, at approximately 10%, suggesting that any drug effect was masked by other beneficial factors in this sample. However, these authors reported that the drug did have a preventive effect in the older subgroup. Kimura *et al.* (2000) found that the cognitive impairment associated with poststroke depression also improved with nortriptyline, but only in those whose mood improved. Lastly, Burns *et al.* (1999) reported that sertraline had a beneficial effect in the treatment of stroke-associated lability of mood and/or pathological crying in the absence of depression.

Psychological treatments for poststroke depression have received little systematic evaluation, although a recent review concluded that cognitive–behavioural therapy (CBT) was most promising (Kneebone and Dunmore 2000). Lincoln *et al.* (1997) described an open study of CBT in 19 depressed patients (recruited from a possible 136)—four recovered and six others derived some benefit. More encouraging have been efforts to assess the impact of practical support for patients and their families. Patients receiving a high level of support tend to have a better prognosis than those who become socially isolated (Glass *et al.* 1993). In one study, counselling and education about stroke and disability improved family function, but counselling was better than education alone (Evans *et al.* 1988). Two controlled trials have examined the effects of a family support worker for stroke victims (Dennis *et al.* 1997; Mant *et al.* 2000). Both found that carers benefited but patients did not.

Conclusions

In this chapter we have set out some principles for liaison old age psychiatry. We have reviewed the effectiveness of a number of initiatives in the organization of services, as well as the published evidence of the benefits of drug and psychological treatments, for medically ill older people with mental disorder. The high prevalence of mental disorder in this vulnerable group and the low referral rate to liaison services suggests a good deal of unmet mental health need in this group. The coexistence of unmanaged mental disorder with physical illness impedes recovery of the latter, delays the patient's discharge from hospital, and affects their long-term survival. Liaison services should be proactive, working with patients most at risk, but also seek to improve the generic mental health skills of general hospital staff. For this to be a realistic possibility, properly funded teams with dedicated staff time are needed. In the years to come, liaison old age psychiatrists may well become involved in the wider issues of clinical ethics. This already includes the assessment of competence and treatment refusal (see Chapter 40), but may soon include the review of the appropriateness of advance directives (Treloar 1999), the propriety of disguising medication in food or drink (Treloar *et al.* 2001), and requests for assisted suicide or euthanasia (Kissane and Kelly 2000).

References

Adshead, F., Day Cody, D., and Pitt, B. (1992). BASDEC: a novel screening instrument for depression in elderly medical inpatients. *British Medical Journal*, **305**, 397.

Allen, N., Ames, D., Ashby, D., Bennetts, K., Tuckwell, V., and West, C. (1994). A brief sensitive screening instrument for depression in late life. *Age and Ageing*, **23**, 213–19.

Ames, D. and Tuckwell, V. (1994). Psychiatric disorders among elderly patients in a general hospital. *Medical Journal of Australia*, **160**, 671–5.

Andersen, G., Vestergaard, K., Riis, J., and Lauritzen, L. (1994*a*). Incidence of post-stroke depression during the first year in a large unselected stroke population determined using a valid standardised rating scale. *Acta Psychiatrica Scandinavica*, **90**, 190–5.

Andersen, G., Vestergaard, K., and Lauritzen, L. (1994*b*). Effective treatment of post-stroke depression with the selective serotonin reuptake inhibitor citalopram. *Stroke*, **25**, 1099–104.

Anderson, D. N. and Philpott, R. M. (1991). The changing pattern of referrals for psychogeriatric consultation in the general hospital: an eight-year study. *International Journal of Geriatric Psychiatry*, **6**, 801–7.

Ardern, M., Mayou, R., Feldman, E., and Hawton, K. (1993). Cognitive impairment in the elderly medically ill: how often is it missed? *International Journal of Geriatric Psychiatry*, **8**, 929–37.

Arfken, C. L., Lichtenberg, P. A., and Tancer, M. E. (1999). Cognitive impairment and depression predict mortality in medically ill older adults. *Journal of Gerontology*, **54**, M152–6.

Arie, T. (1994). Health care of the elderly: the Nottingham model. In *The principles and practice of geriatric psychiatry* (ed. J. R. M. Copeland, M. T. Abou-Saleh, and D. G. Blazer), pp. 883–6.

Arie, T. and Dunn, T. (1973). A 'do-it-yourself' psychiatric-geriatric joint patient unit. *Lancet*, **2**, 1313–16.

Baheerathan, M. and Shah, A. (1999). The impact of two changes in service delivery on a geriatric psychiatry liaison service. *International Journal of Geriatric Psychiatry*, **14**, 767–75.

Benbow, S. M. (1987). Liaison referrals to a department of psychiatry for the elderly 1984–5. *International Journal of Geriatric Psychiatry*, **2**, 235–40.

Benbow, S. M. and Dawson, G. H. (1994). Liaison in old age psychiatry. In *Seminars in Liaison Psychiatry* (ed. E. Guthrie and F. Creed), pp. 220–37. Gaskell, London.

Bergmann, K. and Eastham, E. J. (1974). Psychogeriatric ascertainment and assessment for treatment in an acute medical ward setting. *Age and Ageing*, **3**, 174–88.

Blow, F. C., Brower, K. J., Schulenberg, J. E., Demo-Dananberg, L. M., Young, J. P., and Beresford, T. P. (1992). The Michigan Alcoholism Screening Test—Geriatric Version (MAST-G): a new elderly specific screening instrument. *Alcohol: Clinical and Experimental Research*, **16**, 372.

Borson, S., McDonald, G. J., Gayle, T., Deffenback, M., Lakshminarayan, S., and Van Tuinen, C. (1992). Improvement in mood, physical symptoms, and function with nortriptyline for depression in patients with chronic obstructive pulmonary disease. *Psychosomatics*, **33**, 190–201.

Borson, S., Loebel, J. P., Kitchell, M., Domoto, S., and Hyde, T. (1997). Psychiatric assessment of nursing home residents under OBRA-97: should pre-admission screening and annual review be reformed? *Journal of the American Geriatrics Society*, **45**, 1173–81.

Brainin, M., Bornstein, N. M., Boysen, G., and Demarin, V. (2000). Acute neurological stroke care in Europe: results of the European Stroke Care Inventory. *European Journal of Neurology*, **7**, 5–10.

Brauer, C., Morrison, R. S., Silberzweig, S. B., and Siu, A. L. (2000). The cause of delirium in patients with hip fracture. *Archives of Internal Medicine*, **160**, 1856–60.

British Geriatrics Society. (1995). *The discharge of elderly patients from hospital for community care: a joint policy statement by the British Geriatrics Society, the Association of Directors of Social Services and the Royal College of Nursing*. British Geriatrics Society, London.

British National Formulary. (2000). *British National Formulary 40*. British Medical Association and the Royal Pharmaceutical Society of Great Britain, London.

Burn, W. K., Davies, K. N., McKenzie, F. R., Brothwell, J. A., and Wattis, J. P. (1992). The prevalence of psychiatric illness in acute geriatric admissions. *International Journal of Geriatric Psychiatry*, **8**, 171–4.

Burns, A., Russell, E., Stratton-Powell, H., Tyrell, P., O'Neill, P., and Baldwin, R. (1999). Sertraline in stroke-associated lability of mood. *International Journal of Geriatric Psychiatry*, **14**, 681–5.

Burvill, G. A., Johnson, G. A., Jamrozik, K. D., Anderson, C. S., Stewart-Wynne, E. G., and Chakera, T. M. H. (1995). Prevalence of depression after stroke: the Perth Community Stroke Study. *British Journal of Psychiatry*, **166**, 320–7.

Caraceni, A., Nanni, O., Maltoni, M., Piva, L., Indelli, M., Arnoldi, E., *et al*. (2000). Impact of delirium on the short term prognosis of advanced cancer patients. *Cancer*, **89**, 1145–9.

Chocinov, H. M., Wilson, K. G., Enns, M., and Lander, S. (1994). Prevalence of depression in the terminally ill: effect of diagnostic criteria and symptom threshold judgements. *American Journal of Psychiatry*, **151**, 537–40.

Clarke, D. M., McKenzie, D. P., and Smith, G. C. (1995). The recognition of depression in patients referred to a consultation–liaison service. *Journal of Psychosomatic Research*, **39**, 327–34.

Clément, J-P., Fray, E., Paycin, S., Leger, J-M., Therme, J-F., and Dumont Daniel. (1999). Detection of depression in elderly hospitalized patients in emergency wards in France using the CES-D and the Mini-GDS: preliminary findings. *International Journal of Geriatric Psychiatry*, **14**, 373–8.

Cole, M. G. and Bellavance, F. (1997). Few elderly inpatients who are depressed improve. *Journal of the Canadian Medical Association*, **157**, 1055–60.

Cole, M. G., Fenton, F. R., Engelsmann, F., and Mansouri, I. (1991). Effectiveness of geriatric psychiatry consultation in an acute care hospital: a randomized clinical trial. *Journal of the American Geriatrics Society*, **39**, 1183–8.

Cole, M. G., Primeau, F. J., Bailey, R. F., Bonneycastle, M. J., Masciarelli, F., Engelsmann, F., *et al*. (1994). Systematic intervention for elderly inpatients with delirium: a randomized trial. *Canadian Medical Association Journal*, **151**, 965–70.

Collinson, Y. and Benbow, S. M. (1998). The role of the old age psychiatry consultation liaison nurse. *International Journal of Geriatric Psychiatry*, **13**, 159–63.

Cooper, B. (1987). Psychiatric disorders among elderly patients admitted to hospital wards. *Journal of the Royal Society of Medicine*, **80**, 13–16.

Crisp, A. H. (1968). The role of the psychiatrist in the general hospital. *Postgraduate Medical Journal*, **44**, 267–76.

Currier, M. B., Murray, G. B., and Welch, C. C. (1992). Electroconvulsive therapy for post-stroke depressed geriatric patients. *Journal of Neuropsychiatry and Clinical Neuroscience*, **4**, 140–4.

Dam, M., Tonin, P., De Boni, A., Pizzolato, G., Casson, S., Ermani, M., *et al.* (1996). Effects of fluoxetine and maprotiline on functional recovery in poststroke hemiplegic patients undergoing rehabilitation therapy. *Stroke*, **27**, 1211–14.

Davies, K. N., Burn, W. K., McKenzie, F. R., Brothwell, J. A., and Wattis, J. P. (1993). Evaluation of the Hospital Anxiety and Depression Scale as a screening instrument in geriatric medical inpatients. *International Journal of Geriatric Psychiatry*, **8**, 165–70.

Dennis, M., O'Rourke, S., Slattery, J., Staniforth, T., and Warlow, C. (1997). Evaluation of a stroke family care worker: results of a randomised controlled trial. *British Medical Journal,* **314**, 1071–6.

Denollet, J., Vaes, J., and Brutsaert, D. L. (2000). Inadequate response to treatment in coronary heart disease: adverse effects of type D personality and younger age on 5-year prognosis and quality of life. *Circulation*, **102**, 630–5.

Department of Health. (1995). *NHS responsibilities for meeting continuing health care needs.* HSG (95) 8. Her Majesty's Stationery Office, London.

Draper, B. (2000). The effectiveness of the treatment of depression in the physically ill elderly. *Aging and Mental Health*, **4**, 9–20.

Druss, B. G., Bradford, D. W., Rosenheck, R. A., Radford, M. J., and Krumholz, H. M. (2000). Mental disorders and use of cardiovascular procedures after myocardial infarction. *Journal of the American Medical Association*, **283**, 506–11.

Dunn, N. R., Freemantle, S. N., and Mann, R. D. (1999). Cohort study of calcium channel blockers, other cardiovascular agents, and the prevalence of depression. *British Journal of Clinical Pharmacology*, **48**, 230–3.

Evans, M. (1993). Development and validation of a brief screening scale for depression in the elderly physically ill. *International Clinical Psychopharmacology*, **8**, 329–31.

Evans, M., Hammond, M., Wilson, K., Lye, M., and Copeland, J. (1997). Placebo-controlled treatment trial of depression in elderly psychically ill patients. *International Journal of Geriatric Psychiatry*, **12**, 817–24.

Evans, R. L., Matlock, A. L., Bishop, D. S., Stranahan, S., and Pederson, C. (1988). Family intervention after stroke: does counseling or education help? *Stroke*, 19, 1243–9.

Ewing, J. A. (1984). Detecting alcoholism: the CAGE questionnaire. *Journal of the American Medical Association,* **252**, 608–9.

Farragher, B. and Walsh, N. (1998). Joint care admissions to a psychiatric unit: a prospective analysis. *General Hospital Psychiatry*, **20**, 73–7.

Farrell, K. R. and Ganzini, L. (1995). Misdiagnosing delirium as depression in medically ill elderly patients. *Archives of Internal Medicine*, **155**, 2459–64.

Federoff, J. P., Starkstein, S. E., Parikh, R. M., Price, T., and Robinson, R. G. (1991). Are depressive symptoms non-specific in patients with acute stroke? *American Journal of Psychiatry*, **148**, 1172–6.

Feldman, E., Mayou, R., Hawton, K., Ardern, M., and Smith, E. B. O. (1987). Psychiatric disorder in medical in-patients. *Quarterly Journal of Medicine*, **240**, 301–8.

Finch, E. F., Ramsey, R., and Katona, C. L. (1992). Depression and physical illness in the elderly. *Clinical Geriatric Medicine*, **8**, 275–87.

Folstein, M. F., Folstein, S. E., and McHugh, P. R. (1975). 'Mini-mental state'. A practical method for grading the cognitive state of patients for the clinician. *Journal of Psychiatric Research*, **12**, 189–98.

Forsell, Y. (2000). Do death wishes reflect psychiatric disorder? *Acta Psychiatrica Scandinavica*, **102**, 135–8.

Francis, J., Martin, D., and Kapoor, W. N. (1990). A prospective study of delirium in hospitalized elderly. *Journal of the American Medical Association*, **263**, 1097–101.

Frasure-Smith, N., Lesperance, F., Gravel, G., Masson, A., Juneau, M., Talajic, M., *et al.* (2000). Depression and health-care costs during the first year following myocardial infarction. *Journal of Psychosomatic Research*, **48**, 471–8.

Gainotti, G. Azzoni, A., and Marra, C. (1999). Frequency, phenomenology and anatomical-clinical correlates of major post-stroke depression. *British Journal of Psychiatry*, **175**, 163–7.

Ganzini, L., Smith, D. M., Fenn, D. S., and Lee, M. A. (1997). Depression and mortality in medically ill older adults. *Journal of the American Geriatrics Society*, **45**, 307–12.

Gill, D. and Hatcher, S. (1999). A systematic review of the treatment of depression with antidepressant drugs in patients who also have a physical illness. *Journal of Psychosomatic Research*, **47**, 131–43.

Given, C. W., Given, B., Azzouz, F., Stommel, M., and Kozachik, S. (2000). Comparison of changes in physical functioning of elderly patients with new diagnoses of cancer. *Medical Care*, **38**, 482–93.

Glass, T. A., Matchar, D. B., Belyea, M., and Feussner, J. R. (1993). Impact of social support on outcome in first stroke. *Stroke*, **24**, 64–70.

Gosney, M. (1998). Geriatric oncology. In *Brocklehurst's textbook of geriatric medicine and gerontology* (5th edn) (ed. R. Tallis, H. Fillit, and J. Brocklehurst), pp. 1319–23. Churchill Livingstone, Edinburgh.

Grade, C., Redford, B., Chrostowski, J., Toussaint, L., and Blackwell, B. (1998). Methylphenidate in early poststroke recovery: a double-blind, placebo-controlled study. *Archives of Physical Medicine and Rehabilitation*, **79**, 1047–50.

Health Advisory Service. (2000). *'Not because they are old'. An independent inquiry into the care of older people on acute wards in general hospitals.* Health Advisory Service 2000, London.

Hellbom, M., Brandberg, Y., Glimelius, B., and Sjoden, P. O. (1998). Individual psychological support for cancer patients: utilisation and patient satisfaction. *Patient Education and Counselling*, **34**, 247–56.

Herrmann, C., Brand-Driehorst, S., Buss, U., and Ruger, U. (2000). Effects of anxiety and depression on 5-year mortality in 5,057 patients referred for exercise testing. *Journal of Psychosomatic Research*, **48**, 455–62.

Holmes, J. and House, A. (2000). Psychiatric illness predicts poor outcome after surgery for hip fracture: a prospective study. *Psychological Medicine*, **30**, 921–9.

Hosaka, T. and Aoki, T. (1996). Depression among cancer patients. *Psychiatry and Clinical Neuroscience*, **50**, 309–12.

House, A., Dennis, M., Warlow, C., and Hawton, K. (1989). Emotionalism after stroke. *British Medical Journal*, **298**, 991–4.

Inouye, S. K., Van Dyck, C. H., Alessi, C. A., Balkin, S., Siegal, A. P., and Hawitz, R. I. (1990). Clarifying confusion: the confusion assessment method. *Annals of Internal Medicine*, **113**, 941–8.

Jackson, R. and Baldwin, B. (1993). Detecting depression in elderly medically ill patients: the use of the Geriatric Depression Scale compared with medical and nursing observations. *Age and Ageing*, **22**, 349–53.

Johnston, M., Wakeling, A., Graham, N., and Stokes, F. (1987). Cognitive impairment, emotional disorder and length of stay of elderly patients in a district general hospital. *British Journal of Medical Psychology*, **60**, 133–9.

Katz, I. R., Simpson, G. M., Curlik, S. M., Parmelee, P. A., and Muhly, C. (1990). Pharmacologic treatment of major depression for elderly patients in residential settings. *Journal of Clinical Psychiatry*, **51**(Suppl. 7), 41–57.

Kaufman, B. M. and Bates, A. B. (1990). Factors affecting provision of psychogeriatric care: a survey of geriatricians' views. *Care of the Elderly*, **2**, 25–7.

Kaufmann, M. W., Fitzgibbons, J. P., Sussman, E. J., Reed, J. F. 3rd, Einfalt, J. M., Rodgers, J. K., *et al.* (1999). Relation between myocardial infarction, depression, hostility, and death. *American Heart Journal*, **138**, 549–54.

Kastenbaum, R. (1992). Death, suicide and the older adult. *Suicide and Life-Threatening Behaviour*, **22**, 1–14.

Kimura, M., Robinson, R. G., and Kosier, J. T. (2000). Treatment of cognitive impairment after poststroke depression: a double-blind treatment trial. *Stroke*, **31**, 1482–6.

Kissane, D. W. and Kelly, B. J. (2000). Demoralisation, depression and desire for death: problems with the Dutch guidelines for euthanasia of the mentally ill. *Australia and New Zealand Journal of Psychiatry*, **34**, 325–33.

Kitchell, M. A., Barnes, R. F., Veith, R. C., Okimoto, J. T., and Raskind, M. A. (1982). Screening for depression in hospitalized geriatric medical patients. *Journal of the American Geriatrics Society*, **30**, 174–7.

Kneebone, I. I. and Dunmore, E. (2000). Psychological management of post-stroke depression. *British Journal Clinical Psychology*, **39**, 53–65.

Koenig, H. G. (1998). Depression in hospitalized older patients with congestive heart failure. *General Hospital Psychiatry*, **20**, 29–43.

Koenig, H. G., Meador, K. G., Cohen H. J., and Blazer, D. G. (1988*a*). Depression in elderly hospitalized patients with medical illnesses. *Archives of Internal Medicine*, **148**, 1929–36.

Koenig, H. G., Meador, K. G., Cohen, H. J., and Blazer, D. G. (1988*b*). Detection and treatment of major depression in older medically ill hospitalized patients. *International Journal of Psychiatry in Medicine*, **18**, 17–31.

Koenig, H. G., Shelp, F., Goli, V., Cohen, H. J., and Blazer, D. G. (1989*a*). Survival and health care utilization in elderly medical inpatients with major depression. *Journal of the American Geriatrics Society*, **37**, 599–606.

Koenig, H. G., Goli, V., Shelp, F., Kudler, H. S., Cohen, H. J., Meador, K. G., *et al.* (1989*b*). Antidepressant use in elderly medical inpatients: lessons from an attempted clinical trial. *Journal of General and Internal Medicine*, **4**, 498–505.

Koenig, H., Meador, K. G., Shlep, F., Goli, V., Cohen, H. J., and Blazer, D. G. (1991). Major depressive disorder in hospitalized medically ill patients: an examination of young and elderly male veterans. *Journal of the American Geriatrics Society*, **39**, 881–90.

Koenig, H. G., Cohen, H. J., Blazer, D. G., Medaor, K. G., and Westlund, R. (1992). A brief depression scale for use in the medically ill. *International Journal of Psychiatry in Medicine*, **22**, 183–95.

Koenig, H. G., George, L. K., and Meador, K. G. (1997). Use of antidepressants by nonpsychiatrist in the treatment of medically ill hospitalized depressed elderly patients. *American Journal of Psychiatry*, **154**, 1369–75.

Kok, R. M., Heeren, T. J., Hooijer, C., Dinkgreve, M. A., and Rooijmans, H. H. (1995). The prevalence of depression in elderly medical inpatients. *Journal of Affective Disorders*, **33**, 77–82.

Kugaya, A., Akechi, T., Nakano, T., Okamura, H., Shima, Y., and Uchitomi, Y. (1999). Successful antidepressant treatment for five terminally ill cancer patients with major depression, suicidal ideation and a desire for death. *Supportive Care in Cancer*, **7**, 432–6.

Kurtz, M. E., Given, B., Kurtz, J. C., and Given, C. W. (1994). The interaction of age, symptoms, and survival status on physical and mental health of patients with cancer and their families. *Cancer*, **74**(Suppl. 7), 2071–8.

Kurtz, M. E., Kurtz, J. C., Stommel, M., Given, C. W., and Given, B. (1997). Loss of physical functioning among geriatric cancer patients: relationships to cancer site, treatment, comorbidity and age. *European Journal of Cancer*, **33**, 2352–8.

Kurtz, M. E., Kurtz, J. C., Stommel, M., Given, C. W., and Given, B. A. (2000). Symptomatology and loss of physical functioning among geriatric patients with lung cancer. *Journal of Pain and Symptom Management*, **19**, 249–56.

Lakshmanan, M., Mion, L. C., and Frengley, J. D. (1986). Effective low dose tricyclic antidepressant treatment for depressed geriatric rehabilitation patients. A double-blind study. *Journal of the American Geriatrics Society*, **34**, 421–6.

Lawton, M. P. (1975). The Philadelphia Geriatric Center Morale Scale: a review. *Journal of Gerontology*, **30**, 85–9.

Levkoff, S. E., Evans, D. A., Liptzin, B., Clear, P. D., Lipsitz, L. A., Wetle, T. T., *et al.* (1992). Delirium. The occurrence and persistence of symptoms among elderly hospitalised patients. *Archives of Internal Medicine*, **152**, 334–40.

Lieberman, D., Friger, M., Fried, V., Grinshpun, Y., Mytlis, N., Tylis, R., *et al.* (1999). Characterization of elderly patients in rehabilitation: stroke versus hip fracture. *Disability and Rehabilitation*, **21**, 542–7.

Lincoln, N. B., Flannaghan, T., Sutcliffe, L., and Rother, L. (1997). Evaluation of cognitive behavioural treatment for depression after stroke: a pilot study. *Clinical Rehabilitation*, **11**, 114–22.

Lindberg, G., Bingefors, K., Rantsam, J., Tastam, L., and Melander, A. (1998). Use of calcium channel blockers and risk of suicide: ecological findings confirmed in population based cohort study. *British Journal of Medicine*, **316**, 741–5.

Lipowski, Z. J. (1983). The need to integrate liaison psychiatry and geropsychiatry. *American Journal of Psychiatry*, **140**, 1003–5.

Lipsey, J. R., Robinson, R. G., Pearlson, G. D., Rao, K., and Price, T. (1984). Nortriptyline treatment of post-stroke depression: a double-blind study. *Lancet*, **i**, 297–300.

Loane, R. and Jeffreys, P. (1998). Consultation–liaison in an old age psychiatry service. *Psychiatric Bulletin*, **22**, 217–20.

Luttrell, S., Watkin, V., Livingston, G., Walker, Z., D'Ath, P., Patel, P., *et al.* (1997). Screening for alcohol misuse in older people. *International Journal of Geriatric Psychiatry*, **12**, 1151–4.

Macdonald, A. J. D. and Dunn, G. (1982). Death and the expressed wish to die in the elderly: an outcome study. Age and Ageing, **11**, 189–95.

Mainprize, E. and Rodin, G. (1987). Geriatric referrals to a psychiatric consultation–liaison service. *Canadian Journal of Psychiatry*, **32**, 5–9.

Mant, J., Carter, J., Wade, D. T., and Winner, S. (2000). Family support for stroke: a randomised controlled trial. *Lancet*, **356**, 808–13.

Massie, J. and Holland, J. (1990). Depression and the cancer patient. *Journal of Clinical Psychiatry*, **51**(Suppl. 7), 12–17.

Mayo, N. E., Korner-Bitensky, N. A., and Becker, R. (1991). Recovery time of independent function poststroke. *American Journal of Physical Medicine and Rehabilitation*, **70**, 5–12.

Milstein, A., Barak, Y., Kleinman, G., and Pollack, A. (2000). The incidence of delirium immediately following cataract removal surgery: a prospective study in the elderly. *Aging and Mental Health*, **4**, 178–81.

Moorey, S., Greer, S., Bliss, J., and Law, M. (1998). A comparison of adjuvant psychological therapy and supportive counselling in patients with cancer. *Psychooncology*, **7**, 218–28.

Morris, P. L., Shields, R. B., Hopwood, M. J., Robinson, R. G., and Raphael, B. (1994). Are there two depressive syndromes after stroke? *Journal of Nervous and Mental Disease*, **182**, 230–4.

Mossey, J. M., Knott, K. A., Higgins, M., and Talerico, K. (1996). Effectiveness of a psychosocial intervention, interpersonal counselling, for subdysthymic depression in medically ill elderly. *Journal of Gerontology*, **51**, M172–8.

Murberg, T. A., Bru, E., Aarsland, T., and Sveback, S. (1998). Social support, social disability and their role as predictors of depression among patients with congestive heart failure. *Scandinavian Journal of Social Medicine*, **26**, 87–95.

Murberg, T. A., Bru, E., Sveback, S., Tveteras, R., and Aarsland, T. (1999). Depressed mood and subjective health symptoms as predictors of mortality in patients with congestive heart failure: a two-year follow-up study. *International Journal of Psychiatry in Medicine*, **29**, 311–26.

Newport, D. J. and Nemeroff, C. (1998). Assessment and treatment of depression in the cancer patient. *Journal of Psychosomatic Research*, **45**, 215–37.

Office of National Statistics. (1999). Social Trends 29. The Stationery Office, London.

O'Riordan, T. G., Hayes, J. P., Shelley, R., O'Neill, D., Walsh, J. B., and Coakley, D. (1989). The prevalence of depression in an acute geriatric medical assessment unit. *International Journal of Geriatric Psychiatry*, **4**, 17–21.

Oxman, T. E., Barrett, J. E., Freeman, D. H., and Manheimer, E. (1994). Frequency and correlates of adjustment disorder related to cardiac surgery in older patients. *Psychosomatics*, **35**, 557–68.

Pajarillo, E. J., Sers, A. J., Ryan, R. M., Hradley, B., and Nalven, C. (1997). Consultation–liaison psychiatric nursing in long-term care. *Journal of Psychosocial Nursing and Mental Health Services*, **35**, 24–30.

Palomaki, H., Kaste, M., Berg, A., Lonnqvist, R., Lonnqvist, J., Lehtihalmes, M., *et al.* (1999). Prevention of poststroke depression: 1 year randomised placebo controlled double blind trial of mianserin with 6 month follow up after therapy. *Journal of Neurology, Neurosurgery and Psychiatry*, **66**, 490–4.

Pauser, H., Berstrom, B., and Walinder, J. (1987). Evaluation of 294 psychiatric consultations involving in-patients above 70 years of age in somatic department in a university hospital. *Acta Psychiatrica Scandinavica*, **76**, 152–7.

Pitt, B. and Silver, C. P. (1980). The combined approach to geriatrics and psychiatry: evaluation of a joint unit in a teaching hospital district. *Age and Ageing*, **9**, 33–7.

Poynton, A. (1988). Psychiatric liaison referrals of elderly in-patients in a teaching hospital. *British Journal of Psychiatry*, **152**, 45–7.

Quill, T. E. (2000). Initiating end-of-life discussions with seriously ill patients: addressing the 'elephant in the room'. *Journal of the American Medical Association*, **284**, 2502–7.

Qureshi, K. N. and Hodkinson, H. M. (1974). Evaluation of a ten-question mental test in the institutionalized elderly. *Age and Ageing*, **3**, 152–7.

Ramsay, R., Wright, P., Katz, A., Katz, A., Bielawaski, C., and Katona, C. (1991). The detection of psychiatric morbidity and its effects on outcome in acute elderly medical admissions. *International Journal of Geriatric Psychiatry*, **6**, 861–6.

Rao, R. (2000). Cerebrovascular disease and late life depression: an age old association. *International Journal of Geriatric Psychiatry*, **15**, 419–33.

Ravazi, D., Kormoss, N., Collard, A., Farvacques, C., and Delvaux, N. (1999). Comparative study of the efficacy and safety of trazodone versus clorazepate in the treatment of adjustment disorder in cancer patients: a pilot study. *Journal of Internal Medicine Research*, **27**, 264–72.

Reding, M. J., Orto, L. A., Winter, S. W., Fortuna, I. M., Di Ponte, P., and McDowell, F. H. (1986). Antidepressant therapy after stroke. A double-blind trial. *Archives of Neurology*, **43**, 763–5.

Robinson, R. G. and Starkstein, S. E. (1990). Current research in affective disorders following stroke. *Journal of Neuropsychiatry and Clinical Neurosciences*, **2**, 1–14.

Robinson, R. G., Starr, L. B., Kubos, K. L., and Price, T. (1983). A two-year longitudinal study of post-stroke mood disorders: findings during initial evaluation. *Stroke*, **14**, 736–41.

Robinson, R. G., Schultz, S. K., Castillo, C. Kopel, T., Kosier, J. T., Newman, R. M., *et al.* (2000). Nortriptyline versus fluoxetine in the treatment of depression and in short-term recovery after stroke: a placebo-controlled, double-blind study. *American Journal of Psychiatry*, **157**, 351–9.

Roose, S. P., Laghrissi-Thode, F., Kennedy, J. S., Nelson, J. C., Bigger, J. T. Jr., Pollock, B. G., *et al.* (1998). Comparison of paroxetine and nortriptyline in depressed patients with ischaemic heart disease. *Journal of the American Medical Association*, **279**, 287–91.

Royal College of Physicians. (1992). *Standardized assessment scales for elderly people: Report of the Joint Workshops of the Research Unit of the Royal College of Physicians and the British Geriatrics Society.* Royal College of Physicians, London.

Royal Colleges of Psychiatrists and Physicians. (1999). *The care of older people with mental illness: specialist services and medical training.* Royal College of Psychiatrists, London.

Schein, R. L. and Koenig, H. G. (1997). The Center for Epidemiological Studies—Depression (CES-D) Scale: assessment of depression in the medically ill elderly. *International Journal of Geriatric Psychiatry*, **12**, 436–46.

Schifano, F., Garbin, A., Renesto, V., De Dominicis, M. G., Trinciarelli, G., Silvestri, A., *et al.* (1990). A double-blind comparison of mianserin and maprotiline in depressed medically ill elderly people. *Acta Psychiatrica Scandinavica*, **81**, 289–94.

Schleifer, S. J., Macari-Hinson, M. M., Coyle, D. A., Slater, W. R., Kahn, M., Gorlin, R., *et al.* (1989). The nature and course of depression following myocardial infarction. *Archives of Internal Medicine*, **149**, 1785–9.

Scott, J., Fairbairn, A., and Woodhouse, K. (1988). Referrals to a psychogeriatric consultation–liaison service. *International Journal of Geriatric Psychiatry*, **14**, 131–5.

Sembi, S., Tarrier, N., O'Neill, P., Burns, A., and Faragher, B. (1998). Does post-traumatic stress disorder occur after stroke: a preliminary study. *International Journal of Geriatric Psychiatry*, **14**, 681–5.

Shah, A. (1998). Can depression and depressive symptoms predict mortality at 18-month follow-up in acutely medically ill inpatients over the age of 80 years? *International Journal of Geriatric Psychiatry*, **13**, 240–3.

Shah, A. K., Herbert, R., Lewis, S., Mahendran, R., Platt, J., and Bhattacharyya, B. (1997). Screening for depression among acutely ill geriatric inpatients with a short geriatric depression scale. *Age and Ageing*, **26**, 217–21.

Shah, A., Hoxey, K., and Mayadunne, V. (2000*a*). Suicidal ideation in acutely medically ill elderly inpatients: prevalence, correlates and longitudinal stability. *International Journal of Geriatric Psychiatry*, **15**, 162–9.

Shah, A., Hoxey, K., and Mayadunne, V. (2000*b*). Some predictors of mortality in acutely medically ill elderly inpatients. *International Journal of Geriatric Psychiatry*, **15**, 493–9.

Sheehan, B. and Banerjee, S. (1999). Somatization in the elderly. *International Journal of Geriatric Psychiatry*, **14**, 1044–9.

Sinoff, G., Ore, L., Zlotogorsky, D., and Tamir A. (1999). Short Anxiety Screening Test—a brief instrument for detecting anxiety in the elderly. *International Journal of Geriatric Psychiatry*, **14**, 1062–71.

Starkstein, S. E., Robinson, R. G., and Price, T. R. (1987). Comparison of cortical and subcortical lesions in the production of post-stroke mood disorders. *Brain*, **110**, 1045–59.

Steinhauser, K. E., Christakis, N. A., Clipp, E. C., McNeilly, M., McIntyre, L., and Tulsky, J. A. (2000). Factors considered important at the end of life by patients, family, physicians and other care providers. *Journal of the American Medical Association*, **284**, 2476–82.

Stevens, L. E., de Moore, G. M., and Simpson, J. M. (1998). Delirium in hospital: does it increase length of stay? *Australia and New Zealand Journal of Psychiatry*, **32**, 805–8.

Strain, J. J., Lyons, J. S., Hammer, J. S., Fahs, M., Lebovits, A., Paddison, P. L., *et al.* (1991). Cost offset from a psychiatric consultation–liaison intervention with elderly hip fracture patients. *American Journal of Psychiatry*, **148**, 1044–9.

Sullivan, M., Ormel, J., Kempen, G. I., and Tymstra, T. (1998). Beliefs concerning death, dying, and hastening death among older, functionally impaired Dutch adults: a one-year longitudinal study. *Journal of the American Geriatrics Society*, **46**, 1251–7.

Swanwick, G. R. J., Lee, H., Clare, A. W., and Lawlor, B. (1994). Consultation–liaison psychiatry: a comparison of two service models for geriatric patients. *International Journal of Geriatric Psychiatry*, **9**, 495–9.

Tan, R. S., Barlow, R. J., Abel, C., Reddy, S., Palmer, A. J., Fletcher, A. E., *et al.* (1994). The effect of low dose lofepramine in depressed elderly patients in general medical wards. *British Journal of Clinical Pharmacology*, **37**, 321–4.

Treloar, A. (1999). Advanced directives: limitations upon their applicability in elderly care. *International Journal of Geriatric Psychiatry*, **14**, 1039–43.

Treloar, A. and Macdonald, A. J. D. (1997). Outcome of delirium diagnosed by DSM-III-R, ICD-10 and CAMDEX and derivation of the Reversible Cognitive Dysfunction

Scale among acute geriatric inpatients. *International Journal of Geriatric Psychiatry*, **12**, 609–13.

Treloar, A., Philpot, M., and Beats, B. (2001). Concealing medications in patients' food is legitimate in exceptional circumstances. *Lancet*, **357**, 62–4.

Turner, N. J., Haward, R. A., Mulley, G. P., and Selby, P. J. (1999). Cancer in old age—is it inadequately investigated and treated? *British Medical Journal*, **319**, 309–12.

Unutzer, J., Patrick, D. J., and Diehr, P. (2000). Quality adjusted life years in older adults with depressive symptoms and chronic medical disorders. *International Psychogeriatrics*, **12**, 15–33.

Uwakwe, R. (2000). Psychiatric morbidity in elderly patients admitted to non-psychiatric wards in a general teaching hospital in Nigeria. *International Journal of Geriatric Psychiatry*, **15**, 346–54.

Van de Weg, F. B., Kuik, D. J., and Lankhorst, G. J. (1999). Post-stroke depression and functional outcome: a cohort study investigating the influence of depression on functional recovery from stroke. *Clinics in Rehabilitation*, **13**, 268–72.

Wallace, A. E., Kofoed, A. L., and West, A. N. (1995). Double-blind, placebo-controlled trial of methylphenidate in older, depressed, medically ill, patients. *American Journal of Psychiatry*, **152**, 929–31.

Waller, R. and Hillam, J. (2000). Assessment of depression in older medical inpatients: practice, attitudes and the effect of teaching. *Aging and Mental Health*, **4**, 275–7.

Watson, M., Haviland, J. S., Greer, S., Davidson, J., and Bliss, J. M. (1999). Influence of psychological response on survival in breast cancer: a population-based cohort study. *Lancet*, **354**, 1331–6.

White, A. (1990). Styles of liaison psychiatry: discussion paper. *Journal of the Royal Society of Medicine*, **83**, 506–8.

Wiart, L., Petit, H., Joseph, P. A., Mazaux, J. M., and Barat, M. (2000). Fluoxetine in early poststroke depression: a double-blind placebo-controlled study. *Stroke*, **31**, 1829–32.

Wood, W. R., Vlachonikolis, I., Griffeths, P., and Griffeths, R. A. (1987). The structure of depressive symptoms in the elderly. *British Journal of Psychiatry*, **150**, 463–70.

Wrigley, M. and Loane, R. (1991). Consultation–liaison referrals to the north Dublin old age psychiatry services. *Irish Medical Journal*, **84**, 89–91.

Yesavage, J. A., Brink, T. L., Rose, T. L., Lum, O., Huang, V., Adey, M., *et al.* (1983). Development and validation of a geriatric depression screening scale: a preliminary report. *Journal of Psychiatric Research*, **17**, 37–49.

Zielinski, R. J., Roose, S. P., Devanand, D. P., Woodring, S., and Sackeim, H. A. (1993). Cardiovascular complications of ECT in depressed patients with cardiac disease. *American Journal of Psychiatry*, **150**, 904–9.

III Psychiatric services

20 Principles of service provision in old age psychiatry

Andrew F. Fairbairn

Introduction

The concept of old age psychiatry as a service in its own right is relatively recent. It has not been easy to raise the profile of a service dealing with a sector of the population which is regarded as 'unfashionable' and which also suffers from illnesses—in particular dementia and depression—that are often viewed by the general public as normal phenomena of old age. Provision for the elderly mentally ill—and, equally importantly, for their carers—has not, historically, been a priority.

Changing demographic trends, due to improved health care and other factors, have seen a vast increase in the number of elderly people in society, a figure that will continue to grow for many years to come. Many elderly people will and do lead active, fulfilling lives for many years after they stop paid work. However, the inevitable consequence of a rising population that lives longer is that many more of them manifest symptoms of physical and mental illness which require treatment and, therefore, they become a burden on society and a problem for their families. We have, to some extent, failed to keep up with the shifting demands of the society in which we live.

Doctors who plan a medical career in old age psychiatry will never be short of patients! The fact that many people in our western society are fit and active well into their eighties and nineties is a compliment to health services and to advances in health/social/environmental measures over recent decades. One has only to look at photographs of the Queen Mother on the occasion of her 100th birthday (August 2000) to see how fit a well-preserved centenarian can be. Not all elderly people are so fortunate. We may be living longer than ever before, but as we age we almost inevitably become more frail. We are all familiar with the sadly frequent scenario of a demented or mentally ill elderly person with no-one to support him or her.

So, how has old age psychiatry as a specialty progressed over the years, where do we stand now, and what is the future for all of us—professionals and patients?

Historical context

The creation of geriatric medicine as a specialty in the United Kingdom can be credited to Dr Marjorie Warren, who recognized the need for compassionate, skilled, specialist medical input into National Health Service (NHS) long-term care. Over time, geriatric medicine has become the largest specialty within general internal medicine in the NHS. Old age psychiatry (formerly 'psychogeriatrics') grew out of a similar recognition that patients in long-stay wards in the old psychiatric hospitals deserved particular attention. However, old age psychiatry rapidly developed a multidisciplinary community-oriented approach whilst continuing a commitment to the broad spectrum of care including NHS long-term care (Arie and Jolley 1982).

Amongst the first specialized old age psychiatry services to be created were those at the Maudsley Hospital (London), in Devon, and in Newcastle-upon-Tyne—pioneered by charismatic, entrepreneurial individuals. The original posts in these UK services were filled by general psychiatrists with a special interest in psychogeriatrics and so, fairly rapidly, there was a move towards a full-time commitment to old age psychiatry.

The original formal professional group within the Royal College of Psychiatrists was the Section for the Psychiatry of Old Age. This group pressed for and obtained formal specialty status for old age psychiatry from the Department of Health in 1989. The formal recognition of specialty status, apart from its intrinsic value, has allowed meaningful statistical information to be obtained and has facilitated a focus on specific staffing issues within old age psychiatry.

Although old age psychiatry was created out of general adult psychiatry, it has probably always had a closer clinical working relationship with the specialty of geriatric medicine. It has also had close working relationships over the decades with local social services and a broad spectrum of community services.

The international scene

Old age psychiatry was pioneered in the UK, which can be justifiably proud of this development. However, differing patterns of health care provision in other countries have made the creation of old age psychiatry services elsewhere less straightforward.

Given the link of language, and often the pattern of medical training, Commonwealth countries have generally been most enthusiastic in creating specialist old age psychiatry services. Australia, for example, has now taken the lead as regards innovative service developments.

In relation to Europe, the UK still has the most mature old age psychiatry service. It should be remembered that in many other countries the specialty of neurology takes the leading role in the diagnosis of dementia—an illness which in the UK accounts for between one-half and two-thirds of all referrals to old age psychiatry services (Campbell and Fairbairn 1989). Furthermore, certain countries have geriatric medicine services that are very committed to looking after dementia sufferers.

In developing countries, mental health services for older people are at best embryonic. Nevertheless, some countries (such as India, with 60 million people over the age of 60) are attempting to address the particular needs of old people with mental health problems and not simply rely on geriatric services, such as they may be. In these countries, the strong family commitment to supporting elderly relatives is an admirable act of duty and respect, but it might actually be holding back the development of old age psychiatry services, which the UK would argue are of proven value.

Demographic issues

Major demographic issues are dealt with elsewhere in this book. However, it should be borne in mind that trends in the UK have resulted in an enormous growth in the numbers of older people, particularly those over the age of 80. It should also be remembered that the average age of patients referred to old age psychiatry services is 80+ (Campbell and Fairbairn 1989). It is not the purpose of this chapter to make sociological observations about older people in the UK, but it is worth mentioning that the current old people in Britain are the individuals who fought the Second World War and who, as working adults, paid the taxes that created the National Health Service. Yet they are probably the least demanding sector of the population. Often older people are carers in their own right, and therefore poorly placed to press for improvements in services to support themselves and their dependent relatives (Levin 1997).

The economic strength of a country is the basis on which it funds health care. The NHS has proved immensely good value for money, with health care in the UK taking approximately 6% of GDP (gross domestic product) compared with other European countries that frequently use at least 8% of GDP. The general demographic trend, i.e. the 'rising tide' of older people, is less dramatic in the UK than in any other European Union country (Department of Health 1997, p. 9). Therefore, the UK would seem economically well

Table 20.1 Changes in population in countries who will have more than 15 million people over 60 years of age in 2025

	Rank in 1950	Population aged over 60 1950	1975	2000	2025	Rank in 2025	Magnitude of the increase (1950 to 2025)	
China	1	42.5	73.7	134.5	284.1	1	6.8	China
India	2	31.9	29.7	65.6	146.2	2	4.6	India
USSR	4	16.2	33.9	54.3	71.3	3	4.4	USSR
United States	3	18.5	31.6	40.1	67.3	4	3.6	United States
Japan	8	6.4	13.0	26.4	33.1	5	5.2	Japan
Brazil	16	2.1	6.2	13.9	31.8	6	15.1	Brazil
Indonesia	10	3.8	6.8	14.9	31.2	7	8.2	Indonesia
Pakistan	11	3.3	3.6	6.9	18.1	8	5.5	Pakistan
Mexico	25	1.3	3.1	6.6	17.5	9	13.4	Mexico
Bangladesh	14	2.6	3.3	6.5	16.8	10	6.4	Bangladesh
Nigeria	27	1.3	2.6	6.3	16.0	11	12.3	Nigeria
Italy	9	5.7	9.7	13.5	15.9	12	2.8	Italy
West Germany	6	7.0	12.3	13.3	15.1	13	2.2	West Germany

Reproduced with permission from Kalache (1991). In *Principles and practice of geriatric medicine* (2nd edn) (ed. MSJ Pathy). John Wiley & Sons, Chichester.

placed to address the future health care needs of its elderly population.

In the UK, older people commonly live in older houses which are expensive to repair and to heat. Many are managing financially on the sole basis of the state old age pension, which is less than a student loan for higher education. Many old people live alone, and they are most frequently women—for the simple reason that women tend to survive longer than men (Social Services Inspectorate 1997*b*).

With improved life expectancy and increased social mobility, the children of such older people, in the developed world, do not necessarily live in their local neighbourhood and are therefore poorly placed to act as informal carers for their parents or other family members of the older generation. In addition, these 'children' are most likely to be in their fifties, working in full-time employment, and with teenage families or even their own grandchildren. Despite the logistical difficulties, families are—almost without exception—extremely caring and committed, and will do their utmost to support aged parents and other relatives.

It is worth noting that there are varying patterns of long-term care across Europe, which reflect the culture and history of the different European countries. The Scandinavian countries have the most sophisticated health and social care services, probably due to a national commitment to a high-tax economy in return for a commitment from the state to health and social care (Council of Europe 1995). In the Mediterranean countries, there remains a strong culture of support from within the family, so that the institutionalization of old or otherwise dependent relatives is less likely.

The old Eastern Bloc countries of Europe have in recent years embraced the market economy systems of the West, and also appear to be developing services for their elderly inhabitants that are much more comprehensive than their previous relatively simple, or simplistic, models of institutional care. However, it is only through economic development that such countries can afford to improve their services for older people.

UK health and social services

Funding of health and social services

Funding of the NHS and local authority social services is through the public purse. The actual sums involved are agreed between the Treasury and the Department of Health. Until very recently this was done on an annual basis, and was known as the Public Expenditure Survey, but this 'short-termism' has been improved by the cycle being extended to every 3 years, under the title of the Comprehensive Spending Review. The exact sums given to each locality—district health authorities (including primary care groups and NHS trusts) and local authorities (county/district/city councils)—depend on complex formulas based on population, deprivation indices, and an element of history. However, whilst NHS monies are given directly to districts, funds for local authority social services are channelled through the Department for Environment, Transport and the Regions, which is responsible for local government. This means that centrally identified funding for social services is sent out in block grants to local authorities which provide many other services, such as housing and roads. Local authorities may not therefore divide up their allocations in accordance with centrally intended patterns.

District health services are ultimately accountable to the Department of Health and to health ministers, but social services departments are ultimately accountable to their local council and councillors. This is despite one of the most remarkable—and relatively silent—shifts in the funding of local government that occurred during the last Conservative reign under the leadership of Margaret Thatcher and which has been perpetuated by the current Labour Government. About 20 years ago, 70% of local government funding was raised through local taxation; now only 40% of the funding of local expenditure is raised through the Community Charge (based on housing valuation for home-owners—the old 'rates' system under another name) plus local taxes on businesses. The net result of these shifts is that *total* local expenditure is increasingly under central control, whilst devolved social services budgets may be cut in the game of balancing *local* priorities.

UK community care reforms

Radical changes to the remit and responsibilities of health and social services in relation to community care occurred with the implementation in 1993 of the Community Care Act (Department of Health 1990). The creation of a formal split between 'purchasers' and 'providers' of services had occurred slightly earlier in the NHS, but the Community Care Act attempted to create the same separation in social services. It also gave social services the 'lead role': they now hold both the responsibility and the budget for community provision.

One of the purposes of the Community Care Act was to allow disabled individuals, frequently older people, to continue to live independently for as long as possible in their own homes by creating flexible packages of care to support them there. It is therefore ironic that the 'institutionalization rate' has actually *increased* since the legislation (Audit Commission 1997).

Refreshingly, more recently there have been public concerns about long-term care, which led to the creation of a Royal Commission in 1999. At the time of writing, the Royal Commission has reported and has made two important recommendations. The first is that there should be a National Care Commission set up to monitor standards in long-term care, and the second (by a majority vote) is that both personal and nursing care for old people should be 'free'—i.e. met by public funding. Two of the members of the Royal Commission wrote a minority report recommending that only *nursing* care should be provided free, and it is this minority recommendation that has been accepted by the UK Government in England, Wales, and Northern Ireland. At the time of writing the devolved Scottish Government has undertaken to go along with the Royal Commission majority report

Community care legislation was driven by market economy principles. The rationale was that a particular locality knew its own circumstances best, and that market forces would create the services most suited to local conditions. However, many people had doubts about whether the 'business ethic' could appropriately be applied to health and social services. More importantly, the Community Care Act signified an abandonment of central service planning and hence any application of national standards and norms.

Future funding of services—who should pay?

Who should pay for what services? The current funding of the UK NHS is through general taxation, and therefore health services remain free to all 'consumers' at the point of delivery. Contrary to popular belief, National Insurance deductions from earnings do not constitute a dedicated health tax. Funding for social services has historically come from local authorities (county and district/city councils), although the bulk of local authority funding is now based on grants from central government. This means that social support to individuals continues to be means-tested (i.e. dependent on their income and capital assets), although different local authorities have divergent views on the types of means testing.

That said, there are much broader societal considerations in the funding of the care of older people, particularly those with mental health problems. Recent demographic trends have led economists to describe the 'financial burden' of providing care to older people on a diminishing working population through income tax. When William Beveridge was creating his blueprint for the post-war Labour 'welfare state' in the UK in the 1940s, he looked at male life expectancy (which at that time was, on average, 66 years and 6 months), assumed an active working life of 50 years from the then minimum school-leaving age of 14, and drew a line at the age of 65 for the retirement of men. He anticipated a retirement period of only 18 months before death—whereas it is now perhaps 15 years. *Does this mean that, with increased numbers of fit active individuals aged between 65 and 75, western societies should consider increasing their typical retirement age of 65 to, say, 75?*

Keeping such older people in active employment would mean they would continue to contribute to, rather than become a drain upon, the public purse. This in turn might change views on the balance of state funding versus individual contributions.

If society felt that it valued its older people so much that it wished to relieve them of all financial contribution to their care, then it would seem that this would allow affluent older people to pass their wealth on to the next generation, thus arguably giving unfair advantages to their descendants. *So, should affluent older people pay for their care in whatever setting, including the NHS?*

The balance between central direction and local development

Governments make central policies based on a number of factors. The first is their own political strategies, as exemplified by party manifestos at election time. They also react to public concerns and media pressure.

In the UK, for example, the Department of Health, which is responsible for health and social services in England and Wales, attempts to prioritize health policy issues. Only rarely does formal Parliamentary legislation take place; most central direction is issued in the form of 'guidelines'. These guidelines are often interpreted as having the force of law but generally they have not, although they may attain formal legal status if challenged by Judicial Review. Most of the time, however, government policy is not compulsory, although subsequent failures by local organizations to implement central directives—if exposed as resulting in poor standards of service—will, at least, lead to professional humiliation, and possibly also to a 'media scandal' and consequent public dismay.

Central policy-makers are constantly looking for examples of good service developments. These generally happen in specific localities as the result of imaginative initiatives by local professionals and their employing authorities. The Department of Health, in particular, sees part of its remit as publicizing such innovative moves, in the hope that other local bodies will be inspired to follow suit.

Therefore, the balance between central direction and local development can be described as dynamic. Greater understanding by local services that central government is rather more facilitative than negatively judgmental, might perhaps lead to increased constructive cooperation between the central and local bodies.

The change of government in the UK in 1997, from Conservative to Labour, did lead to a central recognition that health services, in particular, needed national standards and guidelines. To that end National Service Frameworks were introduced. The National Service Framework for Mental Health was published in 1999, but specifically excluded issues to do with the mental health of older people. Shortly afterwards a National Service Framework for Older People was announced, with one task group specifically addressing mental illness. This important document, published in the year 2001, is a framework for high-quality care of older people, including those with mental health problems. The national framework should lead to the creation by local health services, along with their social services partners, of high-quality coordinated and comprehensive provision for older people in every district. Inevitably such frameworks will take some years to implement, but national standards are to be welcomed.

Community-oriented services

Old age psychiatry services in the UK have always been community-oriented. There are many different patterns, a few of which are described below.

Before the recent health and community care reforms, old age psychiatry services often accepted referrals directly from both general practitioners and social workers. Unfortunately, the funding changes following these reforms have led to referrals from social workers becoming much more problematic because general practitioners have to agree to them. A recent survey confirmed general practitioners' lack of diagnostic confidence and therapeutic pessimism in this field (Audit Commission 2000).

Most, but certainly not all, old age psychiatry services, upon accepting a referral, will make the first assessment in the individual's home (Royal College of Physicians and Royal College of Psychiatrists 1998). Typically, this first assessment is carried out by a senior doctor, either a consultant psychiatrist or a specialist registrar in old age psychiatry. Certain services run multidisciplinary allocation meetings, where the most appropriate clinician, not necessarily a psychiatrist, will make the initial assessment and report back to the multidisciplinary team. It is the ethos of old age psychiatry services that such assessments are made quickly. In the vast majority of services it is rare for a referral to wait over a week. Patients referred urgently are seen as soon as possible.

The psychogeriatric day hospital is probably the backbone of more formal assessment. After the initial home assessment, approximately one-third of old people will go on to receive a comprehensive multidisciplinary assessment in the day hospital, whereas only around 6% will require inpatient admission (Campbell and Fairbairn 1989).

Obviously, service styles will vary according to geography and staffing. In densely populated urban settings, it is much easier for medical staff to do home visits. In a rural setting, where a catchment area might be 50 square miles or more, a different approach—for example using community psychiatric nurses (CPNs) to make the initial assessment—might be more appropriate.

Multidisciplinary assessment

The typical multidisciplinary team will consist of a consultant in old age psychiatry, one or more junior doctors, hospital nursing staff, community psychiatric nurses, occupational therapists, attached social workers, and a psychologist. There is also increasing input from the disciplines of physiotherapy and speech therapy. The multidisciplinary team is an integral part of the hospital day and inpatient units, and does not work in isolation in the community. However, in rural settings CPNs may be attached to primary care teams based in GP practices or community hospitals.

Members of the multidisciplinary team get together to communicate and to coordinate their activities on a variety of occasions, typically during case conferences and reviews and formal team meetings. On the one hand, the particular specialist skills of all clinicians need to be respected, but on the other hand recognition needs to be given to the fact that there may be an overlap of skills. Often, it is the team secretary who coordinates the clinical service, and it has often been argued that the secretary is the most crucial member of the team.

In this context, the consultant in old age psychiatry nevertheless has a unique expertise in terms of length of training in both physical and mental health, as well as a breadth of experience, which enables him or her to play a constructive leadership role.

Spectrum of services

The Royal College of Physicians and the Royal College of Psychiatrists have recently published an excellent joint document on the provision of old age psychiatry services, which includes recommended norms for catchment area size, workforce, day places, and inpatient beds (Royal College of Physicians and Royal College of Psychiatrists 1998). (See also Table 20.2.)

The role of the general practitioner and primary care team is vital. They act as the gatekeepers to all secondary specialist services, including of course old age psychiatry, and often—more informally—to other forms of support such as social services and the voluntary sector. The new primary care groups (PCGs, and successor bodies, the primary care trusts, with devolved budgets for purchasing patient care) will serve total populations of around 100 000 people. Therefore, each PCG will typically have on its books about 1000 patients suffering from dementia and a similar number of older people suffering from depression. These significant groups of older people with mental health problems should have their needs addressed by the new PCGs, in conjunction with local social services and with support from secondary hospital-based specialties, i.e. both old age psychiatry and geriatric medicine.

Any psychogeriatric assessment should identify an individual's specific needs and how to address them (Fig. 20.1). Therefore, flexible home-care support should be increasingly available. Home-care provision should cover a wide range of topics—from 'pop-in' checks on safety, through personal assistance with dressing and bathing, to help with practical issues such as cleaning, shopping, and meal preparation. Nowadays such services should be more elastic, and should extend beyond the hours of the traditional working day. If necessary, the elderly person should be left safely in bed during the evening, and support should be available over the weekend.

Other, sometimes apparently low-key, services can often be of great help to a disabled, socially isolated older person. Therefore other forms of visiting support, often run locally by charitable bodies such as Age Concern or the Alzheimer's Society, are very valuable.

A number of remarkably flexible home-care services, such as those provided by the Dementia Care Initiative, demonstrate the potential benefit of intensive domiciliary care (Stirling *et al.* 1996).

Day centres and luncheon clubs provide valuable social contacts for elderly people, and—particularly in relation to dementia sufferers—will allow carers welcome respite. It should be remembered that such community services, if provided by the local authority as opposed to the NHS, are potentially means-tested, the criteria for evaluation being dependent upon the relevant local authority's charging policies. The whole process of means-testing (or indeed any system of charging) can often be an additional hurdle when planning the community care of older people with dementia, who may often lack insight and may therefore be unable to see why they should be in receipt of such services in the first place. Wise social workers working in imaginative social services departments can usually surmount such problems.

With the implementation of the Community Care Act in 1993, social services departments were financially disadvantaged so that they were obliged to reduce, and in many cases entirely cease, their own directly funded provision of services in the shape of day centres and residential care. This shift led to a mushrooming of independent-sector homes, an issue addressed below. Certain old age psychiatry services had in the past a close working liaison with local residential homes, either through routine visits by the consultant in old age psychiatry or through the attachment of a CPN. Such excellent examples of liaison faded as social services closed their residential homes.

Table 20.2 Indicative service levels

General practice

A typical general practice of list size 10 000 will include 1500 people aged 65 and over. These are likely to include around 75 with dementia, 225 with depression (including 30 with severe depression), 30 with psychoses, and others with various less common conditions. Good practice would include: registration of older people with serious mental illness identified during clinical-generated contact or routine surveillance; regular review of health and social status of patients and carers; effective liaison with specialist services, social services, and other agencies including the voluntary and independent sectors.

Service-planning population

A service-planning population of 250 000 will include 37 500 people aged 65 and over. Among these will be approximately 2000 with dementia, 5600 with depression (750 severe), 750 with psychoses, and 750 with other conditions.

An effective old age psychiatry service managed within one provider unit for this population would typically comprise:

- Consultants: 4 whole-time equivalents (w.t.e.)
- Specialist registrar: if able to offer appropriate training
- Trainees: 4 w.t.e. those preparing for careers in psychiatry, medicine, general practice, or other specialty
- Community team: 8 community mental-health nurses, four social workers, clinical psychologists, occupational therapists, physiotherapists, chiropodists, speech therapists, dietitian, pharmacist
- Secretariat: personal secretary for each consultant, administrative, and information staff

Services provided should include:

- Domiciliary and community clinics
- Hospital outpatient clinics
- Day-hospital places: 75–112 distributed appropriately
- Continuing care and respite-care beds: 56–112 distributed appropriately, no more than 20 per unit, best within same unit as day hospital
- Acute assessment and treatment beds: 40–80, no more than 20 per ward in general hospital, with psychiatry and geriatric medicine with all investigative facilities
- Liaison services: with other hospital services, especially geriatric medicine, with general practice and social services
- Educational and supportive activities: medicine, nursing, social work, and other disciplines; carers, voluntary groups, private sector

The service should also have in place a case register and system of audit.

Once the initial assessment of an elderly person has taken place (at home, at a day hospital, or in an inpatient unit) and multidisciplinary assessment has been carried out, the individual may be seen to need continuing institutional care. Long-term care, in the present 'state of the nation', is most likely to be provided in the independent (private and voluntary) sector. The involvement of both the patient and his/her carers in such an important decision on relocation, is paramount. Ironically, therefore, obtaining a place in an independent-sector home has meant that families are often *less* supported by social workers (as agents of the local social services department) in making these very difficult decisions about placement than they would have been when residential homes were directly owned and managed by social services.

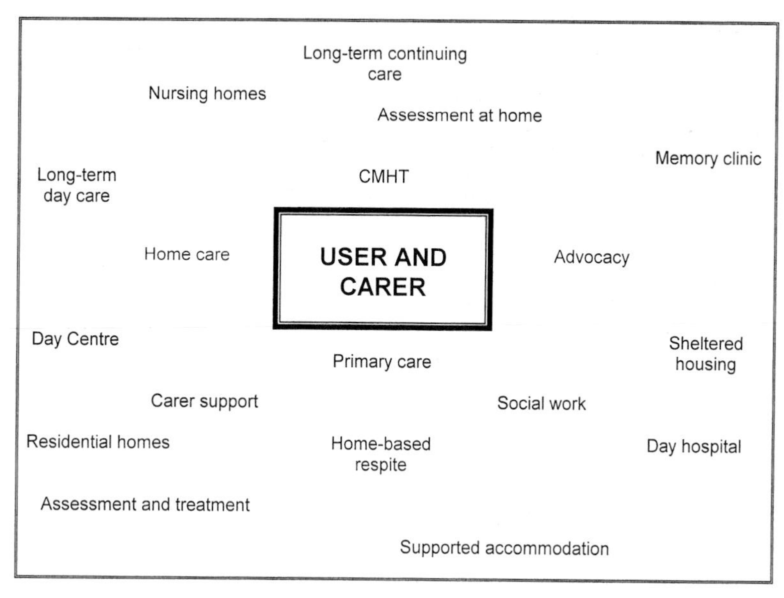

Fig. 20.1 The range of possible services.

The local independent-sector homes will be either residential or nursing homes, but places in both are purchased from social services' budgets (except for the 30% of patients who are self-financing). Homes are regulated by a local inspection team, which is increasingly a joint creation of the district health authority and its social services partners. In many areas there is recognition of the particular needs of behaviourally disturbed dementia sufferers who require a more secure setting, the professional skills of psychiatric nurses, and probably higher staffing levels in any long-term facility. This has led to the development of special 'EMI' (elderly mentally infirm) residential and nursing homes.

The community care legislation gave some less philanthropic district health authorities the opportunity to withdraw funding from NHS continuing care, which was—and still is—free (as it should be) for the most physically and/or psychiatrically disabled patients in all age ranges. In recent years, the Department of Health has issued guidance confirming the commitment of the NHS to such long-stay provision, which, of course, no longer needs to be in a hospital ward but can—indeed should—be in a more *domestic* nursing-home setting (Department of Health 1995).

The balance between standard and specialist services

Most sufferers from mental health problems in old age, particularly those afflicted by dementia, will inevitably be significant 'consumers' of generic health and social services. They will be major users of acute medical beds, orthopaedic services, and a wide range of community facilities provided by social services and the NHS. This means that staff working in generic services need appropriate training and support because of the frequent contact they will have with such 'difficult' elderly people.

Some long-term support services will be required to specialize in dementia care when behavioural aspects of the disease become a particular problem. Often such facilities, be they day centres or residential/nursing homes, carry some kind of euphemistic label—for example, 'EMI' (elderly mentally infirm). The advantage of labelling is the acknowledgement that mentally frail old people have special needs, and that facilities catering for these needs are likely to require enhanced staffing levels and training, and will therefore cost more. The disadvantage of such labelling is the risk of stigma.

At face value, sheltered accommodation should be the *optimal* form of housing for older people. Sheltered accommodation units offer residents a small flat, giving appropriate privacy and dignity, plus the social milieu of the unit as a whole, all monitored by a warden. However, despite the inbuilt safeguards, it often proves difficult in practice to provide intensive support for older people with mental health problems in these blocks of sheltered flats. This may be because dementia sufferers often forget their current domicile and attempt to wander back to past homes, which are more vivid in their memory. Living in a small flat can also be very socially isolating. All in all, the potential of sheltered accommodation has not yet been fully exploited (Audit Commission 2000).

Social services

As outlined above, there has been a major shift over the last decade in government expectations of local social services. The funding basis and accountability of local authorities has changed. Social services departments have largely ceased to provide/fund facilities directly, and now generally 'commission' various forms of care and support for local residents—which remain, however, means-tested.

Social services typically commission and/or provide the services detailed in Table 20.3.

Table 20.3 Services commissioned by social services

Home-care workers
Mobile meals (meals-on-wheels)
Day care
Residential respite care for periods of a few days to a few weeks
Residential care
Nursing-home care

As regards older people, it is generally recognized that close collaboration between health and social services in the commissioning of care, as well as joint working at a clinical level, is vital. To that end the Department of Health and the Social Services Inspectorate have issued a number of guidance documents. *Building bridges* is perhaps the best example in relation to both management and practitioner working (Department of Health 1995). The Social Services Inspectorate, part of the Social Care Division of the Department of Health, regularly issues advice on the mental health of older people and *Assessing older people with dementia living in the community* (Social Services Inspectorate 1996) and *At home with dementia* (Social Services Inspectorate 1997) are two excellent documents.

The Health Act 1999 allows a legal framework for even closer joint working, including joint budgets, but only time will tell if the different patterns of accountability will allow the real creation of unified budgets and truly unified services (Department of Health 1999).

The independent sector

Community care reforms have led to an expansion of independent-sector provision of both residential and nursing homes (Laing 1997). To a lesser extent, the independent sector has become involved in community day care. The term 'independent' in this context covers both private (for profit) and voluntary (charitable) organizations. The independent sector consists of large national companies through a spectrum down to small individually run homes. Traditionally, there has been poor liaison between specialist teams catering for the mental health of older people and independent-sector residential/ nursing homes. The Faculty for the Psychiatry of Old Age and the Independent Healthcare Association have recently issued joint guidelines on good practices and the improvement of links (Royal College of Psychiatrists 1999). In essence, there are three broad recommendations for better joint working. The first is good communication at the time of the transfer of an old person to long-term care, particularly in relation to documentation. Second, there should be a more flexible attitude to support from clinicians in the specialist community multidisciplinary teams. There should be recognition of the valuable expertise of these team members and the ways in which they can contribute to the smooth running and high quality of care in independent-sector homes. Third, there can be an educational role for the multidisciplinary team, using members to contribute to the training of care staff in residential or nursing homes. Table 20.4 lists some points for ensuring good liaison in this area. In addition, there should be continuing team support and review of any placement problems.

A small number of pioneering organizations claim to manage moderately severely, behaviourally disturbed dementia-sufferers in an extremely homely atmosphere using traditional housing (Svanberg *et al.* 1997). Such organizations also advocate the concept of 'shared care'. This means the continuing involvement of informal carers after the admission of a patient to a long-term facility. For example, it might be possible for a daughter to continue some form of personal care for her mother after the mother has been admitted to a residential or nursing home. Larger, profit-making, home-care organizations have traditionally been wary of the involvement of relatives, since they tend to be concerned about legal liability in the event of accidents, and therefore, in general, discourage the participation of informal carers.

It is only a relatively short time since the received wisdom was that dementia sufferers with significant behaviour problems could only be managed in wards in large psychiatric hospitals.

Table 20.4 Features of good liaison with the independent sector

Good, timely written information at the time of admission of a patient.
Named liaison clinician, where resources allow.
Formal and informal multidisciplinary team input into local education and training.
Continuing team support and review of placement problems.

Now the received wisdom is that these people should live in residential and nursing homes with as domestic an atmosphere as possible. As a consequence, the importance of building design has become recognized. The Dementia Services Development Centre at the University of Stirling has been particularly successful in creating building criteria (Chapter 22). Simple signs, colour-coded doors, building layouts that allow some sensible wandering space, are all now commonplace. With modern technology, it should be possible to create 'smart' buildings that increase the freedom of residents, although the technological opportunity should not be used as an excuse to reduce nurse staffing levels and hence the cost of placements. The great bulk of all expenditure on health and social services is tied to staffing and not to expenses of premises or consumables.

Kitwood's concept of 'personhood' and the development of dementia care mapping has not only increased awareness of the need to respect the dignity of dementia sufferers but has also allowed nursing—in particular—to have a raised profile in long-term care (Kitwood 1997). Dementia care mapping allows staff to learn, and consequently the quality of care improves, not only for the individual but in any institution as a whole.

Recently, the particular problems of ensuring that dementia sufferers continue to receive a good diet in residential- and nursing-home care has received attention with the publication of an article in VOICES 1998, giving practical guidance and excellent dietary advice in relation to 'eating well with dementia'.

Voluntary organizations

The Alzheimer's Society and Age Concern are the leading voluntary organizations in the UK dedicated to supporting elderly people, who often have mental health problems. They have an important role in lobbying the government of the day and influencing policy. The Alzheimer's Society has also diversified into significant service provision in certain areas in the country—supplying domiciliary care, sitter services, and specialist day centres.

Both the Alzheimer's Society and other organizations, such as the Alzheimer's Research Trust, now play a vital role in commissioning a broad range of research projects into mental health in old age.

Interface with acute medicine

Since older people with mental health problems are major users of standard health and social services, then it follows that the staff in specialist secondary services—in particular old age psychiatry—should contribute a significant amount of their time to both liaison and education. The liaison role might be in acute medical settings, geriatric medicine and rehabilitation, generic social services provision, and the independent residential and nursing sector. Inevitably there are difficult decisions to be made, when staff are being pulled in all directions, concerning the best 'value for money' in determining where to concentrate the skills of the old age psychiatry multidisciplinary team. For example, it may be that a concentrated spell of liaison and education on, for example, an orthopaedic ward might lead to a reduction in inappropriate discharges back into the community.

The role of old age psychiatry teams in liaising with hospital medical colleagues has become increasingly important in the UK (Anderson and Philpott 1991) (see also Chapter 19). Some services receive one-third of their referrals from hospitals as opposed to the community. Most referrals come from geriatric medicine, but significant others include acute medical wards and orthopaedic departments. To a lesser extent, there is clinical contact with the specialties of neurology and neurosurgery. Liaison is generally consultant-led, but there are a number of services where a liaison nurse is the first point of contact. There are two ways in which old age psychiatry teams can particularly help hospital colleagues. The first is in the identification of psychiatric disorder, particularly depression, and the second is assistance with discharge-planning. The old age psychiatry team tends to be particularly knowledgeable about the availability of local support services, and it is also often well placed to help reduce the pressure for (inappropriately) rapid discharge of elderly inpatients occupying acute hospital beds.

Interface with general psychiatry and learning disability

As indicated above, a number of old age psychiatry services have a strict age-related policy for referrals, typically starting from age 65, but others have a more flexible approach. The more flexible services will inevitably have discussions with general psychiatry colleagues as to which is the most appropriate service to manage a particular individual. The most common area of debate tends to be the 'graduate' population. The second area of clinical overlap is in relation to younger people suffering from dementia. However, it is increasingly likely, as outlined below, that old age psychiatry services will accept responsibility for younger people afflicted by premature dementia.

Old age psychiatry services periodically have an interface with learning disability (formerly mental handicap) services because of the increased incidence of dementia in middle-aged or elderly people with congenital brain damage—particularly sufferers from Down's syndrome (formerly described as mongolism). Thanks to modern medicine, brain-damaged individuals are living much longer than they used to, and one may therefore expect an increasing need for collaboration between old age psychiatry and learning disabilities services in the field of dementia care.

Younger dementia sufferers

Young dementia sufferers are particularly problematic. To suffer dementia in one's forties presents a completely different set of problems to those of an 80-year-old. A 40-year-old may be struggling in employment, be physically fit, and will often have teenage children at home sitting school exams. Younger dementia sufferers are rare enough in any particular district for no clinical service to have felt a particular commitment towards them, hence the national paucity of support for this unfortunate group of patients. That said, there are some notable and praiseworthy exceptions, two particular examples being the respective psychiatric services in Liverpool and Leeds.

The Royal College of Psychiatrists has recently published a policy document on this subject, in which it recognizes that the local clinical lead for younger dementia sufferers is likely to be old age psychiatry, and recommends a highly pragmatic approach to developing care for this patient group (Royal College of Psychiatrists 2000). In essence, the Royal College's recommendation is for two sessions of consultant time, plus the involvement of an experienced CPN, which can then be built on further. This approach should lead to 'something better than nothing' arrangements, which is currently often the case.

A particular uncertainty in terms of service provision for younger dementia sufferers is the emergence of variant Creutzfeldt–Jakob disease (vCJD). CJD proper is a rare and naturally occurring spongiform encephalopathy that typically strikes late in life and is progressive and fatal; vCJD has been linked to the consumption of beef from cattle afflicted with BSE (bovine spongiform encephalopathy) and is likewise fatal, but sufferers are likely to be younger before symptoms appear and are likely to experience a rapid decline. Whilst the prevalence of CJD itself has stayed relatively static for decades, there is no confidence about the future incidence of vCJD. It may well prove necessary for clinicians in old age psychiatry, general psychiatry, neuropsychiatry (if this specialty exists locally), and neurology to agree guidelines for the support of sufferers from vCJD and their families, particularly as these individuals often present psychiatrically at first, and then develop neurological symptoms before becoming physically heavily dependent in advance of death.

Other issues

Psychological approaches

Non-pharmacological approaches to the treatment of mental health problems in older people are just as relevant as with younger people. Nevertheless, the provision of such services is relatively limited. Whilst medical and nursing staff in old age psychiatry may, or may not, have particular expertise in this area, the establishment of a Special Interest Group for the Elderly within the British Psychological Society has been instrumental in increasing/encouraging the number of clinical psychologists committed to working with older people. This is particularly welcome as clinical psychologists can contribute an extra dimension to the treatment of mental health problems in this field.

Services for the functionally ill

Most old age psychiatry services have deliberately not gone down the line of specializing solely in dementia care. However, as the majority of referrals do tend to be for dementia, there is always a risk that sufferers from other problems (depression in particular) may receive less attention than they deserve, despite the considerable evidence that depression is a major problem in residential care and amongst older people in receipt of community services at home (Banerjee and Macdonald 1996; Margallo-Lana *et al.* 2000). There is a historical debate about whether assessment services should have separate 'functional' and 'organic' wards. It is to be hoped that with the modern design of assessment wards a single unit can house both groups and meet their respective needs. With community and residential care services very much geared to dementia sufferers, there is a similar risk that elderly people with functional illness may be difficult to support constructively in the community or to place appropriately, as and when necessary, in long-stay care.

Long-term care and the use of compulsory Mental Health Act powers

The use of the Mental Health Act in the assessment and treatment of older people with mental health problems is far less frequent than it is with the younger population. Nevertheless there is an occasional need for compulsory assessment.

Services should make appropriate arrangements for this.

Paternalism versus autonomy of the individual in service provision

Dementia sufferers, in particular, will incur a loss of insight at some point during the progression of their illness. There is a healthy pressure upon services to listen to the voice of service users, including those with dementia. There is also a healthy emphasis on the **rights** of 'consumers' and their relatives. However, rights only come with responsibilities. Obviously the autonomy of a dementia sufferer should be respected as far as possible, but there comes a point when that autonomy may lead to the person's loss of dignity and to severe stress for his/her informal carers. Although such dilemmas are seen as particularly problematic in the field of services for confused elderly people, they are, in truth, no different from the tensions that any individual in society experiences. As individuals, we all have responsibilities to society and are not irresponsibly autonomous. Service providers also have to accept the additional burden of being responsible to society on behalf of vulnerable patients in their care. Therefore, at some point, a 'paternalistic' judgement may need to be made. In the case of any individual patient, this will hopefully be after due consideration of the options by the professionals and informal carers together. However, very occasionally an apparently authoritarian intervention by the professionals, acting on behalf of society, may be necessary—despite disagreement by the elderly person's relatives or friends.

Even more rarely, but often enough to be an issue, there is an occasional need to enforce long-term care for elderly people under the terms of either a Treatment Order or a Guardianship Order. At the time of the Bournewood case[1] there were concerns that the inability to give informed consent to long-term care might require those with all but the mildest degree of dementia to be *formally detained* under the Mental Health Act so as to clarify their status and rights. Since the House of Lords overturned the Bournewood Judgment, informal admission would now seem to be once again legal, although it is to be hoped that future reviews of the Mental Health Act and of Mental Incapacity legislation may again address the intrinsic problem of patient consent.

The role of memory clinics

Memory clinics are a new growth area in the NHS. They present a new option for the referral of patients with memory problems, and may on occasion be more acceptable to certain patient groups than other forms of assessment for incipient dementia. These clinics tend to be in more academic or research-oriented settings. They can be a useful means of assessing elderly people for the appropriateness of anti-Alzheimer medication and for monitoring the effectiveness of such medication. Memory clinics probably do not address issues of activities of daily living, which only a more comprehensive multidisciplinary assessment—usually in the home—can cover satisfactorily. It remains to be seen whether memory clinics will become a routine part of old age psychiatry services (Audit Commission 2000).

Future prospects

Brain protection units

There is increasing recognition that as we move towards earlier and earlier diagnosis of cerebral impairment—in particular dementia—the next logical step is the concept of a 'brain protection unit', where early investigation of subtle problems might not only reduce or delay the onset of dementia but might also obviate some other costly demands by old people on the NHS, e.g. in respect of falls and fractures.

Unified services between old age psychiatry and geriatric medicine

It is perhaps surprising that, despite the regular clinical contact between the hospital specialties of old age psychiatry and geriatric medicine, the few examples of joint units and services—such as achieved in Nottingham—have not become the norm. It may be that the culture of old age psychiatry is such that a 'mental health service' is felt to be the most appropriate form of provision. However, with the push towards pooled budgets and unified service delivery it is likely that there will be a number of fresh 'service models', experimenting with the combination of old age psychiatry, geriatric medicine, and social services, with the aim of ensuring comprehensive and coordinated support to elderly people in their locality/district.

International growth of services for old people with mental illness

As indicated at the beginning of this chapter, the recognition of dementia as a major health care issue for primarily (but not exclusively) the developed world means that there is likely to be significant international expansion of specialist secondary services in old age psychiatry. It is doubtful whether there will be a 'standard model', given the breadth of services used by dementia sufferers and given the varying sociopolitical approaches in different countries.

The impact of anti-Alzheimer medication on service delivery

It is too early to predict whether the recently licensed drug treatments for Alzheimer's disease will have a significant impact on service provision and costs for dementia sufferers. Research seems to indicate that taking some drugs with or without vitamins may 'delay' the decline in patients with Alzheimer's disease by about 6 months (Chapter 24vii). Simplistically, if prescribed drugs could result in a six-month delay in admission to institutional care, or a six-month delay in the demand for domiciliary services, then anticholinesterase inhibitors might well prove to be highly cost-effective. The design of clinical trials that might answer these complex medical/economic health questions would seem to be extremely difficult, and—once again—the jury appears to be out on this issue and we can only wait and see (Fairbairn 2000).

Subspecialization within old age psychiatry

There are some, including the author, who regret the increasing specialization within hospital medicine in the UK, whilst accepting it as the way of modern life. Therefore it is logical to look beyond the current, confident growth of unified old age psychiatry services in the UK. It may be that there will be the development of subspecialization within old age psychiatry, two possible examples being the growth of specialist liaison services and the creation of memory clinics. How such innovations will affect the current holistic approach of old age psychiatry services to patients remains to be seen.

Commissioning services

District health authorities—and, increasingly, primary care trusts—should now be commissioning mental health services for older people jointly with local social services (Tables 20.5 and

Table 20.5 Commissioning old age psychiatry services

Issues for primary-care groups
1. Old age psychiatry services should be discretely commissioned (not as part of generic mental health commissioning).
2. Awareness of the spectrum of existing local resources, including health, social, voluntary, and independent sectors.
3. Awareness of the eligibility criteria for such services and any potential, or actual deficits.
4. Knowledge of local demography in order to be cognisant of 'local issues'.
5. Consider the opportunity to screen for dementia and depression in primary care.

Table 20.6 Indications for referral of patients with suspected dementia from primary care to specialist old age psychiatry services

1.	Potential treatment with anti-Alzheimer's medication
2.	Accurate diagnosis, particularly of types of dementia
3.	Assessment of risk
4.	Informal carer stress
5.	Behavioural problems
6.	Lack of cooperation with social support packages
7.	Assessment for appropriate care placement or domiciliary social support packages

Table 20.6). Ideally, this should be using a pooled budget.

In order to respond effectively to needs, commissioners will require knowledge of local services including domiciliary support, day-care and respite services, and the spectrum of long-stay care—provided both by the independent sector and by the NHS (Wattis and Fairbairn 1997, p. 21). Local knowledge should allow gaps in services to be identified, and should also give scope for the development of innovative, flexible patterns of local provision (Department of Health 1997, p. 21).

Commissioners will also need to be aware of local eligibility criteria for NHS long-term care (Table 20.7) and ensure that this is consistent with social-care purchased services. There is a requirement for such eligibility criteria to be published locally, and there is a rarely used appeal process for those who feel they have inappropriately been identified as ineligible for continuing NHS care.

Table 20.7 Characteristics of patients in NHS long-term care

1.	Sustained or frequently recurrent difficult behaviour, such as aggression and violence, sexual disinhibition, intractable noisiness, interfering with other residents, persistent absconding.
2.	Physical illness and sensory problems creating needs which cannot be better met in another setting.
3.	Patients with dementia, or other serious psychiatric disorder with failure to cope or rapid deterioration in other settings.

After Wattis and Fairbairn 1996.

Education and training of staff

A recent survey by the Audit Commission of General Practitioners revealed considerable pessimism about the mental health services for older people. The survey indicated that GPs felt they had an inadequate knowledge of mental health problems in old age, especially depression and dementia—above all, dementia. However, there was also a 'therapeutic nihilism' which needs to be addressed: GPs must be convinced that their depressed and confused elderly patients can be helped (Audit Commission 2000) (Table 20.8). Old age psychiatry services should see their role as being educative and supportive to primary care colleagues. The same applies to other health care professionals in the secondary (hospital or specialist) sector. Often the establishment of good liaison arrangements allows a 'quasi-educational culture' to develop.

Perhaps the most important area of concern is the education and training of unqualified staff in the independent care-home sector. Here again old age psychiatry multidisciplinary teams can make an impact. The development of teaching nursing homes may create a beneficial culture, and the development of gerontological nurse specialists to provide skilled nurse leadership in the care-home sector is to be encouraged. Gerontological nurse specialists are senior nurses with at least 2 years comprehensive

Table 20.8 A checklist for when dementia is formally diagnosed

1.	Is the patient to be told?
2.	Relatives to be informed
To either or both:	
3.	Enduring power of attorney information
4.	Testamentary capacity
5.	Consider Attendance Allowance
6.	Telephone number of local Alzheimer's society branch
7.	Local social services telephone number
8.	Helpline number (if locally available)

experience of the care of older people. In large independent organizations they may well be employed by that organization, but other models exist where they are employed by local trusts and work in smaller care homes (Royal College of Physicians and Royal College of Nursing 2000).

Screening of old people in primary care

Resistance to the 'over-75 screen' has resulted in a missed opportunity to identify treatable illness in old age at an early stage. Nevertheless, the development of primary care groups and primary care trusts should provide another opportunity to agree local protocols for screening and for subsequent referral to specialist services. The Joint Report of the Royal College of Physicians and the Royal College of Psychiatrists (1998) recommends that each general practice should compile a simple register of patients who have significant mental health problems in old age (Royal College of Physicians and Royal College of Psychiatrists 1998).

Conclusion

We are the elderly of the future. Although we might sincerely hope that we shall have no need to avail ourselves of the skills of an old age psychiatrist or of any of the associated professionals, it is likely that either we ourselves, or a member of our family, or one of our close circle of friends will, unfortunately, require help or treatment at some stage. So what can and should we hope for?

Patients should receive an efficient service: accurate medical diagnosis followed by effective treatment and appropriate interdisciplinary care and support across a wide spectrum (Table 20.9). And carers? They also require a correct and rapid diagnosis, sensitive handling of the situation, multidisciplinary assistance for the patient, and support for themselves. The patient is the focus of everyone's attention. The territorial interests of professionals are properly irrelevant. Old people with mental health problems and their families can justifiably look to benefit from a 'seamless' service, both efficient and flexible, provided by a broad range of professionals who will retain contact with patients and their informal carers. Where appropriate, treatment will occur within the home setting. Good, sensitive terminal care is essential.

A continued investment of time, money, and people is required to ensure that old age psychiatry will provide a service that delivers the care we all deserve and have a right to receive.

Table 20.9 Use of day hospitals

- Active assessment and treatment of functional illness not requiring inpatient stay
- Accurate diagnosis of subtypes of dementia
- Accurate assessment of behavioural and psychological symptoms of dementia
- To allow coordinated, complex multidisciplinary team work
- As an 'acceptable' method of introducing day support

Notes

1. H. L., a 48-year-old man with autism spent many years in Bournewood Hospital, Chertsey, Surrey, not far from London. In 1994 he went to live with Mr and Mrs E. who cared for him and treated him as one of their family. In July 1997 whilst attending a day centre he became agitated and was re-admitted *informally* (i.e. not under mental health legislation) to Bournewood Hospital. His admission was challenged in court in October 1997 which ruled that he was illegally detained and that he could be legally detained only if admitted under the Mental Health Act. The Court of Appeal upheld this decision on 2nd December 1997 but it was overturned by the House of Lords in 1998.

References

Anderson, D. N. and Philpott, R. M. (1991). The changing pattern of referrals for psychogeriatric consultation in the general hospital: an eight-year study. *International Journal of Geriatric Psychiatry*, 6, 801–7.

Arie, T. and Jolley, D. (1982). Making services work; organisation and style of psychogeriatric services. *The psychiatry of later life* (ed. R. Levy and F. Post), pp. 222–51. Blackwell Scientific, Oxford.

Audit Commission. (1997). *The coming of age*, p. 11. Audit Commission, London.

Audit Commission. (2000). *Forget me not. Mental health services for older people*, pp. 21–4 and 48–50. Audit Commission, London.

Banerjee, S. and Macdonald, A. (1996). Mental disorder in an elderly home care population: associations with health and social service use. *British Journal of Psychiatry*, **168**, pp. 750–6.

Campbell, M. and Fairbairn, A. (1989). Preventing psychogeriatric referrals. *Practitioner*, **233**, 1296–9.

Council of Europe. (1995). Ageing and social protection. *Report from the European Social Security Committee*, pp. 71–9. Council of Europe, Strasbourg.

Department of Health. (1990). *NHS and Community Care Act*. HMSO, London.

Department of Health. (1995). *NHS responsibilities for continuing healthcare needs*. Health Service Guidance, **95**, 8.

Department of Health. (1997). *A handbook on the mental health of older people*. 10307 MHCC 1P Mar 97 SA (13), pp. 9 and 23–7. HMSO, London.

Department of Health. (1999). *The Health Act*. The Stationery Office, London.

Fairbairn, A. F. (2000). The treatment of dementia. *Prescribers Journal*, **40**, 77–85.

Kalache, A. (1991). Ageing in developing countries. In *Principles and Practice of Geriatric Medicine* (2nd edn) (ed. M. S. J. Pathy), pp. 1517–28. Wiley, Chichester.

Kitwood, T. (1997). *Dementia reconsidered: the person first*. Open University Press, Buckingham.

Laing, W. (1997). *Care of elderly people. Market survey* (10th edn). Laing and Buisson. London.

Levin, E. (1997). *Carers: problems, strains and services*, pp. 392–402. Oxford University Press, Oxford.

Margallo-Lana, M., Swann, A., O'Brien, J., Fairbairn, A., Reichelt, K., Potkins, D., *et al.* (2000). Behaviour and psychological symptoms amongst dementia sufferers living in care environment. *International Journal of Geriatric Psychiatry*, **16**, 39–44.

Royal College of Physicians and Royal College of Nursing. (2000). *Care homes report* (In press)

Royal College of Physicians and Royal College of Psychiatrists. (1998). *The care of older people with mental illness, specialist services and medical training. Joint Council Report*, pp. 21–6.

Royal College of Psychiatrists. (1999). *The interface between the NHS and the independent sector in the care of older people with mental illness*. Occasional Paper OP45. RCPsych., London.

Royal College of Psychiatrists. (2000). *Services for younger people with Alzheimer's disease and other dementias*. Occasional Paper. RCPsych., London.

Royal Commission on Long Term Care. (1999). *With respect to old age*. The Stationery Office, London.

Social Services Inspectorate. (1996). *Assessing older people with dementia living in the community*. Department of Health, London.

Social Services Inspectorate. (1997*a*). *At home with dementia. Inspection of services for older people with dementia in the community*. Department of Health, London.

Social Services Inspectorate. (1997*b*). *Older people with mental health problems living alone. Anybody's priority?*, pp. 9–13. Department of Health, London

Stirling, E., Svanberg, R., and Fairbairn, A. F. (1996). Independent living for people with dementia. *Journal of Health and Social Care in the Community*, 33–7.

Svanberg, R., Stirling, E., and Fairbairn, A. F. (1997). The process of care management with people with dementia. *Journal of Health and Social Services*, **5**, 134–6.

VOICES (Voluntary Organisations Involved in Caring for the Elderly) in association with Gardner Merchant Health Care Services (1998). *Eating well for older people with dementia. A good practice guide for residential and nursing homes and others involved in caring for older people with dementia*. Wordwork, London.

Wattis, J. and Fairbairn, A. F. (1996). Towards a consensus on continuing care of older people with mental illness. *International Journal of Geriatric Psychiatry*, **11**, 163–8.

21 Carers' lives

Harry Cayton

Introduction

I didn't plan to be a carer. But when my mother died I couldn't bear to see my father go into a home. Not then anyway. I felt out of my depth a lot of the time at first. And there were moments at three in the morning trying to get him back to bed, unable to console him and with no one to turn to, when I felt it was entirely pointless. There were good times too, when he smiled and recognised me. I learned a lot about human nature especially my own. It certainly changed my life, looking back I think it was for the better but it didn't feel like it at the time.[1]

Carers are not a uniform group; they come from every background and walk of life. They may be daughters or sons, spouses or partners, friends or neighbours. They may have chosen to care or been forced to care, they may be motivated by love or duty, or by that hardest taskmaster of all, a combination of the two. For some, caring becomes a vocation, for others an intolerable burden. When caring is over some are left grieving and debilitated, some wish to share their experience through voluntary work with other carers, and yet others leave it all behind and go on to new lives and interests. It is in the nature of research to look for patterns and generalizations, and patterns there are of course in the lives of carers, but it is important to recognize that, notwithstanding all the generalizations made in this chapter, every individual carer's life and circumstances are their own.

In the decade since 1990 the role and needs of carers have been formally recognized in UK health and social care practice and enshrined in legislation. Whilst many individual carers' experiences remain deeply unsatisfactory and services to support them inadequate, there is no doubt that there has been real progress in understanding and enabling carers. Over this period the tasks performed by carers have, of course, changed very little; indeed Levin's work (Levin and Sinclair 1989) can still stand as having described the basic framework of carers' needs. What has changed has been the attitudes and practice of professionals, first in social care and, more slowly, as part of a more general change in attitudes to users of the health service, among health-care workers. What has also changed is the volume of published research on carers experience and needs. Since the second edition of this book, apart from the changes in law and public policy, there has also been a great deal more experimentation and research on effective interventions to assist carers, particularly those experiencing high levels of distress, and on educating and enabling carers.

It is worth being clear what is meant by the term 'carer'. Carers are those who spend a significant part of their time looking after the health and personal care needs of a partner, relative, friend, or neighbour and may or may not live in the same household. Not everyone who is carrying out that role accepts the term 'carer'.

Carers are unpaid, have no fixed hours, no terms and conditions of employment, and virtually no rights. The term 'carer' is sometimes used casually to denote paid care staff in homes or the community. Paid workers are not included in the term as used here; they are referred to as 'careworkers' to make a useful distinction. Similarly, the term 'informal carer' is not used; there is nothing informal about looking after someone with a mental health problem for 24 hours a day. The word carer is used in this chapter when discussing cited studies, regardless of the term used by the authors of those papers.

There are an estimated 5.7 million carers in the United Kingdom (HM Government 1999). Half of all carers look after someone over 75 years of age. The Carers Recognition and Services Act 1995 defines 'carer' as someone who provides 'a substantial amount of care on a regular basis for another individual'.

Carers' needs of course vary from person to person, but can be categorized in a number of ways. Most obvious is the need for information to enable them to understand the condition of the person for whom they are caring, and for practical help in doing so. Caring is a major emotional and physical challenge for many people, and carers need help with maintaining their own mental and physical health. There is evidence that carers of people with mental health problems such as depression and dementia experience a higher level of stress than those caring for people with physical illnesses (Ory *et al.* 1999). Dementia often combines physical and mental disability.

A range of services has been developed to support carers. However, the availability of such services is limited. Information, self-help, and education opportunities are provided predominantly by the voluntary sector. Other services come from the health service, social services, and the independent sector, often working together. The most widely spread services are carers' groups, home-care services, day-care centres, and short breaks for respite. Although these services exist in most areas, supply rarely matches demand. The Carers Recognition and Services Act gives carers a legal entitlement to an assessment of their needs by social services. The Act does not appear to have had much effect in actually improving support to carers however, as social services are under no obligation to meet assessed needs and may not have the resources to do so (CNA 1997). Indeed, this may reflect a pattern illustrated in this chapter: over the last decade carers' lives and needs have been over-researched, while meeting those needs remains under-resourced.

The social and political context of caring

Carers do not exist independently of the society in which they live, and in recent years significant social and cultural changes have affected their lives. Many of these have come about through the impact of the carers' movement—the voluntary pressure groups which campaign on their behalf, such as the Carers National Association—others through the impact of research in changing professional perceptions and services. These changes have been reflected and reinforced by a series of government initiatives aimed at identifying carers as a significant group within the health and social care system. Carers have become politically important because of their contribution to the economy as unpaid care providers. It has been calculated that carers save the UK state between £15 and £34 billion annually (OPCS 1988). Recognition of carers' value to the state has led to increased acknowledgement of their own health and social care needs.

The most important political step has been the Carers Recognition and Services Act (1995). This private member's bill had all-party support; and for the first time in the UK defined carers in law, and required social service departments to offer them an assessment of their own needs independently of the person for whom they were caring. The Act is more symbolic than practical as social service departments have no duty to provide services to meet carers' needs and no additional resources to back them up. Many carers are unaware of their rights under the Act and it has not been widely implemented (CHSR 1997; CNA 1997). Nevertheless it remains a milestone in the slow progress of the social inclusion of carers. In 1998 the new government published a National Carers Strategy (HM Government 1999). This document, though long on rhetoric and short on resources, confirmed the place of carers as a key element in health and social policy. The National Carers Strategy does set out some targets for services to support carers, including improved government information, involvement in service planning, and new powers for local authorities to provide services for carers, with the focus on respite services. Subsequently they were also given formal acknowledgement in the modernization plan for the National Health Service, which includes in its core principles that the 'NHS will shape its services round the needs and preferences of individual patients, their families and their carers' (HMSO 2000).

The Carers and Disabled Children Act 2000 extends carers' rights to a needs assessment, gives local authorities powers to provide services such as information, emotional support, and skills training direct to carers, and the power to charge for them.

One of the major economic and political issues in the late 1980s was the organization and cost of long-term care for older people. Older people with chronic mental health problems were adversely affected by the programme of closures of NHS continuing-care beds during the 1980s. Over one-third of long-stay beds were closed (ADS 1993*b*). The vast majority of patients were transferred from NHS facilities to private nursing homes. The economic impact of this was to transfer the cost from the state to the individual, from health care free at the point of delivery to means-tested social care. By the middle of the 1990s public concern, particularly on behalf of those home owners who were forced to sell their homes to pay for care, became politically irresistible (Palmer 1993), and in 1997 the new government established a Royal Commission on Long Term Care for the Elderly.

The Royal Commission reported in February 1999. Its main recommendations, backed up by three volumes of detailed research, were: first, that the costs of long-term care should be split between living costs, housing costs, and personal care costs and that personal care should be available and paid for from general taxation; and, second, that a National Care Commission should be established to monitor trends, represent users and carers, and set national standards. The Government published its response in July 2000 (DoH 2000). It rejected the core recommendation of the report that 'personal care' should be made free in care homes and paid for by the health service through taxation.

The Commission particularly noted that the system of means-tested charging for residential and nursing-home care, while long-term care in hospital remained free, discriminated disproportionately against people with dementia who had to pay for their care as opposed to people with cancer who received their care free. The Government was unpersuaded and decided instead to make 'nursing' care free regardless of the setting. At the time of writing the exact definition of nursing care has yet to be decided, but it seems unlikely that this definition will significantly benefit people with dementia in care homes. Indeed, there are fears that the new system, by stressing disability rather than ability, will promote dependency and institutionalization, the opposite of what is intended. Although dementia creates health needs, it is clear that these need not always be met by a qualified nurse. The Government itself estimates that only 35 000 of the 446 000 people in care homes (RCLTC 1999) will benefit from the change. The Scottish Parliament decided, however, to make all personal care free when provided in a care home. The Government established a National Care Standards Commission in 2001, though with a narrower remit than that proposed by the Royal Commission, and agreed to recommendations aimed at encouraging the rehabilitation of those who could return to their own homes.

Between 1998 and 2000 the Audit Commission, which oversees the external audit of local authorities and the National Health Service in England and Wales, carried out a detailed review of services for older people with mental health problems. Its report, *Forget me not; mental health services for older people* (Audit Commission 2000), contains some authoritative recommendations and again stresses the importance of carers in providing care, and in the evaluation and planning of services.

Carers have no specific legal rights or duties in relation to those they care for. They do not even need to be consulted about the medical treatment or other care which the person receives. In

England and Wales lengthy consultation has taken place, first by the Law Commission (Law Commission 1993) and subsequently by the Lord Chancellor's Department (LCD), on changes that might be made to the law relating to people with incapacity and how their interests might be protected (LCD 1997). The idea that carers (in exchange, as it were, for new legal rights to be consulted) might be given a 'duty of care' to act in the best interests of the person they are looking after, was rejected as unworkable and inappropriate as a way of regulating a private relationship. However, the Lord Chancellor's Department has proposed the creation of a 'continuing power of attorney', which would allow a person to appoint an attorney with responsibility for health and care decisions as well and legal and financial powers. This creation of a legal framework for a health care proxy for persons with incapacity has been widely welcomed by patient and carer organizations, but is opposed by some in the medical profession and by 'pro life' religious organizations. The Government has not yet given any indication of its timetable for enacting the necessary legislation. In Scotland, the Adults with Incapacity (Scotland) Act 2000 has been approved by the Scottish Parliament. The Act gives the 'primary carer' the right to be consulted on decisions made within the scope of the Act and also creates a 'welfare power of attorney' with the power to give or withhold consent to decisions made about a person's welfare. In the case of medical treatment, however, two doctors in agreement can override the views of the welfare attorney. Alzheimer Europe, the European federation of family associations, has approved a statement of the legal rights of people with dementia, which sets out the principles of self-determination, maintenance of autonomy, least restrictive environment for care, and the right to appoint financial, legal, and health care attorneys (Alzheimer Europe 2000).

Who are carers, what do they do?

I'm a wife and a mother and a nurse and social worker and driver and cook and home help. I wash and dress and help my husband eat, I get him up in the morning and put him to bed at night. I take him to the toilet and clean up after him when there is an accident. I do this 24 hours a day seven days a week. I have four hours off a week, on Monday and Wednesday when the careworker comes.

To a great extent carers are defined by what they do. As explained in the Introduction the word carers is used in this chapter to apply to family members, partners, close friends, or neighbours who provide regular and substantial support without pay to a dependent person. Carers often, but not necessarily, live in the same home as the person they care for. The Office of Population, Censuses and Surveys in 1988 defined carers as: 'people who are looking after, or providing some regular service for, a sick or handicapped or elderly person living in their own or another household.' This definition was used in a survey of carers in 1985 and again in 1990 and 1995 as part of the general household survey (GHS). The analysis of the latter was published in 1998 by the Office for National Statistics under the title *Informal carers* (Rowlands 1998). The main aim of the questions, which were included in the GHS at the request of the Department of Health, was to provide estimates of the number of people who were providing care for sick, elderly, or handicapped persons. The survey provided a range of useful information.

Rowlands estimated that there were 5.7 million carers. One adult in eight was providing care, and one in six households contained a carer. More women were caring than men: 3.3 million compared to 2.4 million. Where carers were looking after someone in their own household, just over half were caring for a spouse and just over a fifth for parents or parents-in-law. Many of these are older people. Some 18% of respondents said that the person's disability was 'the result of ageing'. This undoubtedly includes many people with dementia, although a further 7% said they were caring for someone with mental disability and another 15% for people with both mental and physical disability. The Department of Social Security looked at family resources in a survey carried out in 1997–8 (DSS 1999). It provided the information about caring in families set out in Table 21.1 below.

In a survey of 3000 carers carried out for the Carers National Association, Henwood (1998)

Table 21.1 Patterns of caring

- Care is provided by 11% of adults; caring is more likely between the ages of 45 and 64 (16%), tailing off after age 75 (7%).
- Two-thirds provide care to someone outside the household. Men are more likely to care for a spouse or partner, women more likely to care for a relative outside of the household. Only 5% of carers looked after more than one person.
- 34% of adult carers are in full-time employment.
- A third of carers lived in households where the main source of income was social security benefits, especially as the number of hours caring increased.
- 26% of those receiving care required continuous help. The likelihood of needing care (5% overall) increased with age (28% of those over 75).

found that 23% were caring for someone with dementia. Of those carers caring for older people, and especially those with mental health problems, a number of studies have shown similar patterns (ADS 1993*a*). The majority of carers are women: in the first instance wives and partners, but also frequently daughters or daughters-in-law. Of those carers who are men (40%) by far the largest proportion are husbands or partners, with a much smaller number being sons. Rowlands reported that the peak age for caring was 45–65 years. The age of carers of people with dementia is unsurprisingly older. One survey by the Alzheimer's Society (ADS 1993*a*) found that 58% of carers of people with dementia were over 65 and that 12% of carers were over 80-years-old. There are of course some young carers who take a significant role in the care of a grandparent or parent with dementia. It is also worth noting that a significant proportion of people with dementia live alone in the community, probably over 150 000 people (ADS 1994), and may be supported by neighbours and friends and by relatives at a distance. However, the vast majority of people with moderate or severe dementia living in the community are cared for by someone living with them in the same home (Schneider *et al.* 1993).

Rowlands provides some comparisons between the results of the GHSs carried out in 1985, 1990, and 1995. She concluded that there was a growing division between those involved in heavy caring responsibilities and those who were largely 'helpers'. She also reported that as 'major care needs do not usually manifest themselves until the age of 75 and older', the increase in the number of carers over the decade was a function of the increase in older people.

Rather less is known about the position of carers in minority ethnic groups, though recently development work has been done by a number of agencies (Patel *et al.* 1998; ICARUS 2000). The age profile of most minority ethnic groups in Britain is different from the indigenous population and differs between groups (Audit Commission 2000). The rate of depression in some groups such as Bengali people and older Somali people is higher than for White British people (Silviera and Ebrahim 1995). Assumptions sometimes made that cultural difference mean that older people and those with mental health problems are cared for within minority ethnic communities are not borne out by studies. According to Brownlee (1991) one-third of Afro-Caribbean elders surveyed had no children living in the UK. Even when an extended family network does exist, caring at home is largely carried out by one person. Knight and McCallum (1998), in a comparison of African-American and White carers of people with dementia in the United States, found that cultural differences did appear to affect both emotional and physical responses to carers' stress. In a study in Liverpool (ICARUS 2000) the authors concluded that the barriers to neurological services experienced by Black and minority ethnic communities were the same as for access to health and social services generally. Patel (Patel *et al.* 1998) has argued more radically that providers should use the minority ethnic community and its norms as the basis for developing new forms of support, rather than trying to make existing services more accessible.

Another group of carers who experience difficulties in accessing support are gay and lesbian carers looking after their partners. They report exclusion from both statutory and voluntary services and that they suffer discrimination on the part of health and social services (Ward 1999):

As a gay man I've found it difficult to find support and information from people who really understand my position...Caring for my partner has meant that I have had to 'come out' to people—social workers, doctors, nursing home staff. There are added difficulties because people may not accept my relationship adding to the sense of isolation.

The tasks involved in caring and their level of difficulty and intensity depend to a great extent on the age and condition of the person being cared for. Depressive illnesses, for example, present different challenges from, say, Pick's disease. Carers for those with dementia face the progressive decline of the person in their care, often over many years, as they themselves get older. Caring tasks therefore become more intense, more intimate, and more complex as time goes on. Carers progress from basic care such as providing companionship, making sure someone is safe, and encouraging them to clean and feed themselves to providing 24-hour nursing care. Caring is therefore not only physically exhausting but emotionally draining as well.

Carers work very long hours. Often they are 'on call' 24 hours a day. Many only receive breaks of a few hours during a week when a home careworker takes over or when the person they care for attends a day-care centre or other activity. Night support is very rarely available, and where it has been it has not been obviously practicable or effective (Watson and Redfern 1997). Many carers therefore experience disturbed sleep, insomnia, and consequent exhaustion (Wilcox and King 1999).

The important role that carers play in the identification of dementia is often overlooked. It is family members who frequently notice the early signs of memory loss or the changes in behaviour that indicate depression or dementia (Aneshensel *et al.* 1995), and it is family members who most frequently press both the person themselves and GPs for a proper assessment and diagnosis (Grace 1994). All too often they report indifference, delay, and ignorance as the response from primary health care (O'Connor *et al.* 1988). The Alzheimer's Society reported in 1995 that in a survey of over 2000 carers 60% said their GP did not offer a memory test, and 42% said the GP did not make a diagnosis. In a parallel study, 71% of GPs reported that they had not received adequate training in the management of dementia (ADS 1995).

My mother's GP was only interested in her physical ailments and refused to help with her mental condition. His diagnosis was unhelpful and he refused to refer her to a specialist even when the family asked him to do so on the advice of social services. He said it would serve no purpose as the NHS had nothing to offer.

Some, including this author, have argued that the introduction of new specific drugs for Alzheimer's disease will improve the response of primary care by giving GPs a specific treatment to offer (Kelly *et al.* 1997). Given that prescription of these drugs in the UK is actively opposed on grounds of cost-effectiveness by many health authorities (Melzer 1998), it is too soon to judge the response. Nevertheless, primary care practitioners should look to family members and carers as active partners in the process of identification and diagnosis. McLoughlin *et al.* (1996) found that spouses and relatives were good at estimating levels of cognitive impairment and that informant data—information given by the carer—was a justified part of clinical practice. They suggest that relying on cognitive tests alone would 'result in an inaccurate portrait of the patient'.

Earlier diagnosis is presenting new dilemmas for the triad of doctor, carer, and person with dementia. The carer's role is crucial in both diagnosis and subsequent care. But the doctor's duty is of course to their patient. Whom to tell and what to tell in the process of diagnosis has become a much debated issue. In the past doctors frequently failed to share the diagnosis with the person with dementia, preferring to tell the carer instead. Rice and Warner (1994) found wide variations in practice by psychiatrists specializing in old age, as far as the giving of information about their condition was concerned. Carers were often happy to collude with this on the assumption that the person concerned would 'not wish to know'. Maguire and Kirby (1996) found that 83% of carers did not wish their relatives to be informed of the diagnosis, although 71% of family members wished to be told if they themselves had Alzheimer's disease. The maintenance of secrecy is no longer ethically sustainable. Earlier diagnosis, the possibility of effective drug treatments, and the need to make legal and financial plans while the person with dementia still has capacity require a realistic sharing of the diagnosis and prognosis with the person themselves. Fearnley *et al.* (1997) argue the case for disclosure of diagnosis on both practical and ethical grounds, and suggest good practice.

The neurologist sent my wife out of the room whilst he informed me of the diagnosis with the obvious implication that she should not know the result. This left me with the awful difficulty of trying to appear normal when I collected her and telling her the first of many lies...From my point of view the decision not to tell has severed the partnership of 40 years where we have faced all our problems together...I feel most strongly that both carer and patient should be present and that the person delivering the diagnosis should be trained to impart the information in a sensitive way.

Carers characterize their own experience in numerous different ways. Therefore it is important to acknowledge that just as the life history and personality of the person with dementia is a key to the manifestation of their illness, so the personality, social skills, and financial security of a carer are essential to their response to the situation in which they find themselves (Hooker *et al.* 1998). Some researchers have gone so far as to suggest it is the carer's personality rather than services that make the difference in enabling carers to cope, and that interventions should concentrate on helping carers to develop coping strategies rather than on providing practical support (Bookwala and Schulz 1998). Mockler *et al.* (1998) found that psychosocial factors influenced the use that carers made of the available mental health services.

Some studies have identified gender differences in the experience of carer stress. McFarland and Sanders (1999) used focus groups to look at the coping skills of men who provided care to women with Alzheimer's disease. Men were found to concentrate on practical tasks of caregiving and to minimize their emotional reaction to caring. Garland and Gray-Amante (1999) argued that women find caring more stressful than men. On the other hand, McKibbin *et al.* (1999) found that wives and daughters who were caring did not smoke or drink alcohol significantly more than population norms in their age group. A Japanese study (Nagatomo *et al.* 1999) found that carers' burden was higher when the person with dementia was a male, a feature the authors attribute to cultural norms of male dominance and aggression. Freyne *et al.* (1999) found that carers of younger people with dementia experienced higher levels of burden than those caring for older people. Perhaps what these and other studies really show us is that it is very difficult to generalize about carers' lives, particularly on the basis of small populations. The number of variables in each carer's situation is so great that the identification of their needs and the mechanisms put in place to support them must be individualized as much as possible. Some people reject the term 'carer' being applied to them at all, preferring to say: I care as a husband, as a daughter, as a friend or partner.

Reference to the role of carer has become commonplace but I wonder if we have acknowledged the change in social relations signified by the change in language...Reference to me as the carer abstracts me from my primary role as husband. Second my wife becomes the 'one to be cared for'. Third the identification of any person as the carer obscures the distinction between effort and achievement. Sometimes, as husband I fail to deliver the care even though I am labelled the carer.

Studies of carers tend to focus, not surprisingly, on those caring for someone full-time at home. Carers also care at a distance, and continue to care for someone when they move into a residential or nursing home. Long-distance carers, of whom many are sons and daughters, have their own difficulties, many of them juggle jobs and relationships and children of their own with caring.

For many carers the transition from full-time caring to sharing the task with careworkers in a care home is a period of great emotional and practical difficulty. The business of finding a high-quality home, which meets the needs of the individual and which is affordable, is time consuming and often difficult. Carers often report feeling guilty that they have failed the person they are caring for; others recognize that it may be the best outcome for both people.

It is not always best to struggle at home. Although it may be hard for carers to admit some people with dementia are best cared for professionally. When my husband was no longer suitable for day care the very caring staff reminded me that I should do what was best for both my husband and me. Those of us who no longer care at home feel no less and grieve no less than those who reject residential care. We have just chosen a different path.

The move into residential care is often precipitated by the sudden deterioration in health of either the person being cared for or the carer (Hope *et al.* 1998). Carers may experience conflicting feelings of relief and guilt when someone moves into a care home (ADS 1997), feelings that are reinforced if careworkers do not allow them the space and time to continue contributing to their partners' or relatives' care.

When my husband developed Alzheimer's I looked after him as long as I could. Then our doctor said for both our sakes he should go into a home. I was most upset but found a lovely home with wonderful care staff. I used to see him at least once a week even though he had no idea who I was. The staff loved him as much as I did. They even gave us a 50th wedding anniversary party, inviting all our friends and relatives.

Dementia has sometimes been described as 'a living death' (Woods 1989). Although this is a metaphor that many would now find unhelpfully negative, it does reflect the slow loss of communication and awareness of the self and other which characterizes dementia. The experience of grief and the need to grieve when someone dies, but who in many ways has already been lost to those who love them, is a problematic one and is a characteristic of the progression of feeling experienced by carers of people with dementia (Almberg *et al.* 2000). Many carers experience what has been called 'anticipatory grief', the process of grieving for someone before they die (Theat *et al.* 1991). Bodnar and Kiecolt-Glaser (1994) found that for some carers grieving continues well beyond the death of the person they had been caring for. Murphy *et al.* (1997) found, in a United States study, that care homes had virtually no policy or practice in supporting families after the death of one of their residents. Considerable improvement is needed in the care of people in the terminal stage of dementia and in supporting their carers through grief and bereavement.

Not all carers are capable of or willing to take on the tasks of caring and to do them in the interests of the person for whom they are caring. Carers and family members do sometimes mistreat or neglect the person they are responsible for. Abuse may be emotional, physical, sexual, or financial. It may arise from a longstanding abusive relationship, from a change in role and power, from stress and inadequacy, or from malice and greed. The Social Services Inspectorate has identified predisposing factors that may lead to abuse, including the behaviour of the person with dementia, the history of family relationships, housing and financial circumstances, carer attitudes and motivation, the carer's own physical and mental health, and the failure of health and social services to meet the carer's needs (DoH 1993). Professionals in contact with carers must be alert to the possibility of neglect or mistreatment and act sensitively but decisively to protect both the person with dementia and the carer. Local authorities in the UK have at their disposal a range of legal powers to protect vulnerable older people and promote their welfare (see also Chapter 37).

Carers' lives

Carers' lives are characterized by loneliness, monotony, frustration, rage, tenderness, anxiety, and love; by small victories and larger defeats; and by the triumph of hope over relentless mental and physical decline.

I retired early to care for my husband Bill, who has Alzheimer's disease. The past three years have been a rollercoaster of emotions—deep love, frustration, anger, self-pity, tenderness, loneliness, fear and isolation.

There has been much descriptive research on carers' lives, too much of it merely repeating or expanding on earlier research such as Levin's (1989), which has so effectively set out the issues. However, it is helpful to see carers' lives as they themselves describe them, remembering all the while that carers are not a homogenous group and that generalizations are inevitably misleading as a guide to how individual caring relationships operate (Hancock and Jarvis 1994).

It is the dislocation of social relationships and networks that seems to figure most prominently.

And another crazy thing about Alzheimer's nobody really wants to talk to you any longer but we can assure everyone we know Alzheimer's is not catching.

Dementia is pre-eminently a social disease as I have argued elsewhere (Cayton 1993). First and foremost it affects the relationship between the person with dementia and their carer. This relationship nearly always has a strong and continuing history—mother and daughter or husband and wife—and it is not only the loss of companionship and the long-time intellectual presence of the other, but the significant change in role which carers can find distressing and difficult to manage.

I don't think you know what it is to be a carer until you've had to wipe your parent's bottom. I had to do it with both my parents when they became incontinent and I don't think it's a role children should be asked to take on. It was really difficult for both of us but you can't have a care assistant in the house all the time if you are caring at home.

For adult children caring for parents the taking on of intimate tasks, such as personal hygiene following incontinence, can be particularly challenging. Amongst older couples where domestic roles may have been quite distinct, husbands may have to learn to cook or to keep house. Wives may have to learn to mend fuses or do repairs. This acquisition of new skills is often viewed positively and is cited by many carers as one of the life-enhancing aspects of caring.

My wife was a cordon bleu cook...for most of our married life I never had to worry about where my next meal was coming from. Now I do it all myself by following the instructions on the packet but she has never refused to eat what I have given her so I can't be too bad.

One skill that is often gender-relevant, particularly amongst older people, is driving. Owning and driving a car has a strong symbolic importance to men, associated as it is with male adulthood and independence. The loss of the ability to drive can therefore have a profound emotional impact, and it can be very difficult to persuade some men to give up driving even when their ability is significantly impaired (Gilley *et al.* 1991). The difficulty is compounded by the fact that dementia damages their insight into their own behaviour. Dubinsky *et al.* (2000) reviewed the literature and concluded that there was significant evidence of the impairment of driving ability even in the early stages of dementia. Loss of the use of a car can have a severe practical impact on quality of life, and when the carer does not drive it can increase the isolation they experience.

Loss of physical mobility, and indeed the capacity to cope with new environments on the part of the person with dementia, means that as the disease progresses it becomes increasingly difficult for the carer to have a holiday either alone or with the person they care for. Carers also find the demands of their role make finding time for their own interests or leisure activities increasingly difficult. Lack of opportunities for holidays not only reduces quality of life but puts carers' health at risk. An Alzheimer's Society survey in 1994 (ADS 1993*a*) found that two-thirds of carers only had a break from caring once a week or less.

One aspect of carers' lives when they are spouses or partners is the inevitable change in their sexual relationship. People with dementia may lose interest in a sexual relationship and become withdrawn at an early stage, while others may show inappropriate sexual behaviours (Archibald 1994). Carers don't lose their own sexual needs or indeed their need for a continuing emotional partnership. Carers may form new relationships even while caring and experience uncertainty and guilt about this. This is an area of their lives where many carers need help, but one they find particularly difficult to talk about.

I am in the 70 plus age range but the body hasn't aged with the calendars! My wife has Alzheimer's and is at a stage where a physical relationship is no longer possible or perhaps advisable. We must accept that sexual activity is a perfectly normal function of our bodies. Unattended these feelings will accumulate and disturb and perhaps become yet another burden.

Comment, explanation, advice and assurance from the medical profession would be useful on this subject but few are likely to approach a GP on this subject.

Not only does the physical and practical impact of caring progressively circumscribe people's lives, reducing mobility, social networks, and community involvement, but the social stigma remains a real barrier for carers and people with dementia.

I discovered very painfully early on that it's a mistake to tell friends because of their reaction. Therefore with most people I live uncomfortably in a sort of double life.

As public awareness of dementia and Alzheimer's disease, especially, have grown, particularly through the identification of public figures such as President Reagan or Dame Iris Murdoch, it might be expected that some of the levels of social exclusion might reduce. Nevertheless the stigma of a diagnosis of dementia remains (Jolley and Benbow 2000), so much so that the Royal College of Psychiatry felt it necessary to launch antidiscrimination campaigns on both depression and dementia in 1996 and 1999, respectively (RCPsych nd).

After isolation, carers most frequently report 'stress' or 'depression' as characteristics of their lives (see Table 21.2). Around one-third of carers have been found to suffer from clinical depression (Coope *et al.* 1995). In one study in London (Livingston *et al.* 1996), 47% of women carers of an older person with dementia were identified as clinically depressed compared with only 3% of carers of a physically disabled older person. Many carers also report high levels of anxiety, sleeplessness, depression, and exhaustion (Levin *et al.* 1989). More recently, Wilcox and King (1999) have looked specifically at sleep disturbance in older women carers.

Table 21.2 Carers reporting stress (%)

Tiredness	66
Depression	40
Stress	70
Loneliness	36
Other	16

There have been a number of attempts made to describe and quantify more precisely the burden that carers experience. Brodaty and Hadzi-Parlovic (1990) found high rates of psychological morbidity in carers of people with dementia. Psychological morbidity in carers was associated with: having an affected person at home; the carer being a spouse; demanding problem behaviours; poor physical health in the carer; social isolation; dissatisfaction with social supports; greater use of psychotropic medication; and a deteriorated marital relationship. There was a vulnerable group of carers who were impaired psychologically, socially, and physically.

Witeratne and Lovestone (1996), Yeatman *et al.* (1993) and Rosenvinge *et al.* (1998) compared psychological morbidity and stress in carers of people with depression and carers of people with dementia. They found higher levels of stress in carers of people with dementia. Researchers (Brodaty and Hadzi-Parlovic 1990; Levin *et al.* 1997) have also tried to identify those factors in the caring situation that are most likely to cause stress for carers and which might be amenable to constructive interventions. Behavioural disturbance, incontinence, and isolation are typically found to be more stressful than cognitive impairment alone. Levin *et al.* (1989) found that levels of strain were associated with particular problems faced by carers. Carers 'experiencing behavioural and interpersonal difficulties and feeling socially restricted were particularly likely to show signs of strain'.

A longitudinal study by Reiss *et al.* (1996) of 213 families caring for people with dementia found that although the degree of cognitive impairment was significantly associated with carer burden at the beginning of the study, this was not the case in later years. Carer personality, they concluded, was a significant factor in whether or not stress was a major problem. Gallaher-Thompson (1994) found that night-time wandering and aggressive behaviours were most likely to predict stress over a period of time, which bears out the findings of Levin and her colleagues.

Recent work by the Alzheimer's Society and others has identified how much normal patterns of eating and diet can be disrupted by dementia and the difficulties of maintaining a normal routine of meals (Alzheimer's Society 2000*a*, VOICES 1998). For many people, meals together are an important part of community and quality of life. Over half of carers (56%) reported that their caring role had had an impact on their own eating patterns and that they ate less healthily. Most cited lack of time and stress or depression as the reasons for this.

Some carers also report physical illness arising from caring. Most commonly this involves muscular strain or back problems (ADS 1994) as a result of moving or lifting the person for whom they are caring. Unsurprisingly, carers of people with dementia, being older themselves, seem more likely to have coexisting physical disabilities of their own such as arthritis or cardiovascular problems. Physical illness on the part of the carer is one of the crucial triggers for the person with dementia being admitted to a care home. Many carers say that the fear of becoming ill themselves and unable to continue caring is a constant cause of anxiety.

'I'm a bit older than my wife and I have angina so I do worry what will happen if I die before she does. I hate to think of her being alone in a nursing home with no one to visit. Our son works abroad you see. It sounds terrible but I sometimes pray that she will die before me.

Literature for carers always urges them to 'take care of themselves' and to pay attention to their own health (Cayton *et al.* 1997; Wilcock, 1999). To what extent this advice is regarded is uncertain. There certainly remains an impression that many carers, perhaps particularly partners, put their caring role above all other considerations and to the detriment of their own mental and physical well-being.

Caring, particularly full-time caring, is likely to have considerable impact on the financial status of the carer and of the household if the carer and person being cared for are living together. Generally, studies have found that caring has a significant impact on income and employment; carers are unlikely to be in paid employment and those carers in paid work have lower earnings, because they work part-time and in lower paid occupations (Parker 1990). Although many carers of older people with mental health problems are themselves over retirement age, one survey (Alzheimer's Disease Society 1993*a*) found that 60% of carers of working age had given up their jobs or taken early retirement to provide full-time care. Women were more likely to have given up work to care than men. Some 41% of carers under the age of 65 had lost their full pension rights through caring.

The difference between carers and non-carers in relation to income are much more marked if, as Hancock and Jarvis (1994) point out, gender, place of residence, and duration and intensity of caring are all taken into account. Carers living as the sole carer with the person they care for and caring for 50 hours a week or more are significantly more likely than others to be in the lowest income groups. Hancock and Jarvis (1994) also point out that full-time caring has a long-term and cumulative impact on finances. Being unable to work means that carers are unable to save or to build up a retirement pension for themselves. People who are currently carers are undoubtedly among the poorest in society. That caring is a path to poverty is clear from the research evidence and from the accounts of carers themselves. In one study, carer households were clustered in the bottom two-fifths of income distribution, with 40% of carers having a gross income of less than £1075 a month in 1994 (Corti *et al.* 1994). Carers National Association research also shows that 77% of carers surveyed in 2000 felt themselves to be worse off financially since they began caring, and over seven in ten had given up work to provide care.

Of course many carers want to work and try to combine work with caring. Levin (1989) found that one-third of carers did more than 10 hours of paid employment each week, and that 60% of adult children and younger carers went out to work. Carers who do work have problems with juggling care and work responsibilities.

The work piles up, we're short of staff and I leave more to my subordinate than I ought to because it's hard to concentrate.

Caring not only reduces earning opportunities and income but increases costs. Special transport arrangements, heating and washing (particularly if there is incontinence), aids and adaptations, home helps, care services, and day care, all cost extra. The cost of residential or nursing-home care for those who have to pay (anyone with assets over £10 000 in 2000) is considerable, from £18 000 a year upwards.

> The social workers tell me that my husband is my responsibility not the state's. If he had cancer he would be given all the medical care he needed by the NHS. When are they going to accept that Alzheimer's disease is a disease not a state of mind? As it is I am going to have to sell our home to fund his care.

Carers have to use their own savings and assets to fund care; over one-quarter were paying over £100 per month at 1993 figures to meet the shortfall in benefits or other state provision (ADS 1993*a*). The social security and benefits system in the UK has, in recent years, been made a little more flexible in relation to carers. However, it remains both inadequate in overall effect and counterproductive in many ways, discouraging part-time working, for instance, or discriminating against those with mental as distinct to physical incapacity. A person with a disability can claim the Attendance Allowance, if under 65 years, or the Disability Living Allowance if over 65. These payments are intended to help with personal care needs and supervision and are not means-tested.

The Invalid Care Allowance is payable to carers who spend at least 35 hours a week looking after someone receiving the Attendance Allowance or Disability Living Allowance, but only if the carer is under 65 years of age and not earning more than £50 per week or in full-time education. According to the Carers National Association (CNA 2000) carers have modest expectations of the social security system. The extension of Invalid Care Allowance to carers over the age of 65 and an end to charging for community services including short breaks would be administratively simple, would benefit many of the poorest carers, and would increase the uptake of support services.

Services for carers

Health and social services exist predominantly for the benefit of the person being cared for. These services do of course benefit carers indirectly. Improvements in a person's health and well-being are of enormous emotional as well as practical value to the carer. So of course are good services, such as expert specialist home care or day care. Good services enhance the quality of life of the person with dementia and make it easier to care for them. Quality services also provide genuine respite for the carer.

> I was sometimes impatient with my mother. Better information would have helped me understand.

Carers mention information as one of their greatest needs in all surveys (Levin 1997; Audit Commission 2000). Clear information both about dementia and about available local services can increase carers' knowledge, reduce stress, and reduce their perception of unmet needs. Reducing carer stress and helping them to cope better may also delay the entry of a person with dementia into a care home.

Information can come from many different sources. The most obvious, the GP, is apparently the least effective. The Audit Commission stated that less than half the carers in its survey reported being asked if they needed any help. It described one site where GPs had refused to give out information leaflets in case they became liable for the accuracy of the information they contained. In one study in Northern Ireland fewer than one in five carers found the information given to them by their GP helpful (Trainor 1997).

It is hardly surprising in this context that both local and national voluntary organizations have been at the forefront of developing and providing information for carers. The Alzheimer's Society and Alzheimer's Scotland in the UK and the Alzheimer's Association in the United States all provide clear, accurate, and appropriate information by telephone and post. The telephone helpline run by the Alzheimer's Society handles over 24 000 calls per year. The largest proportion of calls are from carers, family, and friends, with a quarter being from professionals. Between 1997 and 2000 there was a threefold increase in the number of people who called because they were worried that they themselves might have dementia, and an observable increase in the number of people who had received a diagnosis of

Alzheimer's disease, although this group remains small at less than 1% of the total.[2] The role of the Internet in providing information to carers is considered in the last section of this chapter.

At a local level, information is available from local groups and from generic carers' centres as well as from social services departments. Many groups run regular support groups; self-help meetings of carers providing peer support. Self-help groups can provide an opportunity for carers to share their feelings and experiences, to learn more about dementia and about caring, to talk through problems and listen to and learn from others, and to have a short break from caring (ADI 2000).

Although it might seem to lay people that they are employed primarily to provide community support for people with mental health problems, community psychiatric nurses (CPNs) are very highly regarded by carers for their knowledge, practical advice, and emotional encouragement; and the fact that CPNs regularly make home visits enables carers to talk to them in private and in a relaxed setting. In the UK the Dementia Relief Trust supports a number of pilot projects employing nurses who are specifically trained to support carers (Garland and Garland 1998).

Outreach workers for carers are also available in many areas. Such workers, who may have a social care or nursing background, are trained both in dementia and in carers' support and sometimes counselling. They may be employed by voluntary organizations or by social services. They can make home visits, provide information and advice, and act as an advocate for the carers, helping them to get access to benefits and to local assessments and services both for themselves and for the person they are caring for. This enabling role is one that is very highly valued by carers.

Our support worker was wonderful. She dealt with social services and the consultant and helped us get allowances we didn't know about. And she was just great to talk to when I felt down.

The term 'advocacy' is sometimes used to describe the enabling work that such people do to help carers. However, advocacy workers have a narrower and more specific role: they act to promote the views and wishes of their clients not to advise or inform them, and they work under specific guidelines. Most advocacy projects exist to empower people with disabilities; a small amount of work has been done in developing advocacy with older people in care homes and with people with dementia (Dunning 1995). As most people with dementia and their carers want to stay in their own homes for as long as possible, community-based services are very important. The Community Mental Health Team is usually the core of this, in the UK at least. Such a team is multidisciplinary and provides links to primary care and GPs, as well as to specialist psychiatric assessment and services.

Home-care services are provided for the benefit of the person with dementia or depression rather than for the carer. Nevertheless they are highly valued by carers if they are reliable and flexible and meet the needs of the person with dementia. Good home care builds on the strengths, interests, and abilities of the person with dementia and engages them in as wide a range of activities as possible. Home careworkers may provide personal care such as taking people to the toilet, but that is secondary to their role as someone who provides stimulation and interest for the person they are working with. Surveys suggest that carers would particularly like home care to be available and that there is considerable scope for increasing the supply (Levin *et al.* 1994, Audit Commission 2000).

Day-care services should have a similar objective, the fundamental difference being that rather than having staff going into someone's own home, the person goes out to the day centre where there are opportunities to socialize and to engage in group activities. Day centres are not infrequently called 'clubs'. This is not an avoidance of the care aspect of what they do, but a reflection of their focus on social activity and involvement.

My wife is receiving treatment for her condition and last year the specialist suggested she try a day centre so she would meet people and provide a focal point for some activity. My daughter and I were impressed with the centre but my wife was dead set against it. At the end of June I had a meeting with the new carers' support worker. My wife came with me but frankly she went with an attitude. There was no way she was going to be told what to do. I don't know if it was what the carers' support worker said or how she said it but having listened to us she said that my wife might like to consider going to the day centre we'd visited a year ago. My wife looked up and said 'Yes, it might be worth giving it a try'.

These different forms of care will be appropriate to different people according to their personalities and circumstances. Good care of either kind gives carers a break; a chance to shop, to sleep, see friends, read a book, or pursue their own interests, however briefly. Carers value the time off from caring very highly (Moriaty and Levin 1995). Poor-quality care does not provide the same break, because the carer is anxious about it and because the person returns from the care either disturbed, overstimulated, or unhappy. The availability of day care is also a problem for many people; it is rarely available over the weekend and in some areas not even on every weekday. This means that carers, particularly those who are still working, are unable to rely on care when they need it (Audit Commission 2000).

There are some forms of support aimed at helping carers directly, rather than indirectly. These include therapeutic approaches such as cognitive therapy for depressed carers and structured programmes of carer education.

Cognitive–behaviour therapy is an intervention for depression or anxiety which can be used with individuals or groups. It has been shown to be effective for the carers of people with schizophrenia and has also been applied to depressed carers of people with dementia.

Recently, increasing attention has been paid by researchers to evaluating the effectiveness of interventions of various kinds. Thompson *et al.* (2000) carried out a Cochrane review of 'support for carers of people with Alzheimer's type dementia'.

They examined 10 papers meeting their quality criteria, and found the overall picture to add 'little weight to claims that interventions with carers can exert a quantifiable improvement in outcomes such as quality of life, burden, or improvements in mental health'. They argue that the evidence-base relating to specific interventions is characterized by small, relatively poor-quality studies and recommend larger trials of longer duration, the identification of outcome measures relevant to carers, and more complete reporting of data. Others have criticized this Cochrane review as being too narrow in its scope and requiring revision.

Carers themselves value knowledge of dementia and often ask for educational programmes. A number of researchers have attempted to evaluate the impact on quality of life and carer burden of systematic education programmes. The results are inconclusive. Brodaty *et al.* (1991) reported that the long-term benefits of a 10-day residential training programme for dementia carers were decreased psychological morbidity in carers, higher adjusted survival rates for the people they were caring for, and average savings in care costs of nearly US$6000 per person over the first 39 months. However, in a later paper (Brodaty *et al.* 1994) they reported that a controlled trial of a training programme for carers showed no significant differences between those who had completed the training and the control group on measures of psychological stress, burden, satisfaction with life, well-being, or even knowledge. Graham *et al.* (1997*a*) found that participation in a support group did give carers a greater knowledge of dementia and that more knowledgeable carers experience significantly lower levels of depression (Graham *et al.* 1997*b*). More knowledgeable carers were more likely to have realistic expectations and to feel competent and confident. Jansson *et al.* (1998) examined study circles for carers and volunteer supporters in Sweden. They found that both groups had high levels of satisfaction and increased knowledge, and that the carers had feelings of security and relaxation when their relatives were cared for by the volunteers. On the other hand, a more formal carer education programme implemented in Ireland, although it increased carers' knowledge, had no impact on quality of life or carer burden or well-being (Coen *et al.* 1999).

Changing expectations and changing roles

In the first decade of the twenty-first century, carers, as a group at least, are no longer quite so 'ignored and invisible'. Indeed their importance and their needs are recognized in research, by health and social care practitioners and by local and national government. Carers organizations both nationally and internationally are growing in reputation and influence. This does not mean that all individual carer's lives are easier; for each new carer the experience and the journey though caring is new and personal. The services they need to assist them are still of limited availability and quality. Many carers of people with dementia, however, acknowledge the improvements there have been in public understanding and the public commitment of resources over the last 20 years.

I was just told that my wife was senile and nothing could be done. The doctor didn't want to know. 'Put her in a home', he said. There were no groups or anything like that. Now everyone knows what Alzheimer's is. I don't say carers now have it easy but there is much more information and choice than there was when I started.

In the coming years one of the most significant changes is likely to arise from the earlier diagnosis of Alzheimer's disease and other dementias, and from the impact of pharmaceuticals in maintaining the insight and independence of people with dementia longer into the course of the illness. Although the cholinesterase inhibitors currently available are of limited effectiveness, and indeed are controversial with some doctors, they can have a significant impact on the quality of life of both the person with dementia and their carer.

I'm prepared for the fact that this improvement may be relatively temporary. It will however, for us, have been well worth the additional quality of life it has given us for these years and for the opportunity to prepare ourselves better for whatever the future may hold.

They also raise ethical issues, particularly when taken by people in the middle stages of dementia (Tinker 1997). There are questions which raise possible conflicts between the interests of the person with dementia and those of their carer.

One outspoken member of the NHS when I tackled the subject made a point which made me think. He said, 'Have you considered the moral dimension of asking for a drug which will not cure her but simply slow down and prolong the decline and death? Are you not putting your convenience and ability to look after her above her own real needs?' I am still not sure what the ethical answer is.

People with dementia who are aware of their diagnosis and are able to participate in decisions about their care are already changing the role of carers and attitudes towards them. So too is the theory and practise of 'person-centred care' as developed by Kitwood and others (Kitwood 1997). Person-centred care, which is becoming the orthodoxy in care practice, concentrates on the needs of the person with dementia and on maintaining their independence, individuality, and autonomy for as long as possible.

Kitwood argued that behavioural problems in dementia were best understood as the result of a 'malignant social psychology'. By changing the social environment causing the behavioural disturbance, much of the disability arising from the dementia could be eliminated or reduced. Changing the social environment meant changing the way that carers and careworkers behaved. There is no doubt that this approach has had a profound effect in challenging the negative and defeatist approach to care which had sometimes prevailed previously. However, it follows from Kitwood's social construct that how carers behave may cause or contribute to the ill-effects of dementia, and this has led some to see carers as the problem rather than the solution. Killick (1999) has asserted that carers lack 'emotional and intuitive understanding' of dementia, that they cannot be flexible in their approach because of the history of their relationship with the person they are caring for, and that they are overprotective and dominant. 'Relatives', he says, 'are the least able to cope and the least effective in the caring role'. This view, provocatively expressed, represents an extreme which, in its concentration on the person with dementia, forgets that they too come with relationships, however imperfect, and that older people consistently say that they wish to live in their own homes and to maintain their social networks. Quality of life for older people lies not in the expert care of strangers but in continuity of their environment and social context, choice, and control (Qureshi and Henwood 2000).

A similar perspective is represented by those professionals who argue that people with dementia may need advocates to represent them when their carer fails to act in their interests (Killeen 1996). Of course there are occasions when carers' needs and interests conflict with those for whom they are caring, and the extension of self-determination for people with dementia through earlier and open diagnosis and maintaining drugs may create more situations when this is likely to occur. It is possible to see the views of those like Killick as part of a power struggle between professionals and carers over the lives of people with dementia. It is only in the last decade or so that social workers and therapists have become widely professionally involved in dementia care, and like all new professions dementia specialists have to identify and mark out their territory. Boas (1998) suggests that a whole new range of 'therapies' are being invented to satisfy the needs of workers rather than of people with dementia. It makes careworkers feel important to be providing 'therapy' but in fact the content is less important than 'the human interaction, the companionship of fellow human beings'. There are strong contrasts and conflicts between the view that dementia care is highly skilled and should be entrusted to professionals, and the view that it is common-sense humanity and sensitivity to the lives of others that matters and that family members and carers may bring particular empathy to the task.

Formal programmes of carer training, run by professionals, can be seen as part of the same trend of professionalizing dementia care. Outcome measures such as delay to entry into residential or nursing care and reduced costs to the state are seen by some carers as adding to their burden not relieving it, as an attempt to make them more effective in delivering the state's objective: minimizing the cost of dementia care by using them as cheap labour.

> I'm infuriated being told that if I'm trained as a carer I can care longer and save social services money. Carers have lives too and we should be able to chose not to care if we wish, not be seen as a free service and one which can be trained to be more cost effective.

The increasing focus on the independence and rights of people with dementia, rather than on their dependence on their carers, may be reinforced by developments in new technologies and telemedicine (Fisk 1997). The use of monitored community alarms is already widespread amongst older people and is standard in specialist housing. Responsive telemedicine is also being developed using sensors capable of monitoring people's movements and behaviour patterns, living environments, and physiology. At best, these can be seen as aids to independent living for the person with dementia, as a means of reducing stress for carers, and of enabling people to stay in their own homes much longer. Recently, 'smart houses' (Marshall 2000) have been built incorporating a range of technologies to aid more independent living for people with at least mild dementia. Attempts to develop monitoring systems to protect people who walk about and get lost have been hampered by technical and ethical difficulties. Electronic tagging, however applied, brings about *de facto* restraint (Parkin 1995). Indeed, there are serious ethical problems with all such systems when people with dementia lack the capacity to make judgements or exercise choice. Acceptance of the widespread use of new technologies to support people with dementia and their carers in the community will depend not only on the cost and effectiveness of the devices, but also on the development of guidelines and an ethical consensus around their use.

Information technology is already having a powerful influence on the ability of carers and people with dementia to access information through the Internet. The websites of voluntary organizations, health and research journals, and of the pharmaceutical industry are all readily accessible and free of charge. Increasingly, news groups and chat rooms are being established to provide online information and support for carers.

The general trend towards recognizing the 'expert patient and carer' within the health service and towards seeing them not as the subjects of research but as active participants in it will help in achieving outcomes in health technologies that are generally useful and acceptable (Cayton and Hanley 2001).

The current trend towards the identification and empowerment of carers, greater professional interest in dementia, a concentration on the rights and autonomy of persons with dementia, and towards effective health technologies will all bring about changes in the role of carers. Some of these changes, as I have suggested above, will be contradictory and conflicting. Research will need to concentrate much more on large-scale studies that genuinely test the effectiveness of interventions against outcome measures valued by the carers themselves. Carers' lives seem set to become more complex, but perhaps only a little easier.

Notes

1. All quotations from carers are from letters to or surveys by the Alzheimer's Society. Most have been published in the Society's *Newsletter* or in the reports cited in the references to this chapter. A few are personal communications with the author.
2. Alzheimer's Society helpline annual report. Unpublished.

References

Almberg, B. E., Grafstrom, M., and Winblad, B. (2000). Caregivers of relatives of people with dementia: experiences encompassing social support and bereavement. *Aging and Mental Health*, **4**, 82–9.

Alzheimer's Disease International. (2000). *Starting a self-help group*. ADI, London.

Alzheimer's Disease Society. (1993*a*). *Deprivation and dementia*. Alzheimer's Disease Society, London.

Alzheimer's Disease Society. (1993*b*). *NHS psychogeriatric continuing care beds—a report*. Alzheimer's Disease Society, London.

Alzheimer's Disease Society. (1994). *Home Alone*. Alzheimer's Disease Society, London.

Alzheimer's Disease Society. (1995). *Right from the start; primary health care and dementia*. Alzheimer's Disease Society, London.

Alzheimer's Disease Society. (1997). *Experiences of care in residential and nursing homes; a survey*. Alzheimer's Disease Society, London.

Alzheimer Europe. (2000). *The legal rights of people with dementia*. Alzheimer Europe, Luxemburg.

Alzheimer's Society. (2000*a*). *Food for thought*. Alzheimer's Society, London.

Alzheimer's Society. (2000*b*). *Appraisal of the drugs for Alzheimer's disease; submission to the National Institute for Clinical Excellence (NICE)*. Alzheimer's Society, London.

Aneshensel, C., Perlin, L., *et al.*. (1995). *Profiles in caregiving; the unexpected career*. Academic Press, London.

Archibald C. (1994). *Sexuality and dementia; a guide*. University of Stirling, Stirling.

Audit Commission. (2000). *Forget me not; mental health services for older people*. Audit Commission, London.

Boas, I. (1998). Learning to be rather than do. *Journal of Dementia Care*, **6**, 13.

Bodnar, J. and Kiecolt-Glaser, J. (1994). Carer stress after bereavement; chronic stress isn't over when it's over. *Psychology and Aging*, **9**, 372–80.

Bookwala, J. and Schulz, R. (1998). The role of neuroticism and mastery in spouse caregivers: assessment of and response to a contextual stressor. *Journal of Gerontological Behavioural Psychology*, **53**, 155–64.

Brodaty, H. (2000).

Brodaty, H. and Hadzi-Parlovic, D. (1990). Psychosocial effects on carers living with persons with dementia. *Australian and New Zealand Journal of Psychiatry*, **24**, 351–61.

Brodaty, H., *et al.* (1991). Cost effectiveness of a training programme for dementia carers. *International Psychogeriatrics*, **3**, 11–22.

Brodaty, H., *et al.* (1994). Quasi-experimental evaluation of an educational model for dementia caregivers. *International Journal of Geriatric Psychiatry*, **9**, 195–204.

Brownlee, J. (1991). *A hidden problem? Dementia amongst minority ethnic groups*. DSDC, Sterling.

Cayton, H. (1993). The social consequences of dementia. *The management of Alzheimer's disease* (ed. G. Wilcock), pp. 151–8. Wrightson, London.

Cayton, H. and Hanley, B. (2001). Improving research by involving consumers. *Research and development for the NHS; evidence, evaluation and effectiveness* (ed. M. Baker and S. Kirk). Radcliffe, Abingdon.

Cayton, H., Graham, N., and Warner, J. (1997). *Alzheimer's at your fingertips*. Class Health, London.

CHSR (Centre for Health and Social Research). (1997). *The Carers (recognition and services) Act 1995 and Crossroads care attendant schemes; a baseline survey*. Crossroads, Rugby.

CNA. (1997). *Still battling? The Carers Act one year on*. Carers National Association, London.

CNA. (2000). *Caring on the breadline; the financial implications of caring*. Carers National Association, London.

Coen, R., *et al.* (1999). Dementia carer education and patient behaviour disturbance. *International Journal of Geriatric Psychiatry* **14**, 302–6.

Coope, B., *et al.* (1995). The prevalence of depression in the carers of dementia sufferers. *British Journal of Psychiatry*, **10**, 237–42.

Corti, L., *et al.* (1994). *Caring and employment*. Employment Department Group.

Department of Health. (1993). *Social Services Inspectorate practice guidelines; no longer afraid; the safeguard of older people in domestic settings*. HMSO, London.

Department of Health. (2000). *The NHS plan: the government's response to the Royal Commission on Long Term Care*. The Stationery Office, London.

Department for Social Security. (1999). *Family Resources Survey 1997–8*. The Stationery Office, London.

Dubinsky, R., *et al.* (2000). Practice parameter: risk of driving and Alzheimer's disease (an evidence based review). *Neurology*, **54**, 2205–11.

Dunning, A. (1995). *Citizen advocacy with older people; a code of good practice*. Centre for Policy on Ageing, London.

Fearnley, K., McLennon, J., *et al.* (1997). *The right to know? Sharing the diagnosis of dementia*. Alzheimer Scotland/Mental Health Foundation, Edinburgh.

Fisk, M. (1997). Telemedicine, new technologies and care management. *International Journal of Geriatric Psychiatry*, **12**, 1057–9. [Editorial]

Freyne, A., *et al.* (1999). Burden in carers of dementia patients: higher levels in carers of younger sufferers. *International Journal of Geriatric Psychiatry*, **14**, 784–8.

Gallaher-Thompson, D. (1994). Direct services and interventions for caregivers. In Cantor, D. (ed.). *Family Caregiving*. American Society on Aging, California.

Garland, C. and Garland, J. (1998). A matter of time; supporting the carer. *Journal of Dementia Care*, **6**, 22–3.

Garland, C. and Gray-Amante, P. (1999). Gender differences, family care and dementia. *Generations Review*, **9**, 10–11.

Gilley, D., *et al.* (1991). Cessation of driving and unsafe motor vehicle operation by dementia patients. *Archives of Internal Medicine*, **151**, 941–6.

Grace, J. (1994). Alzheimer's disease; your views. *Geriatric Medicine*, (July). 36–9.

Graham, C., *et al.* (1997*a*). Carers knowledge of dementia and their expressed concerns. *International Journal of Geriatric Psychiatry*, **12**, 470–3.

Graham, C., *et al.* (1997*b*). Carer's knowledge of dementia, their coping strategies and morbidity. *International Journal of Geriatric Psychiatry*, **12**, 931–6.

Hancock, R. and Jarvis, C. (1994). *The long term effects of being a carer*. The Stationery Office, Norwich.

Henwood, M. (1998). *Ignored and invisible: carers experience of the NHS*. Carers National Association, London.

HM Government. (1999). *Caring about carers; a national strategy for carers*. The Stationery Office, Worwich.

HMSO. (2000). *The NHS plan; a plan for investment, a plan for reform* The Stationery Office, Norwich.

Hooker, K., Monaghan, D. J., Bowman, S. R., Frazier, L. D., and Shifren, K. (1998). Personality counts for a lot: predictors of mental and physical health of spouse caregivers in two disease groups. *Journal of Gerontological Behavioural Psychology*, **53**, 73–85.

Hope, T., *et al.* (1998). Predictors of institutionalisation for people with dementia living at home with a carer. *International Journal of Geriatric Psychiatry*, **13**, 682–90.

ICARUS. (2000). *The use of neurological services by Black and ethnic minority communities*. Glaxo Neurological Centre, Liverpool.

Jansson, W., *et al.* (1998). The circle model—support for relatives of people with dementia. *International Journal of Geriatric Psychiatry*, **13**, 674–81.

Jolley, D. and Benbow, S. (2000). Stigma and Alzheimer's Disease: causes, consequences and a constructive approach. *International Journal of Clinical Practice*, **54**, 117–19.

Kelly, C., Harvey, R., *et al.* (1997). Drug treatments for Alzheimer's disease. *British Medical Journal*, **314**, 693–4. [Editorial]

Killeen, J. (1996). Speaking out for Advocacy. *Journal of Dementia Care*, **4**, 22–4.

Killick, J. (1999). Are relatives the last people who should have to care for persons with dementia? *Journal of Dementia Care*, **7**, 11.

Kitwood, T. (1997). *Dementia reconsidered; the person comes first*. Open University Press, Milton Keynes.

Knight, B. and McCallum, T. (1998). Heart rate reactivity and depression in African-American and White caregivers; reporting bias or positive coping? *Aging and Mental Health*, **2**, 212–21.

Law Commission. (1993). *Consultation paper No. 128, mentally incapacitated adults and decision-making; a new Jurisdiction*. HMSO, London.

Levin, E., Sinclair, I., *et al.* (1989). *Families, services and confusion in old age*. Avebury, Aldershot.

Levin, E., *et al.* (1994). *Better for the break*. HMSO, London.

Levin, E. (1997). *Carers: problems, strains and services*. Oxford University Press, Oxford.

Livingston, G., Manela, M., *et al.* (1996). Depression and other psychiatric morbidity in carers of elderly people living at home. *British Medical Journal*, **312**, 153–6.

Lord Chancellor's Department. (1997). *Who decides? Making decisions on behalf of mentally incapacitated adults*. The Stationery Office, London.

McFarland, P. and Sanders, S. (1999). Male caregivers: preparing men for nurturing roles. *American Journal of Alzheimer's Disease*, **14**, 278–82.

McKibbin, C. L., *et al.* (1999). Lifestyle and health behaviours among female family dementia caregivers; a comparison of wives and daughters. *Aging and Mental Health*, **3**, 165–72.

McLoughlin, D., Cooney, C., *et al.* (1996). Carer informants for dementia sufferers: carer awareness of cognitive impairment in an elderly community-resident sample. *Age and Ageing*, **25**, 367–71.

Marshall, M. (2000). *ASTRID. A guide to using technology within dementia care*. Hawker Publications, London.

Melzer, D. (1998). Drug treatments for Alzheimer's disease: lessons for health care policy. *British Medical Journal*, **316**, 762–4.

Mockler, D., Riordan, J. and Murphy, M. (1998). Psychosocial factors associated with the use/non-use of mental health services by primary carers of individuals with dementia. *International Journal of Geriatric Psychiatry*, **13**, 310–14

Moriaty, J. and Levin, E. (1995). How to give carers a break. *Journal of Dementia Care*, **3**, 20–1.

Murphy, K., Hanrahan, P., *et al.* (1997). A survey of grief and bereavement in nursing homes: the importance of hospice grief and bereavement for the end stage Alzheimer's patient and family. *Journal of the American Geriatric Society*, **45**, 1104–7.

Nagatomo, I., *et al.* (1999). Gender of demented patients and specific family relationship of caregiver to patients influence mental fatigue and burdens on relatives as caregivers. *International Journal of Geriatric Psychiatry*, **14**, 618–25.

O'Connor, D., *et al.* (1998). Do general practitioners miss dementia in elderly patients? *British Medical Journal*, **297**, 1107–10.

OPCS. (1988). The General Household Survey. OPCS, London.

Ory, M., *et al.* (1999). Prevalence and impact of caregiving: a detailed comparison between dementia and nondementia caregivers. *Gerontologist*, **39**, 177–85.

Palmer, A. (1993). The price of dementia. *The Spectator*, **270**(8604), 8–10.

Parker, G. (1990). *With Due Care and Attention: a review of research on informal care*. Family Policies Study Centre, London.

Parkin, A. (1995). The care and control of elderly or incapacitated adults. *Journal of Social Welfare and Family Law*, **17**, 431–44.

Patel, N., *et al.* (1998). *Dementia: minority ethnic older people: managing care in the UK, Denmark and France*. Russell House, Lyme Regis.

Petit *et al.* (2000).

Qureshi, H. and Henwood, M. (2000). *Older people's definitions of quality services*. Joseph Rowntree Foundation, York.

Reiss, M., Gold, D., *et al.* (1996). Personality traits as determinants of burden and health complaints in caregiving. *International Journal of Aging and Human Development*, **39**, 257–71.

Rice, K. and Warner, N. (1994). Breaking the bad news. *International Journal of Geriatric Psychiatry*, **9**, 467–71.

Rosenvinge, H., Jones, D. *et al.* (1998). Demented and chronic depressed patients attending a day hospital: stress experienced by carers. *International Journal of Geriatric Psychiatry*, **13**, 8–11.

Rowlands, O. (1998). *Informal carers; an independent study carried out by the Office for National Statistics on behalf of the Department of Health as part of the 1995 General Household Survey*. HMSO, London.

Royal College of Psychiatrists (nd). *Alzheimer's disease and dementia*. Royal College of Psychiatrists, London.

Royal Commission on Long Term Care. (1999). *With respect to old age*. The Stationery Office, London.

Schneider, J., *et al.* (1993). Elderly people with advanced cognitive impairment in England; resource use and costs *Ageing and Society*, **13**, 27–50.

Silviera, E. and Ebrahim, S. (1995). Mental health and the status of elderly Bengalis and Somalis in London. *Age and Ageing*, **24**, 474–80.

Theat, S., *et al.* (1991). Caregivers anticipatory grief in dementia; a pilot study. *International Journal of Aging and Human Development*, **33**, 113–18.

Thompson, C. and Briggs, M. (2000). Support for carers of people with Alzheimer's type dementia. (Cochrane Review). *The Cochrane Library*, Issue 3. Update software, Oxford.

Tinker, A. (1997). Prescribing a hazy future. *Journal of Dementia Care*, **5**, 13.

Trainor, P. (1997). *Debts of love*. Newry and Mourne Health and Social Service Trust, Co Down, NI.

VOICES. (1998). *Eating well for older people with dementia; a good practice guide for residential and nursing homes and others involved in caring for older people with dementia*. Voluntary Organisations Involved in Caring in the Elderly Sector, Potters Bar.

Ward, R. (1999). Waiting to be heard; dementia and the gay community. *Journal of Dementia Care*, **8**, 24–5.

Watkins, M. and Redfern, S. (1997). Evaluation of a new night nursing service for elderly people suffering from dementia. *Journal of Clinical Nursing*, **6**, 485–94.

Wilcock, G. (1999). *Living with Alzheimer's disease and similar conditions; a guide for families and carers*. Penguin books, London.

Wilcox, S. and King A. C. (1999). *Sleep complaints in older women who are family caregivers*. *Journal of Gerontology* (Series B), **54B**, 189–98.

Witeratne, C. and Lovestone, S. (1996). A pilot study comparing psychological and physical morbidity in carers of elderly people with dementia and those with depression. *International Journal of Geriatric Psychiatry*, **11**, 741–4.

Woods, R. (1989). *Alzheimer's disease; coping with a living death*. Souvenir Press, London.

Yeatman, R., Bennetts, K., *et al.* (1993). Is caring for elderly relatives with depression as stressful as caring for those with dementia? A pilot study in Melbourne. *International Journal of Geriatric Psychiatry*, **8**, 339–42.

22 Expect more: making a place for people with dementia

Gareth Hoskins and Mary Marshall

Tensions, dilemmas, challenges, and contradictions

Designing a place for people with dementia is a very complex process. Each built environment will have a particular purpose and a range of users. The needs of the various users will differ, so solutions have to address and respond to a range of needs, some of which will be contradictory. The main users in an establishment caring for people with dementia are the people themselves, their relatives and friends, and the staff. Each will have their own needs and requirements, which have to be considered and understood, and then integrated as far as possible. The same is true for the design of products such as furniture, tableware, curtains, equipment, and fittings. Here we will be mainly considering buildings, but many of the issues can be used to understand the design process more generally. Conflicting needs often arise out of the circumstances discussed below.

Designing for one group's living environment and another group's working environment

For people with dementia for whom the building is a permanent home there needs to be an environment that makes sense as a home. For all of us, a home has private space which expresses the kind of person we are, as well as a place to do all the things we need and want to do such a sleep, eat, be with friends and family, and undertake hobbies and interests. We would expect our homes to be familiar and understandable, as well as being to our taste. For most of us it will have a familiar set of rooms and functions such as a kitchen, a sitting room/lounge, a bedroom, and a bathroom. For most of us home is where we have some degree of control over what happens when. When we are at home we can, with the agreement of the people with whom we live, eat when we want and do pretty much what we want in most respects. On the whole we can choose how we live our lives. People with dementia will usually have had the same experience of their homes as the rest of us, and will have similar expectations if they are to feel 'at home'. Thus the ideal of long-stay care is a fully domestic environment giving people as many opportunities and as much choice as possible. The additional factor for people with dementia is that special efforts may have to be made to ensure it is safe; for example, it will need a stove that cannot be operated unless a staff member is present.

Carers and friends will also have their views on optimal design. They often give a very high priority to safety, having relinquished care because they were no longer able to provide a safe environment at home. They may be very anxious about an environment which is too domestic, with all the potential risks that implies, without always understanding the importance of maintaining familiar activities. They usually need to feel that the building is a pleasant place which is clean, smells nice, and is welcoming to visit. They often like a relatively private place to be with their relative other than the bedroom, and they often appreciate a place where they can make a cup of tea or a snack for themselves and the person with dementia.

For staff, the priorities may be rather different. They will want a building that makes their job as straightforward as possible. They may want to be able to keep an eye on the patients (this word is chosen over 'residents' since the case example in this chapter is a hospital ward). They will want a building that is easy to keep clean, and which makes it as easy as possible to keep the patients clean since many of them will be incontinent. They will want a building where they will not have to walk huge distances to do their job. They will certainly want a building that provides good facilities for them to wash and change and receive training and supervision. Senior staff will want an adequate office. They will, of course, also want what is best for the patients. But it is a work environment for them and a building that makes work more onerous is obviously not ideal.

Staff, in the sense of owners of the building, will want a building that is not too expensive to maintain. Group-care buildings are subject to a lot of wear and tear and the costs of maintenance are often considerable. They will also have to provide a building that meets the various regulations on environmental health and fire safety. They may want a building that offers perceived economies such as an office in the middle of the unit so that unit management staff can do two jobs at once: office work and surveillance. From the point of view of management staff, surveillance of junior staff is as important as surveillance of patients.

The owners of the building have a fundamental role in determining the philosophy of care, which should have a huge impact on the style of the building. They may need to take a view on who do the design decisions belong to: who 'owns' the building on a day-by-day basis? Is it the patients, the relatives, the staff, or themselves?

One of the areas where the conflict of needs is most clearly worked out is in relation to risk and one of the design features which throws this into sharp perspective is kitchens. For many patients a place that does not have an accessible kitchen is obviously not a home in any sense they would understand. Many specialist units have working kitchens where residents can undertake normal domestic tasks (Judd *et al.* 1997), although Gresham (1999) questions whether best use is always made of them. One of the worries often concerns fire regulations, yet with the early involvement of a fire officer this can be resolved. (Dementia Services Development Centre 1998). Some kitchens have taps that are incomprehensible to people with dementia (Stewart 1999), which limits their usefulness as far as normal activities are concerned. Without access to a kitchen many patients, especially women, are deprived of the main activity of their lives.

Designing for a progressive condition

It is easy to make design recommendations which assume that people with dementia are a homogenous group. Yet this is a progressive illness where the needs of people at the beginning and at the end of the disease process are fundamentally different. Most people in the early stages will be able to manage at home, but some people need group care earlier than others for whole sets of reasons such as their behaviour or the capacity of their carer to cope. A familiar environment that enables these people to maintain all their routines and activities is required so they can continue to function at as high a level as possible. Indeed, they may achieve more of their potential than expected if the building provides both reminders and new opportunities.

People in the middle stages are a very disparate group. They will need more support, they may need more surveillance, and they may need higher levels of visual access because they will be less likely to remember what is where. People in the last stages of dementia require very considerable nursing input and a lot of equipment such as special beds and hoists. The patients will be highly dependent and likely to respond mainly to sensory stimulation.

Many settings have to provide for a mixed population in terms of the extent of disability resulting from the dementia. This is often for good reasons, such as maintaining a familiar group of patients and staff to the end, but in terms of optimal design it is problematic.

Designing for very different individuals

We all become more different as we get older. We have different histories, different personalities, different disabilities, different attitudes, different lifestyles, and so on. My idea of a sitting room may be different from your idea of a lounge, illustrating instantly that another way in which we all vary is in terms of class. Some people will have had a good experience of living in groups and be able to live, eat, and spend time in a group. Others will want much more privacy. Traditionally, we have not attempted to provide different units for people with different lifestyles, although this is being piloted in The Netherlands, in Polderburen, a nursing home with several small units (Van Waarde, 2000).

An aspect of design which is slowly emerging in the literature is designing for cultural diversity (Bennett 1997, 2000). People who have changed cultures as adults may well appreciate a familiar design from their past. Thus, for example, people who have come to the UK from Pakistan may well want a design that was popular in Lahore or Peshawar 50 years ago. Bennett has written about the design considerations fro aboriginal Australians, and her processes of consultation could well be replicated with other minority groups. Design considerations related to cultural diversity may not be about the past. They may be about current traditions relating to matters such as religious observance, food preparation, and appropriate activities. Without attention to these matters, the person with dementia may never be able to settle, indeed they may not be able to access the care they need.

Designing for different cohorts

One of the principles of designing for people with dementia is that the building should be 'age appropriate', but there may be as many as 40 years between the oldest and the youngest patients. Their experience of life will have been very different indeed. If the loose assumption is taken that people's most vivid memories of their homes are from the period they were young adults, it is immediately obvious that notions of home can be very different. People who are in their fifties will have been born since the war and will have had much more comfortable homes in the sense of internal sanitation, central heating, electrical goods (including electric kettles), and carpets for example. Those in their eighties will have been born after World War I and into the depression. They may well have had linoleum on the floor instead of carpet, external sanitation, and much cooler houses. They will have been much more likely to have put kettles on the range or on the gas stove.

What is familiar in terms of furniture, fittings, and décor will vary greatly across age ranges. The National Trust performs an invaluable service in maintaining some houses as they were in the 1930s and 1940s. We can all learn what they were like.

A related issue is the fact that buildings (other than family homes) are built to last 30 or 40 years, which means they will housing very different cohorts as time goes on. Most patients today are in their eighties and will have been born in the 1920s, whereas in 30 years time the patients will have been born in the 1950s.

Relatives, staff, and owners of buildings also belong to different cohorts and will have their tastes influenced by their life experience as well.

Designing for different and complex needs

Some people with dementia can have very particular needs. People with challenging behaviour who are fit and active need space and opportunities for constant activities (Coon 1991; Archibald 1997; Pickles 1998). They may need a well-organized outside space to let off steam or to maintain the energetic habits of a lifetime. They may be particularly sensitive to feeling confined so high fences will simply provide an invitation to escape. People with challenging behaviour are often very anxious and restless and may need to be able to see staff at all times. Similarly, staff may want to be able to see patients at all times to ensure they are not doing themselves or other patients any harm. Another less obvious group of people with challenging behaviour are those who are very withdrawn. They may need opportunities to watch without joining in. Places to sit and watch kitchen activities or a busy local street can be much appreciated.

Some people with dementia have complex combinations of dementia with intercurrent illness. They may be people with Huntington's disease or other movement disorders, or complex combinations of the illnesses of old age: affecting hearts, lungs, and joints on the whole. A tiny example shows the design challenge.

Sometimes the needs of someone with arthritis, for example, conflict with the design requirements of dementia. An example of this is the design for a tap. An older person with dementia needs a tap which is familiar: in the UK this means a cross-head tap with separate hot and cold (with temperature controls on the hot), whereas if they also have arthritis they may need a tap which requires little pressure to turn. Fortunately, all modern taps are easier to turn since they are no longer fitted with rubber washers.

There are a complex set of design challenges around the needs of people with a lifetime of disabilities such as those with Down's syndrome (Kerr 1997; Cox and Keady 1999) and dementia, or people who have always had a sensory impairment. Sensory impairment and dementia is a complicated issue since the point at which the impairment was acquired will be very significant. Someone who has always been blind will be able to use cues of touch and sound which can be designed into a building. We do not know if these are effective for someone who is struggling to adapt to impaired vision with the learning impairment resulting from dementia. The needs of people with sensory impairment and dementia are too little understood across the board, not just in design.

Mrs Maxwell has cataracts. When she is tired she gets very anxious because she thinks the blue carpet is water.

Some of the most complex needs are around terminal care (Cox 1996), where there are requirements for equipment and space that conflict with the concept of a familiar environment. Terminal care may be required as a result of dementia but is just as likely to be for some other cause. People with Down's syndrome and dementia who are dying tend to have a lot of fits, which has design implications. There may be a need for special beds for many people who are dying. Quiet and a lack of disturbance caused by noisier patients is usually desirable. Most people who are dying need space for their family and friends nearby.

It is very rare to find units specializing in the care of any one of these groups. They are usually all mixed up, which is a design challenge in itself. The design challenge is eased if the rooms are single and big enough to modify for particular needs. Clusters for small units with different groups of patients may be a way forward, but they are rare at the moment.

Designing for short vs. long stay

Some people need short-stay care because they have a crisis at home, they need to be assessed away from home, or they need to give their carers a break. They need an environment which is immediately understandable and full of multiple cues. There is rarely time to individualize the cues, so it is usually worth having some redundant cues in the hope that one will work. Thus, for example, toilets should have a colour cue such as a red doorframe, a word, a picture, and a landmark nearby.

For all the reasons already listed in this chapter it is impossible to design a unit which is familiar to all patients needing short-stay care, an educated assessment of what will be most familiar to most patients is the best that can be achieved.

Stratheden Hospital in Fife, Scotland, has a psychogeriatric assessment ward in two linked bungalows furnished with solid wood bedroom suites, candlewick bedspreads, and an assortment of old fashioned chairs in the lounges.

This is quite a different approach from patients who are in hospital for a long stay who can reasonably expect a more individualized approach to design. Most units, however, mix the two, which is where the design challenge really bites.

Designing for homeliness

Homeliness means very different things to different people. Some people who have spent their lives in institutions (such as hostels, prisons, or hospitals) will have little understanding of what most of us mean by this.

The manager of a unit for men with alcohol-related brain damage has linoleum on the floors and Formica tables, not because she is motivated by cleanliness but because she says it makes the home very familiar to the residents, many of whom have spent their lives in hostels.

It is not easy to judge what line to take on this issue. Should people with Down's syndrome and dementia who have spent their lives in deprived hospital environments be cared for in such environments at the end of their lives? This could be argued as the environment they find most familiar.

For most people home is a house or apartment with roughly the same combination of rooms. But there are a host of cultural differences; not least whether the prevailing norm is houses or apartments. It is also important to attend to gender issues. A 'home' for an 80-year-old man might have been where he ate and slept, but the most important parts of his life would have been outside the house either at his work or his club or pub. In some communities men and women mix very little.

In the North-West of Scotland where most men were either fisherman or crofters or both, the dementia unit has separate communal space for men and women. The men have their own rather dark room where they smoke and read the papers. They do not mix in the home life of the unit which centres around the kitchen/dining room.

Even within apparently homogenous cultures there will be very different lifestyles. Some people will have had families and will be used to living with other people. Some people are very tidy so will want lots of cupboards, others like a cheerful mess and may want shelves. Some people like a noisy place so will be happy if there is little sound absorption, others like quiet. Taste in décor and pictures will vary hugely. The key question is 'who decides'? Generally speaking it is the staff, with most units reflecting the personality of the manager. Ideally the style of the place should reflect the cultural norms of the locality but this is far from straightforward.

Disentangling staff management issues from design issues

Design will not address some issues such as low morale, poor skills, inadequate staff support, an unstimulating regime, and so on. *Design makes good care easier. It does not make it happen.*

What is good design?

Whether something, be it a place or an item, is considered good design, is often a subjective judgement which is dependent on how that place or item works when we use it, or how it affects us in terms of how we feel or what we experience. The performance is, to a great extent, reliant on the particular circumstances and requirements it aims to address. In terms of dementia care, many hospital units are designed around the operation of managing and caring for people rather than the creation of a place suited to the day-to-day living of an individual. There are many dementia unit guidelines available, with a very high degree of unanimity between them about good design for people with dementia (Calkins 1988; Coons 1991; Centre for Accessible Environments 1998; Cohen and Weisman 1991; Archibald 1997; Judd *et al.* 1997).

The considerations which inform design are not simply the functional use of the place, but a combination of responses to the particular place or surroundings and the needs of all the various groups who will use or interact with the place. Some considerations are evident from the outset, such as particular features of the site—whether it be on a hill or a busy main road. But others have to be worked out through a process of discussion with all the various groups involved, and whose needs have to be drawn out and explained. In addition, designers have to have a really good grasp of the day-to-day operation of the building.

Good design is a process

The challenge for architects is fitting together very different kinds of factors. No one set of factors is sufficient; they all inform the design process. This process is not a linear one where the architect works his or her way through in a straight line step by step, instead, it is a process of going back and forth, up and down until the best possible outcome is arrived at. The following factors have to be considered:

- the people with dementia who will use the building;
- the values and approach of the customer;
- the way the building is to be used over a 24-hour period;
- the key features of the building;
- regulations;
- costings.

Wishes, values, and approach of the customer

Each of these considerations can be assisted by a set of prompts or checklists. The ones here are taken from the strategic brief published by the Glasgow School of Art following the Glasgow 1999 design initiative on dementia. They tend to be worded in the first person to emphasize the centrality of the person with dementia.

It is important to clarify the different understandings about dementia, because if the traditional medical view is held then design has little purpose beyond keeping people warm and comfortable. However, the disability perspective would suggest that design has a crucial role in compensating for the disabilities associated with dementia, and in assisting people to function at the best level.

Like everybody else, people with dementia live in buildings for different lengths of time and for different reasons. Clarifying what these are will assist understanding of who is going to live in the building. The following checklist is provided in the full understanding of its limitations. It is in the first person to demonstrate the importance of putting people with dementia or the centre of the design process:

As a person with dementia using this building I will:

- Live there for the rest of my life regardless of my changing needs, behaviour, or my need for terminal care?
- Live there for the rest of my life regardless of my changing needs, behaviour, or my need for terminal care?
- Live there as long as those who help me can cope?
- Live there for a period of my challenging behaviour?
- Live there for the period of my terminal care?
- Live there only as long as I do not have very challenging behaviour?
- Live there only if I do not disrupt the lives of other people who live there?
- Live there even if I sometimes disrupt the lives of other people who live there?
- Live there only as long as I do not need terminal care?
- Live there only as long as I am active and mobile?
- Live there only to be assessed?
- Live there only while I am receiving treatment for some acute condition or problem?
- Live there only for a brief period to give my carer and me a break from each other?
- Live there for as long as it takes to find me somewhere more suitable?

Note: many places have a mixed group, which presents its own design challenges.

The values and approach of the customer

In gaining further understanding of the customer it is useful to understand their values. One possible checklist for discussion is the set of design principles provided in Judd *et al.* (1997). The question to discuss with the customer for each point is: 'How will this be achieved?'

As a person with dementia I need the building to:

- Compensate for my disability.
- Maximize my independence.
- Enhance my self-esteem and confidence.
- Demonstrate care for those looking after me.
- Be orientating and understandable.
- Reinforce my personal identify.
- Make my relatives and the local community feel welcome.
- Ensure I am not over- or understimulated.

24 Hours of the building

The best way to understand how a building is to be used is to see what is intended to happen through 24 hours in the building. For a customization it is possible to spend time in the unit as it is at present. There is of course the danger of implying that everybody who lives there has the same needs and the same routine, whereas, of course, this is not the case and should never be the case. In obtaining an understanding of how the building is to be used it can be useful to find out whether the customer is happy with what is happening now, or would like the design to make changes possible. A profile of the 24 hours might look like the one from the Glasgow 1999 strategic brief:

What time do people get up?
When and how are relatives and friends involved through the day?
What happens when people get up (baths, showers, dressing)?

Over what time period is breakfast?
How is it organized?
Where?
Who?
How?

Does the dining area need to be near the bedrooms?
What happens after breakfast?
How are drugs organized?
How is laundry in and out organized? How do the cleaners work?
Do people need to be helped to get ready for day care elsewhere?

Are there social, therapeutic and individual activities?
Where are the activities?
What is needed for activities? (flooring, space, storage)
Is there access to garden and for what purpose?
Are there trips out?

Is space required for treatments (occupational therapy, physiotherapy, chiropody, nurse, and doctor)? Are there staff meetings and in what numbers? Is there staff training? (What is required for staff training?)

Where and when do staff have breaks? (What are the requirements for the staff space?)

Lunch: How is it organized? What is required? (Storage of crockery, cutlery, tablecloths etc.) Flooring? Table size and space?

Afternoon: Is anything different from morning?

Evening meal: Is anything different from lunch?

Evening: Are there any special activities/events?

What are the going to bed arrangements?

Night: How much observation and assistance is required during the night?
How much are people with dementia up and about at night?
What activities do people need to be provided with at night?
What is needed to ensure people get an undisturbed night's sleep?

Weekly schedule: Is every day the same? Are there any requirements for religious observations on particular days of the week (space, quiet, altars, music, seasonal changes, and events)?

Cultural issues: Are there special cultural requirements in terms of kitchens, space for prayer, orientation of the building, festivals, laundry/clothing.

Key features

As well as a picture of what currently happens and what the customer would like to happen over 24 hours, a whole set of design features need to be considered. They form a very lengthy list, a sample of which is given here. The full list is given in the Appendix at the end of this chapter.

- Dining space:
- – For each unit?
- – Relation to living space?
- – How many people? Subdivided for people unable to cope with large numbers? Will staff eat alongside the people who live there?
- – What size/shape of tables?

- Alongside unit kitchen/servery or counter?
- Tea/cooking facilities for visitors?
- Storage of cutlery, crockery, tablecloths, etc.?
- Closed or open-fronted cupboards?
- Age-appropriate furniture?
- Toilet off the dining room/just outside the dining room? How many?
- Numbers and location of electric sockets?
- Methods of reducing noise levels?
- Wheelchair access?

Regulations and costings

In addition to considering the approach and intentions of the customer, the way the building is to be used, and the key design features, both regulations and costings are powerfully important factors. Regulations primarily relate to environmental health, fire safety, and registration. The last of these is undergoing major review in the UK as part of the process of setting up national care standards commissions. One of the problems of regulation is the frequent lack of understanding of optimal design for dementia by the regulators. Costs are an obvious consideration. The potential future use of the building has to be taken account of in the design since there may not be an infinite demand for dementia units.

In spite of the way the factors to be considered have been presented here sequentially, the process of design is not a linear one. The architect and the customer constantly revisit the designs as they develop. Ideally the 'customer' should include staff, relatives and the people with dementia themselves

• Good design is helping people to think beyond their particular circumstances and expectations

People often base their expectation on what they feel to be solutions to current needs and the environment and circumstances they are used to. The architect can often bring fresh eyes to assessing needs and developing potential solutions. Architects develop their thinking by actually designing buildings and by looking at a lot of other people's buildings; indeed their concept of research is visiting buildings! A major part of developing a design lies in understanding the requirements of a particular group. This usually comes about through expanding and building upon the initial needs that the customer group express and by asking searching questions about, for example, why certain facilities are needed or why certain operations are carried out in a particular way. It is easy to say that the customer tells the architect the problems and the latter comes up with the solution, but it is much more often a dialogue and a shared problem-solving process.

• Good design is helping people understand what feels good, and why, with examples

There is always a problem about testing out good ideas, since it is always impossible to do a trial building. Some parties to the discussion may be very limited in their ability to read plans. More often it is, the drawings and models that provide the necessary information and impression. Computer renderings are an improvement since they can provide a 3D image; virtual presentation is becoming increasingly available, and provides a walk-through experience

The customer may also have limited experience of other similar buildings. Photographs can help but are no substitute for visits. Visiting other places can be very useful because it provides an opportunity to experience the quality and feeling of a place, which is the result of a complex combination of factors such as space, light, smell, and touch. These sensual qualities are often a major reason for one place feeling better than another, but at the same time they are the most difficult to illustrate.

Balmore Ward, Leverndale Hospital: Case-Study

In 1999 Glasgow was the UK City of Architecture and Design. A major dementia initiative was part of the programme entitled: 'Just another disability; Making design dementia friendly'. Projects included customizations of a hospital ward, a residential home unit, and a council flat as well as a European Conference, a dementia chair (furniture), and numerous publications. All the work was characterized by the active involvement of carers and staff as well as people with dementia where possible. The case study chosen for this chapter is a psychogeriatric assessment ward within a large psychiatric hospital.

The building

Leverndale Hospital, run by Greater Glasgow NHS Trust, is in south Glasgow within a large green site, overlooked by the ruins of the original Victorian hospital. The current hospital comprises ten, single-storey ward units built in the 1970s. Each ward is 'L'-shaped in plan and interlocks with the adjacent ward to allow a connecting route between the ten units.

The case study focused on Balmore Ward, which is an assessment ward where patients come for short periods for care and assessment of their particular needs, following which many move on to longer term care accommodation. The ward can accommodate 30 patients, within a combination of six individual rooms with en-suite toilet facilities and four 6-bed wards, each with a shared wheelchair accessible toilet. This sleeping accommodation is arranged either side of a 30-m long corridor with a fire escape door at one end

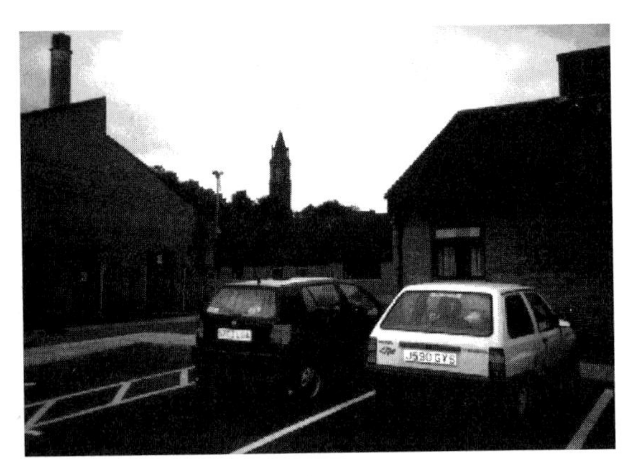

Fig. 22.1(a) Balmore exterior.

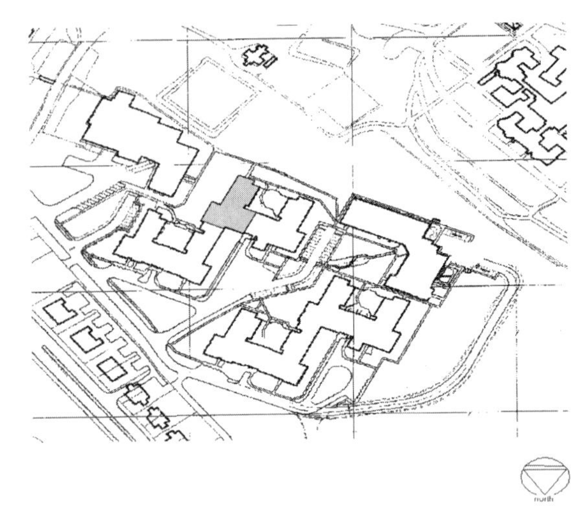

Fig. 22.1(b) Balmore location plan.

and a controlled pass door at the other. The day room, where patients spend most of their time, and the duty room are reached via a short connecting route off this corridor. The day room has one large window and door looking out onto the small garden shared with the adjacent ward. The room is divided in two to form another day area where disruptive patients can sit or visitors can talk in private with their relatives. The internal wall of the day room, opposite the window, has a large glazed screen, looking in to another corridor that connects with the adjacent ward. Staff and visitors can be seen passing along this corridor from the ward entrance, where it links with the recently built communal dining area, again shared with the adjacent ward. The original entrance to the ward has never been used as the access road was never built. The current entrance to the ward is via the service entrance that visitors and patients share with staff, laundry, and deliveries. The environment within the ward is very much that of an institution, with low Artexed ceilings, little natural daylight, and few domestic items of furniture and is supervised by six uniformed staff throughout the day shift. Despite the day room opening on to a garden, this is not used because of supervision difficulties with the challenging behaviour patients from the adjacent ward.

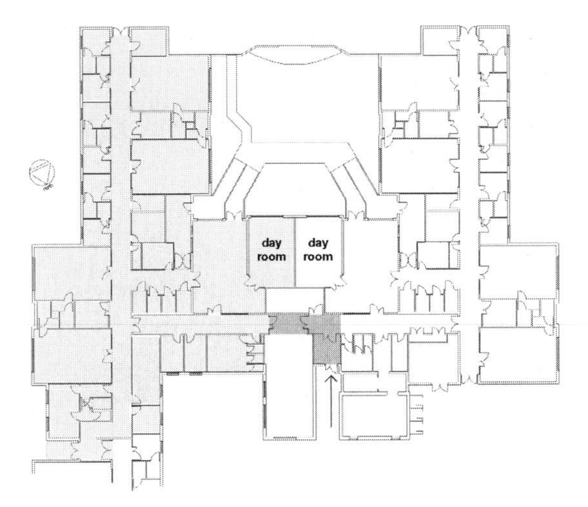

Fig. 22.2 Balmore original layout.

Assessing the issues and developing the brief

A core group of 10 people was established for assessing the issues that should be addressed within the project and to develop a brief for the new design.

The group included the General Manager and administrator for Mental Health within the Trust and an architect from the Trust's Estates Department, representing the economic and policy aspects of the project. Further Trust input was provided by the Senior Clinical Consultant, the Senior Nurse Manager, and the Balmore Ward Manager to represent the staff involved in the day-to-day operation and care within Balmore. Also involved were two members of Glasgow City Council Social Work Department, responsible for the funding and staff allocations within care homes. Input and previous experience was also drawn from a staff nurse involved in a ward customization carried out 2 years before by the Trust.

Alongside the Trust input to the briefing process, was input from visitors, relatives, and patients. This input was brought about through informal discussions between the ward staff and visitors and patients, and by more formal documented consultations carried out by Alzheimer's Scotland. The Alzheimer's Scotland member represented these views within the core group. The final members of the group were architects Nick Domminney and Gareth Hoskins, responsible for developing the brief and the customization design with the group. Prior to the group discussions, Domminney and Hoskins observed the operation of the ward through a series of visits, to gain some understanding of the existing environment and the day-to-day activities within the ward.

Discussions led by the two architects focused on the following areas in turn:

- *The key facts about the current set-up*, i.e. number of patients, number of staff, existing organization, etc.
- *Nature of the existing physical accommodation and environment*, i.e. number of rooms, orientation (which rooms get the sun), where are the entrances, what is the heating like etc.?
- *Understanding the day-to-day operation of the ward*, i.e. when does everyone get up in the morning, what are the staff shifts, is the garden used, how are visitors met?
- *Understanding specifics related to patient care*, i.e. are there any noticeable preoccupations such as wandering, do patients have difficulty in finding their way from sleeping areas to the day room, can they find the toilets, do they prefer to sit near the windows and daylight, is the movement of patients through to the communal dining area disruptive, etc.?

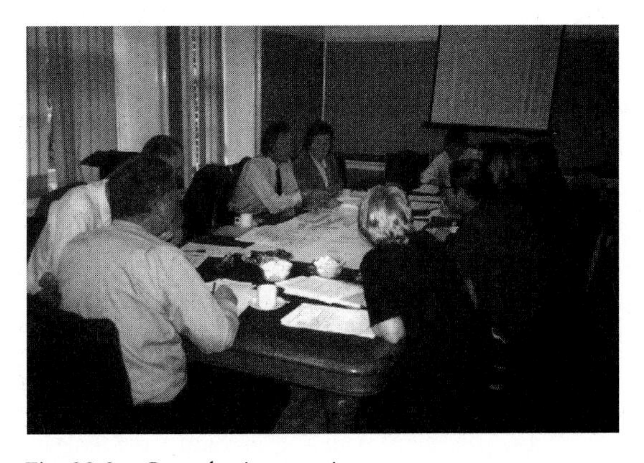

Fig. 22.3 Consultation meeting.

- *Highlighting areas that do not work or issues and concerns within the existing set-up*, i.e. is the lack of a defined entrance difficult in terms of supervision, are there issues over the shared ward spaces etc.?

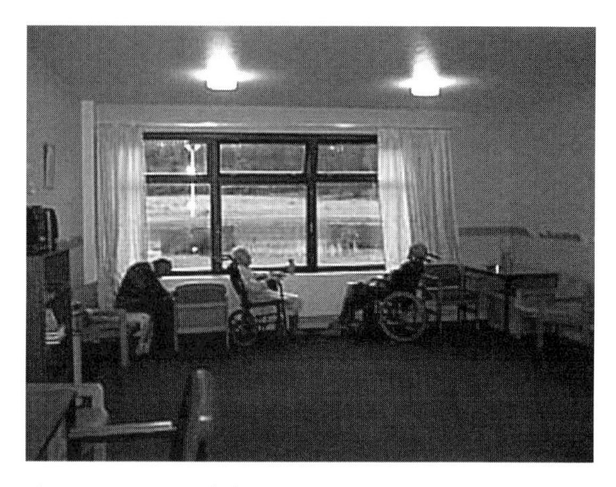

Fig. 22.4 Original dayroom.

The importance of the architects' involvement in assessing the issues and developing the brief became obvious throughout the process, i.e. to draw out issues that might otherwise be difficult to discuss within a hierarchical group, to question areas that might be overlooked or taken for granted due to familiarity, and to begin to suggest options that might not readily be seen by someone who is 'too close' to the issue.

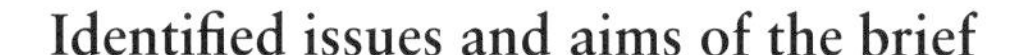

Identified issues and aims of the brief

The assessment process identified a range of issues and highlighted the fact that whilst many of the issues were to do with the physical environment and arrangement, others were issues that could be addressed through changes in management and organization. The key concerns identified are discussed below.

Issue *Size of patient group and overall institutional nature of the ward*—an implicit contradiction in the role of the ward as an assessment ward became evident in terms of realistically assessing a patient's behaviour within an unfamiliar and institutional environment, and amongst strangers in a group much larger than a more familiar everyday family group.

Aim Reduce ward numbers from 30 to 24 patients and reorganise ward to create smaller groupings of patients. Explore ways in which the hospital environment can be reduced and domestic familiarity be introduced without compromising health and safety issues.

Issue *Lack of privacy and individuality for the patients*—arises from the need to share spaces within the communal ward arrangement and the lack of options for places to get away from the group within the existing arrangement. The latter point was a concern both for patients and visitors forced to sit with their relative without privacy within the existing day space.

Aim Attempt to create individual rooms throughout the ward and to rework the existing arrangement to form supervised 'break out' spaces for smaller groups or individuals. Explore the potential for personal items to be brought into the ward.

Issue *Wandering*—was evident within the long corridors, which led to disorientation, frustration and issues of security, when

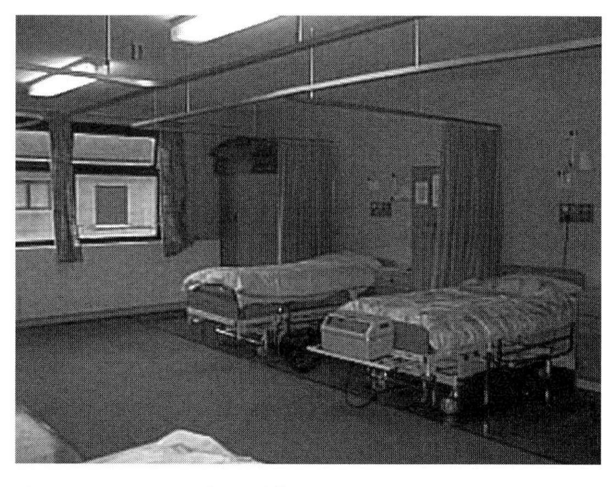

Fig. 22.5 Original ward layout.

patients reached controlled fire doors at either end informing them to 'push'. Patients either became frustrated when the doors were found to be locked with key pads, or they were able to escape the secure confines of the ward by activating the fire doors and alarms. Whilst staff using the corridors could be seen via glazed screens, this caused further frustration as patients attempting to reach them found their way blocked by secure doors.

Aim Explore the possibility of creating circular routes leading through the secure environment of the ward. Relocating fire doors from the ends of corridors and instead creating areas of activity or destinations that patients reach. Explore alternative solutions to the contradiction of ward security and fire escape regulations.

Issues *Disruption and disorientation caused by need to move patients through to communal dining area*—The unfamiliar, institutional nature of the current dining set-up around tables within a poorly lit canteen with food issued from a servery.

Aim Bring meals back into smaller groups within ward. Focus around smaller more intimate, family-scale dining set-ups, allowing a variety of space within day rooms and the potential for activities centred around smaller kitchenettes.

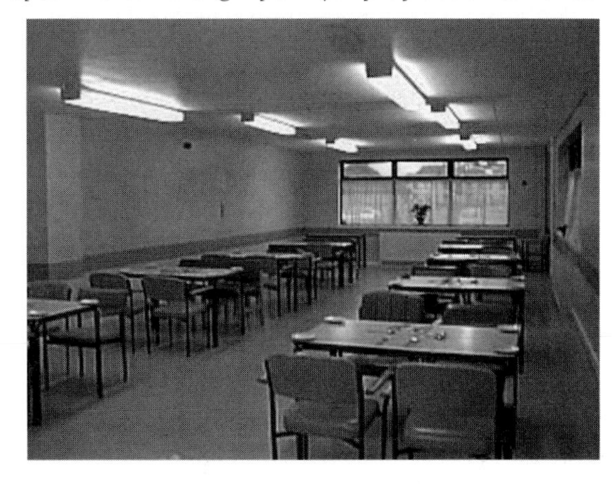

Fig. 22.7 Original dining room.

Issue *Lack of a clear, secure entrance*—The current entrance, shared by staff, patients, relatives, laundry, and refuse is both unclear in terms of access to the ward and offers no control over people leaving or entering the ward.

Aim Create a separate controlled entrance to the ward to maintain security and allow visitors to be greeted by staff.

Issue *Under use of existing garden*—due to poor access and difficulties in shared use with the adjacent challenging-behaviour ward.

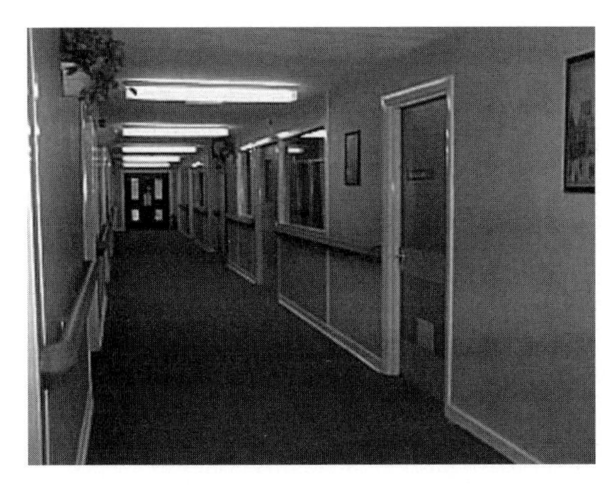

Fig. 22.6 Corridor doors.

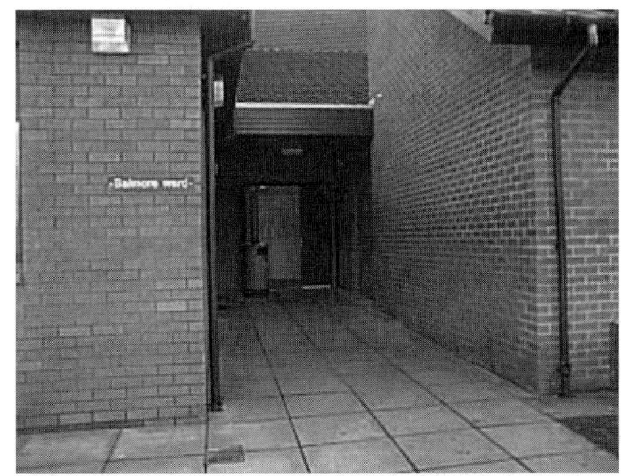

Fig. 22.8 Original entrance.

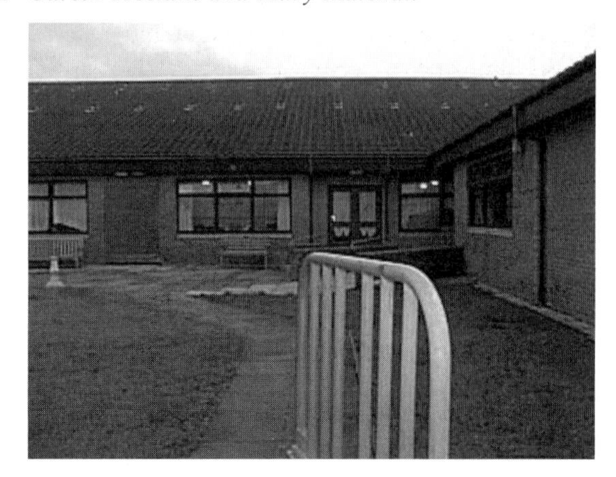

Fig. 22.9 Original garden.

Aims Explore ways of creating a distinct garden area for each ward and increasing connections to this from inside.

Tackling the issues and developing design solutions

Having identified these key issues, a series of possible alterations and reworkings of the ward was explored by the architect team. Through a process of overlaying alternative layouts over the existing plan of the ward and testing how these alterations would affect the spaces by using three-dimensional sketches of the interiors, a set of workable options that addressed the various issues were developed. Organizationally, the options explored ways in which a new entrance might be created, and looked at how the layout of the existing ward might be broken down to create smaller groups and individual rooms for patients. The three-dimensional sketches allowed ways in which the existing spaces might be remodelled to improve the overall environment of the ward.

These options were presented and explained to the client group through a series of simple organizational diagrams, three-dimensional images, and a combination of card and computer models. This combination of methods of presenting the ideas was important in allowing the group to understand the ideas being proposed and to then put forward various questions and suggestions that helped test, develop, and narrow down the options.

An optimum solution and the reality of funding

The responses to the various options led to the decision to investigate an optimum scheme that encompassed all the issues identified, irrespective of cost restraints.

Within the constraints of the footprint of the existing building, the scheme managed to address all the key issues, through the major intervention of removing the existing shared wards and replacing them all with more private and familiar individual bedrooms. The existing single rooms would be retained, and a further 18 built within the ward to replace the accommodation presently provided by the wards. Not only would this allow a greater level of privacy for the individual patients, but the security afforded by the separate rooms would allow people to bring in some of their own furniture, helping improve familiarity, recognition of their personal environment, and hopefully assisting in their assessment.

Generally, single-room accommodation should be provided, with clearly visible en-suite toilet facilities to allow for ease of use and recognition by patients and also to maintain their dignity and privacy when dealing with incontinence. Whilst the existing rooms had en-suite accommodation, the constraints of the available area meant that this was not possible for all the new rooms. A compromise was achieved by grouping small numbers of rooms around new bathroom facilities.

The scheme formed a small courtyard to create the additional area of external wall needed to provide the individual windows planned for each room. Together with this new courtyard, two new day spaces were introduced. These broke up the overall scale of the ward and by grouping the individual bedrooms around these, allowed the overall patient group to be broken down into smaller, more intimate, and familiar-sized groups.

This 'optimum' space proved that it was possible to address the major issues identified by the group. However, the scheme entailed the reworking of a large proportion of the interior of the ward at a cost estimated to be three times the available £150 000 project budget. Without the available funds to explore the option further, the scheme was then reworked to examine how the issues might still be addressed, but in a more financially viable manner.

An affordable solution

The main area of expense within the 'optimum' scheme involved the demolition of the existing wards and rooms and the construction of new individual bedrooms. The scheme was reassessed to explore how the existing wards might be retained to reduce the overall project cost, while achieving some form of improvement in patient privacy and maintaining the essentials of the solutions presented within the 'optimum' scheme.

A revised scheme was developed that retained the wards and addressed the following issues for a reduced figure of £160 000.

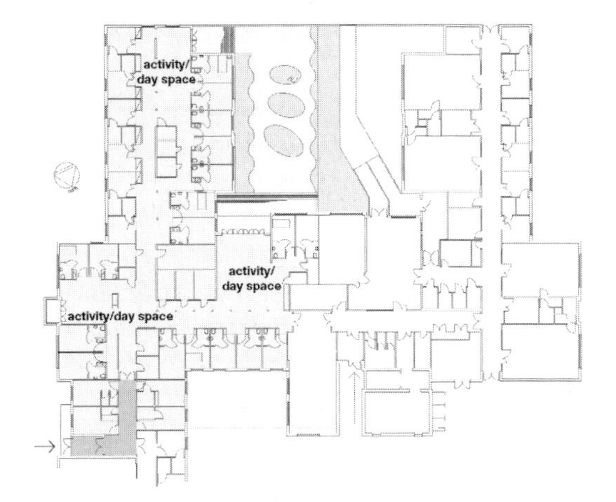

Fig. 22.10(a) Optimum layout.

Providing patient privacy

Without the option of providing an individual room for each patient, the scheme explored how privacy might be provided within the existing 6-bed wards in a more physical manner than the existing bay curtains. As the division of wards to create individual, internal spaces was not permissible, the scheme suggested the installation of purpose-built dressing units to separate each bed from the next. These free-standing units were deliberately designed as familiar pieces of furniture, their wooden surfaces reminiscent of furniture found in a person's home. They incorporate a dressing table, with stools doubling as seating for visitors, shelving for personal items and a wardrobe with hanging space for clothes and wire racks allowing patients to see the garments kept within. A translucent screen ties

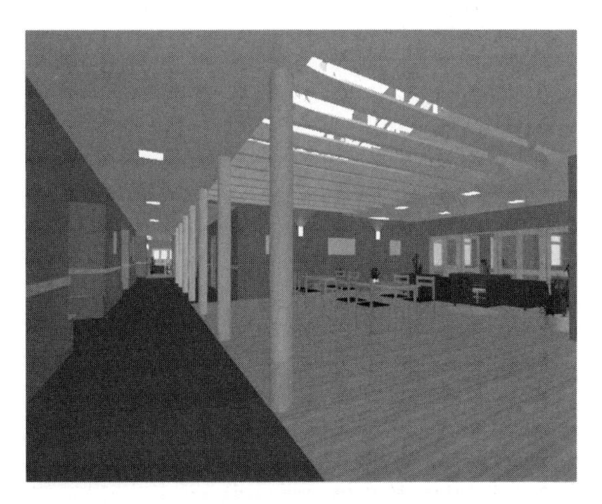

Fig. 22.10(b) Optimum layout interior sketch.

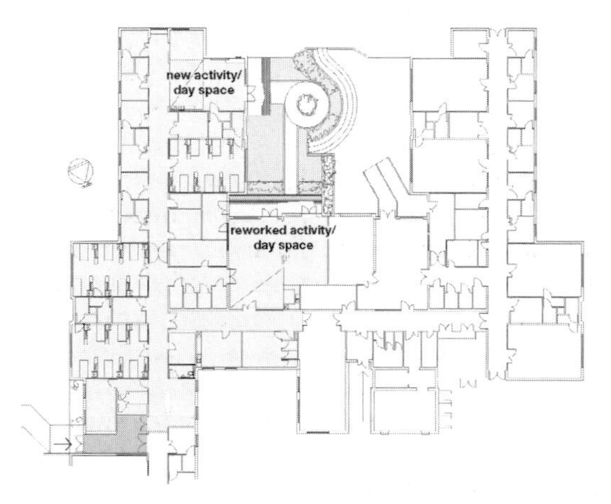

Fig. 22.11 Final layout.

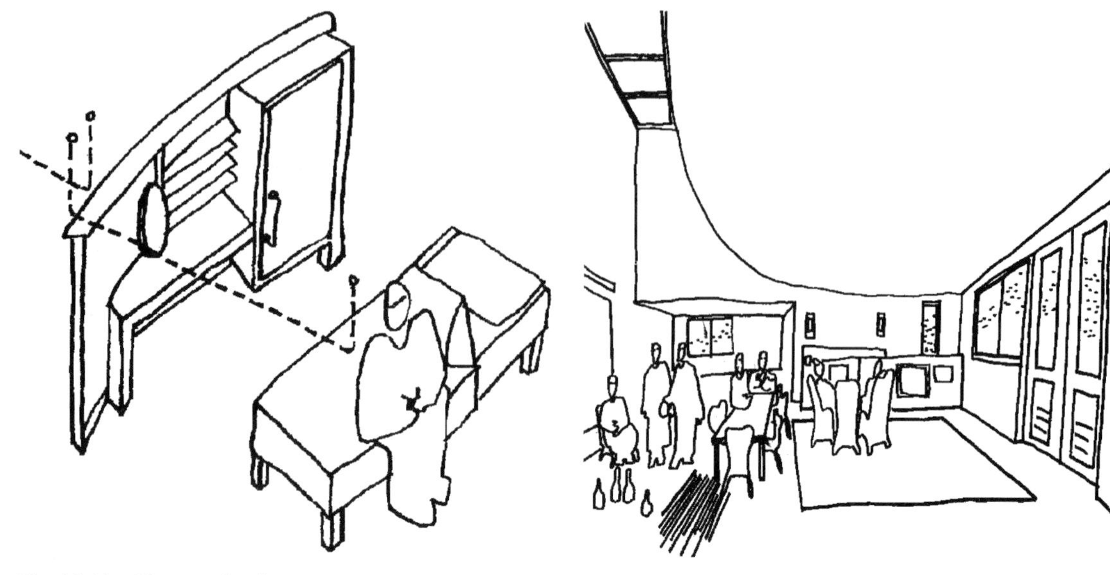

Fig. 22.12 New ward units.

Fig. 22.13 Activities in the new day space.

the pieces together forming the separation between the next bed space and a place for 'garaging' the single enclosing curtain.

Breaking down the scale of the ward and creating family sized areas of activity within

Two further activity/day spaces were introduced within the plan, one at either end of the existing corridor. Combined with the existing day space, these created the potential for the patients living at one end of the ward to use one particular space, thus reducing the numbers within a shared living area to a smaller, more familiar, and manageable group. Whilst staff were initially resistant to this reorganization because it meant splitting staff between the areas, the benefits of reducing numbers and also allowing more activities and mealtimes to be dealt with within these areas was seen as positive. In addition to providing focuses for these smaller patient groups, these new space also created destinations and places of interest and activity at either end of the corridor for those patients wandering within the ward.

Making mealtimes a more positive and less-disruptive experience

In addition to seating space, each of the day areas included an area with a kitchen table and tea point. As meals were brought in, even when served in the existing canteen environment, this allowed the opportunity, through both a physical and operational change, of serving meals within the more familiar and family-scale day space. The kitchen tables and tea point also provide a place, and therefore the opportunity, for further stimulatory activities, such as food making or activities around the table.

Wandering routes, fire escape, and making the garden work

The scheme proposed the removal of the existing pass and fire-escape doors from their current position, clearly visible as the culmination of the views at either end of the corridor. Through discussion with the City Council Building Control Department, a special dispensation ('relaxation') of the regulation was agreed to allow these to be resited to one side of the corridor, doubling as

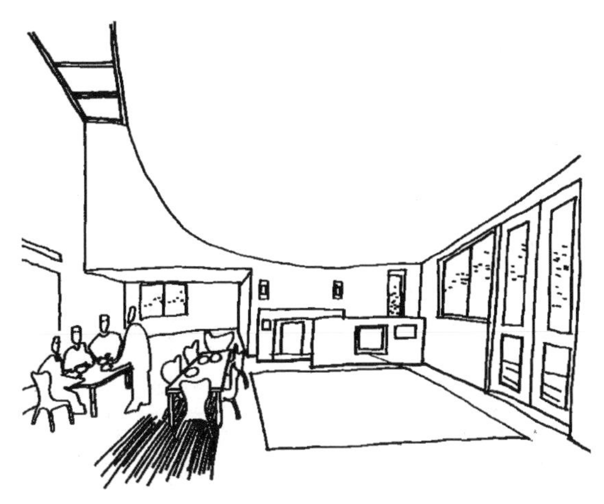

Fig. 22.14 New dining sketch.

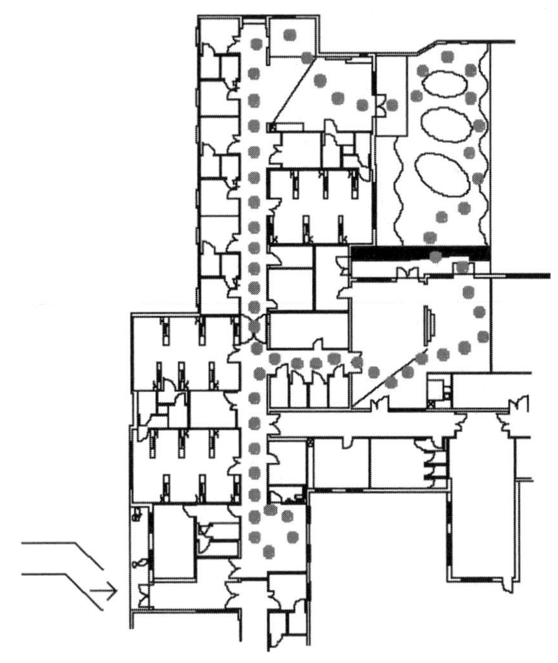

Fig. 22.15(a) Wandering routes.

French doors leading out to the garden. Removing the doors from the direct line of sight lessened the problem of patients walking down a corridor and being faced by a door instructing them to push. To new day areas at the ends of the corridor provide areas where activity is going on. On one hand, this distracts patients from their continual wandering up and down the corridor, and on the other, this offers the opportunity for them to discover something going on that they may take part in. Should they make their way to the relocated doors and open them, they would wander into the secure confines of the garden rather than the current situation of open areas with roads. The scheme also divides the existing garden in two, creating secure areas for both the dementia ward and the challenging-behaviour ward to use. The new garden doors open into a garden, with paths leading through and back into another day space, creating a circular wandering route throughout the ward.

Using daylight, materials, and furniture to create a healthier and more familiar environment

Together with improving access to the secure garden, the scheme suggested the introduction of new windows, lighting, and roof lights, to allow natural daylight into the currently dimly lit

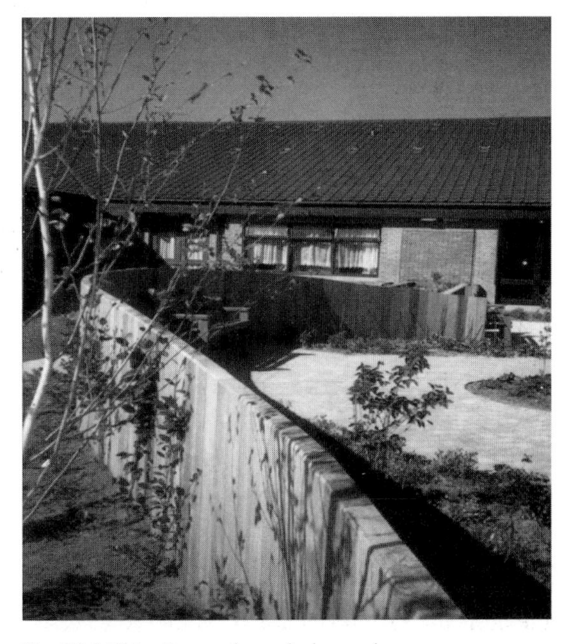

Fig. 22.15(b) Route through the garden.

internal spaces. In addition to improving the daylight within the day spaces, these allow daylight into the corridor and the natural ventilation provided by these features help to remove the stale odours often found in such wards.

The scheme suggested the introduction of more familiar household furniture and fittings, such as bookcases and fireplaces to reduce the institutional nature of the ward environment and create a more domestic feel. Whilst the practicalities of vinyl flooring may be preferred by domestic staff, it is not a material frequently found in people's living rooms. The scheme suggested a maintainable alternative in a laminated timber floor. This provided a cleanable, hard wearing finish that gives a 'warmer' less hospital-like feel within the spaces. Within this it was also possible to define areas for seating by insetting carpets in a similar manner to rugs found within a sitting room. Spaces were repainted and the existing unlined hospital curtains were replaced with a quality fabric of a standard that people would use in their own homes.

Given the difficulty certain patients experience in finding their way between day space and bedroom, various ideas of 'signposting' were explored. Where new rooms were to be formed, niches were to be made at the door to allow familiar items to be placed there to aid patients to recognize their own bedroom. As with the carpet insets within the day spaces, tongues of contrasting colour floor finish from within the bedrooms were continued out to mark the doorways along the length of the corridor.

A clear and secure entrance

The scheme proposed forming a new entrance to the ward to provide a front door for visitors, patients, and staff, separate from the house and back-up services. An existing fire-escape lobby between Balmore Ward and the adjacent Banff Ward provided both the space and the potential to form this new entrance.

Existing entrances to the wards are not manned or supervised, with any security between the ward spaces and outside being provided by baffle locks and alarmed doors. They are also difficult for visitors to find and to orientate themselves, and provide no particular control over who is accessing the ward.

The new entrance is designed to create an obvious, brightly coloured, and clearly lit and signposted front door. The ramped approach leads to a video-controlled entry buzzer allowing staff within the day room at the heart of the ward to monitor access. The doors lead into a new lobby with information and leaflets for visitors, and then on to a new-visits area at the start of the ward. The controlled access allows staff the chance to meet visitors at the entrance, rather than finding them wandering through the ward looking for their relative. The new-visits area has two functions: first, it provides a discrete seating area where staff may talk with visitors, or where visitors may bring their relatives to have some

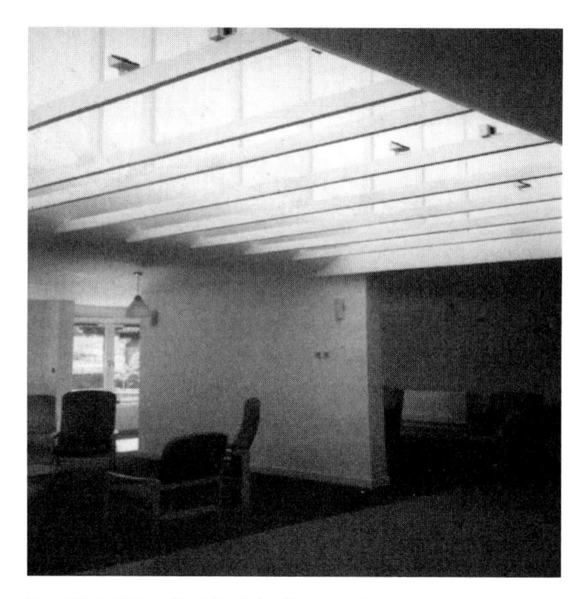

Fig. 22.16(b) Finished daylit new day space.

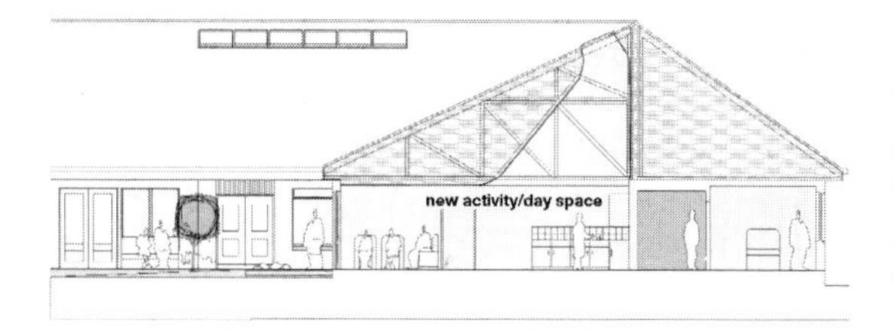

Fig. 22.16(a) Sketch of the daylit new day space.

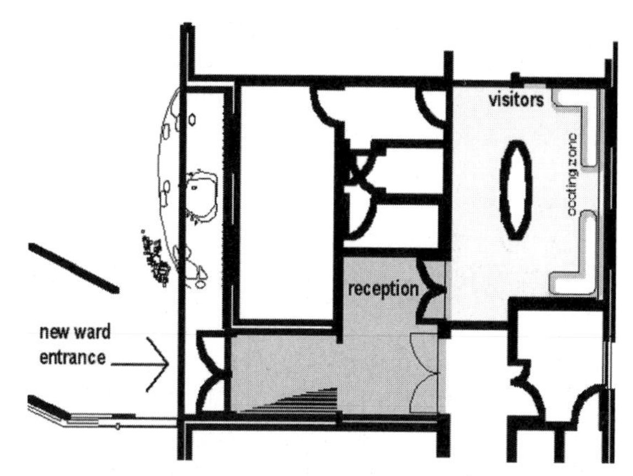

Fig. 22.17(a) Plan of the new entrance.

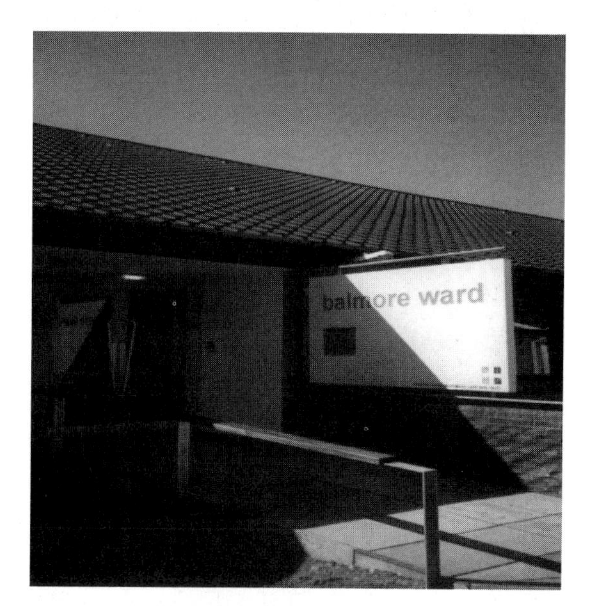

Fig. 22.17(b) Finished new entrance.

privacy from other patients; second, the new space provides a destination at the end of the main corridor for wandering patients, and like the new day room at the opposite end has its eventual entrance/escape doors tucked discreetly to one side. The area was created within the ward by the demolition of two existing rooms that were unused, and it has a new assisted toilet next to it to provide for patients if they are sitting in this area. Whilst the area is partially screened and separated from the main ward by the slatted timber back of a new bespoke seating bench, visitors are still at liberty to meet and walk with relatives throughout the rest of the ward.

A therapeutic and safe garden

The existing garden shared between the two wards was recognized by all as a greatly underused resource, with much missed therapeutic potential.

The revised scheme developed the ideas from the original layouts, to create a division within the garden to form a discrete and secure area for use by each ward. Both the reworked day room and the new day space were provided with new French doors opening out onto timber-deck terraces, continuing the timber floor surfaces of the internal spaces out into the garden. These formed safe level areas where patients could move between inside and out and sit in the fresh air and sun. Both terraces are bounded by timber balustrades to provide a secure edge and to encourage climbing plants to grow over to surround the terraces with colours, textures, and smell. A large brick planter flanks the end of the larger terrace and forms a barrier to the adjacent garden. The planter is set at a level to allow patients to sit beside it and weed and plant within the raised earth border. Paved ramps lead gently down from the two terraces to meet and form a walking route through the garden, and loop through the overall ward. Both paths lead to a large willow tree planted as a central feature of the garden, around which further borders and garden benches are arranged. The circular path around the willow is enclosed by a curving timber wall that again separates the garden from the adjacent ward and acts as a windbreak to shelter the garden. Smaller sitting areas are created throughout the garden, each with a particular surface texture, such as small paving stones or grass, and with different groupings of fragrant plants. In addition to providing an area for patients to walk in and staff to work with them on occupational therapy and physiotherapy activities, the garden also forms a secure place, both for patients managing to open the day room doors and possibly wander unattended, and as a refuge in the event of a fire.

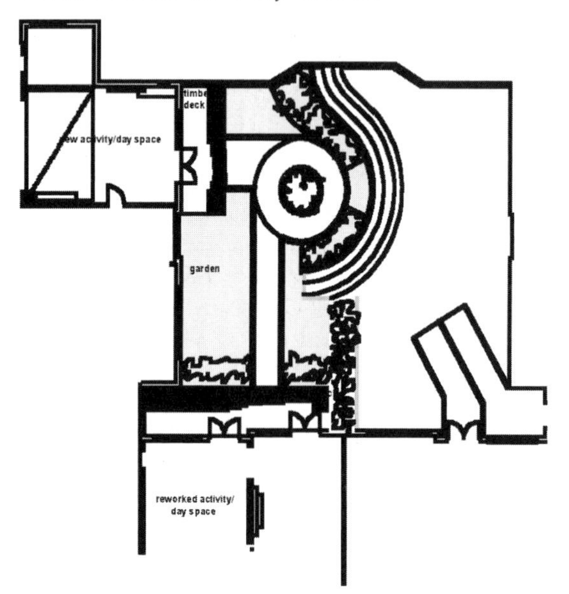

Fig. 22.18(a) Plan of the new garden.

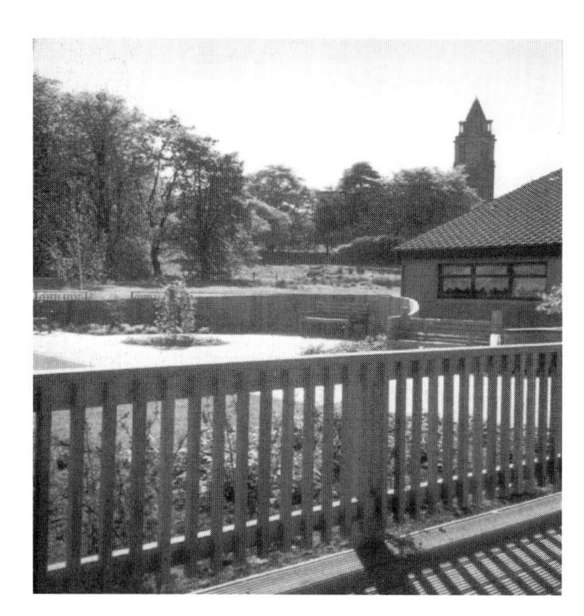

Fig. 22.18(b) Finished new garden.

Making the changes happen within a working ward

A major issue within the project was the implementation of the changes. Much debate focused around the practicalities of moving the patients from the ward to allow the contractors to carry out the work unimpeded and the negative effects on the patients, coupled with the cost of a move to another unfamiliar environment.

The Trust decided the ward should remain in operation throughout the alteration work and that the work should be phased around the daily routine of the patients and staff. The scheme was broken down into several discrete stages, allowing the contractors to work within one defined area whilst the ward continued to operate in a slightly compromised manner in the remaining spaces. Key to the carrying out of the work was the need to maintain patient safety, services, and fire security and escape throughout.

The construction work was broken down into the following stages:

1. *New day room*—one of the existing 6-bed wards was taken out of commission. A secure enclosure was formed around this with

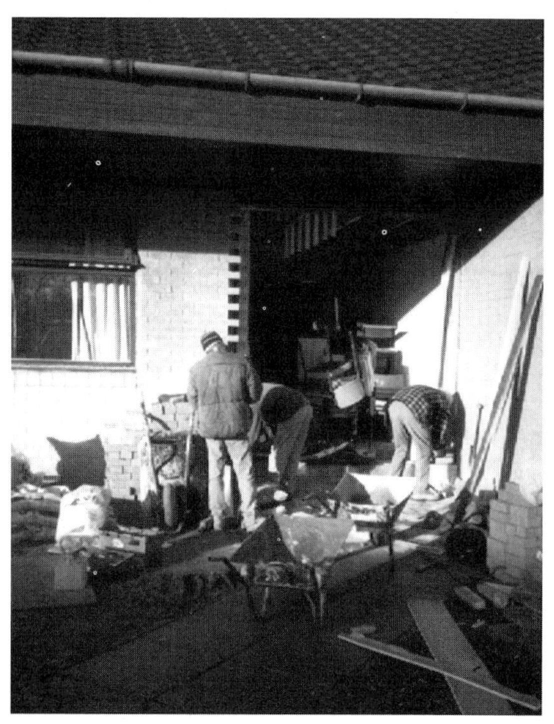

Fig. 22.19 Implementing the proposed changes.

separate access for the contractors to convert the space to the new day room. The patients and staff continued to use the existing day space during this conversion.

2. *New entrance and staff spaces*—the existing escape lobby and staff spaces, all behind the separation of existing secure doors, were reworked to create the new entrance and visits' areas as well as staff space.
3. *Existing day space*—day space use was transferred to the newly completed day space allowing the existing space to be closed off and converted.
4. *Decorations and ward conversions*—the trickiest of the phases involved the contractors working around the daily routine of patients, to fit out and redecorate the existing sleeping areas which had to remain in use throughout. Contractors were required to work within the sleeping areas during the daytime, and in the day spaces during late or evening shifts when the patients were in bed.
5. *Garden*—the reworking of the existing area to form the new garden was relatively simple as it was outside the internal areas being used by the patients and staff. The main concern in terms of phasing the garden was that the shrubs and plants should be planted during early part of the year.
6. *Fire escapes*—as the new garden forms the escape refuge from the ward, it was only possible to take the existing fire escapes out of action (they were to be removed and replaced with the French doors to the garden) once the garden area was complete and secure.

A new environment

The conversion of the ward was completed in the summer of 2000. Daylight now streams into the once dimly lit, claustrophobic spaces, and the garden is beginning to establish itself as an asset in terms of activity and views from the day spaces. The disruption caused by the connecting corridor has been subverted and hidden from the main corridor and day spaces. Patients wandering along this corridor find themselves intrigued by the active spaces they now arrive at. The new roof-lit voids in the ceilings of the day space fill these deep rooms with daylight and allow fresh air to be drawn through the spaces to remove stale odours. Patients now have the opportunity to sit in a variety of spaces, whether around the new fireplaces which have been taken over by ornaments and momentos, or away from the group in the smaller side spaces looking to the hill beyond, or at the kitchen tables next to the new kitchenette. The reworked bedrooms are now more cheerful spaces with the more thoughtful use of light colours and good-quality domestic-type fabrics. The translucent, bed-space units prevent these additional divisions from darkening the ward environment and create privacy and security for patients and their belongings.

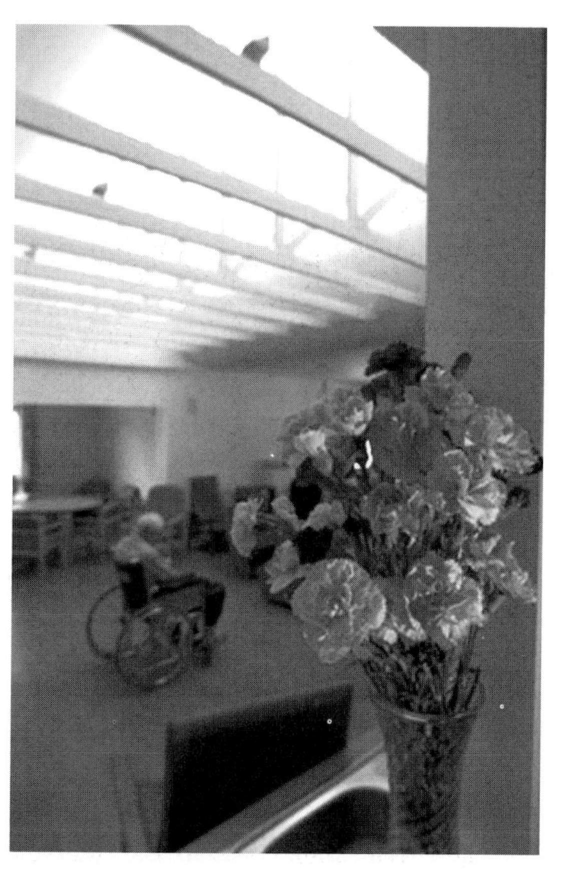

Fig. 22.20 The new day room.

Feedback and lessons

Whilst areas of the reworked ward have been in use since Christmas 1999 as their phased construction has been completed, a considered clinical assessment of the completed environment and changes has not yet been possible.

Ingrained attitudes to the provision of support services, such as catering and laundry have led to difficulty in trying out new arrangements and methods of working centred around the key issue of care. There were also clear difficulties throughout the project. In particular, the constraint of working within an operational ward led to an 8-month programme of work on site, twice the time that would have been required to carry out the works if the ward had been unoccupied. Difficulties in terms of access and working either in cordoned-off areas or around patients also led to difficulties in achieving and maintaining a consistent quality of workmanship throughout.

Despite these issues, patients, visitors, and staff are beginning to register that the changes have resulted in an improvement in the ward environment:

- The general layout and environment is appreciated as being clearer, brighter, and less institutional.
- The day rooms are now perceived as bright and attractive spaces, with patients and staff able to enjoy more views and contact with the outside.
- The two day rooms, and the subspaces within them, allow staff to take distressed or disruptive patients away from the main group of patients to allow them to calm down.
- Within the new day room, the relationship between the main space and the clearly visible toilet has helped patients' awareness and the staff's ability to monitor the space.
- The new kitchenettes within the day rooms have allowed staff and visitors to make refreshments and patients to join in these activities.
- Smells and odours have been noticeably reduced within the day areas through the increased natural ventilation offered by the new opening rooflights.
- The new visits' area is well used, allowing visitors to talk with their relatives in privacy, away from the day spaces.
- The garden is now being well used, with the separation between the garden preventing confrontations between the patients from the dementia ward and the adjacent challenging-behaviour ward. Patients and staff take walks between the day spaces and sit out on the terraces enjoying the smells and colours of the different plants and flowers.
- Whilst the provision is now in place for meals to be taken within the day spaces, staffing and operational issues are still to be agreed by the Trust to enable this to happen.

A noticeable change in patient behaviour has been an increased in activity. Initially this was seen as a cause for concern by the staff. However, with the therapeutic benefits of a stimulating environment on dementia patients, this apparent increase in patient awareness and activity is now being viewed more positively.

Appendix: key features checklist

- **Location:**

- Nature of nearby buildings (e.g. hospital, factories, supermarket, normal homes)
- Close to public transport (visitors and staff)
- Near a post office (regular access required with pension books)
- Near a school (a possible way of involving the community)
- Near a main road (safety concern)
- Near shops (for those able to use places like the betting shop, hairdresser, etc.)
- Near friends and relatives
- Near doctor's surgery

- **Site:**

- Proximity to surrounding buildings
- Size of site: how many floors? (single storey preferred but not always practicable)

- Slope (will affect access to front door layout and access to garden)
- Exposure (will affect aspect and garden)
- Outlook (many people with dementia like to watch activity of some sort from public rooms)

- **Appearance of the building:**

- Like a hotel?
- Like a house in a street?
- Like a row of houses in a street?
- Like a hospital?
- With its own special character, e.g. like a farmhouse
- Familiar to those who live there

- **Garden:**

- Potential for walking, both energetically, and strolling
- Paths which go somewhere
- Need for security, as unobtrusive as possible
- Potential for activities such as growing things, hanging out laundry, sitting in the sun, fiddling in a shed, potting nuts, etc. on a bird table, making things
- Familiar and age-appropriate
- Safe in terms of edible plants, steer people around rather than out
- Orienting
- Views from inside to outside, and vice versa
- Calming, soothing

- **Front door:**

- Like a normal front door or grand entrance?
- Cars and ambulances: access for and movement to and from
- Accessibility: ramps, steps, rails, type of door
- Deliveries
- Lobby: size, seats,
- Is the front door the same for everyone: residents, staff, visitors, deliveries
- Security: bell, knocker, locks
- Will person with dementia answer the door? (need for a camera?)

- **Hallway:**

- Purpose?
- Assists understanding of the building?
- First impression?
- Is a reception area needed?
- Formal and informal areas?

- **Link to living area(s):**

- Are there clusters of grouped, individual living spaces off the hall and, if so, what are the doors to the units intended to express?
- How can you tell what each door in the hall means?
- Does the hallway lead straight into the unit? What should this door look like? Security issues?
- Do people need to see in before they enter? Should the door/doors be glazed?
- Corridors: how can these be avoided?

- **Configuration of living units:**

- How many people in each unit?
- How many units?
- To what extent do they need to link to each other during the day?
- To what extent do they need to link to each other during the night?
- Do people need to go through one unit to get anywhere else?
- Are the same resources available in each unit?

- **Living space:**

- View from windows (to street, garden, car park, school, playground, etc.)?
- How big?
- Fireplace?
- Need for and location of telephone, television, sockets
- Methods of reducing noise levels?
- Numbers of sitting rooms; same or different purpose?
- Separate activity areas?
- Quiet areas?
- Rooms for specific purposes (library, smoking, music)?

- Number of people per sitting room?
- Opportunity to arrange furniture?
- Discrete handrails?
- Importance of access to garden?
- Wheelchair access?
- Need for conservatory?
- Flooring?
- Activity spaces/storage?
- Age-appropriate furniture?
- Toilet off each room/near each door?
- Numbers and location of electric sockets

- **Private living and sleeping space:**

- Ways of making individual doors identifiable to resident?
- Single or shared rooms?
- En-suite toilet facilities?
- Need to see toilet at night?
- Need for shower/bath/hoist?
- External access?
- Extent of window opening?
- Storage requirements?
- If wardrobe provided, how big, more than one? (can be useful to have a second locked one)
- Closed or open-fronted wardrobes/cupboards?
- Need for observation by staff? (glazed door, windows, technology linked to nurse call system, technology linked to PC and alerting staff to behaviour outside normal routine)
- Doors of rooms?
- Space for own furniture (is there to be enough space for personal bed/wardrobe/table?)
- Flooring?
- Phone/TV socket?
- Wallpaper?

- **Private space for specific purposes:**

- Bathrooms: What style of bath? Wet floor? Shower as well as bath? Need for windows in bathroom?
- Storage (does it need to be big enough for spare furniture if a resident brings their own)?
- Treatment?
- Sluice?
- Medication (type of drugs, system used, need for trolley space)?
- Staff office?
- Staff facilities?
- Visitors' room?
- Visitors' sleep-over room?

The next two items need to be considered for all spaces

- **Lighting:**

- Importance of natural light?
- Importance of each light having separate controls?
- Amount of artificial light?
- Style of lighting?
- Variety of lighting?
- External lighting/security lighting?

- **Fittings:**

- Taps: age-appropriate?
- Door handles; age-appropriate?
- Light switches: age-appropriate?
- Locks: which doors have to be locked? How? Locking schedule?
- Handrails?
- Decoration?

References

Archibald, C. (1997). *Specialist dementia units: a practice guide for staff*. Dementia Services Development Centre, Stirling.

Bennett, K. (1997). Cultural issues in designing for people with dementia. In *State of the art in dementia care* (ed. M. Marshall), pp. 164–9. Centre for Policy on Ageing, London.

Bennett, K. (2000). Designing for cultural diversity: an Australian view. In *Just another disability: making design dementia friendly, Conference Proceedings of the European Conference, 1–2 October, 1999* (ed. S. Stewart and A. Pages, pp. 70–81). Just Another Disability, Glasgow.

Calkins, M. P. (1988). *Design for dementia planning: environments for the elderly and the confused*. National Health Publishing, Owings Mills, Maryland.

Centre for Accessible Environments. (1998). *The design of residential care and nursing homes for older people*. Centre for Accessible Environments, London.

Cohen, U. and Weisman, G. D. (1991). *Holding on to home: designing environments for people with dementia*. John Hopkins University Press, Baltimore, MD.

Coons, D. H. (1991). *Specialised dementia units*. John Hopkins University Press, Baltimore, MD.

Cox, S. (1996). Quality care for the dying person with dementia. *Journal of Dementia Care*, **4**, 19–21.

Cox, S. and Keady, J. (ed.). (1999). *Younger people with dementia: planning, practice and development*. Jessica Kingsley, London.

Dementia Services Development Centre. (1998). *Towards a shared understanding: fire regulations and design for dementia Woodgrove, Aberdeen, a cast study*. Dementia Services Development Centre, Stirling.

Gresham, M. (1999). The heart of the home—but how are kitchens used? *Journal of Dementia Care*, 7, 20-23.

Judd, S., Marshall, M., and Phippen, P. (ed.). (1997). *Design for dementia*. Hawker, London.

Kerr, D. (1997). *Down's syndrome and dementia: a practitioner's guide*. Venture Press, Birmingham.

Pickles, J. (1998). *Housing for varying needs, Part 1: houses and flats*. Scottish Homes, Edinburgh.

Stewart, A. (1999). *Thinking about dementia, think about taps*. Dementia Services Development Centre, Stirling.

Van Waarde, H. (2000). Designing for dementia in The Netherlands In *Just another disability: making design dementia friendly, Conference Proceedings of the European Conference, 1–2 October 1999* (ed. S. Stewart and A. Page), 44-52. Just Another Disability, Glasgow.

IV | *Specific disorders*

23 Epidemiology of the dementias of late life

Anthony Jorm

Epidemiology is the study of the distribution of diseases in the population. It includes research describing how frequently diseases occur in the population and the effects of diseases on survival and mortality. Epidemiology also includes studies of subgroups in the population that are at a higher or lower risk of developing diseases. Such research on risk and protection factors may be used to guide preventive efforts, which are the ultimate goal of epidemiology.

A number of dementing diseases occur in later life. However, Alzheimer's disease and vascular dementias overwhelmingly predominate and have been the major focus of epidemiological investigation. For this reason, they are the sole focus of this chapter. The other common dementia of later life, dementia with Lewy bodies, is commonly reported in pathological series, but has not been investigated epidemiologically because of difficulties in its clinical identification within a community sample.

Prevalence and incidence

The prevalence rate of a disease is the number of cases in the population with the disease divided by the number of people at risk. By contrast, the incidence rate refers to the number of new cases arising in a population over a period of time, usually a year. The prevalence rate is determined by both the incidence rate and the average duration of survival after developing the disease. The distinction between prevalence and incidence can be understood using the analogy of a wheat silo, where grains of wheat are pumped in at the top and removed at the bottom. The number of grains of wheat present in the silo at any one time is analogous to the prevalence. The rate at which new grains come into the silo is like the incidence. The average time that grains stay in the silo is analogous to the duration of survival with the disease. The rate at which the grains are removed can be likened to mortality. It is apparent that the amount of wheat in the silo (prevalence) is determined by the rate of in-flow (incidence) and the average time spent in the silo (duration).

Prevalence studies are of practical value in determining service needs for a particular population, but are of less interest theoretically because they combine together incidence and disease duration. A difference between two populations in prevalence could be due to a difference in either the incidence or the duration of disease.

Studies of dementia prevalence

There are two main ways of determining the prevalence of dementia: case register studies and field surveys. Case registers identify cases in contact with services (treated prevalence). Their main limitation is that they miss cases which have not been diagnosed by a service. Some case registers are very comprehensive and include all health services in a region, whereas others are based on hospital services and are more limited in their usefulness. Field surveys involve surveying all individuals, or a random sample of individuals, in a population. While they do cover the cases not in contact with services, there are inevitably refusals. There are also limitations on the amount of clinical investigation that can be carried out, and it may be difficult to implement standard diagnostic criteria developed for clinical situations. A particular difficulty faced by field surveys is defining the boundary separating dementia from normal cognitive ageing. While dementia and normal cognitive ageing appear to be quite distinct in clinical situations, in the community there is a continuum of cognitive functioning and the boundary is a fuzzy one. There are also indefinite boundaries between different levels of severity, usually described as 'mild', 'moderate', or 'severe'. Where these boundaries are set will affect the prevalence rates obtained. For this reason, it is difficult to compare prevalence rates from different studies unless they use exactly the same methodology. Otherwise, any difference in prevalence rates may be real or due to methodological differences. For example, Erkinjuntti *et al.* (1997) examined the rates of dementia in the same sample using six different sets of diagnostic criteria. They found that the percentage with dementia varied from 3.1% using the ICD-10 criteria to 29.1% using DSM-III.

There are now a very large number of prevalence studies in the literature. Fortunately, several meta-analyses have been carried out on pooled data from a number of comparable studies, which makes it easier to summarize this literature. The first of these involved 22 studies published between 1945 and 1985 that gave age-specific prevalence rates (Jorm *et al.* 1987). This meta-analysis found that the actual prevalence rates differed greatly from study to study, but underlying all studies was a consistent trend for prevalence to increase exponentially with age. The prevalence rate for dementia was found to double with every 5.1 years of age. There was a somewhat steeper exponential rise for Alzheimer's disease (doubling every 4.5 years of age) than for vascular dementia (doubling every 5.3 years of age). The implication of these findings was that there is no single set of 'true' prevalence rates. Rather, the prevalence rates found are influenced by the methodology used in a study. However, it is possible to give a summary of age-specific prevalence rates that reflects the average across the studies. These average prevalence rates are shown in Table 23.1.

A subsequent meta-analysis pooled data from 12 European studies carried out between 1980 and 1990 (Hofman *et al.* 1991). This meta-analysis differed from the one by Jorm *et al.* (1987) in that it excluded non-European and older studies. Nevertheless, as shown in Table 23.1, the estimated prevalence rates were strikingly similar to the ones derived by Jorm *et al.* (1987). A pooling of data from more recent European studies by the same group of researchers found similar rates (Lobo *et al.* 2000).

Ritchie and Kildea (1995) carried out a meta-analysis to more precisely estimate prevalence rates at extreme ages. They included nine studies that used DSM-III criteria and included samples of people aged over 80. The rates from these studies are also shown in Table 23.1. Ritchie and Kildea fitted various curves to the data and found

Table 23.1 Prevalence rates (%) for dementia estimated from four different meta-analyses

Age group	Jorm *et al.* (1987)	Hofman *et al.* (1991)	Ritchie and Kildea (1995)	Fratiglioni *et al.* (1999)
60–64	0.7	1.0	—	—
65–69	1.4	1.4	1.5	1.5
70–74	2.8	4.1	3.5	3.0
75–79	5.6	5.7	6.8	6.0
80–84	11.1	13.0	13.6	12.0
85–89	23.6*	24.5*	22.3	—
90–94			33.0	—
95–99			44.8	—

* These rates are for ages 85+

that the rise in prevalence was not exponential over age 95, but showed some levelling off. They found that a modified logistic curve (a logistic curve is S-shaped) provided the best fit to the data. However, as the data in Table 23.1 show, the rates up to age 85 are very close to those of earlier meta-analyses.

The most recent meta-analysis, by Fratiglioni *et al.* (1999), extended the work of Hofman *et al.* (1991) by adding newer European studies as well as studies from other regions of the world. They found similar prevalence rates in various regions, apart from one African study which found much lower rates than other studies. Their summary prevalence rates are also shown in Table 23.1 and are very similar to those of earlier meta-analyses.

Prevalence rates of Alzheimer's disease

There have also been a number of meta-analyses which have focused specifically on Alzheimer's disease. In the first of these meta-analyses, Rocca *et al.* (1991) pooled data from six European studies and found rates of 0.3% at 60–69 years, 3.2% at 70–79 years, and 10.8% at 80–89 years. A pooling of rates from more recent European studies by the same group of researchers gave separate rates for men and women, with higher rates in women, as shown in Table 23.2 (Lobo *et al.* 2000).

A second meta-analysis was carried out by Corrada *et al.* (1995). These authors analysed 15 studies using a logistic model. As in the meta-analysis of dementia prevalence by Jorm *et al.* (1987), they found considerable variability between studies depending on the methodology used. However, there was a consistent underlying age trend, with the risk of developing Alzheimer's disease increasing by 18% for every year of age. Actual prevalence rates for each age were not reported.

The most recent meta-analysis was by the US General Accounting Office (1998) and involved fitting a logistic model to data from 18 studies. This analysis found that the prevalence rates doubled with every 5 years of age up to age 85 and were higher in women than men. Table 23.3 shows the prevalence rates for specific age groups for all levels of severity and for moderate-to-severe cases.

Prevalence rates of vascular dementia

Estimating the prevalence of vascular dementia presents particular problems, mainly because there is no consensus on what diagnostic criteria should be used and how they should be implemented in field surveys (Jorm 2000*a*). Historically, the classification and terminology have changed from chronic hypoperfusion, to multi-infarct dementia (due to large and small strokes), to the broader concept of vascular dementia (which incorporates other types of cerebrovascular disease associated with dementia). As well as this change in terminology over time, there are quite varied diagnostic criteria competing at each point in time. Furthermore, the existing criteria are designed primarily for use in clinical research where a wide range of investigations is possible. However, some types of investigation (e.g. brain imaging) are difficult to implement within the constraints of field studies. The greater

Table 23.2 Prevalence rates (%) for Alzheimer's disease estimated from a pooling of data from European studies by Lobo *et al.* (2000)

Age Group	Males	Females
65–69	0.6	0.7
70–74	1.5	2.3
75–79	1.8	4.3
80–84	6.3	8.4
85–89	8.8	14.2
90+	17.6	23.6

Table 23.3 Prevalence rates (%) for Alzheimer's disease estimated from a meta-analysis by the US General Accounting Office (1998)

	All severity levels		Moderate–severe cases	
Age	Males	Females	Males	Females
65	0.6	0.8	0.3	0.6
70	1.3	1.7	0.6	1.1
75	2.7	3.5	1.1	2.3
80	5.6	7.1	2.3	4.4
85	11.1	13.8	4.4	8.6
90	20.8	25.2	8.5	15.8
95	35.6	41.5	15.8	27.4

the number of clinical investigations carried out when making a diagnosis, the higher the relative prevalence of vascular dementia tends to be. For example, Rocca and Kokmen (1999) have shown that the incidence of vascular dementia by DSM-IV criteria is much higher if vascular imaging lesions are included rather than just clinically evident stroke.

Because of these difficulties, it is only possible to give quite crude estimates of prevalence. Table 23.4 shows the results from a pooling of data from nine European studies (Lobo *et al.* 2000). It can be seen that the prevalence was higher in men up to the age of 84 years, after which it was higher in women. In general, prevalence studies in Western countries find that Alzheimer's disease is more prevalent than vascular dementia, with about 50–70% of total dementia attributable to Alzheimer's disease, compared to 20–30% to vascular dementia (Fratiglioni *et al.* 1999). In East Asian countries, vascular dementia appears to be relatively more common, although more recent studies from those countries show that they are moving toward the Western pattern, with Alzheimer's accounting for 61% and vascular dementia for 31% of total dementia (Fratiglioni *et al.* 1999).

Studies of dementia incidence

Because incidence involves the onset of new cases over a period of time, incidence studies require longitudinal data. Furthermore, new cases are uncommon, so incidence studies require large samples to arrive at stable estimates for specific age groups. Because of these requirements, incidence studies are far less common than prevalence studies.

Prevalence studies face the difficulty of placing the boundary that separates dementia from normal ageing. Incidence studies face the additional problem of estimating the point of onset of a dementing disease. For a slowly progressing dementia, timing the onset will be particularly

Table 23.4 Prevalence rates (%) for vascular dementia estimated from a pooling of data from European studies by Lobo *et al.* (2000)

Age group	Males	Females
65–69	0.5	0.1
70–74	0.8	0.6
75–79	1.9	0.9
80–84	2.4	2.3
85–89	2.4	3.5
90+	3.6	5.8

difficult. In fact, rather than measure the onset of the disease, incidence studies typically measure entry to some stage of severity, such as from normal to mild dementia, or from mild to moderate dementia.

Although incidence studies are much less common than prevalence studies, the number has now cumulated to the point where meta-analyses are possible. The first of these was carried out by Jorm and Jolley (1998) and involved 23 studies. The data from these studies were pooled separately for different regions of the world and for males and females. The incidence rate for both dementia and Alzheimer's disease was found to rise exponentially with age up to age 90, after which there was insufficient data to draw any firm conclusions. There was no sex difference in overall dementia incidence, but females tended to have a higher incidence of Alzheimer's disease at the older ages. East Asian countries had a lower incidence of dementia than European countries and also tended to have a lower incidence of Alzheimer's disease. Tables 23.5 and 23.6 show the results. Data were also analysed on vascular dementia. Although the rates were found to be highly variable from study to study, the underlying trend was for an exponential rise with age up to 90 years. Males were found to have a higher incidence at younger ages, but females tended to catch up at older ages. The higher incidence in males at younger ages may reflect the effects of smoking, with only non-smokers surviving to very old age.

The second meta-analysis was carried out by Gao *et al.* (1998) at the same time as the first, but involved only the 12 studies that used DSM-III or -III-R criteria for dementia and NINCDS-ADRDA criteria for Alzheimer's disease. These authors found that the rise in incidence with age was not exponential, with some slowing of the rate of increase at older ages. Tables 23.5 and 23.6 show their findings for dementia and Alzheimer's disease, respectively. The differences between the two meta-analyses probably occurred because Gao *et al.* (1998) pooled data for different levels of severity and different regions of the world, while Jorm and Jolley (1998) separated them. It can be seen from the tables that the rates obtained by Gao *et al.* (1998) fall in between the rates of Jorm and Jolley (1998) for mild+ and moderate+ dementia. The apparent levelling in incidence may have occurred because of the way in which different levels of severity were mixed in various age groups.

More recently, Fratiglioni *et al.* (2000) pooled incidence data from eight European studies which used the same diagnostic criteria. Table 23.7 shows the results for men and women combined for dementia, Alzheimer's disease, and vascular dementia. An analysis by sex showed that there was little sex difference up to age 80, but a higher incidence in women in very old age. For Alzheimer's disease, the incidence in women was

Table 23.5 Incidence rates (%) for dementia from two meta-analyses

Age group	Europe[a] mild+	Europe[a] moderate+	USA[a] moderate+	East Asia[a] mild+	All cases[b]
55–59	—	—	—	—	0.03
60–64	—	—	—	—	0.11
65–69	0.91	0.36	0.24	0.35	0.33
70–74	1.76	0.64	0.50	0.71	0.84
75–79	3.33	1.17	1.05	1.47	1.82
80–84	5.99	2.15	1.77	3.26	3.36
85–89	10.41	3.77	2.75	7.21	5.33
90–94	17.98	6.61	—	—	7.29
95+	—	—	—	—	8.68

[a]Jorm and Jolley 1998.
[b]Gao *et al.* 1998.

Table 23.6 Incidence rates (%) for Alzheimer's disease from two meta-analyses

Age group	Europe[a] mild+	Europe[a] moderate+	USA[a] mild+	USA[a] moderate+	East Asia[a] mild+	All cases[b]
60–64	—	—	—	—	—	0.06
65–69	0.25	0.10	0.61	0.16	0.07	0.19
70–74	0.52	0.22	1.11	0.35	0.21	0.51
75–79	1.07	0.48	2.01	0.78	0.58	1.17
80–84	2.21	1.06	3.84	1.48	1.49	2.31
85–89	4.61	2.26	7.45	2.60	3.97	3.86
90–94	9.66	4.77	—	—	—	5.49
95+	—	—	—	—	—	6.68

[a]Jorm and Jolley 1998.
[b]Gao *et al.* 1998.

Table 23.7 Incidence rates (%) for dementia, Alzheimer's disease, and vascular dementia in Europe

Age group	Dementia	Alzheimer's disease	Vascular dementia
65–69	0.24	0.12	0.07
70–74	0.55	0.33	0.12
75–79	1.60	0.91	0.35
80–84	3.05	2.18	0.59
85–89	4.86	3.53	0.61
90+	7.02	5.35	0.81

Based on data from Fratiglioni *et al.* 2000.

higher and increased more steeply with age. For vascular dementia, the variation in incidence rates between studies was too large, and the number of cases was too small, to analyse sex differences reliably.

Survival in dementia

Survival after the onset of dementia provides the link between incidence and prevalence. Prevalence will increase if incident (new) cases survive longer. Surprisingly, there is not much data available on the survival of incident cases from population surveys. One study, based on the Rochester (USA) case register, showed that after 5 years the survival of incident cases was 49% compared to an expected figure of 64% for people of the same age and sex; after 10 years, the figures were 16% and 37%, respectively (Schoenberg *et al.* 1981). It is thus clear that dementia reduces survival.

As important as the effect of dementia on survival, is its effect on disability in the population. The Global Burden of Disease study (Murray and Lopez 1996) has focused attention on the importance of disability by quantifying health in terms of disability-adjusted life years (DALYs). This measure combines information on premature death and years lived with disability. A DALY is calculated as the sum of the years of life lost due to premature mortality (YLL) in the population and the years lost due to disability (YLD) for incident cases of the health condition: DALY = YLL + YLD. A Dutch study has shown that from age 55 onwards, men lose an average of 1.2 DALYs from dementia (0.7 years due to mortality + 0.5 due to disability), while women lose 3.1 DALYs (1.9 due to mortality + 1.2 due to disability) (Witthaus *et al.* 1999). A study of the burden of disease in Australia found that dementia accounted for 3.5% of total DALYs in the population and was the sixth most important disease group in terms of burden, being exceeded only by heart disease, stroke, chronic obstructive airways disease, depression, and lung cancer (Mathers *et al.* 2000).

Risk factors for Alzheimer's disease

There are two basic methods of ascertaining risk factors: the cohort or prospective study, and the case-control study. Cohort studies start with a population sample, some members of which have been exposed to a potential risk factor and some not. This sample is followed over time to assess the incidence of the disease in exposed and non-exposed groups. Case-control studies work backwards, by identifying new cases of the disease and comparing them to controls from the same population in terms of exposure to potential risk factors. Cohort studies are considered superior to case-control studies, but are more expensive and time consuming to carry out. Early research on risk factors for Alzheimer's disease relied on case-control studies, but many cohort studies have now become available.

Genetic causes of Alzheimer's disease

There are a number of rare genetic mutations which are known to cause Alzheimer's disease. These mutations affect the amyloid precursor protein gene on chromosome 21 and the presenilin-1 and -2 genes on chromosomes 14 and 1. While of great theoretical importance for an understanding of disease mechanisms, these mutations are less important from a public health perspective since they account for very few cases. Most cases of Alzheimer's disease are thought to have complex causation, involving multiple genetic and environmental factors.

Confirmed risk factors

Only four risk factors for Alzheimer's disease have been confirmed beyond reasonable doubt:

Age

The review of incidence studies above indicated that the incidence of Alzheimer's increases exponentially with age. However, there is controversy about whether the exponential rise continues into extreme old age or whether there is some levelling off.

Family history of dementia.

A meta-analysis of risk factor studies found that first-degree relatives of people with Alzheimer's disease have around 3.5 times the population risk of developing the disorder themselves (van Duijn *et al.* 1991). Family history is a stronger risk factor in cases of early-onset Alzheimer's disease than in late-onset cases. The highest risk occurs in families with rare autosomal dominant mutations. However, the actual percentage risk to a relative of a family member with Alzheimer's disease depends on how long that person lives. Someone with a family history of Alzheimer's disease who only lives to age 50 may have a lower risk than someone with no family history who lives to 100. According to one study, the risk to a first-degree relative is only 1% up to age 60, rising to 5% up to age 70, 16% up to age 80, and 33% up to age 90 (Lautenschlager *et al.* 1996).

APOE genotype

Apolipoprotein E (ApoE) is a plasma protein involved in cholesterol transport and may also have a role in neuronal repair. The *APOE* gene has a polymorphism which affects the risk for Alzheimer's disease. This polymorphism involves three alleles ($\varepsilon 2$, $\varepsilon 3$, and $\varepsilon 4$), with $\varepsilon 3$ being the most common. The $\varepsilon 4$ allele is known to increase the risk for Alzheimer's, while the $\varepsilon 2$ allele decreases risk. The $\varepsilon 4$ allele is unlike the disease-causing mutations discussed above, in that it is not sufficient to produce Alzheimer's disease. A meta-analysis found that, in Caucasians, the $\varepsilon 4/\varepsilon 4$

genotype was associated with 15 times the risk compared to the common *ε3/ε3* genotype, while the *ε3/ε4* genotype was associated with three times the risk (Farrer *et al.* 1997). Having an *ε2/ε2* or *ε2/ε3* genotype reduced the risk by 40%. Although the *APOE* genotype is a risk factor in all ethnic groups examined, the strength of the association appears to be weaker in people of African ancestry. Using data largely from Caucasian samples, it has been estimated that that 60% of Alzheimer's cases over the age of 65 would be avoided if the whole population had the lowest risk APOE genotype (Rubinsztein and Easton 1999).

Down's syndrome

By the age of 40 virtually all people with Down's syndrome have the neuropathological changes of Alzheimer's disease. These early changes are due to having an extra copy of the Aβ precursor protein gene which is on chromosome 21. However, the prevalence of dementia in Down's syndrome is much less than 100%, even by the age of 50 (Zigman *et al.* 1996). The discrepancy between the neuropathology and the clinical picture is not understood. One theory is that clinical dementia is associated with the transition from diffuse to neuritic plaques, and this usually occurs around 50 to 55 years of age in people with Down's syndrome (Schupf 2000).

Possible risk and protection factors

There are also a large number of possible risk and protection factors, which have some evidence to support them but which is not entirely consistent. Only a selection of these possible risk factors are reviewed here.

Other genetic risk factors

Many other candidate polymorphisms have been examined in the hope of finding a risk factor similar to *APOEε4*. One such candidate is the alpha-2 macroglobulin gene which is involved in the clearance of Aβ, one of the neuropathological changes in Alzheimer's disease. While some studies found that a deletion in this gene increased risk (Blacker *et al.* 1998), this association has not been consistently replicated. Another polymorphism which has excited considerable interest involves the regulatory region of the *APOE* gene. This polymorphism has been reported to have an association with Alzheimer's disease independent of *APOEε4* (Bullido *et al.* 1998), but again the effect has not been consistently replicated.

Neurocognitive reserve

A number of studies have found that people with a low level of education have a higher incidence of dementia or Alzheimer's disease, although other studies are negative (Katzman 1993). The association appears to be stronger in populations where there is a high rate of illiteracy or very low levels of education. A possible explanation for these findings is that better educated persons are able to compensate for early cognitive deficits and so the threshold for recognition of dementia is reached at a later stage (Mortimer 1988). Indeed there is some evidence that highly educated persons with dementia have greater brain impairment than would be expected for their level of clinical severity (Stern *et al.* 1992).

Education is related to intelligence and there are other studies indicating that intelligence rather than education is the important factor (e.g. Schmand *et al.* 1997). There is also evidence that demented people with higher premorbid intelligence show greater compensation for cognitive losses (Alexander *et al.* 1997). While the notion that intelligence works via compensation for pathology is widely accepted, this has been challenged by the results of the Nun Study which found a direct association with pathology (Snowdon *et al.* 1996). This study assessed the verbal ability of a group of elderly nuns by analysing the autobiographies they had written as young adults. The autobiographies were analysed for density of ideas and grammatical complexity. Nuns in the study donated their brains for a pathological diagnosis of Alzheimer's disease. Surprisingly, it was found that low verbal ability early in life was associated with greater Alzheimer pathology. Among the nuns who had died while in the study, all those with confirmed Alzheimer's disease had low verbal ability, compared to none of those without Alzheimer's.

Brain reserve is another factor related to intelligence. In normal adults, total brain volume is correlated with IQ scores (Rushton and Ankey 1996). There is also evidence that people with bigger brains have a reduced risk for developing dementia and that they can compensate for Alzheimer pathology (Katzman *et al.* 1988; Schofield 1999). The inter-related data on the protective effects of education, premorbid intelligence, and brain size support the general notion that neurocognitive reserve may provide a protective effect for Alzheimer's and other dementias.

Medical history

It has been found that Aβ can be deposited extensively in the brain following severe head injury, supporting a role for head trauma as a risk factor (Roberts *et al.* 1991). A meta-analysis of early case-control studies found that a history of head trauma with loss of consciousness was 80% more common in Alzheimer's disease cases than in normal controls (Mortimer *et al.* 1991). Head trauma in the 10 years before the onset of dementia was found to be more important as a risk factor than head trauma earlier in life. A weakness of these studies is that a history of head trauma was ascertained by reports of relatives rather than from medical records. It is possible that relatives of people with dementia had a biased recall of such incidents. Prospective studies which have assessed history of head trauma before the onset of dementia, and studies which have used medical records to ascertain head trauma, have generally not found an association with Alzheimer's disease (Breteler *et al.* 1995; Launer *et al.* 1999), although there are some exceptions (Schofield *et al.* 1997).

A meta-analysis of early case-control studies found that a history of depression is a risk factor for Alzheimer's disease (Jorm *et al.* 1991). Studies since that time have had mixed results. However, a more recent meta-analysis has confirmed the association, with a history of depression approximately doubling the risk of Alzheimer's disease and dementia in general (Jorm 2000*b*). There are various hypotheses to explain the association, including depression being a reaction to very early cognitive decline, depression causing subtle cognitive impairments which push the person closer to the threshold for manifesting dementia, and chronic stress leading to hippocampal damage (Jorm 2000*b*).

Medical treatments

Cellular and animal studies suggest that oestrogen may have a beneficial effect on the ageing brain by affecting the metabolism of Aβ, promoting the activity of the cholinergic system, and reducing oxidative stress (Skoog and Gustafson 1999). There is also some epidemiological evidence suggesting that oestrogen replacement therapy in postmenopausal women may have a protective effect against Alzheimer's disease. A meta-analysis of case-control and cohort studies found that oestrogen reduced the risk of Alzheimer's disease by around 30% (Yaffe *et al.* 1998). A limitation of this evidence is that better educated women are more likely to take oestrogen and, as discussed above, education may have a protective effect. Randomized trials of oestrogen replacement therapy provide the best evidence on whether there is a protective effect. A recent trial of oestrogen replacement as a treatment for mild to moderate Alzheimer's disease showed no effect on disease progression (Mulnard *et al.* 2000). However, this is not to say that oestrogen replacement might not have a preventive effect. Currently in the United States, the Women's Health Initiative Memory Study is looking at the effects of oestrogen replacement therapy on the incidence of dementia in over 8000 women (Shumaker *et al.* 1998).

It has been hypothesized that Alzheimer's disease involves a chronic inflammatory state of the brain (McGeer *et al.* 1996). This hypothesis leads to the prediction that individuals taking anti-inflammatory drugs, or having diseases like arthritis which are treated with such drugs, would be protected from Alzheimer's disease. Although the evidence is inconsistent, a meta-analysis of studies on the topic found support for this prediction. Pooled data from case-control studies indicated that arthritis, non-steroidal anti-inflammatory drugs (NSAIDs), and steroids are associated with around half the risk of developing Alzheimer's disease (McGeer *et al.* 1996). Again, randomized controlled trials are needed to convincingly show a protective effect, but the side-effects of these drugs make such trials difficult.

Occupational hazards

The search for occupational hazards associated with Alzheimer's disease has been largely negative, with the exception of work showing a possible association with exposure to electromagnetic fields. Sobel and Davanipour (1996) have hypothesized that electromagnetic fields may upset intracellular calcium homeostasis which may promote the cleavage of Aβ precursor protein into Aβ. They have carried out a series of four case-control studies, which showed that occupations involving high exposure to electromagnetic fields through working with electric motors have around three times the risk of Alzheimer's disease (Sobel *et al.* 1996). However, other studies have not consistently supported this association (Feychting *et al.* 1998; Savitz *et al.* 1998). Future studies need to directly examine exposure to electromagnetic fields rather than inferring such exposure from type of occupation.

Diet

There has been a long scientific interest in aluminium in the water supply as a factor in the development of Alzheimer's disease. As well as naturally occurring aluminium in water, aluminium is added as a flocculent during water treatment. Although aluminium in drinking water supplies only represents around 2.5% of dietary aluminium, it has been hypothesized that this is in a soluble form which has greater bioavailabilty than other dietary aluminium. There is rather mixed evidence from epidemiological studies of aluminium in water as a risk factor for Alzheimer's disease. Some of the early studies reporting an association had poor methodology, identifying Alzheimer's disease via death certificates or other indirect means. However, some more recent studies which are better designed also find an association (e.g. Rondeau *et al.* 2000). Although the accumulated evidence is far from convincing, it is prudent to keep the aluminium content of water as low as practicable (Douglas 1998).

It has been hypothesized that oxidative stress could cause neuronal loss in Alzheimer's disease and that antioxidants are therefore neuroprotective (Behl 1999). Most studies of antioxidants as a protective factor in Alzheimer's disease have used case-control designs, so the results are ambiguous as to whether antioxidant use or intake is a cause or effect of dementia. However, there have also been a small number of prospective studies. Use of vitamin C supplements has been reported to be associated with protection against Alzheimer's disease (Morris *et al.* 1998) and cognitive impairment (Paleologos *et al.* 1998). By contrast, a study of dietary intake of vitamin C found a non-significant trend towards greater cognitive decline (Kalmijn *et al.* 1997). Prospective studies of vitamin E have been largely negative (Kalmijn *et al.* 1997; Perrig *et al.* 1997), although one found a trend towards protection (Morris *et al.* 1998). Randomized controlled trials will provide the ultimate test of whether antioxidants are neuroprotective.

Risk factors for vascular dementia

Risk factors for vascular dementia have received far less attention than risk factors for Alzheimer's disease. The study of risk factors is complicated because there are several different types of vascular dementia, each of which is difficult to diagnose. Furthermore, a number of studies have indicated that vascular risk factors may play a role in Alzheimer's disease (Skoog 2000). The reasons for this association are still unclear.

The most common forms of vascular dementia are multi-infarct dementia, which is due to strokes, and dementia associated with ischaemic white matter lesions. Hospital-based studies show that dementia is a relatively common outcome after stroke, so risk factors for stroke can also be presumed to be risk factors for vascular dementia (Schmidt *et al.* 2000). A review of the evidence on risk factors for dementia associated with stroke concluded that old age is the only confirmed risk factor (Gorelick 1997). However, there is evidence for several other putative risk factors, i.e. race/ethnic group (Orientals, African-Americans), low education, hypertension, cigarette smoking, myocardial infarction, diabetes mellitus, hypercholesterolaemia, and various factors related to the nature and extent of cerebrovascular disease. However, the interesting question becomes whether there are risk factors for dementia following stroke that are independent of those for stroke *per se*. According to an analysis of three studies on this issue, the only factors conferring additional risk were age, non-White race, and diabetes mellitus, suggesting that most of the risk factors are shared with stroke (Schmidt *et al.* 2000). The main risk factor for the ischaemic white matter form of vascular dementia is hypertension (Skoog 1994).

Implications of epidemiological research for prevention

Prevention is often thought of in terms of elimination of disease over an individual's lifespan, as for infectious diseases. However, for chronic diseases of ageing, postponement of disease until later in the lifespan becomes the more feasible goal. Postponement results in more disability-free life years and may also mean that the individual dies before onset would have taken place. It has been estimated that even a delay of one year could produce a large reduction in the number of dementia cases in a population (Brookmeyer *et al.* 1998).

Ideally, prevention would be based on removing the cause or interfering with the pathological mechanism of a disease. For example, fundamental research on Alzheimer's disease might eventually lead to ways of interfering with the cleavage of the Aβ precursor protein into Aβ or with the phosphorylation of tau protein into neurofibrillary tangles. However, even without this understanding, prevention may be possible by modifying risk and protection factors. This is a strategy which has been successful in preventing a number of other major diseases, such as coronary heart disease, lung cancer, and skin cancer. Prevention via risk-factor modification can be aimed at changing exposure in the whole population (such as education campaigns on sun exposure as a risk factor for skin cancer) or targeted specifically at high-risk groups (for example, use of low-dose aspirin to prevent heart attacks and stroke).

With Alzheimer's disease, genetic factors are clearly of great importance, but environmental factors also play some role. Currently, the greatest interest is in the possible protection factors of, for example, anti-inflammatory drugs and oestrogen replacement therapy. Controlled trials will be necessary to confirm whether anti-inflammatory drugs and oestrogen replacement therapy have a protective effect. Any preventive effect on Alzheimer's disease will have to be balanced against the side-effects of these drugs.

Vascular dementia presents the greatest scope for prevention because there are a number of modifiable risk factors, the most important of which is hypertension. Indeed, there is one large-scale controlled trial of antihypertensive drug treatment which indicates the potential for preventing dementia (Forette *et al.* 1998). The Systolic Hypertension in Europe (Syst-Eur) Trial found that antihypertensive medication reduced stroke incidence and had some effect on dementia, with a reduction in incidence of approximately 50% over a 2-year period. Since there were few cases of vascular dementia, most of the effect was due to a lower incidence of Alzheimer's disease. Other preventive trials are ongoing.

While prevention of disease is often a planned activity, there can be major social changes that affect disease incidence in an unplanned way. Of particular interest for dementia are the large rises in levels of education and IQ which are known to have occurred over the past half century in developed countries (Neisser 1997). If neurocognitive reserve is confirmed to protect against the early clinical manifestation of dementia, then these social changes may have important unintended benefits.

References

Alexander, G. E., Furey, M. L., Grady, C. L., Pietrini, P., Brady, D. R., Mentis, M. J. *et al.* (1997). Association of premorbid intellectual function with cerebral metabolism in Alzheimer's disease: implications for the cognitive reserve hypothesis. *American Journal of Psychiatry*, **154**, 165–72.

Behl, C. (1999). Alzheimer's disease and oxidative stress: implications for novel therapeutic approaches. *Progress in Neurobiology*, **57**, 301–23.

Blacker, D., Wilcox, M. A., Laird, N. M., Rodes, L., Horvath, S. M., Go, R. C., *et al.* (1998). Alpha-2 macroglobulin is genetically associated with Alzheimer disease. *Nature Genetics*, **19**, 357–60.

Breteler, M. B. B., de Groot, R. R. M., van Romunde, L. K. J., and Hofman, A. (1995). Risk of dementia in patients with Parkinson's disease, epilepsy, and severe head trauma: a register-based follow-up study. *American Journal of Epidemiology*, **142**, 1300–5.

Brookmeyer, R., Gray, S., and Kawas, C. (1998). Projections of Alzheimer's disease in the United States and the public health impact of delaying disease onset. *American Journal of Public Health*, **88**, 1337–42.

Bullido, M. J., Artiga, M. J., Recuero, M., Sastre, I., Garcia, M. A., Aldudo, J., *et al.* (1998). A polymorphism in the regulatory region of APOE associated with risk for Alzheimer's dementia. *Nature Genetics*, **18**, 69–71.

Corrada, M., Brookmeyer, R., and Kawas, C. (1995). Sources of variability in prevalence rates of Alzheimer's disease. *International Journal of Epidemiology*, **24**, 1000–5.

Douglas, R. (1998). Alzheimer's disease, drinking water and aluminium content. *Australasian Journal on Ageing*, **17**, 2–3.

Erkinjuntti, T., Østbye, T., Steenhuis, R., and Hachinski, V. (1997). The effect of different diagnostic criteria on the prevalence of dementia. *New England Journal of Medicine*, **337**, 1667–74.

Farrer, L. A., Cupples, L. A., Haines, J. L., Hyman, B., Kukull, W. A., Mayeux, R., *et al.* (1997). Effects of age, sex, and ethnicity on the association between Apolipoprotein E genotype and Alzheimer disease. *Journal of the American Medical Association*, **278**, 1349–56.

Feychting, M., Pedersen, N. L., Svedberg, P., Floderus, B., and Gatz, M. (1998). Dementia and occupational exposure to magnetic fields. *Scandinavian Journal of Work Environment and Health*, **24**, 46–53.

Forette, F., Seux, M-L., Staessen, J. A. Thijs, L., Birkenhager, W. H., Babarskiene, M.-R., *et al.* (1998). Prevention of dementia in randomised double-blind placebo-controlled Systolic Hypertension in Europe (Syst-Eur) trial. *Lancet*, **352**, 1347–51.

Fratiglioni, L., De Ronchi, D., and Aguero-Torres, H. (1999). Worldwide prevalence and incidence of dementia. *Drugs and Aging*, **15**, 365–75.

Fratiglioni, L., Launer, L. J., Andersen, K., Breteler, M. M. B., Copeland, J. R. M., Dartigues, J.-F., *et al.* (2000). Incidence of dementia and major subtypes in Europe: a collaborative study of population-based cohorts. *Neurology*, **54** (Suppl. 5), S10–S15.

Gao, S., Hendrie, H. C., Hall, K. S., and Hui, S. (1998). The relationships between age, sex, and the incidence of dementia and Alzheimer disease: a meta-analysis. *Archives of General Psychiatry*, **55**, 809–15.

Gorelick, P. B. (1997). Status of risk factors for dementia associated with stroke. *Stroke*, **28**, 459–63.

Hofman A., Rocca W. A., Brayne C., Breteler M. M. B., Clarke M., Cooper B., *et al.* (1991). The prevalence of dementia in Europe: a collaborative study of 1980–1990 findings. *International Journal of Epidemiology*, **20**, 736–48.

Jorm, A. F. (2000*a*). The epidemiology of vascular dementia: an overview and commentary. In *Cerebrovascular disease and dementia: pathology, neuropsychiatry and management* (ed. E. Chiu, L. Gustafson, D. Ames, and M. F. Folstein), pp. 63–7. Martin Dunitz, London.

Jorm, A. F. (2000*b*). Is depression a risk factor for dementia or cognitive decline? A review. *Gerontology*, **46**, 219–27.

Jorm, A. F. and Jolley, D. (1998). The incidence of dementia: a meta-analysis. *Neurology*, **51**, 728–33.

Jorm, A. F., Korten A., and Henderson A. S. (1987). The prevalence of dementia: a quantitative integration of the literature. *Acta Psychiatrica Scandinavica*, **76**, 465–79.

Jorm, A. F., van Duijin, C. M., Chandra, V., Fratiglioni, I., Graves, A., Heyman, A., *et al.* (1991). Psychiatric history and related exposures as risk factors for Alzheimer's disease: a collaborative re-analysis of case-control studies. *International Journal of Epidemiology*, **20**, S43–S47.

Kalmijn, S., Feskens, E. J. M., Launer, L. J., and Kromhout, D. (1997). Polyunsaturated fatty acids, antioxidants, and cognitive function in very old men. *American Journal of Epidemiology*, **145**, 33–41.

Katzman, R. (1993). Education and the prevalence of dementia and Alzheimer's disease. *Neurology*, **43**, 13–20.

Katzman, R., Terry, R., DeTeresa, R., Brown, T., Davies, P., Fuld, P., *et al.* (1988). Clinical, pathological, and neurochemical changes in dementia: a subgroup with preserved mental status and numerous neocortical plaques. *Annals of Neurology*, **23**, 138–44.

Launer, L. J., Andersen, K., Dewey, M. E., Letenneur, L., Ott, A., Amaducci, L. A., *et al.* (1999). Rates and risk factors for dementia and Alzheimer's disease: results from EURODEM pooled analyses. *Neurology*, **52**, 78–84.

Lautenschlager, N. T., Cupples, L. A., Rao, V. S., Auerbach, S. A., Becker, R., Burke, J., *et al.* (1996). Risk of dementia among relatives of Alzheimer's disease patients in the MIRAGE study: what is in store for the oldest old? *Neurology*, **46**, 641–50.

Lobo, A., Launer, L. J., Fratiglioni, L., Andersen, K., Di Carlo, A., Breteler, M. M. B., *et al.* (2000). Prevalence of dementia and major subtypes in Europe: a collaborative study of population-based cohorts. *Neurology*, **54** (Suppl. 5), S4–S9.

McGeer, P. L., Schulzer, M., and McGeer, E. G. (1996). Arthritis and anti-inflammatory agents as possible protective factors for Alzheimer's disease: a review of 17 epidemiologic studies. *Neurology*, **47**, 425–32.

Mathers, C. D., Vos, E. T., Stevenson, C. E., and Begg, S. J. (2000). The Australian Burden of Disease Study: measuring the loss of health from diseases, injuries and risk factors. *Medical Journal of Australia*, **172**, 592–6.

Morris, M. C., Beckett, L. A., Scherr, P. A., Hebert, L. E., Bennet, D. A., Field, T. S. *et al.* (1998). Vitamin E and vitamin C supplement use and risk of incident Alzheimer disease. *Alzheimer Disease and Associated Disorders,* **12**, 121–6.

Mortimer, J. A. (1988). Do psychosocial risk factors contribute to Alzheimer's disease? In *Etiology of dementia of Alzheimer's type* (ed. A. S. Henderson and J. H. Henderson), pp. 39–52. Wiley, Chichester.

Mortimer, J. A., Van Duijn, C. M., Chandra, V., Fratiglioni, L., Graves, A. B., Heyman, A., *et al.* (1991). Head trauma as a risk factor for Alzheimer's disease: a collaborative re-analysis of case-control studies. *International Journal of Epidemiology*, **20**, S28–S35.

Mulnard, R. A., Cotman, C. W., Kawas, C., van Dyck, C. H., Sano, M., Doody, R., *et al.* (2000). Estrogen replacement therapy for treatment of mild to moderate Alzheimer disease: a randomized controlled trial. *Journal of the American Medical Association*, **283**, 1007–15.

Murray, C. J. and Lopez, A. D. (1996). *The global burden of disease. A comprehensive assessment of mortality and disability from diseases, injuries, and risk factors in 1990 and projected to 2020. Global burden of disease and injury,* Vol. 1. Harvard School of Public Health, Boston.

Neisser, U. (1997). Rising scores on intelligence tests. *American Scientist,* **85**, 440–7.

Paleologos, M., Cumming, R. G., and Lazarus, R. (1998). Cohort study of vitamin C intake and cognitive impairment. *American Journal of Epidemiology*, **148**, 45–50.

Perrig, W. J., Perrig, P., and Stähelin, H. B. (1997). The relation between antioxidants and memory performance in the old and very old. *Journal of the American Geriatrics Society,* **45**, 718–24.

Ritchie, K. and Kildea, D. (1995). Is senile dementia 'age-related' or 'ageing-related'?— evidence from meta-analysis of dementia prevalence in the oldest old. *Lancet*, **346**, 931–4.

Roberts, G. W., Gentlemen, S. M., Lynch, A., and Graham, D. I. (1991). βA4 amyloid protein deposition in brain after head trauma. *Lancet*, **338**, 1422–3.

Rocca, W. A. and Kokmen, E. (1999). Frequency and distribution of vascular dementia. *Alzheimer Disease and Associated Disorders*, **13**(Suppl. 3), S9–S14.

Rocca, W. A., Hofman, A., Brayne, C., Breteler, M. M. B., Clarke, M., Copeland, J. R. M., *et al.* (1991). Frequency and distribution of Alzheimer's disease in Europe: a collaborative study of 1980–1990 prevalence findings. *Annals of Neurology*, **30**, 381–90.

Rondeau, V., Commenges, D., Jacqmin-Gadda, H., and Dartigues, J.-F. (2000). Relation between aluminium concentration in drinking water and Alzheimer's disease: an 8-year follow-up. *American Journal of Epidemiology*, **152**, 59–66.

Rubinsztein, D. C. and Easton, D. F. (1999). Apolipoprotein E genetic variation and Alzheimer's disease. *Dementia and Geriatric Cognitive Disorders*, **10**, 199–209.

Rushton, J. P. and Ankey, C. D. (1996). Brain size and cognitive ability: correlations with age, sex, social class, and race. *Psychonomic Bulletin and Review*, **3**, 21–36.

Savitz, D. A., Checkoway, H., and Loomis, D. P. (1998). Magnetic field exposure and neurodegenerative disease mortality among electric utility workers. *Epidemiology,* **9**, 398–404.

Schmand, B., Smit, J. H., Geerlings, M. I., and Lindeboom, J. (1997). The effects of intelligence and education on the development of dementia. A test of the brain reserve hypothesis. *Psychological Medicine*, **27**, 1337–44.

Schmidt, R., Schmidt, H., and Fazekas, F. (2000). Vascular risk factors in dementia. *Journal of Neurology*, **247**, 81–7.

Schoenberg, B. S., Okazaki, H., and Kokmen, E. (1981). Reduced survival in patients with dementia. A population study. *Transactions of the American Neurological Association*, **106**, 306–8.

Schofield, P. (1999). Alzheimer's disease and brain reserve. *Australasian Journal on Ageing*, **18**, 10–14.

Schofield, P. W., Tang, M., Marder, K., Bell, K., Dooneief, G., Chun, M., *et al.* (1997). Alzheimer's disease after remote head injury: an incidence study. *Journal of Neurology, Neurosurgery and Psychiatry,* **62**, 119–24.

Schupf, N. (2000). Epidemiology of aging and dementia in Down syndrome. *Neurobiology of Aging*, **21**, S138.

Shumaker, S. A., Reboussin, B. A., Espeland, M. A. Rapp, S. R., McBee, W. L., Dailey, M., *et al.* (1998). The Women's Health Initiative Memory Study (WHIMS): a trial of the effect of estrogen therapy in preventing and slowing the progression of dementia. *Controlled Clinical Trials*, **19**, 604–21.

Skoog, I. (1994). Risk factors for vascular dementia: a review. *Dementia*, **5**, 137–44.

Skoog, I. (2000). Vascular aspects in Alzheimer's disease. *Journal of Neural Transmission*, **59**, 37–43.

Skoog, I. and Gustafson, D. (1999). HRT and dementia. *Journal of Epidemiology and Biostatistics*, **4**, 227–52.

Snowdon, D. A., Kemper, S. J., Mortimer, J. A., Greiner, L. H., Wekstein, D. R., and Markesbery, W. R. (1996). Linguistic ability in early life and cognitive function and Alzheimer's disease in late life. *Journal of the American Medical Association*, **275**, 528–32.

Sobel, E. and Davanipour, Z. (1996). Electromagnetic field exposure may cause increased production of amyloid beta and eventually lead to Alzheimer's disease. *Neurology*, **47**, 1594–600.

Sobel, E., Dunn, M., Davanipour, Z., Qian, Z., and Chui, H. C. (1996). Elevated risk of Alzheimer's disease among workers with likely electromagnetic field exposure. *Neurology*, **47**, 1477–81.

Stern, Y., Alexander, G. E., Prohovnik, I., and Mayeux, R. (1992). Inverse relationship between education and parietotemporal perfusion deficit in Alzheimer's disease. *Annals of Neurology*, **32**, 371–5.

United States General Accounting Office. (1998). *Alzheimer's disease: estimates of prevalence in the United States*. United States General Accounting Office, Washington DC.

van Duijn, C. M., Clayton, D., Chandra, V., Fratiglioni, L., Graves, A. B., Heyman, A., *et al.* (1991). Familial aggregation of Alzheimer's disease and related disorders: a collaborative re-analysis of case-control studies. *International Journal of Epidemiology*, **20**, S13–S20.

Witthaus, E., Ott, A., Barendregt, J. J., Breteler, M., and Bonneux, L. (1999). Burden of mortality and morbidity from dementia. *Alzheimer Disease and Associated Disorders*, **13**, 176–81.

Yaffe, K., Sawaya, G., Lieberburg, I., and Grady, D. (1998). Estrogen therapy in postmenopausal women: effects on cognitive function and dementia. *Journal of the American Medical Association*, **279**, 688–95.

Zigman, W. B., Schupf, N., Sersen, E., and Silverman, W. (1996). Prevalence of dementia in adults with and without Down syndrome. *American Journal of Mental Retardation*, **100**, 403–12.

24i Dementia: a twentieth century historical overview

Alistair Burns

Introduction

The word 'dementia' comes from the Latin stem, *demens* which literally means without mind. It first appeared in the vernacular in Blancard's popular dictionary in 1726 (Blancard 1726), defined as 'the extinction of the imagination and judgement'. The adjective, *demented*, was first to be seen in the *Oxford English Dictionary* of 1644. About a century later, it acquired a medical and legal connotation. The French encyclopaedia of 1765 (Diderot and D'Alembert 1765) described the disorder in detail, distinguishing it from delirium and from mania, emphasizing its reversibility and the fact that there were many causes (this 'syndromal' view of dementia is often neglected). By 1900, three types of dementia were recognized—senile, arteriosclerotic, and subcortical. Other related disorders included general paralysis of the insane, dementia praecox, and the cognitive impairment associated with functional psychoses (depression and mania, known as the vesanic dementias, later becoming the pseudodementias). Specific disorders known to give rise to symptoms similar to those of dementia included epilepsy, alcoholism, myxoedema, and lead poisoning.

Alzheimer described a case report at a meeting in 1906 and it was published a year later (Alzheimer 1907). The patient (Auguste D) was 51 when she developed her illness, the same age as Alzheimer was when he died. Her symptoms were of delusions, hallucinations, aphasia, and cognitive impairment. At postmortem, her brain showed neurofibrillary tangles, senile plaques, and arteriosclerotic changes. The presence of neurofibrillary tangles and senile plaques in dementia had been described 5 months previously (Fuller 1907) and plaques had been known to be associated with dementia for 20 years (Beljahow 1889). Delusions and hallucinations had been reported in conjunction with cognitive impairment (see, for example, Marcé 1863). It is clear that Alzheimer felt the novelty in his report was that the features occurred in a young person (Berrios 1994). In 1910, Kraepelin effectively named the disease after Alzheimer in the eighth edition of his handbook (Kraepelin 1910).

Binswanger (1894) was the first to describe the association between a progressive subcortical vascular encephalopathy (PSVE) with focal signs and white matter lesions in the brain. Alzheimer (1898) further defined the syndrome by classifying it into arteriosclerotic brain atrophy, dementia apoplectica (fits associated with cerebral damage followed by cognitive impairment), and perivascular gliosis with PSVE describing Binswanger's disease.

In the century since these early descriptions, and particularly in the last 30 years, there have been significant clinical and scientific advances in our understanding of dementia and its causes. These can be outlined, using Alzheimer's disease as the paradigm, under the following headings: neuropathology, neurochemistry and molecular biology, epidemiology, quantitative assessment, diagnostic criteria, and drug treatment.

Neuropathology, neurochemistry, and molecular biology

A series of classic studies from Newcastle-upon-Tyne in the 1960s showed, for the first time, that there was a significant association between the numbers of senile plaques found at postmortem in the brains of people dying with dementia and the severity of the illness assessed during life (Blessed *et al.* 1968). These studies demonstrated that morphological brain changes had a significant impact on clinical symptomatology, although the cross-sectional nature of the study did not allow causation to be inferred. Major types of dementia were defined (Tomlinson *et al.* 1968), it was shown that the majority of older people with senile dementia had Alzheimer's disease, not arteriosclerosis, and the role of cerebral infarction in the genesis of vascular dementia was postulated (the studies suggested that more than 50 ml of infarcted tissue were necessary for clinical symptoms to appear). The correlation of clinical features and pathological changes was later extended to include neurofibrillary tangles (Wilcock and Esiri 1982) and neuronal synapses (Terry *et al.* 1991).

The acetylcholine deficit in the brains of people dying of Alzheimer's disease has been well documented (Bowen *et al.* 1976) and is one of the most consistent neurochemical changes seen in any disorder (Karczmar 1993). These deficits have been correlated with clinical and pathological features (Perry *et al.* 1978). Although other neurotransmitter abnormalities have been documented, such as deficits in serotonin, catecholamines, and gamma-aminobutyric acid (Proctor *et al.* 2000), current successful treatments for Alzheimer's disease are based on reversing the cholinergic defect.

The development of molecular biology techniques has accelerated our understanding of the pathology of the dementias in general, and Alzheimer's disease in particular. While it had always been accepted that there was a significant familial component to dementia, it was not until the mid-1980s that the linkage of a familial form of the gene to chromosome 21 was proven. The genetics of Alzheimer's disease was revolutionized by a series of observations published in *Science*: it had been known for some time that people with Down's syndrome (the majority of whom had three copies of chromosome 21) developed the pathological changes of Alzheimer's disease; the gene producing the amyloid protein was localized to chromosome 21 at the same time as the linkage of some families with familial Alzheimer's disease was made to the same chromosome; the link seemed obvious (St George Hyslop *et al.* 1987; Tanzi *et al.* 1987; Goldgaber *et al.* 1987). Although the relationship turned out not to be as simple as that predicted, the work acted as a catalyst for the description of the first missense mutation in the β-amyloid (amyloid precursor protein) gene (Goate *et al.* 1991).

Since then, two other mutations have been definitively identified. Sherrington *et al.* (1995) cloned the gene on chromosome 14, the protein product of which is referred to as presenilin-1. Second, Levy-Lahad (1995) reported a similar protein on chromosome 1, termed presenilin-2. These account for the majority of early-onset cases, presenilin-1 being the rarer but particularly aggressive form, with an average age of onset in affected pedigrees of 42 years (van Duijn *et al.* 1994). Both these proteins seem to increase the production of the pathogenic form of β-amyloid. While these discoveries have resulted in major advances in understanding the molecular biology of Alzheimer's disease, it is important to remember that they account for less than 2% of all cases of Alzheimer's disease, and not even the majority of familial autosomal dominant cases.

The discovery of the association between apolipoprotein E and Alzheimer's disease has been a significant advance in that, for the first time, a definable and reproducible biological risk factor for late-onset Alzheimer's disease has been described (Strittmatter *et al.* 1993). The risk ratio for the development of Alzheimer's disease for those with the *β4/β4* allele is about 14, which is one of the strongest associations to be reported for any risk factor. However, it is important to remember that possession of an *β4* allele does not mean that Alzheimer's disease will definitely develop in an individual, nor does its absence confer complete protection.

The genetics of the other major abnormal protein implicated in Alzheimer's disease, tau, which when abnormally phosphorylated contributes to the formation of neurofibrillary tangles, have been described in relation to dementia of the frontal lobe type (Delacourte 1999). An autosomal dominant form of vascular dementia has also been documented—cerebral autosomal dominant arteriopathy with subcortical infarcts and leucoencephalopathy (CADASIL, Dichgans *et al.* 1998).

Epidemiology

The contribution of epidemiology to dementia has been twofold. First, by highlighting the numbers of people affected by the disorder and, second, in uncovering the risk factors for its development using a case-control methodology. Summarized as part of the EURODEM initiative, a meta-analysis of studies confirms that the proportion of people over 65 with dementia is about 10% over the age of 80, rising to 30% over the age of 90 (Hofman *et al.* 1991). The prevalence of Alzheimer's disease is estimated at 11% over the age of 80 (Rocca *et al.* 1991). Vascular dementia is particularly common amongst older women (Skoog *et al.* 1993). The figures for vascular dementia are more difficult to interpret because of the different diagnostic criteria used. However, there is enough evidence to suggest that the prevalence of vascular disease rises steeply with age (in population studies, the prevalence of dementia doubles every 5 years over the age of 60), that it is higher in men, and is slightly less common than Alzheimer's disease (Jorm and Jolley 1998; Jorm 2000).

Risk factors for Alzheimer's disease using a case-control methodology

The known risk factors are age, the presence of Down's syndrome, the possession of an $\beta 4$ allele of the apolipoprotein molecule, and genetic abnormalities in a few familial cases (Hofman *et al.* 1997). Head injury, a past history of depression, and the presence of herpes simplex type 1 virus in the brain have all been implicated as risk factors. Oestrogen replacement, anti-inflammatory medication and arthritis, and smoking have all been suggested as protective factors, although the evidence for the latter is inconclusive. Wine-drinking is protective against the development of Alzheimer's disease, possibly because of its antioxidant effect (Orgogozo *et al.* 1997). A higher level of education also seems to be protective (Stern *et al.* 1994).

Vascular dementia shares the same risk factors as stroke: i.e. previous transient ischaemic attack or stroke, hypertension, diabetes mellitus, hypercholesterolaemia, smoking, heart disease (particularly atrial fibrillation), and a lack of physical exercise.

Quantitative assessment of dementia

A major advance over the last 30 years has been the development of scales which provide a quantitative assessment of dementia. There are now nearly 200 scales which can be applied to assess various aspects of dementia, ranging from the cognitive state, activities of daily living, neuropsychiatric features, carer strain, quality of life, and pleasant events (Burns *et al.* 1999).

The first quantitative measure of cognitive function, the Blessed Dementia scale (Blessed *et al.* 1968), was developed in the Newcastle studies of the 1960s and was used to correlate the severity of the clinical symptomatology with the number of senile plaques seen in the brain at postmortem. It included assessments of activities of daily living and personality change as well as the Mental Test Score, later the Abbreviated Mental Test Score. The Mini-Mental State Examination (MMSE, Folstein *et al.* 1975) is now the most widely used of all the cognitive function scales.

Most published scales have satisfactory validity and reliability and each has its strengths and weaknesses. The development of this multitude of scales has partly been driven by the pharmaceutical industry, in an attempt to measure phenomena in dementia as a prerequisite to assessing change resulting from drug interventions. The ability to measure and assess change in the core features of dementia is crucial to designing effective trials of drugs and other therapies.

The first case described by Alzheimer emphasized that psychiatric symptoms and behavioural disturbances occurred in patients with dementia, a fact all but ignored in studies of dementia until the last 15 years. Since dementia was defined in terms of its effect on cognitive function, so neuropsychological deficits became the focus for research, with the other symptoms being regarded as epiphenomena. The importance of these psychiatric and behavioural aspects of dementia is that they cause significant stress to carers, are amenable to a wide range of pharmacological and non-pharmacological approaches, may be helpful in differential diagnosis, and may shed light on the pathophysiological mechanisms of functional psychiatric disorders (Burns *et al.* 1990*a*). The ability to quantify these features has contributed to their growing importance in the field (Finkel and Burns 2000).

Diagnostic criteria

The development of standardized diagnosis using criteria with satisfactory reliability and validity has been an essential step in the definition of the dementia syndrome. These are two sets of internationally accepted criteria: the Diagnostic and Statistical Manual (DSM; APA 1994), which is the North American system of classification, now in its revised fourth edition (DSM-IVR), and the European-based International Classification of Disease (ICD; WHO 1992), currently in the tenth edition (ICD-10). The definitions have a number of common elements, for example that the disorder should be progressive and should have global effects on higher cortical functions.

The field progressed when operationalized diagnostic criteria for the different causes of dementia were also described. For example, clinical research criteria were suggested for Alzheimer's disease by the NINCDS/ADRDA in 1984 (McKhann *et al.* 1984). These have become the 'gold standard' by which the clinical diagnosis of Alzheimer's disease is made for research purposes. Their reliability and validity have been defined and are excellent (Burns *et al.* 1990*b* Kukull *et al.* 1990).

The clinical criteria for the diagnosis of vascular dementia were first suggested by Hachinski in 1975 with the description of the Hachinski scale (Hachinski *et al.* 1975). This relied mainly on evidence for vascular disease (essentially stroke) and a score was made on a 18-point scale. The original publication showed a clear division between people suffering from primary dementia (Alzheimer's disease) and vascular dementia (termed multi-infarct dementia, following the work of the Newcastle studies referred to earlier). Updates of this original description have been published—the NINCDS/AIREN criteria (Roman *et al.* 1993) and the ADDTC criteria (Chui *et al.* 1992), both of which have satisfactory reliability and validity.

Criteria have also been published for dementia of Lewy body type (McKeith *et al.* 1996) and dementia of frontal lobe type (Neary *et al.* 1998). Operational criteria are also available for mild cognitive impairment (Ritchie and Touchon 2000).

Treatment

A knowledge of the neurochemical changes in Alzheimer's disease prompted the search for treatments. Deficits in the cholinergic system are one of the most consistent found and formed the basis for the majority of currently successful approaches. Lecithin and physostigmine were the subject of trials which showed modest improvement, but the drugs never became part of clinical practice. The anticholinesterase drugs (these inhibit the enzyme that breaks down acetylcholine) are the class of agents that have shown most promise in terms of treatment effect.

Several of these are now in use. Tacrine was the original agent, but hepatotoxicity restricted its use in clinical practice (Eagger *et al.* 1991). Other agents such as donepezil (Aricept, Rogers *et al.* 1996; Burns *et al.* 1999), rivastigmine (Exelon, Rosler *et al.* 1999), and galantamine (Reminyl, Raskind *et al.* 2000; Tariot *et al.* 2000) have now been introduced. Trials have demonstrated that they are effective in the treatment of Alzheimer's disease over 6–12 months. They improve cognition, activities of daily living, and global functioning. Vitamin E has been shown to slow disease progression (Sano *et al.* 1997). It is too early to make firm statements about the prevention of dementia; but it has been demonstrated, in the setting of a clinical trial, that a reduction of blood pressure can decrease the number of people with both Alzheimer's disease and vascular dementia (Forette *et al.* 1998).

Non-pharmacological approaches to the management of dementia have been developed and are often implemented as part of normal clinical practice (Woods and Bird 1998).

Conclusion

Since the first descriptions of Alzheimer's disease and vascular dementia, significant advances have been made in our understanding of these disorders. However, Alzheimer's disease and vascular dementia are a long way from being preventable or even curable conditions. Dementia, because of its inevitable associations with senility and ageing, still does not attract the degree of attention and funding that it should, because of an underlying fear in the public mind. New treatments, the ageing of the population, and a more proactive approach to public understanding of the disease are beginning to have an effect. Awaking professionals from the slumber of therapeutic nihilism is an important step and is beginning. The story of dementia outlined above hopefully sets the scene for the more detailed contributions which follow.

References

Alzheimer, A. (1898). Neuere Arbeiten über die Dementia Senilis und die auf atheromatöser. Gefässerkrankung basierenden Gehirnkrankheiten. *Monatschrift der Psychiatrie und Neurologie*, **3**, 101–15.

Alzheimer, A. (1907). Über eine eigenartige Erkrankung der Hirnrinde. *Allgemeine Zeitschrift für Psychiatrie und Psychisch Gerichtlich Medizin*, **64**, 146–8.

American Psychogeriatric Association (1994). *Diagnostic and statistical manual of mental disorders* (4th edn). APA, Washington DC.

Beljahow, S. (1889). Pathological changes in the brain in dementia senilis. *Journal of Mental Science*, **35**, 261–2.

Berrios, G. (1994). Dementia: historical overview In *Dementia* (ed A. Burns and R. Levy), pp. 5–20. Chapman and Hall, London.

Binswanger, O. (1894). Die Abgrenzung der allgemeinen progessiven Paralyse. *Berliner Klinische Wochenschrift*, **32**, 1103–5, 1137–9, 1180–6.

Blancard, S. (1726). *The physical dictionary* wherein the terms of anatomy, the names and causes of diseases, chirurgical instruments and their use are accurately described. John and Benjamin Sprint. London.

Blessed, G., Tomlinson, B., and Roth, M., (1968). The association between quantitative measures of dementing and senile change in cerebral grey matter of elderly subjects. *British Journal of Psychiatry*, **114**, 797–811.

Bowen, D., Smith, C., White, P., and Davidson, A. (1976). Neurotransmitter related enzymes and indices of hypoxia in senile dementia and other abiotrophies. *Brain*, **99**, 459–96.

Burns, A., Jacoby, R., and Levy, R. (1990*a*). Psychiatric phenomena in Alzheimer's disease. *British Journal of Psychiatry*, **157**, 72–94.

Burns, A., Luthert, P., Levy, R., *et al.* (1990*b*). Accuracy of clinical diagnosis of Alzheimer's disease. *British Medical Journal*, **301**, 1026.

Burns, A., Rossor, M., Hecker, J., Gauthier, S., Petit, H., Möller, H-J., *et al.* (1999). The effects of donepezil in Alzheimer's disease—results from a multinational trial. *Dementia and Geriatric Cognitive Disorders*, **10**, 237–44.

Chui, H., Victoroff, J., Margolin, D. *et al.* (1992). Criteria for the diagnosis of ischaemic vascular dementia. *Neurology*, **42**, 473–80.

Delacourte, A. (1999). Biochemical and molecular characterization of neurofibrillary degeneration in frontotemporal dementias. *Dementia and Geriatric Cognitive Disorders*, **10**(Suppl. 1), 75–9.

Dichgans, M., Mayer, M., Uttner, I., *et al.* (1998). The phenotypic spectrum of CADASIL: clinical findings in 102 cases. *Annals of Neurology*, **44**, 1246–52.

Diderot, D. and D'Alembert, J. (ed.). (1765). *Encyclopédie ou dictionnaire raisonné des sciences, des arts et des métiers*. Vol. 4, pp. 807–8. David le Breton Durand, Paris.

Eagger, S., Levy, R., and Sahakian, B. (1991). Tacrine in Alzheimer's disease. *Lancet*, **337**, 989–92.

Finkel, S. and Burns, A. (2000). Behavioural and psychological symptoms in dementia (BPSD). Clinical Research Update. *International Psychogeriatrics*, **12**, Suppl. 1.

Folstein, M. F., Folstein, S. E., and McHugh, P. R. (1975). Mini-Mental State Examination—A practical method for grading the cognitive state of patients for the clinician. *Journal of Psychiatric Research*, **12**, 189–98.

Forette, F., Seux, M. L., Staessen, J., *et al.* (1998). Prevention of dementia in randomised double blind placebo controlled Systolic Hypertension in Europe (Syst-Eur) trial. *Lancet*, **352**, 1347–51.

Fuller, S. (1907). A study of the neurofibrols in dementia paralytica, dementia senilis. chronic alcoholism, cerebral clues and microcephalic idiocy. *American Journal of Insanity*, **63**, 415–68.

Goate, A., Chartier-Harlin, M., Mullan, M., *et al.* (1991). Segregation of a missense mutation in the amyloid precursor protein gene with familial Alzheimer's disease. *Nature*, **349**, 704–6.

Goldgaber, D., Lernen, M., McBride, O., Saffiotti, U., and Jajdusek, D. (1987). Characterisation and chromosome localization of a cDNA encoding brain amyloid of Alzheimer's disease. *Science*, **235**, 877–80.

Hachinski, V., Iliff, L., Zilka, E., *et al.* (1975). Cerebral blood flow in dementia. *Archives of Neurology*, **32**, 632–7.

Hofman, A., Rocca, W., Brayne, C., *et al.* (1991). Prevalence of dementia in Europe: a collaborative study from 1980–1990. Findings. Eurodem Prevalence Research Group. *International Journal of Epidemiology*, **20**, 736–48.

Hofman, A., Ott, A., Breteler, M., *et al.* (1997). Arthrosclerosis, apolipoprotein E and prevalence of dementia and Alzheimer's disease in the Rotterdam study. *Lancet*, **349**, 151–4.

Hofman, R., Rocca, W., Brayne, C., *et al.* (1991). The prevalence of dementia in Europe. *International Journal of Epidemiology*, **20**, 736–48.

Jorm, A. (2000). Epidemiology: meta-analysis In *Cerebrovascular disease and dementia* (ed, E. Chui, *et al.*), pp. 55–62. Martin Dunitz, London.

Jorm, A. and Jolley, D. (1998). The incidence of dementia: a meta-analysis. *Neurology*, **51**, 728–33.

Karczmar, A. (1993). Brief presentation of the story and present status of the vertebrate cholinergic system. *Neuropsychopharmacology*, **9**, 181–99.

Kraepelin, E. (1910). *Psychiatrie: ein Lehrbuch für Studierende und Ärzte*. Johanan Ambrosius Barth, Leipzig.

Kukull, W., Larson, E., Reifler, B., *et al.* (1990). Inter-rater reliability of Alzheimer's disease diagnosis. *Neurology*, **40**, 257–60.

Levy-Lahad, A., Wijsman, E., Nemens, E., *et al.* (1995). The familial Alzheimer's disease locus on chromosome 1. *Science*, **269**, 970–3.

McKeith, I. G., Galasko, D., Kosaka, K., Perry, E., *et al.* (1996). Consensus guidelines for the clinical and pathologic diagnosis of dementia with Lewy bodies (DLB). *Neurology*, **47**, 1113–24.

McKhann, G., Drachman, D., Folstein, M., *et al.* (1984). Clinical diagnosis of Alzheimer's disease. *Neurology*, **34**, 939–44.

Marcé, L. V. (1863). Recherches cliniques et anatomo-pathologiques sur la démence sénile et sur les différences qui la séparent de la paralysie générale. *Gazette Medicale de Paris*, **34**, 433–5.

Neary, D., Snowden, J. S., Gustafson, L., *et al.* (1998). Frontotemporal lobar degeneration. A consensus on clinical diagnostic criteria. *Neurology*, **51**, 1546–54.

Orgogozo, J. M., Dartigues, J., Lafont, S., *et al.* (1997). Wine consumption and dementia in the elderly. *Revue Neurologique*, **153**, 185–92.

Perry, E., Tomlinson, B., Blessed, G., Bergman, K., Gibson, P., and Perry, R. (1978). Correlation of cholinergic abnormalities with senile plaques and mental test scores in senile dementia. *British Medical Journal*, **214**, 57–9.

Procter, A. (2000). Abnormalities in non cholinergic neurotransmitter systems in Alzheimer's disease In *Dementia* (ed J. O'Brien, D. Ames, and A. Burns), pp. 433–42. Arnold, London.

Raskind, M., Peskind, E., Wessel, T., *et al.* (2000). Galantamine in AD: a six month randomised placebo controlled trial and a six month extension. *Neurology*, **54**, 2261–8.

Ritchie, K. and Touchon, J. (2000). Mild cognitive impairment: conceptual basis and current nosological status. *Lancet*, **355**, 225–8.

Rocca, A., Hoffman, A., and Brayne, E., *et al.* (1991). Frequency and distribution of Alzheimer's disease in Europe; a collaborative study of 1980–1990. Prevalence findings of the Eurodem Prevalence Research Group. *Annals of Neurology*, **30**, 381–90.

Rogers, S. L., Friedhoff, L. T., and the Donepezil Study Group (1996). The efficacy and safety of donepezil in patients with Alzheimer's disease. *Dementia*, **7**, 293–303.

Roman, G., Tatemichi, T., Erkinjuntti, T., Cummings, J., Masdeu, J., and Garcia, J. (1993). Vascular dementia: diagnostic criteria for research studies. *Neurology*, **3**, 250–60.

Rosler, M., Anand, R., Cici-Sain, A., *et al.* (1999). Efficacy and safety of rivastigmine in patients with Alzheimer's disease. *British Medical Journal*, **318**, 633–640.

Sano, M., Ernesto, C., Thomas, R. G., *et al.* (1997). A controlled trial of selegiline, alpha-tocopherol, or both as treatment for Alzheimer's disease. *New England Journal of Medicine*, **336**, 1216–47.

Sherrington, R., Rogaev, I., Liang, Y., *et al.* (1995). Cloning of a gene bearing missense mutations in early onset familial Alzheimer's disease. *Nature*, **375**, 754–60.

Skoog, I., Nilsson, L., Palmartz, B., *et al.* (1993). A population based study of dementia in 85 year olds. *New England Journal of Medicine*, **328**, 153–8.

Stern, Y., Gurland, B., Tatemichi, T. K. Tang, M., Wilder, G., and Mayeux, R. (1994). Influence of education and occupation on the incidence of Alzheimer's disease. *Journal of the American Medical Association*, **271**, 1004–10.

St George Hislop, P., Tanzi, R., Polinsky, R., *et al.* (1987). The genetic defect causing familial Alzheimer's disease—chromosome 21. *Science*, **235**, 885–90.

Strittmatter, W., Saunders, A., Schmechel, D., *et al.* (1993). Apolipoprotein E: high avidity binding to beta amyloid; an increased frequency of type 4 allele in late onset familial Alzheimer's disease. *Proceedings of the National Academy of Sciences of the United States of America*, **19**, 1977–81.

Tanzi, R., Gusella, J., Watkins, P., *et al.* (1987). Amyloid B protein gene. *Science*, **235**, 880–4.

Tariot, P., Soloman, P., Morris, J., *et al.* (2000). A five months randomised placebo controlled trial of galantamine in AD. *Neurology*, **54**, 2269–76.

Terry, R., Masliah, E., Salmon, D., *et al.* (1991). Physical basis of cognitive alterations in Alzheimer's disease:

synapse loss is the major correlate of cognitive impairment. *Annals of Neurology*, **30**, 572–80.

Tomlinson, B., Blessed, G., and Roth, M. (1968). Observations on the brains of non-demented old people. *Journal of the Neurological Sciences*, 7, 331–52.

Van Duijn, C. M., Hendricks, L., Farrer, L. A., Backhovens, H. *et al.* (1994). A population-based study of familial Alzheimer disease: linkage to chromosomes 14, 19 and 21. *American Journal of Human Genetics*, 55, 714–27.

Wilcock, G. and Esiri, M. (1982). Plaques, tangles and dementia. *Journal of the Neurological Sciences*, **56**, 343–56.

Woods, R. and Bird, M. (1998). Non pharmacological approaches to treatment. In *Diagnosis and management of dementia* (ed. G. Wilcock, R. Bucks, and K. Rockwood), pp. 311–31. Oxford University Press, Oxford..

World Health Organisation. (1992). *International classification of diseases—10th revision*. WHO, Geneva.

24ii Alzheimer's disease

Alan J. Thomas and John T. O'Brien

Introduction

Alois Alzheimer wrote his original report (Alzheimer 1907) on a 51-year-old woman (Auguste D) who had suffered an illness involving cognitive impairment and other symptoms including delusions and hallucinations. At postmortem he described the principal neuropathological features, senile plaques and neurofibrillary tangles, of what we now call Alzheimer's disease. This eponymous term was coined by Kraepelin and was initially restricted to a presenile degenerative dementia. After several decades it was conceded that older people with identical symptomatology and pathological features had the same disease and, in fact, formed the great majority of cases. Thus today Alzheimer's disease (AD) refers to a characteristic clinical syndrome that usually occurs in later life and which is associated with the neuropathological findings described in detail in Chapter 5.

Alzheimer's disease and the dementia syndrome

The clinician should proceed through a two-stage process in assessing someone referred with a possible dementia. First he should determine whether or not the patient has the features of the dementia syndrome. Second, if the patient is suffering from a dementia, the clinician should attempt to identify the possible cause. This second stage should not be regarded as merely an interesting exercise in classification as it has important management, prognostic, and therapeutic implications. For not only is it important to identify and treat rarer causes of dementia, such as normal-pressure hydrocephalus or hypothyroidism, it is also important to accurately recognize the dementia subtype. Both typical (McKeith *et al.* 1992) and atypical antipsychotic drugs (Ballard *et al.* 1998) can prove harmful and even fatal to people with dementia with Lewy bodies (DLB); appropriate treatments can slow the advance of vascular dementia (VaD); and, of course, there are now licensed treatments available for AD. This assessment process is described in detail elsewhere (Chapter 9) and here we will focus on the current clinical criteria for diagnosing the dementia syndrome and Alzheimer's disease.

The dementia syndrome

The concept of dementia has developed from a poorly described organic brain syndrome to the present operationally defined syndrome of ICD-10 (World Health Organization 1992) and DSM-IV (American Psychiatric Association 1994). These criteria are summarized in Table 24ii.1. Both these manuals require evidence of multiple cognitive deficits, which must include memory impairment, accompanied by some evidence of a decline in functioning. Typical deficits, in addition to the amnesia, include disorientation, aphasia,

Table 24ii.1 The dementia syndrome (ICD-10 and DSM-IV)

Multiple cognitive deficits (which must include amnesia)
Functional impairment
Clear consciousness
Change from previous level
Long duration (> 6 months)

apraxia, and agnosia and are dealt with below in the section on 'Clinical features of Alzheimer's disease'. These higher cortical deficits must represent a change and occur in clear consciousness (i.e. not occur only during a delirium). ICD-10 adds that the cognitive symptoms and related impairments need to have been present for 6 months to make a confident diagnosis of dementia. Previously, dementia was regarded as a chronic and irreversible condition but the present criteria hedge around this subject, with ICD-10 now saying this is 'usually' the case and DSM-IV demanding it only for its 'Dementia of the Alzheimer's type' criteria. A study of the very similar DSM-III-R criteria (American Psychiatric Association 1987) showed them to have very good inter-rater reliability, with kappa scores of up to 0.7 (Baldereschi *et al.* 1994), but there are some conceptual and practical issues that need to be considered.

Conceptual problems

The placing of memory impairment at the core of the dementia syndrome, and especially the emphasis on it characteristically involving problems with new learning at its onset, ties it very closely to AD. Arguably, it is then something of a self-fulfilling prophecy to find that AD is the commonest cause of dementia. The problem of the requirement for clear consciousness has been highlighted by the recognition of DLB (see Chapter 24iv), in which fluctuation in consciousness is a characteristic feature (McKeith *et al.* 1996). However, fluctuation is also common in vascular dementia (Hachinski *et al.* 1975) and occurs in AD too (Robertson *et al.* 1998). As alluded to above, the previous concept of dementia being irreversible or progressive is not entirely abandoned in the current diagnostic criteria, but is likely to be so soon. Not only are some dementias, including AD, clearly static for periods, but the cholinesterase inhibitors can now symptomatically reverse (at least for short periods) the dementia syndrome in some people with AD and DLB. Also the criteria do not recognize mixed dementia, which is increasingly thought to account for a substantial proportion of cases.

Practical problems

The two major differential diagnoses to be excluded when considering whether cognitive impairment is due to a dementia are depression and delirium. Two kinds of problem can arise at initial assessment. First there may be comorbidity (e.g. delirium often occurs together with dementia) and the contribution of each to the cognitive impairment may not be revealed for some time. Each cause then needs to be dealt with in its own right until the situation becomes clearer. Second, there can be real difficulty in distinguishing the cause at initial presentation. Some cases of delirium are 'subacute' and grumble on for a long period as their underlying cause persists (see Chapters 25 and 26), whilst severe depression in the elderly may manifest itself as marked cognitive impairment (so-called 'depressive pseudodementia'; see Chapter 27). Careful monitoring should clarify the situation with time, but making a confident diagnosis at first presentation is sometimes best avoided.

Sometimes, especially in memory clinics specializing in assessing possible early dementia, a patient is confirmed as having multiple cognitive deficits on testing but does not show any functional impairment in their daily living; such individuals need monitoring but would not, as yet, fulfil the diagnostic criteria for dementia. Similarly, patients are sometimes seen with a clear deficit in only one cognitive domain; again they would not meet dementia criteria but need monitoring, as often they will progress to multiple deficits with functional impairment (i.e. dementia) over time.

Diagnostic criteria for Alzheimer's disease

ICD-10 and DSM-IV criteria

Having confirmed that a patient has the dementia syndrome, the next stage is to try and establish the cause. Since AD causes over 50% of all cases of dementia it has come to be regarded almost as the model for dementia. As such there is still a tendency to diagnose AD by default rather than by the positive identification of the clinical syndrome described below. Table 24ii.2 shows the

Table 24ii.2 Diagnostic criteria for Alzheimer's disease (ICD-10 and DSM-IV)

Fulfil criteria for dementia syndrome
Insidious onset
Gradual progression
No focal neurological signs
No evidence for a systemic or brain disease sufficient to cause dementia

current diagnostic criteria for AD. ICD-10 and DSM-IV both require that dementia due to AD has an insidious onset and a gradual progression. AD cannot be diagnosed if there is a sudden onset, or if there are neurological signs indicating focal brain damage, or if the dementia can be explained by other brain or systemic diseases.

Applying these criteria requires a systematic and thorough assessment: a full history (including from an informant), mental state examination, cognitive examination, physical assessment (including neurological examination), and other investigations. The latter are important because alternative causes include both systemic diseases, e.g. vitamin B_{12} deficiency and hypothyroidism, and brain diseases, e.g. normal-pressure hydrocephalus and stroke. A list of suggested investigations is given in Table 24ii.3.

NINCDS-ADRDA criteria

Both the ICD-10 and DSM-IV criteria for AD are closely related to the more rigorous NINCDS-ADRDA (National Institute of Neurological and Communicative Disorders and Stroke—Alzheimer's Disease and Related Disorders Association) criteria (McKhann *et al.* 1984). These are the widely used research criteria for AD and are shown in the Appendix to this chapter. The McKhann criteria have three levels of certainty for an AD diagnosis: definite AD, probable AD, and possible AD. Definite AD can only be diagnosed at postmortem where tissue evidence confirms AD in someone already recognized as having probable AD. To make a diagnosis of probable AD requires multiple cognitive deficits (including memory) which progressively worsen and occur without disturbance of consciousness in someone with a dementia syndrome. The probable AD diagnosis also requires basic cognitive testing, e.g. the Mini-Mental State Examination (MMSE) (Folstein *et al.* 1975), to demonstrate the deficits and some confirmation of these by other neuropsychological tests. The criteria also set age limits of 45 and 90 years for the onset of the dementia, because of potential difficulties in interpreting cognitive tests in people over 90. There are also similar exclusion criteria to those for ICD-10 and DSM-IV, in that

Table 24ii.3 Recommended investigations in dementia and Alzheimer's disease

Full blood count
Erythrocyte sedimentation rate (ESR) or viscosity
Urea, creatinine, and electrolytes (including calcium)
Liver function tests
Thyroid function tests
Vitamin B_{12} and folate
Syphilis serology
Blood glucose
Cholesterol
Mid-stream urinalysis (MSU)
Chest radiographs
Electrocardiogram
Electroencephalogram (mild diffuse slowing)
CT/MRI scan of the head (may be normal, show generalized atrophy or focal atrophy in medial temporal lobe)
SPET scan—useful in selected cases (bilateral, symmetrical, temporoparietal perfusion)

CT, computed tomography; MRI, magnetic resonance imaging; SPET, single positron-emission tomography.

there must be no disturbance of consciousness and no systemic or brain diseases that could explain the impairment. Where all these criteria cannot be met clinically, e.g. fluctuating course or sudden onset, then a diagnosis of possible AD should be made. The NINCDS-ADRDA criteria have been shown to have a sensitivity and specificity for AD of over 80% (Burns *et al.* 1990*f*; McKeith *et al.* 2000*a*) and very good inter-rater reliability (Farrer *et al.* 1994).

Differential diagnosis

In practice, the exclusion criteria for AD regarding apoplectic onset and focal signs specified in the above criteria usually exclude people who have had a stroke, although other causes, e.g. head trauma or tumour, will also be excluded. Where there is evidence of cerebrovascular disease which is thought likely to contribute to the dementia (usually evidence of stroke clinically or on neuroimaging), then both ICD-10 and DSM-IV state that a double diagnosis of AD and vascular dementia should be made (although many clinicians will refer to this as a 'mixed dementia'). Ideally such a double diagnosis should be made when there is clear evidence of each disease process contributing to the dementia, e.g. someone with AD who subsequently has a stroke and suddenly declines cognitively. However, in clinical practice a more pragmatic decision will often be made based on evidence for both AD and VaD, such that a single pure diagnosis cannot confidently be made. The diagnosis of VaD is dealt with in detail in the next chapter.

The other major differential diagnosis for the dementia syndrome in the elderly is DLB, which is covered in Chapter 24iv. DLB can be diagnosed confidently (probable DLB (McKeith *et al.* 1996)) in the presence of at least two of the three core features (recurrent visual hallucinations, fluctuation, and spontaneous parkinsonism). However, possible DLB (McKeith *et al.* 1996) may be diagnosed when only one of these three features is found, though subjects may meet criteria for possible AD (McKhann *et al.* 1984) as well. Because fluctuation can occur in AD (particularly in moderate and severe dementia) and visual hallucinations are also found (see below), the presence of these features does not necessarily preclude a diagnosis of AD. The situation will often become clearer over time, e.g. the development of parkinsonism, but in any case serious consideration should be given to treating such people with cholinesterase inhibitors. Apart from cognition, symptoms such as delusions, hallucinations, apathy, and agitation are likely to improve (McKeith *et al.* 2000*b*,*c*).

In younger patients frontotemporal dementia should be considered, especially if frontal features are prominent, e.g. primitive reflexes, disinhibition, or marked apathy. This is dealt with in Chapter 23v. Sometimes other rarer causes of dementia, e.g. hypothyroidism or normal-pressure hydrocephalus, may be found in someone with apparent AD. However, it should be remembered that conditions such as hypothyroidism and mild B_{12}/folate deficiency are common and their presence on screening does not necessarily indicate they are solely responsible for the cognitive difficulties. A concomitant diagnosis of AD may still apply, and whether such a decision is correct will reveal itself when the other possible cause of the dementia is treated.

Summary

The diagnosis of AD is a two-stage process. First, clinical evidence for the dementia syndrome is gathered, and depression and delirium are excluded, and, second, the presentation is examined to see if it fits the above AD criteria of insidious onset and gradual progression in the absence of other possible causes. The two main other causes to consider in the elderly are VaD and DLB. Usually a careful assessment allows such distinctions to be made, but sometimes the clinician needs to wait patiently for further evidence as the disease progresses. Such distinctions are important because depression and delirium clearly merit a different kind of treatment from any cause of dementia and, as mentioned above, the three major causes of dementia also carry different treatment implications.

Clinical features of Alzheimer's disease

Cognitive symptoms

These are central to the concept of dementia and AD and are dealt with in detail elsewhere (see Chapters 3 and 9). Here we will just describe the key symptoms and their progression as they are usually encountered in AD in clinical practice. (Note: here we will use aphasia and dysphasia synonymously, although strictly speaking the former refers to complete impairment of language and the latter to partial impairment. The same applies *mutatis mutandis* to apraxia/dyspraxia, alexia/dyslexia, and agraphia/dysgraphia.)

Amnesia

Memory impairment is the classic presenting complaint for AD, although other symptoms, e.g. apathy, subtle personality changes, and dysphasia, are often found early in the illness too. The amnesia typically presents with a history of misplacing and losing objects, forgetting appointments, or repeatedly asking the same question. At this early stage working memory (for example, the ability to repeat back a few words or a list of numbers) is relatively unimpaired. However, the ability to recall such words or numbers a few minutes later is significantly impaired because the earliest deficits in AD are in the process of encoding or laying down new information in the memory stores. This probably results from damage to the hippocampal formation, which is the site of the earliest pathological damage in AD. This failure to lay down new memories can be demonstrated more clearly by tests in which a patient is read a short story and asked to recall it (logical memory tests) or when a long list of words is read and repeated attempts are made to learn the list, e.g. Rey Auditory Verbal Learning Test. Impairment in new learning also leads to the characteristic disorientation in time and place that is prominent even in early AD.

In the early stage of AD the recall of previously learned information remains good, showing that memory retrieval processes remain intact. This results in the characteristic pattern of a failure of new learning (no memory for recent events) combined with clear memories of events earlier in life. As the disease progresses the memory impairment broadens to include retrieval of older memories, and these are typically lost according to Ribot's law (more recent information is lost before more remote events) so that the patient appears to live in the ever-more distant past. As well as these losses in episodic memory (personally related events occurring in a specific situation) there are accompanying losses in semantic memory (facts and vocabulary) and visuospatial memory (remembering pictures or faces).

Aphasia (dysphasia)

Deficits in cortical language production are usually present if they are searched for in the early stages of AD. The earliest manifestation is in word-finding difficulties, in which the patient struggles from time to time to find the correct words to complete sentences. Attempts to cover this up by using circumlocutions are common, and may be cleverly executed by people with premorbid high IQ or people with good social skills so that the deficits are hidden. At this time there is also usually an impairment in the naming of objects (nominal aphasia), this will initially be for the names of less common items rather than the more common objects which are frequently tested, e.g. pen or glasses. Thus asking the patient to name objects in the room, e.g. a video recorder, or parts of objects, e.g. the winder on a watch, may show some nominal aphasia that would not otherwise be revealed. As the AD progresses these deficits worsen and problems in the comprehension of language develop (receptive dysphasia); in addition, the expression of language shows syntactical errors and simplification of sentence structure. Verbal perseveration, in which the patient repeats the same answer to consecutive questions, may occur too. The development of these deficits has serious consequences as the patient now increasingly struggles to understand what is going on around him and to communicate his confusion and distress clearly to others. It should not be assumed that a concurrent loss of all understanding occurs, as patients may still be sensitive to emotional and other non-verbal cues.

As the dementia becomes severe then marked poverty of the content of speech develops, with the repetition of short simple sentences on favourite themes; eventually, mutism may occur. Some patients babble meaningless sounds or repeat words and phrases they hear (echolalia). Progression in language deterioration is not inevitable and many patients remain superficially fluent. They maintain a social discourse that can deceive the unwary about the true extent of their cognitive impairment. Careful attention to their language comprehension and production, however, will invariably reveal a pattern of language impairment including the deficits mentioned above.

Apraxia (dyspraxia)

Dyspraxia is the failure to carry out complex motor tasks due to deficits in the higher cortical control of movement; this is not because of damage to the peripheral sensory or motor systems, or in co-ordination. It typically occurs with cortical deficits in the dominant (usually left) parietal lobe but, as with other cognitive symptoms in dementia, dysfunction in other areas is usually present too. Ideomotor apraxia is the form usually elicited, and refers to the inability of the patient to carry out a motor task to command. Examples include asking the patient: to wave; to demonstrate how he brushes his teeth; or show how he combs his hair. Other common 'dyspraxias' sought by the clinician are dressing dyspraxia and constructional dyspraxia. Strictly speaking these are not dyspraxias as they are not necessarily primarily due to higher motor failure. Dressing dyspraxia refers to the common difficulty patients have in putting their clothes on correctly due to faulty visuospatial processing, which results in them being unable to orientate their body properly in relation to their clothing. It is usually taken to indicate right (non-dominant) parietal lobe damage. Constructional dyspraxia refers to the failure to adequately reproduce a two- (or three-) dimensional drawing, e.g. a star or a clock, or to the similar failure to assemble blocks into the required model. Like dressing, such tasks actually involve multiple cognitive domains (visual, spatial, sensory, motor) but failure is usually taken to indicate right (non-dominant) parietal damage. All these dyspraxias have dire consequences for the patient's ability to carry out many activities of daily living. Cooking, cleaning, and general housework require the ability to carry out motor sequences, as do more basic activities such as eating and using the toilet. Failure in such domains is not primarily due to memory but to dyspraxic losses. Relatives may misunderstand why someone who appears healthy apart from an apparently mild memory impairment should struggle in such areas, so explaining the global nature of dementia can help them understand the true situation.

Agnosia

Agnosia is the failure to correctly interpret a sensory input in the presence of an intact sensory system, and it is common in AD. It is due to cortical damage and can occur in any sensory modality, though visual agnosia is the form usually met in clinical practice. In visual agnosia a patient sees an object but does not recognize it. Perhaps the most well known is prosopagnosia in which the patient fails to recognize a familiar face, and when the face is that of a relative it can be very distressing for all concerned. Other common agnosias include failure to recognize objects around the house, e.g. mistaking the kettle for the teapot or the dustbin for the toilet, and these too can have serious consequences for the patient.

Frontal-executive dysfunction

Damage to the frontal lobes leads to inflexibility in thinking and difficulties in problem-solving, planning, and correctly sequencing behaviour. This is a complex area but one which should none the less be tested for during assessment of dementia. It is dealt with in more detail in Chapter 9. Proverbs have traditionally been used to test how concrete and inflexible someone's reasoning is, but the replies are often very difficult to interpret. 'Similarities and differences' tests involve asking the patient what two objects (e.g. table and chair; shoe and boot) have in common and how they differ. Again these tests can be difficult to interpret but some attempt should be made, especially in someone who appears frontally impaired (e.g. markedly disinhibited). Easier to interpret are verbal fluency tests of frontal lobe function. These involve asking the patient to name as many objects as they can in a category in one minute (e.g. fruit or animals) or asking them to generate as many words as they can think of beginning with the same letter in one minute (e.g. F, A, and S in 'the FAS test'). As a rough guide, a normal subject should produce more than 15 words for each in a minute and less than 10 is clearly abnormal. A third kind of frontal test involves testing the subject's ability to shift from one item to another and this reveals perseverative problems. A sequence of alternating shapes or numbers may be written and the patient asked to continue the sequence. Motor perseveration can be demonstrated using the Luria two-step or three-step tests (in which the subject is asked to copy the examiner in alternately opening and closing the hand or making a fist, then an edge, and then a palm, respectively). In someone who shows any of these 'frontal' features it is particularly important to examine for 'primitive reflexes' (see below).

Other cognitive deficits

Corresponding to the above deficits in spoken language are impairments in reading (dyslexia) and writing (dysgraphia), which can be often identified with simple tests in AD using pen, paper, and reading material. Acalculia (more accurately anarithmetria) is the loss of the ability to do simple sums and can similarly be tested for in a straightforward way. Right/left disorientation may be detected by asking the patient to obey commands such as 'point to the left ear with the right forefinger'.

Non-cognitive symptoms

Psychotic symptoms

As mentioned above, in his original report Alois Alzheimer (Alzheimer 1907) described both delusions and hallucinations in his patient Auguste D, and the emphasis in diagnosis on the cognitive symptoms of dementia can distract from the fact that psychotic symptoms are very common. Table 24ii.4 gives summary estimates of the monthly prevalence in clinical settings (that is, hospital inpatients and day patients, outpatients and other clinic patients) in AD of the most important non-cognitive symptoms derived from the research presented below; lifetime rates will be much higher. Accurately eliciting these mental state phenomena can be difficult in people with dementia and the figures quoted below are derived from interviews with informants, who may overrate some symptoms (e.g. depression) compared with trained observers (Burns *et al.* 1990*c*). The rates of all the psychotic symptoms vary widely depending on, amongst other things, how the phenomena are defined, which patients are sampled, and the time frame over which the survey is conducted. Also it is worth noting that many of the studies were conducted before the accurate recognition of DLB was possible, which

Table 24ii.4 Approximate monthly prevalence of non-cognitive symptoms in Alzheimer's disease

Symptoms	Prevalence (%)
Psychotic	
Delusions	30
Misidentifications	30
Hallucinations	20
Mood	
Depression	25
Euphoria	< 1
Anxiety	30–50
Behavioural	
Apathy	70
Agitation	30
Wandering	20
Physical aggression	20
Verbal aggression	40

has a much higher rate of psychosis, and so the figures for AD are likely to be inflated a little by an admixture of DLB patients.

Delusions

Delusional beliefs are common, can be very distressing to carers, and may contribute to early institutionalization. They are often understandable as attempts by the patient to make sense of his situation, and include beliefs that objects have been stolen, a spouse is unfaithful, or that intruders have been in the house. These beliefs commonly have a paranoid flavour and tend to lack the complexity and systemization of the delusions seen in schizophrenia. The delusions are often short-lived and can therefore be difficult to distinguish from confabulations. For hospital patients the prevalence of delusions in published studies varies from about 25% (Cooper *et al.* 1991) to about 50% (Hirono *et al.* 1998). Burns *et al.* (Burns *et al.* 1990*a*) studied a sample of AD patients in a catchment area and found 16% to have delusions at some point in their illness and 11% to have had them in the previous 12 months. This figure is lower than most studies looking at clinically derived samples. Ballard and Walker (1999) systematically reviewed the literature and found a mean prevalence of delusions of 31% in all clinical settings and 23% in community settings. Burns *et al.* (1990*a*) found that delusions were three times more prevalent in men.

Misidentification syndromes

Misidentification syndromes are sometimes called delusional misidentifications and might be better termed symptoms than syndromes. They are very common in AD, occurring in about 23–30% of sufferers at some time and in about 19% during a single year (Rubin *et al.* 1988; Burns *et al.* 1990*b*). They have been classified as delusions and as hallucinations, depending on how the phenomena are understood. For example, the common assertion by a demented patient that someone else has been in the house, when their family denies such a possibility, could be a paranoid delusional belief or a visual hallucination. In practice it is often not possible to clarify the experience well enough to determine the exact form of the psychotic experience. Another common kind of misidentification is the conviction that a relative or friend is someone else (which may be a Capgras symptom if the misidentified person is accepted as looking exactly the same as their 'double', though this may be difficult to tease out in AD). Commonly a spouse is misidentified as a son or daughter or vice versa, but sometimes the patient believes the misidentified person is a stranger and this may provoke a strong reaction. Other symptoms include beliefs that people or events on the television are actually present in the living room, and the misidentification of the patient's own image in the mirror as that of another person ('mirror sign'). Wrongly believing strangers to have been in the house appears to be the commonest form of misidentification, being found in 12–17%; misidentifying people occurs in about 12%; misidentifying images from the television is found in 6–12%; and misidentifying a mirror image occurs in about 4–7% (Rubin *et al.* 1988; Burns *et al.* 1990*b*). Overall studies show misidentification occurs in 30% of people with AD (Ballard and Walker 1999). Like delusions these misidentification syndromes appear to be more likely to occur in men (Burns *et al.* 1990*b*).

Hallucinations

Hallucinations are less common than delusions and misidentification syndromes. However, study figures here may be underestimates, reflecting an unavoidable bias in the way in which the symptoms are rated. The scores are informant-based and informants will probably be unaware of the full extent of someone else's internal hallucinatory experiences, whilst it seems reasonable to believe that delusions and misidentifications are almost certain to reveal themselves to an informant. Visual hallucinations are commoner than auditory hallucinations and whilst olfactory, gustatory, and tactile hallucinations also occur in AD, they are much rarer. Studies in clinical settings have found prevalence rates for all hallucinations of between 10% (Mega *et al.* 1996) and 40% (Gilley *et al.* 1997) in AD. In their systematic review Ballard and Walker (1999) found mean prevalence rates of 21% for all hallucinations (14% for visual hallucinations and 7% for auditory hallucinations) in clinical settings.

Management of psychotic symptoms in AD

Pharmacological and non-pharmacological interventions may both be of benefit. General health matters should be dealt with, especially sensory deficits which may be exacerbating hallucinations. Increasing the general level of stimulation, e.g. by arranging day care or attendance at a day centre, may be of benefit to someone who has hallucinations or misidentifications. Other interventions can include playing soothing music, using video tapes of familiar figures in conversation, and (for someone with the mirror sign), removing the mirror.

Recent studies have begun to examine whether drug treatments are effective for psychosis in dementia. Antipsychotic drugs have been prescribed empirically for a long time but the 'typical' antipsychotics are likely to produce adverse effects in these vulnerable patients. Most studies have been small or used broad outcome measures such as behavioural change rather than focusing on specific symptoms, but two large randomized controlled trials have shown that treatment produces an improvement in psychotic symptoms in dementia. Katz *et al.* (1999) found psychosis to respond to risperidone (1 mg or 2 mg twice a day) whilst Street *et al.* (2000) similarly found psychosis to respond to olanzapine (5 mg or 10 mg a day). The latter study broke down the data to show that hallucinations (but not delusions) responded to the olanzapine. Encouraging results are emerging from the trials of cholinesterase inhibitors, and retrospective analyses appear to show they too improve psychotic symptoms in AD (Cummings and Masterman 1998). Results from specific trials examining this question are awaited.

Mood changes

Alterations in mood are also extremely common in dementia, with depression being the most common. Here we are concerned with depression occurring during established AD; the relationship of depression to AD as a risk factor is considered below and the concept of 'depressive pseudodementia' is dealt with in Chapter 27.

One problem is in deciding what is meant by the term 'depression'. Even if one separates out studies looking at depressed mood, depressive symptoms, and depressive syndromes this still leaves enormous variability, with rates varying from 0% to 87% for depressed mood (Knesevich *et al.* 1983; Merriam *et al.* 1988); from 0 to 89% for all depressive symptoms (Wragg and Jeste 1989); and from 0% to 30% for depressive syndromes (Burns *et al.* 1990*c*; Teri and Wagner 1991). These rates vary because different populations are sampled, different instruments are used, and different raters make the rating. Problems in the assessment of depressive symptoms also occur, because apathy can easily be mistaken for depression, whilst many depressive symptoms, e.g. poor appetite, weight loss, and sleep disturbance, are also common features of dementia itself.

In a review of studies examining depressive syndromes diagnosed using standardized criteria Ballard *et al.* (1996) found major depression to occur in 21% of dementia sufferers in clinical settings and 13% in the community. No clear association between depression and the severity of dementia has been found, with some studies showing depression to be more common in milder dementia and others showing the opposite.

Depression decreases the quality of life of dementia sufferers, may reduce the duration of survival (Burns *et al.* 1991*c*), and would therefore appear to be important to treat. However, depression and depressive symptoms are usually short-lived in dementia and pharmacotherapy is not without risks, as elderly people with dementia are very prone to adverse effects. Simple social interventions, e.g. befriending or a day centre, should be considered and drug treatment used only if the depression is severe or prolonged. Selective serotonin reuptake inhibitors (Nyth *et al.* 1992), moclobemide (Roth *et al.* 1996), and tricyclic antidepressants (TCAs) (Petracca *et al.* 1996) have all been shown to alleviate depression in dementia, but TCAs should be avoided because they worsen cognitive impairment and are associated with higher drop-out rates (Taragano *et al.* 1997).

Elevation of mood in dementia is much less common and less frequently studied than depression. Burns *et al.* (1990*c*) found only one patient (out of 178) who reported manic symptoms, and only six who had any observable evidence of mania. Other studies have reported higher rates of euphoria (Wragg and Jeste 1989). Anxiety has been much less studied than even euphoria in dementia but, consistent with clinical experience, it is common with studies finding a rate ranging from 30% (Mendez *et al.* 1990) to 50% (Patterson *et al.* 1990).

Behavioural symptoms

Changes in behaviour are common, and an estimate of the monthly prevalence of some of the most important disturbances is given in Table 24ii.4 above.

Apathy

Apathy is diminished motivation and manifests itself as a listlessness in which the patient has lost the drive to engage in activities. It is often confused with low mood and anhedonia, which is a loss of ability to enjoy previously pleasurable activities. Although they may all be present together, they are not the same phenomenon (Levy *et al.* 1998). The distinction is important because carers often think someone with AD is depressed when he has apathy as a part of his dementia. Apathy is probably the most common behavioural change in AD and Mega *et al.* (1996) detected apathy in 72% of outpatients with AD. Apathy is common early in AD, typically becoming more severe as the cognitive impairment worsens. At presentation, apathy is frequently a complaint given by relatives who often misunderstand it as laziness and become frustrated by it. Explaining that apathy is a feature of dementia can remove this misunderstanding and the tension it brings. Failure by paid staff to engage an apathetic patient in some constructive activity is often regarded by relatives as evidence of poor care. Although there are no licensed treatments available at the present time for apathy, there is evidence accumulating that the cholinesterase inhibitors are especially effective in treating this symptom and they may be considered as an intervention (McKeith *et al.* 2000*b*,*c*).

Overactivity

A number of overlapping phenomena involving overactive behaviour are commonly found in AD. The most well known are agitation, which may be defined as painful inner tension associated with excessive motor activity (American Psychiatric Association 1994), and wandering. However, other 'aberrant motor behaviours' are recognized and sometimes measured, e.g. rummaging in drawers and repeatedly taking clothes on and off. All such overactive behaviours tend to become more common with increasing severity of the dementia. Wandering is found in about 20% of people with AD (Burns *et al.* 1990*d*) and the only other available figures for overactive behaviours are for agitation, which is found in about 30% of people with AD (Cohen *et al.* 1993). Several drugs may help such behaviours and, while low-dose antipsychotics are the most widely prescribed, carbamazepine may also be helpful (Tariot *et al.* 1998).

Aggression

Aggression is a major problem in dementia. It is common, and when present causes great distress to the carers and is a common reason for admission to hospital and transfer to residential care. It is open to different definitions and even when verbal aggression (shouting, swearing) is distinguished from physical aggression (punching, kicking, biting, pushing, pinching, etc.) there is still much scope for differences of opinion in each category about what constitutes aggression. Burns *et al.* (1990*d*) defined aggression narrowly as behaviour liable to cause physical injury to others, and still found 20% of their AD subjects to have aggression. Broader definitions naturally lead to higher figures and verbal aggression is usually found to be two to three times more common than physical aggression. Burns *et al.* (1990*d*) found aggression to be much more common in male sufferers of AD. They also found that it became more common with increasing cognitive impairment rising, from 8% in mild AD to 24% in severe AD. Two large randomized controlled trials have demonstrated significant improvement in aggression in severe dementia using risperidone (1 mg and 2 mg twice a day) (Katz *et al.* 1999) and olanzapine (5 mg and 10 mg a day) (Street *et al.* 2000); carbamazepine (at about 300 mg a day) has also been shown to reduce aggression in this population (Tariot *et al.* 1998).

Neurovegetative symptoms

Sleep
Sleep disturbance is another common feature of dementia that can have devastating consequences for carers. It may take the form of frequent wakings, reduced sleep quality, or a disturbance to circadian rhythms. The well-recognized day–night reversal was found to occur in 28% of patients in one study (Reisberg *et al.* 1987), and studies of all forms of sleep disturbance show a prevalence of between 45% and 70% in AD patients (Rabins *et al.* 1982; Merriam *et al.* 1988). To reduce the strain from sleep disturbance the spouse may sleep in another bed or in another room, and psychotropic medication (hypnotics and antipsychotics) is frequently prescribed. Persistent sleep deprivation can eventually lead to exhaustion for the spouse if it persists, especially when it is associated with night wandering. Respite care can then be of great help, although placement in residential care may finally be needed.

Eating
Difficulties with feeding are common in dementia. These tend to progress from initial problems using cutlery with associated spillage of food through to complete dependence on others for feeding. In addition, there may be specific problem behaviours related to eating. Some patients refuse food, whilst others stuff food rapidly and clumsily into their mouths. The latter binge-eating is common, occurring in 10% of people with AD (Burns *et al.* 1990*d*), a figure which is constant for all severities of dementia. It may be part of a wider Klüver–Bucy syndrome, although the full syndrome is rare (Burns *et al.* 1990*d*).

Sexual disinhibition
Sexual disinhibition is also a feature of the Klüver–Bucy syndrome and is another problem which causes great distress to carers. It occurs in about 7% of dementia sufferers, but unlike binge-eating it is rare in mild dementia and increases markedly with dementia severity (Burns *et al.* 1990*d*).

Personality changes

Alterations in personality are ubiquitous in dementia and changes in personality are inseparable from some of the above behavioural changes, e.g. apathy and sexual disinhibition. However, it is important to note that they do occur very early in AD and that 75% of people with mild AD show personality changes (Rubin *et al.* 1987). These may precede the cognitive deficits and are often subtle in form, but none the less they are frequently recognized and commented upon by carers. Such information should be cautiously interpreted, as family and friends are often too closely involved to be able to comment accurately and dispassionately and may either exaggerate or deny any changes. As the AD progresses these initially subtle personality alterations tend to become more evident.

Personality changes not mentioned in the above section on behavioural changes are suspiciousness and disengagement. Suspiciousness is common and was found in 25% of AD subjects (Patterson and Bolger 1994). It may or may not eventually consolidate into frank paranoid delusions; and can cause great friction as repeated accusations are made about the motives and behaviour of well-meaning carers and relatives. Disengagement refers to the detached state of emotional indifference often seen in AD and which is associated with a loss of rapport with other people. The patient is no longer concerned about the feelings of others or affected by their attention or lack of it. Such disengagement can be upsetting to relatives and needs to be distinguished from the low mood of depression.

Physical symptoms

Neurological

Early in AD the neurological examination is usually normal. Focal neurological signs suggest a vascular dementia or other cause of focal damage, whilst extrapyramidal signs indicate DLB. Primitive reflexes, however, may occur early in AD, although their frequency increases as the dementia worsens. Burns *et al.* (1991*a*) found the snout reflex was easily the most common, occurring in 41% of their clinical sample. The grasp reflex was identified in 7% and the palmomental in 2.5%. As the disease progresses, non-specific changes occur in both gait and balance and myoclonic jerks and other seizures may develop. Bilateral non-focal signs (e.g. upgoing plantars) may be seen in the late stage.

Incontinence

Urinary incontinence is a common and well-recognized feature of AD and has been found in 48% of AD subjects (Burns *et al.* 1990*d*), though this figure disguises its strong association with disease severity. Incontinence was found in only 8% of those with mild AD but in 94% of patients with severe AD (Burns *et al.* 1990*d*). This association has important implications in diagnosis as incontinence early in a dementia is characteristic of other dementias, especially frontotemporal dementia and normal-pressure hydrocephalus. Thus the presence of urinary incontinence early in a dementia should lead to a more serious search for possible causes other than AD. It is also vital to consider and exclude other causes of incontinence. Urinary tract infections, especially in women, are a common finding and may be causing the incontinence rather than the dementia. Also the incontinence may result from poor mobility or failure to find the toilet in a strange environment (e.g. when someone has just been admitted to an inpatient unit).

General physical changes

AD is associated with a general physical deterioration, in which the patient loses weight and develops a stooped posture associated with instability and gait abnormalities. Weight loss may be an intrinsic feature of the disease process or secondary to the progressive impairments, which can result in an inadequate consumption of food and fluids. Cronin-Stubbs *et al.* (1997) demonstrated that older people with AD lost weight at over 3.5 times the rate of healthy age-matched controls, a rate of weight loss more severe than in elderly people with cancer. Weight loss was found to be more rapid in the earlier stages of the disease, suggesting it is, at least in part, due directly to the disease process. Whatever the cause, this marked weight loss is likely to contribute to the high mortality of AD.

Summary

Whilst cognitive symptoms are central to the diagnosis of AD, non-cognitive symptoms are arguably of more importance in management. Psychotic and mood symptoms are very common, a cause of distress to both patients and carers, and, in many cases, treatable in their own right. The behavioural disturbances, accompanying personality changes, and neurovegetative symptoms are also much more common than is usually recognized, all of which place great strain on carers. Psychosocial interventions are usually necessary, whilst some of the symptoms (apathy, agitation, aggression, sleep disturbance) may respond to pharmacological treatment. The physical symptoms in AD remind us it is a debilitating condition requiring ongoing assessment and long-term palliative care.

Aetiology of Alzheimer's disease

Identifying risk factors for AD is important for two main reasons. Identification of risk factors and protective factors enables potentially new treatments or public health interventions to be developed. Second, these aetiological factors may throw light on the pathogenesis of AD, stimulating new research which can further our understanding of the disease process leading to new treatment opportunities. Table 24ii.5 summarizes our

Table 24ii.5 Aetiological factors in Alzheimer's disease

Established risk factors	Possible protective factors
Age	Anti-inflammatory medication
Family history	Oestrogen
Down's syndrome	Apolipoprotein $\varepsilon 2$ allele
Apolipoprotein $\varepsilon 4$ allele	High intelligence/education
Autosomal dominant mutations	
Probable risk factors	
Depression	
Hypertension	
Head injury	
Possible risk factors	
Female gender	
Low intelligence/education	
Diabetes	
Smoking	
Aluminium	

present state of knowledge concerning the aetiological factors involved in AD.

Risk factors

Demographic risk factors

Age

It is easily forgotten that old age is the most important risk factor for AD as its prevalence rises rapidly after 60, approximately doubling every 5 years. But for how long does such a rise continue? It is still not clear whether the increase continues indefinitely (so everyone would develop AD if they lived long enough) or tails off. There is evidence that the prevalence of dementia plateaus for people in their nineties and may even drop in the very old (Ritchie and Kildea 1995). However, incidence studies are a better measure of whether age itself is a causal factor in AD and dementia. A meta-analysis of such studies found that the incidence of both AD and dementia continues to increase with increasing age up to age 98, although the rate of acceleration does slow down (Gao *et al.* 1998). Studies of centenarians are clearly difficult to perform, but Blansjaar *et al.* (2000) identified all people over 100 years of age in an area of Holland and managed to assess 15 of these 17 individuals. All were found to be demented, with 12 having a moderate to severe dementia.

Sex

It is well recognized that AD is more common in women, but is female gender an independent risk factor? It could simply be that women live longer than men and consequently are at higher risk, or that they live longer with the illness. Such possibilities might confound prevalence but not incidence studies. One meta-analysis found women to have a higher incidence of AD than men but not a higher incidence of dementia in general (Gao *et al.* 1998). Another meta-analysis found that women tend to have a higher incidence in very old age but not in the younger old (Jorm and Jolley 1998), whilst a pooled analysis of four large prospective studies again found women to be at increased risk for AD and for those over 90 the women's rate was three times higher (Andersen *et al.* 1999). If further research supports such a sex-related risk then it could be related to postmenopausal changes in oestrogens or to an interaction of sex with apolipoprotein E genotype (Gao *et al.* 1998).

Ethnicity

Some studies show the incidence of AD differs in different parts of the world, and in a meta-analysis

Jorm and Jolley (1998) found dementia and AD to have a higher incidence in Europe than in East Asia. However, the way in which dementia is diagnosed shows significant differences even within the same culture, and such differences are likely to be more marked between different cultures and probably dwarf any real differences that may be present. Clearly, studies are needed in which identical methods are applied in a range of countries to determine whether real variations are present.

Genetic risk factors

Family history

Between 25 and 50% of people with AD have an affected relative. Van Duijn *et al.* (1991) conducted a meta-analysis which showed that those with a first-degree relative (parent, sibling, child) with AD had a 3.5-fold increased risk of developing AD. Generally those with an early onset of the disease (before 65 years) show a stronger familial risk, although they account for less than 5% of all AD cases. Conversely, the increased risk is very much less for those whose relatives develop AD in very old age. A number of important genes, which account for some of the genetic contribution, have been identified and are mentioned briefly below (see Chapter 7 for details).

Down's syndrome

Virtually all people with Down's syndrome have the neuropathological features of AD by the age of 40 years (Mann *et al.* 1986), which is probably due to them having a extra copy of the amyloid precursor protein gene located on chromosome 21. However, the prevalence of dementia in people with Down's syndrome is much less than 100% even by age 50, although it is clearly markedly elevated for age (Zigman *et al.* 1996). The reason for this discrepancy between pathology and functional impairment is not understood and complex interactions between maternal age and frequency of the *APOE* ε*4* allele (see below) have been proposed. In addition, the added difficulties of making an accurate clinical diagnosis in this group is likely to contribute to the variable findings.

Apolipoprotein E polymorphism

Apolipoprotein E (ApoE) is a plasma protein involved in lipid transport and its gene is located on chromosome 19 (19q13.2). It has three common alleles: ε*2*, ε*3*, and ε*4*, which in the normal population (in Caucasians) have allele frequencies of about 7%, 77%, and 16%, respectively (Zannis *et al.* 1993). Many studies have shown the ε*4* allele to be much more common in AD subjects, occurring in 30–50% (Roses 1996). A recent meta-analysis found age-adjusted odds ratios for AD of 2.6 for ε*2*/ε*4* heterozygotes, 3.2 for ε*3*/ε*4*, and 14.9 for ε*4*/ε*4* homozygotes (Farrer *et al.* 1997). Thus *APOE* ε*4* alleles have a dose-dependent effect in increasing the risk for AD. Other studies have demonstrated that the increased risk conferred by *APOE* ε*4* is related to it bringing forward the time of onset of AD (Roses 1996). However, these striking findings need to be put in context. Up to 50% of those who are homozygous for ε4 live to beyond 90 without developing AD and about two-thirds of those who develop AD have no ε4 allele (Henderson *et al.* 1995). It should also be noted that there is evidence that the ε2 allele may be protective, as Farrer *et al.* (1997) found an odds ratio for AD of 0.6 for the combined ε*2*/ε*2* and ε*2*/ε*3* genotypes.

Autosomal dominant gene mutations

So far, three genetic loci have been identified with mutations conferring an autosomal dominant pattern of inheritance for AD with almost complete penetrance. These are mutations in the *APP* (amyloid precursor protein) gene on chromosome 21, in the *presenilin-1* gene on chromosome 14, and in the *presenilin-2* gene on chromosome 1. All are associated with early-onset AD (before 65 years) but they account for less than 2% of all AD cases (Farrer *et al.* 1997); they do not seem to be present in even the majority of early-onset familial AD cases (Cruts *et al.* 1998). Their importance lies in the clues they are giving about the pathogenesis of AD. For example, these mutations all lead to an excessive production of the pathogenetic long-chain form of the amyloid beta protein (Ab42) (Hardy 1997), and the protein associated with *presenilin-1* may be an important enzyme (gamma-secretase) involved in producing this Ab42 protein (Saftig *et al.* 1999).

Other gene mutations

It is clear the above genes do not account for all the genetic contribution to AD and researchers are busy trying to identify further important genes. Two genes on chromosome 12 have been proposed as risk factors for AD: the low-density, lipoprotein receptor-related gene (Kang *et al.* 1997) and the alpha-2 macroglobulin gene (Liao *et al.* 1998). Each of these is of interest as they produce proteins which could play an important role in the pathogenesis of AD, but research findings are presently inconsistent for these and the other genes less frequently associated with an increased AD risk.

Intelligence and education

There is evidence that people with lower intelligence and educational attainments have an increased risk of developing AD. Some studies (though not all) have shown that people with a lower level of education have a higher rate of AD or cognitive impairment (Stern *et al.* 1994*b*; White *et al.* 1994; Farmer *et al.* 1995). The most obvious explanation for such findings is that cognitive tests, e.g. the MMSE, are sensitive to education and so poorly educated people cross the thresholds more easily, while better educated people are more able to compensate for their disease impairments and so present later (or not at all if death supervenes). Consistent with this, one functional neuroimaging study showed regional cerebral blood flow to be lower in better educated subjects in the parietal and temporal lobes compared with more poorly educated subjects who had been matched for the severity of their dementia, indicating the former had more advanced disease (Stern *et al.* 1992). However, it appears such parsimonious explanations (intelligent people compensate better and cognitive tests are insensitive to education) may not suffice as there is evidence that low premorbid intelligence, which is correlated with low education, directly influences the pathogenesis of AD. An epidemiological study, which has followed a group of nuns for many years, has shown not only that those nuns with lower verbal ability in early life (a proxy measure of intelligence) had poorer cognitive functioning and a higher rate of AD, but that at postmortem all those with neuropathological evidence of AD had low verbal ability (Snowdon *et al.* 1996). Therefore high intelligence may not just delay presentation through compensatory mechanisms but may actually protect against the pathological process of AD itself, or it may be linked to a more fundamental protective factor.

Depression

It is generally agreed that depression is often a prodromal feature of AD so that those early in their dementing process can appear initially to have a depression. But is depression an independent risk factor for developing dementia or AD? Jorm *et al.* (1991) performed a meta-analysis of four case-control studies and found late-onset AD cases had higher frequencies of treated episodes of depression earlier in life, suggesting depression is a risk factor. Since then some prospective studies have shown depression precedes cognitive impairment and may be a risk factor (Buntinx *et al.* 1996; Devanand *et al.* 1996), whilst others have found it does not predict cognitive decline or dementia (Dufouil *et al.* 1996; Henderson *et al.* 1997; Chen *et al.* 1999). If depression is a risk factor then its effects could be mediated by its association with high cortisol levels and hypothalamic–pituitary–adrenal axis activation, as animal studies have shown such features to be related to hippocampal atrophy (O'Brien 1997). Alternatively, increased vascular pathology associated with depression (Alexopoulos *et al.* 1997) could provide the link, as vascular factors are linked with increased AD (see below).

Vascular disease

Over recent years the debate about the relationship of AD to VaD has been complicated or clarified (depending on your view) by evidence that vascular disease may directly contribute to the pathology of AD. In fact this is far from a new idea, as in his original paper Alois Alzheimer (Alzheimer 1907) described vascular pathology at postmortem in Auguste D. Both apolipoprotein E and homocysteine (discussed elsewhere) are also vascular risk factors and may exert their pathogenic effects in AD via vascular disease. There is good evidence for hypertension as a risk factor for AD. A prospective study examining the effects of blood pressure on dementia found that hypertension 10 and 15 years earlier increased the rate of AD (Skoog *et al.* 1996). In addition, a treatment study, which examined whether treating systolic hypertension in the elderly would reduce the rate of dementia and AD, found that treatment produced a 50% reduction in dementia (mainly AD) over 2 years (Forette *et al.* 1998). Diabetes has also been found to increase the risk of dementia in general (relative risk 1.9) and, more specifically, AD (relative risk 1.9) (Ott *et al.* 1999). A case-control study has found that the use of statins (lipid-lowering agents) substantially reduces the risk of developing dementia, which was presumed to occur via their beneficial effects on vascular disease. However, as with a similar study on oestrogens (see below) the findings could be due to the confounding effects of incipient cognitive impairment and social class, which would make those at high risk of dementia less likely to use statins (Jick *et al.* 2000). Taken together such evidence suggests cerebral ischaemia may be involved in the pathogenesis of AD (Kalaria 2000).

Head injury

A meta-analysis of case-control studies of head injury (with loss of consciousness) showed it to be associated with an 80% increase in risk of AD (Mortimer *et al.* 1991). These early studies used retrospective assessments from relatives (raising the risk of recollection bias); and studies using medical records of head injury have shown no association (Williams *et al.* 1991; Breteler *et al.* 1995). Head injury has been shown to increase Aβ protein deposits in the brain, demonstrating a plausible mechanism for a link between head injury and AD (Roberts *et al.* 1991). It is therefore interesting to note that Mayeux *et al.* (1995) found that head injury is only a risk factor for AD in people with the *APOE* $\varepsilon 4$ allele.

Other possible risk factors

Aluminium

Studies some years ago showed increased aluminium levels in the brains of subjects with AD and also that aluminium is neurotoxic (Crapper *et al.* 1973; Trapp *et al.* 1978). This led to the suggestion that it may play a role in the causation of AD, and epidemiological studies found higher rates of AD in areas with a high aluminium content in the drinking water (Doll 1993). However, other studies did not confirm these early findings and it is clear that aluminium is neither necessary nor sufficient to cause AD (Walton 1991). Interest in this area has waned recently as other factors have now grabbed the limelight.

Smoking

A meta-analysis of case-control studies found smokers had a 20% reduction in AD (Graves *et al.* 1991). A plausible mechanism here is that smoking increases nicotinic receptors in the cortex and this could counteract the cholinergic deficit in AD (see Chapter 6). However, the only prospective study so far has found the opposite, with smokers having twice the risk of AD (Ott *et al.* 1998), and, given the other evidence for vascular factors in AD, smoking is probably best regarded as a risk factor at the present time.

Homocysteine

Another dietary factor implicated in the development of AD is the plasma protein homocysteine, which is also a proposed risk factor for cardiac disease. Some case-control studies have reported high homocysteine levels in AD (Clarke *et al.* 1998; McCaddon *et al.* 1998), but a prospective study found no relationship between homocysteine levels and cognitive impairment (Kalmijn *et al.* 1999).

Herpes simplex virus

One neuropathological study found herpes simplex virus type-1 to be a risk factor for AD in subjects with the *APOE ε4* allele but not in those without it (Itzhaki *et al.* 1997), suggesting an interaction between the virus and the ApoE protein.

Protective factors

Anti-inflammatory medication

A review of case-control studies has suggested that arthritis, non-steroidal anti-inflammatory drugs, and steroids are protective factors for AD, reducing the risk by about 50% (McGeer *et al.* 1996). This fits with current views that AD is associated with an inflammatory response in the brain, because senile plaques are associated with prominent astrocytosis and microglial activation (Dickson *et al.* 1988) and proinflammatory cytokines are increased in the brain in AD subjects (Wood *et al.* 1993). Such changes are believed to contribute to the neuronal damage and dysfunction. In addition, polymorphisms in genes subserving with the immune-inflammatory response, HLA-DR (Curran *et al.* 1997) and interleukin-1α (Du *et al.* 2000), have been associated with increased rates of AD. A dampener for the current enthusiasm about inflammation in AD is a randomized controlled trial examining the effect of prednisone over one year in patients with mild AD which showed no benefits and greater behavioural decline (Aisen *et al.* 2000).

Oestrogen

Another meta-analysis has examined the relationship between hormone (oestrogen) replacement therapy (HRT) and AD and found a 30% reduction in women taking HRT (Yaffe *et al.* 1998). However, there are possible confounds since better educated women tend to use HRT and people with cognitive impairment tend to forget to take their medication. Trials are in progress to examine this issue but initial findings are not optimistic. For example, Mulnard *et al.* (2000) conducted a randomized controlled trial of oestrogen replacement therapy in mild to moderate AD and found no benefits by one year.

Alcohol

Although case-control studies show no association in general between alcohol and AD (Graves *et al.* 1991), a prospective study found wine-drinking was protective for AD—reducing the risk by 80% for moderate drinkers compared with non-drinkers (Orgogozo *et al.* 1997). A mechanism for this protection could involve the antioxidant properties of red wine specifically rather than the alcohol itself. However, at least one prospective study has found an association between heavy alcohol consumption and dementia (Saunders *et al.* 1991), and whether alcohol is a risk factor or a preventive factor, or both, depending on a person's long-term intake, remains unclear.

Summary

At the present time there is clear evidence that age and family history are major risk factors for AD. A few key genes have been identified that are causal in some early-onset cases (*presenilin-1*, *presenilin-2*, and *APP*) and contribute in late-onset cases (Apolipoprotein E). Down's syndrome is the only other well-recognized risk factor and this is mediated via APP. Beyond this, the best current evidence supports depression, hypertension, and head injury as risk factors for AD. There is no conclusive evidence for other risk factors, but there is much current interest in diabetes and other vascular factors and low intelligence/education as risk factors, and in anti-inflammatory drugs and oestrogen as protective factors.

Prognosis of Alzheimer's disease

Until recently no specific treatments were available for AD and so, unlike most other psychiatric disorders, studies of prognosis were largely of the natural history of the condition. However, the introduction of the cholinesterase inhibitors (see Chapter 24vii) has now changed this and in future the effects of these new treatments on prognosis must be considered.

The natural history of Alzheimer's disease

Every old age psychiatrist is familiar with the considerable variability in the pattern, progress, and outcome of AD. All the studies following the natural history of the disease bear this out as they show substantial variations in symptomatology and rates of decline. The practical consequence of this for the clinician is that it makes it very difficult to give accurate predictions to patients or their families about the likely progress of the disease after the diagnosis has been made. Following the introduction of the cholinesterase inhibitors there has been a trend towards earlier diagnosis, which introduces further difficulties because the disease is being picked up at a time when currently available clinical and research experience does not apply. Furthermore, the effects of the drugs themselves in the longer term are unknown. These changes can make prognostic predictions at the present time even more perilous.

However, patients and relatives will continue to seek information on prognosis, and two of the most common outcomes of research interest are time to institutionalization (in some form of residential care) and time to death. Knopman *et al.* (1988) examined time from diagnosis to institutionalization and found that 12% of patients with mild AD were in nursing homes by 1 year and 35% by 2 years. For those severely affected at the outset the figures were 39% at 1 year and 62% at 2 years. Whilst helpful, such figures disguise the fact that certain kinds of symptom (agitation, wandering, aggression, and sleep disturbance) tend to precipitate much earlier institutionalization. These behaviours, which are very distressing for all concerned, are major predictors of early institutionalization (Haupt and Kurz 1993; Bianchetti *et al.* 1995). Time from diagnosis to death is highly variable, with the mean length of survival from diagnosis ranging from 1 year up to 16 years. This is naturally dependent on how early the diagnosis is made, although certain other factors, e.g. age at onset, are also important (see below under 'Predicting rates of decline'). However, studies do give a fairly consistent median survival of 5–6 years (Walsh *et al.* 1990; Heyman *et al.* 1996). Unsurprisingly, patients with the mildest clinical picture at the outset tend to show the longest times to both institutionalization and death.

The cause of death in AD can be difficult to determine. As with other chronic diseases in the elderly many people will die with the disease rather than from it. Since AD is associated with marked weight loss and physical decline (Cronin-Stubbs *et al.* 1997) it is clearly at least a contributory factor to death in many people with advanced disease, although frequently AD is not even mentioned on the death certificate (Burns *et al.* 1990*e*). Whether AD directly causes death is less certain, although it seems plausible as some sufferers do simply fade away without any other obvious cause for death occurring. Many others develop an infection or other complications of immobility and physical debilitation and die of some combination of causes.

Measuring rates of decline

Two kinds of instrument (global rating scales and cognitive scales) have been used to try and measure the rate of decline in patients with AD. The global measures, e.g. the Clinical Dementia Rating Scale (CDR) (Hughes *et al.* 1982), tend to change very slowly over a few years and so are not useful measures of change clinically. The cognitive scales do show significant changes over the course of a year. Some of these are in common use and a knowledge of the research figures may help a clinician to see how rapidly any patient is declining compared with these norms. Thus this could help clarify the prediction of progress and outcome, although the substantial variability should always be borne in mind. The annual rate of change in the Mini-Mental State Examination (MMSE) (Folstein *et al.* 1975) is about 2.5 points a year for moderately affected patients, with higher rates for more severely affected patients and lower rates for milder cases (Salmon *et al.*

1990). Two larger instruments are the CAMCOG (the cognitive component of the Cambridge Mental Disorders of the Elderly Examination (CAMDEX)) and the ADAS-Cog (the Alzheimer's Disease Assessment Scale-cognitive subscale). Burns *et al.* (1991*b*) used the CAMCOG to follow the progress of 110 AD patients. They found a drop of about 12 points in the first year (maximum score 107 with 80/79 as the cut-off for dementia). This included change in every main subsection, but many of the scores were already near the floor at baseline and this instrument appears less useful in more advanced dementia. A couple of studies have used the ADAS-Cog (maximum score 70) and have shown an annual rate of change of 8 to 9 points (Kramer-Ginsberg *et al.* 1988; Yesavage *et al.* 1988).

Predicting rates of decline

Within the rough framework of the above figures for rates of decline and time to institutionalization and death, are there any clinical features which can help sharpen the prediction in individual cases? The severity of the dementia is predictive in that the more severe the dementia the more rapid the rate of decline (Morris *et al.* 1993). Consistent with this, individual rates of decline are non-linear, being slower at the milder stage but accelerating as the dementia progresses (Teri *et al.* 1995). Age of onset is also a recognized predictor of deterioration, with early-onset dementias showing more rapid cognitive and functional decline (Jacobs *et al.* 1994; Teri *et al.* 1995).

Other factors which have been investigated without a clear conclusion include sex, level of education, *APOE* genotype, oestrogen, and NSAIDs.

The study of some key clinical features that may predict outcome has been complicated by the mixing together of patients with AD and DLB in earlier studies. Thus extrapyramidal symptoms were found to predict a more rapid decline in the earlier studies which would have included DLB patients (Miller *et al.* 1991). However, a more recent study in a purer AD group found no association with cognitive decline, but extrapyramidal symptoms were associated with greater functional decline and more rapid institutionalization (Lopez *et al.* 1997). A number of studies have found psychotic symptoms to predict more rapid deterioration, although when groups have been matched for severity of AD at outset the findings on this point have been mixed. Some studies have found psychosis does still predict rate of decline (Chui *et al.* 1994; Stern *et al.* 1994*a*), but others have not (Reisberg *et al.* 1986; Chen *et al.* 1991). One longitudinal study has not found depression to predict decline (Lopez *et al.* 1990) but, unsurprisingly, it has been shown to be associated with greater impairment of activities of daily living (Pearson *et al.* 1989). Both psychotic and depressive symptoms are clinically important regardless of whether they predict deterioration because they increase the suffering of the patients and their carers and, as discussed above, they should be treated in their own right.

The effects of drug treatment on prognosis

As mentioned above, antipsychotic drugs have been shown to adversely affect patients with DLB (Dickson *et al.* 1988; McKeith *et al.* 1992; Ballard *et al.* 1998) but there is some evidence that antipsychotics worsen dementia in AD too. McShane *et al.* (1997) found the use of antipsychotic medication increased the rate of cognitive decline and behavioural disturbance in a mixed group of patients with DSM-III-R dementia. This was not accounted for by DLB subjects, as most of the study patients had AD and there was no association of decline with Lewy body pathology at postmortem. It appears that whilst these widely prescribed drugs do show benefits in the short-term for specific symptoms (as shown above), there is a danger they may worsen patient status overall. At the present time the evidence is that they need close monitoring and regular review, with the aim of discontinuing treatment after 4–6 months to reduce the longer term risks.

What about cholinesterase inhibitors? At the outset here, we should remind ourselves these drugs clearly improve the prognosis of AD in the short-term for the 50–60% who respond to them (see Chapter 24vii). Patients enjoy improved cognitive function, a reduction in disturbed behaviour, and important gains in function in everyday life.

The duration for which such undoubted benefits last is not yet clear but should become so over the next few years. The other main issue to be resolved is the important question as to whether or not these drugs slow down the disease process itself: are they disease-modifying as well as symptomatic treatments? While theoretically they might modify the disease, as cholinergic stimulation may reduce the phosphorylation of tau (a key stage in tangle formation), no reliable data exists for a disease-slowing effect at present. Long-term, open-label treatment studies are somewhat suggestive (Rogers *et al.* 2000), though the comparison groups used in these studies may not be appropriate.

Summary

The pattern and progression of AD is highly variable. Predictors of decline are greater severity of illness and early age of onset, which both predict a more rapid course, and extrapyramidal and psychotic symptoms, which probably do so too. Whilst antipsychotic drugs are of benefit in the short-term in treating some non-cognitive symptoms, their long-term use may worsen the prognosis; cholinesterase inhibitors, on the other hand, improve prognosis in the short term but their effects in the longer term on the disease are unclear at the moment.

Appendix

Appendix 1: NINCDS-ADRDA Criteria for clinical diagnosis of Alzheimer's disease

I The criteria for the clinical diagnosis of PROBABLE Alzheimer's disease include:

dementia established by clinical examination and documented by the Mini-Mental Test, Blessed Dementia Scale, or some similar examination, and confirmed by neuropsychological tests;

deficits in two or more areas of cognition;

progressive worsening memory and other cognitive functions;

no disturbance of consciousness;

onset between ages 40 and 90, most often after age 65; and absence of systemic disorders or other brain diseases that in and of themselves could account for the progressive deficits in memory and cognition.

II The diagnosis of PROBABLE Alzheimer's disease is supported by:

progressive deterioration of specific cognitive functions such as language (aphasia), motor skills (apraxia) and perception (agnosia);

impaired activities of daily living and altered patterns of behaviour;

family history of similar disorders, particularly if confirmed neuropathologically and;

laboratory results of:

normal lumbar puncture as evaluated by standard techniques.

normal pattern or nonspecific changes in EEG, such as increased slow-wave activity, and

evidence of cerebral atrophy on CT with progression documented by serial observation.

III Other clinical features consistent with the diagnosis of PROBABLE Alzheimer's disease, after exclusion of causes of dementia other than Alzheimer's disease, include:

plateaus in the course of progression of the illness;

associated symptoms of depression, insomnia, incontinence, delusions, illusions, hallucinations, catastrophic verbal, emotional, or physical outbursts, sexual disorders, and weight loss;

other neurologic abnormalities in some patients, especially with more advanced disease and including motor signs such as increased muscle tone, myoclonus, or gait disorder;

seizures in advanced disease and;

CT normal for age.

IV Features that make the diagnosis of PROBABLE Alzheimer's disease uncertain or unlikely include:

sudden, apoplectic onset;

focal neurologic findings such as hemiparesis, sensory loss visual field deficits, and incoordination early in the course of the illness and;

seizures or gait disturbances at the onset or very early in the course of the illness.

V Clinical diagnosis of POSSIBLE Alzheimer's disease:

may be made on the basis of the dementia syndrome, in the absence of other neurologic, psychiatric, or systemic disorder sufficient to cause dementia, and in the presence of variation in the onset, in the presentation, or in the clinical course:

Appendix (*Continued*)

may be made in the presence of a second systemic or brain disorder sufficient to produce dementia, which is not considered to be the cause of the dementia and;

should be used in research studies when a single, gradually progressive severe cognitive deficit is identified in the absence of other identifiable cause.

VI Criteria for diagnosis of DEFINITE Alzheimer's disease are:

the clinical criteria for probable Alzheimer's disease and histopathologic evidence obtained from a biopsy or autopsy

VII Classification of Alzheimer's disease for research purpose should specify features that may differentiate subtypes of the disorder, such as:

familial occurrence;

onset before age 65;

presence of trisomy-21 and;

coexistence of other relevant conditions such as Parkinson's disease.

References

Aisen, P. S., Davis, K. L., Berg, J. D., *et al.* (2000). A randomized controlled trial of prednisone in Alzheimer's disease. Alzheimer's Disease Cooperative Study. *Neurology*, **54**, 588–93.

Alexopoulos, G. S., Meyers, B. S., Young, R. C., Campbell, S., Silbersweig, D., and Charlson, M. (1997). 'Vascular depression' hypothesis. *Archives of General Psychiatry*, **54**, 915–22.

Alzheimer, A. (1907). Uber eine eigenartig Erkrankung der Hirnrinde. *Allgemeine Zeitschrift für Psychiatrie und Psychisch Gerichtlich Medizin*, **64**, 146–8.

Andersen, K., Launer, L. J., Dewey, M. E., *et al.* (1999). Gender differences in the incidence of AD and vascular dementia: The EURODEM Studies. EURODEM Incidence Research Group. *Neurology*, **53**, 1992–7.

American Psychiatric Association. (1987). *Diagnostic and statistical manual of mental disorders—third edition revised*. APA, Washington DC.

American Psychiatric Association. (1994). *Diagnostic and statistical manual of mental disorders—fourth edition.* American Psychiatric Association, Washington DC.

Baldereschi, M., Amato, M. P., Nencini, P., *et al.* (1994). Cross-national interrater agreement on the clinical diagnostic criteria for dementia. WHO-PRA Age-Associated Dementia Working Group, WHO-Program for Research on Aging, Health of Elderly Program. *Neurology*, **44**, 239–42.

Ballard, C. G. and Walker, M. (1999). Neuropsychiatric Aspects of Alzheimer's Disease. *Current Psychiatry Reports*, **1**, 49–60.

Ballard, C. G., Bannister, C., and Oyebode, F, (1996). Depression in dementia sufferers. *International Journal of Geriatric Psychiatry*, **11**, 507–15.

Ballard, C., Grace, J., McKeith, I., and Holmes C (1998). Neuroleptic sensitivity in dementia with Lewy bodies and Alzheimer's disease. *Lancet*, **351**, 1032–3.

Bianchetti, A., Scuratti, A., Zanetti, O., *et al.* (1995). Predictors of mortality and institutionalization in Alzheimer disease patients 1 year after discharge from an Alzheimer dementia unit. *Dementia*, **6**, 108–12.

Blansjaar, B. A., Thomassen, R., and Van Schaick, H. W. (2000). Prevalence of dementia in centenarians. *International Journal of Geriatric Psychiatry*, **15**, 219–25.

Breteler, M. M., de Groot, R. R., van Romunde, L. K., and Hofman, A. (1995). Risk of dementia in patients with Parkinson's disease, epilepsy, and severe head trauma: a register-based follow-up study. *American Journal of Epidemiology*, **142**, 1300–5.

Buntinx, F., Kester, A., Bergers, J., and Knottnerus, J. A. (1996). Is depression in elderly people followed by dementia? A retrospective cohort study based in general practice. *Age and Ageing*, **25**, 231–3.

Burns, A., Jacoby, R., and Levy, R. (1990*a*). Psychiatric phenomena in Alzheimer's disease. I: Disorders of thought content. *British Journal of Psychiatry*, **157**, 72–6.

Burns, A., Jacoby, R., and Levy, R. (1990*b*). Psychiatric phenomena in Alzheimer's disease. II: Disorders of perception. *British Journal of Psychiatry*, **157**, 76–81.

Burns, A., Jacoby, R., and Levy, R. (1990*c*). Psychiatric phenomena in Alzheimer's disease. III: Disorders of mood. *British Journal of Psychiatry*, **157**, 81–6.

Burns, A., Jacoby, R., and Levy, R. (1990*d*). Psychiatric phenomena in Alzheimer's disease. IV: Disorders of behaviour. *British Journal of Psychiatry*, **157**, 86–94.

Burns, A., Jacoby, R., Luthert, P., and Levy, R. (1990*e*). Cause of death in Alzheimer's disease. *Age and Ageing*, **19**, 341–4.

Burns, A., Luthert, P., Levy, R., Jacoby, R., and Lantos, P. (1990*f*). Accuracy of clinical diagnosis of Alzheimer's disease. *British Medical Journal*, **301**, 1026.

Burns, A., Jacoby, R., and Levy, R. (1991*a*). Neurological signs in Alzheimer's disease. *Age and Ageing*, **20**, 45–51.

Burns, A., Jacoby, R., and Levy, R. (1991*b*). Progression of cognitive impairment in Alzheimer's disease. *Journal of the American Geriatrics Society*, **39**, 39–45.

Burns, A., Lewis, G., Jacoby, R., and Levy, R. (1991*c*). Factors affecting survival in Alzheimer's disease. *Psychological Medicin*, **21**, 363–70.

Chen, J. Y., Stern, Y., Sano, M., and Mayeux, R. (1991). Cumulative risks of developing extrapyramidal signs, psychosis, or myoclonus in the course of Alzheimer's disease. *Archives of Neurology*, **48**, 1141–3.

Chen, P., Ganguli, M., Mulsant, B. H., and DeKosky, S. T. (1999). The temporal relationship between depressive symptoms and dementia: a community-based prospective study. *Archives of General Psychiatry*, **56**, 261–6.

Chui, H. C., Lyness, S. A., Sobel, E., and Schneider, L. S. (1994). Extrapyramidal signs and psychiatric symptoms predict faster cognitive decline in Alzheimer's disease. *Archives of Neurology*, **51**, 676–81.

Clarke, R., Smith, A. D., Jobst, K. A., Refsum, H., Sutton, L., and Ueland, P. M. (1998). Folate, vitamin B12, and serum total homocysteine levels in confirmed Alzheimer disease. *Archives of Neurology*, **55**, 1449–55.

Cohen, D., Eisdorfer, C., Gorelick, P., *et al.* (1993). Psychopathology associated with Alzheimer's disease and related disorders. *Journal of Gerontology*, **48**, M255–60.

Cooper, J. K., Mungas, D., and Verma, M. (1991). Psychotic symptoms in Alzheimer's disease. *International Journal of Geriatric Psychiatry*, **6**, 721–6.

Crapper, D. R., Krishnan, S. S., and Dalton, A. J. (1973). Brain aluminum distribution in Alzheimer's disease and experimental neurofibrillary degeneration. *Transactions of the American Neurological Association*, **98**, 17–20.

Cronin-Stubbs, D., Beckett, L. A., Scherr, P. A., *et al.* (1997). Weight loss in people with Alzheimer's disease: a prospective population based analysis. *British Medical Journal*, **314**, 178–9.

Cruts, M., van Duijn, C. M., Backhovens, H., *et al.* (1998). Estimation of the genetic contribution of presenilin-1 and -2 mutations in a population-based study of presenile Alzheimer disease. *Human Molecular Genetics*, **7**, 43–51.

Cummings, J. L. and Masterman, D. L. (1998). Assessment of treatment-associated changes in behavior and cholinergic therapy of neuropsychiatric symptoms in Alzheimer's disease. *Journal of Clinical Psychiatry*, **59**, 23–30.

Curran, M., Middleton, D., Edwardson, J., *et al.* (1997). HLA-DR antigens associated with major genetic risk for late-onset Alzheimer's disease. *Neuroreport*, **8**, 1467–9.

Devanand, D. P., Sano, M., Tang, M. X., *et al.* (1996). Depressed mood and the incidence of Alzheimer's disease in the elderly living in the community. *Archives of General Psychiatry*, **53**, 175–82.

Dickson, D. W., Farlo, J., Davies, P., Crystal, H., Fuld, P., and Yen, S. H. (1988). Alzheimer's disease. A double-labeling immunohistochemical study of senile plaques. *American Journal of Pathology*, **132**, 86–101.

Doll, R. (1993). Review: Alzheimer's disease and environmental aluminium. *Age and Ageing*, **22**, 138–53.

Du, Y., Dodel, R. C., Eastwood, B. J., *et al.* (2000). Association of an interleukin 1 alpha polymorphism with Alzheimer's disease. *Neurology*, **55**, 480–3.

Dufouil, C., Fuhrer, R., Dartigues, J. F., and Alperovitch, A. (1996). Longitudinal analysis of the association between depressive symptomatology and cognitive deterioration. *American Journal of Epidemiology*, **144**, 634–41.

Farmer, M. E., Kittner, S. J., Rae, D. S., Bartko, J. J., and Regier, D. A. (1995). Education and change in cognitive function. The Epidemiologic Catchment Area Study. *Annals of Epidemiology*, **5**, 1–7.

Farrer, L. A., Cupples, L. A., Blackburn, S., *et al.* (1994). Interrater agreement for diagnosis of Alzheimer's disease, the MIRAGE study. *Neurology*, **44**, 652–6.

Farrer, L. A., Cupples, L. A., Haines, J. L., *et al.* (1997). Effects of age, sex, and ethnicity on the association between apolipoprotein E genotype and Alzheimer disease. A meta-analysis. APOE and Alzheimer Disease Meta Analysis Consortium. *Journal of the American Medical Association*, **278**, 1349–56.

Folstein, M. F., Folstein, S. E., and McHugh, P. R. (1975). 'Mini-mental state'. A practical method for grading the cognitive state of patients for the clinician. *Journal of Psychiatric Research*, **12**, 189–98.

Forette, F., Seux, M. L., Staessen, J. A., *et al.* (1998). Prevention of dementia in randomised double-blind placebo-controlled Systolic Hypertension in Europe (Syst-Eur) trial. *Lancet*, **352**, 1347–51.

Gao, S., Hendrie, H. C., Hall, K. S., and Hui, S. (1998). The relationships between age, sex, and the incidence of dementia and Alzheimer disease: a meta-analysis. *Archives of General Psychiatry*, **55**, 809–15.

Gilley, D. W., Wilson, R. S., Beckett, L. A., and Evans, D. A. (1997). Psychotic symptoms and physically aggressive behavior in Alzheimer's disease. *Journal of the American Geriatrics Society*, **45**, 1074–9.

Graves, A. B., van Duijn, C. M., Chandra, V., *et al.* (1991). Alcohol and tobacco consumption as risk factors for Alzheimer's disease: a collaborative re-analysis of case-control studies. EURODEM Risk Factors Research Group. *International Journal of Epidemiology*, **20**, S48–57.

Hachinski, V. C., Iliff, L. D., Zilhka, E., *et al.* (1975). Cerebral blood flow in dementia. *Archives of Neurology*, **32**, 632–7.

Hardy, J. (1997). Amyloid, the presenilins and Alzheimer's disease. *Trends in Neurosciences*, **20**, 154–9.

Haupt, M. and Kurz, A. (1993). Predictors of nursing home placement in patients with Alzheimer's disease. *International Journal of Geriatric Psychiatry*, **8**, 741–6.

Henderson, A. S., Easteal, S., Jorm, A. F., *et al.* (1995). Apolipoprotein E allele epsilon **4**, dementia, and cognitive decline in a population sample. *Lancet*, **346**, 1387–90.

Henderson, A. S., Korten, A. E., Jacomb, P. A., *et al.* (1997). The course of depression in the elderly: a longitudinal community-based study in Australia. *Psychological Medicine*, **27**, 119–29.

Heyman, A., Peterson, B., Fillenbaum, G., and Pieper, C. (1996). The consortium to establish a registry for Alzheimer's disease (CERAD). Part XIV: Demographic and clinical predictors of survival in patients with Alzheimer's disease. *Neurology*, **46**, 656–60.

Hirono, N., Mori, E., Yasuda, M., *et al.* (1998). Factors associated with psychotic symptoms in Alzheimer's disease. *Journal of Neurology, Neurosurgery and Psychiatry*, **64**, 648–52.

Hughes, C. P., Berg, L., Danziger, W. L., Coben, L. A., and Martin, R. L. (1982). A new clinical scale for the staging of dementia. *British Journal of Psychiatry*, **140**, 566–72.

Itzhaki, R. F., Lin, W. R., Shang, D., Wilcock, G. K., Faragher, B., and Jamieson, G. A. (1997). Herpes simplex virus type 1 in brain and risk of Alzheimer's disease. *Lancet*, **349**, 241–4.

Jacobs, D., Sano, M., Marder, K., *et al.* (1994). Age at onset of Alzheimer's disease: relation to pattern of cognitive dysfunction and rate of decline. *Neurology*, **44**, 1215–20.

Jick, H., Zornberg, G. L., Jick, S. S., *et al.* (2000). Statins and the risk of dementia. *Lancet*, **356**, 1627–31.

Jorm, A. F. and Jolley, D. (1998). The incidence of dementia: a meta-analysis. *Neurology*, **51**, 728–33.

Jorm, A. F., van Duijn, C. M., Chandra, V., *et al.* (1991). Psychiatric history and related exposures as risk factors for Alzheimer's disease: a collaborative re-analysis of case-control studies. EURODEM Risk Factors Research Group. *International Journal of Epidemiology*, **20**, S43–7.

Kalaria, R. N. (2000). The role of cerebral ischemia in Alzheimer's disease. *Neurobiology of Aging*, **21**, 321–30.

Kalmijn, S., Launer, L. J., Lindemans, J., Bots, M. L., Hofman, A., and Breteler, M. M. (1999). Total homocysteine and cognitive decline in a community-based sample of elderly subjects: the Rotterdam Study. *American Journal of Epidemiology*, **150**, 283–9.

Kang, D. E., Saitoh, T., Chen, X., *et al.* (1997). Genetic association of the low-density lipoprotein receptor-related protein gene (LRP), an apolipoprotein E receptor, with late-onset Alzheimer's disease. *Neurology*, **49**, 56–61.

Katz, I. R., Jeste, D. V., Mintzer, J. E., Clyde, C., Napolitano, J., and Brecher, M. (1999). Comparison of risperidone and placebo for psychosis and behavioral disturbances associated with dementia: a randomized, double-blind trial. Risperidone Study Group. *Journal of Clinical Psychiatry*, **60**, 107–15.

Knesevich, J. W., Martin, R. L., Berg, L., and Danziger, W. (1983). Preliminary report on affective symptoms in the early stages of senile dementia of the Alzheimer type. *American Journal of Psychiatry*, **140**, 233–5.

Knopman, D. S., Kitto, J., Deinard, S., and Heiring, J. (1988). Longitudinal study of death and institutionalization in patients with primary degenerative dementia. *Journal of the American Geriatrics Society*, **36**, 108–12.

Kramer-Ginsberg, E., Mohs, R. C., Aryan, M., *et al.* (1988). Clinical predictors of course for Alzheimer patients in a longitudinal study: a preliminary report. *Psychopharmacology Bulletin*, **24**, 458–62.

Levy, M. L., Cummings, J. L., Fairbanks, L. A., *et al.* (1998). Apathy is not depression. *Journal of Neuropsychiatry and Clinical Neurosciences*, **10**, 314–19.

Liao, A., Nitsch, R. M., Greenberg, S. M., *et al.* (1998). Genetic association of an alpha2-macroglobulin (Val1000lle) polymorphism and Alzheimer's disease. *Human Molecular Genetics*, **7**, 1953–6.

Lopez, O. L., Boller, F., Becker, J. T., Miller, M., and Reynolds, C. Fd. (1990). Alzheimer's disease and depression: neuropsychological impairment and progression of the illness. *American Journal of Psychiatry*, **147**, 855–60.

Lopez, O. L., Wisnieski, S. R., Becker, J. T., Boller, F., and DeKosky, S. T. (1997). Extrapyramidal signs in patients with probable Alzheimer disease. *Archives of Neurology*, **54**, 969–75.

McCaddon, A., Davies, G., Hudson, P., Tandy, S., and Cattell, H. (1998). Total homocysteine in senile dementia of Alzheimer type. *International Journal of Geriatric Psychiatry*, **13**, 235–9.

McGeer, P. L., Schulzer, M., and McGeer, E. G. (1996). Arthritis and anti-inflammatory agents as possible protective factors for Alzheimer's disease: a review of 17 epidemiologic studies. *Neurology*, **47**, 425–32.

McKeith, I., Fairbairn, A., Perry, R., Thompson, P., and Perry, E. (1992). Neuroleptic sensitivity in patients with senile dementia of Lewy body type. *British Medical Journal*, **305**, 673–8.

McKeith, I. G., Galasko, D., Kosaka, K., *et al.* (1996). Consensus guidelines for the clinical and pathologic diagnosis of dementia with Lewy bodies (DLB): report of the consortium on DLB international workshop. *Neurology*, **47**, 1113–24.

McKeith, I. G., Ballard, C. G., Perry, R. H., *et al.* (2000*a*). Prospective validation of consensus criteria for the diagnosis of dementia with Lewy bodies. *Neurology*, **54**, 1050–8.

McKeith, I. G., Del Ser, T., Spano, P., *et al.* (2000*b*). Efficacy of rivastigmine in dementia with Lewy Bodies: results of a randomised placebo-controlled international study. *Lancet*, **356**, 2031–6.

McKeith, I. G., Grace, J. B., Walker, Z., *et al.* (2000*c*). Rivastigmine in the treatment of dementia with Lewy Bodies: preliminary findings from an open trial. *International Journal of Geriatric Psychiatry*, **15**, 387–92.

McKhann, G., Drachman, D., Folstein, M., Katzman, R., Price, D., and Stadlan, E. M. (1984). Clinical diagnosis of Alzheimer's disease: report of the NINCDS-ADRDA Work Group under the auspices of Department of Health and Human Services Task Force on Alzheimer's Disease. *Neurology*, **34**, 939–44.

McShane, R., Keene, J., Gedling, K., Fairburn, C., Jacoby, R., and Hope, T. (1997). Do neuroleptic drugs hasten cognitive decline in dementia? Prospective study with necropsy follow up. *British Medical Journal*, **314**, 266–70.

Mann, D. M., Yates, P. O., Marcyniuk, B., and Ravindra, C. R. (1986). The topography of plaques and tangles in Down's syndrome patients of different ages. *Neuropathology and Applied Neurobiology*, **12**, 447–57.

Mayeux, R., Ottman, R., Maestre, G., *et al.* (1995). Synergistic effects of traumatic head injury and apolipoprotein-epsilon 4 in patients with Alzheimer's disease. *Neurology*, **45**, 555–7.

Mega, M. S., Cummings, J. L., Fiorello, T., and Gornbein, J. (1996). The spectrum of behavioral changes in Alzheimer's disease. *Neurology*, **46**, 130–5.

Mendez, M. F., Martin, R. J., Smyth, K. A., and Whitehouse, P. J. (1990). Psychiatric symptoms associated with Alzheimer's disease. *Journal of Neuropsychiatry and Clinical Neurosciences*, **2**, 28–33.

Merriam, A. E., Aronson, M. K., Gaston, P., Wey, S. L., and Katz, I. (1988). The psychiatric symptoms of Alzheimer's disease. *Journal of the American Geriatrics Society*, **36**, 7–12.

Miller, T. P., Tinklenberg, J. R., Brooks, J. O., and Yesavage, J. A. (1991). Cognitive decline in patients with Alzheimer disease: differences in patients with and without extrapyramidal signs. *Alzheimer Disease and Associated Disorders*, **5**, 251–6.

Morris, J. C., Edland, S., Clark, C., *et al.* (1993). The consortium to establish a registry for Alzheimer's disease (CERAD). Part IV. Rates of cognitive change in the longitudinal assessment of probable Alzheimer's disease. *Neurology*, **43**, 2457–65.

Mortimer, J. A., van Duijn, C. M., Chandra, V., *et al.* (1991). Head trauma as a risk factor for Alzheimer's disease: a collaborative re-analysis of case-control studies. EURODEM Risk Factors Research Group. *International Journal of Epidemiology*, **20**, S28–35.

Mulnard, R. A., Cotman, C. W., Kawas, C., *et al.* (2000). Estrogen replacement therapy for treatment of mild to moderate Alzheimer disease: a randomized controlled trial. Alzheimer's Disease Cooperative Study. *Journal of the American Medical Association*, **283**, 1007–15.

Nyth, A. L., Gottfries, C. G., Lyby, K., *et al.* (1992). A controlled multicenter clinical study of citalopram and placebo in elderly depressed patients with and without concomitant dementia. *Acta Psychiatrica Scandinavica*, **86**, 138–45.

O'Brien, J. T. (1997). The 'Glucocorticoid cascade' hypothesis in man. Prolonged stress may cause permanent brain damage. *British Journal of Psychiatry*, **170**, 199–201.

Orgogozo, J. M., Dartigues, J. F., Lafont, S., *et al.* (1997). Wine consumption and dementia in the elderly: a prospective community study in the Bordeaux area. *Revue Neurologique*, **153**, 185–92.

Ott, A., Slooter, A. J., Hofman, A., *et al.* (1998). Smoking and risk of dementia and Alzheimer's disease in a population-based cohort study, the Rotterdam Study. *Lancet*, **351**, 1840–3.

Ott, A., Stolk, R. P., van Harskamp, F., Pols, H. A., Hofman, A., and Breteler, M. M. (1999). Diabetes mellitus and the risk of dementia: The Rotterdam Study. *Neurology*, **53**, 1937–42.

Patterson, M. B. and Bolger, J. P. (1994). Assessment of behavioral symptoms in Alzheimer disease. *Alzheimer Disease and Associated Disorders*, **8**, 4–20.

Patterson, M. B., Schnell, A. H., Martin, R. J., Mendez, M. F., Smyth, K. A., and Whitehouse, P. J. (1990). Assessment of behavioral and affective symptoms in Alzheimer's disease. *Journal of Geriatric Psychiatry and Neurology*, **3**, 21–30.

Pearson, J. L., Teri, L., Reifler, B. V., and Raskind, M. A. (1989). Functional status and cognitive impairment in Alzheimer's patients with and without depression. *Journal of the American Geriatrics Society*, **37**, 1117–21.

Petracca, G., Teson, A., Chemerinski, E., Leiguarda, R., and Starkstein, S. E. (1996). A double-blind placebo-controlled study of clomipramine in depressed patients with Alzheimer's disease. *Journal of Neuropsychiatry and Clinical Neurosciences*, **8**, 270–5.

Rabins, P. V., Mace, N. L., and Lucas, M. J. (1982). The impact of dementia on the family. *Journal of the American Medical Association*, **248**, 333–5.

Reisberg, B., Ferris, S. H., Shulman, E., *et al.* (1986). Longitudinal course of normal aging and progressive dementia of the Alzheimer's type: a prospective study of 106 subjects over a 3.6 year mean interval. *Progress in Neuro-Psychopharmacology and Biological Psychiatry*, **10**, 571–8.

Reisberg, B., Borenstein, J., Salob, S. P., Ferris, S. H., Franssen, E., and Georgotas, A. (1987). Behavioral symptoms in Alzheimer's disease: phenomenology and treatment. *Journal of Clinical Psychiatry*, **48**, 9–15.

Ritchie, K. and Kildea, D. (1995). Is senile dementia 'age-related' or 'ageing-related'?—evidence from meta-analysis of dementia prevalence in the oldest old. *Lancet*, **346**, 931–4.

Roberts, G. W., Gentleman, S. M., Lynch, A., and Graham, D. I. (1991). beta A4 amyloid protein deposition in brain after head trauma. *Lancet*, **338**, 1422–3.

Robertson, B., Blennow, K., and Gottfries, C. G. (1998). Delirium in dementia. *International Journal of Geriatric Psychiatry*, **13**, 49–56.

Rogers, S. L., Doody, R. S., Pratt, R. D., and Ieni, J. R. (2000). Long-term efficacy and safety of donepezil in the treatment of Alzheimer's disease: final analysis of a US multicentre open-label study. *European Neuropsychopharmacology*, **10**, 195–203.

Roses, A. D. (1996). Apolipoprotein E alleles as risk factors in Alzheimer's disease. *Annual Review of Medicine*, **47**, 387–400.

Roth, M., Mountjoy, C. Q., and Amrein, R. (1996). Moclobemide in elderly patients with cognitive decline and depression: an international double-blind, placebo-controlled trial. *British Journal of Psychiatry*, **168**, 149–57.

Rubin, E. H., Morris, J. C., and Berg, L. (1987). The progression of personality changes in senile dementia of the Alzheimer's type. *Journal of the American Geriatrics Society*, **35**, 721–5.

Rubin, E. H., Drevets, W. C., and Burke, W. J. (1988). The nature of psychotic symptoms in senile dementia of the Alzheimer type. *Journal of Geriatric Psychiatry and Neurology*, **1**, 16–20.

Saftig, P., Hartmann, D., and De Strooper, B. (1999). The function of presenilin-1 in amyloid beta-peptide generation and brain development. *European Archives of Psychiatry and Clinical Neuroscience*, **249**, 271–9.

Salmon, D. P., Thal, L. J., Butters, N., and Heindel, W. C. (1990). Longitudinal evaluation of dementia of the Alzheimer type: a comparison of 3 standardized mental status examinations. *Neurology*, **40**, 1225–30.

Saunders, P. A., Copeland, J. R., Dewey, M. E., *et al.* (1991). Heavy drinking as a risk factor for depression and dementia in elderly men. Findings from the Liverpool longitudinal community study. *British Journal of Psychiatry*, **159**, 213–16.

Skoog, I., Lernfelt, B., Landahl, S., *et al.* (1996). 15-year longitudinal study of blood pressure and dementia. *Lancet*, **347**, 1141–5.

Snowdon, D. A., Kemper, S. J., Mortimer, J. A., Greiner, L. H., Wekstein, D. R., and Markesbery, W. R. (1996). Linguistic ability in early life and cognitive function and Alzheimer's disease in late life. Findings from the Nun Study. *Journal of the American Medical Association*, **275**, 528–32.

Stern, Y., Alexander, G. E., Prohovnik, I., and Mayeux, R. (1992). Inverse relationship between education and parietotemporal perfusion deficit in Alzheimer's disease. *Annals of Neurology*, **32**, 371–5.

Stern, Y., Albert, M., Brandt, J., *et al.* (1994*a*). Utility of extrapyramidal signs and psychosis as predictors of cognitive and functional decline, nursing home admission, and death in Alzheimer's disease: prospective analyses from the Predictors Study. *Neurology*, **44**, 2300–7.

Stern, Y., Gurland, B., Tatemichi, T. K., Tang, M. X., Wilder, D., and Mayeux, R. (1994*b*). Influence of education and occupation on the incidence of Alzheimer's disease. *Journal of the American Medical Association*, **271**, 1004–10. [See comments]

Street, J. S., Scott Clark, W., Cannon, K. S., *et al.* (2000). Olanzapine treatments of psychotic and behavioural symptoms in patients with Alzheimer's disease in nursing care facilities. *Archives of General Psychiatry*, **57**, 968–76.

Taragano, F. E., Lyketsos, C. G., Mangone, C. A., Allegri, R. F., and Comesana-Diaz, E. (1997). A double-blind, randomized, fixed-dose trial of fluoxetine vs. amitriptyline in the treatment of major depression complicating Alzheimer's disease. *Psychosomatics*, **38**, 246–52.

Tariot, P. N., Erb, R., Podgorski, C. A., *et al.* (1998). Efficacy and tolerability of carbamazepine for agitation and aggression in dementia. *American Journal of Psychiatry*, **155**, 54–61.

Teri, L. and Wagner, A. W. (1991). Assessment of depression in patients with Alzheimer's disease: concordance among informants. *Psychology and Aging*, **6**, 280–5.

Teri, L., McCurry, S. M., Edland, S. D., Kukull, W. A., and Larson, E. B. (1995). Cognitive decline in Alzheimer's disease: a longitudinal investigation of risk factors for accelerated decline. *Journals of Gerontology. Series, A., Biological Sciences and Medical Sciences*, **50A**, M49–55.

Trapp, G. A., Miner, G. D., Zimmerman, R. L., Mastri, A. R., and Heston, L. L. (1978). Aluminum levels in brain in Alzheimer's disease. *Biological Psychiatry*, **13**, 709–18.

van Duijn, C. M., Clayton, D., Chandra, V., *et al.* (1991). Familial aggregation of Alzheimer's disease and related disorders: a collaborative re-analysis of case-control studies. EURODEM Risk Factors Research Group. *International Journal of Epidemiology*, **20**, S13–20.

Walsh, J. S., Welch, H. G., and Larson, E. B. (1990). Survival of outpatients with Alzheimer-type dementia. *Annals of Internal Medicine*, **113**, 429–34.

Walton, L. (1991). *Alzheimer's disease and the environment*. Alden Press, Oxford.

White, L., Katzman, R., Losonczy, K., *et al.* (1994). Association of education with incidence of cognitive impairment in three established populations for epidemiologic studies of the elderly. *Journal of Clinical Epidemiology*, **47**, 363–74.

Williams, D. B., Annegers, J. F., Kokmen, E., O'Brien, P. C., and Kurland, L. T. (1991). Brain injury and neurologic sequelae: a cohort study of dementia, parkinsonism, and amyotrophic lateral sclerosis. *Neurology*, **41**, 1554–7.

Wood, J. A., Wood, P. L., Ryan, R., *et al.* (1993). Cytokine indices in Alzheimer's temporal cortex: no changes in mature IL-1 beta or IL-1RA but increases in the associated acute phase proteins IL-6, alpha 2-macroglobulin and C-reactive protein. *Brain Research*, **629**, 245–52.

World Health Organization. (1992). *International classification of diseases and health related problems—*10th revision. World Health Organization, Geneva.

Wragg, R. E. and Jeste, D. V. (1989). Overview of depression and psychosis in Alzheimer's disease. *American Journal of Psychiatry*, **146**, 577–87.

Yaffe, K., Sawaya, G., Lieberburg, I., and Grady, D. (1998). Estrogen therapy in postmenopausal women: effects on cognitive function and dementia. *Journal of the American Medical Association*, **279**, 688–95.

Yesavage, J. A., Poulsen, S. L., Sheikh, J., and Tanke, E. (1988). Rates of change of common measures of impairment in senile dementia of the Alzheimer's type. *Psychopharmacology Bulletin*, **24**, 531–4.

Zannis, V. I., Kardassis, D., and Zanni, E. E. (1993). Genetic mutations affecting human lipoproteins, their receptors, and their enzymes. *Advances in Human Genetics*, **21**, 145–319.

Zigman, W. B., Schupf, N., Sersen, E., and Silverman, W. (1996). Prevalence of dementia in adults with and without Down syndrome. *American Journal of Mental Retardation*, **100**, 403–12.

24iii Vascular dementia

Robert Stewart

Vascular dementia is unfortunately becoming a steadily more uncertain and controversial entity both for clinicians and researchers. In an attempt to unravel some of the confusion it is perhaps worth bearing in mind that this name has two meanings. One is vascular dementia as a 'subject heading' for the broad research field investigating the contribution principally of arterial disease to cognitive decline and, ultimately, dementia. The other is vascular dementia as a diagnostic category, describing cases where dementia is believed to have been caused by vascular disease. Since it is the diagnostic category where most of the controversy lies, this will be considered first.

Problems with the diagnosis

A historical perspective is useful. Throughout the first half of the twentieth century, later onset dementia was generally viewed as an inevitable consequence of ageing and, since atherosclerosis was a popular substrate for ageing, most dementia was therefore assumed to be 'vascular'. Seminal pathological studies in the 1960s and early 1970s challenged this by demonstrating the importance of Alzheimer's disease (AD), previously assumed to be principally a presenile dementia. However, it was also evident that a sizeable proportion of non-Alzheimer dementia was associated with multiple cerebral infarctions and therefore a second 'diagnosis' of multi-infarct dementia arose, later to be subsumed under the more broad category of vascular dementia. This system of subdividing dementia into separate categories has persisted into current diagnostic schedules. For vascular dementia, however, there have been developments since the early pathological studies, suggesting that it is necessary at least to reappraise its usefulness as a diagnosis:

- *Changing cohorts.* The populations of older people who died in the 1960s would have lived through decades when there was little opportunity to prevent or control cerebrovascular disease. More severe and florid pathology would have been expected at postmortem than would be the case (in developed nations) today.
- *New forms of cerebrovascular disease.* Early pathological studies predominantly focused on multiple cortical infarctions. Other more subtle forms of cerebrovascular pathology such as lacunar infarction, white matter disease, vascular amyloid deposition, and microangiopathy have subsequently been highlighted.
- *Advances in neuroimaging.* Clinical diagnostic criteria for multi-infarct or vascular dementia have traditionally relied on a history of vascular risk factors, a history suggestive of recurrent strokes, and examination for neurological deficits predominantly indicative of cortical stroke. Subsequent technological advances now allow *in vivo* identification of subclinical phenomena such as white matter changes and alterations in patterns of perfusion and connectivity (O'Brien 2000).

Vascular dementia as a diagnosis arose in a time when florid cerebrovascular disease was common, severe, and likely to be a primary underlying cause of dementia through multiple cortical infarctions. There was, therefore, some validity in viewing it as a categorical condition. However, this does not necessarily imply indefinite usefulness, particularly where more subtle pathological processes and changes on neuroimaging are identifiable. These factors are common in older age groups, individually are probably not sufficient to cause dementia, and cannot easily be separated or defined as being present or absent. They are better considered as existing across a spectrum of severity and are therefore poorly represented by a categorical diagnostic system. For vascular dementia to be considered as a diagnosis, it would be expected that it represented a discrete syndrome (dementia) with a clear primary cause ('vascular'), as well as having good clinical and clinicopathological reliability. However, it may be challenged as shown below:

- Vascular dementia is described as having a classic 'step-wise' clinical course related to the recurrent stroke episodes assumed to underlie the dementia. However, clinical course has been found to be poor at predicting pathological findings (Fischer *et al.* 1990).
- Dementia following clinical stroke frequently follows an AD-like clinical course and has been found to occur without further infarction in the majority of cases (Tatemichi *et al.* 1994; Kokmen *et al.* 1996).
- Disorders such as hypertension, diabetes, atrial fibrillation, and *in vivo* measures of atherosclerosis appear not only to be risk factors for vascular dementia but also for clinical AD (Stewart 1998).
- Postmortem studies report high rates of mixed cerebrovascular and Alzheimer pathology associated with dementia (Holmes *et al.* 1999). Cerebrovascular disease has been found to be rarely associated with dementia in the absence of Alzheimer pathology (Hulette *et al.* 1997).
- Clinical diagnostic criteria poorly reflect underlying pathology. In particular, NINDS-AIREN criteria for vascular dementia (Román *et al.* 1993) applied clinically were reported to have a high specificity but low sensitivity for vascular pathology at postmortem (Holmes *et al.* 1999). This implies that if a diagnosis of vascular dementia is made there is likely to be cerebrovascular pathology, but also that a substantial proportion of potentially important cerebrovascular pathology will be missed.
- Clinical diagnostic criteria show relatively low inter-rater reliability (Lopez *et al.* 1994; Chui *et al.* 2000). Higher agreement is found where criteria are used such as the Hachinski Ischemic Score (Hachinski *et al.* 1975), which essentially estimates the degree of cerebrovascular disease in the context of dementia. Much lower agreement is found where criteria also involve a judgement as to whether the dementia was caused by cerebrovascular disease. In addition, different diagnostic schedules show poor agreement with each other (Chui *et al.* 2000).
- Operational definitions of dementia have been criticized for focusing excessively on memory impairment and for poorly reflecting cognitive impairment relating to vascular disease, which more often affects non-memory domains such as executive function (Bowler and Hachinski 2000).

In summary, vascular dementia as a diagnosis may underestimate the contribution of vascular pathology to dementia, does not adequately represent mixed pathology, and makes assumptions about causality that may not be biologically valid and which probably underlie the low reliability of diagnostic criteria.

Specific syndromes

If 'vascular dementia' does not represent a discrete and reliably identifiable entity, its continued usefulness as a diagnostic category is questionable. However, particular syndromes are contained within this category which can reasonably be considered as diagnoses. These include genetic disorders such as 'cerebral autosomal dominant arteriopathy with sub-cortical infarcts and leucoencephalopathy' (CADASIL) (Stevens *et al.* 1977). This is a familial disorder manifesting as recurrent strokes (most often lacunar infarcts) usually in the fourth to sixth decades, occurring in the absence of vascular risk factors and associated in most cases with a subcortical dementia and pseudobulbar palsy. The principal underlying pathology is an abnormality in basal smooth muscle cells, predominantly in the media of small cerebral arteries, and underlying mutations have been successfully identified in the *Notch3* gene on chromosome 19 (Joutel *et al.* 1997). Other syndromes of familial

Table 24iii.1 Examples of specific vascular dementia syndromes

Genetic disorders
CADASIL
Hereditary cerebral haemorrhage with amyloidosis—Dutch and Icelandic types
Familial British dementia with amyloid angiopathy
Fabry's disease
Hereditary endotheliopathy with retinopathy, nephropathy, and stroke (HERNS)
Mitochondrial myopathy, encephalopathy, lactic acidosis, and stroke-like episodes (MELAS)
Strategic infarct dementia
Conditions associated with cerebrovascular pathology and secondary dementia
Subdural haematoma
Systemic lupus erythematosus
Polyarteritis nodosa
Buerger's disease
Polycythaemia rubra vera
Neurosyphilis

vascular dementia have been described (Table 24iii.1) and it is likely that, as with AD, further discrete disorders exist which may be explained by specific mutations.

As well as genetic disorders, cases of dementia have been described that appear to have been caused by specific single 'strategic' infarctions, most often within thalamic structures (Tatemichi *et al.* 1992*a*), and which may also be considered as discrete diagnoses. In addition, several non-cardiovascular disorders which may cause secondary dementia do so through their effects on the vasculature (Table 24iii.1).

The epidemiology of vascular and poststroke dementia

Although, as with AD, specific vascular dementia syndromes exist with discrete genetic or environmental causes, they are rare and do not explain most later onset dementia associated with vascular disease. Studies describing the incidence and prevalence of diagnosed vascular dementia have been excellently summarized and reviewed elsewhere (Hebert and Brayne 1995; Desmond 1996; Skoog and Aevarsson 2000). The difficulty is that, if diagnostic criteria have poor inter-rater reliability and poor agreement between different instruments, the generalizability of these studies is limited and, as discussed previously, they may poorly reflect the impact of subclinical cerebrovascular disease as a factor associated with dementia. Estimating the proportion of 'vascular' dementia cases (as opposed to AD, Lewy body dementia, etc.) also generates difficulties. Descriptive data of this kind may merely be illustrating the incidence or prevalence of comorbid stroke in dementia, and therefore are not an adequate way of representing mixed and overlapping pathology. One community-based, clinicopathological study of patients with dementia found a prevalence of clinically defined vascular dementia of 9%. However, on postmortem examination of the same group, infarction was present as a primary pathology in 14% and as a secondary pathology in a further 15% (Holmes *et al.* 1999). Risk factor studies are similarly problematic. Because all cases of vascular dementia have evidence of cerebrovascular disease by definition, any comparison with community controls runs the risk of identifying self-evident risk factors for stroke rather than dementia. An exception to this are studies, which will now be summarized, where case and control groups both have stroke but where those with dementia are compared to those without.

Stroke and dementia

Prospective studies have found that, 3 months after an acute stroke, prevalence rates of dementia are around 20–30% (Tatemichi *et al.* 1992*b*). This represents an approximate ninefold increase in age-adjusted risk (Pohjasvaara *et al.* 1998). Longer follow-up suggests that the relative risk then falls to approximately a twofold increase, which has been found to persist over at least two decades (Kokmen *et al.* 1996). Although strategic infarct dementia syndromes have been described (Tatemichi *et al.* 1992*a*), population-based studies have yet to demonstrate a clear association between stroke location and risk of dementia. Most find hemispheric infarctions to be associated with a higher risk, but show conflicting findings with respect to arterial territories (Censori *et al.* 1996; Pohjasvaara *et al.* 1998; Desmond *et al.* 2000). A study investigating dementia following lacunar infarction also found no association with lesion number or location (Loeb *et al.* 1992). Other factors identified as being associated with a risk of dementia following stroke (albeit not always consistently between studies) are increased age, lower levels of education, previous stroke disease, and vascular risk factors such as diabetes, recent smoking history, and atrial fibrillation (Censori *et al.* 1996; Pohjasvaara *et al.* 1998; Barba *et al.* 2000; Desmond *et al.* 2000). The role of blood pressure is uncertain: most report no association, but one study found that risk of dementia was associated with lower blood pressure and orthostatic changes (Pohjasvaara *et al.* 1998). Disorders associated with hypoxia and ischaemia (such as seizures, arrhythmias, and pneumonia) have also been found to be associated with higher risk of dementia after stroke (Moroney *et al.* 1996).

Although prospective studies following a major stroke represent an important advance in understanding dementia associated with cerebrovascular disease, they may not be generalizable to situations where multiple smaller infarctions have occurred. A differently designed study investigated factors associated with dementia in patients who had suffered multiple cerebral infarctions (Gorelick *et al.* 1993). Independent factors were found to be increased age, lower educational attainment, previous myocardial infarction, recent history of smoking, and lower systolic blood pressure. CT findings additionally associated with dementia were more severe stroke, left cortical infarction, and diffuse enlargement of the lateral ventricle suggesting cerebral atrophy (Gorelick *et al.* 1992).

As has been mentioned earlier, many cases of dementia following stroke appear to follow an AD-like clinical course and to occur without further episodes of infarction (Kokmen *et al.* 1996; Tatemichi *et al.* 1994). Prestroke cognitive decline has been found in many cases (Kase *et al.* 1998), and, on neuroimaging, appears to be associated with atrophic changes rather than early cerebrovascular disease (Pohjasvaara *et al.* 1999). In addition, not only does stroke predict cognitive impairment but cognitive impairment is also associated with a raised risk of future stroke (Ferucci *et al.* 1996), and dementia following stroke predicts further stroke episodes (Moroney *et al.* 1997). Taken together this evidence suggests there is a close (although potentially complex) inter-relationship between stroke and primary degenerative changes underlying many cases of apparent vascular dementia, and that the stroke itself may be a relatively late event in an ongoing process of insidious cognitive decline.

Vascular risk factors and dementia

If clinical stroke is strongly associated with dementia but in many cases does not appear to be the initiating event for cognitive decline, an important consideration is the role of risk factors for cerebrovascular disease that arise earlier in life and which may be precursors of both conditions. Hypertension, a powerful risk factor for cerebrovascular disease, has received particular attention (Stewart 1999). Although, it is only relatively recently that results of prospective studies have begun to clarify the relationship between blood pressure and dementia, it has repeatedly been found that raised blood pressure in mid-life predicts cognitive impairment 10–15 years later (Elias *et al.* 1993; Launer *et al.* 1995; Kilander *et al.* 1998). However, dementia tends to be associated with lower blood pressure in cross-sectional studies of older age groups (Guo *et al.* 1996), including poststroke dementia as mentioned earlier. This 'crossing-over' of association was neatly demonstrated in a Swedish longitudinal study where 80- to 85-year-old participants developing dementia (principally AD) had higher blood pressure 10 years earlier than those without dementia, but lower blood pressure at the time dementia was diagnosed (Skoog *et al.* 1996).

Although raised lipid levels have received less attention than blood pressure as risk factors for dementia, preliminary evidence suggests a similar pattern of association. One study in Finland found that 20–30 years earlier, people with AD had higher recorded levels of cholesterol than controls, but that cholesterol levels had declined in the AD group prior to diagnosis (Notkola *et al.* 1998).

Type-2 (non-insulin-dependent) diabetes has also been found to be a risk factor for dementia (both vascular dementia and AD), particularly in those receiving or requiring insulin treatment (Ott *et al.* 1999). Strong interactions were reported between hypertension and diabetes as predictors of cognitive impairment in one study (Elias *et al.* 1997). However much of the effect of diabetes on the risk of dementia appears to be independent of cerebrovascular disease and may involve other non-vascular pathways or common underlying factors (Stewart and Liolitsa 1999).

Other vascular factors associated with dementia include ECG ischaemia (Prince *et al.* 1994) and atrial fibrillation (Ott *et al.* 1997), as well as measures of peripheral and carotid atherosclerosis (Hofman *et al.* 1997). Early reports that smoking might be protective against AD appear to have arisen because of biased recall and effects on mortality. More recent findings from larger populations have suggested that smoking is, if anything, a risk factor for all types of dementia, although this effect may be restricted to particular subgroups (Ott *et al.* 1998).

Mechanisms of association

What is becoming increasingly apparent is that vascular disorders such as hypertension, diabetes, and dyslipidaemia are associated with an increased risk both of vascular dementia and AD, as diagnosed clinically. One possible explanation is that dementia with subclinical cerebrovascular disease was 'misclassified' as AD in these studies, although, as discussed above, any process that attempts to classify cerebrovascular disease as being present or absent has questionable validity. What is observed is that dementia associated with vascular disease is gradually progressive and not explained by multiple infarctions in many cases. A substantial proportion of subjects with missed infarctions would be required to explain these findings, and this is not supported by neuroimaging data (Ott *et al.* 1999). Other processes must therefore be considered (Fig. 24iii.1). One explanation would be that there are forms of silent cerebrovascular disease which cause a gradually progressive dementia. However, if this was an important phenomenon then substantially more 'pure' vascular dementia would be observed in postmortem series than is generally reported (Hulette *et al.* 1997).

A more likely explanation lies in potential links between vascular disease and AD. These may involve four possible pathways, which of course need not be mutually exclusive:

- Vascular disease may directly induce or accelerate pathological processes underlying AD.
- Cerebrovascular disease and AD may interact in their cognitive effects, influencing the onset of clinical dementia.
- Common factors may underlie both disorders.
- AD may cause or exacerbate cerebrovascular disease.

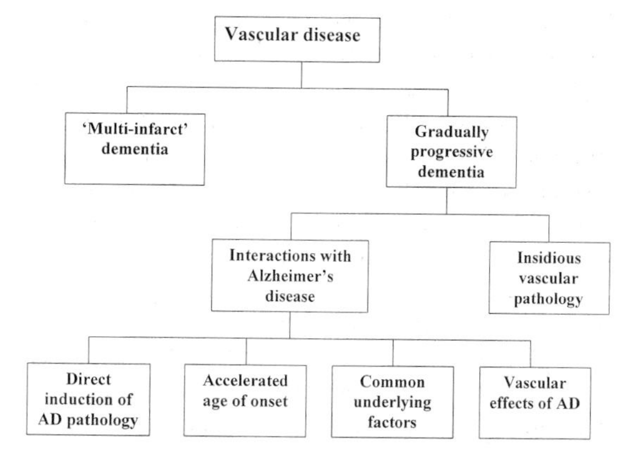

With respect to the first pathway, there are numerous possible ways in which vascular disease may induce or accelerate Alzheimer pathology (Stewart 1998). These include amyloid deposition as a response to ischaemia, links through inflammatory pathways, blood–brain barrier disturbance secondary to cerebrovascular disease and, for diabetes, abnormal protein glycosylation secondary to prolonged hyperglycaemia. However, while these mechanisms are theoretically possible, there is a lack of evidence supporting their involvement. In particular, they predict that increased Alzheimer pathology should be observed at postmortem in association with cerebrovascular disease or vascular risk factors. While one research group have reported this to be the case in non-demented subjects with hypertension or coronary artery disease (Sparks *et al.* 1995, 1996), these findings have yet to be replicated and no increased Alzheimer pathology has been observed in association with diabetes or cerebral infarction (Heitner and Dickson 1997; Snowdon *et al.* 1997).

The second possible pathway suggests that, rather than acting directly on the progression of Alzheimer pathology, vascular disorders accelerate the onset of symptomatic dementia at relatively early stages of comorbid AD. This was observed in a study in the US of elderly nuns who were screened for cognitive function in late life, and a large proportion of whom were followed to postmortem (Snowdon *et al.* 1997). The density of neurofibrillary tangles was found to correlate strongly with previous dementia but showed no association with the presence or absence of cerebral infarction. However, if infarction was present, a lower density of tangles was observed in association with dementia, suggesting the dementia had manifested at an earlier pathological stage. In addition, cerebral infarction was only associated with cognitive impairment if AD pathology was also present. Similar findings were observed in the Oxford OPTIMA study: early Alzheimer pathology was associated with much greater cognitive impairment if cerebrovascular disease was also present (Esiri *et al.* 1999). However, the cognitive impairment associated with later stages of AD did not appear to be influenced by the presence or absence of cerebrovascular disease. One possible explanation is that memory impairment secondary to early AD may be more likely to be noticed as dementia if other cognitive domains are also affected. White matter disease may be important in this respect, in that subtle disruption of frontosubcortical pathways may result in impaired executive function. White matter hyperintensities on magnetic resonance imaging (MRI) are common in older age groups and are associated with vascular risk factors, particularly hypertension (Breteler *et al.* 1994*a*). The pathological basis for these findings on imaging, however, is still controversial. Although they are more common in dementia and, across a population, are associated with relative cognitive impairment (Breteler *et al.* 1994*b*), at an individual level they may be severe without any apparent clinical manifestations (Fein *et al.* 1990). They do not therefore appear to be sufficient in themselves to cause dementia, but may precipitate it in the presence of other pathology such as early AD.

The third possible pathway is via common factors underlying both vascular disease and AD. Vascular risk factors such as hypertension and diabetes are commonly classified as potential 'environmental' risk factors for dementia. However, they are known to have a substantial familial aetiology and it is possible that common genetic factors explain some of their association with AD (Lovestone 1999; Stewart and Liolitsa 1999). Other factors such as diet, physical activity, and personality could also potentially underlie later associations.

A final possible explanation is that AD causes or exacerbates cerebrovascular disease. Even prospective studies cannot conclusively demonstrate the direction of effect where pathological processes may be operating one or two decades before clinical symptoms become manifest. Given that most vascular risk factors manifest in age groups well before dementia starts to become common, it is unlikely that AD initiates hypertension or diabetes for instance. However, deposition of amyloid occurs in cerebral blood vessels as well as the brain parenchyma in AD, and this 'amyloid angiopathy' is associated with both cerebral haemorrhage and small infarctions (Olichney *et al.* 2000). Abnormalities in capillary structure have also been reported in AD (de la Torre and Mussivand 1993). It is therefore possible that the presence of AD may exacerbate or accelerate vascular pathology or render the brain more vulnerable to further insults. Other 'reverse' mechanisms with more direct clinical implications would be the possible effects that early cognitive decline might have on factors such as diet, exercise, and compliance with medication—and therefore on the risk of cerebrovascular events.

Clinical implications

What implications does current research have for clinicians? In theory, these should be numerous since vascular disease is one of few potentially modifiable risk factors for dementia. However, although research attention is increasing in this area, there is woefully little direct evidence at present for the benefit of any intervention to prevent or treat dementia through modifying vascular risk. Despite this, there are particular issues which can be addressed to some extent.

Treatment of dementia

If vascular disease were to cause dementia through the cumulative effect of multiple infarctions, through more gradually progressive cerebrovascular disease, or through direct effects on AD progression, then it is likely that these processes would continue to contribute to the progression of disease after diagnosis. Interventions to halt or slow the progression of vascular disease could therefore be expected at least to prevent further cognitive decline, if not improve cognitive function to some extent. However, as mentioned above, there has been little research into potential interventions. Even for aspirin, only one randomized trial has been published: a pilot study of 70 patients with multi-infarct dementia randomized to aspirin or no additional treatment over 3 years (Meyer *et al.* 1989). Improvement in cognitive scores and cerebral blood flow were noted over the first 2 years in the treatment group. However, the protocol did not involve a placebo and participants were not blind to their allocation. Another study found that men at high risk of cardiovascular disease who had received warfarin or aspirin (as part of a randomized double-blind trial) had better verbal fluency and mental flexibility test scores at the end of a 5-year trial period than those receiving placebo (Richards *et al.* 1997). Cognitive assessment was not carried out at the start of the trial but, since allocation was randomized and groups were similar in many other respects, it is likely that this represents an effect of the intervention. The association with higher cognitive scores was principally in those receiving aspirin rather than warfarin.

Treatment of vascular illness in dementia

In summary, evidence is lacking at present to support the modification of vascular disease as an effective treatment of dementia. However, there is also little evidence at present against such measures. It is perhaps worth considering that the prescription of aspirin or the treatment of hypertension in a patient with dementia and cerebrovascular disease might not only be carried out in the hope of preventing further cognitive decline but also to prevent stroke. Complex ethical issues surround the question of how intensively to treat comorbid disease in individuals with clinical dementia, particularly when the dementia is at an advanced stage. In addition, although there may be no upper age limit for stroke prevention (Staessen *et al.* 2000), the effectiveness of interventions such as blood pressure control has not been assessed in the context of multiple infarction and dementia. However, it is important to bear in mind that, while an acute fatal stroke may be a preferable alternative to end-stage dementia, a non-fatal episode may represent a potentially lengthy period of disability and suffering that might have been prevented.

Iatrogenic dementia?

As has been discussed earlier, although high blood pressure is a risk factor for dementia, blood pressure is frequently lower than average by the time dementia has developed. A concern obviously arises that overzealous correction of blood pressure may itself be a risk factor for dementia (for example, through episodes of hypoperfusion, and ischaemia or infarction in critical 'watershed' zones). However, currently there is little evidence to support this. In the context of randomized clinical trials, blood pressure reduction in hypertension, if anything, has a beneficial effect on risk of dementia (Forette *et al.* 1998), and has not been found to be associated with cognitive decline (Prince *et al.* 1996). Blood pressure is also observed to be progressively lower at increasingly advanced stages of dementia (Guo *et al.* 1996), suggesting that it is a secondary phenomenon and/or a marker of general physical frailty. One observational study of patients with multi-infarct dementia (Meyer *et al.* 1986) suggested that a better clinical course occurred if systolic blood pressure remained within the 'upper limits of normal' (that is 135 to 150 mmHg) compared to lower levels. However, it cannot be concluded whether this observation was explained by blood pressure treatment, factors associated with the dementia, or comorbid disease.

Prevention of dementia

The mechanism or mechanisms by which vascular disease is associated with dementia are of substantial importance in determining the effectiveness of potential interventions. As already discussed, if vascular disease causes dementia through multiple infarcts or through direct effects on AD progression, it would imply that dementia could either be prevented if the intervention is early enough, or at least be stabilized at a later stage. If a common genetic factor explains the association between vascular disease and dementia, there would be no opportunity for prevention or treatment unless the genetic effect could be modified. If vascular disease accelerates the age of onset of dementia in the context of comorbid AD (the mechanism most supported by current pathological evidence), there may be little effect of modifying vascular risk, once dementia was present, on subsequent clinical progression. However, at a population level, there would be ample opportunity to reduce incidence rates of dementia through delaying the age of onset. Because disorders such as hypertension and diabetes have high prevalence rates, even a small increase in the effect on an individual's risk of dementia may translate into a large excess of cases across a population. Relatively little research has attempted to quantify the impact of these disorders, but 9% of new AD cases over 2 years could be attributed to diabetes alone (Ott *et al.* 1999), and the risk of severe cognitive impairment in later life was found to increase by 5% for each 10 mmHg increment (increase) in mid-life systolic blood pressure (Launer *et al.* 1995). It therefore follows that even a small reduction in blood pressure across a population might have a substantial effect on rates of later dementia. Supporting this, one large randomized, placebo-controlled trial of treatment for isolated systolic hypertension in older people found a 50% reduction in the number of cases of dementia (mostly AD) over a 2-year period in the treatment compared to the placebo group (Forette *et al.* 1998). The numbers of cases were, as might be expected, relatively small and further research is clearly required.

Other risk factors for cerebrovascular disease have received less attention. However, two large recent studies have found a negative association between Alzheimer's disease and a previous prescription of cholesterol-lowering agents (Jick *et al.* 2000; Wolozin *et al.* 2000). The association appeared to be specific to statins (HMG CoA-reductase inhibitors) but only for specific agents within this class: a finding that is difficult to explain (Wolozin *et al.* 2000). It remains to be clarified whether these associations are truly causal and, if so, whether any protection conferred is mediated by reduced comorbid vascular disease or is related to specific effects of circulating cholesterol on the progression of Alzheimer pathology (Haley 2000).

What is vascular dementia?

Vascular disease has long been recognized as an important cause of dementia. Renewed recognition of this and of the potential for the prevention or treatment of dementia has resulted in welcome but long-overdue research interest. Vascular dementia as a research field or subject heading is therefore alive and well. The question remains of what to do with the diagnosis. Its continued usefulness is doubted even by those with whose names it is most closely associated, but there is no current consensus as to what should replace it. 'Vascular cognitive impairment' has been suggested in order to move away from a memory-focused assessment (Bowler and Hachinski 2000). However, this still assumes that cerebrovascular disease can be separated out as an underlying cause. For epidemiological research, cognitive decline (deterioration in cognitive test scores over time) is becoming a more favoured outcome measure. This is difficult to apply clinically because of the huge variety of cognitive test batteries (and lack of consensus on which ones to use), because of the uncertainty as to what is 'normal' fluctuation in performance, and because clinical judgements often need to be made without the luxury of a follow-up period. An alternative, at least for clinical purposes, is to consider dementia as the principal diagnosis (expanding the criteria if necessary to include those with a more frontosubcortical picture of impairment) and to include vascular disease as one of several potential predisposing, precipitating, or maintaining factors. This approach is at least in keeping with the tradition of the diagnostic formulation and with the reality of multiple, interacting, and overlapping disorders (and causes for disorders) in older age groups.

References

Barba, R., Martínez-Espinosa, S., Rodríguez-Garcia, E., Pondal, M., Vicancos, J., and Del Ser, T. (2000). Poststroke dementia: clinical features and risk factors. *Stroke*, **31**, 1494–501.

Bowler, J. V. and Hachinski, V. (2000). Criteria for vascular dementia: replacing dogma with data. *Archives of Neurology*, **57**, 170–1.

Breteler, M. M. B., van Swieten, J. C., Bots, M. L., Grobbee, D. E., Claus, J. J., van den Hout, J. H. W., *et al.* (1994*a*). Cerebral white matter lesions, vascular risk factors, and cognitive function in a population-based study: The Rotterdam Study. *Neurology*, **44**, 1246–52.

Breteler, M. M. B., van Amerongen, N. M., van Swieten, J. C., Claus, J. J., Grobbee, D. E., van Gijn, J., *et al.* (1994*b*). Cognitive correlates of ventricular enlargement and cerebral white matter lesions on magnetic resonance imaging. *Stroke*, **25**, 1109–15.

Censori, B., Manara, O., Agostinis, C., Camerlingo, M., Casto, L., Galavotti, B., *et al.* (1996). Dementia after first stroke. *Stroke*, **27**, 1205–10.

Chui, H. C., Mack, W., Jackson, J. E., Mungas, D., Reed, B. R., Tinklenberg, J., *et al.* (2000). Clinical criteria for the diagnosis of vascular dementia. *Archives of Neurology*, **57**, 191–6.

de la Torre, J. C. and Mussivand, T. (1993). Can disturbed brain microcirculation cause Alzheimer's disease? *Neurological Research*, **15**, 146–53.

Desmond, D. W. (1996). Vascular dementia: a construct in evolution. *Cerebrovascular and Brain Metabolism Reviews*, **8**, 296–325.

Desmond, D. W., Moroney, J. T., Paik, M. C., Sano, M., Mohr, J. P., Aboumatar, S., *et al.* (2000). Frequency and clinical determinants of dementia after ischemic stroke. *Neurology*, **54**, 1124–31.

Elias, M. F., Wolf, P. A., D'Agostino, R. B., Cobb, J., and White, L. R. (1993). Untreated blood pressure level is inversely related to cognitive functioning: The Framingham study. *American Journal of Epidemiology*, **138**, 353–64.

Elias, P. K., Elias, M. F., D'Agostino, R. B., Cupples, L. A., Wilson, P. W., Silbershatz, H., *et al.* (1997). NIDDM and blood pressure as risk factors for poor cognitive performance. *Diabetes Care*, **20**, 1388–95.

Esiri, M. M., Nagy, Z., Smith, M. Z., Barnetson, L., and Smith, A. D. (1999). Cerebrovascular disease and threshold for dementia in the early stages of Alzheimer's disease. *Lancet*, **354**, 919–20.

Fein, G., Van Dyke, C., Davenport, L., Turetsky, B., Brandt-Zawadzki, M., Zatz, L., *et al.* (1990). Preservation of normal cognitive functioning in elderly subjects with extensive white-matter lesions of long duration. *Archives of General Psychiatry*, **47**, 220–3.

Ferucci, L., Guralnik, J. M., Salive, M. E., Pahor, M., Corti, M., Baroni, A., *et al.* (1996). Cognitive impairment and risk of stroke in the older population. *Journal of the American Geriatrics Society*, **44**, 237–41.

Fischer, P., Gatterer, G., Marterer, A., Simanyi, M., and Danielczyk, W. (1990). Course characteristics in the differentiation of dementia of the Alzheimer type and multi-infarct dementia. *Acta Psychiatrica Scandinavica*, **81**, 551–3.

Forette, F., Seux, M.-L., Staessen, J. A., Thijs, L., Birkenhager, W. H., Babarskiene, M.-R., *et al.* (1998). Prevention of dementia in randomised double-blind placebo-controlled Systolic Hypertension in Europe (Syst-Eur) trial. *Lancet*, **352**, 1347–51.

Gorelick, P. B., Chatterjee, A., Patel, D., Flowerdew, G., Dollear, W., Taber, J., *et al.* (1992). Cranial computerised tomographic observations in multi-infarct dementia. *Stroke*, **23**, 804–11.

Gorelick, P. B., Brody, J., Cohen, D., Freels, S., Levy, P., Dollear, W., *et al.* (1993). Risk factors for dementia associated with multiple cerebral infarcts. *Archives of Neurology*, **50**, 714–20.

Guo, Z., Viitanen, M., Fratiglioni, L., and Winblad, B. (1996). Low blood pressure, and dementia in elderly people: the Kungsholmen project. *British Medical Journal*, **312**, 805–8.

Hachinski, V. C., Iliff, L. D., Zilhka, E., du Boulay, G. H., McAllister, V. L., Marshall, J., *et al.* (1975). Cerebral blood flow in dementia. *Archives of Neurology*, **32**, 632–7.

Haley, R. W. (2000). Is there a connection between the concentration of cholesterol circulating in plasma, and the rate of neuritic plaque formation in Alzheimer disease? *Archives of Neurology*, **57**, 1410–12.

Hebert, R. and Brayne, C. (1995). Epidemiology of vascular dementia. *Neuroepidemiology*, **14**, 240–57.

Heitner, J. and Dickson, D. (1997). Diabetics do not have increased Alzheimer-type pathology compared with age-matched control subjects. *Neurology*, **49**, 1306–11.

Hofman, A., Ott, A., Breteler, M. M. B., Bots, M. L., Slooter, A. J., van Harskamp, F., *et al.* (1997). Atherosclerosis, apolipoprotein E, and prevalence of dementia and Alzheimer's disease in the Rotterdam Study. *Lancet*, **349**, 151–4.

Holmes, C., Cairns, N., Lantos, P., and Mann, A. (1999). Validity of current clinical criteria for Alzheimer's disease, vascular dementia and dementia with Lewy bodies. *British Journal of Psychiatry*, **174**, 45–50.

Hulette, C., Nochlin, D., McKeel, D., Morris, J. C., Mirra, S. S., Sumi, S. M., *et al.* (1997). Clinical-neuropathological findings in multi-infarct dementia: a report of six autopsied cases. *Neurology*, **48**, 668–72.

Jick, H., Zornberg, G. L., Jick, S. S., Seshadri, S., and Drachman, D. A. (2000). Statins and the risk of dementia. *Lancet*, **356**, 1627–31.

Joutel, A., Vahedi, K., Corpechot, C., Troesch, A., Chabriat, H., Vayssiere, C., *et al.* (1997). Strong clustering, and stereotyped nature of Notch3 mutations in CADASIL patients. *Lancet*, **350**, 1511–15.

Kase, C. S., Wolf, P. A., Kelly-Hayes, M., Kannel, W. B., Beiser, A., and D'Agostino, R. B. (1998). Intellectual decline after stroke: the Framingham Study. *Stroke*, **29**, 805–12.

Kilander, L., Nyman, H., Boberg, M., Hansson, L., and Lithell, H. (1998). Hypertension is related to cognitive impairment. A 20-year follow-up of 999 men. *Hypertension*, **31**, 780–6.

Kokmen, E., Whistman, J. P., O'Fallon, W. M., Chu, C. P., and Beard, C. M. (1996). Dementia after ischemic stroke: a population-based study in Rochester, Minnesota (1960–1984). *Neurology*, **19**, 154–9.

Launer, L. J., Masaki, K., Petrovitch, H., Foley, D., and Havlik, R. J. (1995). The association between midlife blood pressure levels and late-life cognitive function. *Journal of the American Medical Association*, **274**, 1846–51.

Loeb, C., Gandolfo, C., Croce, R., and Conti, M. (1992). Dementia associated with lacunar infarction. *Stroke*, **23**, 1225–9.

Lopez, O. L., Larumbe, M. R., Becker, J. T., Rezek, D., Rosen, J., Klunk, W., *et al.* (1994). Reliability of NINDS-AIREN clinical criteria for the diagnosis of vascular dementia. *Neurology*, **44**, 1240–5.

Lovestone, S. (1999). Diabetes and dementia: is the brain another site of end-organ damage? *Neurology*, **53**, 1907–9.

Meyer, J. S., Judd, B. W., Tawaklna, T., Rogers, R. L., and Mortel, K. F. (1986). Improved cognition after control of risk factors for multi-infarct dementia. *Journal of the American Medical Association*, **256**, 2203–9.

Meyer, J. S., Rogers, R. L., McClintic, K., Mortel, K. F., and Lofti, J. (1989). Randomized clinical trial of daily aspirin therapy in multi-infarct dementia. *Journal of the American Geriatrics Society*, **37**, 549–55.

Moroney, J. T., Bagiella, E., Desmond, D. W., Paik, M., Stern, Y., and Tatemichi, T. K. (1996). Risk factors for incident dementia after stroke. Role of hypoxic and ischaemic disorders. *Stroke*, **27**, 1283–9.

Moroney, J. T., Bagiella, E., Tatemichi, T. K., Paik, M., and Stern, Y. (1997). Dementia after stroke increases the risk of long-term stroke recurrence. *Neurology*, **48**, 1317–25.

Notkola, I.-M., Sulkava, R., Pekkanen, J., Erkinjuntti, T., Ehnholm, C., Kivinen, P., *et al.* (1998). Serum total cholesterol, apolipoprotein E 4 allele, and Alzheimer's disease. *Neuroepidemiology*, **17**, 14–20.

O'Brien, J. T. (2000). Neuroimaging in vascular dementia. In *Cerebrovascular disease and dementia. Pathology, neuropsychiatry and management* (ed. E. Chiu, L. Gustafson, D. Ames, and M. F. Folstein), pp. 145–64. Martin Dunitz, London.

Olichney, J. M., Hansen, L. A., Lee, J. H., Hofsetter, C. R., Katzman, R., and Thal, L. J. (2000). Relationship between severe amyloid angiopathy, apolipoprotein E genotype, and vascular lesions in Alzheimer's disease. *Annals of the New York Academy of Sciences*, **903**, 138–48.

Ott, A., Breteler, M. M. B., de Bruyne, M. C., van Harskamp, F., Grobbee, D. E., and Hofman, A. (1997). Atrial fibrillation and dementia in a population-based study. *Stroke*, **28**, 316–21.

Ott, A., Slooter, A. J. C., Hofman, A., van Harskamp, F., Witteman, J. C. M., Van Broeckhoven, C., *et al.* (1998). Smoking and the risk of dementia and Alzheimer's disease in a population-based cohort study: The Rotterdam Study. *Lancet*, **351**, 1840–3.

Ott, A., Stolk, R. P., van Harskamp, F., Pols, H. A. P., Hofman, A., and Breteler, M. M. B. (1999). Diabetes mellitus and the risk of dementia. *Neurology*, **53**, 1937–42.

Pohjasvaara, T., Erkinjuntti, T., Ylikoski, R., Hietanen, M., Vataja, R., and Kaste, M. (1998). Clinical determinants of poststroke dementia. *Stroke,* **29**, 75–81.

Pohjasvaara, T., Mäntylä, R., Aronen, H. J., Leskalä, M., Alonen, O., Aste, M., *et al.* (1999). Clinical and radiological determinants of prestroke cognitive decline in a stroke cohort. *Journal of Neurology, Neurosurgery and Psychiatry,* **67**, 742–8.

Prince, M., Cullen, M., and Mann, A. (1994). Risk factors for Alzheimer's disease and dementia: a case-control study based on the MRC elderly hypertension trial. *Neurology,* **44**, 97–104.

Prince, M. J., Bird, A. S., Blizard, R. A., and Mann, A. H. (1996). Is the cognitive function of older patients affected by antihypertensive treatment? Results from 54 months of the Medical Research Council's treatment trial of hypertension in older adults. *British Medical Journal,* **312**, 801–4.

Richards, M., Meade, T. W., Peart, S., Brennan, P. J., and Mann, A. H. (1997). Is there any evidence for a protective effect of antithrombotic medication on cognitive function in men at risk of cardiovascular disease ? Some preliminary findings. *Journal of Neurology, Neurosurgery and Psychiatry,* **62**, 269–72.

Román, G. C., Tatemichi, T. K., Erkinjuntti, T., Cummings, J. L., Masdeu, J. C., Garcia, J. H., *et al.* (1993). Vascular dementia: diagnostic criteria for research studies: Report of the NINDS-AIREN International Workshop. *Neurology,* **43**, 1609–11.

Skoog, I. and Aevarsson, O. (2000). Epidemiology of vascular dementia in Europe. In *Cerebrovascular disease and dementia. Pathology, neuropsychiatry and management* (ed. E. Chiu, L. Gustafson, D. Ames, and M. F. Folstein), pp. 15–24. Martin Dunitz, London.

Skoog, I., Lernfelt, B., Landahl, S., Palmertz, B., Andreasson, L., Nilsson, L., *et al.* (1996). 15-year longitudinal study of blood pressure and dementia. *Lancet,* **347**, 1141–5.

Snowdon, D. A., Greiner, L. H., Mortimer, J. A., Riley, K. P., Greiner, P. A., and Markesbery, W. R. (1997). Brain infarction and the clinical expression of Alzheimer disease. *Journal of the American Medical Association,* **277**, 813–17.

Sparks, D. L., Scheff, S. W., Liu, H., Landers, T. M., Coyne, C. M., and Hunsaker, J. C. (1995). Increased incidence of neurofibrillary tangles (NFT) in non-demented individuals with hypertension. *Journal of Neurological Sciences,* **131**, 162–9.

Sparks, D. L., Scheff, S. W., Liu, H., Landers, T. M., Danner, F., Coyne, C. M., *et al.* (1996). Increased density of senile plaques (SP), but not neurofibrillary tangles (NFT), in non-demented individuals with the apolipoprotein E4 allele: comparison to confirmed Alzheimer's disease patients. *Journal of Neurological Sciences,* **138**, 97–104.

Staessen, J. A., Gasowski, J., Wang, J. G., Thijs, L., Hond, E. D., Boissel, J.-P., *et al.* (2000). Risks of untreated and treated isolated systolic hypertension in the elderly: meta-analysis of outcome trials. *Lancet,* **355**, 865–72.

Stevens, D. L., Hewlett, R. H., and Brownell, B. (1977). Chronic familial vascular encephalopathy. *Lancet*; **2**: 1364–5.

Stewart, R. (1998). Cardiovascular factors in Alzheimer's disease. *Journal of Neurology, Neurosurgery and Psychiatry,* **65**, 143–7.

Stewart, R. (1999). Hypertension and cognitive decline. *British Journal of Psychiatry,* **174**, 286–7.

Stewart, R. and Liolitsa, D. (1999). Type 2 diabetes mellitus, cognitive impairment and dementia. *Diabetic Medicine,* **16**, 93–112.

Tatemichi, T. K., Desmond, D. W., Prohovnik, I., Cross, D. T., Gropen, T. I., Mohr, J. P., *et al.* (1992*a*). Confusion and memory loss from capsular genu infarction: a thalamocortical disconnection syndrome? *Neurology,* **42**, 1966–79.

Tatemichi, T. K., Desmond, D. W., Mayeux, R., Paik, M., Stern, Y., Sano, M., *et al.* (1992b). Dementia after stroke: baseline frequency, risks and clinical features in a hospitalised cohort. *Neurology,* **42**, 1185–93.

Tatemichi, T. K., Paik, M., Bagiella, E., Desmond, D. W., Stern, Y., Sano, M., *et al.* (1994). Risk of dementia after stroke in a hospitalised cohort: results of a longitudinal study. *Neurology,* **44**, 1885–91

Wolozin, B., Kellman, W., Ruosseau, P., Celesia, G. G., and Siegel, G. (2000). Decreased prevalence of Alzheimer disease associated with 3-hydroxy-3-methylglutaryl coenzyme A reductase inhibitors. *Archives of Neurology,* **57**, 1439–43.

24iv Dementia in Parkinson's disease and dementia with Lewy bodies (DLB)

Rupert McShane

James Parkinson, in his original description of the shaking palsy, stated that 'The senses and intellect [are] uninjured'. This notion persisted despite the fact that dementia was present in half the cases described by Friederich Lewy in his 1923 monograph on the neuropathology of Parkinson's disease (PD) (Gibb and Poewe 1986). Japanese neuropathologists were the first to describe the presence of 'cortical LBs' (Okazaki *et al.* 1961; Kosaka *et al.* 1976), and the recognition that cortical Lewy bodies (LBs) might be associated with dementia and a characteristic clinical syndrome has led to a more widespread interest from clinicians (Byrne *et al.* 1989; Hansen *et al.* 1990; McKeith *et al.* 1992*a*). Consensus was reached on the clinical criteria for dementia with Lewy bodies (DLB) in 1995 (McKeith *et al.* 1996). It has recently been recognized that the abnormal processing and aggregation of alpha-synuclein (ASN) into filaments is a key event in the pathogenesis of both autosomal dominant PD and sporadic PD (Polymeropoulos *et al.* 1997; Spillantini *et al.* 1997). Similar aggregations are widespread in neurites and axons, particularly in cases with dementia.

What are Lewy bodies?

Lewy bodies are the neuronal inclusion bodies which, when accompanied by the characteristic clinical syndrome of tremor, rigidity, and bradykinesia, define idiopathic Parkinson's disease. In Parkinson's disease they are typically found in the pigmented neurons of the substantia nigra and locus coeruleus, and in the neurons of the cholinergic nucleus basalis of Meynert. Other nuclei are commonly affected in PD: the olfactory bulb, the amygdala, the dorsal nucleus of the vagus. Similar inclusions are also present in multisystem atrophy and amyotrophic lateral sclerosis (motor neuron disease). This family of conditions has been termed 'the alpha-synucleinopathies' because in each of them the characteristic pathology includes abnormal aggregations of alpha-synuclein. Aggregated, filamentous alpha-synuclein is a major constituent of LBs, Lewy neurites, and neuraxonal spheroids. Other constituents of LBs include ubiquitin and neurofilament. The predilection areas for the formation of 'cortical' LBs are the amygdala, cingulate, parahippocampal gyrus, insula cortex, and temporal and frontal neocortex. The finding that many cases of familial AD have LBs in the amygdala and elsewhere suggests that LB formation can be precipitated by abnormalities of amyloid processing (Lippa *et al.* 1998). Nitration of alpha-synuclein due to the formation of free oxygen radicals is a key event in the formation of LBs (Giasson *et al.* 2000). Redox-active iron is sequestered into LBs in the substantia nigra, but not into cortical LBs, and may be involved in protective rather than degenerative mechanisms (Castellani *et al.* 2000).

Prevalence

The prevalence of LBs in elderly people without dementia, extrapyramidalism, or any psychiatric disorder—so-called incidental LBs—is approximately 2% (Smith *et al.* 1991). The rate of LBs in patients with dementia (10–20%) is at least five times higher, suggesting that either LBs are somehow causally related to dementia, or that a process giving rise to dementia may also precipitate the formation of LBs. Unbiased autopsy studies of the prevalence of LBs in dementia are difficult to perform: patients with LBs are likely to be over-represented in autopsy series because of their more rapid decline and death, or because of their interesting symptom profile. In brain-bank series of patients with dementia, 20% of cases have LB pathology in the brainstem. The epidemiologically based Medical Research Council Cognitive Function and Ageing Study found a prevalence of 12% in the first 100 cases of dementia coming to autopsy (Neuropathology Group of MRC CFAS 2001). Although the majority of cases of dementia in which LBs are present do not have clinical PD, dementia in PD is substantially more common than would be expected by chance. The prevalence of dementia in elderly cases of PD is between two and five times that of age-matched controls (Brown and Marsden 1984; Mayeux *et al.* 1992; Tison *et al.* 1995). The relative risk of incident dementia in a given year is approximately 1.7 times that of controls (Marder *et al.* 1995).

Tautological tangles and the cognitive impairment associated with Lewy bodies

DLB is a disease with a short history that has been beset by problems of definition. Attempts at a unifying hypothesis to describe the relationship between PD, dementia, AD, and cortical and brainstem LB pathology have not yet been universally accepted. One reason for this is that at least a few ubiquitinated cortical LBs are found in most cases of PD without dementia (Hughes *et al.* 1993). A simple equation between the presence of cortical LBs and dementia is not therefore possible. Compared to the burden of neurofibrillary tangles in AD, cortical LBs are relatively sparse even in PD with dementia. However, the use of sensitive ASN immunohistochemistry has shown that the presence of a moderate number of cortical LBs does predict dementia in PD (Hurtig *et al.* 2000). A second source of controversy has been the significance of coexisting neurofibrillary tangles and plaques—a debate that was complicated by the use of different definitions of AD.

The simplest approach to the taxonomy is to take a 'lumping' approach: any case with dementia and Lewy bodies is a case of dementia with Lewy bodies (DLB). However, 'splitters' recognize up to four broad patterns of neuropathology associated with cognitive impairment. First, most patients with PD have subtle cognitive impairment. This is characterized by slowed thinking (the so-called 'bradyphrenia' of subcortical dementia), and deficits in visuospatial function, in shifting attention, and in executive function (i.e. the integration of sensory and internally generated signals). Interestingly, subtle extrapyramidalism in the elderly, non-demented population is associated with similar deficits and predicts the onset of dementia rather than PD (Richards *et al.* 1993*a,b*). Whether these deficits reach the point where the patient can be considered to have dementia depends on the definition of dementia, the threshold for which tends to be lower in studies in the US. For example, 69% of patients with PD were found to be demented in the comprehensive epidemiological study of Mayeux *et al.* (1992), whereas the French study of Tison *et al.* (1995), which reported a rather low overall prevalence in the general population (7% in those over 80 years), found a prevalence of 37% in those with PD over 80 years. Cases in which PD precedes dementia by more than a year are excluded from the consensus definition of DLB (McKeith *et al.* 1996), although it is acknowledged that such cases share the clinical features of DLB

A second pattern of pathology is termed 'pure dementia with LB' (or 'diffuse Lewy body dementia' in some schemes). This is defined as dementia occurring in cases with widespread cortical LBs and a heavy burden of Lewy neurites, but no neurofibrillary tangles or senile or neuritic amyloid plaques. It is rare, accounting for less than 5% of cases of DLB.

Two further patterns of DLB occur when Alzheimer's disease (AD) is present as well as cortical LBs. Cases in the first group have clear-cut AD and have been designated by some as 'Lewy body variant of Alzheimer's disease'. In this group, substantial neuritic plaque and tangle pathology is present. However, the burden of tangles found at autopsy is less (i.e. Braak stage 3–4) than that seen in AD without LBs (i.e. Braak stage 5–6). The second group is characterized by AD pathology which is present (distinguishing the group from those with 'pure DLB'), but at levels that are indistinguishable from those of age-matched controls, and which are insufficient for a pathological diagnosis of AD. Tangles may be rare or absent, and plaques are mainly of the non-neuritic variety. The proportion of cases falling into each of these two groups is uncertain because of variations in the criteria applied to define AD in different autopsy series.

There is currently no consensus on the neuropathological criteria for DLB. A system for describing the extent of cortical LBs was devised before the recognition of ASN as a principal component of LBs and Lewy neurites. There is still debate about whether alpha-synuclein is present in non-LB lesions (which would reduce its diagnostic specificity), and it is not clear how many cortical ASN-positive LBs are required to predict the syndrome. The tautology here is that quantitative neuropathological criteria can only be validated against the clinical syndrome—which can only be validated against neuropathological criteria.

Clinical diagnosis of DLB

In the absence of clear aetiological distinctions between the four categories above, a 'lumping' approach to clinical diagnosis is appropriate. There are no pathognomonic clinical signs of DLB and the best available clinical criteria at present are the Consensus Clinical Criteria for DLB (McKeith *et al.* 1996) (Table 24iv.1).

Table 24iv.1 Consensus criteria for probable dementia with Lewy bodies

Two of the following three:
- Persistent visual hallucinations
- Fluctuating deficits of cognitive and functional ability
- Parkinsonism

Most prospective validation studies (Mega *et al.* 1996; Litvan *et al.* 1998; Gomez-Isla *et al.* 1999; Lopez *et al.* 1999; Luis *et al.* 1999; Verghese *et al.* 1999; McKeith *et al.* 2000; McShane *et al.* 2001) have found that the criteria exclude cases without LBs reasonably well (specificities of approximately 80%). The main weakness of the criteria is that they fail to pick up a significant number of cases which turn out to have LBs. Reported sensitivities are typically only 60%, though they reached 80% in a study from Newcastle-upon-Tyne (McKeith *et al.* 2000).

One of the main problems with comparing validation studies is that different neuropathological criteria for DLB are used in different studies. However, many, if not the majority, of these missed cases have concomitant definite AD ('LB variant of AD'). The overall level of cognitive impairment in such cases may be so severe that the distinguishing features—fluctuating attention and hallucinations—become obscured by the overall level of dementia (Verghese *et al.* 1999; McShane *et al.* 2001).

The consensus criteria also included a variety of clinical features which, while not necessary for the diagnosis, were supportive: repeated falls, non-visual hallucinations, systematized delusions (including delusional misidentification), syncope, transient losses of consciousness, and neuroleptic sensitivity. Other features, which are also more common in DLB than other dementias, include depression, reduplicative phenomena such as Capgras syndrome (Ballard *et al.* 1999*b*), more rapid decline (Luis *et al.* 1999), and impaired olfactory function (McShane *et al.* 2001). The originally proposed category of 'possible DLB', defined as the presence of only one of these features, predicts LB pathology at a rate that is no better than chance.

The neuropsychological profile of patients with DLB differs from that of patients with AD in several ways. The visuospatial deficits seen in

DLB are more marked than expected for the overall level of cognitive function. Such deficits are associated with the presence of visual hallucinations, suggesting a higher order deficit in visual processing (Ayre *et al.* 1998). Memory function, particularly recognition memory, is better preserved than in AD. Deficits of attention are common and associated with fluctuation (see below). Verbal fluency and executive function are also impaired. It is not yet known whether the addition of neuropsychological tests to the consensus clinical criteria for DLB will improve their sensitivity. A ratio of praxis score to memory function has been found to distinguish cases with DLB from AD with a specificity of 98% and sensitivity of 33% (or 84% and 63% depending on the cut-off point used) (Ballard *et al.* 1999*a*).

Structural imaging may reveal a degree of atrophy of the medial temporal lobes which is less than expected for the level of cognitive impairment (Barber *et al.* 2000). The dopaminergic deficits in DLB may turn out to be useful diagnostically, since patients with DLB have a reduced density of presynaptic dopamine reuptake protein in the posterior putamen. This can be visualized using specific ligands and SPECT (single photon emission computed tomography) imaging (Walker *et al.* 1999).

The core features of DLB

Fluctuation

It has been suggested in jest that 'dementia with LBs' is a misnomer and the condition should be termed 'delirium with LBs' because fluctuation in attention is a core part of the syndrome of DLB and of delirium. The Newcastle group have recently characterized this fluctuation in more detail (Walker *et al.* 2000*a*,*b*). The amplitude of fluctuation is more marked in DLB than AD and can be assessed by asking the caregiver to give examples of what the patient can do when at their best and when at their worst. A 'One day Fluctuation Assessment Scale' which rates items such as attention, drowsiness, episodes of incoherence, falls, and fluctuation is a potentially useful way of breaking down the various components of 'fluctuation', but it has yet to be neuropathologically validated. Computerized assessments have shown that patients with clinical DLB have marked fluctuations in reaction times over the course of a simple 90-second task. Although highly specific for DLB, this feature was not a sensitive indicator, despite the fact that many of the subjects were selected on the basis that their carers reported fluctuations in cognitive and functional ability. Nevertheless, the test of neuropsychological functioning was validated by showing that second-to-second reductions in EEG activity coincided with periods of slowed reaction times.

These tests have not yet been widely taken up in the clinic situation. However, the point that the fluctuations occur over a short period is useful. In the Oxford Project to Investigate Memory and Ageing, we have found that a simple question about brief fluctuations ('Are there brief periods during 24 hours when he seems much worse and then times when he is quite clear?') was a much better discriminator of those with pathological DLB than a question about longer fluctuations ('Are there episodes lasting days or weeks when his thinking seems quite clear and then becomes muddled?').

What is the aetiology of these brief fluctuations in DLB? Fluctuation is a common sequela of L-dopa treatment in PD, is related to the availability of L-dopa, and is reduced by catechol-*o*-methyl transferase inhibitors such as entacopone. However, many patients with DLB with fluctuations are not taking L-dopa, either because they do not have sufficient parkinsonism symptoms to warrant it, or because the L-dopa exacerbates their hallucinations. Cholinergic mechanisms are probably mainly responsible for the fluctuations of attention in DLB, possibly via thalamic projections. The cholinesterase inhibitor rivastigmine has a clear effect on the overall choice reaction time in patients with DLB; fluctuations during the course of the 90-second task referred to above were markedly less in those taking the drug compared to placebo (McKeith *et al.* 2000).

Parkinsonism

Parkinsonism does not occur until 60% of the dopaminergic neurons in the substantia nigra are lost or dopamine levels in the basal ganglia fall by 80%. LBs rarely, if ever, occur in cortical neurons without being present in at least one of the brainstem nuclei as well. However, cortical LBs not infrequently occur in cases with only mild degeneration of the substantia nigra; which is why parkinsonism is not an invariable feature of DLB and, if it occurs, is often mild.

The pattern of parkinsonism in DLB is similar to that seen in late-onset PD. Unilateral signs and tremor are less common. An impassive expression (facial masking), often associated with a rather staring expression due to a low blink rate, and bradykinesia are more common. Indeed, a presentation of PD with bilateral features or facial masking predicts the onset of dementia and of visual hallucinations (Stern *et al.* 1993; Viitanen *et al.* 1994).

A supporting diagnostic feature of DLB is the presence of neuroleptic sensitivity (McKeith *et al.* 1992*b*). This profound reaction to neuroleptics may take the form of an abrupt worsening of the parkinsonism or of worsened confusion. It occurs both with typical and atypical neuroleptics, though more with the former, and may be more prevalent in DLB than in PD. This may be due to a greater failure in DLB than in PD of postsynaptic dopamine-receptor upregulation in response to the presynaptic dopaminergic deficit. Neuroleptic D_2 antagonists thus occupy a greater proportion of postsynaptic dopamine receptors in DLB than in PD (Piggott 1998).

Visual hallucinations

Visual hallucinations are present in 60–70% of cases of DLB (Klatka *et al.* 1996; Ballard *et al.* 1999*b*). The visual hallucinations are typically of people or animals which often disappear when attention is directly focused on the presumed image. Some patients complain of seeing smoke or fire, or water on surfaces. Detailed, formed visual hallucinations are often preceded by visual illusions or vivid dreams. The illusions commonly take the form of seeing faces or animals in the detailed textures of patterns on furniture, or in trees. Vivid dreams in DLB are associated with rapid eye movement (REM) sleep behaviour disorder. In this condition the normal mechanisms that inhibit muscle activity in REM sleep break down and the patient starts to act out his dreams (Boeve *et al.* 1998).

Patients with isolated visual hallucinations in the absence of cognitive impairment are at increased risk of developing dementia (Ostling and Skoog 1999). Similarly, patients with PD who develop hallucinations are more likely to develop dementia (Stern *et al.* 1993). Whilst they may be made worse by all antiparkinsonian medication, careful enquiry will generally elicit the presence of hallucinations before starting such medication. The link between the Charles Bonnet syndrome (CBS) and DLB is uncertain since there are no substantial neuropathological studies of CBS. CBS is generally thought of as the association of persistent visual hallucinations with visual impairment, in the absence of intellectual impairment. However, advanced age is a consistently reported risk factor for CBS, and detailed neuropsychology suggests that most cases have at least mildly impaired cognitive function (Pliskin *et al.* 1996). These deficits can be stable (Holroyd and Rabins 1996). Poor eyesight makes hallucinations in DLB worse but does not affect their duration (Ballard *et al.* 1995; McShane *et al.* 1995).

Cholinergic deficits are likely to be important in the generation of hallucinations in DLB, since the hallucinations respond to the cholinesterase inhibitor rivastigmine (McKeith *et al.* 2000) and patients with hallucinations have even more severe deficits in cortical cholinergic parameters than those without (Perry *et al.* 1990). Although delusions also respond to rivastigmine, the aetiology of delusions may be different to that of hallucinations because upregulation of the postsynaptic muscarinic receptor is associated with delusions but not hallucinations (Ballard *et al.* 2000*a*).

The management of DLB

What to tell the patient and carer

In explaining the diagnosis, a simple explanation of the condition as 'an overlap between Alzheimer's and Parkinson's disease' is more likely to be useful than detailed explanations of the taxonomy of DLB. It can also be helpful to say that Alzheimer's disease is not an 'all or nothing' diagnosis and that most people have at least a little of the changes of AD. Explaining a 'normal' scan can be complicated. Some carers may be inclined to dismiss the patients' symptoms as wilful or to derive false hope when told that the scan is normal, unless they are clearly told that the investigation is usually insensitive in early cases and is often normal in DLB. One approach is to say that a normal scan indicates that the amount of AD pathology may not be much greater than expected for age, but that this supports the diagnosis of DLB.

The fluctuating nature of the attentional deficits can be perplexing for caregivers, particularly because periods of high functioning indicate that such abilities have not been irretrievably lost. However, this can be a useful lead into a discussion about the maximum potential benefit of medication that can reasonably be expected. A simple explanation for the attentional deficits is that the patient runs out of the 'steam' needed for thinking, because of the cholinergic deficit. The more the patient tries to resolve the muddle, the less they can build up the necessary head of steam to think clearly.

In patients with dementia who have lost insight, it is usually unhelpful for their caregivers to contradict any delusional ideas. However, insight into the illusory nature of hallucinations is very often retained in DLB, particularly in the early stages. In such cases, reassurance that the patient's eyes or imagination are 'playing tricks' with them is useful. An explanation of the progression from vivid dreams, through illusions and plucking at the sheets or picking imaginary threads from the floor, to formed '*de novo*' hallucinations often helps caregivers to make sense of their experience. Since poor eyesight can make visual hallucinations worse it is sensible to maximize the patient's visual acuity. Cataract extraction early in the course may retard the development of hallucinations. Increasing the power and number of light bulbs in the room where the patient typically sits may help, since hallucinations are usually more prominent in low lighting and in the evening. Furniture and curtains with patterns likely to provoke the visual illusions can be covered or replaced with monochromatic, non-patterned material. Paradoxically, illusions are less likely to occur in a new or moderately stimulating environment than in a familiar environment where there is little to occupy the patient's mind. Patients rarely hallucinate when their attention is taken by visitors.

Sometimes it is necessary to advise families about the need to give the patient with bradyphrenia more time to respond or to carry out tasks. The difficulty that the patient has in rapid shifting of attention means that family members should try not to speak more than one at a time or interrupt each other. When this sort of communication occurs in the interview, it can be helpful to point this out gently so that the family understand what is being referred to.

Occasionally, caregivers report that parkinsonism, particularly tremor, improves as cognitive function worsens. This can be explained on the basis of a relatively greater progression of the AD. The worsening cholinergic deficit acts in the same way as giving an anticholinergic drug such as procyclidine.

Drug management

The main target symptoms for drug treatment are parkinsonism, visual hallucinations, delusions, and agitation. However, the most important question in the drug management of DLB, or of psychiatric complications in PD, is not **which** drug to use, but whether to use **any** drug. Reassurance is often sufficient, and it is usually better to start by withdrawing drugs than introducing new ones. One suggested scheme is to withdraw antiparkinsonian drugs from the psychotic PD patient in the following order: anticholinergic, selegiline, dopamine agonists, L-dopa.

As with AD, depression may be the presenting feature of DLB. It needs to be distinguished from the apathy and bradyphrenia of DLB but, when present, should be managed in the usual way. Selective serotonin-reuptake inhibitors (SSRIs) are preferable to tricyclic antidepressants because they are less likely to exacerbate the cholinergic deficits, constipation, and postural hypotension of DLB.

Drugs that relieve psychosis and agitation often cause parkinsonism, and vice versa. There is a risk of neuroleptic sensitivity even with atypical neuroleptics, of which there are no placebo-controlled trials in DLB. A controlled trial of olanzapine for psychosis in PD was stopped early because of worsening parkinsonism (Goetz *et al.* 2000). Open-label studies suggest that, among the atypical neuroleptics, parkinsonism is least likely to occur with clozapine or quetiapine and more likely with risperidone and olanzapine.

L-dopa-exacerbated hallucinations are less common when cholinesterase inhibitors (ChEIs) are co-prescribed. Therefore, one strategy to improve parkinsonism in DLB or in psychotic patients with PD, is to prescribe as high a dose of a ChEI as the side-effects (usually nausea) allow, and then to introduce L-dopa.

There are currently no head-to-head comparisons of ChEIs and neuroleptics. But many would regard the risk of neuroleptic sensitivity to be sufficient to justify the use of ChEIs before neuroleptics for the treatment of psychosis, anxiety, and agitation in DLB. However, the ChEIs have a significant side-effect profile dominated by gastrointestinal effects, such as nausea and vomiting, and they may exacerbate neurovascular instability and falls in patients with DLB (Ballard *et al.* 2000*b*). At the time of writing, rivastigmine is the only ChEI shown to have a beneficial effect in DLB (McKeith *et al.* 2000). In this study, a newly defined cluster of symptoms (visual hallucinations, delusions, anxiety, and apathy) was substantially alleviated. Of those patients taking the active drug 63% had a 30% reduction in symptom scores, compared to 30% on placebo. This effect size was substantially greater than that seen for a functional or global improvement in most of the trials of ChEIs in patients with AD. Thus, patients with DLB appear to be preferential responders. This is not surprising since the principal cholinergic nucleus, the nucleus basalis of Meynert, is in 'double jeopardy' from both LB and neurofibrillary tangle pathology.

Rivastigmine also had a beneficial effect on fluctuations in attention in patients with DLB, as assessed using computerized choice reaction time tasks. This is interesting because it raises the possibility that the ChEIs might also be of value in patients with delirium. If attention is indeed improved across a range of conditions by ChEIs, this would suggest that treatment response may be better predicted by the clinical syndrome than by the presence of LB pathology.

References

Ayre, G., Ballard, C., Pincock, C., Wesnes, K., McKeith, I., and Sahgal, A. (1998). Association between visual hallucinations, neurochemical pathology and cognition in dementia with Lewy bodies. *Journal of Psychopharmacology*, **12**(Suppl. A), A41.

Ballard, C., Bannister, C., Graham, C., Oyebode, F., and Wilcock, G. (1995). Associations of psychotic symptoms in dementia sufferers. *British Journal of Psychiatry*, **167**, 537–40.

Ballard, C., Ayre, G., O'Brien, J., Sahgal, A., McKeith, I. G., Ince, P. G., *et al.* (1999*a*). Simple standardised neuropsychological assessments aid in the differential diagnosis of dementia with Lewy bodies from Alzheimer's disease and vascular dementia. *Dementia and Geriatric Cognitive Disorders* **10**, 104–8.

Ballard, C., Holmes, C., McKeith, I., Neill, D., O'Brien, J., Cairns, N., *et al.* (1999*b*). Psychiatric morbidity in dementia with Lewy bodies: a prospective clinical and neuropathological comparative study with Alzheimer's disease. *American Journal of Psychiatry*, **156**, 1039–45.

Ballard, C., Piggott, M., Johnson, M., Cairns, N., Perry, R., McKeith, I., *et al.* (2000*a*). Delusions associated with elevated muscarinic binding in dementia with Lewy bodies. *Annals of Neurology*, **48**, 868–76.

Ballard, C., O'Brien, J., Barber, B., Scheltens, P., Shaw, F., McKeith, I., *et al.* (2000*b*). Neurocardiovascular instability, hypotensive episodes, and MRI lesions in neurodegenerative dementia. *Annals of the New York Academy of Science*, **903**, 442–5.

Barber, R., Ballard, C., McKeith, I. G., Gholkar, A., and O'Brien, J. T. (2000). MRI volumetric study of dementia with Lewy bodies. *Neurology*, **54**, 1304–9.

Boeve, B. F., Silber, M. H., Ferman, T. J., Kokmen, E., Smith, G. E., Ivnik, R. J., *et al.* (1998). REM sleep behavior disorder and degenerative dementia: an association likely reflecting Lewy body disease. *Neurology*, **51**, 363–70.

Brown, R. G. and Marsden, C. D. (1984). How common is dementia in Parkinson's disease? *Lancet*, **2**, 1262–5.

Byrne, E. J., Lennox, G., Lowe, J., and Godwin-Austen, R. B. (1989). Diffuse Lewy body disease: clinical features in 15 cases. *Journal of Neurology, Neurosurgery and Psychiatry*, **52**, 709–17.

Castellani, R. J., Siedlak, S. L., Perry, G., and Smith, M. A. (2000). Sequestration of iron by Lewy bodies in Parkinson's disease. *Acta Neuropathologica (Berlin)*, **100**, 111–14.

Esiri, M. M., Matthews, F., Brayne, C., and Ince, P. G. The Neuropathology Group of the Medical Research Council

Cognitive Function and Ageing Study (MRC CFAS). *Lancet* (In press.)

Giasson, B. I., Duda, J. E., Murray, I. V., Chen, Q., Souza, J. M., Hurtig, H. I., *et al.* (2000). Oxidative damage linked to neurodegeneration by selective alpha-synuclein nitration in synucleinopathy lesions. *Science*, **290**, 985–9.

Gibb, W. R. and Poewe, W. H. (1986). The centenary of Friederich H. Lewy 1885–1950. *Neuropathology and Applied Neurobiology*, **12**, 217–22. [Review]

Goetz, C. G., Blasucci, L. M., Leurgans, S., and Pappert, E. J. (2000). Olanzapine and clozapine: comparative effects on motor function in hallucinating PD patients. *Neurology*, **55**, 789–94.

Gomez-Isla, T., Growdon, W. B., McNamara, M., Newell, K., Gomez-Tortosa, E., Hedley-Whyte, E. T., *et al.* (1999). Clinicopathologic correlates in temporal cortex in dementia with Lewy bodies. *Neurology*, **53**, 2003–9.

Hansen, L., Salmon, D., Galasko, D., Masliah, E., Katzman, R., DeTeresa, R., *et al.* (1990). The Lewy body variant of Alzheimer's disease: a clinical and pathologic entity. *Neurology*, **40**, 1–8.

Holroyd, S. and Rabins, P. V. (1996). A three-year follow-up study of visual hallucinations in patients with macular degeneration. *Journal of Nervous and Mental Disease*, **184**, 188–9.

Hughes, A. J., Daniel, S. E., Blankson, S., and Lees, A. J. (1993). A clinicopathologic study of 100 cases of Parkinson's disease. *Archives of Neurology*, **50**, 140–8.

Hurtig, H. I., Trojanowski, J. Q., Galvin, J., Ewbank, D., Schmidt, M. L., Lee, V. M., *et al.* (2000). Alpha-synuclein cortical Lewy bodies correlate with dementia in Parkinson's disease. *Neurology*, **54**, 1916–21.

Klatka, L. A., Louis, E. D. and Schiffer, R. B. (1996). Psychiatric features in diffuse Lewy body disease: a clinicopathologic study using Alzheimer's disease and Parkinson's disease comparison groups. *Neurology*, **47**, 1148–52.

Kosaka, K., Oyanagi, S., Matsushita, M., and Hori, A. (1976). Presenile dementia with Alzheimer-, Pick- and Lewy-body changes. *Acta Neuropathologica (Berlin)*, **36**, 221–33.

Lippa, C. F., Fujiwara, H., Mann, D. M., Giasson, B., Baba, M., Schmidt, M. L., *et al.* (1998). Lewy bodies contain altered alpha-synuclein in brains of many familial Alzheimer's disease patients with mutations in presenilin and amyloid precursor protein genes. *American Journal of Pathology*, **153**, 1365–70.

Litvan, I., MacIntyre, A., Goetz, C. G., Wenning, G. K., Jellinger, K., Verny, M., *et al.* (1998). Accuracy of the clinical diagnoses of Lewy body disease, Parkinson disease and dementia with Lewy bodies. *Archives of Neurology*, **55**, 969–78.

Lopez, O. L., Litvan, I., Catt, K. E., Stowe, R., Klunk, W., Kaufer, D. I., *et al.* (1999). Accuracy of four clinical diagnostic criteria for the diagnosis of neurodegenerative dementias. *Neurology*, **53**, 1292–9. [In Process Citation]

Luis, C. A., Barker, W. W., Gajaraj, K., Harwood, D., Petersen, R., Kashuba, A., *et al.* (1999). Sensitivity and specificity of three clinical criteria for dementia with Lewy bodies in an autopsy-verified sample. *International Journal of Geriatric Psychiatry*, **14**, 526–33.

McKeith, I. G., Perry, R. H., Fairbairn, A. F., Jabeen, S., and Perry, E. K. (1992*a*). Operational criteria for senile dementia of Lewy body type (SDLT). *Psychological Medicine*, **22**, 911–22.

McKeith, I., Fairbairn, A., Perry, R., Thompson, P., and Perry, E. (1992*b*). Neuroleptic sensitivity in patients with senile dementia of Lewy body type. *British Medical Journal*, **305**, 673–8.

McKeith, I. G., Galasko, D., Kosaka, K., Perry, E. K., Dickson, D. W., Hansen, L., *et al.* (1996). Consensus guidelines for the clinical and pathological diagnosis of Dementia with Lewy Bodies (DLB): report of the consortium on DLB international workshop. *Neurology*, **47**, 1113–24.

McKeith, I. G., Ballard, C. G., Perry, R. H., Ince, P. G., O'Brien, J. T., Neill, D., *et al.* (2000). Prospective validation of Consensus criteria for the diagnosis of dementia with Lewy bodies. *Neurology*, **54**, 1050–8.

McShane, R., Gedling, K., Reading, M., McDonald, B., Esiri, M. M., and Hope, T. (1995). Prospective study of relations between cortical Lewy bodies, poor eyesight and hallucinations in Alzheimer's disease. *Journal of Neurology, Neurosurgery and Psychiatry*, **59**, 185–8.

McShane, R. H., Nagy, Zs., Esiri, M. M., King, E., Joachim, C., Sullivan, N., *et al.* (2001). Anosmia in dementia is associated with Lewy bodies rather than Alzheimer's pathology. *Journal of Neurology, Neurosurgery and Psychiatry*, **70**, 739–43.

Marder, K., Tang, M. X., Cote, L., Stern, Y., and Mayeux, R. (1995). The frequency and associated risk factors for dementia in patients with Parkinson's disease. *Archives of Neurology*, **52**, 695–701.

Mayeux, R., Denaro, J., Hemenegildo, N., Marder, K., Tang, M. X., Cote, L. J., *et al.* (1992). A population-based investigation of Parkinson's disease with and without dementia. Relationship to age and gender. *Archives of Neurology*, **49**, 492–7.

Mega, M. S., Masterman, D. L., Benson, D. F., Vinters, H. V., Tomiyasu, U., Craig, A. H., *et al.* (1996). Dementia with Lewy bodies: reliability and validity of clinical and pathologic criteria. *Neurology*, **47**, 1403–9.

Neuropathology Group of the Medical Research Council Cognitive Function and Ageing Study (MRC CFAS) (2001). Pathological correlates of late-onset dementia in a multi-centre community-based population in England and Wales. *Lancet*, **357**, 169–75.

Okazaki, H., Lipkin, L. E., and Aronson, S. M. (1961). Diffuse intracytoplasmic ganglionin inclusion (Lewy type) associated with progressive dementia and quadraparesis in flexion. *Journal of Neuropathology and Experimental Neurology*, **20**, 237–44.

Ostling, S. and Skoog, I. (1999). Delusions and hallucinations and their relation to sociodemographic and health variables in non-demented 85-year olds. *Abstracts of the 9th Congress of the International Psychogeriatric Association*, 113.

Perry, E. K., Marshall, E., Perry, R. H., Irving, D., Smith, C. J., Blessed, G., *et al.* (1990). Cholinergic and dopaminergic activities in senile dementia of Lewy body type. *Alzheimer's Disease and Associated Disorders*, **4**, 87–95.

Piggott, M. A., Perry, E. K., Marshall, E. F., McKeith, I. G., Johnson, M., Melrose, H. L., *et al.* (1998). Nigrostriatal dopaminergic activities in dementia with Lewy bodies in relation to neuroleptic sensitivity: comparisons with Parkinson's disease. *Biological Psychiatry*, **44**, 765–74.

Pliskin, N. H., Kiolbasa, T. A., Towle, V. L., Pankow, L., Ernest, J. T., Noronha, A., *et al.* (1996). Charles Bonnet syndrome: an early marker for dementia?. *Journal of the American Geriatrics Society*, **44**, 1055–61.

Polymeropoulos, M. H., Lavedan, C., Leroy, E., Ide, S. E., Dehejia, A., Dutra, A., *et al.* (1997). Mutation in the alpha-synuclein gene identified in families with Parkinson's disease. *Science*, **276**, 2045–7.

Richards, M., Stern, Y., and Mayeux, R. (1993*a*). Subtle extrapyramidal signs can predict the development of dementia in elderly individuals. *Neurology*, **43**, 2184–8.

Richards, M., Stern, Y., Marder, K., Cote, L., and Mayeux, R. (1993*b*). Relationships between extrapyramidal signs and cognitive function in a community-dwelling cohort of patients with Parkinson's disease and normal elderly individuals. *Annals of Neurology*, **33**, 267–74.

Smith, P. E. M., Irving, D., and Perry, R. H. (1991). Density, distribution and prevalence of Lewy bodies in the elderly. *Neuroscience Research Communications*, **8**, 127–35.

Spillantini, M. G., Schmidt, M. L., Lee, V. M., Trojanowski, J. Q., Jakes, R., and Goedert, M. (1997). Alpha-synuclein in Lewy bodies. *Nature*, **388**, 839–40. [Letter]

Stern, Y., Marder, K., Tang, M. X., and Mayeux, R. (1993). Antecedent clinical features associated with dementia in Parkinson's disease. *Neurology*, **43**, 1690–2.

Tison, F., Dartigues, J. F., Auriacombe, S., Letenneur, L., Boller, F., and Alperovitch, A. (1995). Dementia in Parkinson's disease: a population-based study in ambulatory and institutionalised individuals. *Neurology*, **45**, 705–8.

Verghese, J., Crystal, H. A., Dickson, D. W., and Lipton, R. B. (1999). Validity of clinical criteria for the diagnosis of dementia with Lewy bodies. *Neurology*, **53** 1974–82.

Viitanen, M., Mortimer, J. A., and Webster, D. D. (1994). Association between presenting motor symptoms and the risk of cognitive impairment in Parkinson's disease. *Journal of Neurology, Neurosurgery and Psychiatry*, **57**, 1203–7.

Walker, M. P., Ayre, G. A., Cummings, J. L., Wesnes, K., McKeith, I. G., O'Brien, J. T., *et al.* (2000*a*). The Clinician Assessment of Fluctuation and the One Day Fluctuation Assessment Scale. Two methods to assess fluctuating confusion in dementia. *British Journal of Psychiatry*, **177**, 252–6.

Walker, M. P., Ayre, G. A., Perry, E. K., Wesnes, K., McKeith, I. G., Tovee, M., *et al.* (2000*b*). Quantification and characterisation of fluctuating cognition in dementia with Lewy bodies and Alzheimer's disease. *Dementia and Geriatric Cognitive Disorders*, **11**, 327–35.

Walker, Z., Costa, D. C., Ince, P., McKeith, I. G., and Katona, C. L. (1999). In-vivo demonstration of dopaminergic degeneration in dementia with Lewy bodies. *Lancet*, **354**, 646–7. [Letter]

24v Frontotemporal dementia

Lars Gustafson

Introduction

Frontotemporal dementia (FTD) is the second commonest of the early-onset primary degenerative dementias. The clinical picture is caused by degenerative disease predominantly affecting the frontal and temporal lobes. More than 100 years ago, Arnold Pick (1892) pointed out the clinical importance of circumscribed atrophy in these brain regions. Alzheimer (1911) described inflated, ballooned neurons (Pick cells) and argentophilic globes (Pick bodies), in some of these cases with lobar atrophy, later to be named Pick's disease (Onari and Spatz 1926). Pick's disease is, however, rare and during the last two decades attention has been drawn to a much larger group of progressive degenerative FTD lacking the specific neuropathologies of Pick's disease and Alzheimer's disease (AD). In 1994 the Lund–Manchester research groups published clinical and pathological diagnostic criteria for FTD (Brun *et al.* 1994), encompassing three neuropathological conditions: frontal lobe degeneration of non-Alzheimer type (FLD), Pick's disease, and motor neuron disease (MND) with dementia. Two other behavioural syndromes, progressive nonfluent aphasia and semantic dementia, are regarded as belonging to the same clinicopathological spectrum as FTD (Neary *et al.* 1998).

Neuropathology

The common neuropathology of FTD is bilateral frontotemporal degeneration. FLD is characterized by a mild to moderate degeneration of mainly the frontal lobe and by a limited temporal lobe degeneration (Brun 1987, 1993; Neary *et al.* 1988; Knopman *et al.* 1990), characterized by neuronal loss, microvacuolation, and gliosis of the superficial cortical layers. These changes also involve the anterior but rarely the posterior cingulate gyrus, hippocampus, and striate body. The substantia nigra may be moderately affected, and the frontal white matter often shows a mild loss of myelin (Englund and Brun 1987). There are no Alzheimer changes, except mild ones compatible with age, no amyloidosis, and no Pick bodies or inflated neurons in FLD. The cortical atrophy in Pick's disease is severe, circumscribed with a knife-blade appearance of the gyri, more often asymmetrical and also involving the striatum and hippocampus. The pathology in MND with dementia is similar to that of FLD, but in addition there are ubiquitin-positive inclusions in cortical layer II and dentate granule cells, and spinal and bulbar motor system degeneration (Neary *et al.* 1990; Mitsuyama 1993). The histopathology and the pattern of cortical involvement in FTD are strikingly different from those of AD or dementia with Lewy bodies.

Prevalence and epidemiology

Most demographic data concern the group of FTD as a whole, rather than FLD and Pick's disease separately. 'Pure' Pick's disease, as here defined, is rare, with a prevalence of 1–2% in postmortem studies of dementia, compared to a prevalence of 7.5% for FLD and 40–50% for AD (Gustafson 1993). A 20% prevalence rate of FTD among early-onset dementia has been suggested (Neary 1990). FTD was diagnosed in about 5% of 1517 consecutive outpatients with all types of dementia at the Memory clinic in Lille, France

(Pasquier *et al.* 1999). The marked geographic variation in the prevalence of FTD might be due to genetic and environmental factors and to differences in patient selection and diagnostic criteria. The male to female ratio of FLD is 1:1. The prevalence of dementia in patients with MND has been estimated at between 2 and 6% (Lopez *et al.* 1994).

Case 1

The patient was a 52-year-old housewife with three teenagers living at home. Previously a quiet and amiable person, she became uncritically outspoken and tactless even in her contacts with unknown people and markedly unconcerned about her family. The clinical progression was slow, and not until several years later did the family members suspect that the mental changes were caused by a disease. At that time the patient's strange behaviour had caused serious conflicts within the family. The patient was referred to a hospital for medical examination at the age of 55. Neurological examination and EEG were normal. She showed an increased appetite with overeating and rapid weight gain. Her speech was described as aspontaneous, mainly consisting of stereotyped phrases such as, 'May I go now?' She seemed emotionally blunted, with an inadequate smile and lacking in insight, but was well orientated and showed only a slight memory impairment.

At the age of 57 years the patient showed a total amimia, semi-mutism, and a restless pacing. Previously a moderate smoker she was now smoking excessively. She was doubly incontinent. Spatial orientation and facial recognition were, however, preserved and she remained roughly oriented to time. Blood pressure and routine laboratory data were normal, whereas the EEG was slightly pathological with diffuse general slowing. The neuropsychological testing clearly indicated a frontal lobe pattern with reduced vocabulary and verbal fluency, while visuospatial capacity was only slightly below average. Her capacity to write was remarkably spared until the last year of her life. The patient seemed totally unaware of her mistakes in the test situation. Cranial tomography showed only a slight cortical atrophy. Measurement of regional cerebral blood flow (rCBF) showed a total flow level within the normal range, and a marked bilateral focal frontal flow reduction with a slight left-side predominance. The patient died at the age of 59, with a terminal pneumonia caused by dysphagia and aspiration. The patient's mother, at the age of 62 years, had developed a progressive mental deterioration with apathy and mutism. Thus, this middle-aged woman slowly developed a dementia of frontal lobe type with personality changes, a progressive loss of expressive speech, with stereotypy and late mutism. By contrast verbal understanding, writing, spatial orientation, and recognition were comparatively spared. The neuropathological diagnosis was FLD with degeneration in the frontal and anterior temporal lobes and parts of the limbic system.

Clinical course and features

The clinical onset of FTD is insidious and usually between 35 and 70 years of age. The mean age at onset in postmortem verified FLD is 56 ± 7.6 years and the mean duration is of 8 ± 3.4 years (range 3–17 years) (Gustafson 1993). Age at onset in Pick's disease is similar, but the duration is somewhat longer, 9.8 years (range 4.8–21.2 years). Due to the long duration of the disease many FTD patients live until old age. The onset of dementia in MND usually occurs in the sixth decade and the mean duration is about 30 months.

The early stage of FTD is characterized by deterioration of personality, behaviour, and speech rather than by cognitive impairment, although memory failure and a lack of concentration are almost always found. The diagnostic features specified in the Lund–Manchester consensus are presented in Table 24v.1.

Behavioural disorder

Behavioural and emotional changes are always present in FTD. In the early stages they are often non-specific and not easy to recognize as the first manifestations of a dementing illness, which therefore leads to an underestimation of the duration of the disease. Other explanations such as depression, psychosis, conflicts and psychosocial events may be suggested, especially by people who lack previous knowledge of the patient. The patient becomes self-centred with a loss of personal and social awareness, neglects personal hygiene, and shows disinhibition, unpredictability, tactlessness, and even antisocial behaviour. The dysregulation of emotions and

Table 24v.1 The Lund–Manchester clinical criteria for FTD (slightly modified)

Core diagnostic features

Behavioural disorder
- Insidious onset and slow progression
- Early loss of insight into changes of own mental state
- Early loss of personal and social awareness
- Early signs of disinhibition and lack of judgement
- Mental rigidity and inflexibility
- Stereotyped, repetitive, and imitating behaviour
- Hyperorality, oral/dietary changes
- Utilization behaviour
- Distractibility, impulsivity, and impersistence

Affective symptoms
- Depression, anxiety, excessive sentimentality
- Hypochondriasis, bizarre somatic complaints
- Emotional bluntness, apathy, and lack of empathy
- Amimia

Speech disorder
- Progressive reduction of speech output
- Stereotypy of speech, perseveration
- Echolalia
- Late mutism

Spatial orientation, receptive speech, and praxis preserved

Physical signs
- Early primitive reflexes
- Early incontinence
- Late akinesia, rigidity, and tremor
- Low and labile blood pressure

Investigations
- Normal EEG despite clinically evident dementia
- Brain imaging (structural and/or functional): predominant frontal and/or anterior temporal abnormality
- Neuropsychology: profound failure on 'frontal lobe' tests in the absence of severe amnesia, or perceptual spatial disorder

Supportive diagnostic features
- Onset before 65 years of age
- Positive family history of similar disorder in a first-degree relative
- Bulbar palsy, muscular weakness and wasting, fasciculations (motor neuron disease)

behaviour is also seen as tearfulness, inadequate smiling, inappropriate joking, irritability, and restlessness. Easily provoked acts of violence, craving for affection and sexual contacts, impulse buying, shoplifting, and hoarding may lead to social complications, economic problems, divorce, and even suicide in the family. FTD patients also tend to become inattentive and careless in traffic situations, whilst the typical Alzheimer patient is more self-critical and aware of difficulties in driving. A common feature in FTD is stereotyped and perseverative behaviour such as wandering, clapping, humming, and an obsessional preoccupation with daily routines such as washing and locking doors.

In a longitudinal study of dementia, hallucinations and delusions are reported in about 20% of FTD and early-onset AD and in 50% of late-onset AD cases (Gustafson 1993). The hallucinations and delusions in FTD show an important clinical variability and often give the impression of a functional psychosis, with schizophrenia as an early, tentative diagnosis in several cases. This misinterpretation is likely when there is a combination of emotional changes, delusions, and communication problems of frontal lobe type. Visual, auditory as well as tactile, hallucinations are reported in FTD as well as in AD. Hyperaesthesia and severe and long-lasting pain are sometimes reported in FTD.

Restlessness in combination with utilization behaviour (see Chapter 9, p. 000), hyperorality, hypersexuality, and a blunting of drive and emotions are also prevalent in FTD, producing a Klüver–Bucy-like syndrome (Brun and Gustafson 1978; Cummings and Duchen 1981). Hyperorality and changes of oral/dietary behaviour are seen as overeating, food fads, excessive smoking and alcohol consumption, and oral exploration of inanimate objects. The Klüver–Bucy-like syndrome in FTD is usually more complete than in AD, with more hypersexuality and utilization behaviour.

Affective symptoms

Early emotional changes in FTD are described as emotional blunting and shallowness. The patient becomes self-centred, mentally rigid, and inflexible. Elated mood, especially when associated with increased talkativeness and restlessness, may at first sight be mistaken for a hypomanic or a manic state. Slowly developing apathy in combination with sparse mimical movements and verbal aspontaneity may be misdiagnosed as depression. More than one-third of our postmortem-verified FTD patients had been diagnosed as depressed and treated with antidepressant medication during the early stage of the disease. The depressive reactions are mostly transitory. Anxiety and/or hypochondriasis are reported in almost 50% of patients.

The early symptoms of dementia must be judged against information about the patient's premorbid personality, education, cognition, and social background. The premorbid personality is usually judged to be fairly normal, although some FTD cases previously manifested anxiety and restlessness (Gustafson 1987). The emotional features in FTD do not seem primarily related to premorbid personality traits, but rather to the distribution of brain pathology as shown at autopsy and brain imaging (Lebert *et al.* 1995).

Speech disorder

A typical feature of FTD is a progressive loss of expressive speech, described as dissolution of language and '*Sprachverödung*' (van Mansfelt 1954), with late mutism in about 80% of cases. However, even at an advanced stage of the disease, the mute and amimic patient seems to be capable of some understanding and recognition. The speech disorder usually starts as a verbal aspontaneity, with word-finding difficulties and stereotyped comments with frequent repetition of a limited number of phrases. There may be an initial period of increased, unrestrained talking and singing. Imitating behaviour, especially echolalia, is found in about 50% of FTD cases (Gustafson 1993). The patient's handwriting may change in various respects such as magnitude, spelling, and perseveration. These disturbances are usually unlike the dysgraphia in AD. The symptom constellation of palilalia, echolalia, mutism, and amimia (PEMA syndrome of Guiraud) is typical of FTD and rare in AD. By contrast logoclonia is prevalent in AD and uncommon in FTD. Patients with progressive non-fluent aphasia (Snowden *et al.* 1991), characterized by effortful speech production and relative preservation of memory and practical abilities, may develop dementia accompanied by degenerative changes similar to those in FTD, with a predominant involvement of the speech dominant hemisphere.

Physical signs

Patients with FTD are remarkably free from somatic findings even in advanced stages. Neurological signs are generally limited to the presence of primitive reflexes, while akinesia, rigidity, tremor, and dysphagia are late phenomena. Increased muscular tension is more common in AD than in FTD. Lynch *et al.* have linked the syndrome of the disinhibition–dementia–parkinsonism–amyotrophy complex (DDPAC; see Wilhelmsen 1997), also named FTD with parkinsonism, to chromosome 17 (Lynch *et al.* 1994). Low blood pressure, orthostatic hypotension, and syncopal attacks are prevalent in FTD, and also in AD and vascular dementia (Passant *et al.* 1997).

Urinary incontinence, which is reported early in about 50% of FTD cases, is a comparatively late feature in uncomplicated early-onset AD. Generalized epileptic seizures may appear in FTD, although they are less prevalent than in AD; myoclonic twitchings are rare compared to AD.

The clinical picture in MND with dementia is similar to that of FLD, although with a more rapidly aggressive course and physical signs of anterior horn involvement. The mental changes may appear early and sometimes precede the typical neurological features (Mitsuyama 1993).

Investigations

The EEG is judged to be normal or only slightly pathological in most cases of FLD, Pick's disease, and MND with dementia, even when the dementia is clinically evident (Johanneson *et al.* 1977; Gustafson 1987; Pasquier *et al.* 1999). By contrast, the EEG is almost always pathological in AD, even at an early stage.

Brain imaging has greatly improved the recognition of FTD. Computed tomography (CT) and magnetic resonance imaging (MRI) reveal frontal and/or temporal cortical atrophy, sometimes asymmetrical, and more deep white matter lesions than in matched normal controls (Förstl *et al.* 1996; Pasquier *et al.* 1999; Larsson *et al.* 2000). Functional brain imaging using the Xenon-clearance technique (Gustafson *et al.* 1977; Risberg 1987), single photon emission computed tomography (SPECT) (Jagust *et al.* 1989; Miller *et al.* 1993; Frisoni *et al.* 1995; Pasquier *et al.* 1999), and positron emission tomography (PET) has radically improved the early diagnosis of dementia. The frontotemporal flow pathology found in FTD contrasts with the temporal limbic and temporoparietal pathology seen in AD. The flow pattern is, however, not disease-specific but is also found in vascular brain damage, Creutzfeldt–Jakob disease, AD, and in other degenerative diseases with frontal accentuation (Brun and Gustafson 1993).

Neuropsychological testing in FTD shows cognitive deficits suggesting dysfunction of the anterior cortex. Cognition may, however, be difficult to evaluate due to the patient's emotional changes and speech disorder. The early test profile is characterized by slow verbal production and relatively intact reasoning and memory, while intellectual and motor speed are reduced (Neary *et al.* 1988; Johanson and Hagberg 1989; Knopman *et al.* 1989; Pasquier *et al.* 1999). By comparison, patients with early AD show a relatively intact verbal ability and a simultaneous impairment of reasoning ability, verbal and spatial memory dysfunction, dysphasia, and visuospatial dysfunction (Johanson and Hagberg 1989; Frisoni *et al.* 1995). Memory disturbances are found at an early stage of FTD but remote memory and memory for daily events are affected to a lesser extent than in AD. Memory impairment and confabulation may be more prevalent in Pick's disease, because of more severe hippocampal involvement. A short test battery (Elfgren *et al.* 1994) and a screening instrument (Gregory *et al.* 1997) have been developed for discriminating between FTD and AD. Evaluation of the patient's behaviour in the test situation strongly contributes to this differentiation (Johanson and Hagberg 1989; Pachana *et al.* 1996). Receptive dysphasia is found at an early stage only in a minority of FTD cases (mostly Pick cases), and reading and writing may be preserved in FTD even at a late state when the patients have become completely mute.

Differential diagnoses

The clinical neuropsychological and brain imaging differences between FTD and AD have already been touched upon. These differences are often already obvious at an early stage. Patients with frontal ischaemic white matter disease, Binswanger's disease, and strategic infarctions in structures projecting to frontal lobes, may also mimic FTD—especially when developing gradually. Differentiating FTD from Huntington's disease or Creutzfeldt–Jakob disease may be critical when changes of personality and psychotic features dominate the clinical picture and neurological symptoms are less obvious. Patients with progressive supranuclear palsy and progressive subcortical gliosis may also show the clinical and imaging features of a frontal lobe pathology. PSP and corticobasal degeneration are becoming increasingly important because of linkage studies suggesting a linkage to chromosome 17.

Clinical variants and classification of FTD

Early on, clinicopathological subtypes of FTD were suggested on histopathological grounds and on differences in topography, severity, and progression of the degenerative process. Classification based on genetics has been suggested, but the molecular classification of dementia is not yet available (Mann *et al.* 2000). The anteroposterior gradient as well as laterality of the degenerative brain changes influence the clinical picture of FTD. Consequently, different frontal and temporal clinical variants have been described and related to brain dysfunction, as revealed by functional and structural brain imaging (Gregory 1990; Miller *et al.* 1991; Edwards-Lee *et al.* 1997; Didic *et al.* 1998). Van Mansfelt (1954), in a review of 196 cases of Pick's disease reported in the literature, found frontotemporal atrophy in 54%, mainly frontal atrophy in 25%, and predominant temporal atrophy in 17%. Asymmetry was common, with left-side predominance in 46% and right-side predominance in 17%. The clinical similarities between FLD and Pick's disease are important and differential diagnosis on purely clinical grounds is very difficult. Clinical differences can often be explained by variation in the localization and severity of brain pathology against the background of a common pattern of cortical involvement. A problem in attempting to subclassify FTD is that each patient passes through various stages of a changing clinical picture, and that the duration of these stages may vary markedly. The clinical subtypes under discussion today are mainly based on the early clinical manifestations and less on symptoms and treatment problems appearing at later stages of the disease. These points deserve more attention because of the increasing possibilities for early diagnosis and the development of new forms of treatment and care.

The Lund–Manchester consensus (Table 24v.1) is recommended as a guideline for the clinical recognition of FTD. In our clinical work we use a scoring profile based on the three diagnostic assessment scales for the recognition of AD, FTD (Brun and Gustafson 1993), and vascular dementia (Ischemic Score, Hashinski *et al.* 1975).

The several major widely accepted classification systems do not include FTD as a separate entity. The revised fourth edition of the *Diagnostic and statistical manual of mental disorders* (DSM-IV, APA 1994) presents Pick's disease as one of the distinct pathological aetiologies among the dementing processes associated with fronto-temporal brain atrophy. The tenth edition of the *International classification of diseases* (ICD-10, WHO 1992) describes 'dementia in Pick's disease' as a non-Alzheimer degenerative brain disease, but it does not introduce the concepts of frontal lobe dementia or FTD. Guidelines for diagnoses of dementia, such as the NINCDS-ADRDA criteria for the diagnosis of AD (McKhann *et al.* 1984), may easily include FLD and Pick cases in the AD group.

Aetiology

The aetiology and pathogenesis of FLD, Pick's disease, and MND are still unknown. The pattern of degeneration in FTD may be related to selective vulnerability of different brain regions to factors such as oxidative stress, environmental toxins, neurotransmitter dysfunction, and certain mutations. Although there is a tendency for FTD patients to develop hypotension, the pathological changes do not strictly conform to the distribution or type of lesions associated with anoxic or ischaemic lesions. A genetic factor seems most likely, because approximately 50% of FLD cases have a history of a similar disorder in a first-degree relative (Gustafson 1987; Neary *et al.* 1988). Passant *et al.* (1995) described a Swedish family with 11 affected members out of 21 family members in three generations; five cases in the third generation have been verified as FLD. Possible genes have been indicated by mapping to chromosome 3 in a Danish family with dementia of frontal lobe type (Brown *et al.* 1995), and linkage to chromosome 17 and the *tau* gene in families with FTD with parkinsonism (Hutton *et al.* 1998). Characteristic tau phenotypes may distinguish FLD, Pick's disease, corticobasal degeneration, and PSP (Delacourte 1999). The mutations found in AD, Huntington's disease, and MND have not been detected in FLD or Pick's disease. Conflicting results exist concerning the relation of FLD to chromosome 19 and the *APOE* allele pattern (Lehmann *et al.* 2000).

Neurochemical studies of FTD have revealed no systematic alterations in cholinergic markers; but a dopamine decrease and a reduction of serotonin receptors and substance P in the substantia nigra and frontal cortex have been found in Pick's disease (Francis *et al.* 1993). Cerebrospinal fluid analysis has shown reduced somatostatin levels both in FTD and AD, while delta sleep-inducing peptide was significantly reduced in AD and the corticotrophin-releasing factor was significantly reduced in FTD (Edvinsson *et al.* 1993). Prion analysis has so far given negative results in FLD and Pick's disease (Collinge *et al.* 1994).

Treatment and care

The important consequence of an early and specific diagnosis of FTD is that the patient's strange behaviour can be understood and explained, and thereby the family and other carers can be offered support. It also enables FTD to be differentiated from AD, for which pharmacological treatments are now available. The long duration of the dementing process and the awareness of hereditary factors have a strong impact on family members. FTD patients are often restless, impulsive, and stereotyped with a strong need for physical activity. The preserved memory, spatial, and practical abilities should be channelled in a meaningful way rather than restricted. A well-structured programme for daily activities, which takes into account the patient's premorbid personality and interests, may be rewarding and minimize a need for pharmacological treatment. Psychotic features and unpredictable aggressive behaviour should be taken care of by special psychogeriatric or psychiatric services.

References

Alzheimer, A. (1911). Über eigenartige Krankheitsfälle des späteren Alters. *Zeitschrift für die Gesamte Neurologie und Psychiatrie*, **4**, 356–8.

American Psychiatric Association (APA). (1994). *Diagnostic and statistical manual of mental disorders (DSM-IV)*. APA, Washington DC.

Brown, J., Asworth, A., Gydesen, S., Soranden, A., Rossor, M., Hardy, D., *et al.* (1995). Familial non-specific dementia maps to chromosome 3. *Human Molecular Genetics*, **4**, 1625–8.

Brun, A. (1987). Frontal lobe degeneration of non-Alzheimer type. I. Neuropathology. *Archives of Gerontology and Geriatrics*, **6**, 193–207.

Brun, A. (1993). Frontal lobe degeneration of non-Alzheimer type, revisited. *Dementia*, **4**, 126–31.

Brun, A. and Gustafson, L. (1978). Limbic lobe involvement in presenile dementia. *Archiv für Psychiatrie und Nervenkrankheiten*, **226**, 79–93.

Brun, A. and Gustafson, L. (1993). The Lund longitudinal dementia study: a 25-year perspective on neuropathology, differential diagnosis and treatment. In *Alzheimer's disease: advances in clinical and basic research* (ed. B. Corain, K. Iqbal, M. Nicolini, B. Winblad, H. Wasniewski, and P. Zatta), pp. 27–33. Wiley, Chichester

Brun, A., Englund, B., Gustafson, L., Passant *et al* (1994). Clinical and neuropathological criteria for frontotemporal dementia. Consensus statement. The Lund and Manchester Groups. *Journal of Neurology, Neurosurgery and Psychiatry*, **57**, 416–18.

Collinge, J., Hardy, J., Brown, J., and Brun, A. (1994). Familial Pick's disease and dementia in frontal lobe degeneration of non-Alzheimer type are not variants of prion disease. *Journal of Neurology, Neurosurgery and Psychiatry*, **57**, 762.

Cummings, J. L. and Duchen, L. W. (1981). Klüver–Bucy syndrome in Pick's disease: clinical and pathological correlations. *Neurology*, **31**, 1415–22.

Delacourte, A. (1999). Biochemical and molecular characterization of neurofibrillary degeneration in fronto-temporal dementias. *Dementia and Geriatric Cognitive Disorders*, **10**(Suppl. 1), 75–9.

Didic, M., Guisiano, B., de Laforte, C., Ceccaldi, M., and Ponchet, M. (1998). Identification of clinical subtypes of fronto-temporal dementia and cerebral blood flow on SPECT: preliminary results. *Alzheimer's Reports*, 3, 179–85.

Edvinsson, L., Minthon, L., Ekman, R., and Gustafson, L. (1993). Neuropeptides in cerebrospinal fluid of patients with Alzheimer's disease and dementia with fronto-temporal lobe degeneration. *Dementia*, **4**, 167–71.

Edwards-Lee, T., Miller, B. L., Benson, F. D., Cummings, J. L., Russel, G. L., Bonne, K., *et al.* (1997). The temporal variant of fronto-temporal dementia. *Brain*, **120**, 1027–40.

Elfgren, C., Brun, A., Gustafson, L., Johanson, A., Minthon, L., Passant, U., *et al.* (1994). Neuropsychological tests as discriminators between dementia of Alzheimer type and fronto-temporal dementia. *International Journal of Geriatric Psychiatry*, **9**, 635–42.

Englund, E. and Brun, A. (1987). Frontal lobe degeneration of non-Alzheimer type. IV. White matter changes. *Archives of Gerontology and Geriatrics*, **6**, 235–43.

Förstl, H., Besthorn, C., Hentschel F., Geiger-Kabisch, C., Sattel, H., and Schreiter-Gasser, U. (1996). Frontal lobe degeneration and Alzheimer's disease: a controlled study on clinical findings, volumetric brain changes and quantitative electro-encephalography data. *Dementia*, **7**, 27–34.

Francis, P. T., Holmes, C., Webster, M-T., Stratmann, G. C., Procter, A. W., and Bowen, D. M. (1993). Preliminary neurochemical findings in non-Alzheimer dementia due to lobar atrophy. *Dementia*, **4**, 172–7.

Frisoni, G. B., Pizzolato, G., Geroldi, C., Rossato, A., Bianchetti, A., and Trabuceti, M. (1995). Dementia of the frontal type: neuropsychological and (99Tc)-HMPAO SPET features. *Journal of Geriatric Psychiatry and Neurology*, **8**, 42–8.

Gregory, C. (1999). Frontal variant of fronto-temporal dementia: a cross-sectional and longitudinal study of neuropsychiatric features. *Psychological Medicine*, **29**, 1205–17.

Gregory, C. A., Orrell, M., Sahakian, B., and Hodges, J. R. (1997). Can fronto-temporal dementia and Alzheimer's disease be differentiated using a brief battery of tests? *International Journal of Geriatric Psychiatry*, **12**, 375–83.

Gustafson, L. (1987). Frontal lobe degeneration of non-Alzheimer type. II. Clinical picture and differential diagnosis. *Archives of Gerontology and Geriatrics*, **6**, 209–33.

Gustafson, L. (1993). Clinical picture of frontal lobe dementia of non-Alzheimer type. *Dementia*, **4**, 143–8.

Gustafson, L., Brun, A., and Ingvar, D. H. (1977). Clinical neurocirculatory findings in presenile dementia, related to neuropathological changes. *Activitas Nervosa Superior*, **19**, 351–3.

Hachinski, V. F., Iliff, L. D., Zilhka, E., du Boulay, G. H., McAllister, V. L., Marshall, J., *et al.* (1975). Cerebral blood flow in dementia. *Archives of Neurology*, **32**, 632–7.

Hutton, M., Lendon, C. L., Rizzu, P., Baker, M. *et al.* (1998). Association of missense and 5′—splice-site mutations in tau with the inherited dementia FTDP-17. *Nature*, **393**, 702–5

Jagust, W. J., Reed, B. R., Seab, J. P., Kramer, J. H., and Budinger, T. F. (1989). Clinical-psychologic correlations of Alzheimer's disease and frontal lobe dementia. *American Journal of Psychological Imaging*, **4**, 89–96.

Johannesson, G., Brun, A., Gustafson, L., and Ingvar, D. H. (1977). EEG in presenile dementia related to cerebral blood flow and autopsy findings. *Acta Neurologica Scandinavica*, **56**, 89–103.

Johanson, A. and Hagberg, B. (1989). Psychometric characteristics in patients with frontal lobe degeneration of non-Alzheimer type. *Archives of Gerontology and Geriatrics*, **8**, 129–37.

Knopman, D. S., Christensen, K. J., Schut, L. J., Harbaugh, R. E., Reeder, T., Ngo, T., *et al.* (1989). The spectrum of imaging and neuropsychological findings in Pick's disease. *Neurology*, **39**, 362–8.

Knopman, D. S., Mastri, A. R., Frey, W. H., Sung, J. H., and Rustan, T. (1990). Dementia lacking distinctive histologic features. A common non-Alzheimer degenerative dementia. *Neurology*, **40**, 251–6.

Larsson, E-M., Passant, U., Sundgren, P. C., Englund, E., Brun, A., Lindgren, A., *et al.* (2000). Magnetic resonance imaging and histopathology in dementia, clinically of fronto-temporal type. *Dementia and Geriatric Cognitive Disorders*, **11**, 123–4.

Lebert, F., Pasquier, F., and Petit, H. (1995). Personality traits and frontal lobe dementia. *International Journal of Geriatric Psychiatry*, **10**, 1046–9.

Lehmann, D. J., Smith, A. D., Combrinck, M., Barnetson, L., and Joachim, C. (2000). Apolipoprotein E e2 may be a risk factor for sporadic fronto-temporal dementia. *Journal of Neurology, Neurosurgery and Psychiatry*, **69**, 401–9.

Lopez, O. L., Becker, J. T., and De Kosky, S. T. (1994). Dementia accompanying motor neuron disease. *Dementia*, **5**, 42–7.

Lynch, T., Sano, M., Marder, K. S., Bell, K. L., Foster, N. L., Defendini, R. F., *et al.* (1994). Clinical characteristics of a family with chromosome 17-linked disinhibition–dementia–parkinsonism–amyotrophy complex. *Neurology*, **44**, 1878–84.

McKhann, G., Drachmann, D. A., Folstein, M., Katmann, R., Price, D., and Stadlan, E. M. (1984). Clinical diagnosis of Alzheimer's disease: report of the NINCDS-ADRDA Work Group. *Neurology*, **34**, 939–44.

Mann, D., McDonagh, A., Snowden, J., Neary, D., and Pickering-Brown, S. (2000). Molecular classification of the dementias. *Lancet*, **19**, 626.

Miller, B. L., Cummings, J. L., Villanueva-Meyer, J., Boone, K., Mehringer, C. M., Lesser, I. M., *et al.* (1991). Frontal lobe degeneration: clinical, neuropsychological, and SPECT characteristics. *Neurology*, **42**, 1374–82.

Miller, B. L., Chang, L., Mena, I., Boone, K., and Lesser, I. M. (1993). Progressive right fronto-temporal degeneration: clinical, neuropsychological and SPECT characteristics. *Dementia*, **4**, 204–13.

Mitsuyama, Y. (1993). Presenile dementia with motor neuron disease. *Dementia*, **4**, 137–42.

Neary, D. (1990). Dementia of frontal lobe type. *Journal of the American Geriatrics Society*, **38**, 71–2.

Neary, D., Snowden, J. S., Northern, B., and Goulding, P. J. (1988). Dementia of frontal lobe type. *Journal of Neurology, Neurosurgery and Psychiatry*, **51**, 353–61.

Neary, D., Snowden, J. S., Mann, D. M. A., Northen, B., Goulding, P. J., and McDermott, N. (1990). Frontal lobe dementia and motor neuron disease. *Journal of Neurology, Neurosurgery and Psychiatry*, **53**, 23–32.

Neary, D., Snowden, J. S., Gustafson, L., Passant, U., Stuss, D., Black, S., *et al.* (1998). Fronto-temporal lobar degeneration. A consensus on clinical diagnostic criteria. *Neurology*, **51**, 1546–54.

Onari, K. and Spatz, H. (1926). Anatomische Beiträge zur Lehre von der Pickschen umschriebenen Großhirnrinden-Atrophie ('Pickshe Krankheit'). *Zeitschrift Neurologie*, **101**, 470–511.

Pachana, N. A., Brauer-Boone, K., Miller, B. L., Cummings, J. L., and Berman, N. (1996). Comparison of neuropsychological functioning in Alzheimer's disease and frontotemporal dementia. *Journal of the International Neuropsychological Society*, **2**, 505–10.

Pasquier, F., Lebert, F., Amouyel, P., Lavenu, I., and Guillame, B. (1999). The clinical picture of frontotemporal dementia: diagnosis and follow-up. *Dementia and Geriatric Cognitive Disorders*, **10**(Suppl. 1), 10–14.

Passant, U., Warkentin, S., and Gustafson, L. (1995). Functional activation of the frontal lobes: rCBF findings during a word fluency task in normals, in patients with frontal lobe dementia (FLD), and in patients with Alzheimer's disease (DAT). *Journal of Cerebral Blood Flow and Metabolism*, **15/1**, 835.

Passant, U., Warkentin, S., and Gustafson, L. (1997). Orthostatic hypotension and low blood pressure in organic dementia: a study of prevalence and related clinical characteristics. *International Journal of Geriatric Psychiatry*, **12**, 395–403.

Pick, A. (1892). Über die Beziehungen der senilen Hirnatrophie zur Aphasie. *Prager Medizinische Wochenschrift*, **17**, 165–7.

Risberg, J. (1987). Frontal lobe degeneration of non-Alzheimer type. III. Regional cerebral blood flow. *Archives of Gerontology and Geriatrics*, **6**, 225–33.

Snowden, J. S., Neary, D. and Mann, D. M. A. (1991). *Frontotemporal lobar degeneration: Frontotemporal dementia, progressive aphasia, semantic dementia.* Churchill Livingstone, Edinburgh and New York.

Van Mansfelt, J. (1954). Pick's disease. A syndrome of lobar, cerebral atrophy; its clinico-anatomical and histopathological types. *Thesis, Enschede, Utrect.*

WHO (1992). *ICD-10 classification of mental and behavioural disorders. Clinical descriptions and diagnostic guidelines*. World Health Organization, Geneva.

Wilhelmsen, K. C. (1997). Disinhibition–dementia–parkinsonism–amyotrophy complex (DDPAC) is a non-Alzheimer's fronto-temporal dementia. *Journal of Neuronal Transmitters Supplement*, **49**, 269–75.

24vi Neurological dementias

Richard Harvey

Introduction

More than 200 neurological diseases can be associated with progressive cognitive impairment and dementia, all of which present significant diagnostic challenges for the clinician. Many are exceptionally rare, while others have very specific and characteristic physical signs and pathophysiological features. The following chapter briefly summarizes some of the more prominent neurological causes of dementia, particularly those that occasionally present to psychiatrists rather than neurologists. Further details on many rarer causes of dementia can be found in Rossor (2000), and in the references given for each disease covered in this section.

Cerebral vasculitis

This is an inflammatory disorder of cerebral vessels which may be a primary disorder (Wegener's granulomatosis, microscopic polyangiitis, temporal arteritis), or secondary to other systemic diseases (collagen vascular or rheumatological disorders, malignancy, drugs, and infections).

The classic presentation is of progressive multifocal neurological impairment. However, vasculitis may mimic a range of neurological disorders, with symptoms suggesting a cerebral tumour, meningitis, multiple sclerosis, encephalitis, and dementia (Scolding *et al.* 1997), indeed virtually every neurological sign and symptom has been reported at least once!.

Non-focal symptoms such as headache and confusion are, however, the most common initial symptoms. In any patient where a CNS vasculitis is suspected, the first step is to take a thorough history and perform a physical examination to exclude a systemic vasculitis. The physical examination should focus on the skin, eyes, paranasal sinuses, and lungs. A cerebrospinal fluid (CSF) examination is mandatory to exclude infectious and paraneoplasic meningitis.

An elevated erythrocyte sedimentation rate (ESR) or CRP should lead to suspicion. A magnetic resonance imaging (MRI) scan is abnormal in the majority of patients, although changes are not specific. Vasculitis may be visible on ophthalmological examination with video microscopy and low-dose fluorescein angiography. A cerebral biopsy is diagnostic, ideally when directed to lesions visible on MRI.

The potential treatability of this condition is the major reason for invasive investigation. Treatment with steroids, in some cases augmented with immunosuppression, may be dramatically effective (Scolding *et al.* 1997).

Corticobasal degeneration

Corticobasal degeneration (CBD) is a rare form of dementia, with clinical features that are a combination of cognitive impairment and asymmetrical motor symptoms representing dysfunction in both the cortex and the basal ganglia. It is now being increasingly recognized, and is a major differential in the diagnosis of Parkinson's disease.

The disease usually starts after the age of 60 years. Cortical symptoms include dementia, apraxia, dysarthria, speech apraxia, hyperreflexia, and frontal lobe signs. The typical basal ganglia symptoms include parkinsonism (tremor and rigidity) and dystonia.

The clinical presentations are, however, fairly constant. Most patients present with asymmetrical motor symptoms, often described as a stiff hand or arm, or difficulty with writing. Other patients present with cognitive impairment but later develop this asymmetrical apraxia. Nearly all cases have extrapyramidal symptoms in the form of combinations of bradykinesia, 'alien limb', rigidity, tremor, and postural instability; often suggesting a diagnosis of Parkinson's disease. The heterogeneity of the clinical presentation, with initial symptoms of either cognitive or motor problems, result in some patients being referred to neurologists or geriatricians interested in movement disorders, while others are referred to neurologists or psychiatrists interested in dementia.

In a review of consecutive autopsy-diagnosed cases, CBD was usually only one of several differential diagnoses (Boeve *et al.* 1999). Other clinical diagnoses included Parkinson's disease, vascular dementia, atypical Alzheimer's disease, motor neurone disease, Pick's disease, and dementia with Lewy bodies. This heterogeneity is also present neuropathologically, with many cases having neuropathological features of other degenerative dementias as well as CBD.

The diagnosis is based on the history and clinical examination. A structural CT or MRI scan will often show asymmetrical cerebral atrophy (Winkelmann *et al.* 1999). Functional neuroimaging with positron emission tomography (PET) or single photon emission computed tomography (SPECT) will confirm an asymmetrical reduction in cortical metabolism.

Corticobasal degeneration is a slowly progressive dementia, and early signs, such as a limb apraxia, may remain as isolated symptoms for several years before more widespread symptoms appear. There are no specific treatments, and in particular there is no response of the parkinsonian symptoms to L-dopa. The development of dysphagia often marks the onset of the terminal phase of the illness.

The neuropathological diagnosis is based macroscopically on the finding of frontoparietal neuronal loss and gliosis, which is often asymmetrical. Microscopically there are cortical ballooned neurons, degeneration of the substantia nigra, and variable involvement of the subcortical nuclei including the basal ganglia.

Dementia in multiple sclerosis (Feinstein 2000)

Up to half of community-resident multiple sclerosis (MS) patients develop significant cognitive impairment as their illness progresses, and in some cases dementia may be the presenting or major feature.

As MS is a disease of white matter, the dementia associated with MS most commonly has subcortical features. Cognitive function declines as the disease progresses, and remains static when the disease is static. The cognitive impairment is readily detected on neuropsychological testing. Atrophy can be demonstrated on CT or MRI scans, although there is usually no clear correlation between the distribution of atrophy and of the multiple sclerosis plaques.

Dementia in Parkinson's disease

Parkinson's disease (PD) is characterized pathologically by the presence of Lewy bodies in the substantia nigra and other brainstem nuclei. Approximately one-third of PD patients develop dementia as the disease progresses (Mindham 1999), probably as the distribution of Lewy bodies extends from the brainstem to the cortex, although other mechanism have also been suggested.

The clinical features of dementia in PD are, however, very similar to those of patients with dementia with Lewy bodies (DLB). The most common presentation is increasing mental inflexibility in a patient with PD, followed by defects of executive function, marked fluctuation, and in many cases visual hallucinations. The hallucinations are often exacerbated by anticholinergic and dopamine-agonist medications. Management is very similar to that for DLB, and often depends on balancing the need to treat the motor symptoms of PD, while minimizing the side-effects of the treatments in terms of worsened cognition and neuropsychiatric features. Collaboration between the neurologist or geriatrician and the psychiatrist is often the key in providing the best possible care for patients with this disease. Depression is particularly common and should be rigorously identified and treated (Waters 1997).

HIV/AIDS dementia

As many as one-third of patients with the acquired immunodeficiency syndrome (AIDS) eventually develop dementia (Lipton 1997). Human immunodeficiency viral (HIV) dementia is a pervasive neurological disorder with characteristic cognitive, motor, and behavioural symptoms. Cognitive features include mental slowing with impaired consciousness and memory. The motor manifestations include slowed fast limb movements, gait disorder, spasticity, and hyperreflexia. The prominent behavioural changes include apathy and withdrawal.

The disease is most commonly associated with the late manifestations of AIDS, and the patient will usually have evidence of severe immunosuppression, although up to 30% of people who have asymptomatic HIV infection show mild neurological dysfunction.

HIV-associated dementia is a clinical diagnosis, with evaluation directed towards excluding other causes of cognitive impairment. Neuroimaging is important and may show cerebral atrophy, white matter lesions. or evidence of other CNS manifestations of AIDS such as toxoplasmosis or cryptosporidiosis.

Recent anti-HIV triple therapy regimens are effective in treating all manifestations of HIV, including dementia, with treatment being both preventive and symptomatic (Chang *et al.* 1999; Price *et al.* 1999).

Huntington's disease

Huntington's disease (HD) is a hereditary progressive neurological disease characterized by a triad of clinical features: motor symptoms, cognitive impairment, and psychiatric disturbance.

The motor features include abnormalities of voluntary movement (clumsiness, bradykinesia, rigidity, gait disturbance, dysarthria, dysphagia, and saccadic eye movements) and involuntary movement (chorea, dystonia, athetosis, motor restlessness, and myoclonus). The prominence of the chorea usually results in referral to neurologists with an interest in movement disorders, rather than to dementia or memory clinics.

The cognitive deficits relate to impairment of memory, calculation, verbal fluency, visuospatial ability, and frontal executive skills. By contrast, aphasia, apraxia, and agnosia are uncommon in HD. Psychiatrically, patients commonly develop depression and there is a high incidence of suicide. Patients may also become irritable and disinhibited, but are rarely psychotic (Leroi and Michalon 1998).

Diagnosis is based upon the history and examination, particularly in the presence of a family history. Diagnosis can be confirmed by genetic testing showing mutations in the *huntingtin* gene on chromosome 4 (Jones *et al.* 1997).

HD is slowly progressive with death occurring 10–20 years from disease onset, often due to aspiration pneumonia or suffocation. Suicide is also a common cause of death. The later the onset of the disease, the slower is the course. The dementia of HD is untreatable.

Lysosomal storage diseases

The lysosomal storage disorders, Gaucher's disease, Niemann–Pick disease, GM2 gangliosidoses, cerebrotendinous xanthomatosis, and the polysaccharoidoses may all present in late adolescence or early adulthood with dementia. The presentation with dementia is, however, rare and most have other characteristic neurological signs. Kufs' disease and Niemann–Pick disease type-C are the most common to present with dementia (Moser 1998).

Kufs' disease (Ruchoux and Goebel 1997)

Kufs' disease is part of a group of diseases termed the neuronal ceroid lipofuscinoses. The childhood-onset forms are known as Batten's disease. The late-onset form typically starts around 30 years of age.

Onset is usually with dementia, epilepsy, dysarthria, facial dyskinesia, and cerebellar signs. There are also commonly personality and behavioural changes including psychosis. The seizures usually become intractable. Definitive diagnosis is by demonstrating characteristic granular deposits on electron microscopy of skin or cerebral biopsy material.

Niemann–Pick disease type-C (Liscum and Klansek 1998)

The disease is associated with an accumulation of sphingomyelin and other lipids in the liver, spleen, and bone marrow. The type-C variant presents at any time from infancy to adulthood with neurological symptoms and hepatosplenomegaly.

The neurological signs of the disorder are characteristic, with hepatosplenomegaly, ataxia, dementia, dystonia, and supranuclear ophthalmoplegia. The adult-onset disorder progresses more slowly, but can be associated with psychosis. Diagnosis can be made on a bone marrow examination showing 'foam' cells. Elevated levels of sphingomyelin, cholesterol, or glycolipids can also be demonstrated in liver biopsy samples.

Metachromatic leucodystrophy

A disorder of myelin metabolism due to lack of the arylsulphatase A enzyme results in an accumulation of sulphatides which stain with a metachromatic appearance. It is an autosomal recessively inherited disorder.

It is the adult variant of the disease that may present from the mid-teens to mid-70s with peripheral neuropathy, cognitive impairment, and behavioural changes. In particular, there are often frontal lobe deficits and personality changes. Spasticity, emotional lability, and involuntary movements often accompany the dementia. The diagnosis is made by demonstrating reduced arylsulphatase activity in white blood cells. Metachromatic lipid material may also be seen in samples obtained from centrifuged urine or CSF.

Mitochondrial diseases (Suomalainen 1997)

There have been rapid advances in our understanding of mitochondrial function and the identification of specific diseases. A number of these involve cognitive impairment. One of the better characterized mitochondrial syndromes associated with dementia is MELAS (mitochondrial encephalomyopathy, lactic acidosis and stroke-like episodes). In its most common form, it results in stroke-like episodes beginning before 40 years of age, encephalopathy associated with seizures and dementia, lactic acidosis, and the finding of ragged-red fibres on muscle biopsy. A range of mutations in the mitochondrial DNA result in MELAS and other encephalomyopathies

The diagnosis of mitochondrial diseases is not easy. In the family history there may be evidence of maternal inheritance, although the variability, both in the phenotype and severity of the disease, may make this difficult to detect. 'Soft' clinical signs in both the patient and relatives such as headaches, deafness, short stature, ophthalmoplegia, and diabetes may also give clues to the involvement of mitochondrial defects. The pathological hallmarks of mitochondrial diseases are the finding of ragged-red fibres in a muscle biopsy specimen. The ragged-red appearance is due the overproduction of non-functional mitochondria that are also enlarged, distorted, and contain abnormal inclusions. Biochemical analysis of the affected tissue may reveal a specific defect or combination of defects in the respiratory chain enzymes.

Normal-pressure hydrocephalus

Normal-pressure hydrocephalus (NPH) is a term used to describe chronic, communicating adult-onset hydrocephalus. Typically, patients with

NHP have a triad of cognitive impairment, gait disturbance, and urinary incontinence. The cognitive impairment shows a psychomotor slowing with prominent subcortical features. Patients are often apathetic and may appear depressed.

The causes of normal-pressure hydrocephalus include trauma, subarachnoid haemorrhage, and meningitis, although in one-third of cases the condition is idiopathic.

A CT or MRI scan will show enlarged ventricles, and by definition a lumbar puncture will show a normal CSF pressure. Interestingly, in patients with NPH who have undergone long-term CSF pressure monitoring there is good evidence that there are periods of increased CSF pressure, particularly at night (Pleasure and Fishman 1999).

The diagnosis and selection of patients for ventriculoperitoneal shunting is not easy. In particular, patients with evidence of cerebral vascular disease respond poorly to shunting. Success rates for shunting vary widely between centres with some reporting up to 80% success rates; however, in one study of 166 shunted patients, 36% had a poor response and 28% had major complications including infection and subdural haematoma.

There is no good test to establish who will benefit from shunting, although the improvement in gait disturbance following removal of CSF by lumbar puncture gives some indication of the likely value of shunting. Patients with a known cause and a short history, and those in whom imaging shows small cortical sulci and periventricular lucencies, i.e. those in whom an additional degenerative dementia is unlikely, respond best to shunting with respect to the cognitive impairment.

Prion diseases

Prion diseases are very rare, affecting approximately 1 person per million worldwide (Collinge 1997). They arise from the abnormal folding of a normal cellular protein, the prion protein (PrP^{C}) to create a pathological or scrapie isoform (PrP^{sc}). This change in the protein folding pattern may occur rarely as a spontaneous event (sporadic prion disease), or as a result of a mutation in the prion protein gene (familial prion disease). It can also be induced in the normal protein by exposure to the abnormal isoform (transmissible prion disease).

In humans, prion disease may be familial, sporadic, transmissible, or iatrogenic (Table 24vi.1). Iatrogenic prion diseases include the transmission of the disease through the use of pooled human pituitary-derived growth hormone, cadaveric corneal and dura mater grafts, and the use of prion-contaminated neurosurgical and electrophysiological instruments (Brown *et al.* 1994). Additional transmissible forms of the

Table 24vi.1 Human prion diseases

Type	Clinical syndrome	Aetiology
Acquired	Kuru	Cannibalism
	Iatrogenic CJD	Accidental inoculation with human prions (pooled cadaveric growth hormone, corneal transplants, cadaveric dura mater grafts, neurosurgical instruments)
	Variant CJD	Dietary or environmental exposure to pathogenic bovine prion protein
Sporadic	CJD	Spontaneous conversion of normal to pathogenic prion protein
Familial	Familial CJD	Autosomal dominant prion protein gene mutations. These may produce a range of phenotypes; previously known by different names, including: fatal familial insomnia (FFI) and Gerstmann–Straussler–Scheinker disease (GSS)

After Collinge 1997, with permission.

disease include kuru, due to cannibalism, which is now disappearing, and variant CJD (vCJD), transmitted from bovine spongiform encephalopathy (BSE) infected beef.

Diagnosis is based upon the history and characteristic clinical features. The classical clinical triad of CJD is a rapidly progressive dementia, myoclonus, and a periodic EEG. However, the disease is quite variable and in practice only about half of cases have the full triad. Patients usually present (in order of decreasing frequency) with cognitive decline, ataxia, or visual disturbance, either alone or in combination (Table 24vi.2).

Less common presentations include a syndrome resembling a stroke and prominent psychiatric disturbance. Notably, only 1% of sporadic CJD cases in the UK are initially referred to a psychiatrist (source: UK CJD Surveillance Unit). Occasionally there is a history of initial prodromal non-specific symptoms such as headache, fatigue, sleeping difficulties, weight loss, or anxiety (Stewart and Zeidler 1999).

Dementia is invariably present and myoclonus,[1] although rarely a presenting feature, is present at some stage in 80% of cases. Visual abnormalities are also common and include perceptual abnormalities and hallucinations. Unexplained physical pain—lightning or shooting pains—at any stage of the illness may occur, but very rarely.

As the disease progresses there is increasing global cognitive dysfunction, urinary incontinence, ataxia, and dependency, ending ultimately in a bedbound, mute, and unresponsive patient. Terminally, the affected person is rigid, frequently cortical blind, and often with Cheyne–Stokes respiration. The mean duration of illness is 8 months, with only 4% of cases surviving longer than 2 years (Stewart and Zeidler 1999).

Progressive supranuclear palsy (PSP) (Sagar 1998)

PSP (also referred to as the Steele–Richardson–Olsiewski syndrome) is a disease associated with neurodegeneration of the pons, midbrain, dentate and subthalamic nuclei, globus pallidus and nucleus basalis.

Histologically the pathological hallmarks of the disease are neurofibrillary tangles (ultrastructurally distinct from Alzheimer tangles) and gliosis in the absence of senile plaques.

Clinically the syndrome is quite diverse, with a variable age at onset, and with a substantial overlap with other cognitive and movement disorders. The key features in the diagnosis are early downward gaze palsy, symmetrical parkinsonism with ataxia, rigidity, disequilibrium (instability), early falling, and progressive dementia.

Features that support the diagnosis include symmetrical motor symptoms, early gait

Table 24vi.2 Clinical features of CJD at onset and during the course of the illness

Clinical feature	Onset (%)	Course (%)
Cognitive impairment	69	100
Memory loss	48	100
Behavioural abnormalities	29	57
Cerebellar	33	71
Visual	19	42
Pyramidal	2	62
Extrapyramidal	0.5	56
Akinetic mutism	0	75
Seizures	0	19
Myoclonus	1	78
Periodic EEG	0	60

Taken from Stewart and Zeidler 1999 with permission.

disturbance, frequent and early falls, an erect posture, late loss of arm swing, and a 'surprised' facial expression with loss of blinking. Features against a diagnosis of PSP include: visual hallucinations, which suggest DLB; 'alien limb' phenomena, which suggest CBD; and autonomic failure, which suggests multisystem atrophy (MSA).

The correlates of cognitive impairment in PSP are poorly established. There is often no obvious cortical atrophy, ascending dopaminergic systems are spared, although cholinergic projections may be mildly affected. Functional neuroimaging shows marked frontal hypometabolism.

Whipple's disease (Anderson 2000; Swartz 2000)

Whipple's disease is a rare multisystem disorder most commonly presenting in middle-aged men. CNS symptoms occur in 40% of cases.

Core systemic features include malabsorption, weight loss, pyrexia, dementia, polyarthralgia, and lymphadenopathy. The dementia is usually seen in association with ocular palsies and ataxia, or with a hypothalamic syndrome.

CSF examination shows a raised protein level and the presence of oligoclonal bands. PAS-positive cells may be present in the CSF. Diagnosis is by demonstrating the bacilli *Tropheryma whippleii* and abnormal macrophages obtained either from a jejunal or cerebral biopsy. Antibiotic therapy may halt or reverse the disease in some cases.

Wilson's disease (Brewer 2000; Gow et al. 2000)

Wilson's disease is a disorder of copper metabolism found in 30 per million people, and transmitted as an autosomal recessive trait.

It commonly presents with psychiatric symptoms of all types. It also rarely presents as a dementia. Neurological manifestations such as tremor, dystonia, and dysarthria are common. Kayser–Fliesher rings demonstrated in the cornea by slit-lamp examination are diagnostic. Diagnosis can also be confirmed by finding a low serum copper and caeruloplasmin level, with an elevated urinary copper excretion.

Treatment is aimed at first depleting the excessive stores of copper using a chelating agent such as D-penicillamine, and then keeping copper levels low. The rarity of the disease means that few clinicians are familiar with the disease, yet the need for early recognition and treatment are imperative. Maintaining a conscious effort to suspect Wilson's disease in younger patients with cognitive impairment is the key to early diagnosis.

Acknowledgements

Richard Harvey is supported by an Alzheimer's Society Research Fellowship.

Notes

1. The myoclonus in CJD is essentially the same as that seen in AD, although it is an earlier feature and more pronounced.

References

Anderson, M. (2000). Neurology of Whipple's disease. *Journal of Neurology, Neurosurgery and Psychiatry*, **68/1**, 2–5.

Boeve, B. F., Maraganore, D. M., Parisi, J. E., Ahlskog, J. E., Graff-Radford, N., Caselli, R. J., *et al.* (1999). Pathologic heterogeneity in clinically diagnosed corticobasal degeneration. *Neurology*, **53**, 795–800.

Brewer, G. J. (2000). Recognition, diagnosis, and management of Wilson's disease. *Proceedings of the Society for Experimental Biology and Medicine*, **223**, 39–46.

Brown, P., Gibbs, C. J. Jr, Rodgers-Johnson, P., *et al.* (1994). Human spongiform encephalopathy: the National Institutes of Health series of 300 cases of experimentally transmitted disease. *Annals of Neurology*, **35**, 513–29.

Chang, L., Ernst, T., Leonido-Yee, M., Witt, M., Speck, O., Walot, I., *et al.* (1999). Highly active antiretroviral therapy reverses brain metabolite abnormalities in mild HIV dementia. *Neurology*, **53**, 782–9.

Collinge, J. (1997). Human prion diseases and bovine spongiform encephalopathy (BSE). *Human Molecular Genetics*, **6**, 1699–705.

Feinstein, A. (2000). Cognitive dysfunction in multiple sclerosis. In *Dementia* (2nd edn) (ed. J. O'Brien, A. Burns, and D. Ames), pp. 852–59. Arnold, London.

Gow, P. J., Smallwood, R. A., Angus, P. W., Smith, A. L., Wall, A. J., and Sewell, R. B. (2000). Diagnosis of Wilson's disease: an experience over three decades. *Gut*, **46**, 415–19.

Jones, A. L., Wood, J. D., and Harper, P. S. (1997). Huntington disease: advances in molecular and cell biology. *Journal of Inherited Metabolic Disease*, **20**, 125–38.

Leroi, I. and Michalon, M. (1998). Treatment of the psychiatric manifestations of Huntington's disease: a review of the literature. *Canadian Journal of Psychiatry*, **43**, 933–40.

Lipton, S. A. (1997). Neuropathogenesis of acquired immunodeficiency syndrome dementia. *Current Opinion in Neurology*, **10**, 247–53.

Liscum, L. and Klansek, J. J. (1998). Niemann–Pick disease type C. *Current Opinion in Lipidology*, **9**, 131–5.

Mindham, R. H. (1999). The place of dementia in Parkinson's disease: a methodologic saga. *Advances in Neurology*, **80**, 403–8.

Moser, H. W. (1998). Neurometabolic disease. *Current Opinion in Neurology*, **11**, 91–5.

Pleasure, S. J. and Fishman, R. A. (1999). Ventricular volume and transmural pressure gradient in normal pressure hydrocephalus. *Archives of Neurology*, **56**, 1199–200.

Price, R. W., Yiannoutsos, C. T., Clifford, D. B., Zaborski, L., Tselis, A., Sidtis, J. J., *et al.* (1999). Neurological outcomes in late HIV infection: adverse impact of neurological impairment on survival and protective effect of antiviral therapy. AIDS Clinical Trial Group and Neurological AIDS Research Consortium study team. *AIDS*, **13**, 1677–85.

Rossor, M. N. (2000). The dementias. In *Neurology in clinical practice* (ed. W. G. Bradley, R. Daroff, G. Fenichel, and C. D. Marsden), pp. 3–5. Butterworth–Heinemann, New York.

Ruchoux, M. M. and Goebel, H. H. (1997). Diagnostic (clinical and morphological) criteria for adult neuronal ceroid-lipofuscinosis (Kufs' disease), Hôpital de la Salpetrière 'AFM Institut de Myologie', Paris, France, 5 December 1996. *Neuropathology and Applied Neurobiology*, **23**, 262–3.

Sagar, H. J. (1998). Parkinsonian syndromes associated with dementia. In *The dementias* (ed. J. H. Growden and M. N. Rossor), pp. 81–112. Butterworth-Heinemann, Boston.

Scolding, N. J., Jayne, D. R. W., Zajicek, J. P., Meyer, P. A. R., Wraight, E. P., and Lockwood, C. M. (1997). Cerebral vasculitis—recognition, diagnosis and management. *Quarterly Journal of Medicine*, **90**, 61–73.

Stewart, G. and Zeidler, M. D. (1999). Creutzfeldt–Jakob disease: a guide for the old age psychiatrist. *CPD Bulletin in Old Age Psychiatry*, **1**, 67–72.

Suomalainen, A. (1997). Mitochondrial DNA and disease. *Annals of Medicine*, **29**, 235–46.

Swartz, M. N. (2000). Whipple's disease—past, present, and future. *New England Journal of Medicine*, **342**, 648–50.

Waters, C. H. (1997). Managing the late complications of Parkinson's disease. *Neurology*, **49**(Suppl. 1), S49–57.

Winkelmann, J., Auer, D. P., Lechner, C., Elbel, G., and Trenkwalder, C. (1999). Magnetic resonance imaging findings in corticobasal degeneration. *Movement Disorders*, **14**, 669–73.

24vii Specific pharmacological treatments for Alzheimer's disease

Gordon Wilcock

Introduction

A number of treatment approaches for Alzheimer's disease (AD) have been explored over the years, but it was not until the emergence of the cholinergic hypothesis of Alzheimer's disease that a rational approach to treatment began to emerge. Reports in the mid-1970s of substantial reductions in the levels of enzymes responsible for the synthesis of acetylcholine (Bowen *et al.* 1976; Davies and Maloney 1976; Perry *et al.* 1977) led to the hypothesis that it might be possible to develop therapeutic strategies similar to the levodopa treatment approach to Parkinson's disease. It subsequently became clear that a number of other neurotransmitter abnormalities are present in the brain in AD, and these have also formed the basis for therapeutic hypotheses. However, to date the only successful strategy has been that based on the cholinergic hypothesis, which has recently been reviewed by Francis *et al.* (1999).

Early attempts at treatment with lecithin and choline (i.e. precursor loading), produced disappointing results. However, the development of compounds that were effective as cholinesterase inhibitors—thereby preserving the smaller amounts of acetylcholine being produced in the Alzheimer brain—showed sufficient promise for extensive clinical evaluation to be undertaken, and several of these compounds have now been licensed. Even though their benefits are modest, they have proved a major step forward in the pharmacological treatment of people with mild to moderate Alzheimer's disease.

In addition to treatment strategies based upon the neurochemical pathology in Alzheimer's disease, and which produce mainly symptomatic relief, others have been targeted at the fundamental pathology of Alzheimer's disease, i.e. the production of the beta-amyloid protein and the neurofibrillary tangle. Some of these are now coming to the fore, and for some strategies evaluation in early clinical trials is under way.

There have been, in addition, a number of alternative approaches that may prove to be helpful in Alzheimer's disease, but which, if successful, may work through a more general neuroprotective mechanism rather than an anti-plaque or -tangle strategy. Examples include the use of oestrogens, antioxidative treatment, and anti-inflammatory compounds. Finally, the increasing recognition of the role of neurotrophic factors, such as nerve growth factor (NGF), has stimulated interest in exploring a potential role of neurotrophins and similar molecules as neuroprotective agents in AD.

This chapter will provide an overview of the present position of these different therapeutic strategies.

Cholinesterase inhibitors

Pharmacological studies of cholinesterase inhibitors (ChEIs) show that they have a number of different properties, e.g. they can be competitive or non-competitive inhibitors, can vary in the degree of reversibility of their action, and so on. Initially it was felt that these features might affect their clinical utility, but in general, for those that have received a licence, there is little to choose between them on the basis of their pharmacological features.

Tacrine was the first cholinomimetic compound to undergo an extensive clinical evaluation programme, and to gain subsequent approval for its use in some, but not all, countries. Its modest efficacy, albeit limited by its side-effect profile, was clearly established for periods of up to 30 weeks in three pivotal studies (Davis *et al.* 1992; Farlow *et al.* 1992; Knapp *et al.* 1994). This proved that there were modest benefits for some people with mild to moderate Alzheimer's disease, in terms of dose-related improvement in cognition and in a global evaluation of a person's well-being and quality of life. The related compound, velnacrine, was shown to have similar efficacy, but had an unacceptable side-effect profile and did not receive a licence.

Tacrine was prescribed for some 300 000 or so patients worldwide, but arguably its main benefit lies in the fact that it paved the way for the second generation of cholinesterase inhibitors, which have less toxicity. These include donepezil, rivastigmine, metrifonate, and galantamine, amongst others.

Specific ChEIs

Donepezil

Donepezil was licensed in the UK in February 1997, and in many parts of Europe was the first available treatment for mild to moderately severe Alzheimer's disease. Its efficacy was assessed in accordance with regulatory requirements, across a range of modalities, including cognition, global functioning, and ability to undertake activities of daily living (ADL). There has also been an attempt to assess its efficacy in controlling the neuropsychiatric manifestations of Alzheimer's disease, i.e. behavioural difficulties. This drug has probably been the most extensively evaluated of the currently available compounds, and has accumulated some 500 000 patient-days exposure within the various clinical studies. One of the most pivotal studies evaluated the use of donepezil at either 5 mg or 10 mg against placebo, over a 6-month period, in some 473 patients (Rogers *et al.* 1998). The main end-points were an improvement in cognition as shown on the Alzheimer's Disease Assessment Scale-cognitive subscale (ADAS-Cog; Rosen *et al.* 1984) and a general overall clinical assessment using a semi-structured instrument (the CIBIC-Plus). Clinician's Interview Based Impression of Change, with caregiver input, a global assessment measure, which allowed an overall impression of change in four major functional domains: general, cognition, behavioural, and ADL. A quarter of the patients taking the higher, 10 mg, dose improved by 7 points or more on the ADAS-Cog (cf 8% on placebo), indicating they had benefited by at least a 6–12 months' gain in cognitive function when this was compared to their baseline level. On the more general CIBIC-Plus measure, 10% of those on placebo improved compared to 25% receiving donepezil. A responder analysis showed that four patients would need to be treated to gain an improvement in terms of a 4-point change in the ADAS-Cog, compared with 8 for an improvement on the CIBIC-Plus (Allen 1999). There is also some evidence of a continued treatment effect with long-term therapy (Evans *et al.* 2000).

Rivastigmine

Like the other ChEIs, rivastigmine has been shown to be modestly effective in all three major symptom domains of Alzheimer's disease—namely, cognition, activities of daily living, and global functioning—in 30% to 50% of treated patients, depending upon which functional domain is being reported (Corey-Bloom *et al.* 1998; Schneider *et al.* 1998; Rosler *et al.* 1999). It is important to appreciate that, as with all cholinesterase inhibitors, the benefits may include *improvement* in cognition or well-being, or *stabilisation* of the symptomatic deterioration. Some evidence for the latter has been claimed in open-label extension studies.

Galantamine

The most recently licensed cholinesterase inhibitor is galantamine, which is regarded by some as being the first of the third generation of compounds. It differs from the earlier drugs in that it has a dual mode of action; as well as reversibly and competitively inhibiting acetylcholinesterase it also modulates nicotinic acetylcholine receptors. This may prove to be of additional clinical relevance, because activation of presynaptic nicotinic receptors has been shown to increase the release of acetylcholine, and also of other neurotransmitters that are deficient in Alzheimer's disease, such as glutamate. A number of studies of galantamine (Raskind *et al.* 2000; Tariot *et al.* 2000; Wilcock *et al.* 2000) have confirmed its efficacy and tolerability in those patients with mild to moderate Alzheimer's disease. It has been arguably stated that the cognitive benefits of galantamine are at the upper end of the spectrum of benefit experienced with the cholinesterase inhibitors as a group.

During a 6-month, placebo-controlled study, galantamine was shown to alleviate caregiver burden in Alzheimer's disease; indicating that the cognitive and functional benefits of galantamine for the patient are translated into beneficial effects on caregiver burden (Wilcock and Lilienfeld 2000). The time that caregivers needed to spend supervising or assisting patients with Alzheimer's disease was reduced by up to 1 hour a day.

Other cholinesterase inhibitors

There are a number of other compounds under review, including metrifonate and various physostigmine analogues. At the time of writing, these are not available to the clinician, and they will not be discussed further.

General properties of cholinesterase inhibitors

Currently, there is reliable evidence that cholinesterase inhibitors are effective in a significant proportion of people with mild to moderate Alzheimer's disease, and that this is represented in some people by an improvement in cognition, functional ability, etc. Moreover, in some it would appear that treatment with a cholinesterase inhibitor stabilizes that person's symptoms for a variable period. As there is no means of determining who will, or will not, respond to such treatment, a 3-month trial of efficacy would seem justifiable in most people who meet the entry criteria. Some would advocate a longer trial period, i.e. a minimum of 6 months, and there will indeed be some patients for whom it is impossible to determine benefit after a shorter trial.

In general, two to three times as many people in the active treatment arms of studies meet the accepted criteria for efficacy compared with those in the placebo arm, and this ratio is approximately mirrored by the adverse event profile. The latter is mainly what would be expected from cholinergic enhancement, with gastrointestinal tract symptoms being especially prominent. Most of the adverse events experienced occur during the initial, early titration phase of treatment. These events are usually short-lived, and can be successfully treated in most cases with an appropriate antiemetic. Many patients require no treatment, and the majority are adverse event free, or experience only minimal symptoms. The number of patients discontinuing treatment because of adverse events is fewer in clinical practice than in the clinical trials. There is also an emerging picture that cholinesterase inhibitors may help with the management of behavioural problems in people with AD, but this needs to be confirmed in properly conducted studies.

The mechanism of action of cholinesterase inhibitors, including their selectivity and the reversibility of receptor binding characteristics, to some extent determines their potential for adverse interactions with other drugs. This includes some of those used in anaesthetic practice, and possibly others such as ranitidine and cimetidine, although neither of these has proved a significant problem in practice. The side-effect profile and potential for interactions compares favourably with frequently used drugs in elderly patients, such as many of the antidepressants and neuroleptics. Caution should be exercised, however, in those patients with reversible airways disease or in some cardiac conditions such as conduction defects or significant bradycardia.

Choosing the appropriate patients for treatment requires careful consideration. The temptation to undertake a 'therapeutic trial' of a drug in any patient with dementia should be avoided, unless, and until, a benefit for that drug in other conditions, such as Lewy body disease, has been proven. As well as requiring a fairly secure diagnosis of probable Alzheimer's disease, at present the indication for ChEI prescription is only for those patients with mild to moderately severe dementia, but this may change as the outcomes of trials in more severely demented subjects are reported.

When should treatment be stopped in those in whom there has been a favourable response? This is a difficult question, to which only a pragmatic response can be given. Wherever possible, protocols allowing an objective assessment of response in a number of domains should be employed, but in clinical practice it is rarely possible to undertake such a comprehensive approach. Nevertheless, some attempt at objectivity is worthwhile, and for many people this may mean the use of a simple general test of cognition, such as the Mini-Mental State Examination (MMSE), coupled with a global measure formed from the relative's, or other caregiver's, opinion and supplemented by the clinical notes made at earlier consultations. Whenever it looks as if a patient is deteriorating, a phased withdrawal of treatment may reveal whether or not there is still benefit; if the benefit is judged worthwhile, the treatment should be restarted.

In January 2001 in the UK the National Institute for Clinical Excellence (NICE 2001) published guidance for the general use of donepezil, rivastigmine and galantamine in the treatment of Alzheimer's disease, which superseded previous advice. They confirmed that these drugs should be made available in the UK as part of the NHS, as one component in the management of people with mild to moderate Alzheimer's disease. It was suggested that they should be made available to those with an MMSE score above 12, in whom a specialist clinic had made the diagnosis of probable Alzheimer's disease, using tests of cognitive, global, and behavioural functioning, in addition to assessment of activities of daily living. The guidance indicated that compliance should be taken into account, and that in many cases this would need a relative or care-worker who was sufficiently in contact with the patient to be able to monitor compliance.

Although it was suggested that treatment should be initiated in a consultant or specialist clinic, it was accepted that in due course general practitioners might take over prescribing but, if so, under a shared-care protocol with clear treatment end-points.

NICE indicated that an assessment should be made between two and four months after reaching the maintenance dose of the drug, and that continued treatment should be prescribed only where there had been an improvement or no deterioration in the MMSE score, together with evidence of global improvement on the basis of behavioural and functional assessment. NICE further suggested that, once the medication regime is stabilized, there should be reassessments approximately every six months, and that the drug should be continued only while the patient's MMSE score remains above 12, and that the patient's global, functional and behavioural condition suggests that the drug is continuing to have a worthwhile effect. When the MMSE score falls below 12 points, the guidance indicated that the treatment would normally be discontinued, but it did not make this an absolute requirement. The NICE guidance also indicated that the six monthly review should probably be undertaken by a specialist clinic.

This guidance in the UK was welcomed by most working in the field, and also by many of the families of sufferers. It would seem to form a useful basis for the development of a rational prescribing policy for each individual patient, and may well be helpful also outside the UK.

Finally, it is worth remembering that the disappointingly small proportion of people who benefit from these treatments does not necessarily imply that they are not worthwhile. Alzheimer's disease is not a single, homogeneous condition, but the final pathway of a number of heterogeneous factors, both intrinsic and extrinsic. This heterogeneity occurs at genetic, clinical, neurochemical, and neuropathological levels, and may contribute to differing response rates among different patients for a specific therapeutic measure.

Cholinergic agonists

A number of cholinergic agonists, mainly muscarinic receptor agonists, have been evaluated as treatments for Alzheimer's disease. In general, the benefit and adverse event profile has proved disappointing. However, there is some evidence that these agents (e.g. xanomeline, a selective muscarinic agonist) may improve behavioural difficulties such as vocal outbursts and psychotic symptoms (Bodick *et al.* 1997).

Other approaches not specifically directed at the cholinergic system or basic neuropathology of Alzheimer's disease

1. Glutamate modulation has been explored as a possible therapeutic strategy for Alzheimer's disease and other dementias. Memantine is one such drug that may work through this mechanism. It blocks *N*-methyl-D-aspartate (NMDA) receptor channels in the resting state, and has been investigated in large clinical trials in both AD and vascular dementia. It is one of the few compounds so far investigated in more severe dementias, and does appear to hold some promise. The clinical data are currently being evaluated by the licensing authorities.

A number of other compounds, including propentofylline, monoamine oxidase inhibitors such as selegiline, and Hydergine®, piracetam, and other nootropic agents have been evaluated. However, these have given somewhat disappointing results, and are currently not considered front-line drugs for the treatment of any dementia.

2. There has been a lot of controversy about the use of ginkgo-biloba. This is made from extracts of the leaves of the maidenhair tree, and has long been in use in China for a number of different indications, but more recently for cognitive enhancement. It has many potential active ingredients and mechanisms of action: although most studies of its efficacy have been of poor quality, properly constructed double-blind, placebo-controlled trial data is now beginning to emerge. Although there is some evidence of efficacy, the difficulty in identifying and evaluating the active ingredients is likely to cause problems with the regulatory authorities, in terms of it being granted a specific licence as a reimbursable medical treatment. Nevertheless, there is no strong reason for advising patients against trying this, if they feel so inclined, although they should not commit themselves to a lengthy and expensive course of treatment in the absence of any obvious benefit.

3. The use of oestrogen replacement treatment in Alzheimer's disease remains controversial. There is good epidemiological evidence that women of postmenopausal age taking oestrogen preparations may have a reduced or delayed risk of developing dementia (e.g. Tang *et al.* 1996). This led to the hope that it may be a useful adjunctive treatment in those who have already contracted the disease. However, two recent studies, albeit on relatively small numbers of people with Alzheimer's disease, and for a relatively short period, have failed to show any significant benefit (Henderson *et al.* 2000; Wang *et al.* 2000). Further longer term studies on larger numbers of subjects are required. Meanwhile, many clinicians would not advocate the use of oestrogens in this context because of the potential adverse event profile.

4. Antioxidant therapy has also been explored in Alzheimer's disease. This is based upon the premise that cellular respiration produces oxygen derivatives and other free radicals which may be particularly harmful to specific intracellular structures, especially those that are lipid-rich. Under normal circumstances, these radicals are rapidly dealt with by intracellular mechanisms. However, neurons are known to have reduced levels of one important major antioxidant, glutathione, whilst they may have a higher level of oxidative stress related to the very high oxygen consumption of the brain. Whether this is specifically relevant to Alzheimer's disease itself, or, if harmful, has a more general effect upon the background level of neuronal numbers and function, is unclear. The best known antioxidant in relation to Alzheimer's disease is, of course, vitamin E, which is largely based on the study by Sano and colleagues (Sano *et al.* 1997). This study

provided some evidence that the use of vitamin E in high doses may slow the progression of Alzheimer's disease in those who are moderately severely affected. However, this is subject to further scrutiny and we must await the outcome of additional studies.

5. Evidence that an inflammatory process may be present in the brain in Alzheimer's disease (e.g. the association of a number of acute-phase protein markers and cytokines in and around the typical plaques), was one reason for the exploration of anti-inflammatory compounds as therapeutic agents. The other reason is the apparent protection conferred by anti-inflammatory compounds noted in some of the longitudinal studies of ageing. This phenomenon is now well described in the literature, and has stimulated trials of anti-inflammatory drugs in those with the disease. Limited early trials, (e.g. Rogers *et al.* 1993), suggested a possible slowing of the disease process in some subjects with mild to moderate AD, and the outcome of further studies is awaited. Experience with steroids, e.g. prednisone, has, however, proved disappointing. In a recently reported double-blind, randomized control trial of 138 subjects over a 12-month period there was no difference in outcome measures between the treated and the placebo arms of the study, although there was a suggestion that those receiving prednisone declined behaviourally (Aisen *et al.* 2000).

In general, there is a suggestion that a number of potential neuroprotective strategies may be of value. But whether they work at a general level and would be equally helpful in all types of dementia, or whether they have specific actions in Alzheimer's disease, or both, remains to be established, as does the potential magnitude of the benefit if this is genuine.

Strategies designed to rectify the underlying cellular pathology in Alzheimer's disease

More fundamental therapeutic strategies have also been under development, some of which are moving into the phase of early clinical evaluation. These include attempts to try and prevent the deposition of amyloid precursor protein, or accelerate its removal once it has been deposited. Some of these approaches rely upon knowledge gained from our understanding of the genetic contributions to AD, particularly those affecting the presenilin genes, and involve preventing potentially harmful cleaving of the amyloid precursor protein molecule by specific proteases. Other antiamyloid approaches include attempts to try and reduce the damage that it may cause once it has been deposited. One exciting approach has been the theory, gained from experiments with transgenic mice, that it may be possible to generate antibodies against the amyloid beta-peptide, which will lead to clearance of amyloid from the brain or prevent its formation from the peptide. Clinical evaluation of this approach has just started, and we shall have to wait a year or two before we know whether it is beneficial.

The other main pathological lesion in Alzheimer's disease is, of course, the neurofibrillary tangle. This is formed intracellularly through the hyperphosphorylation of microtubule-associated proteins, especially tau. It is possible that strategies to dephosphorylate tau or to reduce the level of abnormal phosphorylation might also be beneficial, and these are also under exploration.

Finally, there is considerable interest in the use of neurotrophic substances (i.e. naturally occurring peptides or proteins) to protect neurons from damage or to augment their natural plasticity. As far as the latter is concerned, nerve growth factor (NGF) is the most likely candidate. A small number of patients has been treated with intracerebroventricular NGF in Sweden, with modest, if any real benefit. However, the dosing pattern and quantity of NGF delivered may not have been optimum and further work in this field is necessary. It is probable that intraparenchymal delivery of NGF into the region of the basal nucleus of Meynert, where most of the cholinergic cells that are important in Alzheimer's disease reside, will be more efficacious than intracerebroventricular delivery, and may also avoid some of the adverse events associated with delivery into the CSF.

References

Aisen, P. S., Davis, K. L., Berg, J. D., Schafer, K., Campbell, K., Thomas, R. G., *et al.* (2000). A randomized controlled trial of prednisone in Alzheimer's disease. *Neurology*, **54**, 588–93.

Allen, H. (1999). Anti-dementia drugs. *International Journal of Geriatric Psychiatry*, **14**, 239–43. [Editorial]

Bodick, N. C., Offen W. W., Levey A. I., *et al.* (1997). Effects of xanomeline, a selective muscarinic receptor agonist, on cognitive function and behavioral symptoms in Alzheimer's disease. *Archives of Neurology*, **54**, 465–73.

Bowen, D. M., Smith C. B., White P., *et al.* (1976). Neurotransmitter-related enzymes and indices of hypoxia in senile dementia and other abiotrophies. *Brain*, **99**, 459–96.

Corey-Bloom, J., *et al.* (1998). A randomised trial evaluating the efficacy and safety of ENA 713 (rivastigmine tartrate), a new acetylcholinesterase inhibitor, in patients with Alzheimer's disease. *International Journal of Geriatric Psychopharmacology*, **1**, 55–65.

Davies, P. and Maloney, A. J. F. (1976). Selective loss of central cholinergic neurones in Alzheimer's disease. *Lancet*, **ii**, 1403.

Davis, K. L., Thal, L. J., Gamzu, E. R., *et al.* (1992). A double-blind, placebo-controlled multicenter study of tacrine for Alzheimer's disease. *New England Journal of Medicine,* **327**, 1253–9.

Evans, M., Ellis, A., Watson, D., and Chowdhury, T. (2000). Sustained cognitive improvement following treatment of Alzheimer's disease with donepezil. *International Journal of Geriatric Psychiatry,* **15**, 50–3.

Farlow, M., Gracon S. I., Hershey L. A., *et al.* (1992). A controlled trial of tacrine in Alzheimer's disease. The Tacrine Study Group. *Journal of the American Medical Association,* **268**, 2523–9.

Francis, P. T., Palmer, A. M., Snape M., and Wilcock G. K. (1999). The cholinergic hypothesis of Alzheimer's disease: a review of progress. *Journal of Neurology, Neurosurgery, and Psychiatry,* **66**, 137–47.

Henderson, V. W., Paganini-Hill, A., Miller, B. L., Elble, R. J., Reyes, P. F., Shoupe, D., *et al.* (2000). Estrogen for Alzheimer's disease in women. Randomized, double-blind, placebo-controlled trial. *Neurology,* **54**, 295–301.

Knapp, J. M., Knopman, D. S., Soloman P. R., *et al.* (1994). A 30-week randomized controlled trial of high-dose tacrine in patients with Alzheimer's disease. The Tacrine Study Group. *Journal of the American Medical Association,* **271**, 985–91.

NICE (2001). *Technology Appraisal Guidance No. 19.* National Institute for Clinical Excellence, London.

Perry, E. K., Gibson, P. H., Blessed, G. *et al.* (1977). Neurotransmitter enzyme abnormalities in senile dementia. Choline acetyl-transferase and glutamic acid decarboxlyase activities in necropsy brain tissue. *Journal of Neurological Science,* **34**, 247–65.

Raskind, M. A., Peskind, E. R., Wessel, T., and Yuan, W. (2000). galantamine in Alzheimer's disease: a six-month randomised, placebo-controlled trial with a 6-month extension. *Neurology*, **54**, 2261–8.

Rogers J., Kirby, L. C., Hempelman, S. R., Berry D. L., McGeer P. L., Kasniak A. W., *et al.* (1993). Clinical trial of indomethacin in Alzheimer's disease. *Neurology,* **43**, 1609–11.

Rogers, S. L., Farlow, M. R., Doody, R. S., Mohs, R., and Friedhoff, L. T. (1998). A 24-week, double-blind, placebo-controlled trial of donepezil in patients with Alzheimer's disease. donepezil Study Group. *Neurology,* **50**, 136–45.

Rosen, W. G., Mohs, R. C., and Davis K. L. (1984). A new rating scale for Alzheimer's disease. *American Journal of Psychiatry*, **141**, 1356–64.

Rosler, M., *et al.* (1999). Efficacy and safety of rivastigmine in patients with Alzheimer's disease: international randomised controlled trial. *British Medical Journal,* **318**, 633–8.

Sano, M., Ernesto, C., Thomas, R. G., Klauber, M. R., Schafer, K., Grundman, M., *et al.* (1997). A controlled trial of selegiline, alpha-tocopherol, or both as treatment for Alzheimer's disease. The Alzheimer's Disease Co-operative Study. *New England Journal of Medicine*, **336**, 1216–22.

Schneider, L., *et al.* (1998). Systematic review of the efficacy of rivastigmine for patients with Alzheimer's disease. *International Journal of Geriatric Psychopharmacology,* **1**(Suppl. 1), S26–S34.

Tang, M. X., Jacobs, D., Stern Y., Marder, K., Schofield, P., Gurland, B., *et al.* (1996). Effect of oestrogen during menopause on risk and age at onset of Alzheimer's disease. *Lancet,* **3448**, 429–32.

Tariot, P. N., Solomon, P. R., Morris, J. C., Kershaw, P., Lilienfeld, S., Ding, C., *et al.* (2000). A 5-month, randomized, placebo-controlled trial of galantamine in AD. *Neurology,* **54**, 2269–76.

Wang, P. N., Liao, S. Q., Liu, R. S., Liu, M. D., Chao, H. T., Lu, S. R., *et al.* (2000). Effects of estrogen on cognition, mood, and cerebral blood flow in AD: a controlled study. *Neurology*, **54**, 2061–6.

Wilcock, G. K. and Lilienfeld, S. (2000). galantamine alleviates caregiver burden in Alzheimer's disease: a 6-month placebo-controlled study. *World Alzheimer Congress July 2000,* Washington DC.

Wilcock, G. K., Lilieufeld, S. and Gaens, E. (2000). Efficacy and safety of galantamine in patients with mild to moderate Alzheimer's disease: multi-centre randomised controlled trial. *British Medical Journal*, **321**, 1445–9.

24viii The management of dementia

Jane Pearce

Introduction

Dementia is a progressive disorder and decline in cognitive function interferes with many aspects of people's lives. Often behavioural disturbance leads to the initial referral. There may be concurrent illnesses, physical or psychological, that may exacerbate the difficulties of coping with or managing the disorder. It is important to screen for these and to treat them. Furthermore, dementia is a source of distress (and problems) both for the individual and for those more closely in contact with the sufferer. Loss of independence in daily living brings with it the involvement of other people as carers to help meet the associated needs. Thus the person-centred approach to the patient has to be integrated with a context-centred (and context-sensitive) approach. Desirable qualities of management therefore include an integrated approach with a central interest in the well-being of the carers as well as in that of the person with the dementia.

The aims of management are to promote the autonomy and well-being of the person with dementia; to support adaptation and maintain and preserve existing function in the sufferer; to assess and define specific problems and identify strategies to deal with them; to treat concurrent illness; and to provide overall care for his or her network of support.

This chapter will focus on the content of management; it will attempt to describe some principles with which to approach management and will describe interventions that have some evidence of efficacy.

Assessment

A process of assessment and reassessment is the basis of management since dementia is a progressive condition. Assessment covers the presenting problem(s), current functional ability of the patient, any risks of harm to the patient or to others, the patient's social circumstances, and the ability of the caregiver to provide the type of care needed. It is also necessary to screen for concurrent physical and psychological conditions. While it is necessary to take a broad approach because of the range of effects that dementia has, it is crucial to focus on specific areas to ensure that, where there are interventions of known efficacy, these are applied.

Definition of presenting problems and current functional ability

This chapter does not focus on the diagnosis itself of dementia. However, it is recommended that any information about prior assessment and investigations should be examined in order to check the robustness of the diagnosis of dementia and to exclude other possible treatable causes. Standardized assessment tools such as the Mini-Mental State Examination (MMSE; Folstein *et al.* 1975) can be used to track the subsequent changes in cognitive function.

In the present chapter we focus on the collection of information about the main presenting problems. The information collected should include precise descriptions of the problems, their nature, and history of their onset.

A number of behaviours lead to morbidity in patients and carers. These include agitation, aggression, sleep disturbance, disruptive vocalization (such as screaming, singing, or shouting), inappropriate control of continence or expression of sexuality, and abnormal patterns of eating and wandering.

Functional activity reflects motor, visual, and other perceptual skills, as well as cognitive competence. It is generally thought of as having two main aspects: first, activities of daily living (ADL) such as basic self-care and self-maintenance skills (washing, bathing, dressing, maintaining continence, eating, transferring, grooming); and, second, the more complex skills that relate to the roles adults perform in order to live independently in the community—the instrumental activities of daily living (IADL). The latter include social and occupational activities that are multifaceted and require organizational and planning skills. A functional assessment is important in order to establish the patient's strengths and weaknesses, and standardized assessment tools are helpful to track changes.

Risk assessment

Risks are common in dementia, and systematic consideration of risk may therefore be valuable. Risk assessment refers to a method of weighing the probability of the range of outcomes that might arise (Vinestock 1996). Relevant questions are:

- Is there a risk of harm?
- If so, what sort of harm, to whom, and what is the likely severity?
- How likely is it to happen?
- How immediate is the risk and how long will it last?
- What factors contribute to the risk?
- How can these factors be modified or managed?

In dementia there are risks of harm occurring both to the patient and to others. The kinds of risk that need to be considered include those arising from activity or disturbed behaviour and those arising from negative or withdrawn behaviour. The risks will change with the progression of the disorder and therefore should be reviewed regularly.

Risks to self may result from specific behaviours, from diminished mastery of the environment, and through vulnerability from the actions of others. Risk related to psychiatric disorder such as the risk of deliberate self-harm also needs to be considered.

Alcohol misuse may already be an aetiological factor for the dementia, but forgetfulness may also lead social drinkers to lose control and thus compound the cognitive losses. An inability or unwillingness to accept help when needed for nutrition and other basic daily needs can result in poor physical health and well-being. Wandering can result in falling or getting lost in unsafe areas. Falls are significantly more common in dementia, and occur particularly to people who have relatively well-preserved functional capability. They are associated with the use of medication, wandering, and current acute confusion and may indicate the need for a greater level of supervision (CHSR 1998). There is a particular risk of falls for patients with Lewy body dementia.

The dependency-needs associated with dementia, and the consequent potential for emotional stress on caregivers, can make the person with dementia more vulnerable to physical, emotional, financial, or sexual abuse and exploitation from those on whom he or she depends (APA 1997). As in elder abuse in general, awareness of the possibility of abuse is important in its detection, and corroborating evidence should be sought where abuse is suspected. Particular vigilance may be indicated where carers are poorly supported, where there is misuse of alcohol, or where there are pre-existing relationship problems (Chapter 37). Complicating factors include the dementia sufferer's limited ability to protest and, sometimes, their reluctance to receive outside help.

Care can often be difficult to deliver. A careworker may be asked to work in a patient's home with a plan to prevent serious self-neglect. The careworker must resist imposing his or her own standards on the client, and has to use sensitivity to achieve the objectives. When the client is reluctant to receive help, more time (such as time to befriend, encourage, and accompany) may be required, although scarcity of staff resources may often make this difficult. Sources of neglect can be subtle and routine, and may also derive from a lack of resources. Likewise, a shortfall in training, time, or manpower may be associated with non-person-centred care.

Risk to others may be posed by aggressive behaviours. Aggression usually occurs in the context of personal care. Verbal aggression is the commonest form and the longest lasting in the course of dementia. Serious aggression is rare, but aggressive resistance and physical aggression are most prevalent among people with more severe dementia and may persist until death (Keene *et al.* 1999). Aggression may pose a risk to carers and other residents in the environment as this group of patients is more likely to be in institutional care. The presence of delusions is an important association with physical violence (Deutsch *et al.* 1991). Indicators of increased risk of dangerous aggression include conflict with others, a previous episode of serious aggression, sudden changes in the environment, as well as psychiatric comorbidity (Hindley and Gordon 2000).

Assessment in the patient's own environment and with information from carers and neighbours is important in identifying the various sources of potential hazards. Examples include fire risks from inappropriate use of electrical appliances and smoking habits, public health risks from a failure to handle refuse and household hygiene, and risks of affray from accusations of theft and trespass made to people around. The risk associated with accidents from driving is considered elsewhere in this book.

Screening for concurrent physical and psychological illness

Concurrent physical disorder is important as it is commonly associated with a deterioration in function or with changes in behaviour. Common aetiologies include acute infections, electrolyte imbalance, metabolic imbalance, heart failure, and the side-effects of medication. Some physical symptoms such as nocturnal dyspnoea and sleep disturbance may trigger behavioural problems; dysuria may trigger inappropriate exposure of genitals, or constipation may trigger inappropriate defaecation. A physical source of pain may trigger noise-making or agitation, aggression or sleep disturbance. Physical discomfort from constipation, hunger, or poor sleep may result in sleep disturbance.

In the person with dementia, a presentation of physical illness may be masked by the lack of complaints about typical symptoms (McCormick *et al.* 1994). Behavioural change may be the most evident feature. Hence screening for common conditions by physical examination and blood and urine tests can be indicated. Liaison with gerontology teams becomes important in informing decisions about the most useful pathways of investigation. This is important when investigation is either invasive or frightening, or if the patient is unable to express his or her wishes.

Finally it is important to consider comorbidity with psychiatric symptoms. This can easily be missed if explicit assessment is not made. Where behaviours are aggressive or agitated, it is particularly important to look actively for signs of psychosis and depression (CHSR 1998).

Carer assessment

Assessment of the social circumstances includes reviewing the caregiver's ability to provide the type of care needed, and the quality and adequacy of the caregiver's own social support systems. This is dealt with in Chapter 21. Changes in the carers' state of health and personal resources, and other stressors in their lives, should be noted. Physical illness in carers may also be important and may too be masked, for example being rationalized as stress or exhaustion.

General principles of management

Management plans

A management plan needs to be developed that addresses the needs for general care related to the patient's functional decline and progressive cognitive loss, and which takes account of any identified risks (core management). When specific problems are present, the plan will include targeted interventions and care (specific management). The desired outcomes of plans and interventions need to be identified and monitored. Carers and family need to be involved in the management plans, and liaison with other services will be necessary.

Core or general care needs can be identified from the assessment of the patient's functional decline and progressive cognitive loss. Interventions can be directed towards adaptation and adjustment. Management plans should deal with overall daily routines, special activities, and the social context of living, including that of carers. The full range of services available locally should be drawn upon, as well as those of specialist dementia services. For the functional impairments, the early needs will be in the domain of advice and monitoring. Useful areas include advice on developing structure and routine in daily life, the adoption of memory aids, suggestions for the reduction in complexity of tasks and activities, optimizing communication, planning safe current and future organization of finances, together with guidance on basic self-care such as nutrition, sleep, and exercise. Plans as such will be very simple but should include regular reviews. As the illness progresses there will be a move towards services that assist and assume greater levels of responsibility for the person's functioning.

The interpersonal needs of the person with dementia may easily be overlooked when he or she becomes a service user. As a person with dementia comes to spend more time out of their own home environment the quality of knowledge about them as individuals can become degraded. The person moving through dementia brings with them their prior tastes, beliefs, values, lifestyle, biography, gender, class, and cultural background. This may be modified by personality changes that occur as a result of the dementia, as well as by the diminished ability to express these characteristics because of specific cognitive losses. Qualities of good care in dementia are described as 'person-centred care' (Kitwood 1997). Promotion of comfort, meeting the need for attachment and feelings of inclusion, meaningful occupation, and maintenance of personal identity have been suggested as the key components of psychosocial care in dementia.

The progression of the disease is associated with progression through different environments and services. There are a number of environmental aspects that will influence their appropriateness for an individual patient's needs. Variables include the physical quality, hygiene, space, and privacy of the accommodation, as well as social aspects of the environment such as access to appropriate social stimulation, support, and care. In general, simplification, availability of activity and company, together with the provision of necessary safety, are positive features of care environments (Lawton *et al.* 1989).

In institutional settings one needs to consider whether the staff are adequately trained to meet the individual patient's needs, in addition to managing the demands from other patients. Commitment to and knowledge of working with dementia is relevant, as is the staff's ability to adapt to change with the progression of the disease (Rovner *et al.* 1996). Staff may or may not have the skills, knowledge, and senior supervision to engage in interventions.

Standard services for dementia in older populations will not necessarily meet needs in an appropriate way for younger-onset patients. Given current service provisions, younger-onset patients with dementia use fewer community services but more institutional care. Financial implications may also be more serious for younger-onset patients: both the patient's and spouse's work may be required to support the family. Opportunities and earning potential are threatened by the dementia, and the loss of one's job may in turn affect pension rights. Moreover, the need for care may mean that both the patient's and the carer's jobs may be threatened. In contrast, where onset is later, patients will already be adjusted to living a life on a pension without paid employment.

Standard service settings designed for the majority may also fail to meet the needs of patients from ethnic minority groups. Dementia contributes to loss of the second language and reversion to the mother tongue may confound the accuracy of diagnosis. In addition, educational and cultural factors, incorrect assumptions about literacy, and the misunderstanding of certain concepts can result in overestimating cognitive loss—while missing other functional reasons for deterioration in a person's function (Bhatnagar and Frank 1997). Some members of ethnic minorities may suffer greater disability from cognitive impairment because of poorer physical health, disadvantaged economic circumstances, or social isolation (Manthorpe and Hettiaratchy 1993). A subgroup may have been exposed to trauma arising from social upheaval, prior displacement (especially among refugees), and other adverse circumstances related to migration. They may feel more isolated from their own community, in particular from younger generations who cannot share their memories. The losses of dementia (in particular loss of control and autonomy) may also trigger the re-emergence of past traumatic experiences (Miesen and Jones 1997).

Ethnosensitive care therefore requires more than the provision of translation services. Liaison workers educated in mental health may play a helpful role when services do not have staff from the similar ethnic background.

Identify desired outcomes of plans and set up methods for monitoring these

Since dementia is a progressive condition, it is essential to develop and regularly review general management plans in the light of the changing capacities of the patient and of the changing burden on carers. Patterns of progression are variable and change in the contextual factors may be unpredictable. However, some changes and future needs can to some extent be anticipated.

Where specific interventions (for example, treatments for cognitive impairment) are being used, clear goals and regular monitoring are needed to evaluate their effectiveness and detect any adverse consequences. Where interventions are more complex and, in particular, where potential risks occur, priorities must first be established. Are the risks assessed to have potentially serious outcomes or are they more minor? Are adverse outcomes thought to be likely or unlikely, and what aspects require an immediate response? The risk assessment should be shared with carers and other workers. Differences of opinion need to be talked through and, when decisions are made, the basis of these should be made clear and understandable.

Plans will depend upon the level of risk. Where the risk is lower, continued monitoring and supervision should be instituted, checking for the occurrence of known triggers and for contributory factors that may increase the risk. Where the risk is higher, it will be necessary to modify or manage the risks, for example by changing the physical or social environment, through caregiving or assistance, or through medication or specific interventions (see below). Often several agencies will be involved and monitoring of service provision is important (SSI 1997). Have the promised services been delivered, and has the patient accepted or refused them? Where risk remains high despite attempts to ameliorate it, compulsion may become necessary. Guardianship under the Mental Health Act may offer an appropriate framework and can be used constructively, for example enabling careworkers to enter a person's home despite initial barriers. Hospital admission may be used to enable further assessment and development of a care plan, and to provide periods of more intensive evaluation with trained staff available 24 hours a day. The Mental Health Act provisions may be needed for such admission when community interventions are unsuccessful, particularly when patients are unable to recognize their need for care and actively refuse help. (See Chapter 36 for further discussion of ethical issues.)

Maintaining liaison

An extended network of care may include primary care, social and personal care services, and mental health teams. Services may include domiciliary, day, or residential care. Exchange of information, opinions, and advice is very important, given the potential complexity of the issues, the number of people involved, and the network of care. In particular, one must balance the needs of the different people involved, reconciling, for example, the patient's best interests and those of the carers. Liaison needs to be especially good when risks are present so that all involved share and understand the concerns, detect increases in risk, and know whom to communicate with about such changes.

Good practice at all stages is characterized by interdisciplinary team working. The 'team' has at its basis the carer who has primary responsibility for direct physical care, the individual with dementia, and family members. There may at times be valid reasons against involving the patient in team planning. However there is evidence to demonstrate that people with dementia can participate in family meetings (Jeffery 1987; Benbow *et al.* 1993). Specific techniques to facilitate communication are described below. For people with dementia who live alone the home carer often becomes one of the most significant people in their life. The home carer may become important in expressing the voice of the patient and in giving the 'user view' (SSI 1997). Their participation in care reviews is therefore very important.

Integration of care is clinically recognized as important. Not all people with a dementia will be under specialist mental health services and primary care may play a key role. When there is use of specialist mental health services, the Care Programme Approach (CPA) has to be applied (Department of Health 1990). CPA requires that the patient have a key worker, that there is full assessment of health and social needs, that a care plan is agreed with the patient and his or her main carers, and that a record is made of unmet needs.

There is only sparse evidence of the effectiveness and efficiency of models of care organization (Melzer *et al.* 1994). Findings on the case management approach for ill older people are contradictory. Reduced hospital admission rates have been found for people with complex health and social needs, but a study of community resource teams (integrated teams providing flexible, tailored care across the range of needs of individuals with dementia) has suggested increased admission rates for those living alone (Melzer *et al.* 1994).

Carer and family involvement

Carers need to be informed of the diagnosis and what to expect in the future. They need to be informed about available services and support and about the principles of care. Carer involvement in the planning for the well-being of the patient is also important. This can be difficult if there is denial or ambivalent relationships, or if the patient is paranoid, makes accusations, or misidentifies the carer.

Ripple effects occur in families, as the change in one set of relationships has implications for other relationships. It is not only the carer–patient relationship that is affected (Garwick *et al.* 1994), but the carer's own relationships with other family members such as adult children and siblings may also be affected. Sometimes the family may be able to serve as an important buffer for a carer and the level of stress he or she carries. Nodal points in the illness such as decisions of whether a person with dementia should move to another residence can be a point of crisis within a family. Carers' emotional needs should therefore be addressed. Management of emotion to enhance mutual support can be valuable, and consistency and continuity of family support networks is a predictor for lower caregiver burden. Carer needs are the subject of a separate chapter and are a central part of the management of dementia.

When dementia is of early onset, the immediate impact on family relationships may include children still living at home. There may be shifts in family relationships with increased closeness to the caregiving parent, sadness at the loss of the affected parent, and a need for more support and genetic counselling (Harvey 1998). Children also experience frustration on seeing that their parents' practical needs are not appropriately met and may want training for themselves in coping with challenging behaviour.

Younger patients are relatively more likely to have frontotemporal and alcohol-related dementias, and hence they more commonly experience focal symptoms such as dysphasia and behavioural disturbance (Seltzer and Sherwin 1983; Harvey 1998). These can be disruptive to family relationships. Sexual relationships may also be more disrupted, with extremes both of loss of sexual intimacy and also, in a minority, of an abnormal increase in sexual drive. The more abrupt and dramatic changes of lifestyle, and the presence of non-cognitive and behavioural symptoms, increase the potential for high carer stress *per se*. In dementia in people with Down's syndrome, the earlier the age of presentation the higher the frequency of behavioural and personality change (Holland *et al.* 2000). Here the family unit may involve older carers and precipitate the need for changes in established caring relationships.

Consideration also has to be given to the wide range of family structures among different ethnic groups and to the wide variation of family groupings within cultures. The notion that ethnic minorities have high levels of family integration is as simplistic as are assumptions about family roles and duties of care among ethnic minorities.

Specific management issues and interventions

Involving the patient

The primary care team is important in identifying the gateway and initiating contact with health and other services. The primary care response to presented problems is shaped by the patient's response to their illness as well as by their family members' concerns and expectations. Referral may result from the concerns of people other than the patient, and a route to assessment should be found that an individual is most comfortable with.

There may be various barriers to accepting referral, particularly where denial or lack of insight is present. Difficulties can also arise when the initial symptomatology disrupts relationships or includes paranoia or anxiety. Mental health teams can support the primary care team in the prereferral stage.

A preliminary risk assessment may be a useful model for planning if there is considerable reluctance on the part of a patient or overzealous concern by friends or neighbours. GP guidelines may be helpful in the prereferral phase in providing indicators of the presence of dementia (CHSR 1998) and a guide to preliminary physical investigation (Haines and Katona 1992). Evidence-based guidelines support the usual clinical practice of the non-use of compulsion; it would be unusual to use mental health legislation to overcome practical difficulties or a lack of cooperation with investigations (RCPsych 1995).

A common point of concern or interest between the patient and referrer needs to be established. Bridges into health care and management may be built through attention to a physical health focus for some, through the investigation offered by a memory clinic for others, while for other people assessment of cognitive function may only be possible once a community psychiatric nurse has built up the person's trust and confidence. A variety of routes of referral and venues for first consultations are needed to provide flexibility and sensitivity to what the patient is willing to accept. Additional barriers may exist for ethnic minority users; training community ethnic-group liaison and link workers may open routes to services.

Disclosure of the diagnosis

There is evidence that health professionals are still reluctant to tell patients their diagnosis. A recent study of current practice and attitudes among geriatricians and old age psychiatrists found that only 40% regularly tell their patients the diagnosis of dementia (Johnson *et al.* 2000). Clinicians have concerns that diagnostic information might result in depression, suicide, or other catastrophic reactions, or that dementia alters the patient's cognition in ways that impair their ability to use information. However, there is no evidence of long-term psychological harm from disclosure.

Patients' preferences may be approximated through insights into the views of their non-demented peers. Most express a wish to be told about the diagnosis (and to be given an opportunity to ask for a second opinion) in order to make decisions about their treatment, care, and affairs and to settle family matters (Erde *et al.* 1988).

Carers of people with dementia may also be reluctant for their affected relative to be informed; however, in most cases the same carers indicated that they would like to be told themselves if they were developing the illness (Maguire *et al.* 1996, Barnes 1997). One should anticipate that carers may sometimes attempt to steer their relative away from such discussion and it is important to consider whether discussion of the diagnosis should be carried out jointly with a carer or alone with the patient.

Disclosure is not a one-off event and needs to be made in the context of the ongoing professional/ patient relationship. Patient-led discussion is applicable in just the same way as it is in discussion of cancer, but adaptation may be needed to compensate for the current level of cognitive impairment. What to tell has to be carefully judged, balancing positive messages against the potential to inflict harm. Consideration should also be given as to how best to assist the patient to participate in (or to maximize involvement in) understanding of future choices, planning (for example, in connection with Power of Attorney), and understanding risks (for example, with driving and the need for supervision).

Some individuals may be helped by discussion of their memory loss in detail, akin to the way they might discuss their loss of ability to move independently (Knight 1986). The problem is perhaps greater for the clinician than for the patient. There is evidence to suggest that patient groups, particularly in the early stages of dementia, may be helpful by providing peer support and may assist with coping and problem-solving (Birnie 1997). Individual psychodynamic work may also be used, again starting early in dementia when facilitation of emotional outlet and grieving for losses can be a realistic goal (Hausman 1992). A number of adaptations can be made to adjust for cognitive impairment.

Genetic counselling should be offered to family members in the case of Huntington's disease, and the experience of running Huntington's disease genetics services may be helpful as and when a predictive test becomes available for Alzheimer's disease.

Communication with the patient

Communication can be affected early on in dementia with receptive or expressive dysphasias. The pragmatics of language (turn-taking and topic management) may also be affected. A reduced ability to communicate has an impact on relationships as well as on the well-being of the patient and on the early stages of management. Specific attention to compensating for functional language loss is relevant to everyone involved. Steps taken will include: attempting to use a calm and organized environment, which is free of distractions; improving sensory input, by maximizing both hearing and vision, and using face-to-face contact or touch when initiating, and during, conversation; simplifying the matters to be discussed, and presenting them as one idea at a time. Orientation to the topic of conversation may help, as may written prompts and reminders. Gestures may remain intact and may be helpful. The person, or those who know her well, can help determine how she can be assisted if she gets 'stuck'. For example, does sentence completion help or make things worse? Reassurance and support need to be given when the person becomes frustrated. The psychological state of a person and their desire to communicate will be important factors.

Speech and language therapists can be of help in providing more information about communication skills and deficits, and in giving advice on maximizing current skills. Helpful techniques include vocabulary access by semantic and/or phonemic cueing, circumlocution, and gesture. Communication strategies have been demonstrated to reduce professional and family carer stress (Ripich 1994).

Maintaining function through pleasurable activities

There are a number of reasons to be concerned about the almost universal problem of the loss of opportunity to engage in pleasurable and rewarding activities. This is important both for the individual and for the carer. Carers who manage to arrange appropriate and enjoyable activities enjoy an improved sense of efficacy and reduced feelings of burden. Interpersonal benefits include maximizing communication. The systemic consequences of a paucity of pleasurable activity include the greater likelihood of a vicious cycle of less communication, lower mood, less participation in any activity, and increased dependence on others.

Teri and Logsdon (1991) have developed a Pleasant Events Schedule. They argue that there is a need for a schedule as it is hard for a carer to be creative all the time; there may be a wide range of people involved in caregiving, and as the disease progresses there needs to be an ongoing process of finding activities within the person's ability. Each activity is rated over the past month for frequency of occurrence, availability, and enjoyability. Ways of increasing selected activities need to be devised and assistance needs to be provided to paid careworkers in planning individualized programmes. Age-appropriate activities should be adapted.

Music and reminiscence therapies may also be helpful. Although there are some methodology problems with the studies, available evidence suggests that music therapy may be beneficial in treating or managing dementia symptoms, and provides sufficient grounds on which to justify further investigation (Koger and Brotons 1999). Reminiscence (the use of silent or vocal recall of events of one's life) may also be beneficial (Spector and Orrell 1998). There is some evidence that, overall, elderly subjects treated with any form of therapy (reality orientation, cognitive training, physical exercise, socialization, reminiscence, and interactive contact or touch) tend to improve (Burckhardt 1987). While these therapies do not have a strong research base, they constitute models for communication and personalizing care and pleasurable experience.

Managing behavioural disturbance

Here we will deal broadly with the general principles for managing a range of psychotic symptoms and behavioural problems. A unified approach is justified because there is frequently overlap in presenting features and some common therapeutic interventions. Although there is some overlap with depression, this will be addressed separately. Associated physical health problems and sources of physical discomfort should also be addressed.

During any specific intervention, or when tackling a concurrent problem, consideration needs to be given to other ongoing aspects of care that might be particularly stretched by the current circumstances. Steps should be taken to maintain the ongoing care plan while the current problem is tackled. Where any medication is used, particular note should be made of side-effect profiles and of the potential to worsen confusion, increase the risk of falls, or reduce mobility. Provision should be made for supervision of correct and safe drug administration.

Delusions and hallucinations are common in dementia, although often they will be transient. They are associated with a number of behavioural symptoms (Ballard *et al.* 1991) and are correlated with entry into institutional care (Steele *et al.* 1990). Simple interventions including distraction, reassurance, and good lighting can be effective. Intervention may be required when the symptoms are more persistent and distressing, or when the resultant behaviours expose either the patient or others to risk. Current evidence (from randomized, placebo-controlled trials) supports the use of atypical antipsychotics such as risperidone because these have fewer extrapyramidal side-effects (De Deyn *et al.* 1999). There is also likely to be a lower risk of tardive dyskinesia. Current general recommendations would be for short-term use at low dose with a view to early reduction and discontinuation. However, there are associations between antipsychotic use and poorer prognosis in the dementias (McShane *et al.* 1997). Typical neuroleptics should not be used where Lewy body disease is suspected because of the neuroleptic sensitivity syndrome. This remains a potential risk with the atypical neuroleptics (McKeith *et al.* 1995). There is now a suggestion that cholinesterase inhibitors may, in some cases, be helpful in ameliorating psychotic and behavioural symptoms (McKeith *et al.* 2000).

Anxiety symptoms can be more difficult to identify because diagnostic features may be masked by the dementia and by the associated cognitive impairment. The study of anxiety in dementia has focused on the subjective, muscular (tension), and autonomic symptoms of anxiety (Ballard *et al.* 1996*b*). It is suggested that there are subgroups of anxious patients with dementia: autonomic and situational anxiety; anxiety with depression; and anxiety with psychotic symptoms. The prevalence of anxiety disorders is 38% among dementia patients (Wands *et al.* 1990). Anxiety disorders are thought to be more common in patients with mild dementia and in patients who retain insight into their condition, although the significance of these associations has not been established (Ballard *et al.* 1994). Little is known about the natural history of anxiety in dementia.

In early dementia, it is possible to treat anxiety with non-pharmacological methods such as relaxation and anxiety management, which allows the actual content of any fears and concerns to be explored. For example, is there fear of losing control or losing the affections of others, or is there experience of stress due to impaired social functioning? Anxiolytic medication may be indicated for short periods when anxiety is associated with agitation, or for carrying out a particular procedure such as tooth extraction. However, the use of these may be limited by the side-effects of sedation, worsening confusion and increasing the risk of falls.

Behaviour-oriented interventions utilize the structure of the ABC analysis of behaviour (Stokes 1990). Analysis is made through observation of the Antecedents and Consequences of each problem Behaviour. While, in principle, antecedent activities should be avoided, frequently these are unavoidable. For example, the use of the toilet or bathing may be associated with aggression. Given the difficulty of new learning in patients with dementia, it is suggested that environmental factors and the behaviours of caregivers should be changed. In a community-based, randomized controlled study a family carers' 'behavioural management strategy' resulted in a reduction in aggression nearing a significant level (Gormley *et al.* 2001). It is of particular interest that carers were able to develop skills in behavioural analysis and were able to devise interventions themselves.

Psychosocial interventions in institutional settings have also been studied (Opie *et al.* 1999). Enriched environments (using artefacts, tape-recordings, paintings, etc.) designed to create 'natural' or 'homelike' settings may be used to reduce agitation, aggression, and wandering into others' rooms. Use of colour or curtains to obscure door handles or mirrors by doors may reduce the frequency of using doors to exit safe areas. Activity programmes with trained volunteers may reduce aggressive incidents in patients whose wandering occurs in the context of boredom and inactivity. Similarly, audiotape material of preferred music, family members' voices, sensory stimulation, and simple exercise may result in reductions in verbally disruptive behaviours.

If the psychosocial or behavioural interventions have limited success, the non-specific use of medication may be appropriate. Indications are acute confusion and serious distress; or behaviour posing a current threat to the patient's or others' health. The use of antipsychotics is shown to provide only a modest improvement in behavioural symptoms in general, but can be successful in treating agitated behaviours and is most effective where there is paranoia with aggressive behaviours (APA 1997). There is a very significant placebo effect. Importantly, however, there are treatment side-effects in over a third of cases (Lanctot *et al.* 1998). At present there are no clear differences in efficacy between individual drugs, and therefore the choice of drug may best be made on the basis of side-effect profiles and the extent to which sedative properties are required.

Alternative medications effective in treating behavioural disturbance include carbamazepine (Tariot *et al.* 1999) and trazodone. (Lebert *et al.* 1994). There is also some evidence to support the use of selective serotonin-reuptake inhibitors (Lebert *et al.* 1994; Aurer *et al.* 1996). Sleep disturbance unresponsive to practical sleep hygiene interventions may warrant the short-term use of hypnotics. There is little to guide choice between agents specifically in dementia; however triazolam is not recommended because of an association with amnesia (APA 1997).

Depression

Depression is a common problem for people during the course of their dementia. It is important as a source of distress not only to the patient but also to carers, and there are associations with entry into residential care and longer hospital stay. In community samples of patients with dementia the prevalence is estimated at 20% (Ballard *et al.* 1996*a*). However, prevalence rates in nursing homes are higher than in the community and raise the question of whether there is improved case detection in these settings. There is some evidence to suggest that depression is more prevalent in patients with less severe dementia

Features of depression in Alzheimer's disease are similar to depression occurring in the absence of cognitive impairment although these features may be masked. First, depression reduces communication skills and performance on independent activities of daily living (Fitz and Teri 1994). The depression may therefore be misidentified as a primary progression of the dementia. Second, patients' responses to enquiry about symptoms and signs of depression can be affected by dementia-related impairment in concentration, memory, and judgement. Third, classic descriptions helpfully remind us that 'depressive ideas are fragmentary and transient' and that the 'mood change is short lived and shallow' (Roth 1955). Finally, features of dementia affecting eating, sleeping, and motor activity may obscure biological symptoms. Diagnosis is more difficult in the presence of more severe cognitive impairment.

However, where there is a personal or family history of depression or recent adverse events such as bereavement or relocation, the likelihood of depression being present is increased (CHSR 1998). Carers' observations of recent changes in activity and behaviour will often be useful. The validity of utilizing a carer observation-based assessment for depression in dementia is demonstrated in the Cornell Scale (a rating scale devised for monitoring the progress of depression in dementia; Alexopoulos *et al.* 1988). Carers assess the behaviour in five domains of function, namely: mood-related signs; behavioural disturbance; physical signs; cyclic functions; and ideational disturbance.

The treatment of depression is covered elsewhere in this book. Consideration should be given to the side-effect profiles of antidepressant and electroconvulsive therapy (ECT) on cognitive function. Cognitive and behavioural strategies have been described for managing depression in dementia (Teri and Gallagher-Thompson 1991). Cognitive strategies are more applicable in patients with mild dementia. Daily thought records can be kept by the patient, and negative thoughts can be challenged in treatment sessions; thus allowing a number of depressive features such as worthlessness and sleep disturbance to be addressed. In the behavioural model, which is applicable in more severe dementia, the carer tracks their relative's mood and the frequency (and duration) of pleasurable activities. Caregiver training is then used to increase the relative's pleasurable experiences and decrease behavioural disturbances that interfere with opportunities for pleasurable experiences (Teri 1994). The efficacy of behavioural treatment in improving mood has been demonstrated in controlled studies (Teri *et al.* 1997; Proctor *et al.* 1999).

Techniques for working with carers and family

It is important for patients that their family and friends adapt to the changes brought about by dementia. Even a family that functions well in terms of its ability to communicate, solve problems, and adapt can be challenged by the changes in function that result from dementia. Providing relevant knowledge may be all that is required for such a family to be able to adapt their usual ways of communicating about problems and to develop their own solutions. In other cases, a family's failed solution to difficulties can be viewed as the problem, but this can be directly tackled through family problem-focused interventions (Herr and Weakland 1979). Some families may lack the resources to tackle certain tasks that arise during times of crisis (for example, the death of a husband carer). At such times conflict of interests (for example, between siblings over finances or priorities) may arise. Poor communication or failure to adapt to changed roles may also lead to inferior outcomes for the patient. Family interventions may be helpful in these situations (Ratna and Davies 1984.). Where there is a pre-existing history of poor family adaptation and function, dementia may become the latest chapter of a long-term struggle for all concerned (Knight 1986). Family therapy may be helpful in this situation. Issues of abuse or neglect may also be addressed through family therapy (Goldstein 1990) and carer stress can usefully be approached using family therapy models (Gilleard *et al.* 1992) (Chapter 17).

Family teams who work with older patients and their families have documented their work with patients who have dementia. There is evidence that family interventions may be successfully applied and helpful, and that dementia does not preclude using these techniques (Benbow *et al.* 1993). A variety of models may be applicable for families who have a relative with dementia. Models described have included family problem-solving (Bonjean 1989), systemic (Benbow *et al.* 1993), and behavioural (Marriott *et al.* 2000).

A number of useful ideas can be taken from family therapy and applied in everyday work with care networks or within the family groupings around the older person with dementia. For example, a family forum to decide how to share care, how to solve a current problem, or simply to impart information and education can be useful. A family forum can also provide an opportunity for professionals to observe family interaction and to assess family coping strategies. It can also provide everyone present with an opportunity to be heard and to face conflicts between family members' own needs and those of the index patient. Emotions of guilt and hostility are common, as are the reactions of avoidance and distancing; these are often associated with tension within relationships.

Managing later stages

The later stages include terminal care, with a resulting shift in emphasis from adaptation to palliative care. General principles from palliative care can usefully be applied (Post and Whitehouse 1995). Terminal care involves an interdisciplinary approach that attends to both the patient's and family's needs. Palliative measures, limited medical intervention, and non-aggressive treatment of infections may be appropriate, but must be combined with a consideration of ethical issues. An important aspect of reassessment is to identify the appropriate time for shifts in the balance of care plans to include palliative principles

In the 11-year longitudinal study of Keene *et al.* (2001), patients with dementia lived an average of 8.5 years, two-thirds dying in a debilitated state, and 76% had spent a mean of 18 months in an institution prior to their death. Over half were hypophagic; one-third were unable to walk, and three-quarters were incontinent of urine. In a retrospective study of the experience of dying with dementia, the most frequent symptoms in the last year of life were mental confusion, urinary incontinence, pain, low mood, constipation, and the loss of appetite (McCarthy *et al.* 1997). These symptoms are comparable to those of patients with cancer, but dementia patients suffered them for longer periods. The high frequency of reports both of pain and of low mood in the last year of life requires further research. This finding is consistent with clinical experience and reminds us of the importance of developing appropriate management strategies.

Carer and family needs during this stage include positive affirmation and good communication with staff in long-term care settings. Carers may need to be given permission to withdraw at this stage (Bonnel 1996). Their personal thoughts and wishes that the person might die should be recognized. They are likely to experience guilt over the active steps they might be taking, for example in making 'tough' decisions about non-aggressive treatment or the withholding of medicines. 'Tough' decision-making could be re-connoted as making positive decisions. Validation of the past caring is important, but may not be offered by staff in long-term care settings who did not know the sufferer or carer personally during the preceding stages of the illness. A communication strategy at this stage requires that one determines what the family's expectations are about the roles, if any, they want to take in planning and about the type of feedback they are hoping for from the care staff. The need for additional family support should also be identified.

References

Alexopoulos, G., Abrams, R. C., Young, R. C., and Shamoian, C. A. (1988). Cornell scale for depression in dementia. *Biological Psychiatry*, **23**, 271–84.

APA (American Psychiatric Association). (1997). Practice guideline for the treatment of patients with Alzheimer's disease and other dementias of late life. *American Journal of Psychiatry*, **154** (Suppl.), 1–39.

Aurer, S. R., Monteiro, J., Turossian, C., Sinaiko, E., Boksyg, J., and Reisbert, B. (1996). The treatment of behavioural symptoms in dementia: haloperidol, thiordazine and fluoxetine: a double blind, placebo-controlled eight month study. *Neurobiology of Aging*, **17**, 652.

Ballard, C. G., Chithiramohan, R. N., Bannister, C., Handy, S., and Todd, N. (1991). Paranoid features in the elderly with dementia. *International Journal of Geriatric Psychiatry*, **6**, 155–7.

Ballard, C. G., Mohan, R. N. C., Patel, A., and Graham. C. (1994). Anxiety disorder in dementia. *Irish Journal of Psychiatry*, **11**, 108–9.

Ballard, C. G., Bannister, C., and Oyebode, F. (1996*a*). Depression in dementia sufferers. *International Journal of Geriatric Psychiatry*, **11**, 507–15.

Ballard, C. G., Boyle, A., Bowler, C., and Lindesay, J. (1996*b*). Anxiety disorders in dementia sufferers. *International Journal of Geriatric Psychiatry*, **11**, 987–90.

Barnes, R. C. (1997). Telling the diagnosis to patients with Alzheimer's disease: relatives should act as proxy for patient. *British Medical Journal*, **314**, 375–6.

Benbow, S. M., Marriott, A., Morley, M., and Walsh, S. (1993). Family therapy and dementia: review and clinical experience. *International Journal of Geriatric Psychiatry*, **8**, 717–25.

Bhatnagar, K. and Frank, J. (1997). Psychiatric disorders in elderly from the Indian sub-continent living in Bradford. *International Journal of Geriatric Psychiatry*, **12**, 907–12.

Birnie, J. (1997). A memory group for older adults. *PSIGE Newsletter*, **59**, 30–3.

Bonjean, M. J. (1989). Solution focussed psychotherapy with families caring for an Alzheimer's patient. *Journal of Psychotherapy and the Family*, **5**, 197–210.

Bonnel, W. B. (1996). Not gone and not forgotten: a spouse's experience of late-stage Alzheimer's disease. *Journal of Psychosomatic Nursing*, **34**, 23–7.

Burckhardt, C. (1987). The effect of therapy on the mental health of the elderly. *Research in Nursing and Health*, **10**, 277–85.

CHSR (Centre for Health Services Research and Department of Primary Care). (1998). *The primary care management of dementia: North of England Evidence–based Guideline Development Project.* CHSR, Newcastle-upon-Tyne.

De Deyn, P. P., Rabheru, K., Rasmussen, A., *et al.* (1999). A randomised trial of risperidone, placebo, and haloperidol for behavioural symptoms of dementia. *Neurology*, **53**, 946–55.

Department of Health. (1990). The Care Programme Approach. *Health Circular-HC (90)23/LASSL(90)11*. HMSO, London.

Deutsch, L. H., Bylsma, F. W., Rovner, B. W., Steele, C., and Folstein, M. F. (1991). Psychosis and physical aggression in probable Alzheimer's disease. *American Journal of Psychiatry*, **148**, 1159–63.

Erde, E. L., Nadal, E. C., and Scholl, T. O. (1988). On truth telling and the diagnosis of Alzheimer's disease. *Journal of Family Practice*, **26**, 401–6.

Fitz, A. E. and Teri, L. (1994). Depression, cognition and functional ability in patients with Alzheimer's disease. *Journal of the American Geriatrics Society*, **42**, 186–91.

Folstein, M. F., Folstein, S. E., and McHugh, P. R. (1975). 'Mini-Mental State': a practical method for grading the cognitive state of patients for the clinician. *Journal of Psychiatric Research*, **12**, 189–98.

Garwick, A. W., Detzner, D., and Boss, P. (1994). Family perceptions of living with Alzheimer's disease. *Family Process*, **33**, 327–40.

Gilleard, C., Lieberman, S., and Peeler, R. (1992). Family therapy for older adults: a survey of professionals' attitudes. *Journal of Family Therapy*, **14**, 413–22.

Goldstein, M. Z. (1990). The role of mutual support groups and family therapy for caregivers of demented elderly. *Journal of Geriatric Psychiatry*, **23**, 117–28.

Gormley, N., Lyons, D., and Howard, R. (2001). Behavioural management of aggression in dementia: a randomised controlled trial. *Age and Ageing*, **26**, 557–80.

Haines, A. and Katona, C. (1992). Dementia in old age. In *Clinical guidelines: occasional paper number* 58, 62–6. Royal College of Psychiatrists, London.

Harvey, R. J. (1998). Young onset dementia: epidemiology, clinical symptoms, family burden, support and outcome. *NHS Executive RFG045*. Imperial College, *Dementia.ion.ucl.ac.uk*.

Hausman, C. (1992). Dynamic psychotherapy with elderly demented patients. In *Care-giving in dementia: research and applications* (ed. G. Jones and B. L. Miesen), pp. 181–98. Routledge, London.

Herr, J. J. and Weakland, J. H. (1979). *Counselling elders and their families: practical techniques for applied gerontology*. Springer, New York.

Hindley, N. and Gordon, H. (2000). The elderly, dementia, aggression and risk assessment. *International Journal of Geriatric Psychiatry*, **15**, 254–9.

Holland, A. J., Hon, J., Huppert, F. A., and Stevens, F. (2000). Incidence and course of dementia in people with Down's syndrome: findings from a population-based study. *Journal of Intellectual Disability Research*, **44**, 138–46.

Keene, J., Hope, T., Fairburn, C. G., and Jacoby, R. (2001). Death and dementia. *International Journal of Geriatric Psychiatry* (In press.)

Keene J., Hope T., Fairburn, C. G., Jacoby, R., Gedling, K., and Ware, C. J. (1999). Natural history of aggressive behaviour in dementia. *International Journal of Geriatric Psychiatry*, **14**, 541–8.

Jeffery, D. (1987). Should you involve an older person about whom there is an issue of cognitive competence in family meetings? *PSIGE* Newsletter, **24**, 8–11.

Johnson, H., Bouman, W. P., and Pinner, G. (2000). On disclosing the diagnosis in Alzheimer's disease: a pilot study of current attitudes and practice. *International Psychogeriatrics*, **12**, 221–9.

Kitwood, T. (1997). The experience of dementia. *Aging and Mental Health*, **1**, 13–22.

Knight, B. (1986). *Psychotherapy with Older Adults*. Sage, Beverly Hills.

Koger, S. M. and Brotons, M. (1999). Music therapy for dementia symptoms. *The Cochrane Library, Issue* 4. Update Software, Oxford.

Lanctot, K. L., Mittman, N., Liu, B. A., Oh, P. I., Einarson, P. R., and Naranjo, C. A. (1998). Efficacy and safety of neuroleptics in behavioural disorders associated with dementia. *Journal of Clinical Psychiatry*, **59**, 550–61.

Lawton, M. P., Brody, E. M., and Saperstein, A. R. (1989). A controlled study of respite services for caregivers of Alzheimer's patients. *The Gerontologist*, **29**, 8–16.

Lebert F., Pasquier, F., and Petit, H. (1994). Behavioural effects of trazodone in Alzheimer's disease. *Journal of Clinical Psychiatry*, **55**, 536–8.

McCarthy, M., Addington-Hall, J., and Altmann, D. (1997). The experience of dying with dementia: a retrospective study. *International Journal of Geriatric Psychiatry*, **12**, 404–9.

McCormick, W. C., Kukull, W. A., van Belle, G., Bowen, J. D., Teri, L., and Larsen, E. B. (1994). Symptom patterns and comorbidity in the early stages of Alzheimer's disease. *Journal of the American Geriatrics Society*, **42**, 517–21.

McKeith, I. G., Harrison, R. W. S., and Ballard, C. G. (1995). Neuroleptic sensitivity to risperidone in Lewy body dementia. *Lancet*, **346**, 699.

McKeith, I. G., Grace, J. B., Walker, S., Byrne, E. J., Wilkinson, D., Stevens, T., *et al.* (2000). Rivastigmine in the treatment of dementia with Lewy bodies: preliminary findings from an open trial. *International Journal of Geriatric Psychiatry*, **15**, 387–92.

McShane, R., Keene, J., Gedling, K., Fairburn, C., Jacoby, R., and Hope, T. (1997). Do neuroleptic drugs hasten cognitive decline in dementia? Prospective study with necroscopy follow up. *British Medical Journal*, **314**, 266–70.

Maguire, C. P., Kirby, M., Coen, R., Coakley, D., Lawlor, B., and O'Neill. D. (1996). Family members' attitudes towards telling the patient with Alzheimer's disease their diagnosis. *British Medical Journal*, **313**, 529–30.

Manthorpe, J. and Hettiaratchy, P. (1993). Ethnic minority elders in the UK. *International Review of Psychiatry*, **5**, 171–8.

Marriott, A., Donaldson, C., Tarrier, N., and Burns, A. (2000). Effectiveness of cognitive-behavioural family intervention in reducing the burden of care in carers of patients with Alzheimer's disease. *British Journal of Psychiatry*, **176**, 557–62.

Miesen, B. M. L. and Jones, G. (1997). Psychic pain resurfacing in dementia. From new to past trauma. In *Past trauma in later life* (ed. L. Hunt, M. Marshall, and C. Rowlings), pp. 142–54. Jessica Kingsley, London.

Melzer, D., Hopkins, S., Pencheon, D., *et al.* (1994). Dementia. In *Health care needs assessment: the epidemiologically based needs assessment reviews*, pp. 303–40. Radcliffe Medical Press, Oxford.

Opie, J., Rossewarne, R., and O'Connor, D. W. (1999). The efficacy of psychosocial approaches to behaviour disorders in dementia: a systematic literature review. *Australian and New Zealand Journal of Psychiatry*, **33**, 789–99.

Post, S. G. and Whitehouse, P. J. (1995). Fairhill guidelines on ethics of the care of people with Alzheimer's disease: a clinical summary. *Journal of the American Geriatrics Society*, **43**, 1423–9.

Proctor, R., Burns, A., Powell, H. S., Tarrier, N., Faragher, B., Richardson, G., *et al.* (1999). Behavioural management in nursing and residential homes: a randomised controlled trial. *Lancet*, **354**, 26–9.

Ratna, L. and Davies, J. (1984). Family therapy with the elderly mentally ill: some strategies and techniques. *British Journal of Psychiatry*, **145**, 311–15.

Ripich, D. N. (1994). Functional communication with AD patients: a caregiver training program. *Alzheimer Disease and Associated Disorders*, **8**, 95–109.

Roth, M. (1955). The natural history of mental disorder in old age. *Journal of Mental Science*, **101**, 281–301.

Rovner, B. W., Steele, C. D, Shmuely, Y., and Folstein, M. F. (1996). A randomised trial of dementia care in nursing homes. *Journal of the American Geriatrics Society*, **44**, 7–13.

RCPsych (Royal College of Psychiatrists). (1995). *Consensus statement on the assessment and investigation of an elderly person with suspected cognitive impairment by a specialist old age psychiatry service*. Council Report CR 49. Royal College of Psychiatrists, London.

Seltzer, B. and Sherwin, I. (1983). A comparison of clinical features of early and late onset primary degenerative dementia. *Archives of Neurology*, **40**, 143–6.

Spector, A. and Orrell, M. (1998). Reminiscence therapy for dementia: a review of the evidence of effectiveness. In *The Cochrane Library*. Update Software, Oxford.

SSI (Social Services Inspectorate). (1997). *Older people with mental health problems living alone. Anybody's priority?* Department of Health, London.

Steele, C., Rovner, B., Chase, G. A., and Folstein, M. (1990). Psychiatric symptoms and nursing home placements of patients with Alzheimer's disease. *American Journal of Psychiatry*, **147**, 1049–51.

Stokes, G. (1990). *Common problems with the elderly confused: screaming and shouting*. Winslow Press, Bicester, Oxon.

Tariot, P. N., Jakimovich, L. J., Erb, R., Cox, C., Lanning, B., Irvine, C., *et al.* (1999). Withdrawal from controlled carbamazepine therapy followed by further carbamazepine treatment in patients with dementia. *Journal of Clinical Psychiatry*, **60**, 684–9.

Teri, L. (1994). Behavioral treatment of depression in patients with dementia. *Alzheimer Disease and Associated Disorders*, **8**, 66–74.

Teri, L. and Gallagher-Thompson, D. (1991). Cognitive-behavioural interventions for treatment of depression in Alzheimer's patients. *The Gerontologist*, **31**, 413–16.

Teri, L. and Logsdon, R. G. (1991). Identifying pleasant activities for Alzheimer's disease patients: the pleasant events schedule-AD. *The Gerontologist*, **31**, 124–7.

Teri, L., Logsdon, R. G., Uomoto, J. M., and McCurry, S. M. (1997). Reducing excess disability in dementia patients: training caregivers to manage patient depression. *Journal of Gerontology*, **52**, 159–66.

Vinestock, M. (1996). Risk assessment. 'A word to the wise'? *Advances in Psychiatric Treatment*, **2**, 3–10.

Wands, K., Merskey, H., Hachinski, V. C., Fishman, M., Fox, F., and Boniferro, M. (1990). A questionnaire investigation of anxiety and depression in early dementia. *Journal of the American Geriatrics Society*, **36**, 535–8.

25 Delirium: the physician's perspective

Neil Stewart and Sebastian Fairweather

Introduction

Acute mental confusion as a presenting symptom holds a central position in the medicine of old age. Its importance cannot be overemphasized, for acute confusion is a far more common herald of the onset of physical illness in an older person than are, for instance, fever, pain, or tachycardia (Hodkinson 1973). Delirium is a common, but under-recognized problem. It is sometimes a harbinger of serious underlying disease, though in other cases there may be a relatively simple cause which may be amenable to treatment. The illness may be short-lived and the prognosis good, particularly if it is managed correctly and care is taken to avoid complications. Recent evidence, however, suggests that delirium may carry a more serious prognosis in terms of cognitive impairment and also physical dependence than was previously thought. We start with an outline of the recognition, assessment, clinical features, and management of delirium. The second part of the chapter will deal with the pathophysiological basis, epidemiology, and causes of delirium.

Definition

Delirium is characterized by a transient and fluctuating global disorder of cognition and attention, a reduced level of consciousness, abnormally increased or reduced psychomotor activity, and a disturbed sleep–wake cycle. This syndrome is normally of abrupt onset (over a few hours) and of relatively short duration (a few days). The global disturbances of cerebral function are shown by:

- an alteration in alertness, arousal, and conscious level—with inability to concentrate and attend, alteration to the sleep–wake cycle, or varying degrees of coma;
- disordered perception and thinking—usually with fear and persecutory overtones;
- motor features—such as tremor or dysarthria;
- autonomic features—such as sweating, tachycardia, penile erection, pupillary abnormalities.

Some characteristic features of delirium are therefore:

- *Its global nature:* Delirium can be thought of as a toxic or metabolic defect affecting most of the central nervous system (though not uniformly). The global defects distinguish it from states brought about by focal (and localized) impairment of cerebral function, or impairment of a specific aspect of cognition, for example such as occurs in transient global amnesia.
- *Fluctuation:* Some degree of fluctuation is so characteristic that the diagnosis must be doubted if variability is not observed.
- *The circumstances of the onset:* Delirium nearly always appears acutely and in the context of a precipitating illness.

Although recognized for centuries, it has only been in the last decades that more formal definitions have been agreed upon within the framework of the *Diagnostic and statistical manual of mental disorders* (DSM-III, -III-R, and -IV) of the American Psychiatric Association and the tenth edition of the World Health

Table 25.1 DSM-IV diagnostic criteria for delirium

A	Disturbance of consciousness (i.e. reduced clarity of awareness of the environment) with reduced ability to focus, sustain, or shift attention.
B	A change in cognition (such as memory deficit, disorientation, language disturbance) or the development of a perceptual disturbance that is not better accounted for by a pre-existing, established, or evolving dementia.
C	The disturbance develops over a short period (usually hours to days) and tends to fluctuate during the course of the day.
D	There is evidence from the history, physical examination, or laboratory findings which suggests the aetiology of the delirium.

Organization *International classification of disease* (ICD-10; WHO 1993) (see Tables 25.1–25.3). The most recent criteria set out in DSM-IV (APA 1994) have evolved from those in DSM-III and DSM-III-R. *Clouding of consciousness* was the primary feature of delirium in the initial definition, but this proved difficult to define and apply accurately in a clinical setting. It was thus replaced by *a reduced ability to maintain attention to external stimuli* (for example, questions must be repeated because attention wanders) *and a reduced ability to shift attention to new external stimuli* (for example, perseverates answer to a previous question). Subsequently diagnostic instruments have been developed for delirium focusing on *inattention* as a major symptom (see later section).

Assessment and recognition

The diagnosis of delirium is entirely clinical; no laboratory or radiological test is pathognomonic, although they may be useful in determining aetiology. The above definitions provide standardization in the diagnosis, which is essential for clinical studies, although these criteria are in a process of evolution and have not been assessed for their diagnostic sensitivity and specificity. There has continued to be disagreement among experts about features essential to the diagnosis (MacDonald *et al.* 1996); and the widespread use of synonyms for the syndrome, such as confusional state, acute brain failure, and

Table 25.2 ICD-10 diagnostic criteria for delirium

Impairment of consciousness and attention
Global disturbance of cognition
Psychomotor disturbance
Disturbance of the sleep–wake cycle
Emotional disturbances

encephalopathy, has also contributed to the difficulties. There are two basic processes in assessing the potentially delirious patient: the first is to decide if the clinical syndrome is delirium, and the second is to identify the underlying cause. Delirium is probably one of the most frequently missed syndromes in the elderly. Like much in medicine, a failure to diagnose frequently results from simply failing to think of the diagnosis as a possibility. To the experienced clinician the sight of an elderly lady immobile for no obvious reason (typically identified as a 'social admission'), untidily slouched in her chair with a bewildered expression on her face, with a slow and variable response to queries, with a hint of dysarthria, a mild tremor and frequent minor jerky movements, all observed while the history is being taken, shrieks delirium. A quick examination of the mental state will either show a much greater cognitive impairment than is first apparent, or direct questions may reveal a frightening array of disordered thoughts. If the diagnosis is to be recognized it is imperative at least to assess basic cognitive function and to obtain a corroborative history of fluctuation in symptoms. The differential diagnosis of delirium includes:

Table 25.3 DSM-III-R diagnostic criteria for delirium

A	Reduced ability to maintain and shift attention to external stimuli.
B	Disorganized thinking, as indicated by rambling, irrelevant, and incoherent speech.
C	At least two of the following: (1) reduced level of consciousness; (2) perceptual disturbances: misinterpretations, illusions, or hallucinations; (3) disturbances of sleep–wake cycle with insomnia or daytime sleepiness; (4) increased or decreased psychomotor activity; (5) disorientation to time, place, or person; (6) memory impairment.
D	Abrupt onset of symptoms (hours to days), with daily fluctuation.
E	Either one of the following: (1) evidence from history, physical examination, or laboratory tests of specific organic aetiological factors; (2) exclusion of non-organic mental disorders, when no aetiological organic factor can be identified.

- dementia;
- acute functional psychosis;
- delusional disorders and acute schizophrenia;
- focal neurological defects

Table 25.4 lists some of the features distinguishing delirium from dementia. Crucial to this distinction is the history (see below).

History

An attempt should be made to obtain a history from the patient, although this will often be unreliable and may be inaccessible; it is therefore important to seek a history from an informant in all cases. A corroborative history may be given by a relative, carer, general practitioner (GP), or someone who knows the premorbid cognitive state of the patient. In hospital, information from the nurses caring for the patient is essential, particularly the observations and comments made by the night staff, as this may be the only time when symptoms are apparent in the early stages or in milder forms of delirium. Specific information should be sought about the abruptness of onset of the illness, fluctuations in the symptoms, evidence of misperceptions, illusions or hallucinations, and level of alertness or drowsiness. It is important to try to determine the premorbid level of cognition and elicit any evidence of longstanding dementia. Specific symptoms suggestive of physical precipitants should also be sought (e.g. fever, pain, cough, dysuria, and so on). An accurate list of drug treatment is vital, including over-the-counter remedies, and whether there have been any recent changes. The inadvertent cessation on admission to hospital of a previously regularly taken benzodiazepine may be the cause of a subsequent florid delirium. A tactful enquiry also needs to be made about alcohol consumption.

Examination

The physical examination of the agitated, hyperalert patient with delirium will be difficult. The detection of physical signs is, however, very important in reaching conclusions about the underlying cause of the delirium, and it is therefore essential to attempt as full an assessment as possible even if this has to be done in a piecemeal way. There are three main facets to the assessment, the clinician should:

(1) examine the mental state of the patient in order to suggest the diagnosis of delirium; then
(2) look for the presence of physical signs associated non-specifically with delirium such as sweating, abnormal movements, tremor, and asterixis; and finally

Table 25.4 Differential diagnosis of delirium and dementia, clinical features

	Delirium	Dementia
Clinical course		
Mode of onset	Acute or subacute (hours or days)	Chronic (usually several years)
Fluctuations	Frequent and rapid (in hours)	Slow changes (months)
Conscious level		
Attention	Markedly reduced	Reduced only in severe cases
Arousal	Increased or decreased	Usually normal
Alertness	Reduced in severe cases	Usually normal
Cognitive changes		
Delusions	Fleeting, poorly systematized	If present often consistent
Hallucinations	Common (usually visual)	Infrequent (both visual and aural)
Orientation	Usually impaired	Impaired in proportion to severity
Motor features		
Abnormal movements	Tremor, asterixis, myoclonus common	Early: dyspraxia common Late: myoclonus especially in prion dementia, also in Alzheimer's disease
Psychomotor activity	Usually abnormal: increased or decreased	Usually normal
Dysgraphia	Usually present	Absent in mild cases
Autonomic features	Abnormalities often present	Normal, except that postural hypotension is common

(3) seek the physical signs associated with the underlying cause of the delirium..

Physical signs associated with the delirium syndrome

The hyperactive, agitated patient may show signs of sympathetic overactivity such as sweating, tremor, pupillary dilatation, dry mouth, tachycardia, and elevated blood pressure. There may be non-specific involuntary movements, for example asterixis, or myoclonus. Dysarthria and dysgraphia will frequently be present. Drawing tasks (see below) may be helpful in assessment.

Physical signs associated with underlying disease

During the general physical examination the following more specific signs of disease, which are associated with delirium, should be sought.

However, it is difficult to give specific advice succinctly. Careful temperature measurement should be made (either on tympanic membrane or rectally) to assess core temperature. Both pyrexia and hypothermia can present with delirium. In a physician's practice, infection is the dominant cause and chest, bladder, kidney, and gallbladder are the commonest sites.

This may also be true for patients developing delirium whilst a psychiatric inpatient. On the other hand, those presenting to a psychiatrist with delirium are more likely to have a covert cause, or the GP would have directed them elsewhere. Therefore look for signs of thyroid disease (facies, tremor, goitre, eye signs) and skin lesions suggesting chronic liver disease (spider naevi, jaundice, etc.). Examination of the skin may also elicit information about cyanosis, anaemia, pigmentation in hyperadrenalism, or pallor and hairlessness in hypopituitarism.

Assessment of mental state

One of the most important parts of the assessment of the mental state is the estimation of cognitive function. Two widely used and accepted methods are the Mini-Mental Status Examination (MMSE) (Folstein *et al.* 1975) and the Abbreviated Mental Test score (AMT) (Hodkinson 1972; Jitapunkul *et al.* 1991). These can be used in the assessment of patients with delirium; and should probably be carried out routinely on all elderly patients on their admission to hospital so that serial results can then be used to assess the changes in cognitive state, which are the hallmark of delirium. Various tests of attention and concentration can be used at the bedside to supplement these cognitive tests, for example trail-following, digit-span, and spelling a simple word backwards. Close clinical observation by experienced staff, with particular attention to fluctuations in alertness, cognition, and orientation, or signs of abnormal perception are also important. Fisher and Flowerdew (1995) found that impairment of the ability to draw a clock-face was a better predictor of the development of postoperative delirium than a low score on the MMSE. They suggest that clock-face drawing is a test of the higher order integration of sensory information and attention, functions that are impaired in delirium. Specific delirium assessment instruments have recently been developed (Trzepacz 1994*a*). These are based on DSM-III and DSM-IV criteria for the diagnosis of delirium and allow bedside testing (possibly by non-medical assessors) in a systematic, standardized, and reproducible way. These instruments also make possible repeat testing to assess change, and the direct comparison of results between testers (see below).

Diagnostic instruments and rating scales

A plethora of diagnostic instruments have been developed for the bedside assessment of delirium, often based on the DSM criteria (see Tables 25.5 and 25.6).

Different tests have been developed for screening, diagnosis, assessment of severity, and evaluation of treatment efficacy (Robertsson 1999). Inouye suggests four essential criteria to determine their usefulness (Inouye 1994):

(1) validated specifically for use in delirium;
(2) capability to distinguish delirium from dementia;
(3) assessment of multiple features of delirium;
(4) feasibility for use in delirious patients.

These instruments are used in allowing standardized assessment, and in the evaluation of the effectiveness of interventions. Their main role is in research practice, although more widespread clinical use might improve the level of recognition of delirium. One of the most commonly used instruments is the Confusion Assessment Method (Inouye *et al.* 1990) (see Table 25.7), which has been shown to be sensitive, specific, and reliable in the detection of delirium. However, if even a simple cognitive test, such as the AMT, were applied more routinely in the initial and subsequent assessment of patients in day-to-day clinical practice, changes in cognitive function could be detected earlier and hence delirium might be diagnosed more quickly and managed more effectively. Prospective studies are needed to evaluate diagnostic criteria and assessment instruments against the 'gold standard' clinical opinion of a specialist. Johnson *et al.* (1992) compared prospective diagnosis by a

Table 25.5 Delirium assessment instruments

Instrument	Basis	Type	Rater	Reference
Confusion Assessment Method	DSM-III-R	Diagnosis	Non-psychiatrist	Inouye 1990
Delirium Symptom Interview	DSM-III	Diagnosis	Non-psychiatrist	Albert 1992
Delirium Rating Scale	—	Diagnosis and severity	Psychiatrist	Trzepacz 1988
Delirium Index	DSM-III-R	Severity	Non-psychiatrist	McCusker 1998
Delirium Assessment Scale	DSM-III	Diagnosis and severity	Non-psychiatrist	O'Keeffe 1994

Table 25.6 Investigations for delirium

Investigation	Underlying problem
Essential/first line[a]	
Pulse + blood pressure[b]	Hypoxia, arrhythmia, cardiac or septic shock
Body temperature	Infection
Full blood count	Anaemia, white cell count in infection
Urea and electrolytes	Uraemia, electrolyte disturbance, especially low Na
Blood glucose/BM stick[b]	Hypoglycaemia, diabetes
ECG[b]	Myocardial infarction, arrhythmia
Blood cultures	Bacteraemia
Urine analysis[b]/culture	Urinary tract infection, diabetes
C-reactive protein	Infection, or inflammatory disorder, e.g. giant-cell arteritis
Chest radiograph	Infection, tumour
Oxygen saturation/pulse oximetry[c]	Heart failure, pulmonary embolus
Second line	
Thyroid function	Hypo- or hyperthyroidism
Serum calcium	(Hypo-) or hypercalcaemia
Drug levels	Lithium, digoxin, anticonvulsants
Oxygen saturation/arterial blood gases	Pulmonary embolus, pneumonia, heart failure
Erythrocyte sedimentation rate	Other inflammatory disorders
Liver function tests	Acute or chronic liver disease
Specific/optional	
Lumbar puncture	If indicated, e.g. meningitis, subarachnoid haemorrhage
EEG	Can help confirm diagnosis if in doubt
Computed tomography of brain	Intracerebral lesion, e.g. stroke, tumour
Vitamin B_{12}/ folate	Deficiency

The first-line tests should be carried out in all cases.
The second-line tests may be indicated in specific circumstances if the history or examination suggest there may be a diagnostic yield.
Specific tests may be indicated in certain circumstances.
[a]It is reasonable to expect these tests to be performed in a psychiatric service, except that cultures might be omitted if the temperature and white cell count are normal and/or a putative cause other than infection is highly likely. It is wise to perform these tests even if alcohol withdrawal is highly likely.
[b]These are the minimal tests one might expect a GP to perform.
[c]Many psychiatric wards will not have the equipment to do this, although it is relatively inexpensive and very easy to perform.

psychiatrist (using DSM-III criteria) and a physician's diagnosis based on a retrospective review of the same case notes. They showed that sensitivity of retrospective diagnosis was low, and concluded that prospective methods of case identification are to be preferred. They also showed that the diagnosis is often made late in the course of delirium, which may contribute to its high mortality and morbidity.

Investigations

The causes of delirium are numerous and varied and it is difficult to provide an exhaustive list of recommended investigations. We have attempted to stratify basic tests in terms of their importance and usefulness, with particular reference to general practice, psychiatry, and internal medicine. It is necessary to repeat here that delirium is frequently a marker of more severe underlying disease than is first apparent, and that it is associated with an appreciable mortality. The physician should therefore consider carefully before electing to manage such a patient without access to the facilities normally available to acute medicine, and should certainly review the patient regularly to determine if transfer to a service with more intensive facilities is appropriate.

Table 25.7 Confusion Assessment Method (CAM)[a]

1	*Acute onset and fluctuating course* This feature is usually obtained from a family member or nurse and is shown by positive responses to the following questions: Is there evidence of an acute change in the patient's mental status from base line? Did the abnormal behaviour fluctuate during the day, i.e. come and go, or increase or decrease in severity?
2	*Inattention* This feature is shown by a positive response to the question: Did the patient have difficulty focusing attention, for example, being easily distractible, or having difficulty keeping track of what was being said?
3	*Disorganized thinking* Was the patients thinking disorganized or incoherent, such as rambling or irrelevant conversation, unclear or illogical flows of ideas, or unpredictable switching from subject to subject?
4	*Altered level of consciousness* This feature is shown by any answer other than *alert* to the following question: Overall how would you rate this person's level of consciousness?: (alert [normal]; vigilant [hyperalert]; lethargic [drowsy, easily aroused]; stupor [difficult to arouse]; coma [unrousable])

[a]The diagnosis of delirium requires the presence of features 1 and 2 and either 3 or 4. Inouye *et al.* (1990).

Clinical features

Lipowski's description of the general clinical features of delirium is clear, concise, and difficult to improve on: delirium is characterized by a global impairment of cognitive processes (thinking, remembering, and perceiving), attentional abnormalities, and a reduced awareness of self and environment. There is defective ability to extract, process, and retain information. The patient's grasp of situations is faulty and there is diminished capacity to act in the customary purposeful, sustained, and goal-directed manner. There are also associated symptoms: emotional and mood disturbance, increased autonomic nervous activity (tachycardia, sweating, dilated pupils, flushed face, elevated blood pressure), involuntary movements, asterixis, dysnomia, dysgraphia, confabulation, and perseveration (Lipowski 1991).

Onset

The onset of symptoms is typically relatively abrupt over a period of hours or days, and often the first symptoms are at night. There is also said to be a prodromal period during which the patient may have a milder form of the syndrome with irritability, and subjective difficulty in thinking clearly. This prodrome may last for days and the symptoms may only be apparent at night (Macdonald 1998).

Duration and course

In the majority of cases the delirium resolves after a few days. There tends to be a delay between recovery from the precipitating acute physical illness and recovery from delirium, and occasionally there are persistent psychological symptoms

Variants: hyperactive, hypoactive, etc.

Lipowski (1991) described three main clinical types of delirium; hyperactive, hypoactive, and a mixed hyperactive/hypoactive variant. The classical picture is the hyperactive and agitated state. This may be commoner in younger people and is also prevalent in withdrawal states, such as withdrawal from alcohol. The hypoactive or somnolent form tends to be more common in older patients and is more difficult to recognize clinically, requiring a higher index of suspicion. The importance of this syndrome can be estimated from the experiences of O'Keeffe and Lavan (1999) who studied 225 admissions to an acute geriatric unit and found 94 patients with delirium; Liptzin and Levkoff (1992) also analysed a group of elderly patients with delirium who had been admitted to hospital with a medical diagnosis (see Table 25.8).

Specific psychological features

Attention/wakefulness

Delirium is commonly described as a disorder of attention, consciousness, or wakefulness. The presence of a wide variety of other symptoms, such as abnormalities of cognition, perception, orientation, and psychomotor alterations, would suggest that the picture is a much more complex one. A deficit in attention or conscious level is, however, integral to the definition and hence to diagnosis of the syndrome as evidenced by the DSM-IV criteria. Therefore the patient with delirium will have difficulty in focusing on a specific task, will be easily distractible, and will not be able to maintain their attention to a task for any length of time. They will also have difficulty with altering the focus of their attention between tasks. These deficits may be fairly obvious in conversation and history-taking, but can be further tested at the bedside with simple tests such as trail-following, spelling words backwards, recounting the months of the year in reverse, etc. Alterations in the level of wakefulness or arousal are again integral to the diagnosis of delirium and clearly have a major bearing on functions of attention. There is almost always alteration in the normal sleep–waking cycle, and this is often reversed, with daytime sleepiness and nocturnal wakefulness. There may be a wide range in the level of arousal—from somnolence or stupor to agitation and hyperactivity (Table 25.9)—and this level may vary and fluctuate over time. These fluctuations and the often subtle nature of the alterations in attention and arousal emphasize the need to observe the patient over time; failure to do this may lead to the diagnosis being missed.

Table 25.8 Delirium: clinical variants (%)

	O'Keeffe	Liptzin
Hyperactive	21	15
Mixed	43	52
Hypoactive	29	19
No disturbance	7	14

Cognition, thinking

Lipowski (1991) has proposed that disorders of thinking in delirium can be categorized under four broad headings: organization or ordering of thoughts; the dynamics or evolution of thoughts over time; the formation of concepts; and the content of thoughts. Disruption of the *organization* of thoughts leads to fragmented and incoherent thinking, inability to process stimuli, and a general inability to think in a structured and goal-directed way. The *stream* of thoughts may be altered, may either be by slowing or by speeding up (Lindesay *et al.* 1990). The ability to grasp

Table 25.9 Degrees of impairment of consciousness in delirium

Mild	Failure to maintain attention, worse under conditions of fatigue, worse in the evening or at night
Moderate	Fluctuation in ability to attend Patient easily distractible Disruption in sleep–wake cycle with sleep at inappropriate times and frequent disturbed nights
Severe	Patient lapses into periods of coma, which often rapidly alternate with periods of increased arousal Attention very difficult to keep
Coma	Unresponsive to all except noxious stimuli

abstract *concepts* is hampered, judgement and logical thought are impaired. The *content* of thought may be influenced by misperception of the surroundings, which may lead to the formation of delusions (fixed abnormal beliefs). These delusions are often fleeting and inconsequential, but if persistent they are likely to take on a persecutory nature, or they may relate to supposed 'bizarre happenings' in the patient's immediate surroundings.

Perception, illusions, hallucinations

Abnormal perceptions can occur in all sensory modalities in delirium (including body shape and image), although they are most commonly visual, or visual and auditory hallucinations (Lindesay *et al.* 1990); they do not have to be present for diagnosis. The hallucinations most commonly take the form of animals, people, or voices.

Vision

Visual hallucinations may range from simple flashes of lights or patterns, to fully formed objects. They are typically of small objects which cannot be described in detail, but are often menacing or associated with fear. Large, fully formed complex and detailed visual hallucinations are not typical in elderly patients, but a reliable systematic analysis of such symptoms in the old is not available to substantiate this claim. Patients will often have insight that their visual experiences are hallucinations, perhaps because they are usually black and white or grey with an ethereal flavour. Illusions and distortions also occur as a result of misinterpretation of the surrounding physical environment, especially in an unfamiliar environment.

Hearing

Altered auditory perception is common. Noises such as the bustle of a general hospital ward may easily be interpreted as menacing. Auditory hallucinations are not rare, but it is very uncommon for them to be fully formed. Well-formed auditory hallucinations point strongly to a functional rather than an organic illness. Even if patients claim to be hearing words they will usually admit that they know intuitively what is said rather than actually hearing the exact words used.

Memory

Memory impairment is common in delirium and includes abnormalities of laying down, retention, and recall. As impairments of perception, attention, and cognition naturally lead to the failure to register and form memories of current events, so there is often amnesia for the period of delirium once recovery has occurred. Short-term and medium-term recall tend to be affected more than remote memory, but in severe cases this may also be abnormal (Macdonald 1990; Trzepacz 1994*b*).

Orientation

Lipowski (1991) states that 'some degree of temporal disorientation at some period during the day is necessary for the diagnosis of delirium'. Errors in orientation with regard to time are likely to be more sensitive indicators of the syndrome than the other facets of orientation, place, and person. The delirious patient is also likely to mistake the unfamiliar for the familiar, thinking that she is at home when in hospital (or both at the same time) or that the doctor is a relative.

Psychomotor

Lipowski describes three separate types of psychomotor behaviour in delirium (Lipowski 1991). These are hyperactive, hypoactive, and a mixed picture with elements of both. Hypoactivity tends to predominate in the elderly patient, with somnolence, reduction in purposeful physical activity, lethargy, slow movements, staring, apathy, and reduced speech. This type of psychomotor disturbance predisposes the patient to pressure-sore formation and hypostatic pneumonia: it is more difficult to recognize clinically and may be associated with more severe underlying disease, a raised mortality rate, and a higher rate of discharge to institutional care (O'Keeffe and Lavan 1999). The hyperactive type, by contrast, is commoner in the younger patient and probably in the syndrome caused by alcohol or drug withdrawal, and it may have a better prognosis. There may be hypervigilance, restlessness, fast or loud speech, irritability, combativeness, anger, wandering, easy distractibility, nightmares, or euphoria, singing, or laughing.

Emotion, mood

Delirium is accompanied for most patients by significant distress, fear, and anxiety. A significant number of patients may also have depression (Macdonald 1990).

Management/treatment

The first step in the management of delirium is obviously to try and prevent its occurrence. As mentioned above, this may be helped by early assessment of the risk factors such as pre-existing cognitive impairment, age, severity of presenting illness, etc. It should be borne in mind that the more vulnerable patient may need only a relatively minor further insult to precipitate delirium, whereas the younger fitter patient with few risk factors will require a correspondingly greater insult (Flacker and Marcantonio 1998). Steps should then be taken to avoid known precipitating factors for delirium (see later) particularly in the high-risk population. Inouye *et al.* (1999) tested this hypothesis with a trial of multicomponent interventions aimed at preventing delirium. Patients admitted to a general medical service were either given routine care, or were managed on a specific unit which had the aim of actively managing six risk factors for delirium: cognitive impairment, sleep deprivation, immobility, visual impairment, hearing impairment, and dehydration. The interventions for risk factors succeeded in reducing the number and duration of episodes of delirium, although there was no effect on the severity or recurrence rates. The authors conclude that primary prevention may be the most effective treatment strategy. Cole *et al.* (1996), however, carried out a meta-analysis of 10 published studies looking at the prevention of delirium in medical and surgical patients. They found some evidence that intensive nursing and prospective management of medical complications may have an effect in reducing the delirium rate. The studies of medical inpatients (of which there were only two, Nagley (1986) and Wanich *et al.* (1992)) showed no preventive effect, although in one the incidence of delirium was negligible and in the other prevalent cases at admission to the unit were unfortunately included in the analysis. However, all the studies examined had significant methodological difficulties and were heterogeneous in terms of study populations and interventions. As the diagnosis is often missed in hospital—in accident and emergency departments, in medical wards, and postoperatively in surgical patients (Flacker and Marcantonio 1998)—it is hardly surprising that management is frequently not ideal.

The second main facet of management after the syndrome has been recognized and diagnosed is a search for the cause and the treatment or correction of this if possible. Assessment by history, examination, and investigation are covered elsewhere.

General care

The general and nursing management of the patient with delirium is important. Attending to the patient's needs, such as nutrition and hydration and early mobilization, is essential. Interdisciplinary working, with involvement of doctors, nurses, physiotherapists, and the patient's family, should also take place. The presence of familiar people, such as friends and relatives, are important for the general orientation of the patient. The nursing environment should be kept as quiet as possible, with minimization of extraneous noise from, say, television and radios, and noisy ward equipment such as pumps, alarms, and bleeps. Efforts should be made to provide visual cues for orientation such as clocks and calendars. Encouraging normal sleep–wake patterns by having ward regimes that avoid waking patients to give them medication, and keeping the ward quiet at normal sleeping times are helpful. The patients should be encouraged to wear their normal spectacles and hearing aids to try to increase awareness of the environment.

The question of where best to manage the delirious patient also arises. This is a complex question and depends on several factors:

1. Is the underlying diagnosis obvious, or is there a need for further investigation to establish the cause?
2. Can the correct treatment for the underlying pathology be given without moving the patient?
3. Can the patient be adequately monitored?
4. Will the patient's condition deteriorate significantly if he or she is admitted to hospital, or will she come to harm by wandering off an open acute ward?

It should be borne in mind that a number of the investigations which are seen as essential may be much more conveniently available in a general hospital, medical inpatient setting. The advantages of admitting the patient to this type of ward from, say, the community or a general psychiatric setting should be balanced against the possible negative effect of a change in the patient's environment and the loss of familiar surroundings and faces, which may exacerbate the delirium.

Iatrogenic complications

The delirious patient is at high risk of iatrogenic complications. Injuries, falls, pressure ulcers, constipation and loss of bladder control, the placement of a urinary catheter, dehydration and undernutrition, and swallowing difficulties leading to aspiration are all potential problems. High levels of nursing and medical surveillance are required to prevent these. Complications may prolong the delirium syndrome, lead to longer hospital stays, potentially increase discharge to institutions, and increase morbidity and mortality.

Removing contributing factors

Apart from treating the underlying physical cause of delirium, close attention should be paid to removing or correcting other metabolic factors such as anaemia, hypoxia, or electrolyte imbalance, which may arise during the illness. Any drugs known to predispose to delirium should be removed, and care should be taken not to introduce new drugs that might exacerbate the syndrome.

Maintaining behavioural control

It is generally recommended that restraint (whether pharmacological or physical) should be avoided, at least initially, in the management of patients with delirium (Flacker and Marcantonio 1998). Treatment of the underlying cause is the most important factor and environmental measures as described above should be implemented. Environmental modification methods are probably underused, particularly in hypoactive patients (Meagher *et al.* 1996). There are very few studies of drug treatments, although benzodiazepines (but see below) or neuroleptics are generally used. Breitbart *et al.* (1996) carried out one of the very few randomized trials in patients with delirium (in the setting of AIDS). They compared haloperidol, chlorpromazine, and lorazepam; haloperidol and chlorpromazine were found to be effective and well tolerated, while lorazepam was less effective in reducing the symptoms of delirium. In all six patients prescribed lorazepam, treatment had to be stopped due to side-effects; these included oversedation, disinhibition, ataxia, and worsening confusion, all of which may be even more likely in the old. In the use of psychotropic drug treatments for delirium the following points should be borne in mind:

- Avoid drugs which may exacerbate or cause delirium, i.e. agents with a central anticholinergic action.
- If alteration in the sleep pattern is prominent, sleep may be promoted by an appropriate dose of a short-acting hypnotic, such as clomethiazole (for the frail patient) or temazepam (in the more robust).
- Episodes of severely disturbed behaviour which are unresponsive to general measures or to specific treatment aimed at correcting the cause (e.g. oxygen in hypoxia), should be treated

only with a major tranquillizer. Drugs such as benzodiazepines may cause disinhibition and make matters worse. Haloperidol is the drug of choice as it has less anticholinergic activity and has minimal effects on respiration and blood pressure. The initial dose should be small (0.5 to 1 mg) and titrated up according to response.
- The management of alcohol and benzodiazepine withdrawal has specific differences which are noted in the next section.

Physical restraint has not been well studied, although there is probably an increase in the rate of falls and injury associated with its use, and there may also be a tendency for the use of restraint to worsen delirium (Inouye 1999).

Management of alcohol-withdrawal delirium (delirium tremens)

Delirium induced by alcohol withdrawal should be regarded as separate from other forms of delirium, mainly due to differences in the management of the condition. A recent meta-analysis (Mayo-Smith 1997) showed that benzodiazepines are effective in relieving the signs and symptoms of alcohol withdrawal, reducing the risk of seizures and of delirium. Clomethiazole has been shown to be more effective than placebo, although there is less randomized trial evidence to support its use rather than benzodiazepines, and the latter may be safer (Hall and Zador 1997). There are two other factors that need be addressed. Nutritional deficiency due to alcoholism necessitates replacement of the B vitamins, particularly thiamine to prevent Wernicke's encephalopathy and the Wernicke–Korsakoff syndrome. It is important to remember that nutritional deficiency may also be present in the non-alcoholic elderly person; if there is any doubt, B vitamins should be given as a routine to the delirious patient. Specific treatment to prevent seizures is also needed, and this should be with a drug that cross-reacts with alcohol, e.g. a benzodiazepine or clomethiazole (Sellers 1988). If seizures occur these should be treated with intravenous diazepam, rather than infusion of clomethiazole (the latter carries a higher risk of respiratory depression as the dose is more difficult to titrate). It should also be noted that phenothiazine treatment may reduce the seizure threshold. Therefore these drugs should not be used in patients whose delirium may be related to alcohol withdrawal, at least not until a drug with cross-tolerance to alcohol can be given (Mayo-Smith 1997). Recently, beta-blocking drugs (particularly ones active in the CNS such as propanolol) and carbamazepine have been used as adjunctive treatments in the alcohol-withdrawal syndrome (Fuller and Gordis 1997), although these agents should be used only in conjunction with alcohol cross-tolerant drugs mentioned above.

Management of benzodiazepine-withdrawal delirium

Dependence may develop after the habitual use of benzodiazepine and other hypnotic and sedative drugs. Their subsequent withdrawal may lead to physical and psychological symptoms, which in severe cases and in the elderly may result in delirium (Busto *et al.* 1986). Consequently, care must also be taken not to stop benzodiazepine medication inadvertently when an elderly person is admitted to hospital, as this has been shown to be a potential cause of delirium (Moss 1991; Moss and Lanctot 1995). The occurrence and timing of any withdrawal symptoms tend to be related to the pharmacological properties of the particular benzodiazepine, and are related to the elimination half-life of the drug: short-acting drugs are more likely to lead to more rapid-onset withdrawal symptoms. Longer acting drugs such as diazepam may cause the onset of withdrawal symptoms to be delayed by up to 1 month after cessation of the drug. There is also some evidence that more severe withdrawal symptoms, such as seizures, may be more likely with the shorter acting agents (Sellers 1988).

Mechanisms of delirium

Neuropathophysiology

The pathophysiology of delirium is still largely obscure. In 1936, Hart wrote that 'of the precise processes by which delirium is mediated we know nothing'. Hart postulated that the impairment of cerebral function underlying the delirium could be produced by a wide range of factors whose connection to the syndrome might be no more specific than that between hemiplegia and its various causes (Lipowski 1991). It has also been suggested that age-related changes in the brain predispose elderly persons to delirium during physiological disturbances that are otherwise tolerated in younger individuals, and that these changes represent an age-associated decline in physiological reserve. Such changes may include reduced blood flow, neuron loss, and reduced levels of neurotransmitters, particularly acetylcholine, norepinephrine (noradrenaline), dopamine, and gamma-aminobutyric acid (GABA) (Flacker 1999*a*). These authors also postulate that the theory of global cerebral impairment should now be revised to take account of disruption of specific neurological pathways and neurotransmitter systems which then lead to delirium. They suggest that there is probably no 'common pathway' in delirium, but rather delirium should be seen as a final common symptom of a variety of situation-specific neurotransmitter abnormalities.

Specific neurotransmitter systems

The cholinergic system

Although a number of neurotransmitter systems have been suggested as playing a role in the pathogenesis of delirium, deficiency of acetylcholine has been the most frequently implicated. It is known that acetylcholine plays an important role in consciousness, that giving drugs having anticholinergic actions (such as atropine) to patients can cause symptoms of delirium, and that certain toxins that have anticholinergic actions may also lead to delirium. The use of anticholinergic agents in the treatment of Parkinson's disease is a common cause of delirium (Cummings 1991); moreover, there is an association between the perioperative use of drugs with anticholinergic activity and postoperative delirium in patients undergoing cardiac surgery (Tune 1981). It has been postulated that reduced numbers of receptors (muscarinic) for acetylcholine in older people may predispose them to delirium. Further support for the role of acetylcholine comes from the use of acetylcholine-agonist drugs such as physostigmine in the treatment of toxin-induced delirium (Flacker 1999*a*). A recent report of the use of donepezil (a cholinesterase inhibitor) possibly leading to the resolution of a delirium in Alzheimer's disease also lends support to this theory (Wengel *et al.* 1998).

Recently an assay for total serum anticholinergic activity has been developed. This has been used to study the anticholinergic effects of drugs commonly prescribed for older patients. The results suggest that, apart from drugs which might be expected to alter acetylcholine receptor function such as atropine, many other drugs also have anticholinergic effects. These include furosemide (frusemide), digoxin, theophylline, warfarin, nifedipine, cimetidine, ranitidine, and prednisolone (Tune 1992). This assay of serum anticholinergic activity has also been used to investigate the hypothesis endogenous anticholinergic substances may be produced during illness. Mach (1995) found that serum anticholinergic activity was higher in patients who were delirious compared to a group of matched controls without delirium on medical wards. They also showed that there was a reduction in serum anticholinergic activity in patients whose delirium resolved. However, Flacker (1999*b*) measured serum anticholinergic activity in a group of nursing-home patients with fever and later at follow-up, and found no difference in levels between patients with and without delirium. But he also showed that at follow-up there was a fall in the level of anticholinergic activity in all the patients, suggesting that the initially raised levels might only be related to the acute febrile illness rather than delirium. More recently, Mussi *et al.* (1999) studied serum anticholinergic activity in patients admitted as medical emergencies to a geriatric service who subsequently developed delirium during their admission. They found that a very high level of serum anticholinergic activity did predict delirium, although levels also tended to be raised, but not by as much, in the patients who did not develop delirium. In summary, there is quite a lot of evidence to relate acetylcholine inhibition to delirium. Further work, particularly on the role of medications such as cholinesterase inhibitors, may elucidate these mechanisms.

Other neurotransmitters

Serotonin may play a role in delirium. It is implicated in mood, wakefulness, and cognition. Supportive evidence for such a role comes from studies of the 'serotonin syndrome', which is characterized by confusion, restlessness, tremor, and sweating and is associated with the use of serotonergic medications such as monoamine oxidase inhibitors (MAOIs) and selective serotonin-reuptake inhibitors (SSRIs) (Sternbach 1991).

Delirium following SSRI withdrawal has been reported (Kasantikul 1995). Haddad (1998) reviewed SSRI discontinuation syndromes and found that confusion and memory problems were reported, although these symptoms were not the most prominent. He found no reported case of delirium in the nine studies reviewed.

Dopamine has also been implicated in the pathophysiology of delirium, with L-dopa being a cause of confusion. Other dopaminergic medications such as pergolide and bromocriptine are prominent causes of delirium (Cummings 1991). GABA would appear to be important in the mediation of the clinical features of hepatic encephalopathy, although probably not in other forms of delirium (Jones *et al.* 1989). Central catecholamine activity may also play a role.

Other potential neural mechanisms

Activity in the hypothalamic–pituitary–adrenal (HPA) axis

Glucocorticoid hormones are necessary for coping with stress, but may have a deleterious effect on mood and memory during prolonged excessive secretion. Abnormalities have been demonstrated in delirium in the 'shut-off' of the HPA axis as tested by the dexamethasone suppression test (Olsson 1999). It has been suggested that this may relate to pathology in the hippocampal formation. O'Keeffe and Devlin (1994) performed dexamethasone suppression tests (1 mg of dexamethasone orally at 2300 hours, with measurements of serum cortisol at 0800 and 1600 hours the following day) on 16 patients—78% of the patients who developed delirium were non-suppressors on the dexamethasone suppression test, compared to 14% of patients without delirium. The authors comment that it is known that some elderly patients, who do not have dementia or depression, fail to suppress cortisol in response to dexamethasone; and they postulate that these patients may be at an increased risk of developing delirium during an acute illness.

Structural changes

Studies using electroencephalography (EEG) and brain imaging to try and elucidate a neuro-anatomical lesion in delirium have generally shown inconclusive and conflicting results (Flacker 1999*a*). Theories include a generalized lesion possibly leading to a global reduction in cerebral oxidative metabolism. This is supported by some EEG studies and could be explained by an overall reduction in acetylcholine production, fitting in with other neurochemical evidence. Other theories suggest limited or localized damage and this has been supported by cases of delirium occurring in stroke, where there is a specific identifiable brain lesion. Imaging studies (CT, SPECT, PET, MRI) have examined the contribution of specific brain areas to delirium, although the number of studies is limited. The frontal cortex, anteromedial thalamus, right basal ganglia, right posterior parietal cortex, and mesobasal temporo-occipital cortex are thought to be particularly important (Trzepacz 1999). There has also been interest in the possibility of an underlying blood–brain barrier (BBB) lesion. Controversy exists over whether normal ageing is associated with a breakdown in the BBB (Rapoport *et al.* 1979). Cerebrovascular and other central nervous system diseases, especially Alzheimer's disease, contribute to an increase in vascular permeability (Glenner 1980; Alafuzoff *et al.* 1983; Elovara *et al.* 1985). This is a ready explanation for the effect of some drugs on the elderly brain, and could potentially explain an increased effect from circulating toxins, such as might result from infection. No such toxin has been identified, but this is at least a possible mechanism. This would not, by itself, however, explain hypoxic delirium.

EEG

The EEG is widely accepted as an ancillary laboratory procedure for the diagnosis of delirium (Koponen 1991). The central nervous system electrical potentials recorded by the EEG are sensitive to alterations in the levels of consciousness and attention. Studies by Romano and Engel (1944) showed increased slow-wave activity and slowing and disruption of the normal alpha rhythm in delirious patients. These changes correlated with the disturbance in consciousness, and the degree of slowing was related to the severity of encephalopathy. However, these changes were not specific for delirium. In 'agitated states', such as might occur in alcohol- or drug-withdrawal delirium, there may be excessive low-amplitude fast activity. The EEG is clearly useful in the diagnosis of non-convulsive status epilepticus, and this may itself present as a delirium-type syndrome. The EEG may also be useful in distinguishing a focal brain pathology (e.g. a tumour) from a generalized lesion such as delirium secondary to a metabolic abnormality. Again this may be a difficult distinction to make clinically. It has also been suggested that the EEG may be a way of distinguishing delirium from dementia. However, Rabins and Folstein (1982) found that although most patients with delirium had diffusely slow EEGs, about one-third of the demented patients also showed this abnormality thus making the test of limited value. The EEG may also be helpful in differentiating delirium from functional or affective disorders such as depression or mania (Brenner 1991).

Epidemiology

Risk and precipitating factors

Risk factors

Some three studies have prospectively assessed a group of elderly patients on medical and surgical wards (who developed delirium during their hospital stay), to try and determine pre-existing factors in those patients which predicted the development of delirium (Schor *et al.* 1992; Inouye *et al.* 1993; O'Keeffe and Lavan 1996; summarized in Table 25.10). Pre-existing visual impairment, cognitive impairment, presentation to hospital with severe illness, and biochemical evidence of dehydration were found by Inouye and colleagues to be independent risk factors for the subsequent development of delirium. Schor looked at medical and surgical patients and also at different patient characteristics. They found that prior cognitive impairment, age more than 80 years, being male, and presentation with a fracture were patient characteristics at baseline that subsequently predicted delirium. In the study by O'Keeffe *et al.*, abnormal serum sodium, pre-

Table 25.10 Risk and precipitating factors

Risk factor	Precipitating factor
Pre-existing cognitive impairment Dehydration Visual and other sensory impairment Severe presenting illness Abnormal serum sodium Presentation with fracture Pre-existing alcohol excess Pre-existing physical dependence in terms of ADL	New drugs started in hospital, particularly opiates or neuroleptics Use of physical restraint Placement of bladder catheter Poor nutrition Intercurrent event: fluid imbalance, GI bleed, pressure ulcer, injury

Schor *et al.* 1993; Inouye *et al.* 1993; O'Keeffe and Lavan 1996.

existing dementia, biochemical evidence of dehydration, and severe underlying illness were found to independently predict incident delirium after admission to an acute medical geriatric unit. More recently, a meta-analysis of risk factors for delirium in medical and surgical inpatients (Elie *et al.* 1998) showed that pre-existing cognitive impairment, underlying severe medical illness, excess alcohol consumption, abnormal serum sodium, and prior physical dependency (determined by ADL) were the most important risk factors.

Precipitating factors

Schor's study and a subsequent study by Inouye and Charpentier (1996) looked at precipitating factors in hospital which led to the development of delirium. Inouye found that the use of physical restraint, the addition of more than three new medications, the use of a bladder catheter, malnutrition (judged by a low serum albumin), or an event such fluid imbalance, bleeding, pressure ulcer, or unintentional injury, all independently predicted the development of delirium. Schor found that the use of opiate analgesia or neuroleptic medication in hospital was a precipitating factor. Inouye and Charpentier (1996) propose that delirium is rarely caused by a single factor, but is a multifactorial syndrome with a complex relationship of baseline vulnerability and precipitating factors.

Incidence/prevalence

Delirium is common, both as a reason for acute emergency admission to hospital, and as one of the most frequent complications of hospitalization in the elderly. The true incidence and prevalence of the syndrome is difficult to ascertain from the available research for several methodological issues (Bucht *et al.* 1999):

- It is a transient disorder of short duration.
- It occurs in the physically ill elderly in whom the diagnosis may be difficult to make.
- The diagnostic criteria have changed with time.
- No reliable and specific diagnostic test or scale has yet been developed.
- Different techniques for finding cases have been used.
- Different patient categories and populations have been studied in various care settings.

Many studies unfortunately fail to distinguish the prevalence (i.e. those presenting with delirium) at admission to hospital from the incidence (i.e. those developing the problem in hospital, having been admitted for some other reason). There is also a separate in-hospital incidence relating to postoperative/procedure/ anaesthetic delirium. In five studies of elderly patients at admission to hospital, mainly to medical wards, between 10% and 42% were found to have delirium (see Table 25.11). A further seven studies, which analysed the incidence of delirium as a new diagnosis during hospital admission in elderly people, found that between 11% and 31% developed this problem (see Table 25.11).

Studies of postoperative delirium tend to be heterogeneous, including patients of various ages and types of surgery, and therefore they are difficult to compare, but one meta-analysis showed a range of between 0 and 74% for the incidence of postoperative delirium (Dyer *et al.* 1995). As the number of elderly patients being admitted to hospital with acute problems increases so delirium is likely to present more commonly.

Prognosis (see Table 25.12)

Cole and Primeau (1993) searched the literature for outcome data from 1980 to 1993 for use in a meta-analysis. They found eight reports, though none of these met the criteria for prognostic studies established by McMaster University. They found that the mean length of hospital stay was 20.7 days, and by 1 month after discharge from hospital 46.5% of patients were in institutional care and 14% had died. At 6-months follow-up, only 54.9% had improved mentally and 43.2% remained in institutions. Compared to unmatched controls, the patients with delirium had a longer

Table 25.11 Incidence and prevalence of delirium

	Population	Age	Assessment	*n*	%	Reference
Prevalence at admission	Medical and surgical	mean 81	Delirium Symptom Interview	325	10.5	Levkoff 1992
	General medical	70+	DSM-III-R	229	16	Francis 1990
	Acute geriatric	60–97	DSM-III-R	184	22	Jitapunkul 1992
	Medical/surgical	65+	CAM	432	15	Pompei 1994
	Acute geriatric	mean 83	Delirium Assessment Scale	225	42	O'Keeffe 1999
Incident after admission	Medicine	60+	DSM-III-R	418	11	Foy 1995
	Acute geriatric	mean 83	DSM-III-R	225	28	O'Keeffe 1996
	Medical and surgical	mean 81	Delirium Symptom Interview	325	31	Levkoff 1992
	General medical	mean 79	CAM	107	25	Inouye 1993
	Medical and surgical	mean 81	DSM-III	291	31	Schor 1992
	General medical	70+	CAM	852	15	Inouye 1999
	General medical	70+	CAM	196	18	Inouye 1996
Postoperative	Meta-analysis, cardiac, orthopaedic and other types surgery			2753	37	Dyer 1995

CAM, Confusion Assessment Method; DSM-III, *Diagnostic and statistical manual of mental disorders*-third edition (R, revised)

Table 25.12 Outcome in delirium

Population	*n*	% Delirium	Follow-up period	Outcomes	Ref. (First author)
General medicine	229	22	2 years Increased dementia	Increased mortality Increased dependency	Francis 1992
General medicine	203	19	3 years	Increased dementia Increased mortality	Rockwood 1999
Acute geriatric	225	42	6 months	Increased length of stay Increased admission long-term care Increased in hospital complications Worse functional decline during hospital stay	O'Keeffe 1997
Medicine and surgery	171*	—	1 year	Increased mortality Increased institutionalization Increased readmission	George 1997
Meta-analysis General medical Surgical Orthopaedic Psychogeriatric	573	—	Up to 12 months	Increased hospital length of stay Increased mortality Increased institutional care at 6 months	Cole 1993
Geriatric	184	22		Increased mortality Increased discharge to institutional care	Jitapunkul 1992

*171 cases with delirium and 95 partially matched case controls.

hospital stay, higher mortality, and higher rates of institutional care. The authors comment that the results may be confounded by dementia or severe physical illness, which were more prevalent in the delirium patients. Subsequently there have been a number of other studies looking at outcome in delirium. O'Keeffe and Lavan (1997), in a study of 225 admissions to an acute geriatric unit, found 94 (42%) patients with delirium. They divided the patients into groups according to the clinical picture: hyperactive, hypoactive, mixed, or neither. The patients in the hypoactive group were more ill at admission and had a longer length of stay compared to the other groups. Jitapunkul *et al.* (1992) studied 184 patients admitted to an acute geriatric unit of whom 22% had delirium. In these delirious patients they found an increased mortality rate in hospital, an increased rate of discharge to institutional care, and an increased number of admissions to hospital prior to the index admission. They found no difference in the length of stay. George *et al.* (1997) followed a group of patients with delirium for 1 year from discharge and compared them with a group of unmatched controls who had been in geriatric wards at the same time as the patients with delirium. They found an increased mortality rate at 6 and 12 months, an increased rate of institutional care, and an increased re-admission rate to hospital in the patients with delirium. Pompei *et al.* (1994) also found that length of stay in hospital and 90-day mortality were higher in patients with delirium. Rockwood *et al.* (1999) followed a cohort of 38 patients who had presented with delirium to a general medicine service. At 3-years follow-up there was an increased risk of death in those with delirium and a higher rate of a new diagnosis of dementia. The authors discuss the reasons why delirium should predict subsequent dementia and suggest there are two underlying factors: either there may be a brain injury as a result of or associated with the episode of delirium, or delirium may be a marker for a subclinical dementing process.

It would appear there may be three distinct outcomes from the delirium syndrome: recovery; persistent symptoms suggestive of continuing delirium; or the development of dementia. A difficulty in interpreting these studies is that the patients with delirium may have had more severe illness than the controls or that they had a degree of dementia prior to the acute illness. In many of the studies patients were assessed for cognitive impairment only at admission. Analysing the role of pre-existing dementia is possible only when studies enrol incident cases who develop delirium while in hospital, having had normal mental function at admission. Even that would not exclude pre-existing subclinical dementia. So in summary, delirium would appear to predict poorer outcomes for hospitalized patients, with increased mortality in hospital, increased mortality over many months and up to 2 years after discharge, and increased disability with increased use of institutionalized care; and although many will make a good or complete recovery, this is by no means the rule. While on the one hand the more recent data on outcome is depressing, on the other it should spur us on to see if aggressive interventions and management of delirium might improve cognitive performance later.

Causes of delirium

The causes of delirium in the elderly are numerous and more than one causative factor is often implicated in each case. The literature describing this area is difficult to interpret and, in particular, the relative frequency of each cause is hard to determine. This is mainly because studies have examined different populations of patients that may not be comparable, for example postoperative hip-replacement patients, acute medical admissions to a district hospital, psychiatric inpatients, or elderly patients seen at a medical day hospital. When one considers the potential causative effects of drug treatments and toxins, the picture becomes even more complicated, because almost any drug can predispose to or contribute to delirium. The literature, often of single case reports, is very large; often both the drug and the underlying condition for which it is being given may be potential causes of delirium; the fluctuating nature of delirium may mean that the removal of the drug may coincide with some spontaneous improvement and therefore be erroneously causatively associated. There is a publication bias for medications which are not expected to be a cause of delirium or which have not been reported before, but these may not reflect the overall prevalence of that drug in the causation of the syndrome in day-to-day practice (MacDonald 1998). Lipowski (1987) proposes dividing the causative organic factors into four broad groups:

(1) primary cerebral disease such as stroke, trauma, infection, epilepsy, or neoplasm;
(2) systemic diseases which affect the brain, e.g. metabolic, infection, cardiovascular, and respiratory diseases;
(3) intoxication with exogenous substances, e.g. medications and poisons;
(4) withdrawal from a substance in an addicted person, in the elderly this would most commonly be alcohol or a hypnotic sedative drug.

The following studies have ranked causative factors. George *et al.* (1997) studied all elderly admissions to a district general hospital and found that the five most common causes of delirium were infection, stroke, drugs, myocardial infarction, and hip fracture. However, we think that while acute focal neurological defects can obviously either

Table 25.13 Causes of delirium

1. *Primary cerebral disease*	
Ischaemia	Especially the transient oedema associated with large cerebral infarcts
Space-occupying lesions	Primary or secondary tumour, subdural,* extradural, subarachnoid, intracerebral haematoma, hydrocephalus,* cerebral abscess*
Infection	Meningitis, encephalitis*
Epileptic	Postgeneralized tonic/clonic convulsions Non-convulsive status epilepticus* (generalized or complex partial) Psychomotor fits* (may be mistaken for delirium)
2. *Systemic disease*	
Hypoxia	Primary respiratory problem, e.g. pneumonia, pulmonary oedema, pulmonary embolism* Secondary to reduced blood oxygen-carrying capacity severe anaemia, carbon monoxide poisoning* Secondary to poor cardiac output, severe CCF, cardiac dysrhythmia*
Metabolic	Renal or hepatic failure,* electrolyte disturbance* (particularly high or low sodium, hypercalcaemia,* hypo- or hyperglycaemia), severe acidosis and hypercapnia*
Endocrine	Myxoedema, thyrotoxicosis, hypopituitarism, hypo- and hyperadrenalism
Vitamin/nutritional	Thiamine deficiency* (Wernicke's encephalopathy), folic and nicotinic acid deficiencies, vitamin B_{12} deficiency*
Infective	Almost any extracerebral infection; most commonly respiratory or urinary
Physical	Hypothermia, hyperthermia, constipation, urinary retention
3. *Intoxication with exogenous substances*	
Drugs	See separate table
Toxins	Domestic and industrial agents
4. *Withdrawal states*	
Alcohol	
Drugs	Those with cross-tolerance with alcohol, particularly benzodiazepines,* but also SSRIs (Kasantikul 1995)

*Indicates conditions which in our experience are reasonably common, yet can be relatively difficult to diagnose.

masquerade or be indistinguishable from delirium, another cause should always be sought, as multiple pathology is not uncommon in the elderly. Furthermore, ascribing delirium to cerebral ischaemia should be a diagnosis of exclusion as so many elderly patients have incidental evidence of cerebral infarction. Rudberg *et al.* (1997) studied medical and surgical admissions to a general hospital and found the five most common causes of delirium to be medication, metabolic abnormality, infection, cardiovascular cause, and neurological cause. Francis *et al.* (1990) found electrolyte imbalance, infection, drug toxicity, metabolic causes, and sensory/environmental factors to be the most important. Some potential causes are listed in Tables 25.13 and 25.14.

Table 25.14 Drugs causing delirium

Class	Drug	Risk
Anticholinergic*	Atropine	High
	Scopolamine	
Benzodiazepines*	Temazepam	High
	Diazepam	Long half-life prolongs effect
Opioid analgesics*	Pethidine	High, particularly pethidine
	Codeine	
	Morphine	
Antipsychotics	Thioridazine*	(NB dose should be restricted)
	Chlorpromazine*	
	Haloperidol	Medium
Antidepressants	Tricyclic* + lithium*	High
	Trazodone	High
	SSRIs	Low
Antiparkinsonian	Anticholinergics*	High, highest risk with anticholinergics
	L-dopa*	
	Bromocriptine*	
	Selegiline	Medium
	Amantadine	
Corticosteroids	Prednisolone	Low
	Desoxymethasone	Medium
Anticonvulsants	Primidone	Medium
	Phenobarbital	
	Phenytoin	High in overdosage
	Valproate	
Antihypertensives	Methyldopa	High, centrally acting agents high
	β-Blocker	Medium, particularly lipid-soluble, CNS-active, e.g. propanolol
	α-Blocker	Medium, e.g. doxasozin
	Ca channel blocker	Low
	ACE inhibitor	Low
	Diuretic	Low
Antiarrhythmic	Lidocaine	High
	Digoxin	High in overdosage
	Quinidine	Medium
H_2 blockers	Cimetidine	Medium
	Ranitidine	Low

Continued

Table 25.14 Drugs causing delirium *contd*

Class	Drug	Risk
Antibiotics	Cephalosporins Penicillins Fluoroquinolones Macrolide	Risk generally low but recognized, difficult to separate from effect of underlying infection Possibly high, especially in the old
NSAID	Indometacin Ibuprofen	Medium to low, paracetamol safer

*Indicates reasonably common culprits in the authors' experience. SSRIs, selective serotonin-reuptake inhibitors; CNS, central nervous system; ACE, angiotensin-converting enzyme; Bowen and Larson 1993; Moore and O'Keeffe 1999; Mermelstein 1998; Cummings 1991; Heckmann *et al.* 2000.

Conclusions

Delirium remains an important, common, and challenging problem for all those looking after elderly patients. It is a frequent presentation of underlying physical disease which is often severe—and treatable. It is unfortunately underdiagnosed, and its causes may not be vigorously enough sought, particularly on general medical and surgical wards. In these settings the cognitive impairment is all too often thought to be chronic, or the subtle symptoms and physical signs are ignored. Delirium represents an overlap between psychiatric and geriatric practice, and as such requires good liaison between these specialities for its effective management. In the future a better understanding of the pathophysiology of the condition might lead to the development of more appropriate and effective specific treatment; further elucidation of risk and precipitating factors may lead to more effective prevention; and systematic research may shed light on the longer term prognosis and the relationship with dementia. The relatively poor prognosis should encourage us to be active, diligent, and detailed in our management of all possible confounding or exacerbating factors. Such an approach will frequently demand good interdisciplinary working.

References

Alafuzoff, I., Adolfson, R., Bucht, G., *et al.* (1983). Albumin and immunoglobulin in plasma and cerebrospinal fluid and blood–cerebrospinal fluid barrier function in patients with dementia of Alzheimer type and multi infarct dementia. *Journal of Neurological Science*, **60**, 465–72.

Albert, M. S., Levkoff, S. E., Reilly, C. H., *et al.* (1992). The delirium symptom interview: an interview for the detection of delirium symptoms in hospitalised patients. *Geriatric Psychiatry and Neurology*, **5**, 14–21.

APA (American Psychiatric Association). (1994). *Diagnostic and statistical manual of mental disorders* (fourth edition). APA, Washington, DC.

Bowen, J. D. and Larson, E. B. (1993). Drug induced cognitive impairment. *Drugs and Ageing*, **3**, 349–57.

Breitbart, W., Marotta, R., Platt, M. M., *et al.* (1996). A double blind trial of haloperidol, chlorpromazine and lorazepam in the treatment of delirium in hospitalised AIDS patients. *American Journal of Psychiatry*, **153**, 231–7.

Brenner, R. P. (1991). Utility of EEG in delirium: past views and current practice. *International Psychogeriatrics*, **3**, 211–29.

Bucht, G., Gustafson, Y., and Sandberg, O. (1999). Epidemiology of delirium. *Dementia and Geriatric Cognitive Disorders*, **10**, 315–18.

Busto, U., Sellers, E. M., Naranjo, C. A., *et al.* (1986). Withdrawal reaction after long term therapeutic use of benzodiazepines. *New England Journal of Medicine*, **315**, 854–9.

Cole, M. G. and Primeau, F. J. (1993). Prognosis of delirium in elderly hospital patients. *Canadian Medical Association Journal*, **149**, 41–6.

Cole, M. G., Primeau, F., and McCusker, J. (1996). Effectiveness of interventions to prevent delirium in hospitalised patients: a systematic review. *Canadian Medical Association Journal*, **155**, 1263–8.

Cummings, J. L. (1991). Behavioural complications of drug treatment in Parkinson's disease. *Journal of the American Geriatrics Society*, **39**, 708–16.

Dyer, C. B., Ashton, C. M., and Teasdale, T. A. (1995). Postoperative delirium. *Archives of Internal Medicine*, **155**, 461–5.

Elie, M., Cole, M. G., Primeau, F. J., *et al.* (1998). Delirium risk factors in elderly hospitalised patients. *Journal of General Internal Medicine*, **13**, 204–12.

Elovara, I., Icen, A., Palo, J., *et al.* (1985). CSF in Alzheimer's disease—studies on blood brain barrier function and intrathecal protein synthesis. *Journal of Neurological Science*, **70**, 73–80.

Fisher, B. W. and Flowerdew, G. (1995). A simple model for predicting post operative delirium in older patients undergoing elective orthopaedic surgery. *Journal of the American Geriatrics Society*, **43**, 175–8.

Flacker, J. M. and Marcantonio, E. R. (1998). Delirium in the elderly: optimal management. *Drugs and Ageing*, **13**, 119–30.

Flacker, J. M. and Lipsitz, L. A. (1999*a*). Neural mechanisms of delirium: current hypotheses and evolving concepts. *Journal of Gerontology: Biological Sciences*, **54A**, B239–246.

Flacker, J. M. and Lipsitz, L. A. (1999*b*). Serum anticholinergic activity changes with acute illness in elderly medical patients. *Journal of Gerontology: Medical Sciences*, **54A**, M12–16.

Folstein, M. S., Folstein, S. E., and McHugh, P. R. (1975). Mini mental state—a practical method for grading the cognitive state of patients for the clinician. *Journal of Psychiatric Research*, **12**, 189–98.

Foy, A., O'Connell, D., Henry, D., *et al.* (1995). Benzodiazepine use as a cause of cognitive impairment in elderly hospital in-patients. *Journal of Gerontology: Medical Sciences*, **50A**, M99-M106.

Francis, J. and Kapoor, W. N. (1992). Prognosis after hospital discharge of older medical patients with delirium. *Journal of the American Geriatrics Society*, **40**, 601–6.

Francis, J., Martin, D., and Kapoor, W. N. (1990). A prospective study of delirium in hospitalised elderly. *Journal of the American Medical Association*, **263**, 1097–101.

Fuller, R. K. and Gordis, E. (1997). Refining the treatment of alcohol withdrawal. *Journal of the American Medical Association*, **272**, 557–8.

George, J., Bleasdale, S., and Singleton, S. J. (1997). Causes and prognosis of delirium in elderly patients admitted to a district general hospital. *Age and Ageing*, **26**, 423–7.

Glenner, G. G. (1980). Myloid deposits and amyloidosis. *New England Journal of Medicine,* **302**, 1283–91.

Haddad, P. (1998). The SSRI discontinuation syndrome. *Journal of Psychopharmacology,* **12**, 305–13.

Hall, W. and Zador, D. (1997). The alcohol withdrawal syndrome. *Lancet*, **349**, 1897–900

Hart, B. (1936). Delirious states. *British Medical Journal*, **2**, 745–9.

Heckmann, J. G., Birklein, F., and Neundorfer, B. (2000). Omeprazole induced delirium. *Journal of Neurology*, **247**, 56–7.

Hodkinson, H. M. (1973). Mental impairment in the elderly. *Journal of the Royal College of Physicians of London*, **7**, 305–17.

Hodkinson, H. M. (1972). Evaluation of a mental test score for assessment of mental impairment in the elderly. *Age and Ageing*, **1**, 233–8.

Inouye, S. K. (1994). The dilemma of delirium: clinical and research controversies regarding diagnosis and evaluation of delirium in hospitalised elderly medical patients. *American Journal of Medicine*, **97**, 278–88.

Inouye, S. K. and Charpentier, P. A. (1996). Precipitating factors for delirium in hospitalised persons. *Journal of the American Medical Association*, **275**, 852–7.

Inouye, S. K., van Dyck, C. H., Alessi, C. A., *et al.* (1990). Clarifying the confusion: the confusion assessment method; a new method for the detection of delirium. *Annals of Internal Medicine*, **113**, 941–8.

Inouye, S. K., Viscoli, C. M., Horwitz, R. I., *et al.* (1993). A predictive model for delirium in hospitalised elderly medical patients based on admission characteristics. *Annals of Internal Medicine*, **119**, 474–81.

Inouye, S. K., Bogardus, S. T., Charpentier, P. A., *et al.* (1999). A multicomponent intervention to prevent delirium in hospitalised older patients. *New England Journal of Medicine*, **340**, 669–76.

Jitapunkul, S., Pillay, I., and Ebrahim, S., (1991). The abbreviated mental test: its use and validity. *Age and Ageing*, **20**, 332–6.

Jitapunkul, S., Pillay, I., and Ebrahim, S. (1992). Delirium in newly admitted elderly patients: a prospective study. *Quarterly Journal of Medicine*, **83**, 307–14.

Johnson, J. C., Kerse, N. M., Gottlieb, G., *et al.* (1992). Prospective versus retrospective methods of identifying patients with delirium. *Journal of the American Geriatrics Association,* **40**, 316–19.

Jones, E. A., Skolnick, P., Gammal S. H., *et al.* (1989). The gamma-aminobutyric acid A (GABA, A) receptor complex and hepatic encephalopathy. Report of NIH conference. *Annals of Internal Medicine*, **110**, 532–46.

Kasantikul, D. (1995). Reversible delirium after discontinuation of fluoxetine. *Journal of the Medical Association of Thailand*, 53–4.

Koponen, H. (1991). Electroencephalographic indices for diagnosis of delirium. *International Psychogeriatrics*, **3**, 249–51.

Levkoff, S. E., Evans, D. A., Liptzin, B., *et al.* (1992). Delirium: the occurrence and persistence of symptoms among elderly hospitalised patients. *Archives of Internal Medicine*, **152**, 334–40.

Lindesay, J., Macdonald, A. and Starke, I. (1990). *Delirium in the Elderly.* Oxford University Press, Oxford.

Lipowski, Z. J. (1987). Delirium (acute confusional states). *Journal of the American Medical Association*, **258**, 1789–92.

Lipowski, Z. J. (1991). *Delirium: acute confusional states.* Oxford University Press, New York.

Liptzin, B. and Levkoff, S. E. (1992). An empirical study of delirium subtypes. *British Journal of Psychiatry*, **161**, 843–5.

McCusker, J., Cole, M., Bellavance, F., *et al.* (1998). Reliability and validity of a new measure of severity of delirium. *International Psychogeriatrics*, **10**, 421–33.

MacDonald (1990).

Macdonald, A. J. D. (1998). Delirium. In *Brocklehurst's textbook of geriatric medicine and gerontology* (5th edn), pp. 685–99. Churchill Livingstone, Edinburgh.

Macdonald, A. J. D. and Treloar, A. (1996). Delirium and dementia; are they distinct? *Journal of the American Geriatrics Society*, **44**, 1001–2.

Mach, J. R., Dysken, M. W., Kuskowski, M., *et al.* (1995). Serum anticholinergic activity in hospitalised older patients with delirium: a preliminary study. *Journal of the American Geriatrics Society*, **43**, 491–5.

Mayo-Smith, M. F. (1997). Pharmacological management of alcohol withdrawal: a meta-analysis and evidence based practice guideline. *Journal of the American Medical Association*, **278**, 144–51.

Meagher, D. J., O'Hanlon, D., O'Mahony, E., *et al.* (1996). The use of environmental strategies and psychotropic medication in the management of delirium. *British Journal of Psychiatry*, **168**, 512–15.

Mermelstein, H. T. (1998). Clarithromycin induced delirium in a general hospital. *Psychosomatics*, **39**, 540–2.

Moore, A. R. and O'Keeffe, S. T. (1999). Drug induced cognitive impairment in the elderly. *Drugs and Ageing*, **15**, 15–28.

Moss, J. H. (1991). Sedative and hypnotic withdrawal states in hospitalised patients. *Lancet*, **338**, 575.

Moss, J. H. and Lanctot, K. L. (1995). Iatrogenic benzodiazepine withdrawal delirium in hospitalised older patients. *Journal of the American Geriatrics Society*, **43**, 1020–2.

Mussi, C., Ferrari, R., and Ascari, S. (1999). Importance of serum anticholinergic activity in the assessment of elderly patients with delirium. *Journal of Geriatric Psychiatry and Neurology*, **12**, 82–6.

Nagley, S. J. (1986). Predicting and preventing confusion in your patients. *Journal of Gerontological Nursing*, **12**, 27–31.

O'Keeffe, S. T. (1994). Rating the severity of delirium: The delirium assessment scale. *International Journal of Geriatric Psychiatry*, **9**, 551–6.

O'Keeffe, S. T. and Devlin, J. G. (1994). Delirium and the dexamethasone suppression test in the elderly. *Neuropsychobiology*, **30**, 153–6.

O'Keeffe, S. T. and Lavan, J. N. (1996). Predicting delirium in elderly patients: development and validation of a risk stratification model. *Age and Ageing*, **25**, 317–21.

O'Keeffe, S. T. and Lavan, J. (1997). The prognostic significance of delirium in older hospital patients. *Journal of the American Geriatrics Society*, **45**, 174-8.

O'Keeffe, S. T. and Lavan, J. N. (1999). Clinical significance of delirium subtypes in older people. *Age and Ageing*, **28**, 115–19.

Olsson, T. (1999). Activity in the hypothalamic–pituitary–adrenal axis and delirium. *Dementia and Cognitive Geriatric Disorders*, **10**, 345–9.

Pompei, P., Foreman, M., and Rudberg, M. A. (1994). Delirium in hospitalised older persons: outcomes and predictors. *Journal of the American Geriatrics Society*, **42**, 809–15.

Rabins, P. V. and Folstein, M. F. (1982). Delirium in dementia: diagnostic criteria and fatality rates. *British Journal of Psychiatry*, **140**, 149–53.

Rapoport, R. I., Ohno, K., and Pettigrew, K. D. (1979). Blood brain barrier permeability in senescent rats. *Journal of Gerontology,* **34**, 162–9.

Robertsson, B. (1999). Assessment scales in delirium. *Dementia and Geriatric Cognitive Disorders*, **10**, 368–79.

Rockwood, K., Cosway, S., Carver, D., *et al.* (1999). The risk of dementia and death after delirium. *Age and Ageing*, **28**, 551–6.

Romano, J. and Engel, G. L. (1944). Delirium. I. Electroencephalographic data. *Archives of Neurology and Psychiatry*, **51**, 356–77.

Rudberg, M. A., Pompei, P., Foreman, M. D., *et al.* (1997). The natural history of delirium in older hospitalised patients: a syndrome of heterogeneity. *Age and Ageing*, **26**, 169–74.

Schor, J. D., Levkoff, S. E., Lipsitz, L. A., *et al.* (1992). Risk factors for delirium in hospitalised elderly. *Journal of the American Medical Association*, **267**, 827–31.

Sellers, E. M. (1988). Alcohol, barbiturate, and benzodiazepine withdrawal syndromes: clinical management. *Canadian Medical Association Journal*, **139**, 113–18.

Sternbach, H. (1991). The serotonin syndrome. *American Journal of Psychiatry*, **148**, 705–13.

Trzepacz, P. T. (1994*a*). A review of delirium assessment instruments. *General Hospital Psychiatry*, **16**, 397–405.

Trzepacz, P. T. (1994*b*). The neuropathogenesis of delirium. *Psychosomatics*, **35**, 374–91.

Trzepacz, P. T. (1999). Update on the neuropathogenesis of delirium. *Dementia and Geriatric Cognitive Disorders*, **10**, 330–4.

Trzepacz, P. T., Baker, R. W., and Greenhouse, J. (1988). A simple rating scale for delirium. *Psychiatry Research*, **23**, 89–97.

Tune, L. E., Namir, D. F., Holland, A., *et al.* (1981). Association of postoperative delirium with raised serum levels of anticholinergic drugs. *Lancet*, **2**, 651–2.

Tune, L., Carr, S., Hoag, E., *et al.* (1992). Anticholinergic effects of drugs commonly prescribed for the elderly: potential means for assessing the risk of delirium. *American Journal of Psychiatry*, **149**, 1393–5.

Van Der Mast, R. C., Fekkes, D., Moleman, P., *et al.* (1991). Is postoperative delirium related to reduced plasma tryptophan? *Lancet*, **338**, 851–2.

Wanich, C. K., Sullivan-Marx, E. M., Gottlieb, G. L., *et al.* (1992). Functional status outcomes of a nursing intervention in hospitalised elderly. *Research Nursing Health*, **8**, 329–37.

Wengel, S. P., Roccaforte, W. H., and Burke, W. J. (1998). Donepezil improves symptoms of delirium in dementia: implications for future research. *Journal of Geriatric Psychiatry and Neurology*, **11**, 159–61.

WHO (World Health Organization). (1993). *The ICD-10 classification of mental and behavioural disorders.* WHO, Geneva.

26 Delirium—the psychiatrist's perspective

James Lindesay

Introduction

Delirium is one of the oldest conditions known to medicine, and one of the least well understood. To the physician it is 'one of the most obscure in the chain of morbid phenomena he has to deal with' (Gallwey 1838), and has too often been ignored or dismissed as a nuisance, rather than valued as an important sign of disturbed physiology. To psychiatrists on the other hand, delirium is an intruder from the world of 'real medicine' with its hard facts and demonstrable causes, and not something that is congenial to their ways of analysis and understanding. The increasing technological sophistication of modern medical practice has, if anything, made physicians and surgeons less tolerant of delirium in their patients, and psychiatrists less confident in their ability to manage the underlying disorders. This is unfortunate, not only because delirium is distressing to the patient, but also because if left untreated it is costly to health services in terms of unnecessarily protracted hospital admissions and adverse outcomes. Delirium is particularly common and problematic in elderly patients, and their needs are best served if there is a good working partnership between physicians and psychiatrists who between them can solve the various and complex medical and management problems. This chapter examines delirium in the elderly population as it presents to psychiatric services, and discusses issues such as screening and management where the psychiatric perspective is helpful.

Epidemiology

The lack of an agreed definition of delirium has been an important obstacle to research into this condition. With the development of rule-oriented diagnostic criteria for mental disorders such as ICD-10 (World Health Organization 1992) and DSM-IV (American Psychiatric Association 1994), this situation has improved, although there are some important differences between these systems so far as delirium is concerned. ICD-10 is the most restrictive, in that the diagnosis of delirium requires disturbances in each of the areas of consciousness, cognition, psychomotor activity, sleep, and emotion. In DSM-IV, the essential criteria for delirium are only disturbed consciousness, cognitive change, and development over a short time. It is subclassified according to its underlying cause, where this is known or likely. These diagnostic systems are all more restrictive than clinical diagnosis, particularly the ICD-10 research criteria (Lipsitz *et al.* 1991); one important consequence of this is that modern studies of delirium using these criteria will include only the most severely ill subjects, and their findings may therefore not apply to the large number of patients whose delirium is relatively partial and transitory.

These problems of definition mean that is difficult to know for certain just how frequently delirium occurs in elderly populations. Most epidemiological studies of delirium in the elderly have been carried out in medical and surgical inpatients. The estimated prevalence and incidence rates of delirium vary considerably between studies; this is because of their different case-definitions of delirium, different case-finding procedures, and differences in the populations studied and the selection criteria used. Prevalence rates between 10% and 30%, and incidence rates between 4% and 53% have been reported (Levkoff *et al.* 1991). Studies using more standardized and comparable definitions of delirium agree more closely: that about 10–16% of elderly medical inpatients are delirious on admission (Francis 1992; Levkoff *et al.* 1992). Some populations such as elderly patients with fractures have consistently higher rates of delirium (Gustafson *et al.* 1988; Schor *et al.* 1992). Studies that have examined the level of awareness by medical and surgical staff of delirium in their patients have found that it often goes undetected, unrecorded, or misdiagnosed (Johnson *et al.* 1992; Bowler *et al.* 1994; Harwood *et al.* 1997).

Another group at increased risk of developing delirium are the elderly residents of nursing homes and other long-term care settings. These people are physically frail, have high rates of psychiatric disorders such as dementia and depression, and are liable to be receiving considerable quantities of medication—much of it psychotropic. Although there have been several studies of psychiatric disorders in nursing-home residents, only a few have included estimates of delirium. Rovner *et al.* (1986) found that 6% of a random sample in one 'intermediate care' facility were suffering from drug-induced delirium; a further 24% were demented and experiencing hallucinations and delusions, and it is likely that a proportion of these were also delirious for other reasons. Sabin *et al.* (1982) found that 25% of cognitively impaired, nursing-home residents had potentially reversible conditions. In a Swedish study of a range of care settings for elderly people, 58% of the nursing-home population were found to have delirium; of these, only 24% had the diagnosis documented (Sandberg *et al.* 1998).

One study that has attempted to estimate the prevalence rate of delirium in the community elderly population suggests that it is less common than in the high-risk groups in hospital, but that there is a marked increase with age. In the Eastern Baltimore Mental Health Survey, carried out as part of the United States Epidemiologic Catchment Area study, the prevalence rate of DSM-III delirium was 0.4% of those aged 18 years and over, 1.1% of those aged 55 years and over, and 13.6% of those aged 85 years and over (Folstein *et al.* 1991). Factors associated with delirium in this study were polypharmacy, visual impairment, diabetes, and structural brain disease. The modern practice of rapid discharge from hospital following medical and surgical procedures is likely to increase the incidence of delirium in the community. The rates of delirium in recently discharged patients and the ability of general practitioners and district nurses to identify it are not known.

The presentation of delirium to psychiatric services

Delirium presents to old age psychiatry services in a number of ways. Many psychiatric disorders and their treatments put elderly patients at risk of developing delirium (see below), and this should always be considered if there is a sudden deterioration in mental state or behaviour in any patient already under the care of the service. Delirium is also an important factor leading to new referrals, not only from settings with high rates of delirium such as hospital wards and nursing homes, but also from the community. In demented individuals, the abrupt decline in function due to a superimposed delirium may result in a crisis or collapse of informal care at home, and the need for specialist assessment and support. Similarly, severely depressed or manic patients may only come to the attention of health services when their self-neglect is so extreme as to cause delirium. Sometimes delirium alone precipitates referral, particularly if it is of the 'hyperactive' variety and associated with disturbed behaviour and psychotic symptoms. This is the usual reason why delirious patients are referred from medical and surgical wards and from nursing homes; 'mad' and disruptive individuals are poorly tolerated in these settings and staff are keen to have the problem solved or removed.

Delirium and other psychiatric disorders

Given the wide range of cognitive, affective, perceptual, and behavioural disturbances that delirium can induce in elderly patients, the differential diagnosis includes most of the other psychiatric disorders that can occur in this age group. However, since many of these disorders and their treatments are themselves potential risk factors for delirium, the possibility of a double diagnosis must always be considered, particularly if there is evidence of physical illness, drug toxicity, or recent drug withdrawal. When there is doubt about the diagnosis, the safest course is usually to investigate and manage the patient as if they were delirious while this issue is resolved.

Dementia

The ability to distinguish between delirium and dementia should be a clinical skill possessed by all doctors, whatever their speciality. Delirium in an elderly patient is an important sign of physical illness and/or iatrogenic poisoning, and its recognition should be followed by a case review and whatever investigations and treatments are necessary to identify and correct the cause. Misdiagnosing a potentially reversible delirium as dementia can have other grave consequences for the patient: for example, if they are deemed unable to return home, they may be moved to institutional care and their possessions disposed of before the delirium resolves and the misplacement becomes apparent.

There are, however, several conceptual and practical difficulties in reliably distinguishing delirium from dementia (Macdonald and Treloar 1996; Lindesay 1999). Most problematically, none of the four essential features of delirium (disturbance of consciousness, disturbances of cognition, rapid onset/fluctuating course, and evidence of cause) is exclusive to this disorder. Disturbance of consciousness is described in Lewy body dementia (Byrne *et al.* 1989; McKeith *et al.* 1990), which is marked by periods of delirium-like deterioration, with fluctuating cognitive impairment, hallucinations and delusions (see Chapter 24iv). These appear to be an integral part of this dementia and not merely an enhanced susceptibility to the external causes of delirium. Disturbance of cognition is clearly non-discriminatory between delirium and any form of dementia. Rapid onset may occur in vascular dementia, and a fluctuating course is seen in both vascular and Lewy body dementias. The cognitive function of patients with dementia may fluctuate during the course of the day (sundowning). The cause of a delirium may not be apparent, particularly in elderly patients with significant pre-existing dementia. Reversibility of cognitive impairment may be the most discriminating feature of delirium (Treloar and Macdonald, 1997*a,b*), but is problematic as a diagnostic criterion since outcome is unknown at the outset of the episode.

In most cases, the most valuable pointer to the correct diagnosis is reliable information about the onset and course of the disorder. Typically, the onset of delirium is abrupt with a short history of cognitive impairment developing over a few days or weeks. In contrast, dementia usually has an insidious onset with evidence of cognitive decline over months and years. Since demented individuals are at a greatly increased risk of developing delirium, a mixed picture is not uncommon: with a recent episode of rapid decline being superimposed on a longstanding process of gradual deterioration. As a rule, any history of rapid deterioration in cognitive function and behaviour in an elderly patient should be regarded as strongly indicative of delirium. The patient's mental state also provides some useful diagnostic clues; in particular, delirium should be suspected if attentional deficits are prominent, if speech is incoherent, thinking is slow and vague, and if there are marked diurnal fluctuations in cognitive impairment and alertness (Treloar and Macdonald 1997*b*). The presence of hallucinations and delusions are less diagnostically specific, as they can occur in dementia as well as in delirium (Burns *et al.* 1990; Treloar and Macdonald 1997*b*). However, they should not be attributed to dementia until the possibility of delirium has been ruled out, particularly if they are pronounced and of recent onset. In most cases, diagnosis is not problematic, so long as the possibility of delirium is considered in the first place. In a few patients, however, there can be genuine diagnostic difficulties: if there is no information about onset and course, the mental state alone may not be sufficiently discriminating; if delirium is prolonged it can come to resemble dementia quite closely; and if any pre-existing dementia is severe, a superimposed delirium may go unnoticed. In difficult cases electro-encephalography (EEG) may be helpful (see Chapter 12). However, the generalized slowing of the alpha rhythm that occurs with ageing and in association with dementia means that its diagnostic value is more limited in the elderly than in younger age groups. A normal EEG in a patient with no apparent cause for delirium would suggest a functional psychiatric disorder.

There are several reasons why elderly people with dementia are at increased risk of developing delirium. There is a non-specific increased vulnerability to physical insult associated with most forms of brain damage, but in addition to this the underlying pathology of the dementia may also specifically predispose the patient to delirium. For example, individuals with vascular dementia may present with delirium following a stroke (Balter *et al.* 1986). Alzheimer's disease is associated with a loss of function of cholinergic systems within the brain, and it is thought that the acute impairment of these systems is also an important aetiological factor in delirium (Trzepacz 1996). Alzheimer's patients are particularly sensitive to the deliriogenic effect of anticholinergic drugs (Sunderland *et al.* 1987). People with dementia living on their own without adequate supervision and support are liable to neglect themselves and to put themselves at risk, for example by wandering at night or misusing medication. As a result, they may become physically ill and delirious, which may be the event which brings their dementia to public notice for the first time.

Depression

Delirium can sometimes be difficult to distinguish from severe depression in elderly patients. Delirium is accompanied by significant affective changes, and while fear is usually regarded as the principal emotion in delirium, depression is also described in up to 60% of delirious elderly inpatients (Beresin 1988). Other features such as agitation, psychomotor retardation, crying, impaired concentration, hallucinations, delusions, diurnal variation in severity, and disturbances of sleep and behaviour also occur in both conditions, and a careful mental state examination is necessary to determine the cause. In general, the cognitive impairment in depression is relatively mild compared to disturbances in mood and behaviour, whereas the reverse is usually the case in delirium. The pattern of diurnal variation also differs. For instance, depressed patients tend to improve towards the end of the day, and delirious patients tend to get worse. However, the 'morning delirium' shown by some patients may cause diagnostic difficulties (Sandberg *et al.* 1998). As with dementia, the history is also helpful; depression usually has a more gradual onset than delirium, and it is often apparent that the presenting clinical picture has developed from a milder depressive episode.

Many elderly depressed patients also suffer from physical illness and self-neglect, so it is not surprising that depression has been found to be associated with delirium in studies of inpatients (Hodkinson 1973; Bergmann and Eastham 1974). Another important factor contributing to this association is antidepressant treatment, particularly with anticholinergic tricyclic drugs; an increased risk of developing delirium following tricyclic drug treatment and electroconvulsive therapy (ECT) is associated with neuroradiological evidence of subcortical disease (Figiel *et al.* 1989, 1990). It may be that depression itself is a risk factor for delirium, particularly in vulnerable individuals. Grief following bereavement may precipitate delirium (Lipowski 1983), and it has been suggested that preoperative depression and anxiety are predictors of postoperative delirium (Berggren *et al.* 1987; Sirois 1988), although not all studies have found this (Millar 1981; Simpson and Kellett 1987; Smith and Dimsdale 1989).

Mania

Mania is much less common than depression in old age, and is often mistaken for delirium.

Patients are hyperactive, agitated, irritable, often disoriented, and may be hallucinating and deluded. There may be a history of manic-depressive illness, but in many cases it is a first episode secondary to organic cerebral pathology such as dementia, stroke, or head injury (Dunne *et al.* 1986; Shulman 1986). Quite often, the clinical picture is a mixed one of 'manic delirium'; elderly manic patients are particularly vulnerable to developing a secondary delirium following self-neglect, dehydration, and exhaustion.

Anxiety

The anxiety disorders that commonly occur in the elderly population are unlikely to be confused with delirium, although the panic of an elderly patient who is phobic of blood or needles and who has been unwillingly admitted to hospital as an emergency might cause diagnostic problems. So far as delirium secondary to anxiety is concerned, it has been suggested that the catecholamines released during autonomic arousal might be able to precipitate a delirium, either directly or by altering cerebral blood flow (Loach and Benedict 1980; Grimley Evans 1982). The regulation of the hypothalamic–pituitary–adrenal axis may also be disturbed in delirium (Olsson 1999).

Paranoid states and schizophrenia

In practice, these conditions rarely present much diagnostic difficulty so far as distinguishing them from delirium is concerned. Attention and orientation are usually intact, delusions are more systematized and lucid than the fragmentary psychotic ideas typical of delirium, and auditory hallucinations are common and visual hallucinations rare, whereas the reverse is the case in delirium. However, if the patient's delusional beliefs involve being poisoned, then they may refuse to eat or drink and so present with a secondary delirium. The anticholinergic drugs used to treat the side-effects of neuroleptic medication are a potent cause of iatrogenic delirium in elderly schizophrenic patients. Catatonic states are occasionally seen in patients with schizophrenia and other disorders such as encephalitis and epilepsy. With psychomotor disturbance, autonomic arousal, hallucinations and delusions are often prominent, but this can be very difficult to distinguish from delirium. EEG may be helpful in establishing the diagnosis.

Other disorders

A number of other conditions in which there are disturbances of cognitive function, perception, mood, and thought, such as amnestic syndromes, temporal lobe epilepsy, epilepsia partialis continua, the Charles Bonnet syndrome (visual hallucinosis in the context of visual pathway disease), and neuroleptic malignant syndrome (NMS), may on occasions be confused with delirium. NMS occurs most commonly in young adults, but elderly cases have been reported (Kellam 1987). Careful history-taking and mental state examination are usually sufficient to establish the diagnosis, but further investigations such as EEG may be necessary in doubtful cases.

Management

Screening for delirium

Before the underlying causes of delirium can be corrected, it is first necessary to recognize that it is present. Floridly disturbed and hyperactive patients are not the problem in this respect; it is the quietly confused and perplexed individual sitting in bed plucking at the blankets who is usually missed on a busy medical or surgical ward. To improve the recognition of delirium in these settings it is necessary to educate the ward staff (both doctors and nurses) about the clinical importance of the condition, and to have in place some routine screening procedures. Teaching ward staff about delirium has been shown to have a positive effect on the rates of detection (Rockwood *et al.* 1994); this might be provided as a formal course of instruction, but it also appears to happen if psychiatrists or psychiatric nurses are regularly involved in medical ward rounds (Bowler *et al.* 1994). The benefit of the latter approach is that the education is then a two-way process, with psychiatric staff also learning something about the medical management of these and other cases.

So far as routine screening arrangements for delirium are concerned, these must not be too onerous and time-consuming; if they are they will not survive the hectic pace of today's acute medical and surgical units. An adequate mental state examination and history on admission is important; as has been pointed out, information about the onset and course of any cognitive impairment is of great diagnostic value. A good initial mental state assessment will also identify those demented and depressed individuals who are at risk of developing delirium as inpatients, and it will provide a crucial baseline against which to compare future assessments. Assessment of attention is important, and this may be tested using digit-span, spelling words backwards, or by a global assessment of patient accessibility during the clinical interview (Anthony *et al.* 1985). Various screening instruments for identifying delirium in inpatients have been developed. Some, such as the Mini-Mental State Examination (Folstein *et al.* 1975) and the Abbreviated Mental Test Score (Hodkinson 1972) are measures of cognitive impairment, and substantial changes in the score over a short period are strongly indicative of delirium. However, these instruments are not diagnostic, and performance is affected by dementia, depression, sensory impairment, age, educational level, and ethnicity. They are also insensitive to the minor or restricted cognitive impairments that occur in early, mild, or resolving delirium. An alternative for use in monitoring such cases is the High Sensitivity Cognitive Screen (Faust and Fogel 1989). Scored clock-drawing tests have also been used to screen for cognitive impairment and to monitor change in delirious patients (Shulman *et al.* 1986; Fisher and Flowerdew 1995). Instruments developed to be more specifically diagnostic of delirium in inpatient settings include the Delirium Rating Scale (Trzpacz *et al.* 1988), the Confusion Assessment Method (Inouye *et al.* 1990), the Delirium Symptom Interview (Albert *et al.* 1992), and the Confusional State Evaluation (Robertsson *et al.* 1997). They appear to perform reasonably well in medical inpatients, but the Delirium Rating Scale has been found to be less efficient in a specifically psychogeriatric population (Rosen *et al.* 1994). Whether screening is carried out by means of structured instruments or less formally by clinical assessment, good communication between medical and nursing staff is essential. Nurses are in contact with patients for much longer periods than doctors, and are in a better position to observe the fluctuations in mental state and behaviour over the course of the day. Communication between shifts is also important; nocturnal disturbance due to disruption of the sleep–wake cycle is commonly seen in delirium, and this information needs to be passed on by the night staff (Treloar and Macdonald 1995).

Another approach to screening for delirium in elderly patients is to focus particular attention on those who are at high risk of developing the disorder. Those with dementia are one important group in this respect, as are those with other chronic brain disorders, such as Parkinson's disease. Certain physical features have also been shown to be predictive of delirium; in a case-note study of inpatients, Levkoff *et al.* (1988) found four independent predictive factors: urinary tract infection, hypoalbuminaemia on admission, a raised white cell count on admission, and proteinuria on admission. Hypoalbuminaemia was also identified as a predictor of delirium by Dickson (1991); it may be an indicator of other disorders such as liver disease, or may have its effect by increasing the unbound serum concentration of toxic drugs (Trzpacz and Francis 1990). Various models for predicting delirium in various elderly inpatient populations have been developed, identifying important predisposing and precipitating factors (Schor *et al.* 1992; Inouye *et al.* 1993; Marcantonio *et al.* 1994; Fisher and Flowerdew 1995; Inouye and Charpentier 1996).

The role of psychiatric services in acute management

The principles of the clinical management of delirium are discussed by Stewart and Fairweather (see Chapter 25). Provided that the underlying cause or causes are promptly identified and treated, and any associated distress and disturbed behaviour is carefully controlled with the short-term use of a safe and potent drug (haloperidol, or one of the newer atypical neuroleptics such as risperidone), most patients should recover without recourse to specialist psychiatric intervention. However, there are some cases where psychiatric involvement is desirable or necessary.

If the diagnosis of delirium is in doubt

If medical staff are uncertain whether a patient's disturbed mental state is due to delirium or some other psychiatric disorder, then a psychiatric opinion should be sought. This can be provided either by a dedicated liaison–consultation service, or by means of specific arrangements between individual medical and psychogeriatric teams.

If other psychiatric disorders are present

Severely depressed or manic patients admitted to medical wards with delirium need their psychiatric disorder treated with the same urgency as their physical debility, and this should be initiated by the psychiatric team who will take over their care once they are well enough to be discharged.

If disturbed behaviour is severely disruptive

Sometimes the behaviour of delirious patients on medical wards is so disruptive that it puts their safety or the safety of others at risk, and cannot be contained without unacceptable sedation or restraint. In such cases the best course may be to transfer the patient to a psychiatric unit, provided that the necessary medical care can be provided there. An alternative might be to arrange for a psychiatric nurse to provide continuous supervision on the medical ward until the problem subsides.

Medicolegal aspects

Delirious patients often present medical staff with tricky ethical and legal problems. If a physically ill and floridly confused individual vigorously refuses to be admitted to hospital, to be examined, investigated, and treated, what is to be done? Delirium is a mental disorder, and in any particular country proper practice will be determined largely by its mental health legislation. In the United Kingdom this is principally set out in the 1983 Mental Health Act (MHA). However, within the UK jurisdiction, the ultimate criterion against which an individual doctor's actions will be judged in law is that of accepted good practice by his or her peers (*Bolam* v *Friern Barnet*). It is important to bear in mind that doctors owe a common law duty of care to their patients, and any necessary action that is performed in their best interests is unlikely to be judged illegal or unethical, provided that it is what most conscientious doctors would do in a similar situation.

To start at the beginning, when is it appropriate to admit an unwilling delirious patient to hospital? If the cause of the delirium is known and can be treated and managed at home, or if the patient is obviously terminally ill, then the wish to stay out of hospital should be respected, provided that this does not impose an unacceptable burden on family and friends. If, however, the delirium requires investigation or treatment in hospital, then involuntary admission will be necessary and this is best achieved by using the provisions of the MHA. Formal admission to hospital under Section 2 of the MHA is usually the most appropriate course; this is always preferable to a simple forced admission or admission under other legislation such as Section 47 of the 1948 National Assistance Act (see Chapter 14), because it provides the patient with important reviews and safeguards, and also allows for both assessment and the treatment that is likely to be required. Although this legislation exists, it is still not used in many cases, either because GPs and physicians are unsure about the status of delirium as a mental disorder (*it is*), or because they believe they cannot admit patients to medical beds under the MHA. The MHA is not clear on the latter point, since it was not drafted with this possibility in mind. In practice, however, the main difficulty is that most general hospitals and acute medical NHS trusts have no bureaucratic provision to administer the MHA, and medical and surgical consultants have no experience of being a 'responsible medical officer' as defined by the MHA. One option in these circumstances is to admit the patient formally to a psychiatric bed and immediately arrange for MHA Section 17 leave, in order for the patient to be admitted to a general hospital bed.

Another problem that doctors and nurses on medical and surgical wards sometimes have to face is the delirious inpatient who suddenly demands to leave, or who makes a dash for the exit. In an emergency, the common law duty of care will justify reasonable restraint and sedation (DHSS 1976), but once the situation has been controlled it is advisable to detain the patient formally under the appropriate Section of the MHA, which makes provision for these cases. Section 5(2) allows for a patient to be detained for up to 72 hours by a registered[1] doctor, and Section 5(4) allows a nurse to detain a patient for 6 hours pending alternative arrangements. These Sections may be used in any ward of any hospital, but Section 5(4) is limited by the requirement that the patient must already be receiving treatment for a mental disorder, and that the detaining nurse must have appropriate psychiatric training. Provided that the patient's delirium has been diagnosed before the emergency then their subsequent treatment will satisfy the terms of the MHA, which is one reason why a policy of regular screening for delirium on medical and surgical wards is a good idea. It will not be practicable to have a psychiatrically trained nurse on every shift on every ward, but ideally there should be someone available within the hospital at all times who can perform this duty when needed. This will be relatively straightforward in general hospitals with psychiatric units, provided there is a good working relationship between medical and psychiatric staff.

Prognosis

Delirium in elderly patients is associated with increased short-term mortality (Francis and Kapoor 1992; Pompei *et al.* 1994). This is due to the severity of the underlying physical illness; if this is controlled, then delirium has only a marginal effect on mortality (Francis *et al.* 1990). The increased short-term morbidity of elderly delirious patients is also reflected in their longer hospital stays and higher rates of discharge to nursing homes (Francis and Kapoor 1992); delirium significantly interferes with the processes of diagnosis, treatment, and rehabilitation (Saravay and Lavin 1994). Increased length of stay and mortality are particularly associated with hypoactive delirium. In general, patients with hyperactive delirium appear to be less severely ill than those with hypoactive delirium; this may be due to differences in the cause of the delirium, or to the fact that hyperactive delirium is more likely to be identified and the causes treated. Hyperactive delirium is associated with falls during the hospital admission, whereas hypoactive delirium is associated with the development of pressure sores; these problems should be anticipated and prevented where possible (O'Keeffe and Lavan 1999).

The long-term outcome of delirium is less clear. Delirium is usually a relatively transient disorder that terminates, in most cases, with either cognitive improvement or death (Rockwood 1989; O'Keeffe and Lavan 1997). However, about one-third of patients have prolonged or recurrent episodes (Levkoff *et al.* 1992; Rockwood 1993). In patients who show continued cognitive decline following recovery from an episode of delirium, this is probably due to the progression of a pre-existing condition such as Alzheimer's disease or cerebrovascular dementia (Koponen and Riekkinen 1993). An episode of delirium occurring while an inpatient, is also a predictor of long-term functional decline following their discharge from hospital (Murray *et al.* 1993). It should be borne in mind that these adverse outcomes may not apply to those patients with mild delirium who would not have met the diagnostic criteria for inclusion in these studies.

Prevention

There are several ways whereby the risks to which elderly people are exposed could be reduced. The aim should be to minimize exposure to the various patient- and hospital-related factors that are known to predispose to delirium (Inouye *et al.* 1993; Inouye and Charpentier 1996). In hospital, the ward environment and routines should aim to avoid unnecessary sensory impairment and sleep deprivation, and support a normal sleep–wake cycle. Non-pharmacological sleep-promotion strategies should be used in preference to hypnotic drugs. It is important to ensure adequate food and fluid intake, and patients should be encouraged to be mobile whenever possible. Careful prescribing is important, particularly in at-risk individuals, avoiding where possible any drugs with known potential to cause delirium, such as anticholinergic agents (tricyclic antidepressants, trihexyphenidyl (benzhexol), procyclidine), tranquillizers and hypnotics with long half-lives, and narcotic analgesics. The drug chart should be regularly reviewed, with the aim of keeping the burden of medication as low as possible. In surgical patients, good pre-, peri- and postoperative care (especially with regard to blood pressure, oxygenation, pain relief, and infection control) will reduce the risk of postoperative delirium (Williams *et al.* 1985; Gustafson *et al.* 1991). A systematic review of the limited evidence-base for systematic interventions to prevent delirium suggests they are of some benefit (Cole *et al.* 1996).

Notes

1. A pre-registration house officer may not do it.

References

Albert, M. S., Levkoff, S. E., Reilly, C., Lipsitz, B., Pilgrim, D., Cleary, P. D., *et al.* (1992). The delirium symptom interview: an interview for the detection of delirium symptoms in hospitalized patients. *Journal of Geriatric Psychiatry and Neurology*, 5, 14–21.

American Psychiatric Association. (1994). *Diagnostic and statistical manual of mental disorders (4th edn).* American Psychiatric Association, Washington, DC.

Anthony, J., Leresche, L., Niaz, U., Von Korff, M. R., and Folstein, M. F. (1985). Screening for delirium in a general medical ward: the tachistoscope and global accessibility rating. *General Hospital Psychiatry*, 7, 36–42.

Balter, R. A., Fricchione, G., and Sterman, A. B. (1986). Clinical presentation of multi-infarct delirium. *Psychosomatics*, **27**, 461–2.

Beresin, E. V. (1988). Delirium in the elderly. *Journal of Geriatric Psychiatry and Neurology*, **1**, 127–43.

Berggren, D., Gustafson, Y., Eriksson, B., Bucht, G., Hansson, L. I., Reiz, S., *et al.* (1987). Post-operative confusion after anaesthesia in elderly patients with femoral neck fractures. *Anaesthesia and Analgesia*, **66**, 497–504.

Bergmann, K. and Eastham, E. J. (1974). Psychogeriatric ascertainment and assessment for treatment in an acute medical setting. *Age and Ageing*, 3, 174–88.

Bolam vs. Friern Barnet Hospital Management Committee (1957). 1 W. L. R., 582.

Bowler, C., Boyle, A., Branford, M., Cooper, S.-A., Harper, R., and Lindesay, J. (1994). Detection of psychiatric disorders in elderly medical inpatients. *Age and Ageing*, **23**, 307–11.

Burns, A., Jacoby, R., and Levy, R. (1990). Psychiatric phenomena in Alzheimer's disease. *British Journal of Psychiatry*, **157**, 72–6.

Byrne, E. J., Lennox, G., Lowe, J., and Godwin-Austin, R. B. (1989). Diffuse Lewy body disease: clinical features in 15 cases. *Journal of Neurology, Neurosurgery and Psychiatry*, **52**, 709–17.

Cole, M. G., Primeau, F., and McCusker, J. (1996). Effectiveness of interventions to prevent delirium in hospitalized patients: A systematic review. *Canadian Medical Association Journal*, **155**, 1263–8.

DHSS. (1976). *The management of violent and potentially violent patients in hospital. Circular HC (76) 11.* HMSO, London.

Dickson, L. R. (1991). Hypoalbuminemia in delirium. *Psychosomatics*, **32**, 317–23.

Dunne, J. W., Leedman, P. J., and Edis, R. H. (1986). Inobvious stroke: a cause of delirium and dementia. *Australian and New Zealand Journal of Medicine*, **16**, 771–8.

Faust, D. and Fogel, B. S. (1989). The development and initial validation of a sensitive bedside cognitive screening test. *Journal of Nervous and Mental Disease*, **177**, 25–31.

Figiel, G. S., Krishnan, K. R., and Nemeroff, C. (1989). Radiologic correlates of antidepressant-induced delirium: the possible significance of basal-ganglia lesions. *Journal of Neuropsychiatry and Clinical Neurosciences*, **1**, 188–90.

Figiel, G. S., Krishnan, K. R., and Doraiswamy, P. M. (1990). Subcortical structural changes in ECT-induced delirium. *Journal of Geriatric Psychiatry and Neurology*, **3**, 172–6.

Fisher, B. W. and Flowerdew, G. (1995). A simple model for predicting postoperative delirium in older patients undergoing elective orthopedic surgery. *Journal of the American Geriatrics Society*, **43**, 175–8.

Folstein, M. F., Folstein, S. E., and McHugh, P. R. (1975). Mini-mental state—a practical method for grading the cognitive state of patients for the clinician. *Journal of Psychiatric Research*, **12**, 189–98.

Folstein, M. F., Bassett, S. S., Romanowski, A. J., and Nestadt, G. (1991). The epidemiology of delirium in the community: the Eastern Baltimore Mental Health Survey. *International Psychogeriatrics*, **3**, 169–79.

Francis, J. (1992). Delirium in older patients. *Journal of the American Geriatrics Society*, **40**, 829–38.

Francis, J. and Kapoor, W. N. (1992). Prognosis after hospital discharge of older medical patients with delirium. *Journal of the American Geriatrics Society*, **40**, 601–6.

Francis, J., Martin, D., and Kapoor, W. N. (1990). A prospective study of delirium in hospitalized elderly. *Journal of the American Medical Association*, **263**, 1097–101.

Gallwey, M. B. (1838). Nature and treatment of delirium. *London Medical Gazette*, **1**, 46–9.

Grimley-Evans, J. (1982). The psychiatric aspects of physical disease. In *The psychiatry of late life* (ed. R. Levy and F. Post), pp. 114–42. Blackwell Scientific Publications, Oxford.

Gustafson, Y., Berggren, D., Brännström, B., Bucht, G., Norberg, A., Hansson, L. I. *et al.* (1988). Acute confusional states in elderly patients treated for femoral neck fracture. *Journal of the American Geriatrics Society*, **36**, 525–30.

Gustafson, Y., Brännström, B., Berggren, D, Ragnarsson, J. I., Sigaard, J., Bucht, G., *et al.* (1991). A geriatric-anesthesiologic program to reduce acute confusional states in elderly patients treated for femoral neck fractures. *Journal of the American Geriatrics Society*, **39**, 655–62.

Harwood, D., Hope, T., and Jacoby, R. (1997). Cognitive impairment in medical inpatients. II Do physicians miss cognitive impairment? *Age and Ageing*, **26**, 37–9.

Hodkinson, H. M. (1972). Evaluation of a mental test score for assessment of mental impairment in the elderly. *Age and Ageing*, **1**, 233–8.

Hodkinson, H. M. (1973). Mental impairment in the elderly. *Journal of the Royal College of Physicians*, **7**, 305–17.

Inouye, S. K. and Charpentier, P. A. (1996). Precipitating factors for delirium in hospitalized elderly persons: predictive model and interrelationship with baseline vulnerability. *Journal of the American Medical Association*, **275**, 852–7.

Inouye, S. K., van Dycke, C. H., Alessi, C. A., Balkin, S., Siegal, A. P., and Horwitz, R. I. (1990). Clarifying confusion: the confusion assessment method. *Annals of Internal Medicine*, **113**, 941–8.

Inouye, S. K., Viscoli, C. M., Horowitz, R. I., Hurst, L. D., and Tinetti, M. E. (1993). A predictive model for delirium in hospitalised elderly medical patients based on admission characteristics. *Annals of Internal Medicine*, **119**, 474–81.

Johnson, J., Kerse, M., Gottlieb, G. L., Sullivan, E., Wonich, C., Kinosian, B., *et al.* (1992). Prospective versus retrospective methods of identifying patients with delirium. *Journal of the American Geriatrics Society*, **40**, 316–19.

Kellam, A. M. P. (1987). The neuroleptic malignant syndrome, so-called: a survey of the world literature. *British Journal of Psychiatry*, **150**, 752–9.

Koponen, H. J. and Reikkinen, P. J. (1993). A prospective study of delirium in elderly patients admitted to a psychiatric hospital. *Psychological Medicine*, **23**, 103–9.

Levkoff, S. E., Safran, C., Cleary, P. D., Gallop, J., and Phillips, R. S. (1988). Identification of factors associated with the diagnosis of delirium in elderly hospitalized patients. *Journal of the American Geriatrics Society*, **36**, 1099–104.

Levkoff, S. E., Cleary, P., Liptzin, B., and Evans, D. A. (1991). Epidemiology of delirium: an overview of research issues. *International Psychogeriatrics*, **3**, 149–67.

Levkoff, S. E., Evans, D. A., Liptzin, B., Cleary, P. D., Lipsitz, L. A., Wetle, T. T., *et al.* (1992). Delirium. The occurrence and persistence of symptoms among elderly hospitalized patients. *Annals of Internal Medicine*, **152**, 334–40.

Lindesay, J. (1999). The concept of delirium. *Dementia and Geriatric Cognitive Disorders*, **10**, 310–14.

Lipowski, Z. J. (1983). Transient cognitive disorders in the elderly. *American Journal of Psychiatry*, **140**, 1426–36.

Lipsitz, B., Levkoff, S. E., Cleary, P. D., Pilgrim, D. M., Reilly, C. H., Albert, M., *et al.* (1991). An empirical study of diagnostic criteria for delirium. *American Journal of Psychiatry*, **148**, 451–7.

Loach, A. B. and Benedict, C. R. (1980). Plasma catecholamine concentrations associated with cerebral vasospasm. *Journal of Neurological Sciences*, **45**, 261–71.

Macdonald, A. J. D. and Treloar, A. (1996). Delirium and dementia: are they distinct? *Journal of the American Geriatrics Society*, **44**, 1001–2.

McKeith, I. G., Perry, R. H., Fairbairn, A. F., Jabeen, S., and Perry, E. K. (1992). Operational criteria for senile dementia of the Lewy body type (SDLT). *Psychological Medicine*, **22**, 911–22.

Marcantonio, E. R., Goldman, L., Mangiore, C. M., Ludwig, L. E., Muraca, B., Haslauer, C. M., *et al.* (1994). A clinical prediction rule for delirium after noncardiac surgery. *Journal of the American Medical Association*, **271**, 134–9.

Millar, H. R. (1981). Psychiatric morbidity in elderly surgical patients. *British Journal of Psychiatry*, **138**, 17–20.

Murray, A. M., Levkoff, S. E., Wetle, T. T., Beckett, L., Cleary, P. D., Schor, J. D., *et al.* (1993). Acute delirium and functional decline in the hospitalized elderly patient. *Journal of Gerontology*, **48**, M81–86.

O'Keeffe, S. and Lavan, J. (1997). The prognostic significance of delirium in older hospital patients. *Journal of the American Geriatrics Society*, **45**, 174–8.

O'Keeffe, S. and Lavan, J. (1999). Clinical significance of delirium subtypes in older people. *Age and Ageing*, **28**, 115–19.

Olsson, T. (1999). Activity in the hypothalamic–pituitary–adrenal axis and delirium. *Dementia and Geriatric Cognitive Disorders*, **10**, 345–9.

Pompei, P., Foreman, M., Rudberg, M. A., Inouye, S. K., Brund, V., and Cassel, C. K. (1994). Delirium in hospitalized older persons: outcomes and predictors. *Journal of the American Geriatrics Society*, **42**, 809–15.

Robertsson, B., Karlsson, I., Styrud, E., and Gottfries, C. G. (1997). Confusional State Evaluation (CSE): an instrument for measuring severity of delirium in the elderly. *British Journal of Psychiatry*, **170**, 565–70.

Rockwood, K. (1989). Acute confusion in elderly medical patients. *Journal of the American Geriatrics Society*, **37**, 150–4.

Rockwood, K. (1993). The occurrence and duration of symptoms in elderly patients with delirium. *Journal of Gerontology*, **48**, 162–6.

Rockwood, K., Cosway, S., Stolee, P., Kydd, D., Carver, D., Jarrett, P., *et al.* (1994). Increasing the recognition of delirium in elderly patients. *Journal of the American Geriatrics Society*, **42**, 252–6.

Rosen, J., Sweet, R. A., Mulsant, B. H., Rifai, A. H., Pasternak, R., and Zubenko, G. S. (1994). The delirium rating scale in a psychogeriatric inpatient setting. *Journal of Neuropsychiatry and Clinical Neurosciences*, **6**, 30–5.

Rovner, B. W., Kafonek, S., Fillip, L., Lucas, M. J., and Folstein, M. F. (1986). Prevalence of mental illness in a community nursing home. *American Journal of Psychiatry*, **143**, 1446–9.

Sabin, T. D., Vitug, A. J., and Mark, V. H. (1982). Are nursing home diagnosis and treatment adequate? *Journal of the American Medical Association*, **248**, 321–2.

Sandberg, O., Gustafson, Y., Brännström, B., *et al.* (1998). Prevalence of dementia, delirium and psychiatric symptoms in various care settings for the elderly. *Scandinavian Journal of Social Medicine*, **26**, 56–62.

Saravay, S. M. and Lavin, M. (1994). Psychiatric comorbidity and length of stay in the general hospital: a critical review of outcome studies. *Psychosomatics*, **35**, 233–52.

Schor, J. D., Levkoff, S. E., Lipsitz, L. A., Reilly, C. H., Cleary, P. D., Rowe, J. W., *et al.* (1992). Risk factors for delirium in hospitalized elderly. *Journal of the American Medical Association*, **267**, 827–31.

Shulman, K. I. (1986). Mania in old age. In *Affective disorders in the elderly* (ed. E. Murphy), pp. 203–16. Churchill Livingstone, London.

Shulman, K. I., Shedletsky, R., and Silver, I. L. (1986). The challenge of time: clock-drawing and cognitive function in the elderly. *International Journal of Geriatric Psychiatry*, **1**, 135–40.

Simpson, C. J. and Kellett, J. M. (1987). The relationship between pre-operative anxiety and post-operative delirium. *Journal of Psychosomatic Research*, **31**, 491–7.

Sirois, F. (1988). Delirium: 100 cases. *Canadian Journal of Psychiatry*, **33**, 375–8.

Smith, L. W. and Dimsdale, J. E. (1989). Postcardiotomy delirium: conclusions after 25 years? *American Journal of Psychiatry*, **146**, 452–8.

Sunderland, T., Tariot, P. N., Cohen, R. M., Weingartner, H., Mueller, E. A., and Murphy, D. L. (1987). Anticholinergic sensitivity in patients with DAT and age-matched controls: a dose-response study. *Archives of General Psychiatry*, **44**, 418–26.

Treloar, A. J. and Macdonald, A. J. D. (1995). Recognition of cognitive impairment by day and night nursing staff among acute geriatric patients. *Journal of the Royal Society of Medicine*, **88**, 196–8.

Treloar, A. and Macdonald, A. J. D. (1997*a*). Outcome of delirium: Part 1. Outcome of delirium diagnosed by DSM-III-R, ICD-10 and CAMDEX and derivation of the Reversible Cognitive Dysfunction Scale among acute geriatric inpatients. *International Journal of Geriatric Psychiatry*. **12**, 609–13.

Treloar, A. and Macdonald, A. J. D. (1997*b*). Outcome of delirium: Part 2. Clinical features of reversible cognitive dysfunction—are they the same as accepted definitions of delirium? *International Journal of Geriatric Psychiatry*. **12**, 614–18.

Trzepacz, P. T. (1996). Anticholinergic model for delirium. *Seminars in Clinical Neuropsychiatry*, **1**, 294–303.

Trzepacz, P. T. and Francis, J. (1990). Low serum albumin and risk of delirium. *American Journal of Psychiatry*, **147**, 675.

Trzepacz, P. T., Baker, R. W., and Greenhouse, J. (1988). A symptom rating scale for delirium. *Psychiatry Research*, **23**, 89–97.

Williams, M. A., Campbell, E. B., Raynor, W. J., Musholt, M. A., Mlynarczyk, S. M., and Crane, L. F. (1985). Predictors of acute confusional states in hospitalized elderly patients. *Research into Nursing and Health*, **8**, 31–40.

World Health Organization. (1992). *International classification of diseases (10th revision)*. World Health Organization, Geneva.

27 Depressive disorders

Robert Baldwin

Introduction

Depression and old age are often regarded as inextricably linked. The litany of losses faced by elderly people is seen as sufficient reason to justify this view, and supportive quotations are not difficult to find. For example, Burton's famous 'after seventy years, all is trouble and sorrow...' comes from his *Anatomy of melancholy* which was published over 300 years ago. In fact though, for contemporary Western people at least, life as an older person is reported by the majority as having turned out be better than hoped for (Harris 1975).

Health professionals mainly see those old people most susceptible to depression, the frail with acute or chronic physical illness or multiple pathology, and who are often living in a residential facility. Under such circumstances distortions are bound to occur with, therefore, an exaggerated view of the extent of depression among old people. The danger is that depressive symptoms may be regarded as so commonplace that older people who develop depressive disorder, which is the topic of this chapter, may be overlooked.

Terms and definitions

In psychiatry, arguments over terminology occur regularly and are subject to fashion. No terminology or method of classifying depression will satisfy everybody. In this chapter 'depressive disorder' will be use to encompass all clinically significant depressions in later life. Table 27.1 employs a classification used by the British Association of Psychopharmacology (Anderson *et al.* 2000).

It has the virtue of being easy to follow. In a major depressive episode there are sufficient symptoms to reach the syndromal threshold. In milder (non-major) depression the symptom count falls just below the threshold and such patients often have quite marked anxiety symptoms. Many patients experiencing psychological reactions to stress fall into this category. There is little evidence that patients with milder depressions respond to antidepressant drug treatment (Anderson *et al.* 2000). Counselling and psychological interventions are the preferred interventions. However, it is insufficient merely to squeeze patients into diagnostic boxes. The number of symptoms, the severity of them, and the resulting disability are all important in weighing up the severity and impact of depression on a person.

Unfortunately other terms which have no agreed meaning are now used regularly in the literature. These include 'subsyndromal depression' and 'minor depression'. In so far as 'subsyndromal depression' has any agreed meaning it denotes depressive disorders in which there are fewer symptoms than are required by DSM or ICD systems of classification (see below). Recent naturalistic studies of mixed-aged patients strongly suggest that much subsyndromal depression is a result of incomplete recovery from a major depressive episode (Judd *et al.* 1998). 'Minor depression', although often used interchangeably with subsyndromal depression, is a construct arising from epidemiological data which suggests a distinct syndrome of low mood, anhedonia, retardation, poor concentration, and poor perceived health in some older people (Blazer 1991). There is insufficient data to provide clear treatment guidelines for minor depression. 'Dysthymia' is a form of chronic depression (of at least 2 years' duration), often with episodes of major depression. Because its incidence is considered highest in younger adults it has received less attention than major depression. However, evidence, from community surveys and patients referred to psychiatrists, shows that it is by no means uncommon (Kivela and Pahkala 1989; Devanand *et al.* 1994). 'Adjustment disorder', a form of milder depression, is characterized by its proximity to a major traumatic event, its self-limiting nature, and its time course, generally less than 6 months.

The current major classification systems are DSM-IV (American Psychiatric Association 1994) and ICD-10 (World Health Organization 1993). The criteria for DSM-IV are summarized in Table 27.2 and for ICD-10 in Tables 27.3 and 27.4. Note that in DSM-IV a complaint of depression is not a necessary requirement. This may be especially relevant when considering elderly people, as will be discussed.

In addition, a fifth character (F32.01) may be added to specify the presence of a 'somatic syndrome', as shown in Table 27.4.

The somatic syndrome (Table 27.4) is not mandatory for diagnosis and appears to be an attempt to retain some aspects of older terms such as 'endogenous' depression and melancholic depression. Although they employ different terms, DSM-IV and ICD-10 have moved much closer to agreement concerning the classification of affective disorders.

An issue related to nomenclature is the use in research of structured, and hence standardized, methods of recording mental states. Inter-rater reliability is good, but the instruments are not always very discriminating. For example, distinguishing bereavement from depression can be problematic, a point which is usefully made in DSM-IV (see Table 27.2E). An important development in terms of epidemiological research has been the introduction of computerized diagnostic algorithms, such as AGECAT. This system generates diagnostic categories derived from the Geriatric Mental Status Schedule, which is a computerized structured psychiatric schedule (Copeland *et al.* 1986). Some of the original terms are perhaps a little out of date, but they appear to

Table 27.1 Classification of mood disorders

Classification	DSM-IV code	ICD-10 code
Major depression	Major depressive episode, single episode or recurrent (296)	Depressive episode, severe (F32.2), moderate (F32.1), or mild with at least 5 symptoms (F32.0);[1] recurrent depressive disorder current episode severe (F33.2), moderate (F33.1), or mild with at least 5 symptoms (F33.0)[1]
Milder depression	Depressive disorder not otherwise specified (311)	Depressive disorder, mild with four symptoms (F32.0).[1] Recurrent depressive disorder current episode mild with four symptoms[1] (F33.0); mixed anxiety and depressive disorder (F41.2)
	Adjustment disorder with depressed mood/mixed anxiety and depressed mood (309)	Adjustment disorder: depressive reaction/mixed anxiety and depressive reaction (F43.2); other mood (affective disorders (F38)
Dysthymia	Dysthymia (300.4)	Dysthymia (F34.1)

[1] For a list of symptoms see Table 27.3. Must include at least two of (i) depressed mood, (ii) loss of interest or pleasure, (iii) decreased energy or increased fatiguability.

Table 27.2 DSM-IV criteria for major depressive episode

A. Five or more of the following symptoms have been present during the same 2-week period and represent change from previous functioning; at least one of the symptoms is either (1) depressed mood or (2) loss of interest or pleasure.

Note Symptoms that are clearly due to a general medical condition are not included, nor are mood-incongruent delusions or hallucinations

(1) Depressed mood most of the day, nearly every day, as indicated by either subjective report (e.g. feels sad or empty) or observation made by others (e.g. appears tearful).
(2) Markedly diminished interest or pleasure in all, or almost all, activities most of nearly every day (as indicated by either subjective account or observation made by others).
(3) Significant weight loss when not dieting or weight gain (e.g. a change of more than 5% of body weight in a month), or decrease or increase in appetite nearly every day.
(4) Insomnia or hypersomnia nearly every day.
(5) Psychomotor agitation or retardation nearly every day (observable by others, not merely subjective feelings of restlessness or being slowed down)
(6) Fatigue or loss of energy nearly every day.
(7) Feelings of worthlessness or excessive or inappropriate guilt (which may be delusional) nearly every day (not merely self-reproach or guilt about being sick).
(8) Diminished ability to think or concentrate or indecisiveness, nearly every day (either by subjective account or as observed by others).
(9) Recurrent thoughts of death (not just fear of dying), recurrent suicidal ideation without a specific plan, or a suicide attempt, or a specific plan for committing suicide.

B. The symptoms do not meet the criteria for a mixed episode.

C. The symptoms cause clinically significant distress or impairment in social, occupational, or other important areas of functioning.

D. The symptoms are not due to the direct physiological effects of a substance (e.g. a drug of abuse, a medication) or a general medical condition (e.g. hypothyroidism).

E. The symptoms are not better accounted for by bereavement, i.e. after the loss of a loved one, the symptoms persist for longer than 2 months or are characterized by marked functional impairment, morbid preoccupations with worthlessness, suicidal ideation, psychotic symptoms, or psychomotor retardation.

Specifiers can be coded for *severity* (mild, moderate, or severe); *psychosis* (mood-congruent or mood-incongruent delusions or hallucinations) and *remission* (partial or full).

correlate very well with the DSM and ICD classifications (Copeland *et al.* 1990, 1992).

Epidemiology

Studies of elderly populations consistently demonstrate that the prevalence of *depressive symptoms* far exceeds that of *depressive episode.* Some classic research from Newcastle-upon-Tyne (Kay *et al.* 1964) found a prevalence of about 10% for depression in community residents, although only 1.3% met the criteria for what would correspond nowadays to a depressive episode. In a cross-national comparison (Gurland *et al.* 1983), levels of 'pervasive depression' were found in 13% of New York elderly residents and 12.4% of Londoners. Point prevalence for the past month of 'manic depressive/depressive disorder', akin to depressive episode, was 1.3% and 2.5%, respectively. Copeland *et al.* (1987), using AGECAT, found similar rates in the city of Liverpool: 11.3% for 'diagnostic syndrome cases' but only 3% qualifying as cases of what they termed 'depressive psychosis', which is close in meaning

Table 27.3 ICD-10 depressive episode

A. The syndrome of depression must be present for at least 2 weeks; no history of mania; and not attributable to organic disease or psychoactive substance

Mild depressive episode

B. At least *two* of the following *three* symptoms must be present:
(1) Depressed mood to a degree that is definitely abnormal for the individual, present for most of the day and almost every day, largely uninfluenced by circumstances, and sustained for at least 2 weeks.
(2) Loss of interest or pleasure in activities that are normally pleasurable.
(3) Decreased energy or increased fatiguability.

C. An additional symptom or symptoms from the following (at least *four*):
(1) Loss of confidence or self-esteem.
(2) Unreasonable feelings of self-reproach or excessive and inappropriate guilt.
(3) Recurrent thoughts of death or suicide, or any suicidal behaviour.
(4) Complaints or evidence of diminished ability to think or concentrate, such as indecisiveness or vacillation.
(5) Change in psychomotor activity, with agitation or retardation (either subjective or objective).
(6) Sleep disturbance of any type.
(7) Change in appetite (decrease or increase) with corresponding weight change.

Moderate depressive episode

As above but at least *six* of the symptoms under C.

Severe depressive episode

All *three* from Section B and *at least five* from Section C (*eight* symptoms in total).

Severe cases may be further subdivided according to the presence or otherwise of psychosis and/or stupor.

Table 27.4 Somatic syndrome of ICD-10

At least 4 of:
(1) Marked loss of interest or pleasure
(2) Lack of emotional reaction to events or activities normally producing a response
(3) Wakening in the morning 2 hours or more before the usual time
(4) Depression worse in the morning
(5) Objective evidence of marked psychomotor retardation or agitation
(6) Marked loss of appetite
(7) Weight loss (5% of body weight in the past month)
(8) Marked loss of libido

to major depressive disorder. The Liverpool researchers make the further point that levels of both depressive symptoms and depressive illness show no consistent positive correlation with levels of social disturbance and deprivation. Indeed, rates of depressive disorder seem to be similar in New York, London, and Liverpool, despite clear differences in socioeconomic factors. However, in moving beyond the English-speaking world, quite large differences become apparent. In the nine-centre EURODEP (European Collaborative Depression programme) programme, cases deemed appropriate for some level of intervention ranged between 8.8% in Iceland and 23.6% in Munich. The overall prevalence was 12.3% (Copeland *et al.* 1999).

A word of caution is necessary. Much epidemiological research samples relatively small numbers of the very elderly, and extrapolation to the fastest growing sector of the ageing population may be inaccurate. However, Morgan *et al.* (1987), using a stratified sample, found similar rates in both the over 75s and those between 65 and 74 years. Nonagenarians seem to be an indestructible breed. Some evidence suggests that they, in contrast to 'younger' elderly, have lower rates of depressive symptoms (Lindesay *et al.* 1989). Finally, depressive symptomatology is usually more prevalent among women than among men in later life; for example in the EURODEP programme the averages were 14.1% for women and 8.6% for men. Possibly this difference may be less marked for more severe forms of depression (Lindesay *et al.* 1989). In summary then, between 10 and 15% of elderly people in the community have some degree of *depressive symptomatology* at a given time, but only about 3% have a *depressive episode.*

This discrepancy between depression as a symptom and as a psychiatric diagnosis requires additional explanation. Studies at Duke University, using a modification of DSM-III, (Blazer and Williams 1980), found a prevalence of depressive disorder of 14.7%, which could be subdivided into 6.5% of people who were regarded as having 'dysphoric' disorders secondary to health problems and a further 3.7% who had major depressive disorder (depressive episode). Only half of the latter group were regarded as having 'primary' disorders, the remainder having evidence of cognitive impairment or 'thought disorder'. A final 4.5% were judged to have 'simple dysphoria': a category focused on by other researchers (Gillis and Zabow 1982). Nowadays, these subsyndromal states might come under the umbrella of subsyndromal depression, either as 'minor' depression or dysthymia. Thinking has altered, in that the depressive states identified in these studies of the 1980s were regarded as having much in common with (depressive) personality disorder, whereas now they are regarded as disorders in their own right and worthy of intervention. This is an important shift, based largely on the findings from epidemiological studies which have shown distinct patterns of depression in older people that DSM-IV and ICD-10 fail to recognize, and the increasing evidence that 'minor' depression is certainly not trivial but is associated with a considerable morbidity and impact on health care systems (Beck and Koenig 1996). Further support for this comes from Kivela *et al.* (1989), who identified a dysthymic group which did not meet DSM-III criteria for major depression, and showed that this group's depression was just as severe as a comparison group with major depression.

Although depressive symptoms (subsyndromal depression, minor depression, or dysthymia) are common in old age, arguably more common than among younger adults, there is no evidence that depressive episode also increases in prevalence with advancing age. While some have found a fairly constant prevalence of depressive episode across the adult lifespan (Gurland 1976; Blazer and Williams 1980; Lindesay *et al.* 1989), even into extreme old age (Heeren *et al.* 1992), the influential North American Epidemiologic Catchment Area (ECA) studies found a decrease with age. A spirited critique of the ECA survey suggests that possibly the methodology and sampling—which contained no reports of cases in institutions where the prevalence of depression is likely to be high, and which excluded those with physical illness—may have led to an underestimate of depression in the elderly subsample (Snowdon 1990). For example, cases of phobia exceeded those of affective disorder, a finding that certainly does not accord with clinical experience (see below), suggesting these phobias may have been the leading symptoms of depressive illness which was unrecognized by the rigid interview system. However, Henderson and colleagues (1993) have reported rates of major depressive episode similar to the ECA findings. They comment that this may be because they strictly applied the DSM and ICD diagnostic criteria. Once again, current thinking has it that older age is associated with depressive disorders not identified by the rigid criteria of current operational classification.

Is ageing *per se* a risk factor for depression? Robert *et al.* (1997) used DSM-IV criteria to assess depression in an epidemiologically derived cohort of patients. Their conclusion was that healthy older people are at no greater risk of depression than anyone else. Any apparent age effect was attributable to physical health problems.

One intriguing finding from the ECA studies (Robins *et al.* 1984) was that the elderly subjects, who had passed through the period of maximum risk for depression, nevertheless had a lower lifetime prevalence of depression than those in middle life. Obviously impaired recall among the older group or selective mortality of those with earlier depression cannot be ruled out. Otherwise another possible interpretation is that the elderly of tomorrow may prove to be at higher risk for affective illness than those of today.

Prevalence varies by location. Milder depression (see Table 27.1) was found in a third of elderly patients attending their general practitioner (GP) in the United Kingdom (McDonald 1986). However, a lower figure was found in a North America study (Callaghan *et al.* 1994) using stricter criteria, although the rates were still high at 17.1% baseline and 18.8% 9 months later. In hospitalized elderly patients the prevalence ranges between 12 and 45%, with an average of about 20% for depressive episode (Koenig *et al.* 1988; Jackson and Baldwin 1993). Most disturbing of all perhaps is the discovery of 'significantly depressed mental state' in almost two-fifths of residents in local authority homes (Ames *et al.* 1988).

Depressive disorder in old age often coexists with cerebral disease and many studies exclude such cases. Allen and Burns (1995) reviewed published data and calculated a prevalence of moderate to severe depressive disorder in patients with Alzheimer's disease at 20%, higher than in aged-matched community residents. Depression is probably more common in vascular as opposed to Alzheimer-type dementia (Allen and Burns 1995).

Clinical presentation

Past literature has emphasized certain aspects of depressive disorder that are thought to be typical of old age. These include a preponderance of somatic complaints (De Alarcon 1964), excessive hypochondriasis (Gurland 1976), and greater agitation (Winokur *et al.* 1973) compared to younger patients; more frequent delusions (Hordern *et al.* 1963); a more 'endogenous' picture (for a review see Blazer *et al.* 1986); and an increased likelihood of presentations coloured by confusion. These findings have tended to create a stereotype of depressive disorder in old age. However, earlier studies were often conducted solely on inpatients. The 'typical' picture may simply be a reflection of more severe illness and therefore not representative of contemporary old age psychiatry. Indeed, even Post (1972), who observed inpatients, recorded that only about one-third of his elderly depressed inpatient sample could be classified as 'typical' cases.

Perhaps not surprisingly then, few of the 'typical' features of late life depression have withstood the scrutiny of modern research. Two main approaches have been adopted: first, to compare patients with depression in later life with younger adult depressives; second, to compare early- versus late-onset depressions in later life (60 years being the most commonly adopted cut-off point). Regarding the former, Blazer *et al.* (1986) controlled for symptoms which might fortuitously increase with age independent of depression. They found that older community subjects, characterized according to DSM criteria, reported more somatic symptoms, had more thoughts about death, and a non-significantly increased preoccupation with the wish to die compared with depressed younger persons. Surprisingly, it was the younger rather than the older depressives who reported more memory problems. There was no support for the notion of a special 'masked' depression occurring in old age. In another iconoclastic study, this time from Italy (Musetti *et al.* 1989), 70 community-dwelling patients over the age of 65 were compared with 330 under that age using DSM-III-R criteria for depressive episode. No special clinical features differentiated the older from the younger group; in fact, the older ones tended to exhibit more retardation than agitation. In Gurland's study (Gurland 1976), only hypochondriasis was more common in older people. A recent study (Brodaty *et al.* 1991) found that elderly depressives were more agitated than younger adult depressives and were more 'endogenous'. Their depressions also tended to be more severe. However, when homogeneous groups were compared (for example, melancholic subtype only), almost all differences disappeared.

Brodaty's group also reported more delusions among elderly as opposed to younger adult depressives. Elsewhere Meyers *et al.* (1988) have argued that delusions occur more frequently in late-onset depression and that this implicates cerebral ageing as an aetiological factor. However, others have not confirmed that a later age of onset is associated with a higher prevalence of delusions (Nelson *et al.* 1989; Baldwin 1992), and, in any case, delusional depressive disorder is a rare disorder among elderly people in the community (Kivela and Pahkala 1989).

The second distinction, early versus late age of onset in older depressed patients, seems a more promising approach, as symptomatic differences might reflect different disease subtypes associated with the ageing brain. The results to date have been disappointing. Thus, apart from the well-known lower prevalence of a family history of affective disorder among late-onset elderly depressives, Conwell *et al.* (1989) could find few clinical differences. Likewise, Brodaty *et al.* (1991) found that late- and early-onset elderly depressives were similar in almost all phenomenological aspects.

However, where studies try to examine whether there are characteristic symptoms in old age depression by using strict diagnostic criteria, such as those outlined earlier, they risk 'defining away' any peculiarities of young versus old depression, leaving only those features which are the same at all ages. The argument thus becomes circular, unless research can demonstrate that older depressives do indeed experience symptoms not currently included in the standard classifications and descriptions of mood disorders. Evidence in favour of this is beginning to emerge. Prince *et al.* (1999) used the 'EURO-D' scale in 14 countries to compare symptoms of depression. A factor analysis of the scale revealed two factors representing the main classes seen in older people. One they called 'affective suffering', characterized by depression, tearfulness, and a wish to die; this was associated with female gender. A second was a 'motivation' factor, comprising loss of interest, poor concentration, and anhedonia; this showed a positive correlation with age.

A gap in research concerns possible differences in the symptomatic presentation of depressive disorder between the old and the very old, or 'old-old', i.e. those over 80 years of age. This is of course the age group which is expected to expand at the fastest rate. There is little systematic data, but a study of very old, nursing-home residents found that reduced interest, irritability, and social withdrawal were common symptoms (Burrows *et al.* 1994).

Lack of motivation and apathy are features of 'vascular depression'. The hypothesis is that damage to end-arteries supplying subcortical striatopallidothalamocortical pathways, disrupts neurotransmitter circuitry involved in mood regulation and may thus cause or predispose to depression. The onset is typically in later life and the presentation comprises apathy, reduced depressive ideation (such as guilt), increased psychomotor retardation, and cognitive impairment, notably poor executive function (Alexopoulos *et al.* 1997).

Diagnostic difficulties

There is then some truth in the adage that 'depression is depression at any age', at least in terms of its clinical presentation. Rather, there are factors that may modify the expression of depressive disorder in the elderly. Some of these arise from the ageing process itself; some are due to differences between generations in how psychological and physical health are perceived; other differences occur because of the frequent overlap of depressive symptoms and physical illness. Some of these factors may accentuate certain aspects of the clinical picture, whilst others may mask the diagnosis. The factors leading to an altered presentation of depression in older people are summarized in Table 27.5.

A common difficulty arises from associated physical ill-health, leading to overlapping

Table 27.5 Factors which influence how depressive disorder presents in old age

Overlap of physical and somatic psychiatric symptoms
Minimal expression of sadness
Somatization or disproportionate complaints associated with physical disorder
Neurotic symptoms of recent onset
Deliberate self-harm (especially medically 'trivial' attempts)
'Pseudodementia'
Depression superimposed upon dementia
Accentuation of abnormal personality traits
Behaviour disorder
Late-onset alcohol dependency syndrome

symptoms. DSM-IV takes an aetiological approach to mood symptoms; that is to say, symptoms which the clinician thinks are due to physical illness (for example, reduced appetite) should be discounted when diagnosing depression. In practice this may not be easy. An individual with active rheumatoid arthritis may experience insomnia, fatigue, and poor appetite equally from his or her physical illness or an associated depression. Matters can, however, often be clarified if attention is paid to the following. First, the history may indicate, on closer enquiry, that some symptoms are new. For example, early morning wakening may emerge from a background of more generalized sleep disturbance due to pain. Second, for those with limited mobility or exercise tolerance, questions about energy and activity must be appropriate: 'Do you feel tired even when resting?'; not 'Have you no energy?' Third, patients who dismiss depression as purely 'understandable' because of ill-health can easily wrong-foot an inexperienced clinician. A history not only from the patient but also from an informant is thus essential. It may demonstrate, for example, a recent decline in interests at a time of static physical health. Cohen-Cole and Stoudemire (1987) provide a useful overview of the problems of diagnosing depression in the presence of major physical illness. Many would agree with their view that whereas exclusive criteria are necessary for research, clinicians may well wish to take a more inclusive approach to DSM criteria to avoid missing depression in complex cases.

Depressive disorder may be overlooked because elderly people tend to minimize feelings of sadness (Georgotas 1983), presumably reflecting a cohort of people brought up not to bother their doctors with emotional difficulties. Therefore it is very important to enquire carefully about two areas: anhedonia (an inability to experience pleasure) and depressive thoughts, such as reduced self-esteem, guilt, worthlessness, and suicidal ideation. The author well remembers an elderly gentleman with abdominal pain for which his surgeon could find no explanation and whose family were pressing hard for a laparotomy. When asked about depressed mood he snarled angrily, 'That's what everyone is trying to say: of course I get fed up but it's this pain that does it. I'm not depressed.' Yet enquiry revealed that he was eating poorly, had lost more than 9 kg in weight, felt no interest or pleasure in anything, and had thought of putting his head in the gas oven because he felt a burden to his family. His pain disappeared after 3 weeks' antidepressant medication.

This introduces two further ways in which the presentation of old age depression may be modified. A *pain* with no medical explanation, as in the above case, may occasionally have its origin in undiagnosed depression. The history is the key. Similar is Post's observation that occasional cases of severe tinnitus are relieved when an underlying depression is treated (Post 1982). More common though is the presentation of an elderly person beyond reassurance who has physical complaints disproportionate to known pathology. Again the key is a good history, especially noting recent changes in pain threshold, plus a thorough physical review.

A serious error is to take neurotic symptoms of recent onset at face value. The sudden emergence of severe anxiety, obsessive-compulsive phenomena, hysteria, or hypochondriasis in an elderly person not previously prone to such disorders should lead to a careful search for depressive disorder, which is the usual cause (Baldwin 1988*a*). Likewise, at all degrees of severity of depression, anxiety is a common accompanying symptom (Post 1972). If it dominates the clinical picture the unwary may miss underlying depressive disorder. Perhaps least pardonable is to dismiss an act of deliberate self-harm because the medical consequences appear to be trivial. There is no reliable correlation between the medical severity of deliberate self-harm and any associated psychiatric seriousness. The severity of depression is not a reliable guide either, as most elderly patients who kill themselves while depressed have moderate rather than severe depression (Barraclough 1971). Suicide is covered later. Elderly people rarely take 'manipulative' overdoses. Most have serious depressive disorder and *all* require psychiatric referral. More difficult to characterize is the concept of depression presenting as 'subintentional' suicide. These individuals are profoundly withdrawn, reject assistance, refuse food, and suffer severe weight loss, which in combination with inactivity may even lead to a peroneal nerve palsy (Massey and Bullock 1978). However, patients who 'turn their face to the wall' are a heterogeneous group, some of whom may be severely depressed but others not clearly so. The author's views are tempered by experiences of a few such cases referred by geriatricians, these patients were not obviously suffering from physical illness, but, on postmortem examination, they had occult carcinomas.

Lishman (1987) describes 'pseudodementia' as 'a number of conditions [in which] a clinical picture resembling organic dementia presents for attention yet physical disease proves to be little if at all responsible'. It is, in many respects, an unsatisfactory term, but one which seems here to stay, although other terms such as 'dementia of depression' have been proposed (Pearlson *et al.* 1989).

'Pseudodementia' is used in several different ways. The first and least satisfactory use is when an elderly person, usually clearly depressed, fails to pass a routine 'bedside' screening test for dementia. Since dementia is defined clinically and not on the basis of screening tests, this usage is not acceptable.

The second use is to a characterize a particular clinical presentation of severe depressive disorder coloured by confusion. Post (1982) has summarized this. The patient's informants are invariably aware of memory impairment and can usually date the onset accurately, unlike the onset of dementia which is much more insidious. Patients often complain at length about their memory, and occasionally other cognitive difficulties, again unlike most people with dementia. Questions about cognitive function often lead to 'don't know' responses, sometimes accompanied by considerable irritation, in contrast to those with dementia who simply try their best but are inaccurate. Patients with pseudodementia convey a great deal of despair, often non-verbally, during the interview. The history is often short and sometimes a previous personal or family history of depression is uncovered. Nursing observation may reveal insomnia, diurnal mood change, and the chance comment to suggest depressive ideation, for example, 'I've nowhere to live'; 'I'm ruined'. These patients are often perplexed and inaccessible. Post argues that depressive pseudodementia should only be diagnosed in patients who *can* be tested, rather than those who appear confused but are inaccessible and hence not really testable.

Third, the term 'pseudodementia' is sometimes applied to an obviously depressed patient who is found to have demonstrable cognitive impairment. After reviewing the literature, Reynolds *et al.* (1988*a*) found this to be so in 10–20% of depressed elderly patients. Usually any impairment is circumscribed, as in an amnesia, but attentional deficits may be severe enough to lead to global impairment. However, specific deficits in higher cortical function not secondary to poor attention, such as aphasia, agraphia, acalculia, etc. are rarely present; where they are clearly detectable, then the case is almost certainly one of organic mental impairment with secondary depression

Post (1982) argues that depressive 'pseudodementia' is a term with limited clinical utility: for severe depressive symptoms require treatment, whether or not it is thought that dementia is present. Perhaps then the term serves its purpose best by acting as a reminder that sometimes patients who appear demented are in fact suffering from severe depression.

'Depression on dementia' refers to the superimposition of depression on an established dementia. It should not be confused with the American term 'double depression' in which a depressive episode is superimposed on chronic dysthymia.

Less discussed in the literature, but readily recognizable to clinicians working with elderly mentally ill people, is depression presenting as a 'disorder of behaviour'. Pitt (1982), drawing upon his long experience, points to certain patterns. These include presentations with food refusal, 'incontinence' (for example, a perverse ability to eliminate in almost any place other than the toilet, unlike the incontinence of dementia), screaming, and outwardly aggressive behaviour. Often the location is a residential- or nursing-home facility and the context one of resented dependency. The history is crucial. The immediate history is best given by one of the care staff who knows the resident well. It is important to find out from other sources whether there has ever been a past history of affective disorder. The checklists in Tables 27.1 and 27.2 are useful, but so too is a history of a recent change in behaviour. Besides the disruptive behaviours described by Pitt, other quieter problems, such as social withdrawal and loss of interest in self and the environment, may occur.

Likewise, depressive illness may lead to an accentuation of premorbid personality traits. Such individuals are often well known for their flamboyant displays. The advent of depressive disorder may lead to dramatic theatricality and ceaseless importuning, sometimes to several agencies simultaneously, for example social services, primary care, and the local Accident and Emergency Department. The key is find out what changes have occurred in the light of the patient's known premorbid personality traits. An escalation in the disruptive behaviour of such an individual might herald the onset of depression. Other behavioural problems may occur as 'markers' of depressive disorder in older people. They include shoplifting, and alcohol-dependence syndrome acquired for the first time in later life.

Last, a complaint of loneliness from an individual who has hitherto coped quite well alone, usually accompanied by a request to be rehoused, should lead to a high index of suspicion with regard to depressive disorder.

Cognitive impairment in old age depressive disorder

This will be considered from both a neuropsychological and a clinical perspective. Neuropsychologically, there seems to be reasonable agreement that both memory and speed of information processing are impaired in depression (Caine 1981; McAllister 1981). An important question is whether such deficits are qualitatively different from those seen in other psychiatric or neurological conditions. For example, it has been argued that the memory failure caused by depression is most evident on effortful tasks involving sustained motivation and active processing operations (Weingartner *et al.* 1981), and that this differentiates depression from dementia in later life (Weingartner *et al.* 1982).

However, memory deficits are not confined to elderly depressives, although they are arguably more severe (Austin *et al.* 1992). In an elegant study, Abas *et al.* (1990) found that 70% of depressed patients (mean age 70 years) had deficits in memory and in measures of cognitive slowing. Although none suffered from dementia as judged clinically (that is a global impairment of cognitive function), the severity of some of the individual impairments was equivalent to a group of patients with Alzheimer's disease (AD). Nevertheless, as already discussed, cortical dysfunction such as aphasia and apraxia, which are common in AD, rarely if ever occur as features of a primary mood disorder. Additionally, in the study of Abas and colleagues, the memory dysfunction of the two groups differed qualitatively. So, for example, poor memory associated with depression usually improves with cueing, suggesting that the problem is one of unreliable retrieval of memories which have been laid down. In AD, deficits are common at the earliest (registration) stage of memory, so that the information is not merely difficult to access but non-existent.

The pattern of cognitive disturbance—memory and attentional deficits with low effort—has led to speculation that depressive illness is associated with subcortical dysfunction. Attractive though this theory is, it is neither unique to older patients (Austin *et al.* 1992) nor has precise equivalence been demonstrated between observed neuropsychological impairment in later life depression and that seen in idiopathic Parkinson's disease, with its known subcortical pathology (Fleminger 1991; Sahakian 1991). Thus, if there is a 'neurology of depression' (Coffey 1987) in the elderly, its anatomy is as yet unknown, although recent imaging data (Dolan *et al.* 1992) suggest that the parts of the brain involved in the cognitive disorder of AD are different from those associated with cognitive impairment in major depression. This is discussed later.

Turning to the clinical perspective, there are two pertinent questions: whether depression-associated cognitive impairment: (1) is reversible; and (2) presages future dementia. The study by Abas *et al.* (1990) found that disordered attention and information processing persisted in around a third of their elderly subjects after successful treatment of their depression. In an uncontrolled study, Kral and Emery (1989) reported that 39 of 44 elderly patients originally diagnosed as cases of depressive pseudodementia had developed the typical picture of AD after a median period of follow-up of 8 years. Again the index affective disorder had improved with treatment. More recently Alexopoulos *et al.* (1993) followed 57 depressed patients annually for an average of 3 years. They subdivided the group according to whether or not 'reversible dementia' was present. This they defined as a dual diagnosis of DSM-III-R major depression plus DSM-III-R dementia with, in addition, remission of dementia after improvement of the depression. Using survival analysis, there was an almost fivefold increase in the risk of developing dementia over approximately 3 years for those originally presenting with 'reversible dementia'. This is at odds with naturalistic studies of depressive disorder in later life which do not show a higher than expected rate of new dementia (Murphy 1983; Baldwin and Jolley 1986). However, these studies specifically excluded patients who had cognitive impairment at the index assessment. Furthermore, in both the study of Alexopoulos and colleagues and that of Kral and Emery (1989) one cannot rule out the possibility that some of those studied were already demented at presentation, even though their cognitive function improved temporarily with depression treatment, or that referral bias resulted in an over-representation of such cases. Nevertheless, these studies suggest that when a patient presents with depressive disorder and also has significant cognitive impairment at initial assessment then they are at high risk for later dementia; whether or not their impairment reverses with treatment; they should be closely followed up. In summary, in some elderly patients depression will be a prodrome of a dementing illness.

Alexopoulos *et al.* (1993) were unable to identify clinical predictors of eventual dementia, but neuropsychological and imaging data were not systematically recorded at baseline. Reding *et al.* (1985) found that the presence of cerebrovascular, extrapyramidal, or spinocerebellar disorder, and the development of confusion on treatment with low doses of tricyclic drugs were the best baseline predictors of future dementia in their series, although the setting—a dementia clinic—may have resulted in a biased sample.

In summary, depression in the elderly is frequently associated with subtle cognitive dysfunction that persists in a minority, and may reflect disruption to subcorticofrontal brain circuits or, in a subgroup which is as yet not readily characterized clinically, may be a harbinger of irreversible dementia. Practically, patients who present with obvious cognitive impairment when depressed (or with a Mini-Mental State Examination score of below 24) should be closely followed up after recovery as they appear to have a higher risk for later dementia.

Aetiology

Aetiology is often subdivided into risk factors (vulnerability to depression), precipitating factors, and features which maintain depression (perpetuating factors). Maintaining factors are more relevant to management and will be discussed later. Lastly, there are factors which protect (or 'buffer') against depression. As has been mentioned, although it is very often assumed that age itself is a risk factor for depression, for physically healthy older individuals this is not so (Robert *et al.* 1997).

Predisposing factors

Genetic susceptibility

The genetic contribution to depressive disorder decreases with age. Hopkinson (1964) reported that the risk to first-degree relatives of probands with depressive disorder was 20% where onset was early, but only 8% where onset had been late. Others have confirmed this (Mendelwicz 1976).

Gender and civil status

Depression in all age groups is more common in women, and this is no less true in later life, with a ratio of approximately 70:30 female:male. In a Finnish study of elderly people (Kivela *et al.* 1988), higher rates of depression were found in those who were widowed or divorced.

Neurobiological risk factors

This is a complex area. The main changes and how they differ between ageing and depression are shown in Table 27.6. With regard to the amine theory of depression there are difficulties in attributing the direction of cause and effect in depression. Amine changes may predispose to depression or be altered as a consequence of it. Perhaps not surprisingly no clear consensus has emerged in respect of amine changes in later life depression. However, some biological changes associated with ageing are similar to those seen in depression. Thus, both normal ageing and depression are associated with decreased brain concentrations of serotonin, dopamine, norepinephrine (noradrenaline) and some metabolites, and increased monoamine oxidase-B (MAO-B) activity (Veith and Raskind 1988; Karlsson 1990). Although there has been extensive research on platelet markers in affective disorders (MAO activity, [^{3}H]imipramine binding sites, platelet α_2-adrenergic binding), few studies have included older depressed patients. Limited evidence suggests that platelet MAO activity may correlate with severity and with certain symptoms (for example, anhedonia) more than with specific subtypes such as early- versus late-onset depression (Schneider 1992). Platelet [^{3}H]imipramine binding may differentiate primary from secondary (organic) depression (Schneider 1992).

There is no convincing evidence that levels of neuropeptides, which may act as neurotransmitter modulators, alter with age (Leake and Ferrier 1993).

A variety of neuroendocrine changes are associated with ageing (Veith and Raskind 1988; and for a comprehensive review see Schneider 1992). The exact site of these effects is not clear but may involve changes at the cortical, limbic, hypothalamic, or pituitary level. Depression in all age groups is associated with hyperactivity and dysregulation of the hypothalamic-pituitary-adrenal (HPA) axis. Ageing is associated with increasing cortisol levels and cortisol non-suppression (Alexopoulos *et al.* 1984).

Schneider (1992) has speculated that normal ageing is associated with enhanced limbic-HPA axis activity, perhaps related to neuronal degeneration in the hippocampus; and that the latter may be exacerbated by raised glucocorticoid secretion, caused either by depression or repeated stressful life events or both (the 'feed-forward cascade'; Sapolsky *et al.* 1986). In support, Krishnan (1991) reported reduced T_1 spin-lattice relaxation times in the hippocampus, as measured by magnetic resonance imaging (MRI), in a group of depressed patients compared to controls. The effect was particularly striking for elderly patients and was suggestive of tissue damage. The thyroid-stimulating hormone (TSH) response to administered thyroid-releasing hormone (TRH) is less age-dependent, but is not specific for depression and is quite variable in ageing persons (Targum *et al.* 1992).

Table 27.6 Neurotransmitter changes in depression and ageing: direction of change in key markers

Markers	Ageing	Depression
MHPG (NA)	↓	↑
β-receptors	↓	↑
α_2-receptors	↓ or normal	↑
5-HIAA (5-HT)	↑	↑
5-HT_2 receptors	↓	↑
HVA (DA)	↓	↓
MAO-B	↑	↑
Acetylcholine	↓	?

↑, Increased; ↓, decreased; NA, noradrenaline; DA, dopamine; MHPG, 3-methoxy-4-hydroxyphenylglycol; 5-HIAA: 5-hydroxy-indoleacetic acid; HVA: homovanilic acid; MAO-B: monoamine oxidase-B.

Recent studies of corticotropin-releasing hormone (CRH) have shown that CRH-mRNA levels in the paraventricular nucleus of elderly depressed patients are higher than the levels in Alzheimer's disease patients (also elevated), and very much higher than the normal controls (Raadsheer *et al.* 1995). This has led to speculation that hyperactivation of paraventricular CRH neurons may contribute to the aetiology of late-life depression

In summarizing this area of research, Schneider (1992) concludes that none of the neurochemical markers or neuroendocrine challenge tests mentioned are sufficiently sensitive or specific to be of clinical use in depressions of old age. However, meagre though the evidence is, the direction of reported changes is similar to depression in younger adult life.

Slowing of the alpha waves is the most common electroencephalographic (EEG) change recorded after the age of 60. Increases in waking alpha-rhythm amplitude have been reported consistently in depression (Schneider 1992) and can be distinguished from those seen in normal ageing and dementia. EEG variables measured during sleep show similar changes in both depression and normal ageing (Veith and Raskind 1988). These include similarities in night-time wakefulness, decreased slow-wave sleep, total rapid-eye movement (REM) sleep, and REM latency. Using discriminant function analysis, Reynolds *et al.* (1988*b*) found that four EEG sleep variables correctly differentiated depressed from demented elderly patients in 80% of cases. Lastly, Reynolds *et al.* (1990) showed that REM sleep deprivation produced different effects in elderly depressed patients, a comparison group with dementia, and normal controls; suggesting that depression psychopathology may accentuate age-related changes in sleep architecture.

Depression in old age and structural brain changes

More than 30 years ago, Felix Post wrote: '...subtle cerebral changes may make ageing persons increasingly liable to affective disturbance' (Post 1968). Recent renewed interest in this hypothesis has several strands. The first, the altered role of genetics, has been discussed. The relevance is that a reduction in the role of a key risk factor such as this ought to lead to a reduced prevalence of depression in later life. Since this does not seem to be the case, it suggests that something else, perhaps subtle brain damage, may be offsetting it. Second, biological and clinical markers have been described which may distinguish early- from late-onset depressions. These include a lower sedation threshold to barbiturates, both before and after treatment (Cawley *et al.* 1973); latency in auditory cortical evoked responses midway between demented patients and controls (Hendrickson *et al.* 1979); and a higher than expected rate of death from vascular causes (Kay and Bergmann 1966; Murphy *et al.* 1988).

The third source of evidence to support Post's hypothesis comes from neuroimaging. Jacoby and Levy (1980), using computed tomography (CT), compared findings over time in three groups: normal elderly controls, patients with senile dementia, and a group with depressive disorder. A subgroup of 9 of the original 41 depressed patients were identified as having ventricular enlargement, suggesting atrophy of the brain. They were characterized by being older, having a later age of onset of depression, a more 'endogenous' clinical picture, and a higher death rate from extracerebral causes at 2 years than the other 32 patients with depression (Jacoby *et al.* 1981). Ventricular dilatation has been associated with: cognitive dysfunction (Pearlson *et al.* 1989; Abas *et al.* 1990) which often runs true in future episodes of depression (Pearlson *et al.* 1989), a poor response to tricyclic drugs (Young *et al.* 1988), and an increase in mortality (Jacoby *et al.* 1981); suggesting that it is a meaningful finding.

More recent research using MRI has largely confirmed the CT findings with regard to atrophy, and has extended them. The literature has been summarized (Baldwin 1993; O'Brien *et al.* 1996). In brief, several recent studies (Coffey *et al.* 1990; Zubenko *et al.* 1990; Churchill *et al.* 1991; Rabins *et al.* 1991) have identified an unexpectedly high rate of particular brain changes (periventricular hyperintense areas, subcortical white matter lesions, and subcortical grey matter lesions, especially in the basal ganglia) in the brains of elderly depressed patients compared to age-matched control subjects.

The significance of these changes is controversial. First, it is unclear whether atrophy is a risk factor for depression or whether depression causes atrophy. For example, atrophy may be caused by hypercorticolism (O'Brien *et al.* 1996), and also by rather more mundane factors such as malnutrition and weight loss (Swayze *et al.* 1996). Though white matter change is commoner in elderly depressed patients, it is not confined to them or even to depression itself (Dolan *et al.* 1986; Morris and Rapaport 1990). Furthermore, white matter change is strongly age-related (Zubenko *et al.* 1990), and there are no normative data from community-dwelling older people. Many consider that these brain abnormalities are caused by vascular disease, giving rise to the so-called 'vascular depression hypothesis' of late-onset depressive disorder which is described below.

Functional brain changes in depression have also been reported. Bench *et al.* (1992) reported focal abnormalities in regional cerebral blood flow (rCBF) using positron emission tomography (PET) in middle-aged and elderly depressives. Reduced rCBF was found in the left anterior cingulate gyrus and left dorsolateral prefrontal cortex. However, additional abnormalities were apparent in a depressed subgroup with coexistent cognitive impairment—reduced flow to the left anterior medial prefrontal gyrus and increased flow to the cerebellar vermis. The cingulate gyrus shows the greatest functional decrease in rCBF with age (Martin *et al.* 1991), which lends some support to a biological basis for a proportion of depressions arising in later life. Furthermore, the dissociation in rCBF between depression-associated cognitive impairment and that seen in depression without such impairment is of particular interest to an understanding of depressive pseudodementia in elderly patients. Different functional pathways are presumably involved.

Single photon emission tomography (SPET) is a more readily accessible technique. Studies of elderly depressed patients are few, but they do support a general reduction in cerebral perfusion mainly, but not exclusively, to the frontal cortex (Sackeim *et al.* 1990; Upadhyaya *et al.* 1990; Philpot *et al.* 1993). Furthermore, the presence and severity of white matter hyperintensity as visualized on MRI correlates with reduced measures of subcortical white matter perfusion (Kobari *et al.* 1990). Although the direction of cause and effect is not clear, the evidence is suggestive that some of the MRI lesions visualized in late-life depressions may lead to functional brain disturbance.

There are methodological problems associated with SPET (Philpot *et al.* 1993), and no studies to date have assessed changes in perfusion longitudinally to establish whether abnormalities reflect state changes in depression or are trait phenomena. Finally, it is possible that dynamic imaging changes are diagnostically non-specific and instead are associated with certain types of psychopathology, for example delusions (Dolan *et al.* 1992). Functional MRI (David *et al.* 1994) may help resolve some but not all of these issues; however, there are no data at present for late-life depressive disorder.

Postmortem data on elderly depressed patients are sparse. Bowen *et al.* (1989) reported subtle serotonin receptor loss in a small series of autopsies of patients who had major depression in late life.

Two studies have demonstrated more neuronal loss in the locus coeruleus of demented patients with depression compared with those without depression (Zubenko and Moossy 1988; Forstl *et al.* 1992), suggesting a distinct pathological substrate for depression in these patients.

The vascular depression hypothesis (Table 27.7)

This hypothesis is based on a number of premises (which are discussed in more detail by Alexopoulos *et al.* 1997). First, patients with vascular disease have a high rate of depression. Second, diseases affecting blood vessels, such as stroke, hypertension, and diabetes, are associated with frequent white matter hyperintensities (WMH). Third, neurological diseases affecting the subcortex are associated with a high rate of depression. Fourth, late-onset depression may be

Table 27.7 Vascular depression hypothesis

Premises	Proposed features
• Vascular disorders are associated with depression	• Mainly late-onset
• Hyperintensities on MRI are associated with vascular disorder	• Reduced depressive ideation
• Subcortical disease is associated with depression	• Reduced insight
• Late-onset depression is associated with greater vascular disease and vascular risk	• More overall morbidity
• Late-onset depression is associated with more deep white matter abnormality than early-onset depression in later life	• Apathy and retardation
	• More cognitive impairment (particularly executive dysfunction)
	• Poorer recovery

associated with higher rates of vascular disease and vascular risk factors compared to early-onset depression in late life (Baldwin and Tomenson 1995) and with higher rates of WMH (Figiel *et al.* 1991; Greenwald *et al.* 1996). Conversely, if depressed patients with vascular disease are excluded from study, WMH is no more common in depressed patients than among healthy controls (Miller *et al.* 1994).

In 'vascular depression' damage to end-arteries supplying subcortical striatopallidothalamocortical pathways disrupts neurotransmitter circuitry involved in mood regulation and may thus cause or predispose to depression, even in the absence of genetic predisposition or significant psychosocial precipitants (Fujikawa *et al.* 1997).

However, as indicated, the significance of WMH is controversial and they may be found in a wide variety of non-vascular disorders such as hyodrocephalus, multiple sclerosis, Alzheimer's disease, and in normal ageing. Two recent studies of late-life depression (Kumar *et al.* 1997; Lyness *et al.* 1998) failed to demonstrate any relationship between cerebrovascular disease risk factors and depression severity, symptomatology, or brain volume measures. So, it cannot be assumed uncritically that visualized brain changes are caused by end-artery disease. Whether 'vascular' or not in aetiology, there is evidence implicating WMH and subcortical pathology in late-life depression with: subtypes of late-life depression such as psychotic depression and 'minor' depression; the presence of particular symptoms (reduced depressive ideation and increased psychomotor retardation); greater cognitive impairment; greater physical morbidity; a greater risk of ECT-induced delirium; and a poorer outcome to antidepressant treatment (summarized by Baldwin 1999).

The vascular hypothesis, although unproven, is an important aetiological concept as it lends itself to hypothesis-driven research that can be supported by modern neuroimaging techniques. It also has important implications for the treatment of depression. These include whether agents to reduce the risk of end-artery occlusion, such as aspirin, may be of use, as well as rehabilitative strategies designed to counter brain-based apathy and lack of motivation.

In summary, although elderly people share with younger adults many factors aetiologically relevant to depression, there is increasing evidence that structural change, perhaps vascular in nature, renders some people in later life vulnerable to depression.

Physical ill-health and depression

Community studies (Kennedy *et al.* 1990; Beekman *et al.* 1995; Prince *et al.* 1998) have shown a close association between the onset of depression and physical ill-health. Physical impairment may provoke a depressive disorder, which may in turn increase the degree of disability associated with the original physical impairment (Prince *et al.* 1998).

There are several mechanisms whereby physical disorder may lead to depression. The dementias, stroke, and Parkinson's disease are all associated with depression. Specific brain-based aetiologies have been proposed and some discussion of particular disorders follows later in this chapter. These more biologically oriented explanations may help us to understand how a depressive episode may arise in the setting of a particular medical (usually neurological) disorder. They are less helpful in clarifying the onset of depressive symptoms, which occur commonly in many illnesses, including non-neurological ones. The wide range of medical conditions, as well as hearing and visual deficits, which are associated with depression, as summarized in Table 27.8(a) (Eastwood and Corbin-Rifat 1987), suggests that the meaning of the illness for the sufferer is as important as the precise body system involved (Murphy 1982). Recently, Prince *et al.* (1998) have shown that handicap, the disadvantage in society imposed by a physical impairment and ensuing disability, is a key risk factor for depression in older people at home.

The highest prevalence of depressive disorders in older people is found in residential and nursing homes, medical wards for the elderly and among older people in receipt of extensive home care support (Ames 1988; Banerjee *et al.* 1996). The usual explanation is that this simply reflects the concentration of disablement found in these settings. However, the concept of handicap provides another perspective, as handicap is as much a societal issue as a medical one. Thus some care settings may lead to a disadvantage by depriving people of benefits which might be available to others with a similar level of disability who live in settings where more care, aides and adaptations are provided. Some care settings may therefore be aetiological agents for depression. This has implications for prevention.

Reference has already been made to specific diseases, some with occult presentation, which may predispose to severe depression (see Table 27.8(a)).

Medication

A large number of medications with effects on the central nervous system (Table 27.8(b)) has been associated with precipitating or perpetuating depression in later life. Probably these are

Table 27.8(a) Medical conditions that may cause organic depression

Medical conditions	
Endocrine/metabolic	**Occult carcinoma**
Hypo-/hyperthyroidism	Pancreas
Cushing's disease	Lung
Hypercalcaemia	
Subnutrition	**Chronic infections**
Neurosyphilis	Brucellosis
Pernicious anaemia	Neurocysticercosis
	Myalgic encephalomyelitis
Organic brain disease	AIDS
Cerebrovascular disease/stroke	
CNS tumours	
Parkinson's disease	
Alzheimer's disease and vascular dementia	
Multiple sclerosis	
Systemic lupus erythematosus	

Table 27.8(b) Central-acting drugs that may cause organic depression

Anti-hypertensive drugs	**Anti-parkinson**
Beta-blockers	L-dopa
Methyldopa	Amantadine
Reserpine	
Clonidine	
Tetrabenazine	
Nifedipine	
Psychiatric drugs	
Neuroleptics	
Benzodiazepines	
Steroids	
Analgesic drugs	**Miscellaneous**
Opioids	Sulfonamides
Indomethacin	Oral contraceptives
	Digoxin

implicated more in 'minor' than major depression. The true estimate is unknown but is almost certainly higher than generally recognized (Dhondt and Hooijer 1995).

Personality

Surprisingly little has been written about personality and depression. Roth (1955) believed that those with late-onset depressive disorder had more robust personalities than those with recurrent depression arising earlier in life. Reporting in 1972, Post too noted that severe depression was associated with less premorbid personality dysfunction than milder depression. However, differentiating features of the current illness from features of the premorbid personality can be very difficult, and even informants often provide biased accounts. Even so, both Bergmann (1978) and Post (1972) note that patients with predominantly neurotic symptom profiles of depression were often categorized as anxiety-prone individuals. Bergmann (1978), basing his argument on the influential work of Bowlby, suggests that perhaps satisfactory attachment behaviour in early life is a necessary prerequisite to adaptive coping, rather than non-adaptive anxiety, in the face of the very real threats that accompany old age. Furthermore, Post (1972) noted that obsessional traits were over-represented in his inpatient group. More structured techniques of assessing personality, for example derived from DSM-III (Abrams *et al.* 1987), suggest that personality dysfunction, especially of the 'avoidant' and 'dependent' types, is associated with late-life depression. Murphy (1982) found that a lifelong lack of a capacity for intimacy, in other words a personality variable, seemed to be a risk factor for depression in later life.

Social supports and intimacy

Some of the vulnerability factors for depression identified by Brown and Harris (1978) in their influential research are not relevant to the elderly. One potentially relevant one—loss of mother before 11 years of age—was not confirmed by Murphy (1982) in her study of depressed elderly patients.

Expressed differently, Murphy's data on the lack of capacity for intimacy suggests that a confidant may act as a buffer against those social losses implicated in the aetiology of depressive illness. However, not all research is in complete agreement over the issue of confidants. Thus, Henderson *et al.* (1986) found that elderly depressed people living at home did not report a lack of intimate relationships, although they did lack relationships of more diffuse support. The investigators used a different instrument from Murphy's so that direct comparison is difficult. In another study (Emmerson *et al.* 1989) it was men who more often reported poor or no confiding relationships. Indeed, so striking was the effect of an absence of a confidant that it almost eclipsed severe life events in the aetiology of depressive disorder, although life events were by no means unimportant. Further evidence that there may be gender differences in either the perception or availability of intimacy comes from a large Finnish study. Pahkala (1990) found that only females reported a relationship between (lack of) perceived intimacy with their spouse and depression.

The area is a difficult one. First, there is no consensus on the meaning or measurement of intimacy. Second, distinctions between objective and subjective measures of support are not always made. Subjective reports of support are liable to be influenced by lowered mood. Objective measures may not be capable of differentiating which 'supports' are healthy and which are not.

As a footnote, the increased realization in recent years that childhood sexual abuse often has severe and long-lasting damaging effects, including depression, should not be overlooked when treating elderly patients. One patient who presented to the author with a late-onset depressive disorder coloured by frequent panic attacks and nightmares revealed for the first time (to a female member of the team) that she had been abused by her brothers 60 years earlier. This became an important focus of her treatment.

Precipitating factors

Life events

A common-sense view is that life events are an obvious cause of depression in old age. However, if it were the case that adversity alone is sufficient to 'explain' depression then eventually all old people ought to fall victims to it. Since clearly the majority do not, how are we to understand the role of major life events in the aetiology of depression? As early as 1962 Post pointed out that around two-thirds of the patients studied by him had experienced a likely precipitating factor, usually an actual or threatened loss. Since then life events research has moved on from simple checklists to more sophisticated tools. The seminal work of Brown and Harris (1978) found that only the most severely threatening life events were related to depression. Extending the methodology of Brown and Harris to the elderly, Murphy (1982) found that 48% of a population of 119 people suffering from depressive disorder, as opposed to 23% of a control group, had experienced at least one severe life event in the preceding year. The events were threatening and often involved loss—such as the death of a loved one, life-threatening illness in somebody close, major financial problems, and enforced, peremptory removal from one's home. In addition, major social difficulties (as distinct from abrupt life events) lasting for 2 years or more were also significantly associated with depression.

Although Murphy's findings concerning life events were broadly in line with Brown's and Harris's younger subjects, one major difference that emerged was the conspicuous role of poor physical health among the elderly depressed group. This took the form of either a grave illness of recent onset, or a longer term seriously disabling one. A word of caution is necessary though. About 25% of Murphy's control group had experienced a major adverse event without the development of depression. Therefore, the relationship of depression to life events is only a statistical one. Not all adverse events are followed by depression; not all depressions are preceded by adverse life events. Thus an adverse life event and the onset of depressive disorder occurring within the same individual are not necessarily causally linked. Establishing the role of a major event for an individual patient rests on an adequate understanding of that person, based on a good history-taking. Otherwise, an uncritical acceptance of an adverse life event as a trigger for depression may result in a serious underlying organic illness being missed. Such was the near fate of a depressed, recently retired school teacher. A chest radiograph resulted in an abrupt change of emphasis in treatment—from retirement counselling to a pneumonectomy! That said, Table 27.9 lists the more typical antecedents and stressors associated with late-life depressive disorder.

Caregiving

This deserves special attention as a risk factor of depression, as there are opportunities for prevention, identification, and treatment. In one study (Ballard *et al.* 1996), 25% of carers of people with dementia were depressed, and many had persistent symptoms. Factors associated with depression in carers were depression and problem behaviours in the designated patient.

Management

Assessing the patient

Checklists of symptoms, as in ICD and DSM, are helpful, but from what has been discussed so far it is clear that a number of factors may modify clinical presentation in the older depressed patient,

Table 27.9 Precipitating factors in depression of later life

Life-events	Chronic stress
1. Bereavement	1. Declining health and mobility; dependence
2. Separation	2. Sensory loss, cognitive decline
3. Acute physical illness	3. Housing problems
4. Medical illness or threat to life of someone close	4. Major problems affecting family member
5. Sudden homelessness or having to move into an institution	5. Marital difficulties
6. Major financial crisis	6. Socioeconomic decline
7. Negative interactions with family member or friend	7. Problems at work; retirement
8. Loss of 'significant other' (including a pet)	8. Caring for a chronically ill and dependent family member

sometimes quite dramatically. A comprehensive history from both patient and informant often helps clarify areas of uncertainty in difficult cases. Evidence of whether there has been a recent change or not is often crucial. Other details include a family and personal history of depression. A full drug and alcohol history (sometimes only ascertained with certainty by conducting the assessment at the patient's home) must be obtained. Alcohol depresses mood when taken to excess. Treatment and response in previous depressive episodes, where relevant, should be clarified. Information about major adverse life events, for example bereavement and other losses such as ill-health, should be documented, along with the individual's previous capacity to cope with stressful situations and difficulties. This is a matter of personality. Personality traits may be difficult to assess but they are important in setting a realistic target for therapy. For example, an individual with longstanding dysthymic disorder may become severely depressed and require treatment, but restitution to a previous state of gloom is more realistic than trying to help the patient attain perfect happiness. Availability and (if possible) quality of supports from family, friends, neighbours, and both statutory and voluntary sectors are further important points to address in the history. These points are of aetiological relevance but they are also important in management.

A full mental state examination is necessary and care must be taken to elicit severe depressive symptomatology such as suicidal ideation and delusional phenomena. Evidence of cognitive impairment should be carefully documented so that comparisons can be made after recovery. Routine neuropsychiatric testing is not usually warranted unless dementia is suspected, and even then the findings might be equivocal. It is useful though to incorporate a screening measure such as the Mini-Mental State Examination (Folstein *et al.* 1975) into one's assessment. This samples several cognitive domains and not just memory. A physical examination should also be carried out. Ill-health is often the trigger for severe depression and is linked closely to prognosis. Also, depressive disorder may be precipitated by a large number of occult medical conditions and drugs (see Tables 27.8(a) and (b)) If implicated in the aetiology of a case of depression then the term 'organic depressive episode' is used in ICD-10. The mood symptoms may be just as severe as in an non-organic case but a clear aetiological role must be established for the disease or drug before the term is used. If in spite of these steps key elements of the assessment cannot be clarified, then admission will be needed, either as an inpatient or to a psychiatric day hospital where skilled psychiatric nursing observations will be needed.

Laboratory investigation should include haemoglobin and red blood cell indices, which may point to a possible vitamin B_{12} deficiency or alcohol excess. Vitamin B_{12} estimation should be undertaken in a first episode of depression. At the same time, folate levels should also be checked. It does not take long for undernutrition to develop in severe depression, and the folate level may be correspondingly low. Urea and electrolyte estimations are important for similar reasons. A low serum potassium level will lead to electroconvulsive therapy (ECT) being delayed; an elevated calcium level is occasionally associated with depression, as in primary hyperparathyroidism (Peterson 1968) or metastatic cancer. The guiding principle is an awareness that elderly people have less physiological reserve. Severe depression in a 75-year-old subject may lead to quite serious metabolic derangement that would be unlikely in a fit 40-year-old. Thyroid function testing should be performed because of the well-known association of depression with hypothyroidism, which may be overlooked in the elderly, and because 'apathetic hyperthyroidism' can be mistaken for depression. Table 27.10 summarizes those investigations appropriate for a first episode of depression and for a recurrence.

Regarding the electroencephalogram (EEG) there are no diagnostic changes specific to depression on the standard 12-lead EEG. The main benefit of an EEG clinically is to help differentiate depression from an organic brain syndrome. Other changes are discussed under 'Aetiology'.

Neuroimaging in affective disorders is largely performed to rule out a space-occupying lesion. However, O'Brien *et al.* (1994) found good discrimination between Alzheimer's disease and depressive illness using measures of temporal lobe atrophy on MRI. New technologies may eventually lead to their more routine use in depressive disorder. Currently though, a brain scan is only carried out in depressed patients if clinically indicated; for example, an atypical history with neurological symptoms, such as headache or visual change, or unexpected neurological findings.

Hypercorticolism is a well-known feature of depressive disorder. The dexamethasone suppression test (DST) measures activity of the hypothalamic-pituitary-adrenal axis. Non-suppression of cortisol after ingestion of dexamethasone is common in depression, and once seemed promising as a diagnostic tool for depression (Carroll *et al.* 1981). Unfortunately the DST has not lived up to expectations in general, and in old age psychiatry in particular the situation is even more complicated. Non-suppression gradually increases with age alone, particularly after 75 years (Blazer 1989) and the DST does not differentiate between dementia and depression in any reliable manner (Spar and Gerner 1982).

Tritiated-imipramine binding to platelets has been found to be altered in depressive illness. The lower numbers of binding sites in depressed patients seems relatively independent of age and less susceptible to interference by cognitive impairment (Nemeroff *et al.* 1988), giving it an advantage over the DST. However, this is still a research investigation. Clearly there is no test which can diagnose depression in late life, or is any real substitute for a proper history and mental state examination.

Another approach to diagnosis is the use of screening questionnaires. The most widely used rating instruments in depression are the Zung

Table 27.10 Investigations for depression in later life

Investigation	First episode	Recurrence
Full blood count	Yes	Yes
Urea and electrolytes	Yes	Yes
Calcium	Yes	Yes
Thyroid function	Yes	If indicated, or more than 12 months previously
Vitamin B_{12}	Yes	If indicated, or more than 12 months previously
Folate	Yes	If indicated by nutritional state
Liver function	Yes	If indicated (e.g. alcohol abuse)
Syphilitic serology	If neurologically indicated	Only if not already done
CT (brain)	If clinically indicated	Only if indicated
EEG	If clinically indicated	Only if indicated

Depression Rating Scale, which may require adjustment of its cut-off for 'caseness' in older people (Zung 1967), and the Beck Depression Inventory (Beck *et al.* 1961). Neither of these was designed specifically for use with elderly people and both use a multiple-choice format which some elderly people find confusing. For this reason rating scales that have been validated in older people are preferred. These include the Brief Assessment Schedule Depression Cards (BASDEC) (Adshead *et al.* 1992); the SelfCARE(D), which has been used in community surveys (Bird *et al.* 1987); and the Geriatric Depression Scale (GDS) (Yesavage *et al.* 1983). The BASDEC is unusual in comprising a 19-item deck of cards requiring yes/no responses. It is useful where privacy is hard to ensure, as on a medical ward, or where the person has significant expressive language problem, as pointing to either 'yes' or 'no' cards is all that is required.

The GDS is the most widely used self-rating scale. It avoids questions concerning physical depressive symptomatology, which are often poor discriminators between depression and physical ill-health, and instead focuses on the cognitive aspects of depressive disorder. It also has a simple 'yes/no' format. In the United Kingdom, the GDS has been endorsed for hospital use by the Royal College of Physicians and the British Geriatric Society (Royal College of Physicians 1992) and in primary care by the Royal College of General Practitioners (Williams and Wallace 1993).

Even so, the full version has 30 questions (Table 27.11) and the original validation was carried out on a physically fit group of patients with depressive disorder, some of whom were as young as 55 years. A cut-off score of 11 or above indicates probable depression. The same cut-off was found to give satisfactory sensitivity and specificity in hospitalized elderly patients with concurrent medical illness (Koenig *et al.* 1988; Jackson and Baldwin 1993). It loses specificity in severe dementia (Burke *et al.* 1989) but seems to perform reasonably well in dementia of mild to moderate severity (O'Riordan *et al.* 1990). New scales, for example the Cornell Scale for Depression in Dementia (Alexopoulos *et al.* 1988), have been introduced to address this difficult area. The latter incorporates information from a carer.

Shorter versions of the GDS have been introduced, including a 15-item version (Table 27.11) and a 4-item one, which utilizes questions 1, 3, 8, and 9 (Katona and Katona 1997).

It is important to place screening questionnaires in their proper context. They do not 'make' a diagnosis. In fact, their use requires careful thought. False-positives are bound to occur and could result in increased referrals to psychiatric services with all the ensuing worry and possible stigma. The answer is to ensure that non-psychiatrically trained personnel using scales such as the GDS are given proper training in their use and adequate support. With this proviso, instruments such as the GDS may have a useful role in settings such as geriatric wards and nursing homes where the prevalence of depressive disorder is high and detection generally poor. For example, Rapp and Davis (1989) demonstrated poor knowledge of the key features of depression in elderly patients among junior medical staff on geriatric wards. Not surprisingly, the rate of detecting depressive illness by these doctors was very low (only 2 cases out of 23 identified by the authors). Rapp and Davis argue that the routine use of a scale such as the GDS would improve the detection of depression in medical wards considerably. They contrast the lack of use of such scales for depression with the routine use by physicians of screening instruments for dementia. Of course even successful detection does not guarantee adequate treatment, but where detection rates improve treatment generally improves too.

Pharmacotherapy

Principles of prescribing

Alterations in pharmacodynamics and kinetics with age mean that many, but not all, antidepressants should be given in lower dosages with advancing years. Furthermore, greater interindividual variation in drug-handling can lead to unpredictable patterns of response and side-effects, especially with the older drugs. For the older antidepressants, in particular, the adage 'start low—go slow' is apt. Probably related to pharmacodynamics, older people often take

Table 27.11 Geriatric Depression Scale

Instructions: Choose the best answer for how you have felt over the past *week*.

1.	**Are you basically satisfied with your life?**	No
2.	**Have you dropped many of your activities and interests?**	Yes
3.	**Do you feel your life is empty?**	Yes
4.	**Do you often get bored?**	Yes
5.	Are you hopeful about the future?	No
6.	Are you bothered by thoughts you can't get out of your head?	Yes
7.	**Are you in good spirits most of the time?**	No
8.	**Are you afraid something bad is going to happen to you?**	Yes
9.	**Do you feel happy most of the time?**	No
10.	**Do you often feel helpless?**	Yes
11.	Do you often get restless and fidgety?	Yes
12.	**Do you prefer to stay at home, rather than going out and doing new things?**	Yes
13.	Do you frequently worry about the future?	Yes
14.	**Do you feel you have more problems with your memory than most?**	Yes
15.	**Do you think it is wonderful to be alive now?**	No
16.	Do you often feel down-hearted and blue (sad)?	Yes
17.	**Do you feel pretty worthless the way you are?**	Yes
18.	Do you worry a lot about the past?	Yes
19.	Do you find life very exciting?	No
20.	Is it hard for you to start on new projects (plans)?	Yes
21.	**Do you feel full of energy?**	No
22.	**Do you feel that your situation is hopeless?**	Yes
23.	**Do you think most people are better off (in their lives) than you are?**	Yes
24.	Do you frequently get upset over little things?	Yes
25.	Do you frequently feel like crying?	Yes
26.	Do you have trouble concentrating?	Yes
27.	Do you enjoy getting up in the morning?	No
28.	Do you prefer to avoid social gatherings (get-togethers)?	Yes
29.	Is it easy for you to make decisions?	No
30.	Is your mind as clear as it used to be?	No

Notes: (1) Answers refer to responses which score '1'; (2) bracketed phrases refer to alternative ways of expressing the questions; (3) questions in bold comprise the 15-item version. Cut-off scores for possible depression: ≥ 11 (GDS30); ≥ 5 (GDS15); ≥ 2 (GDS4).

longer to respond to treatment than younger patients. Whereas in younger people 4 weeks might be regarded as an adequate trial of therapy, 6 or even 8 weeks is more realistic in older people.

The type of depression is important. First, there is good evidence that psychotic depression requires either a combined approach with both antidepressant and antipsychotic drugs or ECT (Baldwin 1988*b*). Second, there is some evidence that at the more severe end of the spectrum, tricyclic antidepressants are more effective than selective serotonin-reuptake inhibitors (Roose *et al.* 1994). Third, current antidepressants are only indicated for major depressive episode. However, there is an emerging literature, not yet large enough to make definite recommendations, that they may be effective in so-called minor depression.

Antidepressants can be classified as in Table 27.12.

With 19 antidepressants listed in Table 27.12 (at the time of writing reboxetine is not recommended for elderly patients because of insufficient efficacy data) it is important to have a general principle when faced with such a large choice. It is therefore best to match the antidepressant to the patient, taking account of tolerability, safety, side-effects, drug interactions, and contraindications. Although newer antidepressants, especially the selective serotonin-

Table 27.12 Classification of antidepressants

Class	Examples
Older tricyclics	Secondary amines (nortriptyline, desipramine) Tertiary amines (imipramine, amitriptyline, dosulepin (dothiepin), clomipramine)
Newer tricyclics	Lofepramine
Atypical antidepressants	Trazodone, nefazodone, mianserin
Monoamine oxidase inhibitors (non-reversible) (MAOIs)	Phenelzine
Reversible inhibitors of monoamine oxidase A (RIMAs)	Moclobemide
Selective serotonin-reuptake inhibitors (SSRIs)	Fluvoxamine, fluoxetine, paroxetine, sertraline, citalopram
Noradrenaline and specific serotonin enhancers (NASSe)	Mirtazapine
Noradrenaline reuptake inhibitors (NARI)	Reboxetine
Serotonin/noradrenaline-reuptake inhibitors (SNRI)	Venlafaxine

reuptake inhibitors (SSRIs) are often recommended as first-line treatment for depressive disorder in older people, it is unwise to dismiss the tricyclics out of hand. Argument for the virtual abandonment of tricyclics in favour of newer drugs on safety grounds, notably in overdosage (Beaumont 1989), seem to place drug profiles ahead of clinical considerations. It may lead to a complacent attitude to suicide risk, which must be properly managed. Nevertheless, the point is well made that casual, often half-hearted and poorly supervised prescribing of potentially lethal drugs such as tricyclic drugs is to be deplored (Beaumont 1989).

Special considerations

Sometimes it is difficult to pigeon-hole patients into one category of depression or another. If this is the case, it can be helpful to see the patient several times over a period of a few weeks or to enlist a community psychiatric nurse (CPN) to assess the patient over a period of time. In some patients, particularly those with milder symptoms involving a clear triggering life event, depression resolves spontaneously. An alternative to this 'wait and see' approach is to conduct a therapeutic trial of an antidepressant. Once antidepressants have been prescribed at the therapeutic dosage the patient's mood should be reassessed not less than 3–4 weeks later. At that point if there has been a response, or a partial response, the antidepressant should be continued with a review of the dosage to ensure it is optimal. If there has been little or no response at 3–4 weeks the antidepressant should be changed or augmentation introduced. This is discussed later (see 'resistant depression'). At all stages of treatment, the tolerability, side-effects, compliance, and the possibility of psychosocial influences that may maintain the patient in an invalid role should be monitored. Lastly, although controlled trials are lacking, the best results come from combining drug treatment with psychological intervention (Chiu *et al.* 1999; Reynolds *et al.* 1999).

Some of the symptoms of bereavement overlap with those of depressive illness, so this provides a good example of how to weigh up symptoms which may or may not require pharmacological treatment. Clayton (1982) makes some important points. First, the clinician always has a duty to relieve suffering. Where this takes the form of severe and enduring affective symptoms arising during bereavement then short-term relief with pharmacotherapy may be justified. It is also not uncommon for specific symptoms, for example insomnia, to be treated with an hypnotic for a matter of a few weeks. Longer use obviously risks dependency, but there is also a concern that centrally-acting drugs given for long periods might cause sufficient befuddling as to interfere with the natural processes of bereavement. The decision to treat will invariably be based on the particulars of the case. However, certain features point more clearly towards depressive disorder and hence to a consideration of antidepressants. First, the bereaved individual may have begun to make progress over the first few months only to slip back for no apparent reason. Second, the presence of suicidal thoughts, pervasive guilt (not merely remorse over what more might have been done to prevent death), retardation, and 'mummification' —maintaining grief by keeping everything unchanged—suggest the presence of depressive disorder.

Antidepressants should not be prescribed in a manner that renders the patient passive. Although there has been a decided move away from medical paternalism over recent decades, this is probably less true for elderly people, many of whom remain somewhat in awe of their doctors. Numbers of them will discreetly throw their antidepressants into the rubbish bin or retain them neatly in their bottles or sealed packages, rather than risk offending the doctor by saying they do not consider tablets to be the answer to their depression. Building a partnership with the patient is therefore crucial. This begins with an explanation that depression warranting treatment with tablets is an illness, and that it is common, treatable, and not a sign of moral weakness. Many patients need reassurance that the tablets they will be asked to take are not addictive, and that depression is not 'senility' or a harbinger of dementia. They should be involved in the treatment. They need to be told, in layman's terms, why they should not expect immediate results. They and the clinician should agree on a plan of treatment. For example, a patient should be informed that antidepressants will relieve their depressive symptoms, but that further help to manage anxiety or address a bereavement, for example, is also indicated. Nowadays, almost all psychiatrists specializing in the care of older people work as part of a multidisciplinary team. A 'key worker' from this team should be appointed who can coordinate the care delivered and act as a point of contact for the patient and family. Besides then being multimodal, the treatment of later life depression should also be multidisciplinary.

Efficacy

Numerous antidepressant drug trials have demonstrated the superiority of antidepressants over placebo, but most of these have been conducted on younger patients. The National Institutes of Health (NIH) Consensus Development Panel on Depression in Late Life (Schneider *et al.* 1994, p. 181) found only a few double-blind, placebo-controlled trials, mostly of the traditional tricyclics. Numbers of those aged over 65 completing double-blind trials of antidepressant drugs were: nortriptyline (229); amitriptyline (181); doxepin (66); imipramine (53). These are modest numbers. Gerson has summarized the position with regard to the older antidepressants in the elderly: 'Drugs are clearly superior to placebo; they show comparable therapeutic efficacy, about 50% improvement in Hamilton scores versus 20–25% improvement on placebo; and all of them have undesirable side-effects' (Gerson 1985).

Studies of newer antidepressants have involved comparison against established drugs, such as the older tricyclics, mianserin or trazodone. Few have included a placebo arm and it is unlikely that any future drug trials will do so, because it is improbable that ethical committees will sanction such studies given the known superiority of medication over placebo. The published literature suggests that the newer drugs are as effective as the older ones, and this is supported by a meta-analysis of antidepressants in older people which concluded that efficacy was similar across all classes of antidepressants (Mittman *et al.* 1997).

However, research sponsored by drug companies usually excludes the typical patient seen by old age psychiatrists—the very old and frail. When side-effect profiles of the older tricyclic reference compounds are compared with newer drugs used in elderly people, we see not so much a dramatic reduction in side-effects with the latter but a different, possibly more benign, pattern. For example, Cohn *et al.* (1990) compared sertraline with amitriptyline in elderly patients over 8 weeks: 161 versus 80 patients, respectively. The mean age was 71 years. Some 28% of those treated with sertraline compared to 35% treated with amitriptyline withdrew because of side-effects. The difference, whilst significant, is rather modest and the figures indicate a high level of drug intolerance in both groups. Now 16 years on, and with a host of newer antidepressants, the perceptive remark of Gerson (1985) still holds true: '...the choice of drug is based on side-effect profiles and potential drug-drug interactions rather than on degree of therapeutic efficacy'.

The main mode of action for the most commonly available antidepressants is listed in column two of Table 27.15. This is not an exact science. For example, tricyclics act on more than one neurotransmitter system; they are certainly not pure norepinephrine (noradrenaline) reuptake inhibitors. The tricyclic clomipramine is in fact a potent serotonin reuptake inhibitor. Lofepramine is metabolized to desimipramine, a secondary amine tricyclic antidepressant.

Moclobemide is as effective as traditional tricyclics and tetracyclics (De Vanna al 1990; Tiller *et al.* 1990). It also compares favourably with SSRIs (Bocksberger *et al.* 1993) when used in elderly people, and, like SSRIs, requires no dose adjustment for age. It does not need dietary intervention. Venlafaxine is the first of another new class of antidepressant, serotonin and norepinephrine reuptake inhibitor (SNRI). It is, in effect, a 'belt and braces' drug, causing re-uptake inhibition in both noradrenergic and serotonergic systems. A study comparing it to dosulepin (dothiepin) in subjects aged over 64 showed similar response rates—60% in each arm (Mahapatra and Hackett 1997). Its side-effect profile is similar to that of the SSRIs, although both hypertension and postural hypotension may occur in older patients. Like most of the SSRIs, dosages require no adjustment for older patients. Mirtazapine is another interesting new agent as it appears to enhance both noradrenergic and serotonergic function via antagonism at the presynaptic α_2 receptor. Differences in pharmacodynamics and kinetics are minimal with age. One acute treatment trial against amitriptyline in older patients showed comparable effect and tolerability (Hoyberg *et al.* 1996). The side-effect profile is similar to tricyclics; weight gain and sedation can be troublesome, although initially useful when the patient has a poor appetite and has lost a considerable amount of weight. Nefazodone is an inhibitor of serotonin reuptake and also blocks postsynaptic 5-HT_2 receptors. Dose adjustment for older patients may be needed. There are few data pertaining to older depressed patients. Sedation can be a problem but sexual dysfunction is rare, making it a useful alternative to SSRIs in this respect.

L-tryptophan is not an effective antidepressant on its own. However, it had an important role as an adjunctive therapy in treatment-resistant depression until its withdrawal because of an association with the eosinophilic-myalgic syndrome. It can still be prescribed, subject to certain restrictions.

Efficacy in special patient groups

Elderly patients with dementia

Reifler *et al.* (1989) reported improvement in depression in 28 elderly patients with underlying Alzheimer's disease in a trial of imipramine, mean dosage 80 mg, lasting 8 weeks, but comparable improvement was also noted in a placebo group! Of the newer drugs, Hebenstreit *et al.* (1991) demonstrated significant therapeutic efficacy of moclobemide (400 mg) over placebo in 726 elderly patients with unspecified dementia who were also depressed. Postma and Vranesic (1985) described 10 depressed patients with dementia who responded well to moclobemide at a much lower dose (maximum 225 mg). A significant response rate was also reported by Roth *et al.* (1996) in a large sample size of 511 using moclobemide against placebo in patients with and without dementia. Of note, some improvement in cognitive function was seen in patients who were depressed with low baseline cognitive function. Similar findings have been reported for the SSRI citalopram (Nyth *et al.* 1992). The study of Reifler *et al.* (1989) highlights how high the placebo rate is for recovery of depressive symptoms in dementia. The practical message seems to be that moderate and severe depressive symptoms should be treated with antidepressants in those with dementia, but in milder cases it is often better to offer support to the patient and carers; in many cases the symptoms will improve within a month.

Depression associated with general systemic disease

There is no evidence that antidepressants are effective in patients with acute physical illness (Chiu *et al.* 1999). However, they are more effective in chronic stable illness in the elderly, although poor tolerability occurs in about a third of cases (Lipsey 1984). To emphasize the point, Koenig *et al.* (1989) had to abandon a proposed drug trial using nortriptyline in physically ill older patients because virtually all of them had contraindications or were intolerant of the drug.

If the newer antidepressants have anything to offer it is surely in the area of patients seriously compromised by physical illnesses which preclude treatment with traditional drugs. Yet there is little systematic evaluation of them in this setting. The SSRI fluoxetine was found to be more effective than placebo in one recent study; and interestingly it was as effective or possibly even more effective the more severe the underlying physical condition (Evans *et al.* 1997). The drug was well tolerated in a range of serious medical disorders, many grave. However, Roose *et al.* (1994) found that 22 depressed patients (mean age of 73 years) with heart disease responded less well to fluoxetine than 42 comparable patients treated with nortriptyline (mean age 70). Indeed only 5 of the 22 fluoxetine-treated patients responded; those with melancholic subtype of major depression (the majority) did especially poorly. The number of drop-outs in each group was similar.

So although the newer antidepressants appear to have a niche here, their advantage in physically compromised patients is not all that convincing.

Depression in people living in residential and nursing homes

The detection and management of depression in frail elderly people in residential and nursing homes is often poor. In a placebo-controlled study of nortriptyline a significant effect was seen, but a third of those entered could not tolerate the drug (Katz *et al.* 1990). In an open-labelled study of SSRIs in a similar setting, which included very old subjects, the response rate to major depression was poor in subjects with depression complicating dementia (Trappler and Cohen 1998). Given the high prevalence of depressive symptoms in care settings and the high rate of intolerance to older antidepressants it would seem prudent to avoid the oldest antidepressants and proceed cautiously with newer agents such as the SSRIs.

Side-effects

The cardiotoxicity of tricyclic drugs has probably been exaggerated. Minor electrocardiographic ischaemia, an uncomplicated myocardial infarct at least 3 months old, or even heart failure, provided it is stable (Glassman *et al.* 1983), are not of themselves definite contraindications. Nevertheless, a tricyclic should not be given to patients with a known tendency to either a tachy- or bradyarrhythmia, bundle-branch block, those with abnormal QT interval syndromes (Cohen-Cole and Stoudemire 1987), or where heart failure is poorly controlled. Newer drugs have been shown to be safer in healthy subjects, but some trials exclude the elderly and very few studies have been conducted on people with heart disease. In the absence of such information it is unwise to assume uncritically that newer antidepressants are totally safe in patients with heart disease.

The main problem when tricyclics are given to the elderly is that they often cause postural hypotension, which may lead to unpleasant dizziness or dangerous falls. Secondary amine tricyclics are generally safer in this respect than tertiary drugs. Those with poor left ventricular function are most at risk, as are patients taking diuretics, on antihypertensive medication, or with left bundle-branch block. Lying and standing blood pressure should be measured before starting treatment. In the USA an electrocardiogram is recommended prior to treatment with tricyclics. Delirium is an occasional problem, more so in medically compromised patients.

The main side-effects of the older tricyclics are summarized in Table 27.13.

Lofepramine has minimal anticholinergic effects and a good safety record, although there has been some concern about occasional disturbance of liver function (Committee on Safety of Medicines 1988).

Of the atypical antidepressants, mianserin again has few anticholinergic or adverse cardiovascular effects, at least in normal individuals, but it is quite sedative. Unfortunately, concerns over blood dyscrasias necessitating regular blood counts make it inconvenient to use. Trazodone, another novel non-tricyclic drug, also has sedative properties and a good safety record, making it a useful alternative. There have been occasional reports of priapism.

The side-effects of the SSRIs are shown in Table 27.14.

The main metabolite of fluoxetine is clinically active and remains so for approximately a week, possibly longer for older patients. Obviously this is important in anticipating side-effects, although it also makes fluoxetine a *de facto* sustained-release preparation, a sort of 'depot' antidepressant; however, it is not licensed for use in this way. It also means that the drug must be discontinued for at least 5 weeks before an older monoamine oxidase inhibitor can be used.

Some members (thus far fluoxetine, fluvoxamine, paroxetine, and to some degree citalopram) have proved to be inhibitors of hepatic enzymic oxidation (cytochrome P450 2D6—debrisoquine hydrochloride (Crewe *et al.* 1992)). These drugs can alter the pharmacokinetics of other, hepatically oxidized drugs, leading to drug interactions. Drugs metabolized by this enzyme, and hence likely to be affected by these new antidepressants are: tricyclic antidepressants and trazodone; neuroleptics; lipophilic beta-blockers (e.g. metoprolol); some antiarrhythmics, and triazolobenzodiazepines, such as alprazolam. About 7% of Caucasians lack P450 2D6 because of a genetic mutation. The combination of a tricyclic with an SSRI was recently quite popular but is not without risk of elevating tricyclic levels into the toxic range. A particular problem arises from the long half-lives of fluoxetine and its main metabolite.

For moclobemide the side-effect profile seems relatively benign, although nausea, dizziness, headache, agitation, and insomnia may occur. The latter two side-effects may require the co-prescription of a benzodiazepine for the first 2 weeks of treatment. The dosage should be halved if cimetidine is used; and dosages of ibuprofen should be reduced. Codeine and pethidine analgesia should be avoided and care must be taken with co-prescriptions of tricyclics and

Table 27.14 Side-effects of SSRIs

Nausea (around 15%)
Diarrhoea (around 10%)
Insomnia (5–15%)
Anxiety/agitation (2–15%)
Sexual dysfunction (up to 30% in younger people)
Headache
Weight loss

Table 27.13 Tricyclic side-effects

Anticholinergic	Antihistaminic	Antiadrenergic
Dry mouth	Oversedation	Postural hypotension
Blurred vision	Weight gain	
Constipation		
Urinary retention		
Cardiotoxicity		
Delirium		

SSRIs. Few interactions have been reported though (Amrein 1992). A wash-out period of around 4–5 half-lives of the drug and any active metabolite is advised when transferring from a tricyclic or SSRI to moclobemide (but not from moclobemide to a tricyclic or SSRI).

Behavioural toxicity (affecting vigilance, reaction times, etc.) has been largely ignored among elderly people. Now that so many older people drive and pursue other activities demanding high levels of vigilance, this must be taken more seriously. Sherwood and Hindmarch (1993) found that among five commonly prescribed antidepressants lofepramine, fluoxetine, and paroxetine had more favourable profiles with respect to measures of skilled performance, thought to reflect everyday activities, than amitriptyline and dosulepin (dothiepin). Very little is known about behavioural and cognitive toxicity in relation to blood levels. However, age-related changes in the metabolism of these drugs (including the increased variability in serum levels among older subjects compared to younger ones), the greater likelihood of being on concurrent medication causing adverse reactions, and the increased susceptibility of the elderly brain to delirium are all reasons why such toxicity may be more common in elderly depressives. In one study, patients with antidepressant levels in excess of 450 ng/ml were very much more likely to develop adverse behavioural or cognitive changes than those within the therapeutic range (Meador-Woodruff *et al.* 1988). The adverse events were mainly subacute delirious states or psychomotor agitation.

A profile of side-effects by three biochemical systems for the main antidepressants in use in Great Britain is shown in Table 27.15.

The adage 'start low—go slow' is especially appropriate when using tricyclic antidepressants. Suggested *starting* doses are given in Table 27.15, in accordance with *British national formulary* guidelines.

Initial anticholinergic symptoms often subside after a few days and dosages of tricyclic agents can be increased every four or five days. For tricyclic antidepressants the effective dose in the elderly is roughly half the adult dose (Table 27.15). However, depression at all ages is frequently undertreated and sometimes elderly patients will require dosages as high as younger ones, if tolerated. The dose-response curve of imipramine is linear, so that if there is no benefit at 75 mg the dose can be increased to tolerance; the dose-response relationship is less clear with amitriptyline. Nortriptyline has a 'therapeutic window' reflected in serum levels of between 80 and 120 ng/ml (Schneider *et al.* 1994, p. 246). Some of the newer antidepressants, such as mianserin, most of the SSRIs, venlafaxine, mirtazapine, and moclobemide often require no dose adjustment in older people. Patients and relatives should be warned that the antidepressant effects may not be apparent for 10 to 14 days, otherwise compliance is less likely.

Psychotic (delusional) depressive disorder rarely responds to an antidepressant alone and requires either an antidepressant/neuroleptic combination or ECT (Baldwin 1988*b*).

A successful outcome is unlikely if little no response at all has occurred within 4 weeks, assuming adequate dosage and compliance (Table 27.16). Most responders will have improved within 3 to 4 weeks of being on a therapeutic dosage of the chosen antidepressant. For tricylics, serum monitoring may help determine compliance. If no worthwhile improvement has occurred most clinicians switch to an antidepressant from another class, although augmentation or even ECT is preferable if the patient is severely depressed. If, however, some improvement has occurred it is worth persisting for another 2–4 weeks, provided the patient is involved in the discussion, is supported by the clinical team, and his or her condition does not warrant more urgent intervention. Elderly depressed patients take longer to recover. One study (Georgotas and McCue 1989) found still further improvement when the treatment course was extended to 9 weeks. If this strategy is ineffective then the next choices are either to give ECT or to augment with lithium therapy. The use of depression severity scales, such as the Montgomery Asberg Depression Rating Scale or the Hamilton Rating Scale for Depression, could strengthen this approach by documenting degrees of improvement (or lack of it). Continuation treatment will be discussed later.

Table 27.15 Side-effect profiles and dosages of the main antidepressants available in the UK

Drug	Main mode of action	Anticholinergic	Antihistaminic	α_1-adrenergic block	Starting dose (mg)	Average daily dose (mg)
Amitriptyline	NA++ 5-HT+	++++	++++	++++	25–50	75–100
Imipramine	NA++ 5-HT+	+++	++	+++	25	75–100
Nortripyline	NA++ 5-HT+	+++	++	++	10 tds	75–100
Dosulepin	NA++ 5-HT+	+++	++	++	50–75	75–125
Mianserin	α_2	0/+	+++	0/+	30	30–90
Lofepramine	NA++ 5-HT+	+	+	+	70–140	70–210
Trazodone	5-HT_2	0	+++	+	100	300
Fluvoxamine	5-HT	0/+	0/+	0	50–100	100–200
Sertraline	5-HT	0/+	0	0	50	50–100
Fluoxetine	5-HT	0/+	0	0	20	20
Paroxetine	5-HT	0/+	0	0	20	20–30
Citalopram	5-HT	0/+	0	0	20	20–40
Moclobemide	MAO	0/+	0	0	300	300–400
Venlafaxine	NA+ 5-HT++	0/+	0	0/+	75	150
Mirtazepine	α_2 5-HT_2	0	++	0	30	30
Nefazodone	5-HT_2	0	+	+	50 bid	200

Numbered + to ++++ by degree of effect; NA, noradrenaline (norepinephrine); 5-HT, 5-hydroxytryptamine (serotonin). tds, three times a day; bid, twice a day

Table 27.16 Strategy for initiating and continuing antidepressants

- If little or no response (< 25% change in symptoms) by 4 weeks:
  - Increase the dose *OR* if dosage optimal
  - Change to another antidepressant (switch class)
- If partial response (25–50% change in symptoms) by 4 weeks:
  - Increase dose (if possible)
  - Carry on for a further 2–4 weeks
- If little further improvement:
  - Augment *OR*
  - Switch to another class
- At any stage ECT may be the preferred option

Electroconvulsive therapy (ECT)

Unfortunately ECT remains a controversial treatment, largely from its misuse several decades ago. However since its introduction in 1938, ECT has remained the most effective treatment for depression, with a recovery rate of approximately 80% in acute-phase treatment. It is as effective in older people as any other age group and is effective and well tolerated in the 'old-old' (Tew *et al.* 1999). ECT is the treatment of choice for patients whose lives are threatened by food and/or fluid refusal, profound retardation, or suicidal behaviour. It is highly effective for delusional (psychotic) depression (Baldwin 1988*a*). Both anaesthetic technique and the delivery of the electrical impulse have improved over recent years.

Symptoms predicting a positive response to ECT are similar at all ages, generally favouring patients with melancholic symptomatology (guilt, agitation, marked loss of interest, worthlessness, and delusions), but in addition older depressed patients with marked anxiety appear to respond (Benbow 1989). Patients with dementia and depression can be given ECT (Godber *et al.* 1987) but post-ECT delirium is a greater risk

Experts are divided regarding electrode placement. Some prefer unilateral electrode placement to avoid the risk of memory problems in older patients. Others argue that unilateral placement is less effective than bilateral and that, in any case, memory impairment, whilst measurably worse with bilateral treatment, may not be of clinical significance (Benbow 1989). A compromise is to start with unilateral placement and continue with bilateral if there has been no response after four to six treatments.

The contraindications to ECT are all relative. If it is given as a life-saving procedure it may be used even if hazardous physical illness is present, although the patient's physical condition should be optimized and the anaesthetist must be a senior clinician. It is best avoided within 3 months of a stroke or myocardial infarction or if pulmonary reserve (as assessed on pulmonary function testing) is gravely compromised. Since most complications are cardiovascular (Benbow 1989) uncontrolled hypertension or heart failure and a predisposition to serious arrhythmia should be carefully assessed and treated. Aortic or carotid aneurysms also require careful assessment. Cerebral oedema from, say, a tumour, should first be treated with steroids. Because they bind irreversibly to receptors, monoamine oxidase inhibitors should be discontinued at least 10 days prior to commencement of ECT, although in emergencies anaesthetists are unlikely to insist on this. A cardiac pacemaker is not a contraindication, provided the patient is totally insulated and no-one touches him or her during the electrical impulse. Careful physical examination remains the most important method of screening (Abramczuk and Rose 1979) with referral, as appropriate, to relevant specialists.

Benzodiazepines should either be discontinued or reduced to the lowest dose possible because of their anticonvulsant effect. The advice of the local consultant psychiatrist responsible for ECT should be obtained if the patient is receiving antidepressants or lithium, as different departments have different policies.

Pharmacological treatment of resistant depression

At least a third of patients fail to respond to monotherapy, as defined by 4–6 weeks of a single antidepressant in a therapeutic dosage (Dinan 1993). Guscott and Grof (1991) have proposed a systematic approach in which key questions are posed before augmentation regimes or electroconvulsive therapy (ECT) are contemplated (Table 27.17). Thus, the diagnosis should be reviewed; for example, an older depressed patient quietly harbouring psychotic thoughts will not recover with an antidepressant alone. Treatment adequacy, duration of treatment (at a therapeutic dose), compliance with treatment, psychosocial reinforcers, and side-effects should all be re-evaluated, (Table 27.17) taking an overview of the patient. Improvement on a rating scale may not go hand in hand with social and functional recovery.

The stepped-care part of this approach rests on the clinician using a framework of treatment based on logical, evidence-based protocols. There is insufficient evidence to confidently recommend one strategy over another. However, those recommended include increasing the dosage, particularly for the tricyclics, changing from one class of antidepressant to another (for example, a tricyclic to an SSRI or *vice versa*), augmentation with various agents (lithium (see below) being the one with the most evidence), combining a tricyclic with a neuroleptic, ECT, or, *in extremis*, psychosurgery. Class-switching remains the most popular strategy, although controlled trial data are remarkably sparse. The best evidence is for ECT and lithium augmentation. All the commonly prescribed antidepressants can be combined with lithium, but there is a risk of a serotonin syndrome with SSRIs

Lithium augmentation

Although ECT remains the most effective remedy for severe depression, lithium augmentation has become an accepted alternative for the management of resistant cases (reviewed by Baldwin 1996). Of published studies some reported response rates of only 20% and 23%, much lower than open studies of younger adults. There have been no double-blind, placebo-controlled trials of augmentation therapy in elderly patients. The issue of the optimum dose of lithium in lithium augmentation has not been settled. In the absence of clear evidence it is best to keep within a range of 0.35 to 0.7 mmol/l for serum lithium concentrations.

Foster (1992) reviewed the use of lithium in elderly patients and found that non-toxic side-effects are common. For example, polydipsia occurred in 50–74%, polyuria 25–58%, tremor 33–58%, dry mouth 53%, nausea 33%, and memory impairment 33%. Of concern was Foster's finding that the frequency of acute lithium toxicity appears to be in the range of 11 to 23% for elderly patients.

Monoamine oxidase inhibitors

Georgotas *et al.* (1983) gave phenelzine (15–75 mg per day) to 20 elderly patients with refractory depression and obtained a 65% recovery rate. This was an unusually chronically ill group and

Table 27.17 A systematic approach to resistant depression

- Is the diagnosis correct?
- Was treatment adequate (duration, dose, compliance)?
- Has a stepped-care pharmacological approach been used?
- Has the outcome been measured appropriately?
- Has medical and/or psychiatric comorbidity been addressed?
- Are there factors in the treatment setting (including psychosocial reinforcers) that have been overlooked?

Taken from Guscot and Grof 1991 with permission.

many older patients cannot tolerate MAOIs. Likewise, the once fashionable combination of a heterocyclic antidepressant with a MAOI is potentially dangerous and has never been tested in an elderly patient group. Whether the newer reversible MAOI, moclobemide, will prove to be helpful in resistant cases remains to be seen.

Combination therapies: SSRI plus a tricyclic

This combination was quite fashionable. Seth *et al.* (1992) gave a fluoxetine/nortriptyline combination to eight, mainly elderly, refractory depressives. All improved. However, as has been discussed, both fluoxetine and the tricyclics are hepatically demethylated. Fluoxetine (and other SSRIs) competitively inhibits this process so there is a danger of toxic tricyclic levels developing. This effect may be aggravated and prolonged by the very long half-life of fluoxetine's main metabolite. Also, if there is benefit to the combination it may merely result from the increased serum level of the tricyclic agent. Newer antidepressants such as venlafaxine, with their dual role, are now a more logical choice.

L-Tryptophan augmentation

L-Tryptophan has not been validated as a combination therapy in the elderly. It can now be prescribed again subject to certain restrictions. In the United Kingdom these are:

(1) refractory depression (of duration greater than 2 years);
(2) available only to a hospital specialist;
(3) only to be used as adjunctive treatment;
(4) failed standard treatment;
(5) regular blood tests after 3 months and then 6 monthly, if given long term (with Merck's own 'OPTICS' monitoring).

Psychological approaches to management

Counselling

This may well be more appropriate for managing depressive symptoms accompanying change, stress, threat or loss to the individual. A good example is that of bereavement, and it is worthwhile having at least one member of the team trained in bereavement work. However, depressive disorder should first be optimally treated.

Psychotherapy

Cognitive-behavioural therapy (CBT) (Koder *et al.* 1996) and interpersonal psychotherapy (IPT) (Frank *et al.* 1993) are the two most widely advocated forms of psychotherapy in elderly patients with depression, including carers looking after a person with dementia. In CBT the aim is to counter automatic negative habits of thinking about oneself, the environment, and the future. In IPT the focus is on relevant social issues such as interpersonal conflict, grief, and role transition. There is now a sufficient evidence-base for the effectiveness of psychological interventions such as CBT or IPT for them to be recommended routinely in the management of depressive disorder in older people, either alone in mild cases or adjunctively in more severe cases (Scogin and McElreath 1994; Koder, *et al.* 1996; Cuijpers 1998; Reynolds *et al.* 1999).

There is evidence too that psychotherapeutic techniques can be applied to elderly depressed patients in the group situation as well as individually. Some believe this approach to be more effective than individual work with the elderly, but not all experts agree about the desirable composition of the group—for example, whether a group of elderly depressed persons is more or less effective than a group with a mix of diagnoses. In one study (Steuer *et al.* 1984) two groups of patients with depressive disorder were compared. One received a psychodynamic approach and the other a cognitive-behavioural one. At 9 months both groups had improved by an equivalent amount, suggesting little to choose between the treatment types. Jarvik *et al.* (1982) studied two groups with a mean age of 67 years. One was treated with standard tricyclic antidepressants and the other given either dynamic or cognitive-behavioural therapy, both in groups. Although both groups fared better than a third placebo group, more of those treated with antidepressants enjoyed complete remissions. Yost *et al.* (1986) provide comprehensive practical guidance for those wishing tc work with groups with the elderly. Psychotherapy is most effective when combined with antidepressant medication.

The style of individual work with older patients may need some modification. The standard '50-minute hour' can be shortened if fatigue and poor concentration are genuine difficulties. Given the decline in semantic processing which occurs with ageing, the frequent occurrence of deafness, and proportionately greater memory problems associated with old age depressions, it may be necessary to rely more on repetition and writing things down. The goals of therapy should be explicit and some advocate a more active role by the therapist (Busse and Pfeiffer 1977).

Life review

Erik Erikson's views on the life cycle have stimulated interest in a psychology of ageing, rather than a prophecy of decline. Life review (Butler 1963) has grown out of this. Although its aims are to achieve a resolution of one's life cycle as an integrated and positive experience, it could seriously backfire with depressed patients who are excessively preoccupied with the past. Nevertheless, those experienced with the techniques—genealogies, autobiographical records, 'pilgrimages', etc.—may find them useful adjuncts in selected cases.

The place of these therapies in relapse prevention is not fully defined, but the evidence is promising. For example, Reynolds *et al.* (1999) found that monthly IPT given in the continuation phase of treatment was more effective than routine care, and the combination of IPT with maintenance antidepressant therapy was the most effective of all.

Anxiety management

This is another behavioural approach that can be helpful in depression, although it is more relevant when patients are recovering or have recovered from depression but are left with residual anxiety. Techniques may involve progressive relaxation, either alone with a commercial tape, or in groups such as those often supervised in a psychiatric day hospital. Another problem, which is probably under-recognized, is that of phobic avoidance of normal activities after a prolonged episode of depression. Specific graded tasks under the supervision of an occupational therapist or psychologist can be extremely helpful. These patients are also occasionally encountered on geriatric wards where they may be labelled as having 'lost confidence'.

Family work

'Far and away the most important agency supporting the psychogeriatric patient at home is the family' (Pitt 1982). Not only may a dysfunctional family contribute to the onset of depressive illness, but the family is often critical in ensuring a successful outcome in treatment. Beginning with the psychiatric history, information must be sought concerning the nature, frequency, and, (albeit subjective) quality of family interactions. Current stresses within the family, attitudes towards having a member with psychiatric disturbance, and tolerance of particular depressive symptoms, such as agitation, are important. During treatment the family often serve as the 'ears' of the clinical team alerting them to, say, suicidal thoughts not declared to the clinician, or as its 'hands' in assuming responsibility for monitoring medication.

Interventions with families vary in complexity. Often the first step is to give straightforward information about the nature of the illness. Granted that clinicians in the past have tended to link affective disorder with dementia, it is hardly surprising that relatives often jump to the same conclusion. Relatives may feel hurt and guilty by remarks uttered by a depressed patient with low self-esteem and feelings of rejection, unless the nature of altered thinking in depression is explained to them. Simple behavioural techniques to modify negative thoughts or behaviours, such as perpetual remarks related to hopelessness or constant demands for attention, can take some pressure off families and, likewise, graded activity aimed at countering withdrawal may lessen the family's own sense of despair.

Sometimes the roles adopted by different family members can subtly undermine recovery or unwittingly collude with the patient's more maladaptive behaviours. This then demands more attention to the dynamics of the family. The next step is to engage a member of the clinical team, such as a social worker, psychiatric nurse, or psychologist, to carry out more detailed interviews with members of the family. As the family is often spread out over some distance from the patient it may be necessary to carry out a number of separate interviews, if practicable, or at least several phone calls. After this some of the key family roles will become clearer.

Formal *family therapy* can be offered to families with an elderly depressed member if it is thought that family dynamics are a factor in perpetuating depressive illness. However, it is dangerous to merely regard elderly depressed patients as simply 'markers' of family pathology in a way analogous to a child's disordered conduct. Certainly there may be much family disturbance by the time a request for medical help has been received, but the patient's illness should not be lost sight of; for it can be difficult to disentangle cause and effect. The first step has to be the optimal treatment of the elderly patient's depressive disorder. Unless this is maintained as a goal, behaviour arising from the depressive illness may be wrongly attributed to family dysfunction. Most experienced clinicians can recall cases where more rigorous treatment for depression led to better family coping in the face of pressure to 'deal with' family dysfunction.

This point has also been emphasized from a family therapist's standpoint. Benbow and colleagues (Benbow *et al.* 1990), using a systemic family therapy model applied within an old age psychiatry service suggest that '...in the majority we feel that simple treatment of the illness presented will enable the family to resolve their problems and move on'. In their experience, some preparatory work is often helpful where an older family member is the presenting patient. This includes treatment of a mood disorder, where relevant, perhaps time attending a day hospital, attention to health issues, or involvement with other members of the team. They emphasize how family therapy can compliment other strategies, including drug treatment of depression. In their view family therapy can be of considerable help to the minority of patients where, as management proceeds, family issues increasingly dominate the agenda, or where 'routine' treatment causes increasing difficulties for the family.

There has been no formal evaluation of the efficacy of family therapy in families with a depressed elderly patient. Nevertheless, Benbow *et al.* (1990) provide a useful overview of the principles they use, based on an adaptation of the life cycle, and illustrate them by use of case histories.

Having obtained the relevant family background, a single 'diagnostic' family interview carried out by two people from the team can clarify many issues and is well within the abilities of most multidisciplinary teams working in old age psychiatry. A useful function of working in this more formal way with families is to encourage a consistent approach towards the elderly depressed person. This avoids counter-therapeutic behaviour by various family members, but implies that, in some cases, the 'family' may need to be extended to include involved professional helpers. For example, district nurses and primary care physicians may undermine, albeit unwittingly, attempts by others to achieve a coherent treatment strategy.

Marital therapy

This utilizes skills from several of the therapies described above, and it may become a more delineated form of family work, in which case it is best if therapists work in pairs. Unresolved conflicts may be resurrected by a depressive disorder. Fear of a future relapse and the responsibilities that go with suicidal ideation may also be a focus of therapy.

Social treatments

This brief resumé of treatment should, by now, have conveyed one obvious fact: the treatment of elderly patients with depressive disorder demands skills from a range of disciplines. As with dementia, a multidisciplinary approach is essential. Given this, the psychiatric day hospital, where resources are concentrated, is an appropriate place to treat elderly patients with depressive disorder: either from the beginning of contact, or after discharge from inpatient care in more severe cases.

The day hospital also serves a useful function as a 'bridge' between psychiatric services and the community. This is especially relevant to social aspects of management. For example, poor housing, poverty, high local rates of crime, and other indices of deprivation are important prognostic considerations (Murphy 1983), and sometimes a change to better circumstances can be crucial to recovery. Generally, though, it is best to defer discussion of issues such as rehousing until after recovery of depression: the patient's view often changes.

Whether or not a direct attempt to alter the social network of a depressed patient reduces the risk of a future relapse is a key question. The small amount of research to draw upon will be discussed under 'Prevention', but a number of psychiatric services offer informal after-care support groups for recovered depressives. They are usually run by two people and tend to be practically oriented rather than psychodynamic; anecdotally, they seem to be effective.

Prognosis

The outcome of depression can be expressed either as the 'natural history', based on aggregated data obtained from large numbers of patients, or as an outcome for a particular patient, based on various predictive variables. It is fair to say that we know much more about the former than the latter (Jablensky 1987).

Natural history

In his classic studies, Post (1962, 1972) found that around 60% of elderly depressed patients requiring hospitalization had, after up to 6 years' follow-up, either remained well or experienced relapses followed by full recovery. Interestingly, the advent of tricyclic antidepressants during the period between these two studies appeared to make little difference to outcome, although selective entry of more 'difficult' cases into the later study may have been a factor in this. The task of summarizing naturalistic studies of prognosis has been made easier by two meta-analyses: the first by Cole (1990) and the updated one by Cole and Bellavance (1997). The latter covered the period from 1955 to 1993, and comprised 16 hospital-based studies (n = 1487) and 5 community-based ones (n = 249). They selected only those studies involving at least 20 patients and a minimum follow-up period of 12 months. Table 27.18 summarizes the findings of their meta-analysis of hospital-based studies. The category 'other' included patients who had died or who were demented prior to ascertainment of outcome.

Taken together, whether in the short term (24 months or less) or longer term (more than 24 months), about 60% either remained well or remain well but had further relapses and/or recurrences that were treatable. However, about 1 in 5 patients can be expected to develop chronic symptomatology.

Table 27.18 Meta-analysis of prognosis studies

	Studies < 24 months (%)		Studies > 24 months (%)	
Prognosis category	Results	Combined results	Results	Combined results
Well	25–68	43.7	18–34	27.3
Relapse with recovery	11–25	15.8	23–52	32.5
Continuously ill	3–69	22.5	7–30	14.2
Other	8–40	22.5	23–39	30.9

After Cole and Bellavance 1997.

These outcomes are better than for community-dwelling older people and patients on medical and surgical wards, where only about 1 in 5 patients recover (Cole and Bellavance (1997). In these groups low rates of detection and undertreatment have been consistently reported, which may explain this discrepancy (Jackson and Baldwin 1993; Green *et al.* 1994; Koenig *et al.* 1997).

Comparative outcome

A common misconception is that late-life depression has a worse outcome than at other times of life. Table 27.19 summarizes the comparative findings from six recent studies. All show outcomes in the elderly as good as or better than for younger depressed patients.

Problems of all the published studies include the small numbers and the lack of treatment data. For example, in Murphy's study, few patients were given ECT—16% of the total, compared with 48% in that of Baldwin and Jolley (1986). Even more puzzling is that only 13 out of 30 deluded patients were treated with ECT, although it is often regarded as being particularly effective for such cases. Outcome cannot be divorced from treatment adequacy which may, therefore, have been a factor in the poor prognosis of this group.

Mortality

Though rates for relapse and chronicity vary quite considerably, there is a little more uniformity regarding mortality. In Murphy's study of 124 patients (Murphy 1983), the mortality at 1 year was 14%, and in a further follow-up at 4 years (Murphy *et al.* 1988) it was 34%. These are much above that expected, assuming, roughly, a 5% year-on-year mortality in this group. In some cases, for example the study of Rabins *et al.* (1985), it exceeded that expected by a factor of 2.5 times, chiefly due to cardiovascular causes, an excess also reported by Murphy *et al.* (1988). The common-sense explanation, that those with higher mortality had worse initial health, is unlikely to be the whole answer. In the study of Murphy *et al.* (1988), two groups were compared: a group with depression and an age- and sex-matched control group from the community. The groups were then matched for levels of physical illness, with the finding that the depressed group still had statistically higher mortality.

Table 27.19 Comparative outcome of depression, older versus younger patients

Study	Age (*n*)	Findings
Meats *et al.* 1991	65+ (56) Under 65 (24)	At 1 year: 68% of older patients are well compared to 50% of younger ones
Brodaty *et al.* (1993)	18–39 (104) 40–59 (77) 60+ (61)	No significant differences at 1 and 4 years
Hinrichsen (1992)	60+ (127)	72% recovery at 1 year; not significantly different from NIH study of mixed-aged patients
Hughes *et al.* (1993)	60+ (46) under 65 (67)	Elderly group had greater improvement on depression score (CES-D) than younger group
Reynolds *et al.* (1994)	32 elderly; mean age 67 with recurrent depression patients.	80% recovery with combined pharmacotherapy and psychotherapy; same as previously studied mid-life
Alexopoulos *et al.* (1996)	Old–mean age 75 (63) Young–mean age 55 (23)	Time to recovery, using survival analysis. 60% of both groups recovered at 6 months.

Prognostic factors

Which variables best predict outcome? As a generalization they may be divided into *general factors* and those relevant to *clinical features of the disorder* (Table 27.20). Adverse factors of a general kind include chronic stress associated with poor environment, crime and poverty, becoming a victim of crime, poor perceived (but not necessarily tangible) social support, and supervening serious physical ill-health. Surprisingly few features of the illness itself can be directly linked with a poorer prognosis. From my own review of the literature the following are suggestive: a slow or incomplete recovery, three or more previous episodes, severity of illness and duration of onset exceeding 2 years, and organic cerebral pathology, either coarse (Post 1962) or more subtle changes (Jacoby *et al.* 1981).

Other outcomes

Other aspects of outcome are the use of resources by elderly depressives and social outcomes. Regarding the former, Murphy and Grundy (1984) demonstrated in a London hospital that, compared to younger depressives, the elderly used roughly 1.5 more bed days. Anyone who has treated elderly physically ill depressives, many of whom live on their own and cannot be discharged partially recovered, will not be surprised at this. Another factor is that more cases are likely to be delusional in later life and this has been shown to be associated with slower recovery (Baldwin 1988*b*). Little is known about social recovery. Post (1962) used various methods of classifying outcome, including five social categories. However, in his view the progress of the illness was in most instances more important than social circumstances. He therefore abandoned measures of social outcome in favour of measures of the course of symptoms. Others too (for example, Hughes *et al.* 1993) have found that psychosocial factors exert less influence on older patients than younger ones in terms of recovery. Nevertheless, there is an important gap in our knowledge. To what extent do previously depressed elderly people resume their normal activities; how many are relocated into alternative, usually residential, accommodation as a result of depression?

In summary, the immediate prognosis for an episode of depressive illness in later life is good. In the longer term only about 25% will remain completely well. These patients seem to be characterized as having responded well and rapidly to conventional treatments and are notable for their physical fitness (Baldwin and Jolley 1986). For approximately 60% of all patients the longer term prognosis is quite good, in that they will either remain well (as above) or have relapses that can be successfully treated. About 7–10% seem, sadly, resistant to all conventional therapies and up to one-third will improve but will be left with some

Table 27.20 Poor outcome factors

Disorder—clinical features
Slower initial recovery
More severe initial depression
Duration > 2 years
Three or more previous episodes (for recurrence)
Previous history of dysthymia
Psychotic symptoms
Extensive deep white matter and basal ganglia grey matter brain disease
Coarse brain disease (e. g. dementia)
General factors
Chronic stress associated with poor environment, crime, and poverty
A new physical illness
Becoming a victim of crime
Poor perceived (but not necessarily tangible) social support

disabling symptoms such as anxiety and hypochondriasis. Little is known about this latter group. Finally, relapses are common and occur relatively early on: two-thirds occurred within the first 18 months of follow-up in the study of Godber *et al.* (1987). Careful follow-up, especially during this period, is therefore essential. Lastly, these naturalistic studies do not support the view that patients with depression have a higher than expected rate of dementia, an important point to emphasize both to patient and carer.

The ultimate tragedy in terms of outcome is of course suicide. This is covered in Chapter 28.

Prevention

Primary prevention

Because *depressive symptomatology* appears to increase in older age groups, common sense suggests that strategies to promote positive, adaptive change around the critical period of retirement ought to prevent some of this distress. This, in part, is the rationale of pre-retirement counselling and, in Britain, the University of the Third Age. Whether the same logic can be applied to the prevention of *depressive disorder* (especially major depression) is unclear. Some individuals seem especially at risk. Those who lack the capacity for intimacy have already been mentioned (Murphy 1983). Anecdotally, anxiety-prone personalities and/or those with obsessional traits are further vulnerable groups.

Specialist mental health professionals have an important role in education. Those most vulnerable to depression—lonely isolated older people with disability and handicap, often in receipt of maximum home-care packages (Banerjee *et al.* 1996)—will often be in touch with a home help, a warden, or a district nurse. This is where targeting education about detection would be best placed. Yet training in recognition is often minimal, although some organizations such as Age Concern do work closely with health care staff to ensure basic training of their volunteers. Targeting staff who work in high-risk groups, such as residential-care establishments, would also be helpful. Ultimately these problems become public health issues. For it is only through a shift away from ageist attitudes and the acceptance that depression in later life is neither natural nor inevitable that the threshold for recognizing depressive illness will be altered. This was the emphasis of the 'Defeat depression' campaign of the UK Royal College of Psychiatrists in the 1990s, which included an initiative with elderly patients, including a special leaflet for carers and patients. The implementation of postgraduate training programmes aimed at general practitioners is another way of improving detection via the 'filter' of primary care.

Awareness of organizations that can help is also clearly important. These include:

- *CRUSE*—CRUSE House, 126, Sheen Road, Richmond, Surrey TW9 1UR; tel. 0208 940 4818;
- *MIND*—National Association for Mental Health, 15–19 Broadway, London E15 4BQ; tel. 0208 519 2122;
- Depression Alliance—35 Westminster Bridge Rd, London SE1 7JB; tel. (admin.) 0207 633 0557, tel. (helpline) 020 7633 0101;
- Help The Aged and Age Concern— any local office.

Secondary prevention

Depressive illness at any age is a condition that is prone to recur. There are three aspects to prevention—treatment adequacy; prophylaxis, and planned after-care—and these are discussed below.

Treatment adequacy

This first aspect has been touched upon earlier. To summarize: there is evidence that late-life depressive illness is undertreated in primary care (Gurland *et al.* 1983; MacDonald 1986). In specialist settings the evidence is based, less directly, on the observation that studies which either have not specified treatments or have used them sparingly are associated with a worse prognosis than those offering standard treatments energetically applied. Persistence pays. Flint and Rifat (1996) showed that sequential regimes of antidepressant therapy eventually produced improvement or recovery in over 80% of their patients. Furthermore, the increased mortality associated with depressive disorder may, in part, be linked to undertreatment. Thus, cardiovascular mortality is reportedly higher in elderly men with inadequately treated depression (Avery and Winokur 1976) and higher in elderly women not given ECT when compared to those who had received it (Babigian and Guttmacher 1984).

Prophylaxis

The second aspect of secondary prevention is prophylaxis. Depression treatment is conventionally subdivided into acute phase, relapse prevention (continuation phase), and prevention of recurrence (prophylaxis). Acute treatment has already been discussed. The optimum duration of *continuation* treatment is not truly known. The standard 6 months recommended for younger patients is probably too short—Flint (1992) calculated the maximum risk period for relapse and recurrence to be 2 years. My own practice is to continue treatment for a minimum of 12 months and then reassess the risk. This seems to be in keeping with recent guidelines as well (Anderson *et al.* 2000).

Since, as discussed, at best only about one-quarter of patients with depressive illness in later life will remain completely well in the long term, currently there is interest in the prevention of relapse and recurrence. In an open study of nortripyline (mean dosage 50 mg) in the *maintenance treatment* of 27 recovered elderly depressed patients, 85% were relapse-free over 12 months and 81.5% at 18 months (Reynolds *et al.* 1989). In a double-blind, placebo-controlled trial, it was found that maintenance dosulepin (dothiepin), 75 mg daily, was associated with a 2.5 times reduction in relapse/recurrence over 2 years (OADIG 1993). Both these studies used the statistical technique of survival analysis to assess outcome. In the OADIG study, the benefit of prophylaxis was irrespective of whether the index episode was the first or a recurrence.

Given these findings, plus the high rate of recurrence and relapse among elderly depressed patients, there is an argument for indefinite prophylactic treatment of major depression in elderly patients. But which drug should be used and at what dosage? The influential Pittsburgh group (Frank *et al.* 1990) has found in mixed-aged patients that the maintenance dose of antidepressant should be kept as close as possible to that which got the patient better. There are difficulties with the long-term use of tricyclics, notably weight gain and dental decay. Do the newer antidepressants offer prevention against recurrence with fewer side-effects? In a small open-label study (Feighner and Cohn 1985), patients were continued on fluoxetine or doxepin. Both were equally effective in preventing relapse over 48 weeks. Clearly studies of the benefits of SSRIs and other new antidepressants in the prevention of relapse and recurrence of depression in older patients are needed. Given the higher costs of the newer antidepressants, it is in this area that cost-benefit questions are particularly pertinent. A different view is that since some of those in the OADIG study who were in the placebo group remained well, there will be a risk of overtreatment if there were to be a blanket policy of prophylaxis, with its attendant risks in a group whose susceptibility to unwanted drug effects is liable to increase with ageing. Clearly identifying those patients who would benefit most from prophylactic medication is an important task for future research. Those with two or more recurrences in the past 2 years, serious ill-health, chronic social difficulties, or very severe depressive symptoms are the most obvious candidates based on current (limited) knowledge (Table 27.20).

Medical, i.e. drug, prophylaxis is not the only means of prevention. For example, Ong *et al.* (1987) were able to demonstrate that a support group for discharged elderly depressives, run by a social worker and a community psychiatric nurse, resulted in a significant reduction in relapses and readmissions over a 1-year period. Reynolds *et al.* (1999) have provided convincing evidence for combined psychotherapy and drug treatment as optimal maintenance treatment, and Watereus *et al.* (1994) have showed that a psychiatric nurse can be deployed with effect in the treatment and prevention of recurrence.

Lastly, maintenance ECT may benefit a few patients who experience frequent relapses despite drug intervention. Although there is very little research, in one small series it was helpful (Mirchandani *et al.* (1994). Treatments are usually spaced at between 2 and 4 weeks.

Planned after-care

Without planned after-care relapses and recurrences are likely to go undetected (Sadavoy and Reiman-Sheldon 1983), even though further treatment is often successful (Godber *et al.* 1987). Old age psychiatrists are busy people and after-care does not have to be provided entirely by them. Often a community psychiatric nurse, a social worker or health visitor specializing in the elderly, or an interested general practitioner may be called upon.

Tertiary prevention

Diseases do not always get better. An arteriopath who comes to limb amputation would feel justifiably angry if health agencies abandoned him on the grounds that his illness 'only' had social implications. Yet such is the plight of depressives who fail to improve. Evidently clinicians allow their failures to slip quietly away—out of sight and out of mind.

The needs of such patients are poorly understood. Some people benefit from a change to more supportive living circumstances such as residential care; for others physical health difficulties become the most important issue in worsening depression (Baldwin and Jolley 1986). What is clear is that the burden of care upon families is considerable. Troublesome symptoms include importuning hypochondriacal complaints, but 'negative' features such as lack of interest, poverty of conversation, and withdrawal are also problematic. The mental health of carers suffers and, at the very least, health professionals should feel some commitment to them. Often the emphasis must be on basic explanations and on simple directions about how to manage particular behaviours. It may also mean supportive work to enable guilt to be worked through. Although respite care is usually associated with dementia, occasionally there is a case for it in those with resistant depression to allow the relative(s) a break. Sometimes it also helps to halt a cycle of poor relationships which can develop between patient and carer.

Depression and physical symptomatology

Those engaged in old age psychiatry are constantly challenged by the admixture of physical and psychiatric disorder in their patients. Indeed, for many it is a chief fascination of the specialty. This applies as much to depressive disorders as to the organic psychosyndromes. The overlap of depressive and physical symptomatology is a mine for the clinically curious, as well as being of immense practical importance. There are various ways of understanding this overlap.

Physical symptoms arising out of depressive illness

Excessive concern with health may be associated with physiological changes due to ageing or disease, with physical disease in peers or peer expectations (for example, concerning the regularity of bowel habit), as an illness behaviour to maintain certain roles and patterns, or as part of a psychiatric disorder such as depressive disorder. Hypochondriasis, a morbid fear of bodily illness, in depressive illness is common. Sometimes these preoccupations can become delusional, occasionally achieving grotesque proportions. For example, one patient dismissed the author and instead requested an undertaker, for she believed herself dead and was convinced that her flesh had rotted. Hypochondriacal complaints arising in the setting of a depressive disorder are often quite distinct from symptoms that might be expected from a physical pathology which is known to be present (Kramer-Ginsberg *et al.* 1989). A careful evaluation of both mood and actual health is thus required.

Sometimes a known physical illness, previously tolerated, becomes unbearable when depressive disorder develops. This has already been discussed, as has the less common situation of depression presenting as an actual physical complaint, for which no physical cause can be found. The mechanism underlying these presentations include the known tendency for depression to lower the pain threshold, although it is interesting that antidepressants often relieve chronic pain whether or not depression is present. The notion of chronic pain as a depressive 'equivalent' is controversial and is probably an oversimplification. Any aetiological model will need to address a number of factors, including personality, interpersonal factors, and family dynamics, as well as depressed mood or some putative 'equivalent' to it. Regardless of causation it is always worth enquiring carefully for depressive symptomatology where chronic pain is present, for this is often the most treatable aspect. One survey of chronic pain in the elderly found that depression was significantly associated with pain but that both were undertreated (Roy and Thomas 1986).

Particular difficulties arise in treatment when patients fail to comply with psychotropic medication because of their persistent attribution of all symptoms to physical illness. Time must be set aside to spell out carefully the nature and extent of any actual physical illness present and its likely effects. Sometimes too, it is necessary to examine the ways in which both the patient and his or her family understand illness and its consequence, in order to understand what might be the rewards of invalidism. An elderly patient may use physical illness and physical symptomatology to foster dependence, often in the face of social isolation. Sometimes, after the depressive component has been treated adequately, these issues linger and impede functional recovery, in which case inpatient or day-patient admission may be the only way to achieve progress. Such cases demand a consistent staff approach and a behavioural programme with appropriate rewards, or at the very least a carefully structured day to promote useful activity.

Physical illness leading to depressive symptoms

In recent years much energy has been expended on demonstrating links between depression and particular physical illnesses. In fact the literature is growing in a manner which suggests that a great many illnesses, both acute and chronic, are associated with depressive symptoms. In only a minority does this reach the intensity of a depressive illness. Mention has already been made of the interesting notion that depression in later life may be associated with subtle brain abnormalities. What then should be made of the relationship between depression and major neurological disorders (excluding dementia which has been mentioned earlier)? Most research has been conducted on patients with stroke and idiopathic Parkinson's disease, both of which are especially relevant to elderly people, in whom they reach their maximum incidence.

Over the years a plethora of articles concerning poststroke depression has emerged from the Johns Hopkins School of Medicine in Baltimore, USA. One of the many findings was of an association between the incidence of depressive disorder, including major depression, and the proximity of the stroke lesion to the anterior pole of the left hemisphere (Robinson *et al.* 1984). Although intriguing, the work has been criticized on the grounds of patient selection and location, the way in which rating instruments were used, and the fact that lesions close to the left anterior pole are found only in a minority of strokes if patients from the community and not just the hospital are included (House 1987). Also, although between on-third and one-fifth of poststroke survivors may suffer depression of all grades of severity, it is by no means agreed that this is higher than in other patients with chronic disabling illnesses (House 1987).

A number of other neurotransmitter systems are disrupted in Parkinson's disease besides the dopamine pathways. In relation to depression, which is the most frequent mental change in Parkinson's disease, it has been suggested that serotonin deficiency may be an important predisposing factor (Mayeux *et al.* 1986). However, although depressive symptoms occur in around 40% of patients with the disease, probably only a minority amount to major depressive disorder. Moreover, there is disagreement as to whether this prevalence is, in any case, above that found in other disabling conditions such as rheumatoid arthritis (Gotham A-M, *et al.* 1986) and chronic obstructive pulmonary disease in older people (Yohannes *et al.* 1998). As far as *life-time risk* for depressive disorder is concerned the risk may be as high as 40%, so it certainly represents considerable morbidity. Parkinson's disease serves as a useful model for exploring the links between psychiatry and physical illness. For example, the manner in which ECT not only benefits lowered mood but also the motor changes of Parkinson's disease is of considerable neurobiological interest.

Other factors, besides biochemical ones, are associated with depression in Parkinson's disease: these include motor disability, change in symptom severity, coping styles, perception of self and of the illness, and the level of practical and emotional support available (Baldwin and Byrne 1989). Distinctions such as 'reactive' versus 'endogenous' or 'biogenic' versus 'psychogenic' are, therefore, oversimplifications. This is not to undermine the possible role of neurochemical factors, for an intriguing finding, which is a feature of some other subcortical diseases such as Huntington's chorea, is that a sizeable minority, perhaps a fifth or so, of Parkinson's patients experience their first depressive illness before the onset of any neurological symptoms. For most patients with a physical illness accompanied by depression, there will be a complex interplay of factors in the causation of the depression: some of these factors are directly related to underlying illness, some are more to do with the individual, and others are environmental or social in nature.

Organic depressive disorder has been covered earlier, and clearly a number of illnesses, some of which are not obvious at first presentation, may be involved in triggering depression. Furthermore, even for manifest diseases, treatment may sometimes precipitate depression. Nowadays probably steroids and non-selective beta-blockers are the main offenders—and alcohol abuse should always be considered.

The headings used in this section are not meant to imply fixed causal relationships. An association undoubtedly exists between depression and physical illness which is not based on chance alone (Murphy and Brown 1980). Thus Kay and Bergmann (1966) in a case-controlled study of community-dwelling old people and found that chronic (but not acute) physical illnesses proved to be significantly more common in elderly men with affective disorder than among elderly people who were mentally well. Moreover, at 3–4 years' follow-up, almost half of elderly men with affective disorder from the original sample had died—a highly significant difference from the control subjects. Such findings are not consistent with the view that the association between chronic physical illness and depression is merely due to the chance association of two relatively common problems in elderly people: physical disease and affective disorder.

Strict divisions along the lines of physically induced depression or psychologically induced physical disorder have not in the past proved very helpful. They risk a rehearsal of the sterile mind-body dualism of earlier times. A model based on interactions rather than causal relationships lends itself to multivariate analysis (Eastwood and Corbin-Rifat 1986) and also fits in with modern, eclectic, psychiatric practice.

Conclusions

Depressive disorder is the most common mental health problem of older people. It can be difficult to diagnose because of physical comorbidity which can mask depression and age-associated factors that modify its clinical presentation. It is important to rule out organic factors in aetiology, including alcohol and iatrogenic drugs, and to give as much attention to optimizing physical ill-health as to treating psychiatric symptoms. New research suggests that brain abnormalities, most likely vascular in nature, contribute to the onset of depressive disorder in late-onset depression. Treatment should be multimodal and multidisciplinary, with the aim of complete recovery and not simply improvement. Persistence pays—using a range of treatments, the great majority of patients will recover. Keeping patients well is more of a challenge. Treatment (including psychological therapies wherever available) should be continued for at least 12 months. Many patients who could benefit from long-term maintenance therapy do not receive it. With optimum management the prognosis is at least as good as that for any other time of adult life.

References

Abas, M. A., Sahakian, B. J., and Levy, R. (1990). Neuropsychological deficits and CT scan changes in elderly depressives. *Psychological Medicine*, **20**, 507–20.

Abramczuk, J. A. and Rose, N. M. (1979). Pre-anaesthetic assessment and the prevention of post-ECT morbidity. *British Journal of Psychiatry*, **134**, 582–7.

Abrams, R. C., Alexopoulos, G. S., and Young, R. C. (1987). Geriatric depression and DSM-III-R personality disorder criteria. *Journal of the American Geriatrics Society*, **35**, 383–6.

Adshead, F., Day Cody, P., and Pitt, B. (1992). BASDEC: a novel screening instrument for depression in elderly medical inpatient. *British Medical Journal*, **305**, 397.

Alexopoulos, G. S., Young, R. C., and Kocsis, J. H. (1984). Dexamethasone suppression test in geriatric depression. *Biological Psychiatry*, **19**, 1567–71.

Alexopoulos, G. S., Abrams, R. C., Young, R. C., and Shamoian, C. A. (1988). Cornell Scale for depression in dementia. *Biological Psychiatry*, **23**, 271–84.

Alexopoulos, G. S., Meyers, B. S., Young, R. C., Mattis, S., and Kakuma, T. (1993). The course of geriatric depression with reversible dementia: a controlled study. *American Journal of Psychiatry*, **150**, 1693–9.

Alexopoulos, G. S., Meyers, B. S., Young, R. C., Kakuma, T., Feder, M., Einhorn, A., *et al.* (1996). Recovery in geriatric depression. *Archives of General Psychiatry*, **53**, 305–12.

Alexopoulos, G. S., Meyers, B. S., Young, R. C., Campbell, S., Silbersweig, D., and Charlson, M. (1997). 'Vascular depression' hypothesis. *Archives of General Psychiatry*, **54**, 915–22.

Allen, N. H. P. and Burns, A. (1995). The non-cognitive features of dementia. *Reviews in Clinical Gerontology*, **5**, 57–75.

American Psychiatric Association (APA). (1994). *Diagnostic and statistical manual Version IV*. APA, Washington DC.

Ames, D., Ashby, D., Mann, A. H., and Graham, N. (1988). Psychiatric illness in elderly residents of part III homes in one London borough: prognosis and review. *Age and Ageing*, **17**, 249–56.

Amrein, R., Guntert, T. W., Dingemanse, J., Lorscheid, T., Stabl, M., and Schmidt-Burgk, W. (1992). Interactions of moclobemide with concomitantly administered medication: evidence from pharmacological and clinical studies. *Psychopharmacology*, **92**, 106(Suppl.), S24–S31.

Anderson, I. M., Nutt, D. J., and Deakin, J. F. W. (2000). Evidence-based guidelines for treating depressive disorders with antidepressants: a revision of the 1993 British Association for Psychopharmacology guidelines. *Journal of Psychopharmacology*, **14**, 3020.

Austin, M-P., Ross, M., Murray, C., O'Carroll, R. E., Ebmeier, K. P., and Goodwin, G. M. (1992). Cognitive function in major depression. *Journal of Affective Disorders*, **25**, 21–30.

Avery, D. and Winokur, G. (1976). Mortality in depressed patients treated with electroconvulsive therapy and antidepressants. *Archives of General Psychiatry*, **33**, 1029–37.

Babigian, H. M. and Guttmacher, L. B. (1984). Epidemiologic considerations in electroconvulsive therapy. *Archives of General Psychiatry*, **41**, 246–53.

Baldwin, R (1988*a*). Late life depression—under-treated? *British Medical Journal*, **296**, 519.

Baldwin, R. (1988*b*). Delusional and non-delusional depression in late life: evidence for distinct subtypes. *British Journal of Psychiatry*, **152**, 39–44.

Baldwin, R. C. (1992). The nature, frequency and relevance of depressive delusions. In *Delusions and hallucinations in old age* (ed. C. Katona and R. Gaskell Levy), pp. 97–114. Royal College of Psychiatrists, London.

Baldwin, R. C. (1993). Late life depression and structural brain changes: a review of recent magnetic resonance imaging research. *International Journal of Geriatric Psychiatry*, **8**, 115–23.

Baldwin, R. C. (1996). Treatment resistant depression in the elderly: a review of treatment options. *Reviews in Clinical Gerontology*, **6**, 343–8.

Baldwin, R. C. (1999). The aetiology of depression in late life. *Advances in Psychiatric Treatment*, **5**, 435–42.

Baldwin, R. C. and Byrne, E. J. (1989). Psychiatric aspects of Parkinson's disease. *British Medical Journal*, **299**, 3–4.

Baldwin, R. C. and Jolley, D. J. (1986). The prognosis of depression in old age. *British Journal of Psychiatry*, **149**, 574–83.

Baldwin, R. C. and Tomenson, B. (1995). Depression in later life: a comparison of symptoms and risk factors in early and late onset cases. *British Journal of Psychiatry*, **167**, 649–52.

Ballard, C. G., Eastwood, C., Gahir, M., and Wilcock, G. (1996). A follow-up study of depression in the carers of dementia sufferers. *British Medical Journal*, **312**, 947.

Banerjee, S., Shamash, K., Macdonald, A. J. D., and Mann, A. H. (1996). Randomised controlled trial of intervention by psychogeriatric team on depression in frail elderly people. *British Medical Journal*, **313**, 1058–61.

Barraclough, B. M. (1971). Suicide in the elderly. In *Recent developments in psychogeriatrics* (ed. D. W. K. Kay and A. Walk), pp. 87–97. Headley Bros, Kent.

Beaumont, G. (1989). The toxicity of antidepressants. *British Journal of Psychiatry*, **154**, 454–8.

Beck, D. A. and Koenig, H. G. (1996). Minor depression: a review of the literature. *International Journal of Psychiatry in Medicine*, **26**, 177–209.

Beck, A. T., Ward, C. H., Mendelson, M., Mock, J. E., and Erbaugh, J. (1961). An inventory for measuring depression. *Archives of General Psychiatry*, **4**, 561–71.

Beekman, A. T. F., Deeg, D. J. H., Smit, J. H., and Van Tilburg, W. (1995). Predicting the course of depression in the older population: results from a community-based study in the Netherlands. *Journal of Affective Disorders,* **34**, 41–9.

Benbow, S. B. (1989). The role of electroconvulsive therapy in the treatment of depressive illness in old age. *British Journal of Psychiatry,* **155**, 147–52.

Benbow, S., Egan, D., Marriott, A., Tregay, K., Walsh, S., Wells, J., *et al.* (1990). Using the family life cycle with later life families. *Journal of Family, Therapy,* **12**, 321–40.

Bench, C. J., Friston, K. J., Brown, R. G., Scott, L. C., Frackowiak, R. S. J., and Dolan, R. J. (1992). The anatomy of depression—focal abnormalities of cerebral blood flow in major depression. *Psychological Medicine,* **22**, 607–15.

Bergmann, K. (1978). Neurosis and personality disorder in old age. In *Studies in geriatric psychiatry* (ed. A. D. Isaacs and F. Post), pp. 41–75. Wiley, Chichester.

Bird, A. S., Macdonald, A. J. D., Mann, A. H., and Philpot, M. P. (1987). Preliminary experiences with the SelfCARE(D). *International Journal of Geriatric Psychiatry,* **2**, 31–8.

Blazer, D. (1989). Affective disorders in late life. In *Geriatric psychiatry* (ed. E. Busse and D. Blazer), pp. 369–401. Cambridge University Press, Cambridge.

Blazer, D. (1991). Clinical features of depression in old age: a case for minor depression. *Current Opinions in Psychiatry,* **4**, 596–9.

Blazer, D. and Williams, C. V. (1980). Epidemiology of dysphoria and depression in an elderly population. *American Journal of Psychiatry,* **137**, 439–44.

Blazer, D., George, L., and Landerman, R. (1986). The phenomenology of late life depression. In *Psychiatric disorders in the elderly* (ed. P. E. Bebbington and R. Jacoby), pp. 143–52. Mental Health Foundation, London.

Bocksberger, J. P., Gachoud, J. P., Richard, J., and Dick, P. (1993). Comparison of the efficacy of moclobemide and fluvoxamine in elderly patients with a severe depressive episode. *European Psychiatry,* **8**, 319–24.

Bowen, D. M., Najlerahim, A., Proctor, A. W. *et al.* (1989). Circumscribed changes of the cerebral cortex in neuropsychiatric disorders of later life. *Proceedings of the National Academy of Sciences, USA,* **86**, 9504–8.

Brodaty, H., Peters, K., Boyce, P., Hickie, I., Parker, G., Mitchell, P., *et al.* (1991). Age and depression. *Journal of Affective Disorders,* **23**, 137–49.

Brodaty, H., Harris, L., Peters, K., Wilhelm, K., Hickie, I., Boyce, P., *et al.* (1993). Prognosis of depression in the elderly: a comparison with younger patients. *British Journal of Psychiatry,* **163**, 589–96.

Brown, G. W. and Harris, T. O. (1978). *The social origins of depression.* Tavistock, London.

Burke, W. J., Houston, M. J., Boust, S. J., and Roccaforte, W. H. (1989). Use of the Geriatric Depression Scale in dementia of Alzheimer type. *Journal of American Geriatrics Society,* **37**, 856–60.

Burrows, A. B., Satlin, A., and Salzman, C. (1994). Depression in a long-term care facility: clinical features and discordance between nursing assessments and patient interviews. *Journal of the American Geriatrics Society,* **43**, 1118–22.

Burvill, P. W., Hall, W. D., Stampfer, H. G., and Emmerson, J. P. (1991). The prognosis of depression in old age. *British Journal of Psychiatry,* **158**, 64–71.

Busse, E. G. and Pfeiffer, E. (1977). *Behaviour and adaptation in later life* (2nd edn). Little, Brown, Boston.

Butler, R. N. (1963). The life review: an interpretation of reminiscence. *Psychiatry,* **26**, 65–76.

Caine, E. D. (1981). Pseudodementia. *Archives of General Psychiatry,* **38**, 1359–64.

Callaghan, M. C., Hui, S. L., Nienaber, N. A., Musick, B. S., and Tierney, W. M. (1994). Longitudinal study of depression and health services use among elderly primary care patients. *Journal of the American Geriatrics Society,* **42**, 833–8.

Carroll, B. J., Feinberg, M., Greden, J. F., Tarik, A. J., Albal, A. A. A., Haskett, R. F., *et al.* (1981). A specific laboratory test for the diagnosis of melancholia. *Archives of General Psychiatry,* **38**, 15–22.

Cawley, R. H., Post, F., and Whitehead, A. (1973). Barbiturate tolerance and psychosocial functioning in elderly depressed patients. *Psychological Medicine,* **8**, 39–52.

Chiu, E., Ames, D., Draper, B., and Snowdon, J. (1999). Depressive disorders in the elderly: a review. In *Depressive disorders* (ed. Maj and N. Sartorius), pp. 313–63. Wiley, Chichester.

Churchill, C. M., Priolo, C. V., Nemeroff, C. B., Krishnan, K. R. R., and Breitner, J. C. S. (1991). Occult subcortical magnetic resonance findings in elderly depressives. *International Journal of Geriatric Psychiatry,* **6**, 213–16.

Clayton, P. J. (1982). Bereavement. In *Handbook of affective disorders* (ed. E. S. Paykel), pp. 403–15. Churchill Livingstone, Edinburgh.

Coffey, C. E. (1987). Cerebral laterality and emotion. The neurology of depression. *Comprehensive Psychiatry,* **28**, 197–219.

Coffey, C. E., Figiel, G. S., Djang, W. T., and Weiner, R. D. (1990). Subcortical hyperintensity on magnetic resonance imaging: a comparison of normal and depressed elderly subjects. *American Journal of Psychiatry,* **147**, 187–9.

Cohen-Cole, S. A. and Stoudemire, A. (1987). Major depression and physical illness: special considerations in diagnosis and biologic treatment. *Psychiatric Clinics of North America,* **10**, 1–17.

Cohn, C. K., Shrivastav, A. R., Mendels, J., Cohn, J. B., Fabre, L. F., Claghorn, J. L., *et al.* (1990). Double-blind, multicenter comparison of sertraline and amitriptyline in elderly depressed patients. *Journal of Clinical Psychiatry,* **12**(Suppl. B), 28–33.

Cole, M. G. (1990). The prognosis of depression in the elderly. *Canadian Medical Association. Journal,* **143**, 633–40.

Cole, M. G. and Bellavance, F. (1997). The prognosis of depression in old age. *American Journal of Geriatric Psychiatry,* **5**, 4–14.

Committee on Safety of Medicines. (1988). *Current problems.* 23rd September. CSM, London.

Conwell, Y., Nelson, J. C., Kim, K. M., *et al.* (1989). Depression in late life: age of onset as marker of subtype. *Journal of Affective Disorders,* **17**, 189–95.

Copeland, J. R. M., McWilliam, C., Dewey, M. E., Forshaw, D., Shiwach, R., Abed, R. T., *et al.* (1986). The early recognition of dementia in the elderly: a preliminary communication from a longitudinal study using the GMS (community version/9—AGECAT package). *International Journal of Geriatric Psychiatry,* **1**, 63–70.

Copeland, J. R. M., Dewey, M. E., Wood, N., Searle, R., Davidson, I. A., and McWilliam, C. (1987). Range of mental illness among the elderly in the community: prevalence in Liverpool using the GMS-AGECAT package. *British Journal of Psychiatry,* **150**, 815–23.

Copeland, J. R. M., Dewey, M. E., and Griffiths-Jones, H. M. (1990). Dementia and depression in elderly persons: AGECAT compared with DSM-III and pervasive illness. *International Journal of Geriatric Psychiatry,* **5**, 47–51.

Copeland, J. R. M., Davidson, I. A., Dewey, M. E., Gilmore, C., Larkin, B. A., McWilliam, C., *et al.* (1992). Alzheimer's disease, other dementias, depression and pseudodementia: prevalence, incidence and three-year outcome in Liverpool. *British Journal of Psychiatry,* **161**, 230–9.

Copeland, J. R. M., Beekman, A. T. F., Dewey, M. E., Hooijer, C., Jordan, A., Lawlor, B. A., *et al.* (1999). Depression in Europe: geographical distribution among older people. *British Journal of Psychiatry,* **174**, 312–21.

Crewe, H. K., Lennard, M. S., Tucker, G. T., Woods, F. R., and Haddock, R. E. (1992). The effect of selective serotonin reuptake inhibitors on cytochrome P4502D6 (CYP2D6) activity in human liver microsomes. *British Journal of Clinical Pharmacology*, **34**, 262–5.

Cuijpers, P. I. M. (1998). Psychological outreach programmes for the depressed elderly: a meta-analysis of effects and dropouts. *International Journal Geriatric Psychiatry,* **13**, 41–8.

David, A., Blamire, A., and Breiter, H. (1994). Functional magnetic resonance imaging. *British Journal of Psychiatry,* **164**, 2–7.

De Alarcon, R. D. (1964). Hypochondriasis and depression in the aged. *Gerontology Clinic,* **6**, 266–77.

Devanand, D. P., Nobler, M. S., Singer, T., Kiersky, J. E., Turret, N., Roose, S. P., *et al.* (1994). Is dysthymia a different disorder in the elderly? *American Journal of Psychiatry,* **151**, 1592–9.

De Vann, A. M., Kummer, J., Agnoli, A., Gentili, P., Lorizio, A., and Anand, R. (1990). Moclobemide compared with second-generation antidepressants in elderly people. *Acta Psychiatrica Scandinavica*, **Suppl. 360**, 64–6.

Dhondt, A. D. F. and Hooijer, C. (1995). Iatrogenic origins of depression in the elderly: is medication a significant aetiological factor in geriatric depression? Considerations and a preliminary approach. *International Journal of Geriatric Psychiatry,* **10**, 1–8.

Dinan, T. G. (1993). A rational approach to the non-responding depressed patient. *International Clinical Psychopharmacology,* **8**, 221–3.

Dolan, R. J., Calloway, S. P., Thacker, P. F., and Mann, A. H. (1986). The cerebral cortical appearance in depressed subjects. *Psychological Medicine,* **16**, 775–9.

Dolan, R. J., Bench, C. J., Brown, R. G., Scott, L. C., Friston, K. J., and Frackowiak, R. S. J. (1992). Regional cerebral blood flow abnormalities in depressed patients with cognitive impairment. *Journal of Neurology, Neurosurgery, and Psychiatry,* **55**, 768–73.

Eastwood, M. R. and Corbin-Rifat, S. L. (1986). The relationship between physical illness and depression in old age. In *Affective disorders in the elderly* (ed. E. Murphy), pp. 177–86. Churchill Livingstone, Edinburgh.

Eastwood, R. and Corbin-Rifat, S. (1987). Hearing impairment, mental disorder and the elderly. *Stress Medicine,* **3**, 171–4.

Emmerson, J. P., Burvill, P. W., Finlay-Jones, R., and Hall, W. (1989). Life events, life difficulties and confiding relationships in the depressed elderly. *British Journal of Psychiatry*, **155**, 787–92.

Evans, M. E., Hammond, M., Wilson, K., Lye, M., and Copeland, J. (1997). Placebo-controlled treatment trial of depression in elderly physically ill patients. *International Journal of Geriatric Psychiatry,* **12**, 817–24.

Feighner, J. P. and Cohn, J. B. (1985). Double-blind comparative trials of fluoxetine and doxepin in geriatric patients with major depressive disorder. *Journal of Clinical Psychiatry*, **46**, 20–5.

Figiel, G. S., Krishnan, K. R. R., Doraiswamy, P. M., Rao, V. P., Nemeroff, C. B., and Boyko, O. B. (1991). Subcortical hyperintensities on brain magnetic resonance imaging: a comparison between late age onset and early onset elderly depressed subjects. *Neurobiology of Aging,* **12**, 245–7.

Fleminger, S. (1991). Depressive motor retardation. *International Journal of Geriatric Psychiatry,* **6**, 459–68.

Flint, A. J. (1992). The optimum duration of antidepressant treatment in the elderly. *International Journal of Geriatric Psychiatry*, **7**, 617–19.

Flint, A. J. and Rifat, S. L. (1996). The effect of sequential antidepressant treatment on geriatric depression. *Journal of Affective Disorders*, **36**, 95–105.

Folstein, M. F., Folstein, S. E., and McHugh, P. R. (1975). 'Mini-Mental State': a practical method for grading the cognitive state of patients for the clinician. *Journal of Psychiatric Research*, **12**, 185–98.

Forstl, H., Burns, A., Luthbert, P., Cairns, N., Lantos, P., and Levy, R. (1992). Clinical and neuropathological correlates of depression in Alzheimer's disease. *Psychological Medicine*, **22**, 877–84.

Foster, J. R. (1992). Use of lithium in elderly psychiatric patients: a review of the literature. *Lithium*, **3**, 77–93.

Frank, E., Kupfer, D. J., Perel, J. M., Cornes, C., Jarrett, D. B., Malliger, A. G. *et al.* (1990). Three-year outcomes for maintenance therapies in recurrent depression. *Archives of General Psychiatry*, **47**, 1093–9.

Frank, E., Frank, N., Cornes, C., Imber, S. D., Miller, M. D., Morris, *et al.* (1993). Interpersonal psychotherapy in the treatment in the late-life depression. In *New applications of interpersonal psychotherapy* (ed. G. L. Klerman and M. M. Weissman), pp. 167–98. American Psychiatric Association, Washington, DC.

Fujikaw, A. T., Yanai, I., and Yamawaki, S. (1997). Psychosocial stressors in patients with major depression and silent cerebral infarction. *Stroke*, **28**, 1123–5.

Georgotas, A. (1983). Affective disorders in the elderly: diagnostic and research considerations. *Age and Ageing*, **12**, 1–10.

Georgotas, A. and McCue, R. (1989). The additional benefit of extending an antidepressant trial past seven weeks in the depressed elderly. *International Journal of Geriatric Psychiatry*, **4**, 191–5.

Georgotas, A., Friedman, E., McCarthy, M., Mann, J., Krakowski, M., Siegel, R., *et al.* (1983). Resistant geriatric depressions and therapeutic response to monoamine oxidase inhibitors. *Biological Psychiatry*, **18**, 195–205.

Gerner, R. H. (1985). Present status of drug therapy of depression in late life. *Journal of Affective Disorders* (Suppl. 1), S23–S31.

Gillis, L. S. and Zabow, A. (1982). Dysphoria in the elderly. *South African Medical Journal*, **62**, 410–13.

Glassman, A. H., Johnson, L. L., Giardin. A. E. V., Walsh, B., Roose, S. P., and Couper, TB. (1983). The use of imipramine in depressed patients with congestive heart failure. *Journal of the American Medical Association*, **250**, 1997–2001.

Godber, C., Rosenvinge, H., Wilkinson, D., and Smithies, J. (1987). Depression in old age: prognosis after ECT. *International Journal of Geriatric Psychiatry*, **2**, 19–24.

Gotham, A-M., Brown, R. G., and Marsden, C. D. (1986). Depression in Parkinson's disease: a quantitative and qualitative analysis. *Journal of Neurology, Neurosurgery, and Psychiatry*, **49**, 381–9.

Green, B. H., Copeland, J. R. M., Dewey, M. E., Sharm. A. V., and Davidson, I. A. (1994). Factors associated with recovery and recurrence of depression in older people: a prospective study. *International Journal of Geriatric Psychiatry*, **9**, 789–95.

Greenwald, B. S., Kramer-Ginsberg, E., Krishnan, K. R. R., Ashtari, M., Aupperle, P. M., and Patel, M. (1996). MRI signal hyperintensities in geriatric depression. *American Journal of Psychiatry*, **153**, 1212–15.

Gurland, B. J. (1976). The comparative frequency of depression in various adult age groups. *Journal of Gerontology*, **31**, 283–92.

Gurland, B., Copeland, J., Kuriansky, J., Kelleher, M., Sharpe, L., and Dean, L. L. (1983). *The mind and mood of aging*. Haworth Press, New York.

Guscott, R. and Grof, P. (1991). The clinical meaning of refractory depression: a review for the clinician. *American Journal of Psychiatry*, **148**, 695–704.

Harris, D. (1975). *The myth and reality of aging in America*. The National Council on Aging, Washington, DC.

Hebenstreit, G. F, Baunhackl, U., Chan-Palay, V., Gruner, E., Kasas, A., Katschnig, H., *et al.* (1991). The treatment of depression in geriatric depressed and demented patients by moclobemide: results from the international multicenter double-blind placebo-controlled trial. In *Proceedings of the Fifth Congress of the International Psychogeriatric Association*, Rome, p. 31.

Heeren, T. H., Van Hemert, A. M., Lagaay, A. M., and Rooymans, G. M. (1992). The general population prevalence of non-organic psychiatric disorders in subjects aged 85 years and over. *Psychological Medicine*, **22**, 733–8.

Henderson, A. S., Grayson, D. A., Scott, R., Wilson, J., Rickwood, D., and Kay, D. W. K. (1986). Social support, dementia and depression among the elderly living in the Hobart community. *Psychological Medicine*, **16**, 379–90.

Henderson, A. S., Jorm, A. F., MacKinnon, A., Christensen, H., Scott, L. R., Korten, A. E., *et al.* (1993). The prevalence of depressive disorders and the distribution of depressive symptoms in later-life: a survey using Draft ICD-10 and DSM-III-R. *Psychological Medicine*, **23**, 719–29.

Hendrickson, E., Levy, R., and Post, F. (1979). Averaged evoked responses in relation to cognitive and affective state of elderly psychiatric patients. *British Journal of Psychiatry*, **134**, 494–501.

Hinrichsen, G. A. (1992). Recovery and relapse from major depressive disorder in the elderly. *American Journal of Psychiatry*, **149**, 1574–9.

Hopkinson, G. (1964). A genetic study of affective illness in patients over 50. *British Journal of Psychiatry*, **110**, 244–54.

Hordern, A., Holt, N. F., Burt, C. G., and Gordon, W. F. (1963). Amitriptyline in depressive states: phenomenology and prognostic considerations. *British Journal of Psychiatry*, **109**, 815–25.

House, A. (1987). Mood disorders after stroke: a review of the evidence. *International Journal of Geriatric Psychiatry*, **2**, 211–21.

Hoyberg, O. J., Maragakis, B., and Mullin, J. (1996). A double-blind multi-centre comparison of mirtazepine and amitriptyline in elderly depressed patients. *Acta Psychiatrica Scandinavica*, **93**, 184–90.

Hughes, D. C., DeMalie, D., and Blazer, D. G. (1993). Does age make a difference in the effects of physical health and social support on the outcome of the major depressive episode. *American Journal of Psychiatry*, **150**, 728–33.

Jablensky, A. (1987). Prediction of the course and outcome of depression. *Psychological Medicine*, **17**, 1–9.

Jackson, R. and Baldwin, B. (1993). Detecting depression in elderly medically ill patients: the use of the Geriatric Depression Scale compared with medical and nursing observations. *Age and Ageing*, **22**, 349–53.

Jacoby, R. J. and Levy, R. (1980). Computed tomography in the elderly, 3: affective disorder. *British Journal of Psychiatry*, **136**, 270–5.

Jacoby, R. J., Levy, R., and Bird, J. M. (1981). Computed tomography and the outcome of affective disorder: a follow-up study of elderly patients. *British Journal of Psychiatry*, **139**, 288–92.

Jarvik, L. S., Mintz, J., Steuer, J., and Gerner, R. (1982). Treating geriatric depression: a 26 week interim analysis. *Journal of the American Geriatrics Society*, **30**, 713–17.

Judd, L. L., Akiskal, H. S., Maser, J. D., Zeller, P. J., Endicott, J., Coryell, W., *et al.* (1998). A prospective 12-year study of subsyndromal and syndromal depressive symptoms in unipolar major depressive disorders. *Archives of General Psychiatry*, **55**, 694–700.

Karlsson, I. (1990). 5-HT reuptake inhibition in the elderly. In *Proceedings of the 17th CINP Congress* (ed. A. I. Yamashit, M. Toru, and A. J. Coppen), pp. 99–100. Raven Press, New York.

Katona, A. C. L. E. and Katona, A. P. M. (1997). Geriatric Depression Scale can be used in older people in primary care. *British Medical Journal*, **315**, 1236. [Letter]

Katz, I. R., Simpson, G. M., Curlik, S. M., Parmelee, P. A., and Muhly, C. (1990). Pharmacologic treatment of major depression for elderly patients in residential care settings. *Journal of Clinical Psychiatry*, **51**(Suppl. 4), 41–7.

Kay, D. W., Beamish, P., and Roth, M. (1964). Old age mental disorders in Newcastle-upon-Tyne, Part I: a study of prevalence. *British Journal of Psychiatry,* **110**, 146–58.

Kay, D. W. K. and Bergmann, K. (1966). Physical disability and mental health in old age: a follow-up of a random sample of elderly people seen at home. *Journal of Psychiatric Research*, **10**, 3–12.

Kennedy, G. L., Kelman, H. R., and Thomas, C. (1990). The emergence of depressive symptoms in late life: the importance of declining health and increasing disability. *Journal of Community Health*, **15**, 93–103.

Kivela, S-L. and Pahkala, K. (1989). Dysthymic disorder in the aged in the community. *Social Psychiatry and Psychiatric Epidemiology*, **24**, 77–83.

Kivela, S-L., Pahkala, K., and Laippala. P. (1988). Prevalence of depression in an elderly Finnish population. *Acta Psychiatrica Scandinavica*, **78**, 401–13.

Kivela, S-L., Pahkala, K., and Eronen, P. (1989). Depressive symptoms and signs that differentiate major and atypical depression from dysthymic disorder in elderly Finns. *International. Journal of Geriatric Psychiatry*, **4**, 79–85.

Kobari, M., Meyer, J. S., and Ichijo, M. (1990). Leukoaraiosis, cerebral atrophy and cerebral perfusion in normal aging. *Archives of Neurology*, **47**, 161–5.

Koder, D-. A., Brodaty, H., and Anstey, K. J. (1996). Cognitive therapy for depression in the elderly. *International. Journal of Geriatric* Psychiatry, **11**, 97–107.

Koenig, H. G., Meador, K. G., Cohen, H. J., and Blazer, D. (1988). Depression in elderly hospitalised patients with medical illness. *Archives of. Internal Medicine*, **148**, 1929–36.

Koenig, H. G., Goli, V., Shelp, F., Kudler, H. S., Cohen, H. J., Meador, K. G., *et al.* (1989). Antidepressant use in elderly medical patients: lessons from an attempted clinical trial. *Journal of General Internal Medicine*, **4**, 498–505.

Koenig, H. G., George, L. K., Peterson, I., and Pieper, C. F. (1997). Depression in medically ill hospitalised older adults: prevalence, characteristics, and course of symptoms according to six diagnostic schemes. *American Journal of Psychiatry*, **154**, 1376–83.

Kral, V. A. and Emery, O. B. (1989). Long-term follow-up of depressive pseudodementia of the aged. *Canadian. Journal of Psychiatry,* **34**, 445–6.

Kramer-Ginsberg, E., Greenwald, B. S., Aisen, P. S., and Brod-Miller, C. (1989). Hypochondriasis in the elderly depressed. *Journal of the American Geriatrics Society*, **37**, 507–10.

Krishnan, K. R. R. (1991). Organic basis of depression in the elderly. *Annual Review of Medicine,* **42**, 261–6.

Kumar, A., Miller, D., Ewbank, D., Yousen, D., Newberg, A., Samuels, S., *et al.* (1997). Quantitative anatomical measures and comorbid medical illness in late-life depression. *American Journal of Geriatric Psychiatry*, **5**(1), 15–25.

Leake, A. and Ferrier, I. C. (1993). Alterations in neuropeptides in aging and disease. *Drugs and Aging*, **3**, 408–27.

Lindesay, J., Briggs, K., and Murphy, E. (1989). The Guy's/Age Concern survey: prevalence rates of cognitive impairment, depression and anxiety in an urban elderly community. *British. Journal of Psychiatry,* **155**, 317–29.

Lipsey, J. R., Robinson, R. G., Pearlson, G. D., Rao, K., and Price, T. R. (1984). Nortriptyline treatment of post-stroke depression: a double-blind study. *Lancet*, **333**, 297–300.

Lishman, W. A. (1987). *Organic psychiatry*, 2nd edn. Blackwell, Oxford.

Lyness, J. M., Caine, E. D., Cox, C., King, D. A., Conwell, Y., and Olivares, T. (1998). Cerebrovascular risk factors and late-life major depression. *American. Journal of Geriatric Psychiatry*, **6**, 5–13.

McAllister, T. W. (1981). Cognitive functioning in the affective disorders. *Comprehensive Psychiatry*, **22**, 572–86.

MacDonald, A. J. D. (1986). Do general practitioners 'miss' depression in elderly patients? *British Medical Journal,* **292**, 1365–7.

Mahapatra, S. N. and Hackett, D. (1997). A randomised, double-blind, parallel-group comparison of venlafaxine and dothiepin in geriatric patients with major depression. *International Journal of Clinical Practice,* **51**, 209–13.

Martin, A. J., Friston, K. J., Colebatch, J. G., and Frackowiak, R. S. J. (1991). Decreases in cerebral blood flow with normal aging. *Journal of Cerebral Blood Flow and Metabolism*, **11**, 684–9.

Massey, E. W. and Bullock, R. (1978). Peroneal palsy in depression. *Journal of Clinical Psychiatry*, **287**, 291–2.

Mayeux, R., Stern, Y., Williams, J. B. W., Cote, L., Frantz, A., and Dyrenfurth, I. (1986). Clinical and biochemical features of depression in Parkinson's disease *American. Journal of Psychiatry,* **143**, 756–9.

Meador-Woodruff, J. H., Akil, M., Wisner-Carlson, R., and Grunhaus, L. (1988). Behavioural and cognitive toxicity related to elevated plasma tricyclic antidepressant levels. *Journal of Clinical Psychopharmacology*, **8**, 28–32.

Meats, P., Timol, M., and Jolley, D. (1991). Prognosis of depression in the elderly. *British Journal of Psychiatry,* **159**, 659–63.

Mendelwicz, J. (1976). The age factor in depressive illness: somogenetic considerations. *Journal of Gerontology*, **31**, 300–3.

Meyers, B. S., Greenberg, R., and Alexopoulos, G. (1988). Age of onset and studies of late-life depression. *International. Journal of Geriatric Psychiatry*, **3**, 219–28.

Miller, D. S., Kumar, A., Yousem, D. M., and Gottlieb, G. L. (1994). MRI high-intensity signals in late-life depression and Alzheimer's disease *American. Journal of Geriatric Psychiatry*, **2**, 332–7.

Mirchandani, I. C., Abrams, R. C., Young, R. C., and Alexopoulos, G. S. (1994). One-year follow-up continuation convulsive therapy prescribed for depressed elderly *patients. International. Journal of Geriatric Psychiatry*, **9**, 31–6.

Mittman, N., Herrmann, N., Einarson, T. R., Busto, U. E., Lanctot, K. L., Liu, B. A., *et al.* (1997). The efficacy, safety and tolerability of antidepressants in late life depression: meta-analysis. *Journal of Affective Disorders*, **46**, 191–217.

Morgan, K., Dallosso, H. M., Arie, T., Byrne, E. J., Jones, R., and Waite, J. (1987). Mental health and. psychological well-being among the old and very old at home. *British Journal of Psychiatry,* **150**, 801–7.

Morris, P. and Rapaport, S. I. (1990). Neuroimaging and affective disorder in late-life: a review. *Canadian. Journal of Psychiatry,* **35**, 347–54.

Murphy, E. (1982). Social origins of depression in old age. *British Journal of Psychiatry,* **141**, 135–42.

Murphy, E. (1983). The prognosis of depression in old age. *British Journal of* Psychiatry, **142**, 111–19.

Murphy, E. and Brown, G. W. (1980). Life events, psychiatric disturbance and physical illness. *British Journal of Psychiatry,* **136**, 326–38.

Murphy, E. and Grundy, E. (1984). A comparative study of bed usage by younger and older patients with depression. *Psychological Medicine*, **14**, 445–50.

Murphy, E., Smith, R., Lindesay, J., and Slattery, J. (1988). Increased mortality rates in late-life depression. *British Journal of Psychiatry,* **152**, 347–53.

Musetti, L., Perugi, G., Soriani, A., Rossi, V. M., Cassano, G. B., and Akiskal, H. P. (1989). Depression before and after age, 65: a re-examination. *British Journal of Psychiatry,* **155**, 330–6.

Nelson, J. C., Conwell, Y., Kim, K., *et al.* (1989). Age at onset in late-life delusional depression. *American. Journal of Psychiatry,* **146**, 785–786.

Nemeroff, C. B., Knight, D. L., Krishnan, R. R., Slotkin, T. A., Bissette, G., Melville, M. L., *et al.* (1988). Marked reduction in the platelet-tritiated imipramine binding sites in geriatric depression. *Archives of General Psychiatry*, **45**, 919–23.

Nyth, A. L., Gottries, C. G., Lyby, K., Smedegaard Andersen, L., Gylding Sabroe, J., Kristensen, M., *et al.* (1992). A multicenter clinical study of citalopram and placebo in elderly depressed patients with and without concomitant dementia. *Acta Psychiatrica Scandinavica*, **86**, 138–45.

O'Brien, J. T., Desmond, P., Ames, D., Schweitzer, I., Tuckwell, V., and Tress, B. (1994). The differentiation of depression from dementia by temporal lobe magnetic resonance imaging. *Psychological Medicine*, **24**, 633–40.

O'Brien, J. T., Ames, D., Schwietzer, I. (1996). White matter changes in depression and Alzheimer's disease, a review of magnetic resonance imaging findings. *International. Journal of Geriatric Psychiatry*, **11**, 681–94.

Old Age Depression Interest Group. (1993). How long should the elderly take antidepressants? A double blind placebo-controlled study of continuation/prophylaxis therapy with dothiepin. *British Journal of Psychiatry,* **162**, 175–82.

Ong, Y-L., Martineau, F., Lloyd, C., and Robbins, I. (1987). Support group for the depressed elderly. *International. Journal of Geriatric Psychiatry*, **2**, 119–23.

O'Riordan, T. G., Hayes, J. P., O'Neill, D., Shelley, R., Walsh, J. B., and Coakley, D. (1990). The effect of mild to moderate dementia on the Geriatric Depression Scale and on the General Health Questionnaire. *Age and Ageing*, **19**, 57–61.

Pahkala, K. (1990). Social and environmental factors and depression in old age. *International. Journal of Geriatric Psychiatry*, **5**, 99–113.

Pearlson, G. D., Rabins, P. V., Kim, W. S., Speedie, L. J. Moburg, P., Burns, A., *et al.* (1989). Structural brain CT changes and cognitive deficits with and without reversible dementia ('pseudodementia'). *Psychological Medicine*, **19**, 573–84.

Peterson, P. (1968). Psychiatric disorders in primary hyperparathyroidism. *Journal of Clinical Endocrinology, and Metabolism*, **28**, 1491–5.

Philpot, M. P., Banerjee, S., Needham-Bennett, H., Campos Costa, D., and Ell, P. J. (1993). -^{99}mTc-HMPAO single photon emission tomography in late life depression: a pilot study of regional cerebral blood flow at rest and during a verbal fluency task. *Journal of Affective Disorders*, **28**, 233–40.

Pitt, B. (1982). *Psychogeriatrics*, 2nd edn. Churchill Livingstone, Edinburgh.

Post, F. (1962). *The significance of affective symptoms in old age*. Maudsley Monographs, **10**. Oxford University Press, London.

Post, F. (1968). The factor of ageing in affective disorder. In *Recent developments in affective disorders* (ed. A. Coppen and A. Walk), Royal Medico-Psychological Association Publication No. 2. Headley Bros, Kent.

Post, F. (1972). The management and nature of depressive illnesses in late life: a follow-through study. *British Journal of Psychiatry*, **121**, 393–404.

Post, F. (1982). Functional disorders. In *The psychiatry of late life* (ed. R. Levy and F. Post), pp. 176–221. Blackwell, Oxford.

Postma, J. U. and Vranesi, C. D. (1985). Moclobemide in the treatment of depression in demented geriatric patients. *Acta Therapeutica*, **11**, 1–4.

Prince, M. J., Harwood, R. H., Thomas, A., and Mann, A. H. (1998). A prospective population-based cohort study of the effects of disablement and social milieu on the onset and maintenance of late-life depression. The Gospel Oak Project VII. *Psychological Medicine*, **28**, 337–50.

Prince, M. J., Reischies, F., and Beekman, A. T. F. (1999). Development of the EURO-D scale—a European Union initiative to compare symptoms of depression in 14 European centres. *British Journal of Psychiatry*, **174**, 330–8.

Raadsheer, F. C., Joop, J., Van Heerikhuize, J. J., and Lucassen, P. J. (1995). Corticotropin-releasing hormone mRNA levels in the paraventricular nucleus of patients with Alzheimer's disease and depression. *Archives of General Psychiatry,* **152**, 1372–6.

Rabins, P. V., Harvis, K., and Koven, S. (1985). High fatality rates of late-life depression associated with cardiovascular disease. *Journal of Affective Disorders*, **9**, 165–7.

Rabins, P. V., Pearlson, G. D., Aylward, E., Kumar, A. J., and Dowell, K. (1991). Cortical magnetic resonance imaging changes in elderly patients with major depression. *American Journal of Psychiatry,* **148**, 617–20.

Rapp, S. R. and Davis, K. M. (1989). Geriatric depression: physicians' knowledge, perceptions, and diagnostic practice. *The Gerontologist*, **29**, 252–7.

Reding, M., Haycox, J., and Blass, J. (1985). Depression in patients referred to a dementia clinic. *Archives of Neurology*, **42**, 894–6.

Reifler, B. V., Teri, L., Raskind, M., *et al.* (1989). Double-blind trial of imipramine in Alzheimer's disease patients with and without depression *American Journal of Psychiatry*, **146**, 45–9.

Reynolds, C. F., Hoch, C. C., Kupfer, D. J., Buysse, D. J., Houck, P. R., Stack, J. A., *et al.* (1988*a*). Bedside differentiation of depressive pseudodementia from dementia. *American Journal of Psychiatry,* **145**, 1099–103.

Reynolds, C. F., Kupfer, D. J., Houck, P. R., Hoch, C. C., Stack, J. A., Berman, S. R., *et al.* (1988*b*). Reliable discrimination of elderly depressed and demented patients by electroencephalographic sleep data. *Archives of General Psychiatry*, **45**, 258–64.

Reynolds, C. F., Perel, J. M., Cornes, C., and Kupfer, D. J. (1989). Open-trial maintenance pharmacotherapy in late-life depression: survival analysis. *Psychiatric Research*, **27**, 225–31.

Reynolds, C. F., Buysse, D. J., Kupfer, D. J., Hoch, C. C., Houck, P. R., Matzzie, J., *et al.* (1990). Rapid eye movement sleep deprivation as a probe in elderly subjects. *Archives of General Psychiatry*, **47**, 1128–36.

Reynolds, C. F., Frank, E., Perel, J. M., Miller, M. D., Cornes, C., Rifai, A. H., *et al.* (1994). Treatment of consecutive episodes of major depression in the elderly. *American Journal of Psychiatry,* **151**, 1740–3.

Reynolds III, C. F., Frank, E., Perel, J. M., Imber, S. D., Cornes, C., Miller, M. D., *et al.* (1999). Nortriptyline and. interpersonal psychotherapy as maintenance therapies for recurrent major depression: a randomized controlled trial in patients older than 59 year. *Journal of the American Medical Association*, **281**, 39–45.

Robert, R. E., Kaplan, G. A., Shema, S. J., and Strawbridge, W. J. (1997). Does growing old increase the risk for depression?. *American Journal of Psychiatry*, **154**, 1384–90.

Robins, L. N., Helzer, J. E., Weissman, M. M., Orvaschel, H., Gruengerg, E., Burke, J. D., *et al.* (1984). Lifetime prevalence of specific psychiatric disorders in three sites. *Archives of General Psychiatry*, **41**, 949–58.

Robinson, R. G., Kubos, K. L., Starr, L. B., Rao, K., and Price, T. R. (1984). Mood disorders in stroke patients: importance of location of lesion. *Brain*, **107**, 81–93.

Roose, S. P., Glassman, A. H., Attia, E., and Woodring, S. (1994). Comparative efficacy of selective serotonin reuptake inhibitors and tricyclics in the treatment of melancholia. *American Journal of Psychiatry,* **151**, 1735–9.

Roth, M. (1955). The natural history of mental disorder in old age. *Journal of Mental Science*, **101**, 281–301.

Roth, M., Mountjoy, C. Q., and Amrein, R. (1996). Moclobemide in elderly patients with cognitive decline and depression: an international double-blind placebo-controlled study. *British Journal of Psychiatry,* **168**, 149–57.

Roy, R. and Thomas, M. (1986). A survey of chronic pain in an elderly population. *Canadian Family Physician*, **32**, 513–16.

Royal College of Physicians and. British Geriatric Society. (1992). *Standardised assessment scales for elderly people,* Report of the Joint Workshops of the Research Unit of the Royal College of Physicians and the British Geriatric Society, London Royal College of Physicians.

Sackeim, H. A., Prohovnik, I., Moeller, J. R., Brown, R. P., Apter, S., Prudic, J., *et al.* (1990). Regional cerebral blood flow in mood disorders: 1. Comparison of major depressives and normal controls at rest. *Archives of General Psychiatry*, **47**, 60–70.

Sadavoy, J. and Reiman-Sheldon, E. (1983). General hospital geriatric psychiatric treatment: a follow-up study. *Journal of the American Geriatrics Society*, **31**, 200–5.

Sahakian, B. J. (1991). Depressive pseudodementia in the elderly. *International Journal of Geriatric Psychiatry*, **6**, 453–8.

Sapolsky, R., Krey, L., and McEwen, B. (1986). The neuroendocrinology of stress and aging: the glucocorticoid cascade hypothesis. *Endocrine Review*, **7**, 284–301.

Schneider, L. S. (1992). Psychobiologic features of geriatric affective disorders. *Clinics in Geriatric Medicine*, **8**, 253–65.

Schneider, L. S., Reynolds, C. F., Lebowitz, B. D., and Friedhoff, A. J. (1994). *Diagnosis and treatment of depression in late life*. American Psychiatric Press, Washington DC.

Scogin, F. and McElreath, L. (1994). Efficacy of psychosocial treatments for geriatric depression: a quantitative review. *Journal of Consulting and Clinical Psychology*, **62**, 69–74.

Seth, R., Jennings, A. L., Bindman, J., Phillips, J., and Bergmann, K. (1992). Combination treatment with noradrenalin and serotonin reuptake inhibitors in resistant depression. *British Journal of Psychiatry,* **161**, 562–5.

Sherwood, N. and Hindmarch, L. (1993). A comparison of five commonly prescribed antidepressants with particular reference to their behavioural toxicity. *Human Psychopharmacology*, **8**, 417–22.

Snowdon, J. (1990). The prevalence of depression in old age. *International Journal of Geriatric Psychiatry*, **5**, 141–4.

Spar, J. E. and Gerner, R. (1982). Does the dexamethasone suppression test distinguish dementia from depression? *American Journal of Psychiatry*, **139**, 238–40.

Steuer, J. L., Mintz, J., Hammen, C. L., Hill, M. A., Jarvik, L. F., McCarley, T., *et al.* (1984). Cognitive-behavioral and psychodynamic group psychotherapy in treatment of geriatric depression. *Journal of Consulting and Clinical. Psychology*, **52**, 180–9.

Swayze, V. W., Anderson, A., Arndt, S., Rajerethinam, R., Fleming, F., Sato, Y., *et al.* (1996). Reversibility of brain tissue loss in anorexia nervosa assessed with a computerised Talairach, 3-D proportional grid. *Psychological Medicine*, **26**, 381–90.

Targum, S. D., Marshall, L. E., and Fischman, P. (1992). Variability of TRH test responses in depressed and normal elderly subjects. *Biological Psychiatry*, **31**, 787–93.

Tew, J. D., Mulsant, B. H., Haskett, R. F., Prudic, J., Thase, M. E., Crowe, R. R., *et al.* (1999). Acute efficacy of ECT in the treatment of major depression in the Old-Old. *American Journal of Psychiatry*, **156**, 1865–70.

Tiller, J., Maguire, K., and Davies, B. (1990). A sequential double-blind controlled study of moclobemide and mianserin in elderly depressed patients. *International Journal of Geriatric Psychiatry*, **5**, 199–204.

Trappler, B. and Cohen, C. I. (1998). Use of SSRIs in 'very old' depressed nursing home residents. *American Journal of Geriatric Psychiatry*, **6**, 83–9.

Upadhyaya, A. K., Abou-Saleh, M. T., Wilson, K., Grime, S. J., and Critchley, M. (1990). A study of depression in old age using single photon emission tomography. *British Journal of Psychiatry*, **157**(Suppl. 9), 76–81.

Veith, R. C. and Raskind, M. A. (1988). The neurobiology of aging: does it predispose to depression? *Neurobiology of Aging*, **9**, 101–17.

Waterreus, A., Blanchard, M., and Mann, A. (1994). Community psychiatric nurses for elderly: well-tolerated, few side effects and effective in the treatment of depression. *Journal of Clinical Nursing*, **3**, 299–306.

Weingartner, H., Cohen, R. M., Murphy, D. L., Martello, J., and Gerdt, C. (1981). Cognitive processes in depression. *Archives of General Psychiatry*, **38**, 42–7.

Weingartner, H., Cohen, R. M., Bunney, W. E., Ebert, M. H., and Kaye, W. (1982). Memory-learning impairments in progressive dementia and depression. *American Journal of Psychiatry*, **139**, 135–6.

Williams, E. I. and Wallace, P. (1993). Health checks for people aged 75 and over. *British Journal of Geriatric Practice*, Occasional Paper number 59.

Winokur, G., Morrison, J., Clancy, J., *et al.* (1973). The Iowa 500 familial and clinical findings favour two kinds of depressive illness. *Comprehensive Psychiatry*, **14**, 99–107.

World Health Organization. (1993). *The ICD-10 Classification of Mental and Behavioural Disorders: Research Criteria*. WHO, Geneva.

Yesavage, J. A., Brink, T. L., Rose, T. L., and Lum, O. (1983). Development and validation of a geriatric depression screening scale: a preliminary report. *Journal of Psychiatric Research*, **17**, 37–49.

Yohannes, A. M., Roomi, J., Baldwin, R. C., and Connoly, M. J. (1998). Depression in elderly outpatients with disabling chronic obstructive pulmonary disease. *Age and Ageing*, **27**, 155–60.

Yost, E. B., Beutler, L. E., Corbishley, M. A., and Allender, J. R. (1986). *Group cognitive therapy: a treatment approach for depressed older adults*. Pergamon Press, New York.

Young, R. C., Nambudiri, D., Alexopoulos, G. S., and Roe, R. (1988). Ventricular-brain ratio and response to nortriptyline in geriatric depression. *Annual Meeting, Society of Biological Psychiatry*. [Abstract]

Zubenko, G. S. and Moossy, J. (1988). Major depression in primary dementia: clinical and neuropathological correlates. *Archives of Neurology*, **45**, 1182–6.

Zubenko, G. S., Sullivan, P., Nelson, J. P., Belle, S. H., Huff, J., and Wolf, G. L. (1990). Brain imaging abnormalities in mental disorders of late life. *Archives of Neurology*, **47**, 1107–11.

Zung, W. W. K. (1967). Depression in the normal aged. *Psychosomatics*, **8**, 287–92.

28 Suicide in older persons

Daniel Harwood

A common view amongst lay people is that a suicide in an older person is likely to be a rational act in response to unbearable or terminal physical illness. In fact, most self-inflicted deaths are the end result of a complex interplay of biological, psychological, and social factors. Although clinicians on their own cannot make a significant impact on national suicide rates, they need some knowledge of these risk factors for suicide in order to understand the sources of distress in the patients they work with and to inform the management of the suicidal patients under their care.

Suicidal behaviour occurs in a spectrum ranging from thoughts of hopelessness through indirect self-destructive behaviour and deliberate self-harm to completed suicide. As will become evident, apparently trivial acts of self-harm occurring in older people can be indicators of high suicidal intent and serious psychiatric disorder.

Suicidal ideation

Feelings of hopelessness are common in older people: of a sample of people aged 65 and over in Dublin, 15.5% said they had felt life was not worth living in the month prior to the interview (Kirby *et al.* 1997). Serious suicidal thoughts are less common: only 3.3% of this sample had felt an actual wish to die. Suicidal thoughts in samples of older people in the community are usually associated with psychiatric disorder, or psychiatric symptoms, especially depression (Forsell *et al.* 1997). However, physical disability, pain, sensory impairments, institutionalization, and single marital status are all associated with suicidal thinking in the elderly, even when depression has been controlled for (Jorm *et al.* 1995; Forsell *et al.* 1997).

Indirect self-destructive behaviour

Older people may be especially prone to behaviours, which, although not directly suicidal, still increase the chance of dying, such as refusing food with the aim of starving, or not taking prescribed medication. This 'indirect self-destructive behaviour' is more common in institutional settings, and may be a substitute for overt suicidal acts in physically ill and dependent people (Nelson and Farberow 1980). Indirect self-destructive behaviours are particularly frequent amongst women and the very old (Osgood *et al.* 1991).

Deliberate self-harm

The high suicidal intent of most acts of deliberate self-harm in older people contrasts with the higher frequency and more heterogeneous nature of these acts in younger people (Draper 1996). In developed countries, drug overdose is the commonest method of self-harm in older people, with hypnotics, analgesics, and antidepressants the usual drugs chosen (Draper 1996). The absolute number of deliberate self-harm episodes in the elderly is higher in women in a 3:2 ratio, but *rates* in men and women are similar because there are fewer men than women in the older population. Other demographic risk factors associated with deliberate self-harm in the elderly include single or divorced marital status, and, possibly, low socioeconomic group (Draper 1996).

Older people attempting suicide are more likely to have a psychiatric illness than younger patients (Merrill and Owens 1990). Over half will have a depressive disorder, with alcohol abuse in 5–32% and other psychiatric disorders in around 10%. A minority, probably less than 14%, will have no psychiatric illness (Draper 1996). Personality factors associated with attempted suicide in the elderly have been under-researched, although it seems likely that personality disorder is much rarer than in the younger self-harm population.

Non-psychiatric risk factors for self-harm in the elderly have not been well studied. Grief, especially after spousal bereavement, and interpersonal problems, are consistently found to be associated with self-harm in the elderly (Draper 1996). Physical illness was found to be a contributory factor in only 18% of one series of attempted suicides in older people (Pierce 1987). Social isolation may be more important in old compared with young suicide attempters (Nowers 1993).

A recent British study found the rate of repetition of self-harm in a cohort of older deliberate self-harm patients was 5.4% annually, lower than for younger age groups. However, the rate of *completed suicide* (around 6% during the 2–5 year follow-up period) was higher than for younger deliberate self-harm patients. The factors predicting later suicide were male gender, a psychiatric history prior to the index attempt, and persistent depression being treated by a psychiatric team (Hepple and Quinton 1997).

Suicide

Epidemiology

In England and Wales, suicide rates in older people fell by half between 1985 and 1996 (Hoxey and Shah 2000; McClure 2000), a trend mirrored by many other industrialized countries (Pritchard 1996). However, the suicide rate in very old men (those over 85) has either remained static or increased over the same period (Pritchard 1996; Kelly and Bunting 1998), and in most countries of the world suicide rates are still highest in older people (De Leo 1997).

Suicide rates show dramatic international variations. Rates in older people are very high in Hungary, Lithuania, and other central and eastern European countries, with low rates in southern Europe (World Health Organization, 1998).

Suicide rates are subject to *period effects*. World War II, the change over from toxic coal gas to safer North Sea gas (Murphy *et al.* 1986), and restrictions on barbiturate prescribing (Nowers and Irish 1988) all led to reductions in the suicide rate in older people in the UK. Lindesay (1991) noted that suicide rates tend to be higher in those age groups that constitute larger proportions of the population, and predicted a rise in suicide rate as the 'baby boom generation' ages.

Older men are more likely to die through suicide than older women. In the US, older male suicides outnumber female by 4:1 (Bharucha and Satlin 1997), in the UK the ratio is nearer 3:1 (Hoxey and Shah 2000; Harwood *et al.* 2000), whereas in Hong Kong rates in older men and women are similar (Yip *et al.* 1998). Marriage is a protective factor against suicide, with rates higher in the divorced and single (Smith *et al.* 1988; Harwood *et al.* 2000). Widowers are at a much greater risk of suicide than widows (Li 1995). Suicide rates in older immigrants to the UK are influenced by their country of origin (Raleigh and Balarajan 1992), and in the USA rates are higher in older Whites than non-Whites (Moscicki 1995).

Method of suicide

In general, elderly men adopt more violent methods than women, which may partly account for the sex difference in rates. Shooting is the commonest method in the USA (Kaplan *et al.* 1996, 1997). Drug overdose (more common in women) and hanging (more common in men) are the commonest methods in the UK (Cattell and Jolley 1995; Harwood *et al.* 2000), with paracetamol, combination analgesics, and antidepressants the three most frequent drug classes implicated in the latter study.

Risk factors

Neurobiology

The study of the neurobiology of suicide in older people is fraught with methodological problems

(Conwell *et al.* 1995). The most consistent research findings in the biology of suicidal behaviour are the associations with underactivity of the serotonin system and low serum cholesterol (Jones *et al.* 1990; Träskman-Bendz and Mann 2000).

Psychiatric disorder

Over 70% of older people who commit suicide are suffering from a psychiatric illness at the time of death, and between 44 and 87% are suffering from depression (Conwell 1997). Case-control studies using both deceased and living control groups have confirmed depressive disorder as a risk factor for suicide in older people (Conwell *et al.* 2000; Harwood *et al.* 2001). Depression is more frequently associated with suicide in older people than younger age groups (Conwell *et al.* 1996). Chronic depression and a first episode late in life may be indicators of an increased suicidal risk (Shah and De 1998).

Rates of alcohol misuse in older suicide victims are higher in the USA than Britain where studies show rates of 10% or lower (Barraclough 1971; Harwood *et al.* 2001). Schizophrenia is found in less than 10% of older suicides (lower rates than for younger age bands), and anxiety disorders are rarely found (Conwell *et al.* 1996; Conwell *et al.* 2000; Harwood *et al.* 2001). The rates of dementia found in psychological autopsy studies of older suicide victims are similar to the general population rates of these disorders (Harwood *et al.* 2001). However, this finding may mask a possible increased risk of suicide in *early* dementia, particularly if depressive symptoms are also present (Rohde *et al.* 1995; Draper *et al.* 1998).

Personality

Around 15% of suicides in people 60 years and over are associated with a personality disorder diagnosis (Henriksson *et al.* 1995; Harwood *et al.* 2001), lower rates than those found in samples of younger suicide victims. However, an additional 28% may have significant accentuation of personality traits, most notably anankastic and anxious traits. These two personality traits were found to be predictors of suicide in a case-control analysis (Harwood *et al.* 2001) a finding consistent with research in the USA showing a link between suicide in old age and low 'openness to experience' (methodical, rigid, and emotionally restricted traits) (Duberstein *et al.* 1994).

Physical illness

The most frequent type of life event preceding suicide in an older person is a physical illness (Heikkinen and Lönnqvist 1995). In 84% of one sample of older suicide victims, medical illness was considered a stressor at the time of death (Carney *et al.* 1994). Physical illness may lead to suicide through causing functional limitation, which was found to be a predictor of suicide in a recent case-control study (Conwell *et al.* 2000). Pain was noted to be important factor in around 20% of suicides in older people in another recent study (Purcell *et al.* 1999). Comorbid psychiatric disorders contribute to the risk of suicide in the medically ill (Conwell *et al.* 1990; Horton-Deutsch *et al.* 1992). Specific conditions associated with an increased suicide risk include cancer (particularly in the first year after diagnosis), stroke, multiple sclerosis, and epilepsy (Stenager and Stenager 2000). Unfortunately, the suicide risk associated with common cardiovascular and respiratory disorders has not been well researched.

Social factors and life events

Suicide is rare in residential care (Osgood *et al.* 1991). Research findings conflict as to whether living alone is a risk factor for suicide in older people (Shah and De 1998). Social isolation is an important factor in some cases, although a Finnish study found levels of social contact prior to death to be similar in old and young suicide victims (Heikkinen and Lönnqvist 1995). In the UK, areas of social deprivation, especially with high levels of social fragmentation, have higher suicide rates in all age bands, including those over 65 years old (Whitley *et al.* 1999). Bereavement may be no more common as a precipitant to suicide in the elderly than in younger age groups (Heikkinen and Lönnqvist 1995), but the death of a spouse increases the risk of suicide in older men in the first year after bereavement (Bunch 1972; Li 1995). Poverty (Rao 1991), elder abuse (Conwell 1995), and interpersonal conflict or financial problems (Heikkinen and Lönnqvist 1995) have all been cited as risk factors for suicide in older people.

Rational suicide

Around 20% of suicides in older people are not associated with psychiatric disorder, and undoubtedly some of these are rational acts in response to insoluble life problems. However, there is a concern that the suicidal wishes of older people may be assumed to be rational when in fact they are coloured by depressive illness (Conwell and Caine 1991).

Suicide prevention in older people

Risk assessment

Using established risk factors to assess suicide risk in an individual tends to produce many false-positive predictions, which is due to the high prevalence of many of the risk factors but the relatively low rate of suicide. Risk assessment in clinical practice should adopt a more individualized approach with a thorough interview covering suicidal intent and details of past suicide attempts (Morgan *et al.* 1998).

Suicide prevention

The greatest potential for reducing suicide rates lies in limiting the availability of the means of self-destruction (Lewis *et al.* 1997). In the USA where most suicides in older people are inflicted by gunshot (Kaplan *et al.* 1996, 1997), the obvious measure to reduce rates would be stringent gun control. In most European countries where overdose is more common, limiting the use of drugs frequently implicated in suicide might help (Dennis and Lindesay 1995; Harwood *et al.* 2000). Combination analgesics should be avoided in the elderly because of their limited effectiveness (Po and Zhang 1997) and high lethality in overdose. Deaths through antidepressant overdose could be reduced by exercising caution in the prescription of cardiotoxic antidepressants (notably amitriptyline and dosulepin (dothiepin); Henry *et al.* 1995), particularly if the patient does not have a carer who can supervise the medication.

Another approach to suicide prevention is the targeting of high-risk groups. An Italian study demonstrated that a service involving an alarm system to access help and regular telephone support seemed to reduce the suicide rate in a population of socially isolated elderly people (De Leo *et al.* 1995).

About 50% of older suicide victims contact their general practitioner (GP) in the month before death (Vassilas and Morgan 1994; Harwood *et al.* 2000), so the identification and treatment of depression by GPs is often advocated as a method of trying to reduce the suicide rate in older people. In a group of older suicide victims who had visited their family physician in the month before death, the doctor had identified psychiatric symptoms in most cases, but less than half of those with a psychiatric disorder were offered treatment (Caine *et al.* 1996). Clearly, there remains scope for the education of GPs in the detection and treatment of depression in the elderly, especially in those with comorbid medical conditions. Only about 25% of older people dying through suicide have been in contact with a psychiatric team in the year before death (Harwood *et al.* 2000). However, psychiatric services have a role in preventing suicides by improving the overall care offered to high-risk patients, especially older deliberate self-harm patients (Pierce 1987). Multidisciplinary audit of cases of suicide known to the psychiatric services is a useful way of highlighting possible deficits in local services. In the UK, the National Confidential Inquiry, an ambitious national audit of suicides occurring whilst under psychiatric care, has recently published its report. This makes 31 recommendations, which include an overhaul of the care programme approach, better training in risk assessment for all mental health workers, changes to the structure of some inpatient units, and more effective information exchange (Appleby *et al.* 1999). The clergy are under-recognized as an important source of psychological support for many older people. A recent paper from the USA advocated better education of ministers about suicide in older people (Weaver and Koenig 1997). The International Psychogeriatric Association has recently launched an International Suicide Prevention Programme to try and implement some of the measures discussed above.

References

Appleby, L., Shaw, J., and Amos, T. (1999). *Safer services: Report of the National Confidential Inquiry into Suicide and Homicide by People with a Mental Illness.* Department of Health, London.

Barraclough, B. M. (1971). Suicide in the elderly. *British Journal of Psychiatry* (special supplement 6), 87–97.

Bharucha, A. J. and Satlin, A. (1997). Late-life suicide: a review. *Harvard Review of Psychiatry*, **5**, 55–65.

Bunch, J. M. (1972). Recent bereavement in relation to suicide. *Journal of Psychosomatic Research*, **16**, 361–6.

Caine, E. D., Lyness, J. M., and Conwell, Y. (1996). Diagnosis of late-life depression: preliminary studies in primary care settings. *American Journal of Geriatric Psychiatry*, **4**(Suppl. 1), 545–50.

Carney, S. S., Rich, C. L., Burke, P. A., and Fowler, R. C. (1994). Suicide over 60: the San Diego study. *Journal of the American Geriatrics Society*, **42**, 174–80.

Cattell, H. and Jolley, D. J. (1995). One hundred cases of suicide in elderly people. *British Journal of Psychiatry*, **166**, 451–7.

Conwell, Y. (1995). Elder abuse—a risk factor for suicide? *Crisis*, **16**, 104–5.

Conwell, Y. (1997). Management of suicidal behavior in the elderly. *The Psychiatric Clinics of North America*, **20**, 667–83.

Conwell, Y. and Caine, E. D. (1991). Rational suicide and the right to die: reality and myth. *New England Journal of Medicine*, **325**, 1100–3.

Conwell, Y., Caine, E. D., and Olsen, K. (1990). Suicide and cancer in late life. *Hospital and Community Psychiatry*, **41**, 1334–9.

Conwell, Y., Raby, W. N., and Caine, E. D. (1995). Suicide and aging II: the psychobiological interface. *International Psychogeriatrics*, **7**, 165–81.

Conwell, Y., Duberstein, P. R., Cox, C., Herrmann, J., Forbes, N. T., and Caine, E. D. (1996). Relationships of age and axis I diagnoses in victims of completed suicide: a psychological autopsy study. *American Journal of Psychiatry*, **153**, 1001–8.

Conwell, Y., Lyness, J. M., Duberstein, P., Cox, C., Seidlitz, L., DiGiorgio, A. and Caine, E. D. (2000). Completed suicide among older patients in primary care practices: a controlled study. *Journal of the American Geriatrics Society*, **48**, 23–9.

De Leo, D. (1997). Suicide in late life at the end of the 1990s: a less neglected topic? *Crisis*, **18**, 51–2.

De Leo, D., Carollo, G., and Dello Buono, M. (1995). Lower suicide rates associated with a Tele-help/Tele-check service for the elderly at home. *American Journal of Psychiatry*, **152**, 632–4.

Dennis, M. S. and Lindesay, J. (1995). Suicide in the elderly: the United Kingdom perspective. *International Psychogeriatrics*, **7**, 263–74.

Draper, B. (1996). Attempted suicide in old age. *International Journal of Geriatric Psychiatry*, **11**, 577–87.

Draper, B., MacCuspie-Moore, C., and Brodaty, H. (1998). Suicidal ideation and the 'wish to die' in dementia patients: the role of depression. *Age and Ageing*, **27**, 503–7.

Duberstein, P. R., Conwell, Y., and Caine, E. D. (1994). Age differences in the personality characteristics of suicide completers: preliminary findings from a psychological autopsy study. *Psychiatry*, **57**, 213–24.

Forsell, Y., Jorm, A. F., and Winblad, B. (1997). Suicidal thoughts and associated factors in an elderly population. *Acta Psychiatrica Scandinavica*, **95**, 108–11.

Harwood, D. M. J., Hawton, K., Hope, T., and Jacoby, R. (2000) Suicide in older people: mode of death, demographic factors, and medical contact before death in one hundred and ninety-five cases. *International Journal of Geriatric Psychiatry*, **15**, 736–43.

Harwood, D. M. J., Hawton, K., Hope, T., and Jacoby, R. (2001) Psychiatric disorder and personality factors associated with suicide in older people: a descriptive and case-control study. *International Journal of Geriatric Psychiatry*, **16**, 155–65.

Heikkinen, M. E. and Lönnqvist, J. K. (1995). Recent life events in elderly suicide: a nationwide study in Finland. *International Psychogeriatrics*, **7**, 287–300.

Henriksson, M. M., Marttunen, M. J., Isometsä, E. T., Heikkinen, M. E., Aro, H. M., Kuoppasalmi, K. I., *et al.* (1995). Mental disorders in elderly suicide. *International Psychogeriatrics*, **7**, 275–86.

Henry, J. A., Alexander, C. A., and Sener, E. K. (1995). Relative mortality from overdoses of antidepressants. *British Medical Journal*, **310**, 221–4.

Hepple, J. and Quinton, C. (1997). One hundred cases of attempted suicide in the elderly. *British Journal of Psychiatry*, **171**, 42–6.

Horton-Deutsch, S. L., Clark, D. C., and Farran, C. J. (1992). Chronic dyspnea and suicide in elderly men. *Hospital and Community Psychiatry*, **43**, 1198–203.

Hoxey, K. and Shah, A. (2000). Recent trends in elderly suicide rates in England and Wales. *International Journal of Geriatric Psychiatry*, **15**, 274–9.

Jones, J. S., Stanley, B., Mann, J. J., Frances, A. J., Guido, J. R., Träskman-Bendz, L., *et al.* (1990). CSF 5-HIAA and HVA concentrations in elderly depressed patients who attempted suicide. *American Journal of Psychiatry*, **147**, 1225–7.

Jorm, A. F., Henderson, A. S., Scott, R., Korten, A. E., Chirstensen, H., and Mackinnon, A. J. (1995). Factors associated with the wish to die in elderly people. *Age and Ageing*, **24**, 389–92.

Kaplan, M. S., Adamek, M. E., and Geling, O. (1996). Sociodemographic predictors of firearm suicide among older white males. *Gerontologist*, **36**, 530–3.

Kaplan, M. S., Adamek, M. E., Geling, O., and Calderon, A. (1997). Firearm suicide among older women in the US. *Social Science and Medicine*, **44**, 1427–30.

Kelly, S. and Bunting, J. (1998). Trends in suicide in England and Wales 1982–1996. *Population Trends*, **92**, 29–41.

Kirby, M., Bruce, I., Radic, A., Coakley, D., and Lawlor, B. A. (1997). Hopelessness and suicidal feelings among the community dwelling elderly in Dublin. *Irish Journal of Psychological Medicine*, **14**, 124–7.

Lewis, G., Hawton, K., and Jones, P. (1997). Strategies for preventing suicide. *British Journal of Psychiatry*, **171**, 351–4.

Li, G. (1995). The interaction effect of bereavement and sex on the risk of suicide in the elderly: an historical cohort study. *Social Science and Medicine*, **40**, 825–8.

Lindesay, J. (1991). Suicide in the elderly. *International Journal of Geriatric Psychiatry*, **6**, 355–61.

McClure, G. M. G. (2000). Changes in suicide in England and Wales 1960–1997. *British Journal of Psychiatry*, **176**, 64–7.

Merrill, J. and Owens, J. (1990). Age and attempted suicide. *Acta Psychiatrica Scandinavica*, **82**, 385–8.

Morgan, G., Buckley, C., and Nowers, M. (1998). Face to face with the suicidal. *Advances in Psychiatric Treatment*, **4**, 188–96.

Mościcki, E. K. (1995). Epidemiology of suicide. *International Psychogeriatrics*, **7**, 137–48.

Murphy, E., Lindesay, J., and Grundy, E. (1986). 60 years of suicide in England and Wales: a cohort study. *Archives of General Psychiatry*, **43**, 969–76.

Nelson, F. L. and Farberow, N. L. (1980). Indirect self-destructive behavior in the elderly nursing home patient. *Journal of Gerontology*, **35**, 949–57.

Nowers, M. (1993). Deliberate self-harm in the elderly: a survey of one London borough. *International Journal of Geriatric Psychiatry*, **8**, 609–14.

Nowers, M. and Irish, M. (1988). Trends in the reported rates of suicide by self poisoning in the elderly. *Journal of the Royal College of General Practitioners*, **38**, 67–9.

Osgood, N. J., Brant, B. A., and Lipman, A. (1991). *Suicide among the elderly in long-term care facilities.* Greenwood Press, New York.

Pierce, D. (1987). Deliberate self-harm in the elderly. *International Journal of Geriatric Psychiatry*, **2**, 105–10.

Po, A. L. W. and Zhang, W. Y. (1997). Systematic overview of co-proxamol to assess analgesic effects of addition of dextropropoxyphene to paracetamol. *British Medical Journal*, **315**, 1565–71.

Pritchard, C. (1996). New patterns of suicide by age and gender in the United Kingdom and the Western World 1974–1992; an indicator of social change? *Social Psychiatry and Psychiatric Epidemiology*, **31**, 227–34.

Purcell, D., Thrush, C. R. N., and Blanchette, P. L. (1999). Suicide among the elderly in Honolulu county: a multiethnic comparative study (1987–1992). *International Psychogeriatrics*, **11**, 57–66.

Raleigh, V. S. and Balarajan, R. (1992). Suicide levels and trends among immigrants in England and Wales. *Health Trends*, **24**, 91–4.

Rao, A. V. (1991). Suicide in the elderly: a report from India. *Crisis*, **12**, 33–9.

Rohde, K., Peskind, E. R., and Raskind, M. A. (1995). Suicide in two patients with Alzheimer's disease. *Journal of the American Geriatrics Society*, **43**, 187–9.

Shah, A. and De, T. (1998). Suicide and the elderly. *International Journal of Psychiatry in Clinical Practice*, **2**, 3–17.

Smith, J. C., Mercy, J. A., and Conn, J. M. (1988). Marital status and the risk of suicide. *American Journal of Public Health*, **78**, 78–80.

Stenager, E. N. and Stenager, G. (2000). Physical illness and suicidal behaviour. In *The international handbook of suicide and attempted suicide* (ed. K. Hawton and K. van Heeringen), pp. 405–20. Wiley, Chichester.

Träskman-Bendz, L. and Mann, J. J. (2000). Biological aspects of suicidal behaviour. In *The international handbook of suicide and attempted suicide* (ed. K. Hawton and K. van Heeringen), pp. 65–77. Wiley, Chichester.

Vassilas, C. A. and Morgan, H. G. (1994). Elderly suicides' contact with their general practitioner before death. *International Journal of Geriatric Psychiatry*, **9**, 1008–9.

Weaver, A. J. and Koenig, H. (1996). Elderly suicide, mental health professionals, and the clergy: a need for clinical collaboration, training and research. *Death Studies*, **20**, 495–508.

Whitley, E., Gunnell, D., Dorling, D., and Smith, G. D. (1999). Ecological study of social fragmentation, poverty, and suicide. *British Medical Journal*, **319**, 1034–7.

World Health Organization (1998). *1996 World health statistics manual.* WHO, Geneva.

Yip, P. S. F., Chi, I., and Yu, K. K. (1998). An epidemiological profile of elderly suicides in Hong Kong. *International Journal of Geriatric Psychiatry*, **13**, 631–7.

29 Manic syndromes in old age

Kenneth I. Shulman and Nathan Herrmann

Classification issues

The title of this chapter deliberately uses the broader and generic notion of 'syndrome' to label the heterogeneous clinical conditions under review. Mania or hypomania is fundamental to the diagnosis of bipolar disorder as conceived in DSM-IV (American Psychiatric Association 1994). Within this context, 'bipolarity' is considered a primary mood disorder. Further refinement into bipolar I, II, or even III depends on the severity of manic symptomatology or the ease with which episodes are precipitated, i.e. whether they are spontaneous or drug-induced. The available evidence suggests that the primary form of bipolarity is heavily influenced by genetic (familial) factors (Goodwin and Jamison 1990).

However, the very high levels of comorbidity within the elderly population cloud the diagnostic picture (Shulman 1997*a*). DSM-IV has established a category of 'mood disorder due to a general medical condition' (293.83), with the prescription that 'the disturbance is the direct physiologic consequence of a general medical condition'. Given the high prevalence of neurological and medical comorbidity in old age (described below), the issue of 'direct physiologic consequence' becomes difficult indeed. The extent to which the clinician can be sure that an episode of mania is causally related to associated medical conditions is questionable. Hence, the assumption of an aetiological relationship is even more precarious.

Outside the formal DSM and ICD classification system, is the widely held concept of secondary mania (Krauthammer and Klerman 1978). This category also implies that cerebral organic factors are responsible for the syndrome. Supporting factors include a close temporal relationship between the medical/neurological condition and the manic syndrome, negative prior history or family history, and a distinction from delirium. Furthermore, the neurological literature uses the term 'disinhibition syndrome' in a way that is virtually identical to the psychiatric notion of mania, and which has similar implied conditions that underlie the clinical syndrome. Finally, the concept of a 'bipolar spectrum' (Akiskal 1986) has considerable merit when applied to the elderly. Affective vulnerability (inherited or acquired) may be expressed through temperament in adult life, and in late life may interact with a variety of cerebral organic factors to produce a manic syndrome.

Nosology remains at the heart of our understanding of disorders that have 'manic expression'. Diagnostic terms are inextricably linked to the understanding of the nature, pathogenesis, and aetiology of these syndromes. The uncertainty and fuzziness that pervades our current classification should be a stimulus for further clarification based on the best available data. Indeed, the practical question of management and prognosis will follow from our use of diagnostic terminology.

This chapter will critically review the literature on mania in late life by describing its epidemiology, pathogenesis, comorbidity, and management. Based on the available evidence, a summary of the essential determinants of manic syndromes in old age will be presented. A classification of subtypes of mania is proposed as a basis for further research into the cause of these syndromes as well as their effective management. Hopefully, this approach will help to improve the current confusion around classification, and enhance our capacity to understand these conditions.

Epidemiology

Methodological concerns confound the data regarding the prevalence and incidence of mania in old age. Some of the concerns are inherent in identifying individuals with mania in the community who, similar to paranoid patients, are not readily amenable to interview or cooperation with community surveys. Compounding these problems is the diagnostic uncertainty described above. Interestingly, the clinical features of mania in older people do not differ from those in younger people, except for the higher prevalence of cognitive dysfunction (Broadhead and Jacoby 1990). While clinical symptoms in an elderly cohort are similar to those in a mixed-age population they tend toward lesser severity and intensity in the former.

Opposite trends apply to age and bipolarity for published hospital admission rates and community prevalence. Relatively high 'treated prevalence'[1] (4–8%) has been reported for inpatient psychogeriatric units (Yassa *et al.* 1988), while, in a national survey, first admission rates for mania showed a modest increase for the extremes of old age (Spicer *et al.* 1973; Eagles and Whalley 1985). Specialized psychogeriatric units report significant numbers of elderly people with bipolar disorder, approximately 7–10 admissions per year (Shulman and Post 1980; Yassa *et al.* 1988; Shulman *et al.* 1992). In contrast, the Epidemiologic Catchment Area (ECA) study shows a negligible prevalence of mania in over-65-year-olds in the community (< 0.1%), down from a high of 1.4% in young adults (Weissman *et al.* 1991). Other studies of elderly cohorts also support the conclusion that there is a significant decrease in the community prevalence of mania at the extreme end of the lifespan (Tsuang 1978; Weeke and Vaeth 1986; Snowdon 1991).

So, where have all the young bipolars gone? Some suggest the influence of a relatively high mortality rate from natural causes, suicide in the long-term course of bipolar disorders, as well as 'burn out' over a long-term course (Winokur 1975; Snowdon 1991). Given the very early age of onset of the majority of bipolar disorders (early twenties), prospective follow-up studies are not easily conducted and the dependence on retrospective data makes this question an ongoing challenge.

Age of onset

Age of onset has been viewed as an important variable that could distinguish the subtypes of mania, and hence lead to an improved understanding of its pathogenesis and aetiology (Young and Klerman 1992). However, the cut-off age used for 'late onset' has been variable (Yassa *et al.* 1988). Wylie *et al.* (1999) have suggested that, in a sample of mixed-age patients, the *median age* at onset could reasonably be used to set the cut-off point between early and late onset. In their sample of elderly bipolar patients (over 60 years of age), the median age of onset was 49 years, which in turn was influenced by the cut-off for the age considered 'elderly'. Most studies have used age 65 as the benchmark for old age, and in such samples the late-onset cut-off point would probably then be in the early to mid-fifties. This was the case in a study in which the mean age of the elderly patients with bipolar disorder was 70 and the mean age of their first psychiatric hospitalization was 55 (the median age was not reported) (Shulman *et al.* 1992). While no clear convention for 'late onset' in the elderly has been established, an age of at least 50 years would seem a reasonable marker for future use. In the study by Wylie *et al.* (1999), using a cut-off point of 49 years, the late-onset group of elderly bipolar patients were found to have more psychotic features and to demonstrate an increase in cerebrovascular risk factors (see Fig. 29.1). At the time of discharge, outcome as measured by the Brief Psychiatric Rating Scale (BPRS), Mini-Mental State Examination (MMSE), and Global Assessment was not significantly different between the early- and late-onset cases. An increase in vascular comorbidity was also found in a sample of elderly bipolar patients (mean age 74 years) using a cut-off of 50 years for age at onset (Hays *et al.* 1998). Late-onset subjects were reported to have more psychosocial supports and also less family history of psychiatric problems. However, their results do show a very high proportion of patients with a positive family history, 83% for late onset and 88% for early onset—a difference that is not significant. Previous attempts to link age of onset with a family history of mood disorder have produced

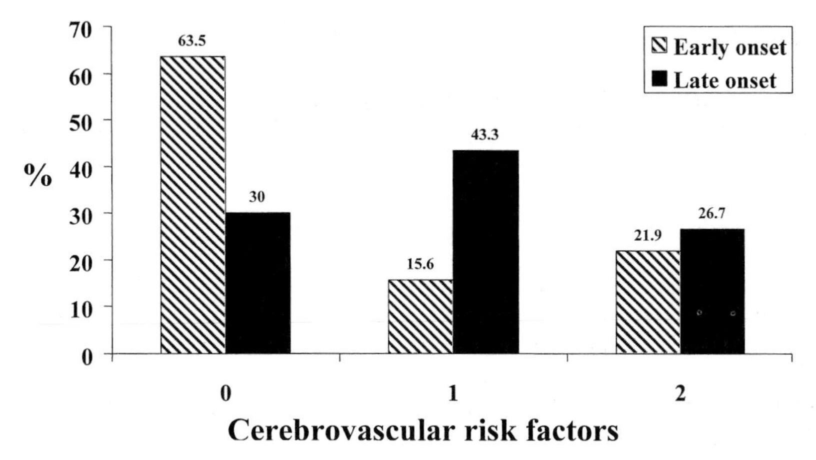

Fig. 29.1 Cerebrovascular risk factors in old age bipolar disorder. (Adapted with permission from Wylie *et al.* 1999.)

inconsistent results. With the most recent data from Hays *et al.* (1998), results have ranged from 24% to 88% for the presence of a positive family history (Glasser and Rabins 1984; Stone 1989; Broadhead and Jacoby 1990; Snowdon 1991; Shulman *et al.* 1992). The usual methodological issues arise with respect to the rigor of investigation and the criteria for a positive family history of psychiatric disorder (i.e. use of only first-degree relatives). Within the elderly bipolar group, a trend towards a higher rate of a positive family history exists in those with an earlier age of onset (Stone 1989; Hays *et al.* 1998), while the converse holds true for those with comorbid neurological disorders. The latter group are associated with very late-onset bipolarity (Snowdon 1991; Shulman *et al.* 1992; Tohen *et al.* 1994). However, even in the neurological subgroup of patients, significant prevalence rates of 30% apply for a positive family history in first-degree relatives.

The 1-year incidence rates reveal that almost 20% of the first admissions of patients with bipolar disorders in Finland occurred after the age of 60, with the peak admission rates being in middle age (Rasanan *et al.* 1998). This contrasts with the age of onset determined by episode rather than by hospitalization, in which community surveys found a very early age of onset of about 20 years. This is consistent with the earlier paradox reported in the Epidemiology section of this chapter, in which community and hospital prevalence rates moved in opposite directions. Community-based samples such as the ECA Study (Weissman *et al.* 1991) and the US National Comorbidity Study (Kessler *et al.* 1997) report the mean age of onset of bipolarity as 21 years. In mixed-age studies of manic inpatients, the mean age of onset is higher at 30 years (Goodwin and Jamison 1990; Tohen *et al.* 1990). With this early onset of bipolarity in the general population, it is noteworthy that very few elderly bipolar inpatients experienced their first mania before the age of 40 (Snowdon 1991; Shulman *et al.* 1992). One could conclude that the early-onset, community-based, bipolar patients burn-out or die by old age, and that the late peak in first admissions for mania represents a subgroup of neurologically based manic syndromes most often requiring hospitalization because of their severity (psychosis) or associated vascular risk factors. Further studies must carefully isolate age and onset as separate variables for analysis.

Neurological comorbidity and pathogenesis

While the neurological and psychiatric literature have operated independently, a confluence of findings has resulted (Shulman 1997*b*). Whether one uses the term 'disinhibition syndrome' which the neurologists prefer (Starkstein and Robinson

1997) or 'secondary mania' (Krauthammer and Klerman 1978), both clinical features and neurological findings are similar. Moreover, individual case reports and small case series tend toward a predominance of heterogeneous right hemisphere lesions (Starkstein *et al.* 1990; Strakowski *et al.* 1994; Verdoux and Bourgeois 1995; Carroll *et al.* 1996; Steffens and Krishnan 1998). Similarly, Sackeim *et al.* (1982) noted that pathological laughing was associated with right-sided lesions while left-sided lesions tended to produce pathological crying.

Still in this vein, Pearlson (1999) has observed that 'normal mood is dependent on the integrity of the frontal, limbic, and basal ganglia circuit'. Indeed, it has been argued that this is a functional system (known as the orbitofrontal circuit) which integrates sensory input with motivational states (Zald and Kim 1996). Evidence supporting the hypothesis that the right-sided orbitofrontal circuit mediates manic syndromes comes from a variety of sources. Disinhibition of sexuality and oral behaviour (Klüver–Bucy syndrome) are associated with bitemporal lesions (Kling and Steklis 1976).

A preponderance of basal temporal lesions was found in patients who developed a manic episode in the first year following head injury (Jorge *et al.* 1993). This is consistent with the hypothesis that the inferior surface of the skull is more likely to be damaged in injuries (Starkstein and Robinson 1997). Furthermore, patients with frontotemporal dementias distinct from Alzheimer's disease are more likely to manifest disinhibition (Neary *et al.* 1988). Indeed in those cases of dementia with disinhibition, the decrease in metabolic activity was greater in the orbitofrontal circuit than in parietal areas (Kumar *et al.* 1990; Starkstein *et al.* 1994). Moreover, in an elegant synthesis of the available data, Starkstein and Robinson (1997) have suggested that disinhibition syndromes in secondary mania are produced because of lesions disrupting connections within the orbitofrontal circuit. The frontal lobes modulate motivational and psychomotor behaviour; limbic connections modulate emotions; while the biogenic amine nuclei in the hypothalamus, amygdala, and brainstem modulate instinctive behaviours.

In a recent comprehensive review of published case reports involving focal unilateral cortical lesions, the trend towards right-sided lesions for mania and pseudomania was confirmed (Braun *et al.* 1999) (see Fig. 29.2).

In specific studies of mania in old age, the association with heterogeneous neurological disorders was high (36%) compared to age- and sex-matched cases of depression (8%) (Shulman *et al.* 1992). Within the manic group, a subgroup with a first affective episode of mania was even more likely to present with coarse neurological abnormalities (71%) than elderly patients with multiple episodes of bipolar disease (28%). Very late-onset mania is strongly associated with neurological comorbidity as well as high mortality due to cerebrovascular disease (Tohen *et al.* 1994). Out of 14 such patients, 10 were found to have comorbid neurological disorders, largely due to cerebral infarctions (Tohen *et al.* 1994).

Lesions and disorders associated with secondary mania include head injuries (Jorge *et al.* 1993); endocrine conditions (Sweet 1990; Lee *et al.* 1991; Ur *et al.* 1992); HIV infection (Lyketsos *et al.* 1993); and epilepsy (Carroll *et al.* 1996). However, reports of right-sided cerebrovascular lesions dominate the literature (Jampala and Abrams 1983; Robinson *et al.* 1988; Fawcett 1991; Isles and Orrell 1991; Cummings 1993; Carroll *et al.* 1996).

The high prevalence of cerebrovascular disease associated with mania led Steffens and

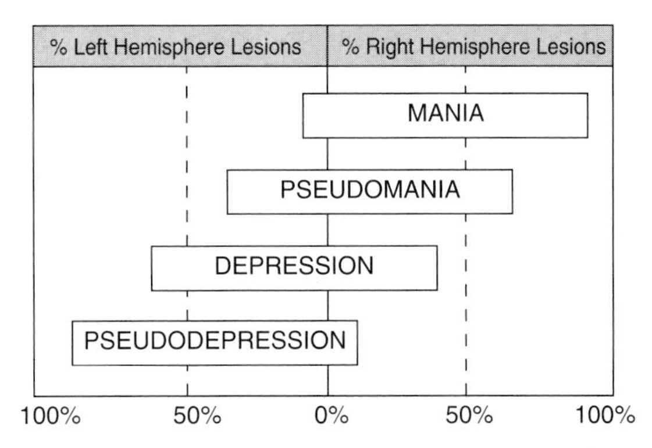

Fig. 29.2 Focal unilateral cortical lesions. (Taken from Braun *et al.* 1999.)

Krishnan (1998) to propose a vascular subtype of mania similar to the subtype of vascular depression proposed by Alexopoulos *et al.* (1997). The vascular subtype of mania fits the data found in studies of elderly patients with bipolar disorder. This subtype is defined by a manic syndrome in the context of cerebrovascular disease, based on clinical or neuroimaging findings, with further evidence of neuropsychological impairment. Clinical evidence can include stroke, a transient ischaemic attack (TIA), or focal signs, while positive neuroimaging includes hyperintensities or silent cerebral infarctions. Impairment of cognition is most common in the area of memory or executive function. Further support of this subtype includes late onset, a switch to mania shortly after the onset of vascular disease, a negative family history, and impairment of independent activities of daily living (IADL).

Significant cognitive dysfunction has been a consistent finding in most studies of mania in late life (Stone 1989; Broadhead and Jacoby 1990; Berrios and Bakshi 1991; Dhingra and Rabins 1991). This reflects the neurological comorbidity described above, especially when associated with cerebrovascular disease (Steffens and Krishnan 1998). Spicer *et al.* (1973) had hypothesized that the increase in first admission rates for mania late in life was a reflection of an increased prevalence of dementia in this subpopulation. However, none of the studies that have followed the course of mania in old age have found dementia to be more common than in age-matched controls. None the less, in the light of recent findings by Alexopoulos *et al.* (1993) with respect to pseudodementia and major depression, longer follow-up may be necessary to confirm or refute this concern.

Neuroimaging research

It is apparent that the recent research in neuroimaging has helped to clarify the nature more than the localization of brain lesions (Shulman 1997*a*). The findings on neuroimaging studies tend towards a preponderance of subcortical hyperintensities, decreased cerebral blood flow, and evidence of silent cerebral infarctions. Young *et al.* (1999) conducted an analysis of computerised tomography in 30 geriatric manic patients and compared them to age-matched controls. The manic patients showed greater cortical sulcal widening, and the authors suggested a need for further investigation of brain structure in geriatric mania. The increase in subcortical (basal ganglia) hyperintensities found in the elderly bipolar population is largely localized to the inferior half of the frontal lobe (McDonald *et al.* 1991; Woods *et al.* 1995). More recently, McDonald *et al.* (1999) further investigated the finding of an increase in white matter hyperintensities in elderly patients with bipolar disorder. In their recent study, they also found an increase in subcortical white matter hyperintensities, but this did not correlate with clinical evidence of cerebrovascular disease. Indeed, controlling for age, the late-onset older bipolar patients had the same numbers of hyperintensities in deep white matter and subcortical grey nuclei as did young bipolar patients and early-onset older bipolar patients. The authors conclude that the evidence supports the hypothesis that neuroanatomical changes in the brains of people with mania are present early in life.

The association of hyperintensities with risk factors such as hypertension, arteriosclerotic heart disease, and diabetes mellitus strengthens the relationship of mania to cerebrovascular pathology. Delayed-onset mania has been associated with a high prevalence of silent cerebral infarctions on neuroimaging (Kobayashi *et al.* 1991; Fujikawa *et al.* 1995). The highest proportion of silent cerebral infarctions occurred in late-onset mania when compared to a group of age-matched depressive patients. Indeed, the proportion of manic patients over the age of 60 with silent cerebral infarctions was more than 20%. These patients also had a relatively low incidence of a family history in first-degree relatives, consistent with the notion of secondary mania. These neuroimaging findings provide additional support for the proposal of a vascular subtype of mania (Steffens and Krishnan 1998).

Clinical course and outcome

Specific studies of elderly bipolar patients reveal that by and large they experience a relatively late age of onset at approximately 50 years, with half of the index patients first hospitalized for the treatment of depression (Stone 1989; Broadhead and Jacoby 1990; Snowdon 1991; Shulman *et al.* 1992). Another striking finding is the fact that a very long latency (mean 15 years) precedes the onset of first mania in those elderly bipolar patients whose first episode was depression (Shulman and Post 1980; Shulman *et al.* 1992). Within this subgroup, almost one-quarter of the patients experienced a latency of at least 25 years between the first episodes of depression and mania. In contrast to the conclusion of Perris (1966) that three consecutive depressive episodes could define unipolar depression, about half of the elderly patients with bipolar disorder whose first episode is depression also go on to experience at least three distinct depressions before mania becomes manifest (Shulman and Post 1980; Stone 1989; Snowdon 1991). It is this apparent 'conversion' to a bipolar diagnosis after many years of a unipolar course that highlights the importance of the cerebral-organic changes and comorbid neurological disorders described below.

Although the diagnosis of bipolar disorder is dependent upon a single episode of mania, most of the elderly bipolar patients experienced a clinical course that was characterized by both depressive and manic episodes. However, a small subgroup (12%) met strict criteria for a course of unipolar mania (Shulman and Tohen 1994). This group experienced at least three distinct manic episodes without major depression, with a minimum period of 10 years' follow-up from the time of their first hospitalization for a manic episode. Interestingly, the age of onset for this subgroup was significantly lower (41 years) compared to the mean of 65 years for elderly manics. These 'unipolar' manic patients were among the very few elderly patients whose illness began early in life. This suggests that this unique clinical course is worthy of further investigation with regard to differences in genetic vulnerability as well as pathogenesis.

The long-term clinical outcomes in elderly bipolar patients have been reported by Berrios and Bakshi (1991), Dhingra and Rabins (1991), and Shulman *et al.* (1992). In two of these studies, a mean of 6 years' follow-up data is available and a comparison group of elderly depressives was utilized (Dhingra and Rabins 1991; Shulman *et al.* 1992). Prognosis seems to be better than the original finding by Roth (1955), as 72% of patients still alive were considered symptom-free and were living independently (Dhingra and Rabins 1991). In this latter study, however, about one-third of the original cohort had died at follow-up and a significant decline in cognition was reported in a similar proportion of patients. Shulman *et al.* (1992) found a significant difference in mortality in the elderly manic group. Half of the elderly manics had died at a mean 6-year follow-up, compared to only one-fifth of age- and sex-matched elderly depressives. Using a depressive comparison group, Berrios and Bakshi (1991) also found that the manic patients were less likely to respond to treatment and to suffer from a higher prevalence of cerebrovascular disease with cognitive dysfunction, leading to persistent disturbances in behaviour and psychosocial functioning. In summary, elderly manic patients experience high rates of mortality and morbidity, reflecting the underlying CNS pathology found in association with these syndromes.

Determinants of bipolarity in old age

There appear to be four broad factors that have relevance to the manifestation of manic syndromes in old age:

1. Despite the general pattern of less genetic loading in later onset disorders and in those associated with neurological disorders, this subgroup still has a very significant familial prevalence of mood disorder (50–85%) in first-degree relatives (Shulman *et al.* 1992; Hays *et al.* 1998). Clinical experience also suggests that affective vulnerability may not be based solely on genetic factors, but also on the psychological sequelae of early loss and early trauma

in childhood and adolescence. This merits evaluation in future studies of bipolarity late in life. Paradoxically, one suspects that it is the losses of early life that are more relevant to affective disorder in old age than the ubiquitous losses associated with old age.

2. Degenerative changes associated with normal ageing may be a significant factor in the apparent conversion of 'latent' bipolarity—i.e. middle-aged depressives who become manic after many years—and multiple episodes of unipolar depression. Other determinants, however, must also be present to elicit a manic syndrome.
3. Heterogeneous brain lesions are associated with mania late in life, with a predominance of cerebrovascular disease including silent cerebral infarctions as well as more obvious strokes. Chronic alcoholism, brain tumours, and a variety of metabolic conditions have also been implicated.
4. The localization of lesions to the right hemisphere and specifically to the orbitofrontal circuit also seems to be critical for the manifestation of mania in old age. While not rare, manic syndromes are certainly uncommon in comparison to depression in old age. Thus, localization of CNS pathology to the right-sided orbitofrontal circuit in association with a vulnerability to mood disorder constitute the necessary pathogenetic mechanism(s) for the development of mania in the elderly.

Management

This review will focus only on those features of the management of bipolar disorder that are unique to the elderly. Most fundamental is the high prevalence of neurological morbidity in manic syndromes in old age, and hence the need to search assiduously for evidence of localizing neurological signs and symptoms. A careful history searching for evidence of head injury, cerebrovascular disease, and related risk factors is essential in light of the data available for bipolar disorder in old age. Indeed, neuroimaging has been considered an essential component of the investigation for elderly manic patients (Van Gerpen *et al.* 1999). Another common feature in old age is the narrow therapeutic range of pharmacological therapies for mood stabilizers and antimanic agents (Shulman and Herrmann 1999).

Mood stabilizers

Lithium

Lithium continues to be the most commonly used mood stabilizer in old age (Head and Dening 1998). This may be a cohort effect because the elderly bipolar population was started on lithium before the introduction of the newer mood-stabilizing agents, particularly sodium valproate. Unfortunately, there are no randomized controlled trials for the use of lithium either in acute mania or as maintenance therapy in late life (Himmelhoch *et al.* 1980; Shulman and Post 1980; Janicak 1993). Lithium must be used with considerable caution in the geriatric population as it is eliminated exclusively by the kidneys (Hardy *et al.* 1997). Normal declines in renal function including creatinine clearance and the glomerular filtration rate (GFR) will clearly affect the pharmacokinetics of lithium. Other factors include a decrease in the volume of distribution and marked intraindividual variability (Hardy *et al.* 1987). In their study of the pharmacokinetics of lithium in older people, lithium was excreted at a rate approximately half that in younger patients. Because of the marked change in renal function and pharmacokinetics, only half the adult dose should be prescribed.

From a pharmacodynamic perspective, sensitivity is also increased in old age (Shulman and Herrmann 1999). Adverse reactions and toxicity at 'normal' adult serum levels have been reported (Roose *et al.* 1979; Smith and Helms 1982; Murray *et al.* 1983). However, under well-controlled conditions in a specialized geriatric clinic, lithium is reported to be safe and well tolerated (Parker *et al.* 1994). None the less, concerns remain, depending on the patient population. Stoudemire *et al.* (1998) studied a medically ill, elderly population who received lithium as an augmenting agent and found relatively poor tolerability.

Some controversy continues to revolve around the appropriate maintenance dose for lithium use in old age. Recommendations have varied from lower maintenance serum levels of 0.5 mmol/l (Shulman *et al.* 1987) to higher levels associated with better outcome (Young 1996; Chen *et al.* 1999). Clinical experience and the high comorbidity found in elderly manic patients does suggest caution and the need for better data on recommended serum levels.

The adverse effects of lithium include a wide range of systemic reactions especially affecting the central nervous system (Shulman and Herrmann 1999). These include lithium-induced tremor, aggravation of parkinsonian tremor, and spontaneous extrapyramidal symptoms. A recent community study found that almost one-third of elderly patients taking lithium were on thyroid replacement therapy or else had elevated levels of thyroid-stimulating hormone (Head and Dening 1998).

Drug interactions with lithium continue to be of concern; particularly thiazide diuretics which can decrease lithium clearance significantly, thereby increasing the serum lithium levels and the potential for toxicity. Other medications of concern include angiotensin-converting enzyme (ACE) inhibitors and non-steroidal anti-inflammatory drugs (NSAIDs) such as indometacin (Shulman and Herrmann 1999).

Anticonvulsants

Valproic acid or divalproex has emerged as a significant and viable alternative to lithium carbonate for mood stabilization. Within the elderly population, only case reports (McFarland *et al.* 1990; Risinger *et al.* 1994) and case series (Kando *et al.* 1996; Noaghiul *et al.* 1998; Jeste *et al.* 1999; Mordecai *et al.* 1999) are available. Early indications are that valproate is indeed an effective and well-tolerated mood stabilizer in an elderly population. Noaghiul *et al.* (1998) studied 21 elderly manic patients and rated the majority as much improved. In this study, the average mean dose of divalproex was 1400 mg per day with an average serum level of 72 mg/l. In another retrospective study, Chen *et al.* (1999) found lithium to be more effective for classic mania, while response rates for mixed mania were similar for lithium and valproate. This is in contrast to the findings of Bowden *et al.* (1996) in a mixed-age population. Single case reports reflect valproate's usefulness in elderly rapid-cycling bipolar patients (Gnam and Flint 1993) or as a combination agent with lithium carbonate (Schneider and Wilcox 1998; Goldberg *et al.* 2000).

Based upon these reports of elderly patients with mania, as well as elderly dementia patients treated for agitation (Porsteinsson *et al.* 1997; Herrmann 1998), valproic acid appears to be well tolerated. The main side-effects have included sedation and gastrointestinal disturbance, which can be modulated by dosage reduction (Shulman and Herrmann 1999). Potential adverse reactions can occur because of drug interactions. Valproate is highly protein-bound and a weak inhibitor of cytochrome P450 2D6. Accordingly, it could inhibit the metabolism of tricyclic antidepressants and displace diazepam from protein binding sites thus increasing plasma concentrations (Janicak 1993).

These authors' clinical experience suggests that valproic acid in the form of divalproex is a very reasonable alternative mood stabilizer and is well tolerated at mean dosages ranging between 1000 and 1500 mg daily. The value of monitoring serum levels is unclear, though one retrospective series suggested greater effectiveness was associated with increased serum levels (Niedermier and Nasrallah 1998). Further systematic studies will be necessary to confirm these positive initial clinical impressions.

Carbamazepine, another widely used mood stabilizer, has had less exposure in an elderly population, with only a few case reports (Schneier and Kahn 1990; Kellner and Neher 1991). As with other mood-stabilizing agents, there has been no controlled trial of its use in elderly populations. Because it is a potent inducer of cytochrome P450 2D6 and is highly protein-bound, it has the potential for drug interactions (Janicak 1993). Clinical experience also suggests that it can be highly neurotoxic in the elderly population, hence recommendations have suggested maintaining relatively low serum levels below 9 μg/ml (Young 1996). Tariot *et al.* (1998) have recommended the use of carbamazepine for the treatment of agitation in dementia patients, suggesting that it is well tolerated. Drug interactions in the elderly include those that can increase plasma levels of carbamazepine: fluoxetine, cimetidine, erythromycin, and calcium-channel blockers. Conversely, carbamazepine may decrease the plasma concentration and half–lives of alprazolam, haloperidol, theophylline, and warfarin.

A number of isolated case reports involve the newer anticonvulsant agents. Gabapentin was successfully used to treat an elderly bipolar patient who was tolerant of neither lithium or valproate (Sheldon *et al.* 1998). Two recent case studies of gabapentin included a subsample of elderly patients (Ghaemi *et al.* 1998; Cabras *et al.* 1999). Lamotrigine was added to divalproex in the treatment of a rapid-cycling, elderly bipolar patient (Kusumakar and Yatham 1997); and in an open-label trial of treatment in refractory bipolar disorder, a number of elderly patients appeared to tolerate lamotrigine (Calabrese *et al.* 1999). Clearly, more clinical experience and trials are required to establish the safety and efficacy of these newer agents.

Other treatments

Those typical antipsychotics commonly used as adjunct treatments for bipolar disorder can cause significant side-effects, including anticholinergic effects, orthostatic hypotension, and extra-pyramidal symptoms (Naranjo *et al.* 1995). In contrast, atypical antipsychotics including risperidone, olanzapine, and quetiapine appear to be better tolerated and produce fewer extra-pyramidal symptoms, including tardive dyskinesia, and are increasingly being used for elderly manic patients (Jeste *et al.* 1999). Tohen *et al.* (1999) have suggested that the atypical antipsychotics such as olanzapine have mood-stabilizing properties. Some support for this claim is given by a report of three elderly manic patients who were successfully treated with clozapine having previously been refractory to both lithium and valproate (Shulman *et al.* 1997). There is a single case report of verapamil, a calcium-channel blocker, successfully treating a 66-year-old manic patient (Gash *et al.* 1992). In a final alternative-treatment note, Mukherjee *et al.* (1994) highlight the fact that electroconvulsive treatment may also be effective and well tolerated in elderly patients suffering from mania.

Summary

As a means of organizing the available evidence and data on manic syndromes in old age, we propose four distinct subtypes that may have heuristic value for further investigation:

1. *Primary bipolar disorder*. This includes early-onset bipolar patients who remain symptomatic into old age and require ongoing management. While relatively few of these individuals appear in studies of hospitalized elderly manic patients, a community or outpatient sample may reveal a different pattern.
2. *Latent bipolar disorder*. This subgroup consists largely of middle-aged onset depressives who 'convert' to mania later in life after a long latency and multiple depressive episodes. It is postulated that this conversion may be due to cerebral organic factors including normal degenerative changes and drug-induced mania.
3. *Secondary mania (disinhibition syndromes)*. This group consists mainly of very late-onset manic syndromes without a prior history and a lower familial disposition, or in association with neurological or other systemic medical disorders.
4. *Unipolar mania*. This relatively small subgroup appears to have an earlier age at onset compared to other elderly bipolar patients, with persistence of manic-only episodes into old age. The element of chronic frontal disinhibition may also be relevant, but requires further study.

Future research

Retrospective studies have yielded sufficient data to propose hypotheses for future research, which now needs to use prospective studies incorporating neuroimaging and neuropsychological testing. Specific attention to frontal lobe function and the role of disinhibition in manic syndromes will be particularly relevant. Inevitably, an integrative model will be best suited to further our understanding of mania not only in old age but also in younger bipolar patients.

Finally, it will be useful to determine whether there is a differential response to mood stabilizers or antipsychotics by mania subtype. Specifically, do manic syndromes associated with neurological comorbidity require long-term stabilization or can we treat these conditions with short-term antipsychotics? Is valproate as effective as lithium in old age? Prospective systematic multicentre trials will be necessary to obtain meaningful information to inform clinical practice.

Notes

1. This is an epidemiological term which reinforces the potential selection bias for manic patients who are admitted to or registered in hospital and hence represent 'treated prevalence'.

References

Akiskal, H. (1986). The clinical significance of the 'soft' bipolar spectrum. *Psychiatric Annals*, **16**, 667–71.

Alexopoulos, G. S., Meyers, B. S., Young, R. C., *et al.* (1993). The course of geriatric depression with 'reversible dementia': a controlled study. *American Journal of Psychiatry*, **150**, 1693–9.

Alexopoulos, G. S., Meyers, B. S., Young, R. C., Kakuma, T., Silbersweig, D., and Charlson, M. (1997). Clinically defined vascular depression. *American Journal of Psychiatry*, **154**, 562–5.

American Psychiatric Association. (1994). *Diagnostic and statistical manual of mental disorders, 4th edition (DSM-IV)*. APA, Washington, DC.

Berrios, G. E. and Bakshi, N. (1991). Manic and depressive symptoms in the elderly: Their relationships to treatment outcome, cognition and motor symptoms. *Psychopathology*, **24**, 31–8.

Bowden, C. L., Janicak, P. G., Orsulak, P., Swann, A. C., Davis, J. M., Calabrese, J. R. *et al.* (1996). Relation of serum valproate concentration to response in mania. *American Journal of Psychiatry*, **153**, 765–70.

Braun, C. M. J., Larocque, C., Daigneault, S., and Montour-Proulx, I. (1999). Mania, pseudomania, depression, and pseudodepression resulting from focal unilateral cortical lesions. *Neuropsychiatry, Neuropsychology, and Behavioural Neurology*, **12**, 35–51.

Broadhead, J. and Jacoby, R. (1990). Mania in old age: A first prospective study. *International Journal of Geriatric Psychiatry*, **5**, 215.

Cabras, P. L., Hardoy, J., Hardoy, M. C., and Carta, M. G. (1999). Clinical experience with gabapentin in patients with bipolar or schizoaffective disorder: results of an open-label study. *Journal of Clinical Psychiatry*, **60**, 245–8.

Calabrese, J. R., Bowden, C. L., McElroy, S. L., Cookson, J., Andersen, J., Keck, P. E., *et al.* (1999). Spectrum of activity of lamotrigine in treatment-refractory bipolar disorder. *American Journal of Psychiatry*, **156**, 1019–23.

Carroll, B. Y., Goforth, H. W., Kennedy, J. C., and Dueño, O. R. (1996). Mania due to general medical conditions: frequency, treatment, and cost. *International Journal of Psychiatry in Medicine*, **26**, 5–13.

Chen, S. T., Altshuler, L. L., Melnyk, K. A., Erhart, S. M., Miller, E., and Mintz, J. (1999). Efficacy of lithium vs valproate in the treatment of mania in the elderly: a retrospective study. *Journal of Clinical Psychiatry*, **60**, 181–6.

Cummings, J. L. (1993). Frontal-subcortical circuits and human behavior. *Archives of Neurology*, **50**, 873–80.

Dhingra, U. and Rabins, P. V. (1991). Mania in the elderly: a five-to-seven year follow-up. *Journal of the American Geriatrics Society*, **39**, 582–3.

Eagles, J. M. and Whalley, L. J. (1985). Ageing and affective disorders: the age at first onset of affective disorders in Scotland, 1996–1978. *British Journal of Psychiatry*, **147**, 180.

Fawcett, R. G. (1991). Cerebral infarct presenting as mania. *Journal of Clinical Psychiatry*, **52**, 352–3.

Fujikawa, T, Yamawaki, S., and Touhouda, Y. (1995). Silent cerebral infarctions in patients with late-onset mania. *Stroke*, **26**, 946–9.

Gash, A. J., Cole, A. J., and Bray, G. P. (1992). Case report: efficacy of verapamil in an elderly patient with mania unresponsive to neuroleptics. *International Journal of Geriatric Psychiatry*, **7**, 913–15.

Ghaemi, S. N., Katzow, J. J., Desai, S. P., and Goodwin, F. K. (1998). Gabapentin treatnment of mood disorders: a preliminary study. *Journal of Clinical Psychiatry*, **59**, 426–9.

Glasser, M. and Rabins, P. (1984). Mania in the elderly. *Ageing*, **13**, 210–13.

Gnam, W. and Flint, A. J. (1993). New onset rapid cycling bipolar disorder in an 87 year old woman. *Canadian Journal of Psychiatry*, **38**, 324–6.

Goldberg, J. F., Sacks, M. H., and Kocsis, J. H. (2000). Lithium augmentation of divalproex in geriatric mania. *Journal of Clinical Psychiatry*, **61**, 304.

Goodwin, F. K. and Jamison, K. R. (1990). *Manic-depressive illness*. Oxford University Press, New York.

Hardy, B. G., Shulman, K. I., MacKenzie, S. E., Kutcher, S. P., and Silverberg, J. D. (1987). Pharmacokinetics of lithium in the elderly. *Psychopharmacology*, 7, 153–8.

Hardy, B. G., Shulman, K. I., and Zucchero, C. (1997). Gradual discontinuation of lithium augmentation in elderly patients with unipolar depression. *Journal of Clinical Psychopharmacology*, **17**, 22–6.

Hays, J. C., Krishnan, K. R. R., George, L. K., and Blazer, D. G. (1998). Age of first onset of bipolar disorder: demographic, family history, and psychosocial correlates. *Depression and Anxiety*, 7, 76–82.

Head, L. and Dening, T. (1998). Lithium in the over-65s: who is taking it and who is monitoring it? *International Journal of Geriatric Psychiatry*, **13**, 164–71.

Herrmann, N. (1998). Valproic acid treatment of agitation in dementia. *Canadian Journal of Psychiatry*, **43**, 69–72.

Himmelhoch, J. M., Neil, J. F., May, S. J., Fuchs, C. Z., and Licata, S. M. (1980). Age, dementia, dyskinesis, and lithium response. *American Journal of Psychiatry*, **137**, 941–5.

Isles, L. J. and Orrell, M. W. (1991). Secondary mania after open-heart surgery. *British Journal of Psychiatry*, **159**, 280–2.

Jampala, V. S. and Abrams, R. (1983). Mania secondary to left and right hemisphere damage. *American Journal of Psychiatry*, **140**, 1197–9.

Janicak, P. G. (1993). The relevance of clinical pharmacokinetics and therapeutic drug monitoring: anticonvulsants, mood stabilizers and antipsychotics. *Journal of Clinical Psychiatry*, **54**(Suppl. 9), 35–41.

Jeste, D. V., Lacro, J. P., Bailey, A., Rockwell, E., Harris, M. J., and Caligiuri, M. P. (1999). Lower incidence of tardive dyskinesia in risperidone compared with haloperidol in older patients. *Journal of the American Geriatrics Society*, **47**, 716–19.

Jorge, R. E., Robinson, R. G., Starkstein, S. E., Arfndt, S. V., Forrester, A. W., and Geisler, F. H. (1993). Secondary mania following traumatic brain injury. *American Journal of Psychiatry*, **150**, 916–21.

Kando, J. C., Tohen, M., Castillo, J., and Zarate, C. A. (1996). The use of valproate in an elderly population with affective symptoms. *Journal of Clinical Psychiatry*, **57**, 238–40.

Kellner, M. B. and Neher, F. (1991). A first episode of mania after age 80. *Canadian Journal of Psychiatry*, **36**, 607–8.

Kessler, R. C., Rubinow, D. R., Holmes, C., Abelson, J. M., and Zhao, S. (1997). The epidemiology of DSM-III-R bipolar I disorder in a general population survey. *Psychological Medicine*, **27**, 1079–89.

Kling, A. and Steklis, H. D. (1976). A neural substrate for affiliative behavior in nonhuman primates. *Brain Behaviour and Evolution*, **13**, 216–38.

Kobayashi, S., Okada, K., and Yamashita, K. (1991). Incidence of silent lacunar lesions in normal adults and its relation to cerebral blood flow and risk factors. *Stroke*, **22**, 1379–83.

Krauthammer, C. and Klerman, G. L. (1978). Secondary mania: manic syndromes associated with antecedent physical illness or drugs. *Archives of General Psychiatry*, **35**, 1333–9.

Kumar, A., Schapiro, M. D., Haxby, J. V., Grady, C. L., and Friedland, R. P. (1990). Cerebral metabolic and cognitive studies in dementia with frontal lobe behavioral features. *Journal of Psychiatric Research*, **24**, 97–109.

Kusumakar, V. and Yatham, L. N. (1997). Lamotrigine treatment of rapid cycling bipolar disorder. *American Journal of Psychiatry*, **154**, 1171–2.

Lee, S., Chow, C. C., Wing, Y. K., Leung, C. M., Chiu, H., and Chen, C. (1991). Mania secondary to thyrotoxicosis. *British Journal of Psychiatry*, **159**, 712–13.

Lyketsos, C. G., Hanson, A. L., Fishman, M., Rosenblatt, A., McHugh, P. R., and Treisman, G. J. (1993). Manic syndrome early and late in the course of HIV. *American Journal of Psychiatry*, **150**, 326–7.

McDonald, W. M., Krishnan, K. R. R., Doraiswamy, P. M., and Blazer, D. G. (1991). Occurrence of subcortical hyperintensities in elderly subjects with mania. *Psychiatry Research*, **40**, 211–20.

McDonald, W. M., Tupler, L. A., Marsteller, F. A., Figiel, G. S., DiSouza, S., Nemeroff, C. B., *et al.* (1999). Hyperintense lesions on magnetic resonance images in bipolar disorder. *Biological Psychiatry*, **45**, 965–71.

McFarland, B. H., Miller, M. R., and Straumfjord, A. A. (1990). Valproate use in the older manic patient. *Journal of Clinical Psychiatry*, **51**, 479–81.

Mordecai, D. J., Sheikh, J. I., and Glick, I. D. (1999). Divalproex for the treatment of geriatric bipolar disorder. *International Journal of Geriatric Psychiatry*, **14**, 494–6.

Mukherjee, S., Sackeim, H. A., and Schnur, D. B. (1994). Electroconvulsive therapy of acute mania episodes: a review of 50 years' experience. *American Journal of Psychiatry*, **151**, 169–76.

Murray, N., Hopwood, S., Balfour, D. J. K., Ogston, S., and Hewick, D. S. (1983). The influence of age on lithium efficacy and side effects in out-patients. *Psychological Medicine*, **13**, 53–60.

Naranjo, C. A., Herrmann, N., Mittmann, N., and Bremner, K. E. (1995). Recent advances in geriatric psychopharmacology. *Drugs and Aging*, 7, 184–202.

Neary, D., Snowden, J. S., Northern, B., *et al.* (1988). Dementia of frontal lobe type. *Journal of Neurology, Neurosurgery and Psychiatry*, **51**, 353–61.

Niedermier, J. A. and Nasrallah, H. A. (1998). Clinical correlates of response to valproate in geriatric inpatients. *Annals of Clinical Psychiatry*, **10**, 165–8.

Noaghiul, S., Narayan, M., and Nelson, J. C. (1998). Divalproex treatment of mania in elderly patients. *American Journal of Geriatric Psychiatry*, **6**, 257–62.

Parker, K. L., Mittmann, N. Shear, N. H., Herrmann, N., Shulman, K. I., Silver, I. L., *et al.* (1994). Lithium augmentation in geriatric depressed outpatients: a clinical report. *International Journal of Geriatric Psychiatry*, **9**, 995–1002.

Pearlson, G. D. (1999). Structural and functional brain changes in bipolar disorder: a selective review. *Schizophrenia Research*, **39**, 133–40.

Perris, C. (1966). A study of bipolar (manic depressive) and unipolar recurrent psychoses (IX). *Acta Psychiatrica Scandinavica*, **194** (Suppl.), 1–189.

Porsteinsson, A. P., Tariot, P. N., and Erb, R. (1997). An open trial of valproate for agitation in geriatric neuropsychiatric disorders. *American Journal of Geriatric Psychiatry*, **5**, 344–51.

Rasanan, P, Tiihonen, J., and Hakko, H. (1998). The incidence and onset-age of hospitalised bipolar affective disorder in Finland. *Journal of Affective Disorders*, **48**, 63–8.

Risinger, R. C., Risby, E. D., and Risch, S. C. (1994). Safety and efficacy of divalproex sodium in elderly bipolar patients. *Journal of Clinical Psychiatry*, **55**, 215.

Robinson, R. G., Boston, J. D., Starkstein, S. E., and Price, T. R. (1988). Comparison of mania with depression following brain injury: causal factors. *American Journal of Psychiatry*, **145**, 172–8.

Roose, S. P., Bone, S., Haidorfer, C., Dunner, D. L., and Fieve, R. R. (1979). Lithium treatment in older patients. *American Journal of Psychiatry*, **136**, 843–4.

Roth, M. (1955). The natural history of mental disorder in old age. *Journal of Mental Science*, **101**, 281–301.

Sackeim, H. A., Greenberg, M. S., Weiman, A. L., Gur, R. C., Hungerbuhler, J. P., and Geschwind, N. (1982). Hemispheric asymmetry in the expression of positive and negative emotions. *Archives of Neurology*, **39**, 210–18.

Schneider, A. L. and Wilcox, C. S. (1998). Divalproex augmentation in lithium-resistant rapid cycling mania in four geriatric patients. *Journal of Affective Disorders*, **47**, 201–5.

Schneier, H. A. and Kahn, D. (1990). Selective response to carbamazepine in a case of organic mood disorder. *Journal of Clinical Psychiatry*, **51**, 485.

Sheldon, L. F., Ancill, R. J., and Holliday, S. G. (1998). Gabapentin in geriatric psychiatry patients. *Canadian Journal of Psychiatry*, **43**, 422–3.

Shulman, K. I. (1997*a*). Neurologic co-morbidity and mania in old age. *Clinical Neuroscience*, **4**(1), 37–40.

Shulman, K. I. (1997*b*). Disinhibition syndromes, secondary mania and bipolar disorder in old age. *Journal of Affective Disorders*, **46**, 175–82.

Shulman, K. I. and Herrmann, N. (1999). The nature and management of mania in old age. *Psychiatric Clinics of North America*, 22(3), 649–65.

Shulman, K. and Post, F. (1980). Bipolar affective disorder in old age. *British Journal of Psychiatry*, **136**, 26–32.

Shulman, K. I. and Tohen, M. (1994). Unipolar mania reconsidered: evidence from an elderly cohort. *British Journal of Psychiatry*, **164**, 547–9.

Shulman, K. I., MacKenzie, S., and Hardy, B. (1987). The clinical use of lithium carbonate in old age. *Journal of Progress in Neuro-Psychopharmacology and Biological Psychiatry*, **11**, 159–64.

Shulman, K. I., Tohen, M., Satlin, A., Mallya, G., and Kalunian, D. (1992). Mania compared with unipolar depression in old age. *American Journal of Psychiatry*, **142**, 341–5.

Shulman, R. W., Singh, A., and Shulman K. I. (1997). Treatment of elderly institutionalised bipolar patients with clozapaine. *Psychopharmacology Bulletin*, **33**, 113–18.

Smith, R. E. and Helms, P. M. (1982). Adverse effects of lithium therapy in the acutely ill elderly patient. *Journal of Clinical Psychiatry*, **43**, 94–9.

Snowdon, J. (1991). A retrospective case-note study of bipolar disorder in old age. *British Journal of Psychiatry*, **158**, 484–90.

Spicer, C. C., Hare, E. H., and Slater, E. (1973). Neurotic and psychotic forms of depressive illness: evidence from age-incidence in a national sample. *British Journal of Psychiatry*, **123**, 535–41.

Starkstein, S. E. and Robinson, R. G. (1997). Mechanism of disinhibition after brain lesions. *Journal of Nervous Mental Disorder*, **185**, 108–14.

Starkstein, S. E., Mayberg, H. S., Berthier, M. L., Fedoroff, P., Price, T. R., and Robinson, R. G. (1990). Mania after brain injury: neuroradiological and metabolic findings. *Annals of Neurology*, **27**, 652–9.

Starkstein, S. E., Migliorelli, R., Teeson, A., *et al.* (1994). The specificity of cerebral blood flow changes in patients with frontal lobe dementia. *Journal of Neurology, Neurosurgery and Psychiatry*, **57**, 790–6.

Steffens, D. C. and Krishnan, K. R. R. (1998). Structural neuroimaging and mood disorders. Recent findings, implications for classification, and future directions. *Biological Psychiatry*, **43**, 705–12.

Stone, K. (1989). Mania in the elderly. *British Journal of Psychiatry*, **155**, 220–4.

Stoudemire, A., Hill, C. D., Lewison, B. J., Marquardt, M., and Dalton, S. (1998). Lithium intolerance in a medical-psychiatric population. *General Hospital Psychiatry*, **20**, 85–90.

Strakowski, S. M., McElroy, S., Keck, P., and West, S. (1994). The co-occurrence of mania with medical and other psychiatric disorders. *International Journal of Psychiatry in Medicine*, **24**, 305–28.

Sweet, R. (1990). Case of craniopharyngioma in late life. *Journal of Neuropsychiatry*, **2**, 464–5.

Tariot, P. N., Eerb, R., Podgorski, C. A., Cox, C., Patel, S., Jakimovich, L., *et al.* (1998). Efficacy and tolerability of carbamazepine for agitation and aggression in dementia. *American Journal of Psychiatry*, **155**, 54–61.

Tohen, M., Waternaux, C. M., and Tsuang, M. T. (1990). Outcome in mania: a four year prospective follow-up study utilising survival analysis. *Archives of General Psychiatry*, **47**, 1106–11.

Tohen, M., Shulman, K. I., and Satlin, A. (1994). First-episode mania in late life. *American Journal of Psychiatry*, **151**, 130–2.

Tohen, M., Snager, T. M., McElroy, S. L., Tollefson, G. D., Chengappa, R., Daniel, D. G., *et al.* and the Olanzapine HGEH Study Group. (1999). Olanzapine versus placebo in the treatment of acute mania. *American Journal of Psychiatry*, **156**, 702–9.

Tsuang, M. T. (1978). Suicide in schizophrenics, manics, depressives, and surgical controls. *Archives of General Psychiatry*, **35**, 153–5.

Ur, E., Turner, T. H., Godwin, T. J., *et al.* (1992). Mania in association with hydrocortisone replacement for Addison's disease. *Postgraduate Medicine*, **68**, 41–3.

Van Gerpen, M. W., Johnson, J. E., and Winstead, D. K. (1999). Mania in the geriatric patient population: a review of the literature. *American Journal of Geriatric Psychiatry*, **7**, 188–202.

Verdoux, H. and Bourgeois, M. (1995). Manies secondaires a des pathologies organiques cerebrales. *Annals of Medical Psychology*, **153**, 161–8.

Weeke, A. and Vaeth, M. (1986). Excess mortality of bipolar and unipolar manic-depressive patients. *Journal of Affective Disorders*, **11**, 227–34.

Weissman, M. M., Bruce, M. L., Leak, P. J., *et al.* (1991). Affective disorders. In *Psychiatric disorders in America: The Epidemiologic Catchment Area Study* (ed. L. N. Robins and D. A. Regier), pp. 53. Free Press, New York.

Winokur, G. (1975). The Iowa 500: heterogeneity and course in manic depressive illness (bipolar). *Comprehensive Psychiatry*, **16**, 125–31.

Woods, B. T., Yurgelun-Todd, D., Mikulis, D., and Pillay, S. S. (1995). Age-related MRI abnormalities in bipolar illness: a clinical study. *Biological Psychiatry*, **38**, 846–7.

Wylie, M. E., Mulsant, B. H., Pollock, B. G., Sweet, R. A., Zubenko, G. S., Begley, A. E., *et al.* (1999). Age at onset in geriatric bipolar disorder. *American Journal of Geriatric Psychiatry*, **7**, 77–83.

Yassa, R., Nair, V., Nastase, C., *et al.* (1988). Prevalence of bipolar disorder in a psychogeriatric population. *Journal of Affective Disorders*, **14**, 197–201.

Young, R. C. (1996). Treatment of geriatric mania. In *Mood disorders across the life span* (ed. K. I. Shulman, M. Tohen, and S. P. Kutcher), pp. 411–25. Wiley-Liss, New York.

Young, R. C. and Klerman, G. L. (1992). Mania in late life: focus on age at onset. *American Journal of Psychiatry*, **149**, 867–76.

Young, R. C., Nambudiri, D. E., Jain, H., de Asis, J. M., and Alexopoulos, G. S. (1999). Brain computed tomography in geriatric manic disorder. *Biological Psychiatry*, **45**, 1063–5.

Zald, D. and Kim, S. W. (1996). Anatomy and function of the orbital frontal cortex: I anatomy, neurocircuitry, and obsessive-compulsive disorder. *Journal of Neuropsychiatry and Clinical Neuroscience*, **8**, 125–38.

30 Neurotic disorders

James Lindesay

Introduction

Although neurotic disorders in elderly people are common, distressing, and treatable, they have traditionally been neglected relative to other psychiatric disorders in old age, and to neuroses in younger adults. However, as psychogeriatric services develop, as the primary care sector becomes increasingly involved in the commissioning and delivery of mental health services, and as elderly people themselves become more demanding of equitable treatment, the needs of this group are becoming apparent. The growing literature reflects this: there has in recent years been a steady increase in the number of research papers, reviews, and textbooks addressing anxiety and neurotic disorders in old age. However, as this chapter makes clear, there is still much that we do not know about these interesting and important conditions.

The concept of neurosis

The term 'neurosis' was originally coined in the eighteenth century to describe a group of conditions such as hysteria, melancholia, and epilepsy that were thought at that time to be due to pathology of the peripheral nerves (Cullen 1784). By the mid-nineteenth century this model had largely been abandoned, and attention moved to factors such as constitution and environment, with neurosis regarded as the consequence of adverse external agents acting on 'degenerate' and 'nervous' temperaments. In general terms this model still underlies our current thinking, but the unitary, dimensional concept of neurosis yielded in the second half of the twentieth century to a system of specific diagnostic categories based upon patterns of symptoms. This process was driven by the growth of biological psychiatry, clinical dissatisfaction with psychoanalysis, and the natural human need for clinicians, researchers, and service planners to deal with 'cases' (Lindesay 1995*a*). Current nosological thinking in this twenty-first century is still embodied in the tenth edition of the *International classification of diseases* (ICD-10) (World Health Organization 1992) and the fourth edition of the *Diagnostic and statistical manual of mental disorders* (DSM-IV) (American Psychiatric Association 1994) (Table 30.1). ICD-10 still contains a vestigial remnant of the earlier approach in its reference to 'neurotic, stress-related and somatoform disorders'; in DSM-IV, however, all mention of neurosis and the neurotic has been expunged.

Although unfashionable, and difficult to accommodate in descriptive classifications, the broad dimensional concept of neurosis is not obsolete (Andrews 1996). Tyrer (1989, 1990) has reviewed the evidence in favour of a general neurotic syndrome, pointing out that there is considerable comorbidity between the specific neurotic categories, and between them and other disorders such as depression. These categories are also unstable over time, and the effectiveness of treatments appears to be relatively independent of diagnosis. The dimensionality of these disorders is particularly apparent in community and primary care populations; latent trait analysis of psychological symptoms in both younger and older adults identifies independent but related dimensions of depression and anxiety underlying the manifest symptomatology (Goldberg *et al.* 1987; Mackinnon *et al.* 1994). An individual's symptoms during any particular episode are determined by pre-existing vulnerability, the particular factors precipitating that episode

Table 30.1 Modern classifications of neurotic disorders (ICD-10 and DSM-IV)

ICD-10		DSM-IV	
Mood disorders		**Mood disorders**	
F34:	*Persistent mood disorders*	*Depressive disorders*	
	Dysthymia	300.4:	Dysthymic disorder
Neurotic, stress-related, and somatoform disorders			
F40:	*Phobic anxiety disorders*	**Anxiety disorders**	
.0:	Agoraphobia	300.01:	Panic disorder without agoraphobia
.1:	Social phobia	300.21:	Panic disorder with agoraphobia
.2:	Specific phobia	300.22:	Agoraphobia without history of panic disorder
		300.23:	Social phobia
F41:	*Other anxiety disorders*	300.29:	Specific phobia
.0:	Panic disorder	300.3:	Obsessive–compulsive disorder
.1:	Generalized anxiety disorder	309.81:	Post-traumatic stress disorder
.2:	Mixed anxiety and depressive disorder	300.02:	Generalized anxiety disorder
F42:	*Obsessive–compulsive disorder*	293.89:	Anxiety disorder due to a general medical condition
		292.89:	Substance-induced anxiety disorder
F43:	*Reaction to severe stress, and adjustment disorders*		
.0:	Acute stress reaction		
.1:	Post-traumatic stress disorder		
.2:	Adjustment disorders		
F44:	*Dissociative disorders*	**Dissociative disorders**	
.0:	Dissociative amnesia	300.12:	Dissociative amnesia
.1:	Dissociative fugue	300.13:	Dissociative fugue
.2:	Dissociative stupor	300.14:	Dissociative identity disorder
.3:	Trance and possession states	300.6:	Depersonalization disorder
.4:	Dissociative motor disorders		
.5:	Dissociative convulsions		
.6:	Dissociative anaesthesia and sensory loss		
F45:	*Somatoform disorders*	**Somatoform disorders**	
.0:	Somatization disorder	300.81:	Somatization disorder
.1:	Undifferentiated somatoform disorder	300.11:	Conversion disorder
.2:	Hypochondriacal disorder	300.7:	Hypochondriasis
.3:	Somatoform autonomic dysfunction	300.7:	Body dysmorphic disorder
.4:	Persistent somatoform pain disorder	307.80:	Pain disorder associated with psychological factors
F46:	*Other neurotic disorders*	307.89:	Pain disorder associated with both psychological factors and a general medical condition
.0:	Neurasthenia condition	300.81:	Undifferentiated somatoform disorder
.1:	Depersonalization-derealization syndrome		

(destabilization factors), and the steps taken by the patient or the doctor to manage it (restitution factors). Most of the current diagnostic categories such as phobic disorder, dissociative disorder, or somatoform disorder result from various maladaptive attempts by patients to reduce their symptoms (Goldberg and Huxley 1992). The importance of the dimensional approach to these disorders is that it formulates them as longitudinal processes rather than just as cross-sectional episodes; this perspective is particularly important in elderly patients who often present with many years of illness experience. It also integrates the depressive component of many neurotic disorders, something that categorical classifications have never been able to do satisfactorily.

Modern nosologies are probably most appropriate in their categorization of obsessive–compulsive disorder (OCD) as a distinct disorder, although its current classification with the anxiety disorders may be inappropriate. Although a proportion of OCD patients also develop significant symptoms of depression and anxiety, it is a relatively persistent and stable diagnosis; it shows an early and specific response to treatment with serotonergic drugs, and the placebo response rate is much lower than occurs in depression and anxiety. OCD appears to have more in common with neurodevelopmental disorders such as Gilles de la Tourette's syndrome; Insel (1992) has suggested that it is due to impairment of a specific neuronal circuit involving the orbitofrontal cortex, basal ganglia, substantia nigra, and ventrolateral pallidum. This is in contrast to other anxiety disorders, which are thought to be due to disturbances in the frontal cortex–amygdala–septum–hippocampus system which mediates fear (Gray 1982).

Epidemiology

Neurotic disorders are uncommon primary diagnoses in hospital inpatient, outpatient, and casualty populations (Thyer *et al.* 1985; Schwartz *et al.* 1987), but as comorbid disorders their prevalence in clinical populations is significant (Hocking and Koenig 1995). The picture is rather different in primary care settings, where there is a steady accumulation of chronic psychiatric cases of all types in older age groups (Shepherd *et al.* 1981). However, there is a marked decline in the rate of new consultations with increasing age, with new cases after the age of 65 years being only about 10% of all cases in that age group (Shepherd *et al.* 1981; Cooper 1986). These falls in the prevalence and incidence of neurotic disorders with age in clinical populations are not simply due to falls in the general population (see below), but to non-presentation by patients and non-recognition by clinicians; one recent study of anxiety in elderly attenders at an inner-city general practice found very high rates of generalized anxiety and agoraphobia (Krasucki *et al.* 1999). Neurotic disorders do not pass easily through the various 'filters' on the pathway to psychiatric care (the subject's decision to consult, detection of disorder, psychiatric referral, admission to a hospital bed) (Goldberg and Huxley 1980); factors such as the age and sex of the subject, the severity of the disorder, and the doctor's attitudes are all important impediments. However, these patients may instead be referred inappropriately to non-psychiatric specialist services for investigation and treatment (Beitman *et al.* 1991; Blazer *et al.* 1991). Over the last three decades a number of epidemiological studies of elderly community populations have provided information about the rates of neurotic disorder in this age group, through the use of standardized methods and operationalized diagnostic criteria. These methodological developments have greatly improved the reliability and comparability of the results, but the different rates found using different criteria indicates that their validity is still questionable. For example, in the United States Epidemiologic Catchment Area (ECA) Study, the overall one-month prevalence of DSM-III phobic disorder was 4.8% (Regier *et al.* 1988), but in studies using the Geriatric Mental State (GMS)/ AGECAT system, diagnostic syndrome cases of phobic neurosis were very rare (Copeland *et al.* 1987). Most of these discrepancies are probably due to differences in the diagnostic criteria used, particularly the rules governing severity thresholds and hierarchies of disorders (Lindesay and Banerjee 1993).

Table 30.2 summarizes the findings of the ECA study so far as DSM-III categories related to neurotic disorder in the elderly population are concerned. Overall, lifetime prevalence rates decreased with age, although this decline was least apparent in phobic disorder and somatization disorder; phobic disorder was the commonest psychiatric disorder identified in women over 65 years of age, and the second commonest after cognitive impairment in men. Females had higher period prevalence rates than males for phobic disorder, panic disorder, generalized anxiety disorder, and somatization disorder, and higher lifetime prevalence rates of obsessive–compulsive disorder and somatization disorder. Most elderly subjects with neurotic disorders had developed them before their fifties, but elderly cases of phobic disorder, panic

Table 30.2 Prevalence and incidence rates of specific DSM-III mental disorders (ECA study)

		Males	Females	Total
One-month prevalence (%)[a]				
Dysthymia	65+	1.0	2.3	1.8
	all ages	2.2	4.2	3.3
Phobic disorder	65+	2.9	6.1	4.8
	all ages	3.8	8.4	6.2
Panic disorder	65+	0.0	0.2	0.1
	all ages	0.3	0.7	0.5
Obsessive–compulsive disorder	65+	0.7	0.9	0.8
	all ages	1.1	1.5	1.3
Somatization	65+	0.0	0.2	0.1
	all ages	0.0	0.2	0.1
Generalized anxiety disorder	65+	—	—	1.9*
	45–64	—	—	3.1*
Annual incidence per 100 person-years of risk[b]				
Phobic disorder	65+	2.66	5.52	4.29
	all ages	2.33	5.38	3.98
Panic disorder	65+	0.00	0.07	0.04
	all ages	0.30	0.76	0.56
Obsessive–compulsive disorder	65+	0.12	1.00	0.64
	all ages	0.39	0.92	0.69

[a]Regier *et al.* 1988; Blazer *et al.* 1991. [b]Eaton *et al.* 1989. *6-month prevalence.

disorder, and obsessive–compulsive disorder tended to be of later onset. Incidence rates of most neurotic disorders fell with age in both sexes, but this was least apparent for phobic disorder and OCD (Robins and Regier 1991). The Longitudinal Aging Study Amsterdam also used the Diagnostic Interview Schedule (DIS/DSM-III, and has reported similar prevalence rates to the ECA study for phobic disorder, panic disorder, and OCD (Beekman *et al.* 1998). However, at 7.3%, the rate of generalized anxiety disorder was rather higher. Within their sample (aged 55–85 years), there was little evidence of a change of rates of these disorders with age.

Not surprisingly, given the more stringent case definitions employed, the prevalence rates of neurotic disorders in studies using the GMS/AGECAT system are lower than those found by DIS/DSM-III (Table 30.3). However, a significant proportion had subcase levels of 'Anxiety, phobic and obsessional neurosis'. Age and sex differences for the case and subcase AGECAT categories were less consistent than those found by the ECA study using DSM-III criteria. A 3-year follow-up of the Liverpool sample found an incidence rate for neurotic disorders of 4.4/1000 per year (Larkin *et al.* 1992). In their view, the findings supported the idea of a general neurotic syndrome, with the majority of affected subjects having a prolonged course and variations in the predominance of different symptoms over time.

Another study of neurotic disorders in elderly community populations is the Guy's/Age Concern Survey; this looked at anxiety disorders using the Anxiety Disorder Scale which employed non-hierarchical, non-judgemental diagnostic criteria,

Table 30.3 One-month prevalence rates (%) of GMS/AGECAT neurotic disorders

	Male		Female	
	case	subcase	case	subcase
Anxiety neurosis	0.2	18.5	1.7	16.9
Phobic neurosis	0.0	3.7	1.2	5.6
Obsessional neurosis	0.0	2.4	0.2	1.4
Hypochondriacal neurosis	0.5	0.2	0.5	0.2

Taken from Copeland *et al.* 1987 with permission.

validated against clinical diagnosis (Lindesay *et al.* 1989). The overall 1-month prevalence was 10% for phobic disorders, and 3.7% for generalized anxiety; rates were higher in women than in men, although this was only statistically significant for phobic disorders. No subject met the DSM-III criteria for panic disorder. Another community survey using the same instrument found very similar prevalence rates of anxiety disorders (Manela *et al.* 1996). Phobic disorders in the Guy's/Age Concern sample were examined further in a case-control study (Lindesay 1991); cases had more neurotic symptoms than controls and higher rates of previous psychiatric disorders. Some one-third of the cases had their onset after the age of 65 years. Phobic subjects reported higher rates of contact with their general practitioners, but only a minority were receiving any form of treatment for their anxiety.

One interesting finding of the ECA study was that elderly subjects also had lower lifetime prevalence rates of depression and neurotic disorders than did younger groups; it is unclear whether this is a genuine cohort phenomenon or merely the result of a survivor effect or non-recall of past illness episodes by older adults (Klerman 1988). In a review of epidemiological studies over the lifespan, Jorm (2000) concludes there is evidence that old age may reduce the risk of anxiety and depression. However, other risk factors modify this effect, and it is difficult to separate ageing from cohort effects in cross-sectional studies. If there is an age effect, it may be the result of decreased emotional responsiveness, increased emotional control, or psychological immunization to stress. The relationship between anxiety disorders and age has also been reviewed by Krasucki *et al.* (1998).

Little is known about the longer term course and outcome of neurotic disorders in old age. In the 3-year follow-up study of Larkin *et al.* (1992), only 20% of the re-interviewed elderly people had improved. In their review of studies of general adult populations, Marks and Lader (1973) concluded that 41–59% of cases of 'anxiety neurosis' (generalized anxiety and panic) were recovered or much improved at 1- to 20-years follow-up. Noyes and Clancy (1976) found that 33% of their patient sample was unchanged or worse at 5-year follow-up, and that a later age of onset of anxiety was a predictor of poor outcome, particularly in men. In a 35-year follow-up of former panic patients, Coryell (1984) found there was an excess mortality in this group. In particular, male patients had a higher rate of deaths from cardiovascular disease. Follow-up studies of general adult phobic populations have produced similar results, with about half of the subjects showing at least some improvement (Roberts 1964; Agras *et al.* 1972). A Scandinavian follow-up study of inpatients with 'pure' anxiety neurosis found an increased risk of suicide and unnatural deaths in subjects who died before the age of 70 years (Allgulander and Lavori 1991). Suicide rates were also higher than expected in those patients with anxiety and/or depressive neurosis who survived until 71 years of age. Among this group, both men and women with 'pure' anxiety neurosis had a higher than expected mortality due to cardiac causes.

Transcultural epidemiology

Evidence regarding the epidemiology of anxiety disorders in late life across different cultures and ethnic groups is still very limited, with most of it coming from studies of immigrant groups in Western populations. In the ECA study, phobic disorders were more prevalent in the Black and Hispanic groups aged 65 years and older, and the prevalence of panic disorder increased with age in Hispanic females, in contrast to the other groups. Rates of generalized anxiety did not appear to differ (Robins and Regier 1991). In the UK, a study of elderly immigrant Gujarati Asians found that they had lower rates of simple phobia than the indigenous elderly population (Lindesay *et al.* 1997). Research in this area is fraught with methodological difficulties, however, and more work is needed.

Associated factors

Biological

To date, there has been little research into the biological aspects of neurotic disorders in the elderly population, and much has to be inferred from studies of younger subjects, and studies of elderly depressed patients where there is information about 'neurotic' subgroups. There are important limitations to much of this research: the subject samples are usually highly selected and unrepresentative; the study designs are rarely longitudinal; and 'old age' is always defined chronologically rather than biologically. In the absence of markers of biological age, however, it is not possible to determine to what extent ageing is and of itself a biological risk factor for neurotic disorders in late life (Philpott 1995).

Genetics

Studies of the inheritance of neurotic disorders suggest that, while there is a significant genetic component to vulnerability to these disorders as a group, it is not disorder-specific, and it is environmental factors which determine the particular form of illness that patients develop (Andrews *et al.* 1990; Kendler *et al.* 1992). There is, however, some evidence that the genetic heritability of OCD and panic disorder may be more specific (Marks 1986; Torgersen 1990). Genetic factors contribute to the heritability of personality traits that confer vulnerability to developing neurotic disorders, such as fearfulness and neuroticism (Goldsmith and Gottesman 1981; Bouchard *et al.* 1990), and to measures of arousal such as the galvanic skin response (Marks 1986). There is an association between neurotic disorder in elderly community populations and below-average intelligence (Nunn *et al.* 1974); this vulnerability factor is presumably also under a degree of genetic control. The contribution of genetic factors to affective disorders diminishes with age, but it is not known if this is also true of neurotic disorders.

Brain structure and function

There have been many structural and functional neuroimaging studies of elderly patients with affective disorders (see Chapter 12), but they provide only limited information about neuroses. The implication of computed tomography (CT) studies is that patients with milder forms of depression and higher anxiety scores are more likely to have normal scans (Jacoby and Levy 1980; Alexopoulos *et al.* 1992). Magnetic resonance imaging (MRI) studies have shown that elderly depressed patients have more subcortical grey and white matter lesions (Coffey *et al.* 1990), but it is not known if this is also true for patients with neurotic disorders. Studies of poststroke anxiety disorders show that the distribution of lesions differs from that in patients with poststroke affective disorders, but they are not consistent as to location; for example, Sharpe *et al.* (1990) found anxiety to be related to the size of left hemisphere lesions, whereas Castillo *et al.* (1993) found pure anxiety states to be associated with right hemisphere lesions. Astrom (1996) has reported that in the acute phase following a stroke, generalized anxiety disorder (GAD) with depression was associated with left hemispheric lesions on CT, whereas GAD alone was associated with right hemispheric lesions. GAD was not related to frontality of lesion, lesion volume, subcortical versus cortical lesion, or cerebral atrophy. At 3-year follow-up, cerebral atrophy on a repeat CT scan was associated with both anxiety and depression.

A few functional neuroimaging studies have been carried out with younger neurotic subjects. A small study of phobic patients found a fall in regional cerebral blood flow (rCBF) in occipital and posterior temporal regions when they were exposed to their feared stimulus. Social phobia has been associated with dysfunction of the striatal dopaminergic system in a single photon emission computed tomography (SPECT) study (Tiihonen *et al.* 1997). In OCD, the induction of obsessional thoughts resulted in increased rCBF in the right caudate nucleus and right orbitofrontal cortex in two studies (McGuire *et al.* 1994; Rauch *et al.* 1994), but others have found this disorder to be associated with reduced caudate nucleus rCBF (Machlin *et al.* 1991; Rubin *et al.* 1992). Lucey *et al.* (1995) found that the obsessive–compulsive and anxious-avoidant dimensions of OCD were associated with functionally distinct rCBF patterns. Factors such as hyperventilation and hypocapnia have an important influence on rCBF in anxious patients, and need to be controlled for (Mountz *et al.* 1989). Abnormalities of caudate nucleus metabolism in OCD have also been found using positron emission tomography (PET) (Baxter *et al.* 1992). In a PET study of GAD, Wu *et al.* (1991) found that provocation of anxiety was associated with a relative increase in basal ganglia metabolism, and that benzodiazepines reduced metabolism in this area, as well as in cortical and limbic areas. Metabolic changes in these areas were also correlated with changes in anxiety scores following administration of a placebo.

Psychosocial

There is considerable evidence that psychosocial factors such as prolonged adversity, life events, early experiences, and social relationships have an important influence on the onset and course of neurotic disorders at all ages. Protective factors and those determining recovery have been less extensively studied, but these also need to be identified and understood if these disorders are to be effectively treated and prevented (Lindesay 1995*b*).

Adversity

At all ages, there is a clear relationship between psychological ill-health and indicators of social adversity such as low occupational class, unemployment, poor housing, overcrowding, and limited access to amenities such as transport (Harris 1988; Champion 1990). In the elderly population, the evidence for this association is strongest in those studies using dimensional scales for measuring anxiety and depression (Himmelfarb and Murrell 1984; Kennedy *et al.* 1989, 1990). The relationship between adversity and categorical definitions of cases is less clear; in the ECA study there was no association between DSM-III affective disorders and socioeconomic variables, and among neurotic disorders, only generalized anxiety was associated with low household income. Phobic disorders in the elderly population are associated with urban domicile in some studies (Walton *et al.* 1990; Blazer *et al.* 1991) but not others (Beekman *et al.* 1998); this may not be an indicator of adversity so much as of poor social networks. Beekman *et al.* (1998) found an association between DSM-III anxiety disorders and lower levels of education. It would appear that adversity increases levels of distress, but may be less important as an aetiological factor in the development of more severe disorders.

There are several ways in which social adversity causes psychological ill-health in elderly people; for example, through increased levels of physical illness, and higher rates of adverse life events. Brown and Harris (1978) identified poor self-esteem as an important mediator between adverse social circumstances and psychiatric disorder in their study of young women. It is not clear whether this is applicable to elderly people, since self-esteem appears to be very resilient in late life (Baltes and Baltes 1990). It may be that those who have endured a lifetime of hardship will be better equipped to cope with adversity in old age than those for whom it is a new experience (Fillenbaum *et al.* 1985).

Life events

Adverse life events are a significant class of provoking agent which determine the onset of some psychiatric disorders in vulnerable individuals. The best evidence comes from studies using investigator-rated events (Brown and Harris 1978, 1989); most studies have been carried out in young adults, although Murphy (1982) has shown the importance of life events in relation to depression in elderly people. It is the meaning of the event to the individual, rather than its severity, that appears to be important (Brown *et al.* 1987), and different types of event in terms of their particular meaning may provoke the onset of different disorders. Loss events lead to depression, and threatening events to anxiety (Brown 1993). Positive 'fresh start' and 'anchoring' events have also been shown to contribute to recovery in younger patients with depression and anxiety, respectively (Brown *et al.* 1992; Brown 1993). Only some life events are followed by disorder, and only some disorders are preceded by life events, so in the individual case the presence of a preceding life event does not mean there are no other aetiologically important factors, and these should always be looked for (Murphy 1986).

Some classes of life event, such as bereavement, retirement, and institutionalization, are commoner in old age than at other time of life, but their psychological impact is still under-researched. Bereavement appears to take the same form and follow the same course in old age as it does earlier in life, with only a minority developing a psychiatric disorder (Blazer 1982). It has been suggested that the 'timeliness' of some losses in old age may reduce their impact (Zisook *et al.* 1987; Davis 1994); in one study, the only significant predictor of persistent grief in elderly men was the unexpectedness of their spouses' death (Byrne and Raphael 1994). It is not known if psychiatric morbidity following bereavement is more or less common in elderly people compared to other age groups. Significant anxiety following bereavement in old age may be associated with the subsequent persistence of depression (Prigerson *et al.* 1996*a*). Retirement is the event that defines the beginning of 'old age' for many people, and while most do not consider it to be stressful, some individuals react with increased levels of depression and anxiety. Factors such as early retirement due to ill-health or redundancy, lower income, lower educational attainment, and reduced social contacts are associated with higher levels of postretirement stress and dissatisfaction (Fillenbaum *et al.* 1985). Institutionalization is a profound loss event, and one that is experienced by a particularly physically and mentally vulnerable part of the elderly population. Most studies have been of established residents, and while many have shown them to have a poor quality of life and a high level of depression, it is not possible to distinguish between the impact of the transitional process and the effect of the institutional environment. Longitudinal studies suggest that factors such as preadmission vulnerability, the degree of difference between home and institution, and the choice and control the individual has in the admission process are important determinants of subsequent well-being (Tobin and Liebermann 1976).

Exposure to extreme catastrophe can cause significant psychological disturbance, and because of the close relationship of these stress reactions to acute or continuing trauma they are now classified as specific diagnoses in DSM-IV and ICD-10, notably post-traumatic stress disorder (PTSD). Little is known about the long-term effect of severely traumatic experiences, although PTSD can persist for many years. Its onset may also be delayed, sometimes manifesting itself for the first time in old age following retirement or an adverse life event (Scaturo and Hyman 1992; Kaup *et al.* 1994). Many people, now elderly, were exposed to severe trauma as service personnel and civilians during the Second World War, and it appears that what we now call PTSD was common then and has been persistent. In one study of US ex-prisoners of war, 67% had suffered from PTSD following traumatic exposure, and only 27% had fully recovered (Kluznik *et al.* 1986). Another recent study of 800 World War II prisoners of war found that 80% had persistent nightmares, and that those who had been imprisoned for longer periods and who had been subjected to more severe stress were more likely to meet the diagnostic criteria for PTSD (Guerrero and Crocq 1994). Traumatic wartime experiences have an enduring effect on a significant minority of older people, particularly more vulnerable groups such as psychiatric patients or those in long-term care (Rosen *et al.* 1989; Hermann and Eryavec 1994), and health professionals need to be aware of this when making assessments. Now that PTSD sufferers are eligible for financial compensation, increasing numbers of veterans are coming forward for diagnosis and treatment, and psychiatric services will need to develop better strategies for dealing with this problem.

Early experience

Experiences such as early parental loss and physical and sexual abuse in childhood are significant vulnerability factors for depression and other psychiatric disorders in adult life, although their significance in old age has not been extensively studied. Depression is associated with early maternal loss in young women (Brown and Harris 1978), but Murphy (1982) found no relationship between depression and parental loss in her elderly sample. So far as anxiety disorders are concerned, studies have shown a link between early parental loss and phobic disorders, particularly agoraphobia, in both young adulthood and old age (Faravelli *et al.* 1985; Tweed *et al.* 1989; Lindesay 1991). Generalized anxiety has also been linked with early parental loss in men (Zahner and Murphy 1989). Most interest has focused on maternal loss, but there is some evidence that anxiety disorders may be related more to the loss or departure of the father (Finlay-Jones 1989; Lindesay 1991). It appears that it is not so much parental loss that is important, so much as associated experiences such as prior marital conflict or subsequent inadequate care (Tennant *et al.* 1982). Presumably these experiences affect the developing personality and result in particular cognitive habits and 'defence styles' (Pollock and Andrews 1989) that determine the responses to adverse events and experiences in later life. In a study of 50 elderly spousal carers of terminally ill patients, childhood adversity, together with paranoid, histrionic, or self-defeating personality styles, directly increased the odds of having a DSM-III anxiety disorder (Prigerson *et al.* 1996*b*). Beekman *et al.* (1998) found that external locus of control was a significant vulnerability factor for anxiety disorders in their community sample.

Case 1

A 77-year-old widow developed generalized agoraphobia following a mugging in the street. In addition, she had a severe but untroublesome mouse phobia which had persisted since childhood. There was no other formal psychiatric history, but she described herself as 'a lifelong worrier' who always responded to threats and challenges by avoiding them. She attributed this tendency to her disrupted childhood; her father died when she was a baby and her mother was hospitalized for long periods, with the result that the patient had spent most of her early years in children's homes.

The possible role of abuse in childhood in determining vulnerability to psychiatric disorder in old age is still unexplored; one small study has suggested a link between childhood sexual abuse and panic disorder in old age (Sheikh *et al.* 1994).

Relationships

Cross-sectional studies usually show a relationship between psychological ill-health and reduced levels of social support. However, it is not clear from these whether psychiatric disorder leads to social withdrawal, or whether lack of social relationships increases vulnerability to disorder. On this point, follow-up studies are inconsistent in their findings; Blazer (1983) found that depression was associated with increased levels of social support 13 months later, whereas Oxman *et al.* (1992) found that reduced social support was associated with increased depression at 3-year follow-up. The quality of social relationships is as important as the quantity, and it appears to be the lack of an intimate confidant that particularly increases a person's vulnerability to depression in old age (Murphy 1982; Blazer 1983; Kennedy *et al.* 1989). Of course, the lack of a confidant in old age may reflect a longstanding difficulty in forming and sustaining close relationships, and Murphy (1986) has argued that it is this that increases vulnerability to life events. Regarding the association between anxiety and either the presence or absence of intimate relationships, the evidence is mixed. Some studies have not found a relationship (Finlay-Jones 1989; Lindesay 1991), but in the Longitudinal Aging Study Amsterdam anxiety disorders were associated with smaller contact networks and loneliness (Beekman *et al.* 1998).

Physical illness

Neurotic disorders in old age are associated with increased mortality and physical morbidity in community populations (Kay and Bergmann 1966; Lindesay 1990; Beekman *et al.* 1998), and in both psychiatric and medical patients (Bergmann 1971; Burn *et al.* 1993). There are several reasons why neurotic and physical disorders are linked in old age, as discussed below.

Physical illness causing neurotic disorders

The onset of physical illness is an important life event that most elderly people have to negotiate at some time, and in most it will evoke some degree of anxiety and sadness, particularly if it is painful, life-threatening, or disabling. In some, this response may be sufficiently severe to qualify as an adjustment disorder (Pitt 1995), and in a few vulnerable individuals it may trigger the onset of an anxiety or depressive disorder. For example, mild, chronic anxiety symptoms are relatively common following myocardial infarction in old age (Peach and Pathy 1979), and in a few cases this can develop into a severe and disabling 'cardiac neurosis', often focused on somatic anxiety symptoms such as palpitations. Such anxiety about physical illness can have important behavioural consequences: the onset of agoraphobia after the age of 65 years is attributed in most cases to the experience of a physical health event such as a myocardial infarct, a fracture, or elective surgery (Lindesay 1990). These and other traumatic experiences, such as falls or muggings, probably play a similar aetiological role to that of panic attacks in younger adults in precipitating loss of confidence, fear, and avoidance in vulnerable individuals. The fear of falling associated with balance disorders and mobility problems appears to be a common cause of disabling secondary avoidance in older adults (Marks 1981; Isaacs 1992). Since the experience of physical health events is an important precipitant of agoraphobia in old age, the identification and rehabilitation of elderly medical and surgical patients at risk may be an effective preventive strategy.

Case 2

An active 81-year-old widow with no previous history of psychiatric disorder sustained a minor injury after falling off a bus as it pulled away. She made a full physical recovery, but in the year following this accident she gradually lost confidence in going out by herself, and eventually became totally housebound unless accompanied by her daughter. She also developed severe episodes of free-floating anxiety associated with thoughts of the accident, and mild depression secondary to her isolation and restricted mobility, Her anxiety disorder only came to the attention of the health services because a psychiatric report was required to support her claim against the bus company.

A number of studies have examined the prevalence and course of anxiety following specific physical illnesses. Anxiety disorders are common following stroke, both in the acute phase and at medium- to long-term (1–5 years) follow-up (Sharp *et al.* 1990; Burvill *et al.* 1995; Astrom 1996; Schultz *et al.* 1997), with prevalence figures ranging from 5 to 28%. Agoraphobia is the most common disorder in this population (9–20%), followed by GAD. Studies of the 1- to 3-year outcome of poststroke anxiety disorders show that only around 25–50% have resolved at 12 months. A non-resolution of symptoms at 12 months is associated with a chronic course and poor functional outcome over 3 years. The presence of comorbid depression not only adversely affects the responsiveness to treatment but also increases mortality. Follow-up studies of patients with acute myocardial infarction have also reported that depression and anxiety independently predict a higher rate of subsequent cardiac events (Frasure-Smith *et al.* 1995).

It is not only acute episodes of physical ill health that provoke anxiety and fear in elderly people. Chronic disability due to conditions such as arthritis and sensory impairment is also associated with high rates of subjective anxiety and avoidance (Kay *et al.* 1987; Lindesay 1990; Beekman *et al.* 1998), perhaps because they heighten the individual's sense of vulnerability to and gravity of the consequences of possible future adverse events.

Physical illness mimicking neurotic disorders

A number of physical disorders may present with apparently neurotic symptoms in old age, and these are considered in the discussion of the differential diagnosis of neurotic disorders below.

Neurotic disorders mimicking physical illness

Neurotic disorders at all ages are associated with a variety of somatic symptoms such as palpitations, dysphagia, nausea, altered bowel habit, paraesthesia, and pain. It is a common clinical impression that the somatization of psychological distress is more often seen in elderly patients, but to some extent this may be due to a selection bias, since it is the individuals who complain of physical symptoms of anxiety and depression who will be most likely to make it through the 'filters' and present to medical services. Anxious and depressed elderly people are also more likely to be concerned about trivial physical problems, which will lead them to consult their doctors. The somatization of anxiety in elderly patients is discussed further below.

Neurotic disorders causing physical illness

Neurotic disorders may cause physical illness through direct or indirect effects on bodily function. Most important in this respect are the higher rates of damaging behaviours such as smoking and alcohol abuse. Among younger adults, phobic anxiety is commoner in smokers than non-smokers (Haines *et al.* 1980); if anxious, avoidant individuals are more likely to be (or have been) smokers, it may be that the increased rates of cardiovascular and respiratory illness observed in association with anxiety disorders in elderly people are a result of this. In the Northwick Park heart study, phobic anxiety was strongly related to subsequent ischaemic heart disease in men aged 40–64 years (Haines *et al.* 1987). However, smoking did not explain the association in this sample, and it is suggested that anxiety-related hyperventilation might cause coronary artery spasm, or that subjects with phobic anxiety might have exaggerated hormonal responses to myocardial infarction.

Clinical assessment and diagnosis

It is evident from the epidemiology and associations of neurotic disorder in old age that health professionals need to become more alert to the possibility of these conditions in their patients, and aware of the ways in which they may present. These disorders have psychological and somatic symptoms, and are often associated with particular disturbances of behaviour. For the most part, these are similar to those seen in younger adults, but there are some important differences in how they manifest themselves.

Psychological symptoms

The depressive symptomatology that may accompany neurotic disorders is described in Chapter 27. So far as anxiety is concerned, patients' preoccupations are usually focused on topics that are of concern to most elderly people, such as physical illness, finances, crime, and the family. The fears and phobias described by elderly people are similar to those found in younger adults: animals, heights, enclosed spaces, public transport, going out of doors (Lindesay *et al.* 1989). Severe anxiety about death appears to be less common than might be supposed in this age group, perhaps because elderly people are more familiar with it (Kay 1988). Clinically important worries and fears in elderly people are often dismissed as reasonable simply because of the patient's age. In fact, an elderly person's perception of their vulnerability is determined more by factors such as physical disability and the availability of social support, and it is these rather than age that should be taken into account when judging the reasonableness of fears.

The clinical features of OCD in elderly patients are broadly similar to those seen in younger adults (Kohn *et al.* 1997). It is rare for obsessional symptoms to appear for the first time in old age, although cases have been reported (Bajulaiye and Addonizio 1992). More often, cases that present in old age are longstanding disorders that have never been adequately assessed or treated (Jenike 1989). Some late-onset cases may be due to external factors, such as adverse life events, that weaken an elderly individual's resistance to longstanding subclinical obsessionality (Colvin and Boddington 1997). It is important therefore that all elderly people receive a thorough evaluation and the benefit of modern treatments as and when they present to psychogeriatric services (Austin *et al.* 1992). In old age, the late appearance of apparently obsessional orderliness and preoccupation with routines may presage the onset of dementia, particularly if the frontal lobe is involved (Neary 1990). Obsessional symptoms may also appear at any age following head injury or cerebral tumour; in such cases, apparently obsessional and stereotypic behaviour is not preceded by mounting anxiety nor followed by a release of tension.

Somatic symptoms

The somatic symptoms of anxiety in elderly people are also similar to those occurring at other ages. These include the full range of autonomic symptoms, muscular tension pains, motor restlessness, globus hystericus, dyspnoea, and the effects of hyperventilation. In elderly patients, however, they may be wrongly attributed by both the patient and the doctor to physical illness, with the result that their significance is missed and the patient is subjected instead to unnecessary investigations and treatments. Careful enquiry into the circumstances surrounding the onset of the symptoms, and the accompanying mood, is usually sufficient to determine their origin. Most elderly patients who misattribute the symptoms of psychological distress to physical illness will readily accept the real cause when it is explained to them, but a minority are extremely resistant and will meet the criteria for a somatization disorder. In these individuals, the somatization of psychological disturbance will usually have started early in life, but they may have been skilled at avoiding psychiatrists in their youth and adulthood, only presenting to psychiatric services for the first time in old age. They are usually accompanied by a voluminous medical history of negative investigations, unhelpful treatments, and complicating iatrogenic problems. Studies of clinical populations suggest that somatization disorder is a chronic condition and does not ameliorate substantially with age (Pribor *et al.* 1994). However, it was not identified in the elderly (65 years and over) subjects in the ECA study (Myers *et al.* 1984). This may reflect the difficulty of identifying somatic complaints without an organic basis in a population where physical disorders are relatively common. Alternatively, as they age, patients with somatization disorder may transfer their concern to genuine organic symptoms—they graduate from being somatizers to being 'heartsink' patients.

In contrast to patients with somatization, who have multiple physical complaints and who demand relief from their distress, the focus of hypochondriacal patients is usually restricted to one or two body organs or systems. Typically, they are preoccupied with the possibility of serious illness, and their demand is for investigation rather than treatment. In elderly patients, primary hypochondriasis is usually longstanding; if it presents for the first time in old age it is more likely to be a secondary manifestation of depression or anxiety.

Hysterical symptoms in elderly patients are an important exception to the general rule that neurotic symptoms in old age have the same diagnostic significance as in younger adults. As Bergmann (1978) has said, 'it is best to assert dogmatically that primary hysterical illness does not begin in old age'; apparently dissociative symptoms are usually due either to underlying undiagnosed physical illness, or the release of old hysterical tendencies in vulnerable personalities by organic cerebral pathology or functional psychiatric disorder.

Case 3

A 65-year-old man whose wife was dying of dementia was admitted to hospital following the appearance of dysphasic symptoms similar to his wife's when he was particularly distressed. Physical examination was normal, and his illness was initially diagnosed as a dissociative disorder, but further investigation revealed that he was suffering from neurosyphilis, and his condition greatly improved following treatment.

Panic in old age may also be a significant cause of misdiagnosed somatic symptoms. Despite the considerable amount of research that has been carried out into panic in recent years, very little is known about this condition in the elderly population. Cross-sectional epidemiological studies suggest that it is rare, and a number of explanations have been put forward to account for this (Flint *et al.* 1996). However, its prevalence may be underestimated by survey methodology, given the chronic episodic nature of the disorder. The limited evidence from case reports (Frances and Flaherty 1989; Luchins and Rose 1989), volunteer samples (Sheikh *et al.* 1991), and non-psychiatric patient populations (Katon 1984; Beitman *et al.* 1991) suggest that panic in old age is less common than in early adulthood, is commoner in women and widows, and late-onset cases are less severe in terms of symptoms and secondary avoidance than those whose disorder started earlier in life. Elderly panic patients tend not to present to psychiatric services (Thyer *et al.* 1985; Kenardy *et al.* 1990), but because of the prominent physical symptoms they may be referred instead for investigation and treatment to cardiologists, neurologists, and gastroenterologists. In a study of cardiology patients with chest pain and no evidence of coronary artery disease, one-third of those aged 65 years and over met the diagnostic criteria for panic disorder (Beitman *et al.* 1991). At all ages, there is extensive comorbidity between panic disorder and somatization disorder (Boyd *et al.* 1984), and patients with panic are often misdiagnosed by their GPs as chronic somatizers (Katon 1984). In late-onset cases, the possibility of depression or an iatrogenic cause such as dopamine-agonist treatment for Parkinson's disease should be considered.

A common somatic symptom of anxiety in elderly patients is delayed or interrupted sleep due to worry and nightmares, and this is often the presenting complaint in those who seek medical help. Daytime tiredness is common in those with generalized anxiety, and specific fears or rituals associated with bedtime may interfere with the sleep routines of phobic and obsessional patients. As a group, patients with sleep disturbance due to a neurotic disorder often have problems with chronic hypnotic, sedative, and alcohol abuse. The effective management of disturbed sleep is an important aspect of the care of these patients (see below).

Behaviour disturbance

The psychological and somatic symptoms of anxiety and depression can have important adverse behavioural consequences. Many of the neurotic responses to somatic symptoms discussed above can be understood as forms of abnormal illness behaviour. Another important behavioural consequence of anxiety and panic is the phobic avoidance of feared objects and situations. Lifelong avoidance is unlikely to present as a problem in old age unless a change in circumstances makes this avoidance impossible, such as the death of a spouse who used to do the shopping. Late-onset agoraphobic avoidance is more likely to be restricting, but if it is rewarded with the provision of domiciliary services and well-meaning family support, it will not present as a problem. Sometimes cases present as a family problem if the patient becomes overdependent on others for support.

Chronic psychological distress may also lead to the use and abuse of sedative drugs and alcohol. As a group, elderly people are among the heaviest consumers of psychotropic drugs, particularly repeat prescriptions of benzodiazepine tranquillizers and hypnotics (Catalan *et al.* 1988). Less is known about the extent of alcohol abuse as a result of anxiety and depression in old age, but about one-third of elderly alcohol abusers appear to have started late in life as the result of 'stress' (Rosin and Glatt 1971; Gurnack and Thomas 1989). An eating disorder may re-emerge in old age as a maladaptive coping strategy in an individual who is having difficulty adjusting to their old age (Bowler 1995).

Assessment scales

Over the years, a wide range of instruments have been used to identify and measure anxiety in elderly patients. However, there are very few scales available that have been specifically developed for use with the elderly population. In a recent compendium of instruments for use in old age psychiatry there was no scale for the assessment of primary anxiety disorders, compared with over 15 scales for depression (Burns *et al.* 1999). Recently however, some elderly-specific instruments have been developed, such as the 10-item Short Anxiety Screening Test (SAST) in medical inpatients and outpatients (Sinoff *et al.* 1999), the four-item FEAR in elderly primary care attenders (Krasucki *et al.* 1999), and RAID (Rating Anxiety in Dementia scale) in elderly patients with dementia (Shankar *et al.* 1999).

Differential diagnosis

Depression

In view of the extensive comorbidity between neurotic disorders and depression, and the fact that depressive symptoms are often an integral component of the neurotic disorder, it is not useful to consider them as strict diagnostic alternatives. Using data from three ECA sites to study the effect of DSM-III hierarchical exclusion criteria, Boyd *et al.* (1984) found that agoraphobia was 15 times commoner, and panic disorder 19 times commoner, in subjects with major depression. In studies of elderly subjects using GMS/AGECAT, anxiety disorders were 20 times more likely to occur in depressed than non-depressed subjects (Kay 1988). Elderly subjects with phobic disorders report an increased history of depression compared to controls (Lindesay 1990). Clinical experience suggests that late-onset anxiety in elderly patients is nearly always associated with some degree of depression, but it should be borne in mind that it is the currently or previously depressed cases who will be more likely to present or be known to services.

The possibility that anxious, hypochondriacal, and obsessional individuals are also depressed (and vice versa) should always be considered, since treating one part of the problem may not alleviate the other (Blazer *et al.* 1989). For example, if an elderly person is depressed because of the restrictions imposed by agoraphobia, it is not sufficient to prescribe antidepressants without attending to the underlying cause. Certain clinical features such as pronounced hypochondriasis, anhedonia, guilt, agitation, or panic attacks are highly indicative of associated depression requiring treatment in its own right. Comorbid anxiety may have an adverse effect on treatment outcome, reducing responsiveness to antidepressants and increasing discontinuation rates. Persistence of anxiety following remission of the depression is associated with quicker relapse (Flint and Rifat 1997*a,b*).

Case 4

A 79-year-old man was referred to the local psychiatric service by his general practitioner for assessment of an anxiety state, which had developed following a minor head injury the previous year. His principal complaints were severe anxiety with both subjective and somatic symptoms, panic attacks at night, and generalized agoraphobic avoidance associated with a fear of falling. On examination, however, it was apparent that he was also severely depressed, with early morning wakening, hypochondriacal delusions, and auditory hallucinations urging him to commit suicide. He was admitted to hospital and, following treatment with an antidepressant, the depression, subjective anxiety, and panic all resolved. He was discharged home, but at follow-up he remained agoraphobic. This required further outpatient treatment with a programme of graded desensitization.

Dementia

Krasucki *et al.* (1998) have suggested that anxiety disorders may predispose to cognitive impairment in later life, resulting in a 'diagnostic shift' towards the latter that might explain the observed decline in the prevalence of anxiety disorders with age. This idea remains speculative, although there is some epidemiological evidence to support an association, at least in the case of generalized anxiety (Manela *et al.* 1996). It is certainly true that in the early stages dementia may reveal itself through symptoms such as anxiety or obsessionality (Wands *et al.* 1990; Ballard *et al.* 1994); however, it should be borne in mind that anxiety alone can impair performance on tests of cognitive function. In the later stages, anxiety may be a cause of agitated behaviour. Anxiety in demented patients may be associated with depressive or psychotic symptoms, or with concerns about the implications of the disorder and its impact on social functioning (Ballard *et al.* 1996). Studies have yet to examine the possibility that the neurodegenerative process in Alzheimer's disease is itself a cause of anxiety.

The reported prevalence of anxiety symptoms/disorders in subjects with dementia ranges from 3% to 38% (Wands *et al.* 1990; Forsell and Winblad 1997). Whether the prevalence of anxiety in demented individuals is higher than in age-matched controls is unclear, but the evidence suggests that it is rates of symptoms rather than disorders that are elevated. There appears to be no correlation between anxiety and the severity of cognitive impairment, but the expression of anxiety may change as the dementia progresses; in more severely demented patients anxiety may manifest itself as agitation. Patients with vascular dementia may be more prone to develop anxiety symptoms than those with Alzheimer's disease (Sultzer *et al.* 1993).

Dementia also puts a considerable strain on carers, and their rates of anxiety symptoms and disorders have been consistently found to be significantly higher than controls (Dura *et al.* 1991; Russo *et al.* 1995). One study has found that carers' subjective competence is related to their neuroticism and the behaviour problems in the patient, but not to the formal support and help they receive (Vernooij-Dassen *et al.* 1996).

Delirium

Although delirium in the elderly is usually relatively 'quiet', affected individuals are sometimes terrified by their hallucinations and imagined persecutions, and may present as panic rather than delirium. Panic attacks are uncommon in old age, and the abrupt onset of terror should be regarded as a sign of delirium until proved otherwise, particularly if there is evidence of cognitive impairment and the individual is physically ill. Careful examination of the mental state and a history from an informant will usually determine the presence or absence of other features of delirium, such as attentional deficits, fluctuating level of consciousness, and perceptual disturbances. Very occasionally, anxiety itself may induce delirium in vulnerable individuals (see Chapter 26).

Paranoid states and schizophrenia

Occasionally, the fear and anxiety accompanying a functional psychosis may be mistaken for a simple anxiety state. However, a careful history and examination will usually reveal the underlying psychotic experiences and beliefs. Peculiar hypochondriacal preoccupations can sometimes be difficult to distinguish from monosymptomatic delusional disorders.

Physical illness

In view of the important association between neurotic disorders and physical illness in old age, assessment should always include a thorough physical examination to exclude any primary physical cause of the neurotic symptoms. Some of the physical causes of neurotic symptoms in elderly patients are listed in Table 30.4. In particular, a number of important cardiovascular, respiratory, and endocrine disorders may present atypically with anxiety or depression and little else in this age group. A physical cause for neurotic symptoms should be considered if there is no psychiatric history, and no sufficient current stress in the patient's life to account for the mental disturbance. Anxiety symptoms can also be caused by prescribed drugs such as oral hypoglycaemics and corticosteroids, or by substances such

Table 30.4 Physical causes of neurotic symptoms in the elderly

Cardiovascular	**Neurological**
myocardial infarction	head injury
cardiac arrhythmias	cerebral tumour
orthostatic hypotension	dementia
mitral valve prolapse	delirium
	epilepsy
Respiratory	migraine
pneumonia	cerebral lupus erythematosus
pulmonary embolism	demyelinating disease
emphysema	vestibular disturbance
asthma	subarachnoid haemorrhage
left-ventricular failure	CNS infections
hypoxia	
chronic obstructive airways disease	**Dietary and drug related**
bronchial carcinoma	caffeine
	vitamin deficiencies
Endocrine and metabolic	anaemia
hypo- and hyperthyroidism	sympathomimetics
hypo- and hypercalcaemia	dopamine agonists
Cushing's disease	corticosteroids
carcinoid syndrome	withdrawal syndromes
hypoglycaemia	akathisia
insulinoma	digoxin toxicity
phaeochromocytoma	fluoxetine
hyperkalaemia	
hypokalaemia	
hypothermia	

Taken from Pitt 1995 with permission.

as caffeine and over-the-counter preparations containing sympathomimetics (Lader 1982). Drug withdrawal is also likely to lead to anxiety if the patient is physically dependent. Similarly, the erratic use of very short-acting hypnotics, such as triazolam, may cause rebound withdrawal during the day. In patients with a physical cause for their neurotic symptoms, these usually remit with treatment of the underlying disorder.

Management

Despite the greater clinical awareness of neurotic disorders in elderly patients nowadays, many still go unrecognized and untreated. In the minority who do receive treatment, this usually takes the form of medication with anxiolytic and hypnotic drugs, and few patients receive any form of psychological intervention (Lindesay *et al.* 1991). This over-reliance on drugs and the neglect of alternatives is unfortunate, since the latter are probably much safer and may well be more effective in the long-term management of neurotic symptoms in this age group. Krasucki *et al.* (1999) have recently reviewed the treatment of anxiety disorders in elderly patients.

Since most cases of neurotic disorder in elderly patients are seen in the primary care and general medical settings, this is where the focus of identification and treatment should be. Specialist psychogeriatric services have only a limited role to play in the management of these patients, particularly in the long term, but they are a valuable source of expertise and should aim to offer advice and education to primary care and general hospital staff in appropriate management strategies. For example, one group of patients who are mismanaged by most health professionals are the 'heartsink' group with longstanding mood disturbance and hypochondriacal preoccupations, persistent insomnia, and dependence on anxiolytic and hypnotic medication. While it is probably optimistic to hope for complete cure in such cases, there is much that can be done, provided that there is a firm and consistent strategy. In the first place, there should be a single individual (ideally the general practitioner) responsible for coordinating the various aspects of care, and this should be made clear to all concerned, particularly the patient and their family. Two important functions of the coordinating practitioner are to rationalize existing medication and to ensure that the patient does not receive unnecessary investigations or treatments. If somatic complaints are a particular problem, the patient should be offered regular check-ups rather than consultation on demand. There is little point in engaging in battles over the cause of complaints; the best approach is simply to express understanding of the patient's distress, agree that they need help, and reassure them that they are being cared for. Once a reasonably positive relationship is established, it may eventually be possible to engage the patient in an examination of cognitions and dynamics.

Case 5

A 72-year-old woman was referred to the local psychogeriatric service by her exasperated GP. She and her husband had been patients of the practice for many years, both attending regularly with an ever-changing repertoire of non-specific somatic complaints. The routine of joint attendance at the surgery to complain and collect their repeat prescriptions for night sedation had been broken by the sudden death of her husband from a heart attack the year before. Subsequently, her demands on the practice escalated to the point where she was telephoning the GP at his home at night to demand home visits. When these were refused, she started to importune the neighbours and on one occasion was taken to casualty following a collapse in the street. The psychogeriatrician's opinion was that this severe exacerbation of her longstanding anxiety state was a bereavement reaction, complicated by anger against the GP over the death of her husband. Following a joint meeting of the patient, the GP, and the psychogeriatrician, it was agreed that the GP would undertake to physically examine the patient and listen to all complaints once a week, provided that no other demands were made. The GP was also instructed in appropriate strategies for addressing the patient's anxious and angry thoughts. After two months, the frequency of these contacts were reduced to once a month, and the patient agreed to attempt a gradual withdrawal of her night sedation.

Psychological treatments

Cognitive–behavioural

Cognitive–behaviour therapy (CBT) for neurotic disorders is of proven benefit in younger adults, but its effectiveness has only recently begun to be evaluated in elderly patients. However, individual case-reports and small case-series of successful treatments in elderly patients with phobic disorders and OCD (Thyer 1981; Woods and Britton 1985; Downs *et al.* 1988; Colvin and Boddington 1997) show that this approach can be successfully applied to this age group (see Chapter 11). CBT has also been evaluated in elderly patients with depression, prolonged grief, generalized anxiety, and panic with encouraging results (Thompson *et al.* 1987; King and Barrowclough 1991; Radley *et al.* 1997). CBT involves both the cognitive and behavioural approaches to conceptualizing and modifying the disturbances in thinking and behaviour that characterize neurotic disorders. Although theoretically distinct, they are in practice rarely carried out in isolation, and procedures such as anxiety management training draw heavily on both models (Woods 1995). Cognitive therapy involves identifying, evaluating, controlling, and changing the negative thoughts, cognitive distortions, and false attributions that occur in anxiety and depression. For example, in an elderly anxious patient this might involve challenging the misattribution of autonomic anxiety symptoms to physical disease, or the automatic thoughts about vulnerability that maintain agoraphobic avoidance. In behaviour therapy, on the other hand, it is the concepts of conditioning, reinforcement, and avoidance that underlie clinical strategies such as desensitization for phobic disorders and habituation for obsessional rumination. CBT may be carried out both individually and in groups. The advantages of groups are that they are more cost-effective, and they also harness useful peer support which often persists after the formal treatment has finished (Zerhusen *et al.* 1991). However, it can be difficult and time-consuming to assemble groups in which the members are sufficiently similar to ensure they work well together and do not exclude or scapegoat particular individuals. While the principles of applying CBT to elderly patients are the same as for younger adults, the goals and techniques may need to be adapted in some cases, for example if there is significant physical disability or cognitive impairment (Woods 1995; Koder 1998). It has been suggested that elderly patients are less psychologically minded and so are less likely to be able to use CBT, but there is no good evidence to support this; factors such as education and sociocultural background are probably more important in this respect. CBT may also be effective in lowering the risk of relapse by reducing underlying vulnerability factors such as neuroticism and locus of control (Andrews 1996).

Psychodynamic

As Martindale (1995) has pointed out, some knowledge of psychodynamics is of great value when assessing elderly patients, particularly if their disorders involve difficulties in negotiating the developmental issues of late life, or the inappropriate and maladaptive use of defence mechanisms. Formal psychodynamic treatments and techniques, particularly in group settings, are also useful in the treatment of neurotic disorders in elderly patients. These are discussed in depth in Chapter 16.

Physical treatments

Medication has an important role in the treatment of neurotic disorders in elderly patients, but much current practice is still insufficiently careful, rational, or discriminating. Before starting an elderly patient on any psychotropic medication there are a number of important factors to consider. First, will it have an adverse effect on the patient's physical condition? Someone with respiratory failure may be killed by a respiratory depressant such as a benzodiazepine. The anticholinergic and quinidine-like effects of tricyclic antidepressants will exacerbate problems such as glaucoma and urinary retention, and can be very dangerous in patients with cardiovascular disease. Second, will the medication interact with any other drugs (including alcohol) the patient is taking? Third, what are the pharmacokinetics and pharmacodynamics of the patient? Drug handling by the body is very variable in elderly individuals (Braithwaite 1982), and prescribed doses need to be titrated accordingly. Last, but not least, is the patient likely to take the drugs as prescribed? The risk of suicide must also be taken into consideration.

Benzodiazepines

Although clinical fashion has turned against the use of benzodiazepines in recent years, they are still prescribed in considerable quantities as tranquillizers and hypnotics to elderly patients. Certain patient groups, such as those in long-term care, are particularly likely to receive these drugs (Gilbert *et al.* 1988). Important problems associated with the prolonged use of benzodiazepines include dependence, memory impairment, poor motor coordination, depression of respiratory drive, and paradoxical excitement (Tyrer 1980; Curran 1986; Fancourt and Castleden 1986). Elderly people are particularly sensitive to these adverse effects, and the accumulation of drugs with long elimination half-lives also leads to drowsiness, delirium, incontinence, falls, and fractures. In one study of elderly hospitalized patients, benzodiazepines were found to account for 29% of new episodes of acute confusion (Foy *et al.* 1995). Surprisingly little controlled research has been conducted into the therapeutic effect of benzodiazepines in elderly patients, and most practice is guided by studies in younger adults and by anecdotal clinical experience (Salzman 1991). Despite these problems, there is still a place for benzodiazepines in the management of transient, short-term anxiety symptoms in elderly patients. Drugs with short half-lives and no active metabolites, such as oxazepam, are to be preferred, although it should be borne in mind that patients on such drugs are at greater risk of developing withdrawal symptoms on discontinuation. The long-term use of benzodiazepines should be avoided, and established users weaned off their medication when possible (Higgitt 1988).

The commonest and least justifiable reason why elderly patients are given benzodiazepines is because they complain of insomnia. Quite often, this complaint is merely concern over normal changes in the quantity and pattern of sleep that occur with increasing age (Reynolds *et al.* 1985), and explanation and reassurance are usually all that is required. Where there is an underlying cause for the sleep disturbance, such as depression, pain, or breathlessness, it is this rather than the sleeplessness that should be treated. Psychophysiological insomnia due to tension and worry at bedtime is best managed in the first instance with a programme of advice on sleep hygiene (Bramble 1995) to help the patient establish a regular sleep routine. A hypnotic should only be prescribed if this is ineffective, or if the insomnia is transient.

Antidepressants

If there is any evidence of depression associated with the patient's neurotic disorder, then a trial of a 6–8-week course of antidepressant medication is indicated. Generalized anxiety and panic also respond to antidepressant drugs. Tricyclics are effective, but their use is limited by the risks they pose to physically ill patients, and their toxicity in overdose; an important exception in this respect is lofepramine (Dorman 1988). The introduction of the selective serotonin-reuptake inhibitors (SSRIs) has transformed the treatment of depression in old age, because they can be used safely even in severely physically ill and suicidal patients (Evans and Lye 1992). Drugs with serotonin-reuptake inhibiting activity also have a specific effect in OCD, and are effective in elderly patients (Jenike 1985; Austin *et al.* 1991). Monoamine oxidase inhibitors (MAOIs) are relatively well tolerated by elderly patients, although their use has declined in recent years. A specific MAO-B inhibitor, moclobemide, has recently been introduced which has much less peripheral activity than the older MAOIs, and therefore there is less need for dietary restrictions. Whether or not it has any particular role in the treatment of neurotic disorders is not known. The use of antidepressant medication is discussed in more detail in Chapter 27.

Neuroleptics

A short course of a conventional neuroleptic drug, such as haloperidol or zuclopenthixol, may be used to control severe anxiety in elderly patients, most effectively when it is due to psychotic experiences, as in delirium. However, the risk of disabling extrapyramidal side-effects such as parkinsonism and tardive dyskinesia associated with these drugs, even in low doses, means that they are not indicated for the long-term management of anxiety in old age. The new generation of 'atypical' neuroleptics, such as risperidone, have a much reduced incidence of side-effects, and are to be preferred if long-term management with this group of drugs is unavoidable.

Beta-blockers

These drugs are sometimes used to control the sympathetic somatic symptoms of anxiety where these are particularly troublesome (Kathol *et al.* 1980). However, they are contraindicated in patients with asthma, chronic obstructive airways disease, sinus bradycardia, and heart failure. These restrictions, together with side-effects such as nightmares and insomnia, limit their usefulness in elderly patients.

Antihistamines

Antihistamine drugs such as hydroxyzine have long been used as anxiolytics in elderly patients. Their effect is probably due primarily to their sedative action. They are relatively safe, although hypotension can be a problem. They have a role in patients where respiratory depressant drugs are contraindicated.

Buspirone

Buspirone is a recently introduced azapirone anxiolytic, which acts differently from the benzodiazepines and has no cross-tolerance with them. Its pharmacokinetics, safety, and efficacy in elderly patients are similar to those in younger adults (Robinson *et al.* 1988), and its short-term use is not associated with rebound, dependence, or abuse (Lader 1991). It appears to be well tolerated by elderly patients receiving treatment for chronic medical conditions (Bohm *et al.* 1990). Unlike other anxiolytics, it takes about 2 weeks to become effective, so it has a limited role in the management of acute anxiety states. It is indicated for severe, chronic generalized anxiety (Feighner 1987), and in patients where there is a risk of dependence and abuse.

Barbiturates

The use of barbiturates and related drugs such as meprobamate and glutethimide has declined considerably, but there are still a few elderly people who are being maintained on these preparations. Their use is associated with many serious problems, notably physical dependency, dangerous withdrawal states, delirium, and paradoxical excitement. They are a very effective means of suicide. No patient should ever be started on a sedative or hypnotic barbiturate, and established users should be carefully weaned off these drugs. Barbiturate withdrawal should be covered with a reducing regime of phenobarbital to prevent fits.

The cost of neurotic disorders

At all ages, patients with neurotic disorders are high consumers of all types of health services (Leon *et al.* 1995; Kennedy and Schwab 1997). In a study of elderly patients in the UK, it was estimated that the mean cost per month of community care for an individual without mental health problems was £32.52, compared with £86.96 for those with anxiety, £85.93 for depression, and £194.70 for dementia. The total estimated UK health care cost due to anxiety in old age was £750 million. (Livingston *et al.* 1997).

Conclusions

Our knowledge of neurotic disorders in the elderly population has improved considerably in recent years, but there is still much to be learned about their origins, course, and outcome; about their impact on other disorders and upon health services generally, and about the effectiveness of different treatment strategies. Elderly people are a very diverse group exposed to a wide range of physical, environmental, and psychosocial factors that determine vulnerability to, onset of, and recovery from neurotic disorders, and further study of this age group will almost certainly enhance our understanding of these conditions at all ages.

References

Agras, W. S., Chapin, N., and Oliveau, D. C. (1972). The natural history of phobia: course and prognosis. *Archives of General Psychiatry*, **26**, 315–17.

Alexopoulos, G. S., Young, R. C., and Shindeldecker, R. D. (1992). Brain computed tomography findings in geriatric depression and primary degenerative dementia. *Biological Psychiatry*, **31**, 591–9.

Allgulander, C. and Lavori, P. W. (1991). Excess mortality among 3302 patients with 'pure' anxiety neurosis. *Archives of General Psychiatry*, **48**, 599–602.

American Psychiatric Association (1994). *Diagnostic and statistical manual of mental disorders* (4th edn). American Psychiatric Association, Washington.

Andrews, G. (1996). Comorbidity in neurotic disorders: the similarities are more important than the differences. In *Current controversies in the anxiety disorders* (ed. R. M. Rapee), pp. 3–20. Guilford Press, New York.

Andrews, G., Stewart, G., Allen, R., and Henderson, A. S. (1990). The genetics of six neurotic disorders: a twin study. *Journal of Affective Disorders*, **19**, 23–9.

Astrom, M. (1996). Generalized anxiety disorder in stroke patients. A 3-year longitudinal study. *Stroke*, **27**, 270–5.

Austin, L. S., Zealberg, J. J., and Lydiard, R. B. (1991). Three cases of pharmacotherapy of obsessive–compulsive disorder in the elderly. *Journal of Nervous and Mental Disease*, **179**, 634–5.

Bajulaiye, R. and Addonizio, C. (1992). Obsessive–compulsive disorder arising in a 75-year-old woman. *International Journal of Geriatric Psychiatry*, **7**, 139–42.

Ballard, C. G., Mohan, R. N. C., Patel, A., and Graham, C. (1994). Anxiety disorder in dementia. *Irish Journal of Psychological Medicine*, **11**, 108–9.

Ballard, C. G., Boyle, A., Bowler, C., and Lindesay, J. (1996). Anxiety disorders in dementia sufferers. *International Journal of Geriatric Psychiatry*, **11**, 987–90.

Baltes, P. B. and Baltes, M. M. (1990). Psychological perspectives on successful aging: the model of selective optimization with compensation. In *Successful aging* (ed. P. B. Baltes and M. M. Baltes), pp. 1–34. Cambridge University Press, Cambridge.

Baxter, L., Schwartz, J., Bergman, K. S., Phelps, M., Guze, B., and Gerner, R. (1992). Caudate glucose metabolic rate changes with both drug and behaviour therapy for obsessive–compulsive disorder. *Archives of General Psychiatry*, **49**, 681–9.

Beekman, A. T. F., Bremmer, M. A., Deeg, D. J. H., Van Balcom, A. J. L. M., Smit, J. H., De Beurs, E., *et al.* (1998). Anxiety disorders in later life: a report from the Longitudinal Aging Study Amsterdam. *International Journal of Geriatric Psychiatry*, **13**, 717–26.

Beitman, B. D., Kushner, M., and Grossberg, G. T. (1991). Late onset panic disorder: evidence from a study of patients with chest pain and normal cardiac evaluations. *International Journal of Psychiatry in Medicine*, **21**, 29–35.

Bergmann, K. (1971). The neuroses of old age. In *Recent developments in psychogeriatrics* (ed. D. W. K. Kay and A. Walk), pp. 39–50. Headley Bros, Ashford.

Bergmann, K. (1978). Neurosis and personality disorder in old age. In *Studies in geriatric psychiatry* (ed. A. D. Isaacs and F. Post), pp. 41–75. John Wiley and Sons, Chichester.

Blazer, D. G. (1982). Late life bereavement and depressive neurosis. In *Depression in late life* (ed. D. G. Blazer). C. V. Mosby and Co., New York.

Blazer, D. G. (1983). The impact of late-life depression on the social network. *American Journal of Psychiatry*, **140**, 162–6.

Blazer, D. G., Hughes, D. C., and Fowler, N. (1989). Anxiety as an outcome symptom of depression in elderly and middle-aged adults. *International Journal of Geriatric Psychiatry,* **4**, 273–8.

Blazer, D. G., George, L. K., and Hughes, D. (1991). The epidemiology of anxiety disorders: an age comparison. In *Anxiety in the elderly* (ed. C. Salzman and B. D. Lebowitz), pp. 17–30. Springer, New York.

Bohm, C., Robinson, D. S., Gammans, R. E., Shrotriya, R. C., Alms, D. R., Leroy, A. *et al.* (1990). Buspirone therapy in anxious elderly patients: a controlled clinical trial. *Journal of Clinical Psychopharmacology*, **10**, (Suppl. 3), 47–51.

Bouchard, T. J., Lykken, D. T., McGue, M., Segal, N. L., and Tellegen, A. (1990). The Minnesota study of twins reared apart. *Science*, **250**, 223–8.

Bowler, C. (1995). Eating disorders. In *Neurotic disorders in the elderly* (ed. J. Lindesay), pp. 193–204. Oxford University Press, Oxford.

Boyd, J. H., Burke, J. D., Gruenberg, E., Holzer, C. E., Rae, D. S., George, L. K., *et al.* (1984). Exclusion criteria of DSM-III: a study of co-occurrence of hierarchy-free syndromes. *Archives of General Psychiatry*, **41**, 983–9.

Braithwaite, R. (1982). Pharmacokinetics and age. In *Psychopharmacology of old age* (ed. D. Wheatley), pp. 46–54. Oxford University Press, Oxford.

Bramble, D. (1995). Sleep and its disorders. In *Neurotic disorders in the elderly* (ed. J. Lindesay), pp. 227–243. Oxford University Press, Oxford.

Brown, G. W. (1993). Life events and psychiatric disorder: replications and limitations. *Psychosomatic Medicine*, **55**, 248–59.

Brown, G. W. and Harris, T. O. (1978). *Social origins of depression.* Tavistock, London.

Brown, G. W. and Harris, T. O. (ed.) (1989). *Life events and illness.* Unwin Hyman, London.

Brown, G. W., Bifulco, A., and Harris, T. O. (1987). Life events, vulnerability and onset of depression: some refinements. *British Journal of Psychiatry*, **150**, 30–42.

Brown, G. W., Lemyre, L., and Bifulco, A. (1992). Social factors and recovery from anxiety and depressive disorders: a test of the specificity hypothesis. *British Journal of Psychiatry*, **161**, 44–54.

Burn, W. K., Davies, K. N., McKenzie, F. R., Brothwell, J. A., and Wattis, J. P. (1993). The prevalence of psychiatric illness in acute geriatric admissions. *International Journal of Geriatric Psychiatry*, **8**, 175–80.

Burns, A., Lawlor, B., and Craig, S. (ed.) (1999). *Assessment scales in old age psychiatry.* Martin Dunitz, London.

Burvill, P. W., Johnson, G. A., Jamrozik, K. D., Anderson, C. S., Stewart-Wynne, E. G., and Chakera, T. M. H. (1995). Anxiety disorders after stroke: results from the Perth Community Stroke Study. *British Journal of Psychiatry*, **166**, 328–37.

Byrne, G. and Raphael, B. (1994). A longitudinal study of bereavement phenomena in recently widowed elderly men. *Psychological Medicine*, **24**, 411–21.

Castillo, C. S., Starkstein, S. E., Federoff, J. P., Price, T. R., and Robinson, R. G. (1993). Generalised anxiety disorder after stroke. *Journal of Nervous and Mental Disease*, **181**, 102–8.

Catalan, J, Gath, D. H., Bond, A., Edmonds, G., Martin, P., and Ennis, J. (1988). General practice patients on long-term psychotropic drugs: a controlled investigation. *British Journal of Psychiatry*, **152**, 399–405.

Champion, L. (1990). The relationship between social vulnerability and the occurrence of severely threatening life events. *Psychological Medicine*, **20**, 157–61.

Coffey, C. E., Figiel, G. S., Djang, W. T., and Weiner, R. D. (1990). Subcortical hyperintensity on magnetic resonance imaging: a comparison of normal and depressed elderly subjects. *American Journal of Psychiatry*, **147**, 187–9.

Colvin, C. and Boddington, S. J. A. (1997). Behaviour therapy for obsessive–compulsive disorder in a 78-year old woman. *International Journal of Geriatric Psychiatry*, **12**, 488–91.

Cooper, B. (1986). Mental illness, disability and social conditions among old people in Mannheim. In *Mental health and the elderly* (ed. H. G. Häfner, N. Moschel, and N. Sartorius), pp. 35–45. Springer, Berlin.

Copeland, J. R. M., Dewey, M. E., Wood, N., Searle, R., Davidson, I. A., and McWilliam, C. (1987). Range of mental illness among the elderly in the community: prevalence in Liverpool using the GMS-AGECAT package. *British Journal of Psychiatry*, **150**, 815–23.

Coryell, W. (1984). Mortality after thirty to forty years. Panic disorder compared with other psychiatric illnesses. In *Psychiatry update* (ed. L. Grinspoon). American Psychiatric Association, Washington, DC.

Cullen, W. (1784). *First lines of the practice of physic.* Reid and Bathgate, Edinburgh.

Curran, H. V. (1986). Tranquillising memories: a review of the effects of benzodiazepines on human memory. *Biological Psychiatry*, **23**, 179–213.

Davis, A. (1994). Life events in the normal elderly. In *Principles and practice of geriatric psychiatry* (ed. J. R. M. Copeland, M. T. Abou-Saleh, and D. G. Blazer), pp. 106–114. Wiley, Chichester.

Dorman, T. (1988). The management of depression and the use of lofepramine in the elderly. *British Journal of Clinical Practice*, **42**, 459–64.

Downs, A. F. D., Rosenthal, T. L., and Lichstein, K. L. (1988). Modelling therapies reduce avoidance of bath-time by the institutionalised elderly. *Behaviour Therapy*, **19**, 359–68.

Dura, J. R., Stukenberg, K. W., and Kiecolt-Glaser, J. K. (1991). Anxiety and depressive disorders in adult children caring for demented parents. *Psychology and Aging*, **6**, 467–73.

Eaton, W. W., Kramer, M., Anthony, J. C., Dryman, A., Shapiro, S., and Locke, B. Z. (1989). The incidence of specific DIS/DSM-III mental disorders: data from the NIMH Epidemiologic Catchment Area program. *Acta Psychiatrica Scandinavica*, **79**, 163–78.

Evans, M. E. and Lye, M. (1992). Depression in the physically ill; an open study of treatment with the 5-HT reuptake inhibitor fluoxetine. *Journal of Clinical and Experimental Gerontology*, **14**, 297–307.

Fancourt, G. and Castleden, M. (1986). The use of benzodiazepines with particular reference to the elderly. *British Journal of Hospital Medicine*, **V**, 321–5.

Faravelli, C., Webb, T., Ambonetti, A., Fonessu, F., and Sessarego, A. (1985). Prevalence of traumatic early life events in 31 agoraphobic patients with panic attacks. *American Journal of Psychiatry*, **142**, 1493–4.

Feighner, J. P. (1987). Buspirone in the long-term treatment of generalized anxiety disorder. *Journal of Clinical Psychiatry*, **48**(Suppl.), 3–6.

Fillenbaum, G. G., George, L. K., and Palmore, E. B. (1985). Determinants and consequences of retirement among men of different races and economic levels. *Journal of Gerontology*, **40**, 85–94.

Finlay-Jones, R. (1989). Anxiety. In *Life events and illness* (ed. G. W. Brown and T. O. Harris), pp. 95–112. Unwin Hyman, London.

Flint, A. J. and Rifat, S. L. (1997*a*). Two-year outcome of elderly patients with anxious depression. *Psychiatry Research*, **66**, 23–31.

Flint, A. J. and Rifat, S. L. (1997*b*). Anxious depression in elderly patients. Response to antidepressant treatment. *American Journal of Geriatric Psychiatry*, **5**, 107–15.

Flint, A. J., Cook, J. M., and Rabins, P. V. (1996). Why is panic disorder less frequent in late life? *American Journal of Geriatric Psychiatry*, **4**, 96–109.

Forsell, Y. and Winblad, B. (1997). Anxiety disorders in non-demented and demented elderly patients: prevalence and correlates. *Journal of Neurology, Neurosurgery and Psychiatry*, **62**, 294–5.

Foy, A., O'Connell, D., Henry, D., *et al.* (1995). Benzodiazepine use as a cause of cognitive impairment in elderly hospital inpatients. *Journal of Gerontology*, **50**, M99–106.

Frances, A. and Flaherty, J. A. (1989). Elderly widow develops panic attacks, followed by depression. *Hospital and Community Psychiatry*, **40**, 19–23.

Frasure-Smith, N., Lesperance, F., and Talajic, M. (1995). The impact of negative emotions on prognosis following myocardial infarction: is it more than depression? *Health Psychology*, **14**, 388–98.

Gilbert, A., Quintrell, L. N., and Owen, N. (1988). Use of benzodiazepines among residents of aged-care accommodation. *Community Health Studies*, **12**, 394–9.

Goldberg, D. and Huxley, P. (1980). *Mental illness in the community.* Tavistock, London.

Goldberg, D. and Huxley, P. (1992). *Common mental disorders: a bio-social model.* Tavistock/Routledge, London.

Goldberg, D. P., Bridges, K., Duncan-Jones, P., and Grayson, D. (1987). Dimensions of neurosis seen in primary care settings. *Psychological Medicine*, **17**, 461–70.

Goldsmith, H. H. and Gottesman, I. I. (1981). Origins of variation in behavioural style; a longitudinal study of temperament in young twins. *Child Development*, **52**, 91–103.

Gray, J. (1982). *The neuropsychology of anxiety.* Oxford University Press, Oxford.

Guerrero, J. and Crocq, M. (1994). Sleep disorder in the elderly: depression and PTSD. *Journal of Psychosomatic Research*, **38**(Suppl. 1), 141–50.

Gurnack, A. M. and Thomas, J. L. (1989). Behavioural factors related to elderly alcohol abuse: research and policy issues. *International Journal of Addictions*, **24**, 641–54.

Haines, A. P., Imeson, J. D., and Meade, T. W. (1980). Psychoneurotic profiles of smokers and non-smokers. *British Medical Journal*, **280**, 1422.

Haines, A. P., Imeson, J. D., and Meade, T. W. (1987). Phobic anxiety and ischaemic heart disease. *British Medical Journal*, **295**, 297–9.

Harris, T. O. (1988). Psychosocial vulnerability to depression. In *Handbook of social psychiatry* (ed. S. Henderson and G. Burrows). Elsevier, Amsterdam.

Hermann, N. and Eryavec, G. (1994). Posttraumatic stress disorder in institutionalized World War II veterans. *American Journal of Psychiatry*, **151**, 324–31.

Higgitt, A. (1988). Indications for benzodiazepine prescriptions in the elderly. *International Journal of Geriatric Psychiatry*, **3**, 239–49.

Himmelfarb, S. and Murrell, S. A. (1984). The prevalence and correlates of anxiety symptoms in older adults. *Journal of Psychology*, **116**, 159–67.

Hocking, L. B. and Koenig, H. G. (1995). Anxiety in medically ill older patients: a review and update. *International Journal of Psychiatry in Medicine*, **25**, 221–38.

Insel, T. R. (1992). Neurobiology of obsessive–compulsive disorder: a review. *International Clinical Psychopharmacology*, **7**(Suppl. 1), 31–3.

Isaacs, B. (1992). *The challenge of geriatric medicine*, pp. 84–5. Oxford University Press, Oxford.

Jacoby, R. and Levy, R. (1980). Computed tomography in the elderly. 3. Affective disorder. *British Journal of Psychiatry*, **136**, 270–5.

Jenike, M. A. (1985). *Handbook of geriatric psychopharmacology*. PSG, Littleton, Mass.

Jenike, M. A. (1989). *Geriatric psychiatry and psychopharmacology: a clinical approach*. Mosby Year Book, St Louis.

Jorm, A. F. (2000). Does old age reduce the risk of anxiety and depression? A review of epidemiological studies across the adult life span. *Psychological Medicine*, **30**, 11–22.

Kathol, R. G., Noyes, R., Slyman, D. J., Crowe, R. R., Clancy, J., and Kerbor, R. (1980). Propanolol in chronic anxiety disorders. A controlled study. *Archives of General Psychiatry*, **37**, 1361–5.

Katon, W. J. (1984). Chest pain, cardiac disease and panic disorder. *Journal of Clinical Psychiatry*, **51**, 27–30.

Kaup, B. A., Ruskin, P. E., and Nyman, G. (1994). Significant life events and PTSD in elderly World War II veterans. *American Journal of Psychiatry*, **2**, 239–243.

Kay, D. W. K. (1988). Anxiety in the elderly. In *Handbook of anxiety*, Vol. 2: *Classification, etiological factors, and associated disturbances* (ed. R. Noyes, M. Roth, and G. D. Burrows), pp. 289–310. Elsevier, Amsterdam.

Kay, D. W. K. and Bergmann, K. (1966). Physical disability and mental health in old age. *Journal of Psychosomatic Research*, **10**, 3–12.

Kay, D. W. K., Henderson, A. S., Wilson, J., Rickwood, D., and Grayson, D. A. (1986). Dementia and depression among the elderly living in the Hobart community: the effect of diagnostic criteria on the prevalence rates. *Psychological Medicine*, **15**, 771–88.

Kay, D. W. K., Holding, T. A., Jones, B., and Littler, S. (1987). Psychiatric morbidity in Hobart's dependent aged. *Australian and New Zealand Journal of Psychiatry*, **21**, 463–8.

Kenardy, J., Oei, T. P. S., and Evans, L. (1990). Neuroticism and age of onset for agoraphobia with panic attacks. *Journal of Behaviour Therapy and Experimental Psychiatry*, **21**, 193–7.

Kendler, K. S., Kessler, R. C., Heath, A. C., and Eaves, L. J. (1992). Major depression and generalized anxiety disorder. Same genes, (partly) different environments? *Archives of General Psychiatry*, **49**, 716–22.

Kennedy, B. L. and Schwab, J. J. (1997). Utilization of medical specialists by anxiety disorder patients. *Psychosomatics*, **38**, 109–12.

Kennedy, G. J., Kelman, H. R., and Thomas, C. (1989). Hierarchy of characteristics associated with depressive symptoms in an urban elderly sample. *American Journal of Psychiatry*, **146**, 220–2.

Kennedy, G. J., Kelman, H. R., and Thomas, C. (1990). The emergence of depressive symptoms in late life. The importance of declining health and increasing disability. *Journal of Community Health*, **15**, 93–104.

King, P. and Barrowclough, C. (1991). A clinical pilot study of cognitive-behavioural therapy for anxiety disorders in the elderly. *Behavioural Psychotherapy*, **19**, 337–45.

Klerman, G. (1988). The current age of youthful melancholia: evidence for increase in depression among adolescents and young adults. *British Journal of Psychiatry*, **152**, 4–14.

Kluznik, J. C., Speed, N., Van Valkenberger, C., and McGraw, R. (1986). Forty-year follow-up of United States prisoners of war. *American Journal of Psychiatry*, **143**, 1443–5.

Koder, D. (1998). Treatment of anxiety in the cognitively impaired elderly: can cognitive-behaviour therapy help? *International Psychogeriatrics*, **10**, 173–82.

Kohn, R., Westlake, R. J., Rasmussen, S. A., Marsland, R. T., and Norman, W. H. *et al.* (1997). Clinical features of obsessive-compulsive disorder in elderly patients. *American Journal of Geriatric Psychiatry*, **5**, 211–5.

Krasucki, C., Howard, R., and Mann, A. (1998). The relationship between anxiety disorders and age. *International Journal of Geriatric Psychiatry*, **13**, 79–99.

Krasucki, C., Ryan, P., Ertan, T., Howard, R., Lindesay, J., and Mann, A. (1999). The FEAR: A rapid screening instrument for generalized anxiety in elderly primary care attenders. *International Journal of Geriatric Psychiatry*, **14**, 60–8.

Lader, M. (1982). Differential diagnosis of anxiety in the elderly. *Journal of Clinical Psychiatry*, **43**, 4–9.

Lader, M. (1991). Can buspirone induce rebound, dependence or abuse? *British Journal of Psychiatry*, **159**(Suppl. 12), 45–51.

Larkin, A. B., Copeland, J. R. M., Dewey, M. E., Davidson, I. A. Saunders, P. A., Sharma, V. K., *et al.* (1992). The natural history of neurotic disorder in an elderly urban population. Findings from the Liverpool Longitudinal Study of Continuing Health in the Community. *British Journal of Psychiatry*, **160**, 681–6.

Leon, A. C., Portera, L., and Weissmann, M. M. (1995). The social costs of anxiety disorders. *British Journal of Psychiatry*, **27**(Suppl.), 19–22.

Lindesay, J. (1990). The Guy's/Age Concern Survey: physical health and psychiatric disorder in an urban elderly community. *International Journal of Geriatric Psychiatry*, **5**, 171–8.

Lindesay, J. (1991). Phobic disorders in the elderly. *British Journal of Psychiatry*, **159**, 531–41.

Lindesay, J. (1995*a*). Introduction: the concept of neurosis. In *Neurotic disorders in the elderly* (ed. J. Lindesay), pp. 1–11. Oxford University Press, Oxford.

Lindesay, J. (1995*b*). Psychosocial factors. In *Neurotic disorders in the elderly* (ed. J. Lindesay), pp. 56–71. Oxford University Press, Oxford.

Lindesay, J. and Banerjee, S. (1993). Phobic disorders in the elderly: a comparison of three diagnostic systems. *International Journal of Geriatric Psychiatry*, **8**, 387–93.

Lindesay, J., Briggs, K., and Murphy, E. (1989). The Guy's/Age Concern Survey: prevalence rates of cognitive impairment, depression and anxiety in an urban elderly community. *British Journal of Psychiatry*, **155**, 317–29.

Lindesay, J., Jagger, C., Hibbett, M., Peet, S., and Moledina, F. (1997). Knowledge, uptake and availability of health and social services among Asian Gujarati and White elderly persons. *Ethnicity and Health*, **2**, 59–69.

Livingston, G., Manela, M., and Katona, C. (1997). Cost of care for older people. *British Journal of Psychiatry*, **171**, 56–9.

Lucey, J. V., Costa, D. C., Blanes, T., Busatto, G. F., Pilowsky, L. S., Takei, N., *et al.* (1995). Regional cerebral blood flow in obsessive–compulsive disordered patients at rest: differential correlates with obsessive–compulsive and anxious-avoidant dimensions. *British Journal of Psychiatry*, **167**, 629–34.

Luchins, D. J. and Rose, R. P. (1989). Late-life onset of panic disorder with agoraphobia in three patients. *American Journal of Psychiatry*, **146**, 920–1.

McGuire, P. K., Bench, C. J., Frith, C. D., Marks, I. M., Frakowiak, R. S. J., and Dolan, R. J. (1994). Functional anatomy of obsessive–compulsive phenomena. *British Journal of Psychiatry*, **164**, 459–68.

Machlin, S. R., Harris, G. J., Pearlson, G. D., Hoehn-Saric, R., Jeffrey, P., and Camargo, E. E. (1991). Elevated, medial-frontal cerebral blood flow in obsessive–compulsive patients: a SPECT study. *American Journal of Psychiatry*, **148**, 1240–2.

Mackinnon, A., Christiansen, H., Jorm, A. F., Henderson, A. S., Scott, R., and Korten, A. E. (1994). A latent trait analysis of an inventory designed to detect symptoms of anxiety and depression using an elderly community sample. *Psychological Medicine*, **24**, 977–86.

Manela, M., Katona, C., and Livingston, G. (1996). How common are the anxiety disorders in old age? *International Journal of Geriatric Psychiatry*, **11**, 65–70.

Marks, I. M. (1981). Space phobia: a pseudo-agoraphobic syndrome. *Journal of Neurology, Neurosurgery and Psychiatry*, **44**, 387–91.

Marks, I. M. (1986). Genetics of fear and anxiety disorders. *British Journal of Psychiatry*, **149**, 406–18.

Marks, I. and Lader, M. (1973). Anxiety states (anxiety neurosis): a review. *Journal of Nervous and Mental Disease*, **156**, 3–18.

Martindale, B. (1995). Psychological treatments II: psychodynamic approaches. In *Neurotic disorders in the elderly* (ed. J. Lindesay), pp. 114–37. Oxford University Press, Oxford.

Mountz, J. M., Modell, J. G., Wilson, M. W., Curtis, G. C., Lee, M. A., Schmaltz, S., *et al.* (1989). Positron emission tomographic evaluation of cerebral blood flow during state anxiety in simple phobia. *Archives of General Psychiatry*, **46**, 501–4.

Murphy, E. (1982). Social origins of depression in old age. *British Journal of Psychiatry,* **141**, 135–42.

Murphy, E. (1986). Social factors in late life depression. In *Affective disorders in the elderly* (ed. E. Murphy), pp. 79–96. Churchill Livingstone, London.

Myers, J. K., Weissman, M. M., Tischler, G. I., Holzer, C. E., Leaf, P. J., Orvaschel, H., *et al.* (1984). Six-month prevalence of psychiatric disorders in three communities: 1980–1982. *Archives of General Psychiatry*, **41**, 959–967.

Neary, D. (1990). Dementia of frontal lobe type. *Journal of the American Geriatrics Society,* **38**, 71–2.

Noyes, R. and Clancey, J. (1976). Anxiety neurosis: a 5-year follow-up. *Journal of Nervous and Mental Disease*, **162**, 200–5.

Nunn, C., Bergmann, K., Britton, P. G., Foster, E. M., Hall, E. H., and Kay, D. W. K. (1974). Intelligence and neurosis in old age. *British Journal of Psychiatry*, **124**, 446–52.

Oxman, T. E., Berkman, L. F., Kasl, S., Freeman, D. H., and Barratt, J. (1992). Social support and depressive symptoms in the elderly. *American Journal of Epidemiology*, **135**, 356–68.

Peach, H. and Pathy, J. (1979). Disability of the elderly after myocardial infarction. *Journal of the Royal College of Physicians*, **13**, 154–7.

Philpot, M. (1995). Biological factors. In *Neurotic disorders in the elderly* (ed. J. Lindesay), pp. 72–96. Oxford University Press, Oxford.

Philpot, M. and Levy, R. (1987). A memory clinic for the early diagnosis of dementia. *International Journal of Geriatric Psychiatry*, **2**, 195–200.

Pitt, B. (1995). Neurotic disorders and physical illness. In *Neurotic disorders in the elderly* (ed. J. Lindesay), pp. 46–55. Oxford University Press, Oxford.

Pollock, C. and Andrews, G. (1989). The defense style associated with specific anxiety disorders. *American Journal of Psychiatry*, **146**, 455–60.

Pribor, E. F., Smith, D. S., and Yutzy, S. H. (1994). Somatization disorder in elderly patients. *American Journal of Geriatric Psychiatry*, **2**, 109–17.

Prigerson, H. G., Shear, M. K., Newsom, J. T., *et al.* (1996*a*). Anxiety among widowed elders: is it distinct from depression and grief? *Anxiety*, **2**, 1–12.

Prigerson, H. G., Shear, M. K., Bierhals, A. J., *et al.* (1996b). Childhood adversity, attachment and personality styles as predictors of anxiety among elderly caregivers. *Anxiety*, **2**, 234–41.

Radley, M., Redston, C., Bates, F., Pontefract, M., and Lindesay, J. (1997). Effectiveness of group anxiety management with elderly clients of a community psychogeriatric team. *International Journal of Geriatric Psychiatry*, **12**, 79–84.

Rauch, S. L., Jenike, M. A., Alpert, N. M., Baer, L., Breiter, H. C., Sarage, C. R., *et al.* (1994). Regional cerebral blood flow measured during symptom provocation in obsessive–compulsive disorder using oxygen 15-labelled carbon dioxide and positron emission tomography. *Archives of General Psychiatry*, **51**, 62–70.

Regier, D. A., Boyd, J. H., Burke, J. D., Rae, D. S., Myers, J. M., Krammer, M., *et al.* (1988). One-month prevalence of mental disorders in the United States. *Archives of General Psychiatry*, **45**, 977–86.

Reynolds, C. F., Kupfer, D. J., Taska, L. S., Hoch, C. C., Spiker, D. G., Sewitch, D. E., *et al.* (1985). EEG sleep in elderly depressed, demented and healthy subjects. *Biological Psychiatry*, **20**, 431–42.

Roberts, A. H. (1964). Housebound housewives—a follow-up study of a phobic anxiety state. *British Journal of Psychiatry*, **110**, 191–7.

Robins, L. and Regier, D. (ed.). (1991). *Psychiatric disorders in America*. The Free Press, New York.

Robinson, D., Napoliello, M. J., and Shenck, L. (1988). The safety and usefulness of buspirone as an anxiolytic drug in elderly versus young patients. *Clinical Therapeutics*, **10**, 740–6.

Rosen, J., Fields, R. B., Hand, A. M., Falsettie, G., amd Van Kammen, D. P. (1989). Concurrent posttraumatic stress disorder in psychogeriatric patients. *Journal of Geriatric Psychiatry and Neurology*, **2**, 65–9.

Rosin, A. J. and Glatt, M. M. (1971). Alcohol excess in the elderly. *Quarterly Journal of Studies on Alcohol*, **32**, 53–9.

Rubin, R. T., Villanueva-Meyer, J., Anath, J., Trajmar, P. G., and Mena, I. (1992). Regional xenon^{133} cerebral blood flow and cerebral technetium^{99m} HMPAO uptake in unmedicated patients with obsessive–compulsive disorder and matched control subjects: determination by high-resolution single-photon emission computed tomography. *Archives of General Psychiatry*, **49**, 695–702.

Russo, J., Vitaliano, P. P., Brewer, D. D., Katon, W., and Becker, J. (1995). Psychiatric disorders in spouse caregivers of care recipients with Alzheimer's disease and matched controls: a diathesis-stress model of psychopathology. *Journal of Abnormal Psychology*, **104**, 197–204.

Salzman, C. (1991). Pharmacologic treatment of the anxious elderly patient. In *Anxiety in the elderly* (ed. C. Salzman and B. D. Lebowitz), pp. 149–73. Springer, New York.

Scaturo, D. J. and Hayman, P. M. (1992). The impact of combat trauma across the family life cycle: clinical considerations. *Journal of Trauma and Stress*, **5**, 273–88.

Schultz, S. K., Castillo, C. S., Kosier, J. T., and Robinson, R. G. (1997). Generalized anxiety and depression: assessment over 2 years after stroke. *American Journal of Geriatric Psychiatry*, **5**, 229–37.

Schwartz, G. M., Braverman, B. G., and Roth, B. (1987). Anxiety disorders and psychiatric referral in the general medical emergency room. *General Hospital Psychiatry*, **9**, 87–93.

Shankar, K. K., Walker, M., Frost, D., and Orrell, M. W. (1999). The development of a valid and reliable scale for rating anxiety in dementia. *Aging and Mental Health*, **3**, 39–49.

Sharpe, M., Hawton, K., House, A., Molyneux, A., Sandercock, P., Bamford, J., *et al.* (1990). Mood disorders in long-term survivors of stroke: associations with brain lesion location and volume. *Psychological Medicine*, **20**, 815–28.

Sheikh, J. I., King, R. J., and Barr Taylor, C. (1991). Comparative phenomenology of early-onset versus late-onset panic attacks: a pilot survey. *American Journal of Psychiatry*, **148**, 1231–3.

Sheikh, J. I., Swales, P. J., Kravitz, J., Bail, G., and Barr Taylor, C. (1994). Childhood abuse history in older women with panic disorder. *American Journal of Geriatric Psychiatry*, **2**, 75–7.

Shepherd, M., Cooper, B., Brown, A. C., and Kalton, G. (1981). *Psychiatric illness in general practice*. Oxford University Press, London.

Sinoff, G., Ore, L., Zlotogorsky, D., and Tamir, A. (1999). Short Anxiety Screening Test: a brief instrument for detecting anxiety in the elderly. *International Journal of Geriatric Psychiatry*, **14**, 1062–71.

Sultzer, D. L., Levin, H. S., Mahler, M. E., High, W. M. and Cummings, J. L. (1993). A comparison of psychiatric symptoms in vascular dementia and Alzheimer's disease. *American Journal of Psychiatry*, **150**, 1806–12.

Tennant, C., Bebbington, P., and Hurry, J. (1982). Social experiences in childhood and adult psychiatric morbidity: a multiple regression analysis. *Psychological Medicine*, **12**, 321–7.

Thompson, L. W., Gallagher, D. E., and Breckenridge, J. S. (1987). Comparative effectiveness of psychotherapies for depressed elderly. *Journal of Consulting and Clinical Psychology*, **55**, 385–90.

Thyer, B. A. (1981). Prolonged in-vivo exposure therapy with a 70 year old woman. *Journal of Behaviour Therapy and Experimental Psychiatry*, **12**, 69–71.

Thyer, B. A., Parrish, R. T., Curtis, G. C., Nesse, R. M., and Cameron, O. G. (1985). Ages of onset of DSM-III anxiety disorders. *Comprehensive Psychiatry*, **26**, 113–22.

Tiihonen, J., Kuikka, J., Bergstrom, K., Lepola, U., Koponen, H., and Leinonen, E. (1997). Dopamine reuptake site densities in patients with social phobia. *American Journal of Psychiatry*, **154**, 239–42.

Tobin, S. S. and Liebermann, M. A. (1976). *Last home for the aged*. Jossey-Bass, San Francisco.

Tweed, J. L., Schoenbach, V. J., George, L. K., and Blazer, D. G. (1989). The effects of childhood parental death and divorce on six-month history of anxiety disorders. *British Journal of Psychiatry*, **154**, 823–8.

Tyrer, P. (1980). Dependence on benzodiazepines. *British Journal of Psychiatry*, **137**, 576–7.

Tyrer, P. (1989). *Classification of neurosis*. Wiley, Chichester.

Tyrer, P. (1990). The division of neurosis: a failed classification. *Journal of the Royal Society of Medicine*, **83**, 614–16.

Torgersen, S. (1990). Comorbidity of major depression and anxiety disorders in twin pairs. *American Journal of Psychiatry*, **147**, 1199–202.

Vernooij-Dassen, M. J., Persoon, J. M., and Felling, A. J. (1996). Predictors of sense of competence in caregivers of demented persons. *Social Science and Medicine*. **43**, 41–9.

Walton, V. A., Romans-Clarkson, S. E., Mullen, P. E., and Herbison, G. P. (1990). The mental health of elderly women in the community. *International Journal of Geriatric Psychiatry*, **5**, 257–63.

Wands, K., Merskey, H., Hachinski, V. C., Fisman, M., Fox, H., and Boniferro, M. (1990). A questionnaire investigation of anxiety and depression in early dementia. *Journal of the American Geriatrics Society*, **36**, 535–8.

Woods, R. T. (1995). Psychological treatments I: behavioural and cognitive approaches. In *Neurotic disorders in the elderly* (ed. J Lindesay), pp. 97–113. Oxford University Press, Oxford.

Woods, R. T. and Britton, P. G. (1985). *Clinical psychology with the elderly*. Croom Helm/Chapman Hall, London.

World Health Organization. (1992). *International classification of diseases* (10th revision). WHO, Geneva.

Wu, J. C., Buchsbaum, M. S., Hershey, T. G., Hazlett, E., Sicotte, N., and Johnson, J. C. (1991). PET in generalised anxiety disorder. *Biological Psychiatry*, **29**, 1181–99.

Zahner, G. E. P. and Murphy, J. M. (1989). Loss in childhood: anxiety in adulthood. *Comprehensive Psychiatry*, **30**, 553–63.

Zerhusen, J. D., Boyle, K., and Wilson, W. (1991). Out of the darkness: group cognitive therapy for the elderly. *Journal of Psychosocial Nursing*, **29**, 16–20.

Zisook, S., Shuchter, S. R., and Lyons, L. E. (1987). Predictors of psychological reactions during the early stages of widowhood. *Psychiatric Clinics of North America*, **10**, 355–68.

31 Psychiatric aspects of personality in later life

Klaus Bergmann

Introduction

Personality is a vague and scientifically soft concept, like the proverbial elephant, hard to define but easy to recognize when you see it. The clinician will acknowledge the great variation with which different patients face up to loss, illness, brain damage, and social stress in old age. Diagnostic labels such as 'dementia', 'depression', and 'paranoid psychosis' sometimes seem to explain only a little of what transpires in any individual clinical encounter, although highly significant relationships may exist between diagnosis, mortality, morbidity, and measures of institutionalization and other types of care received. An acknowledgement of the importance of personality is the proviso that has sometimes been made that 'successful' treatment can mainly be expected in those of previously good personality. Those falling outside this group, however, form a distressingly large proportion of our patients. Many important issues such as compliance with treatment, acceptance of help, relating to carers, and making adaptive decisions are often determined by the patient's personality, as well as by the more precisely definable diagnostic features of psychiatric illness.

The importance of personality factors can be intuitively recognized, but is perhaps even harder to understand and evaluate in older patients than in our younger ones. Questions that confound the issue include: what is the effect of ageing on personality and what is the effect of personality on ageing? How much is what we ascribe to ageing the result of a cohort effect in populations subject to different historical, social, and cultural influences rather than true effects of ageing? Another point, which is rarely considered, is the social contribution to the concept of what defines old age; the receipt of pensions and benefits, retirement from work, and other special provisions related to reaching a certain age. In earlier times older people were likely to be defined by the advent of severe illness, or indigent poverty. Otherwise they continued to work up to the time of death.

Personality changes with ageing

There is a popular assumption that any change in personality with age must be a negative or deleterious one. Such stereotypes exist even among those who might be assumed to take a dispassionate and professional view of such changes. The example quoted by Neugarten (1977) illustrates this tendency. She reviewed a number of aspects of personality function, which had been investigated in older populations, and divided these into negative, neutral, and positive aspects of personality in old age. These are shown in below:

(1) *Negative*
  (a) egocentricity
  (b) dependency
  (c) dogmatism
  (d) rigidity
(2) *Neutral*
  (a) risk-taking
  (b) perceived locus of control
  (c) self-concept
  (c) self-image

(3) *Positive*
   (a) happiness
   (b) morale
   (c) reminiscence
   (d) dreams and daydreams

Negative or neutral views predominate over positive ones. Professionals who care for older people, often at times of stress and in the presence of severe mental and physical ill health, are also inclined to take a predominantly decremental view of the changes they perceive in their elderly clients or patients. What changes in personality are truly related to ageing and how has this been studied?

There are two ways of looking at the changes of personality with ageing. First, at the changes in various personality traits—do they become more marked or less prominent? Second, what developmental processes take place in the personality. The latter approach is more closely linked with the concept of adjustment in later life and will be considered in that context.

The argument over whether one would expect personality to change with ageing or after an initial period of formative development, to remain relatively stable and constant over most of the lifespan, is one that merits attention. Many theoretical considerations might make one support the concept of a stability of personality throughout life. For example, a dynamic view of personality formation, that the most important determinants of personality were formed after a critical period in early life, would lead one to favour the concept of stability. An opposing view, such as that emphasizing the importance of genetic and early constitutional factors, could also lead one to support stability.

Schaie and Parham (1976) discuss these issues in detail and point out that personality traits can be divided into three groups; biological, cultural, and those with both cultural and biological contributions. They also point to the operation of the cohort effect in the field of personality studies, as well as those on the effects of ageing on intelligence. It could be argued that much cross-sectional research of personality and ageing reflects changes which represent our value judgements concerning the beliefs and attitudes of previous generations. Examples of this may include the so-called age-related changes such as 'rigidity', 'conservatism', and 'narrowness of outlook'. Schaie and Parham (1976) suggest that their results show that in a longitudinal study of several age cohorts, while there are clear cross-sectional differences between different cohorts, 'the change, however, is a function of specific early socialization experiences, commonly shared generation specific environmental impact and particular socio-cultural transitions that may affect individuals at all ages'. They conclude that stability of traits 'is the rule rather than the exception'. Neugarten (1977), summing up a number of studies, generally supports the idea of the stability of personality with age; the only changes of any consistency being an increase of introversion with age.

Leon *et al.* (1979), reporting a 30-year longitudinal study, also favour the stability model and point out that some changes found, which might have been ascribable to hypochondriasis and depression in younger groups, appeared to be more related to an appropriate reaction to real ill-health.

Adjustment and concepts of successful ageing

Adjustment in old age is a difficult idea as definitions are subjectively tinged by the values and philosophy of various investigators, and in many so-called research studies there exists a circularity in which the variables used to define and those employed to rate adjustment are often so close to each other that correlations 'proving' these theories are largely spurious. An example of this is the Kansas City study carried out by Neugarten *et al.* (1964) concluding, 'the integrated personalities and those high on ego qualities are high on measures of life adjustment'. However, the typologies derived from studies of the Kansas City sample are worth quoting as they illustrate the result of such investigations. Neugarten, following the multivariate analysis of many personality and self-concept questionnaires, derives five components:

(1) zest vs. apathy;
(2) resolution and fortitude;
(3) goodness of fit between desired and achieved goals;
(4) positive self-concept;
(5) mood tone.

In general, the arguments around the empirical studies of personality and adjustment to ageing have centred on the conflict between 'activity' and 'disengagement' models of adjustment (Cummings *et al.* 1990). The activity theories of ageing state the most common-sense and, on the surface, the most valid view. This asserts that the successfully adjusted older person is fully engaged in life, with many interests, has a high level of social contacts and involvement, and generally behaves like a slightly more wrinkled younger person!

Havighurst (1963) developed a 'Life Satisfaction Rating Scale', which judges adjustment on a largely internal criterion centring on the way that the older person feels about himself and his life. Such a scale has proved useful and remains one of the best measures of its kind. The work of Havighurst and colleagues also suggests that the activity concept of adjustment in old age seems to relate best to measures of life satisfaction.

The disengagement theory was definitively presented by Cummings and Henry in their book (1961). The theory is based on the perception of the changing social and family role that ageing brings, and suggests that disengagement from involvement, dissolution of bonds, and greater concentration on the inner world is an adaptive response. It brings greater satisfaction, a degree of personal liberation, and a greater freedom to please oneself. Havighurst, Neugarten, and Tobin (1968) reviewing these conflicting views suggest that, for the majority of older people, the activity view of adjustment in ageing seems to be the most appropriate, but for a minority of older people disengagement as a style of adjustment seems to be valid. Perhaps the resources available to the older person make some differences. Also, health, financial security, lifelong educational and cultural experiences, and the expectations of other age groups may be as important in determining adjustment in old age as internally determined personality factors.

Dynamic concepts of adjustment in ageing are more difficult to fit into an empirical experimental context, but at least Erikson's developmental view is of help in understanding the particular tasks an older person faces in adjusting to the processes of ageing. By placing concepts of adjustment in old age within a lifespan context, it emphasizes the need not to judge older people by the same criteria as those that are relevant in earlier life. Erikson outlined the psychosocial tasks of adult life by the following criteria: 'intimacy' versus 'isolation' in young adult life; 'generativity' versus 'stagnation' in mid-life; and 'integrity' versus 'despair' in old age (Erikson 1959).

An important empirical study of adjustment in old age is that of Thomae (1976). It deals with a longitudinal investigation of two cohorts of subjects comprising 220 people born between 1890–1895 and between 1900–1905. The variables studied reflecting aspects of personality were activity and mood. Social, historical, and personal stress factors were examined. More than half the subjects had a stable or increasing level of activity and this stability was highly correlated with 'subjectively experienced intensive and positive contacts with friends'. Generational differences also interacted with differences in social class, gender, and marital status. Mood was 'apparently less influenced by family of origin and the development in childhood than by specific experiences in later adolescence and adulthood' (Lehr 1986).

An attempt to define adjustment in old age as various modes of adjustment is reported from the Newcastle random samples of patients seen at home and supplemented by various hospital and institutional samples (Savage *et al.* 1977). The investigators employed a variety of measures of cognitive function, personality structure, and self-concept and derived four descriptive groups: the 'Normal', the 'Introverted', the 'Perturbed', and the 'Mature'.

The 'Normal' group, 54% of the sample, were described as more intense and apprehensive than younger groups. They were rather wary and somewhat rigid, but they were also shrewd, analytic, and calculating.

The 'Introverted' group, 19.5% of the sample, were sober, taciturn, and reserved. 'Self restraint and serious-mindedness typify the group, along with sensitivity to others and some tension in themselves'.

The 'Perturbed' group, 11% of the sample, were seen as difficult to get along with, emotionally unstable, and uncontrolled. 'Being in a state of inner turmoil,' also characterized this group. They were the most likely to be psychiatrically ill.

The 'Mature' group, 16% of the sample, were highly self-sufficient and resourceful people. They were shrewd, worldly, and tough-minded. They showed a higher degree of activity and life satisfaction than both the introverted and the perturbed.

The effects of personality disorder on adjustment and coping mechanisms

Patients with depressive disorder who had already received acute treatment but who no longer met the research and diagnostic criteria for major depressive disorder were the subject of an investigation by Abrams *et al.* (1998). Total personality disorder scores were inversely associated with measures of functioning, sociability, and the presence of a satisfying relationship. The authors suggest that this group who showed residual malfunction after treatment for major depression, may need a special therapeutic regime.

Crisis intervention in depressed patients with personality disorder reveals a poorer 2-year outcome. However, subjects with personality disorder who showed a better working alliance and increased insight at the termination of crisis intervention had a more favourable prognosis (Andreoli *et al.* 1993).

A study of hospital utilization in veterans with psychiatric problems also addressed the effect of personality disorder (Williams *et al.* 1998). Hospital utilization was found to be related to the psychiatric diagnosis, marital status, and various personality factors. Factors relating to social disadvantage also played a role: the diagnoses most significantly associated with increased hospital utilization included passive aggressive personality traits and antisocial personality disorder.

It appears that the coping mechanisms, which usually help patients to maintain themselves in the community and to recover from illness, are substantially impaired by the presence of personality disorders.

Personality and physical health

The relationship between personality and physical health is an important one, though none of the studies available can distinguish between the effect of illness on various aspects of personality and the effects of various personality variables on the onset of illness.

Longitudinal studies are most useful in demonstrating relationships between personality traits, initially demonstrated, and the subsequent advent of ill health. The second Duke longitudinal study of community-resident elderly subjects (Rusin and Siegler 1975), showed that those subjects dropping out of the longitudinal study, mainly because of illness and death, were more anxious and neurotic than those subjects who were long-term survivors.

Costa *et al.* (1983), reporting the Baltimore Longitudinal Study, reached similar conclusions. A cross-sectional study of interest (Himmelfarb and Murrell 1984) described a community sample of 713 males and 1338 females. The authors found that the highest correlation with abnormally high anxiety levels was physical ill health. High anxiety levels were significantly correlated with nine illnesses, including: high blood pressure, neurological disorders, urological disorders, heart trouble, stomach ulcers, hardening of the arteries, stroke, and diabetes. It was also of interest that anxiety was significantly correlated with not having physical health needs met for more than 6 months. There must be at least good presumptive evidence that adequate and prompt attention to physical illness is likely to be an important factor in the maintenance of good mental health in old age.

A survey of African-American older community residents (Gao *et al.* 2000) reported on 1970 non-demented respondents. Using informant-based measures of personality change, derived from the CAMDEX, the following questions were put: 'Have you noticed any changes in his/her personality?', 'Has he/she become more irritable?', 'Has he/she become more stubborn?' and 'Does he/she show less concern for others?'

A positive answer to these questions was taken to indicate personality change. The main factors predicting personality change in this sample were poor activities of daily living (ADL) function, physical disability, and a history of cancer.

These results are of interest. They suggest that one link between the advent of personality change and physical ill health is the degree to which day-to-day functioning is affected by illness.

Chronic neurotic personality problems in old age

Much energy can be expended on arguing whether a person who suffers from neurotic symptoms over a long period has a personality disorder or a neurotic illness. Comparing prevalence studies of neurotic and personality disorders in old age, Scandinavian authors such as Essen-Moller (1956) can find only 1.4% of neurotic illness in their sample, and 10.6% of personality disorders. On the other hand, Kay *et al.* (1964) found 8.9% of subjects with neurotic illness and only 3.6% suffering from personality disorder. Such differences are likely to be the results of diagnostic conventions rather than any fundamental differences, especially as the combined proportions of both groups are much the same for the two samples. Neurotic personality disorder and chronic neurotic disorder will therefore be considered together in this section. Chronic neurotic disorder is associated with prominent personality problems throughout life, and what happens to such people when they encounter old age is often viewed with a pessimistic eye.

Old, chronically neurotic people are considered to be like themselves, only more so! Old age is said to distort and exaggerate previously restrained and moderated psychopathological tendencies. Objective studies do *not* tend to confirm such findings. Ernst (1959) in a long-term, follow-up study of a population of neurotic outpatients, from a psychiatric clinic, concluded that even the most severe hysterical conversion or dissociative states did not persist in that form for more than 5 years. Depressive reactions remitted over time and only anxiety tended to persist. Ciompi (1969) in his extended catamnestic studies also tended to confirm the amelioration of neurotic symptoms in later life. Even for more malignant obsessional states Pollit (1957) found amelioration with time.

Bergmann (1978) reporting a group of long-standing neurotic subjects from a community random sample, found considerable disruption and disturbance in their earlier life, but a relatively good enjoyment of life in old age in spite of the persistence of quite marked neurotic symptoms. They appeared to be active, not lonely, not particularly isolated, and indeed more active than the normal subjects—perhaps an example of Butler's concept of counterphobic overactivity (1968).

Examples of case histories which illustrate some aspects of this amelioration, will be briefly outlined below.

Case 1

A 79-year-old lady was, in her youth, the first woman in the city to win a scholarship to Cambridge University. She could not take it up because of a crippling phobic anxiety state, which rendered her largely housebound. Her social life was restricted and she remained single, living with relatives. In old age she was crippled with arthritis but cheerful, intellectually active, reading, listening to music and enjoying the company of quite a few friends; accepting life with fortitude and enjoyment.

Case 2

Another example is that of a 67-year-old woman. She suffered great anxiety in earlier adult life from fears of sexuality, of having children, and of financial insecurity. She quarrelled with her husband as to who should buy the contraceptive sheaths, both refusing to do so. As she grew older her children left home, sexual activity ceased, and she became financially more secure. Currently, she still suffered from moderately severe intermittent tension symptoms but she led an active life, was sociable, and had many interests, keeping very active. Her relationship with her husband had greatly improved.

It would appear that in later life for people such as these, that as issues of sexuality, competition in the outside world, and heavy responsibility for others receded, other neurotic substitutes were not necessarily found. On the contrary, often for the first time, they were able to make the best of their lives and obtain satisfaction in a number of ways. For some older neurotic personalities, at least, the exaggeration of their earlier psychopathology did not appear to take place.

Another question that may be asked is what effect on neuroticism and psychosomatic disorders in old age does severe stress in earlier life have? Research on a population of Israeli Holocaust survivors compared to age- and sex-matched controls who had emigrated before 1939 sheds some light on this (Carmil and Carel 1986; Aviram *et al.* 1987). Their findings are, however, ambiguous. On the one hand, the prevalence of psychosomatic illnesses was no different between the two groups, but on the other hand the Holocaust population had a slightly higher degree of emotional distress 40 years after their traumatic experiences. If one took the need for antihypertensive therapy as an indicator of longstanding stress then no significant difference between the two groups was found.

In a similar study, from Australia, soldiers who had been Japanese prisoners of war were compared to ex-combatants in the South-East Asian theatre of war who had not been captured (Tennant *et al.* 1986). This revealed more current depressive and anxiety disorders and a greater prevalence of psychiatric illness overall during the postwar period in the former group. The index group also showed a higher incidence of duodenal ulcer, but otherwise their physical health did not differ significantly from the control group; neither did their age-adjusted mortality. In conclusion, it seemed that these powerful stresses of earlier life had a significant effect on the victims of these experiences but it was not as remarkable as one might have expected.

The epidemiology of personality disorder

Older surveys in which clinical judgement and semi-structured interviews were used to obtain a diagnosis, yielded prevalences of personality disorder. However, such results depended on individual diagnostic conventions and were not comparable to each other (Table 31.1).

Table 31.1 Prevalence of neurosis and personality disorder in 7 community studies (n = 3054)

Diagnosis	Mean (%)	Range (%)
Neurosis	6.2	1.4–10.6
Personality disorder	5.8	2.2–12.6
Total	12.0	7.4–17.6

Adapted from Simon 1980 with permission.

For example, the Newcastle-upon-Tyne survey of 1964 (Kay *et al.* 1964) yielded a relatively lower prevalence of personality disorder (3.2%) and a higher one for the diagnostic categories subsumed by neurosis (9.4%). Bergmann (1971) found that a primary diagnosis of personality disorder occurred in about 6% of a further random sample of respondents from Newcastle-upon-Tyne who were over 65 years of age (n = 300). The two diagnostic groupings identified were 'paranoid and hostile' and 'inadequate'. Conversely, the Swedish surveys (Essen-Moller *et al.* 1956) tended to assign a diagnosis of personality disorder (10.6%) in preference to neurosis (1.4%). A follow-up study of this population (Hagnell *et al.* 1994) examined the point prevalence of psychopathic personality disorder. The diagnosis predominated in men and was higher in those who were under 60 years than in the older group (8.9% and 2.9%, respectively). Aggressive and explosive subgroups were not found in the older respondents. These estimates were clinically meaningful but were not comparable with other studies. It is, however, of interest to note that when the prevalence of personality disorder and the prevalence of neurosis for these samples are added up the sums obtained are very comparable (12.5% in the British sample and 12% in the Swedish sample). This finding suggests that the differences between such surveys has more to do with the conventions employed in making the diagnosis rather than true differences in prevalence.

The advent of standardized questionnaires such as the GMSS and the later computer-assisted programs such as AGECAT (Saunders 1993) provided reliable, repeatable, and valid results. Hence, the prevalence of major categories of psychiatric disorder in old age could be compared to other studies and cross-national comparisons could be made.

However, the detection of personality disorders on the same basis was not possible. Personality disorders have indistinct boundaries and are difficult to detect using such questionnaires. Categorical definitions of all the major types of personality disorder are available in the DSM-III-R and DSM-IV manuals. However, many types of personality disorder are better delineated by dimensional descriptions; but dimensional psychological tests of personality are lengthy, time-consuming, and difficult to employ on a large number of subjects in the community. The advent of a simple questionnaire, the DIS, based on the DSM-III nosology, gave a boost to the collection of large-scale community samples. Under the auspices of the ECA program a 6-month prevalence in three communities was carried out (Myers *et al.* 1984). A number of diagnostic categories indicative of personality disorder were included. Among these categories was 'antisocial personality,' the average prevalence of which in the three districts for male subjects over 65 was 1.1%. For younger males between 18 and 44 years of age it was 2.2%. No diagnosis of antisocial personality was made in any of the groups of females over 65 years of age. Personality disorders did not feature among the four most frequent DSM-III diagnoses for males or females over 65 years of age.

In spite of the availability of the DIS, which is a valid and reliable questionnaire, there seems to be a barrier to the study of personality disorder in large-scale, random, community samples. Only the more gross forms of personality disorder, such as psychopathy and antisocial personality, emerge, and other clinically meaningful entities are very difficult to uncover.

The study of personality disorder in clinical settings presents a greater opportunity to apply more specific questionnaires and delineate other aspects of personality disorder with clinical relevance. A commonly accepted classification of personality disorder for such studies is that described by DSM-III-R and DSM-IV.

The prevalence of personality disorder in various settings

The community

A total of 100 male and 100 female elderly subjects attending a senior citizens' community centre volunteered to complete the more-detailed SIDP-R 160-item questionnaire, in an attempt to delineate the presence of personality disorder (PD) in the community (Ames and Molinari 1994). The nosological categories were those outlined in DSM-III-R. Some 13% of this community sample was categorized as having a diagnosis of personality disorder; both men and women with PD had a significantly higher record of prior mental health consultations. When the prevalence of PD in this cohort was compared with a younger sample the latter had a higher prevalence. However, there were greater percentages of paranoid, schizoid, and narcissistic PDs in the older sample and fewer antisocial, passive aggressive, or borderline PDs.

Primary care

The problems of personality disorder do not figure greatly in general practice studies. Schizophrenia, depression, and organic mental disorders are more likely to be the cause of crises requiring action. However, a general practice study in which personality questionnaires were employed within 12 practices was reported by Hueston *et al.* (1999). Unfortunately there was only a 38% response rate and the informant-based diagnoses could not be definitive. People had to be judged to be 'at high risk' for personality disorder. The at-risk patients were compared to those not at risk and were found to be of poorer health status in seven out of the eight categories employed. They were also noted to have had more outpatient, emergency, and inpatient visits in the previous 6 months. A significant proportion of this population was in the older age groups.

The indication is that personality disorder can and does influence other health factors of importance in the general practice setting.

Outpatients

Molinari and Marmion (1993) applied DSM-III-R-based criteria for personality disorder. They found that in 'geropsychiatric' outpatients 58% met the criteria for a diagnosis of personality disorder, but compared to a sample of younger patients they had a significantly lower prevalence. Golomb *et al.* (1995) could find no significant differences between two groups of people aged 21–44 years and 45–64 years, but point out that the seventh, eighth, and ninth decades might begin to reveal differences.

Hospital inpatients

The prevalence of personality disorder among first admissions to a psychiatric hospital of a nationwide cohort was reported by Kastrup (1985). The prevalence of personality disorder as a primary diagnosis for patients over 64 years of age was very low (0.8% for men and 2.8% for women).

A large inpatient sample reported by Fogel and Westlake (1990) reviewed Axis II diagnoses in 2322 psychiatric inpatients with an Axis I diagnosis of depression, and found there was a diminution in the Axis II diagnoses of personality disorder in those patients over the age of 64 compared to younger patients, the prevalence being 11.2% and 17.1%, respectively. There was, however, an excess of compulsive personality disorders in the older group, and they comprised 45% of older patients with an Axis II disorder.

Somewhat different findings were reported by Ames and Molinari (1994). A total of 100 male and 100 female geropsychiatric inpatients, in two different units, were assessed employing the SIDP-R. The questionnaire revealed a higher prevalence of PD than did the Axis II diagnoses of the psychiatrists, and over half the patients were judged to have one or more PD diagnoses. More elderly men were diagnosed as having PD, and the older patients did not have a lower prevalence than younger patients. Older patients were more likely to be placed within the 'Odd,' paranoid-schizoid, cluster and younger ones within the 'Dramatic,' borderline histrionic, cluster.

The relationship between various Axis I diagnoses and Axis II diagnoses was reported by Kunic *et al.* (1994); here, 13% of all patients received a diagnosis of personality disorder (PD). The rate of comorbid PD varied from 6% for patients with organic disorders to 24% for patients with major depression. There was no significant relationship between various PD clusters and any particular Axis I diagnoses. The negative correlation between PD and the Mini-Mental State Examination (MMSE) suggested that a standardized informant questionnaire might have yielded more PD diagnoses in patients with organic psychiatric disorders.

A meta-analysis of 11 studies of personality disorder in those over 50 years (Abrams and Horowitz 1996) aimed to provide prevalence data from a large pooled sample. The number of subjects in any study ranged between 3 and 547. The overall prevalence of PD was 10% compared to 21% prevalence in subjects under the age of 50 years. The settings within which these data were collected varied widely as did the prevalences within those settings. This study raises more questions than answers but the authors do point out directions in which further research might move.

Although it is difficult to draw definitive conclusions from the studies in epidemiology and prevalence so far carried out, some general impressions can be outlined:

- A primary diagnosis of personality disorder is rare both in community and hospital samples.
- There is some evidence to suggest that personality traits may have adverse affects even on elderly community residents.
- Nosologically the older patient suffers less from problems of aggression, and impulse control and antisocial traits are less evident.
- Institutional settings, especially those with a higher prevalence of Axis I psychiatric diagnoses also reveal a higher proportion of various types of personality disorder.
- It is not clear to what extent comorbidity magnifies or exaggerates the manifestation of personality disorder. It is probable that the reported prevalence of personality disorder in patients with organic brain disorder might be increased by the use of the valid informant questionnaires.

Deviations of personality in old age

This section could have been concerned with a wide range of deviations of personality, which seem to become evident in older people, but it is worth emphasizing that not all deviant personality traits seen in older people are of concern to the clinician. Eccentrics with strange hobbies or fanatically pursued interests are often reported to their own doctors and thence to a psychiatrist because they are 'abnormal'. Some criterion has to be adopted to avoid labelling these people as patients and, worse still, offending against their autonomy. More important and more common are those people who are natural isolates. They have what can be termed the 'Miller of Dee' syndrome:

> I care for nobody no not I, if nobody cares for me.
>
> *Love in a Village*, Isaac Bickerstaff, 1735–1812.

Empirical research in this area was carried out by Lowenthal (1964; Lowenthal and Boler 1965). She differentiated between 'pure isolates' and semi-isolates, and concluded that the former were not characterized significantly by psychiatric breakdown. Townsend (1957) also makes the distinction between 'isolates' and 'desolates'. Bergmann (1978) in a factor-analytic study of the components of loneliness distinguished three groups: (1) the isolated lonely; (2) the non-isolated lonely; (3) the non-lonely isolates. The last group had the temperament and the capacity to live alone.

Personality problems strongly affecting others

> O wad some Pow'r the giftie gie us,
> To see ourselves as others see us!
> It would frae money a blunder free us,...
>
> *To a Louse*, Robert Burns, 1759–1796.

Senile self-neglect or squalor (Diogenes syndrome)

It is appropriate to start with the above quotation, as the two major personality problems to be discussed in this section are senile self-neglect, ineptly named the *Diogenes syndrome*, and hypochondriasis. It is a characteristic of patients exhibiting these personality problems that either they are unaware anything is wrong or that they are in strong disagreement with others as to the nature of what is wrong.

They often cause others to suffer far more than they themselves do. The psychiatrist may be called in because someone else can no longer stand the situation and, 'Something must be done'. This is a difficult ethical position for the psychiatrist, who is called upon to take action. Some sort of value judgement has to be made, but an understanding of the nature of these conditions, the social norms of the society in which the patient lives, and the stresses faced by the carers, all have a part in reaching an informed decision.

Self-neglect in old age is not uncommon and forms part of the picture of many dementing illnesses and of some functional psychotic disorders. What characterizes the 'Senile self-neglect syndrome' is the presence of very gross self-neglect unaccompanied by any psychiatric disorder sufficient to account for the squalor in which the patients exist. It can be said that patients with Senile self-neglect syndrome never suffer with a psychiatric condition sufficient to account for the presenting picture, although some early organic cerebral impairment or mild depressive symptoms may be present and yet permit a diagnosis of Senile Self-Neglect Syndrome. An illustrative case is described below:

Case 3

The social services received a request from their housing department. One of their tenants was complaining that a foul smelling liquid resembling urine was leaking through their ceiling. The man upstairs was a 68-year-old single reclusive bachelor who had not responded to his neighbour's requests and complaints. After a preliminary contact, a social worker requested a psychiatric interview to assess whether there were grounds for removing this man under a Section of the Mental Health Act. The man was lying in a filthy bed soaked in ammoniacal urine, stained with faecal smears. By his bed was a plastic bowl overflowing with urine, which had soaked into the rug and also into the floor. His room was dirty and smelly and he himself was unkempt and in a generally neglected state, although not malnourished.

His mental state was remarkably intact. He spoke clearly and coherently, was not depressed or paranoid. He was fully oriented and mentally alert with a good memory for recent events. Physically he was fully mobile and not complaining of any pain or malaise. When the appalling conditions were pointed out to him and its effect on the downstairs neighbours was explained he showed little concern. It was emphasized to him that something had to be done to which he replied, ' Alright I'll do something on Monday'. He was bland, smiling, and could not understand the concern and sense of urgency of other people. Few grounds could therefore be found for invoking the Mental Health Act, and action had to be taken under the appropriate Section (47) of the Public Health Act.

Psychiatric and geriatric medical studies on this condition have been carried out (Macmillan and Shaw 1966; Clarke *et al.* 1975). Both emphasize the large number of cases with no evidence of formal psychiatric disorder, and their hypothesis is that senile self-neglect was a manifestation of a certain type of personality reacting to stress and loneliness. Post (1982) suggested that such people are best seen as the end-stage of a personality disorder manifesting itself in the form of senile reclusiveness.

All studies agreed that the prognosis of such cases was not good. Rehabilitation by a period of training and supervision during inpatient care was followed inevitably by relapse into the previous squalid and degrading conditions. Day-care on an indefinite basis may maintain such patients for a longer period, but often some form of institutional or residential care becomes necessary. It is the intractable nature of so many cases that brings the explanation of a personality reaction to stress into some doubt. Why is it so impossible, even when stresses appear to be remedied, to re-establish adequate and independent self-care, even with social support?

A case report (Orrell *et al.* 1989) has suggested that frontal lobe impairment, without evidence of dementia, may play a part. This study also indicated that certain tests of frontal lobe function may be of use not only in arriving at a diagnosis but in elucidating some of the mechanisms which could mediate the development of this type of condition. Brain imaging may also have a part to play in reaching an understanding of the neuroanatomical background of the Senile self-neglect syndrome.

Hypochondriasis

The *Oxford English dictionary* defines the hypochondriac as, 'chiefly characterized by the unfounded belief that he is suffering from some serious bodily illness'. But for the older person such a definition is unsatisfactory because they may suffer not only from one but several serious illnesses, and yet exhibit hypochondriasis. A more acceptable definition is that formulated by Pilowsky (1978):

> Hypochondriasis is a form of illness behaviour in which the individual experiences and manifests a degree of concern over his state of health, which is out of proportion to the amount considered appropriate to the degree of objective evidence for the presence of disease.

The first requirement, therefore, before any definition of a hypochondriacal state can be reached, is a thorough assessment of the patient's physical status. Too often the elderly hypochondriac has an unfortunate habit of dying of the disease he has not got! Furthermore, only those with some experience of examining the older patient, with an awareness of the presence of multiple pathology and an understanding of the older person's pattern of reacting to disease, can make the judgement as to whether any individual is exhibiting hypochondriacal behaviour.

Hypochondriasis can be divided into primary and secondary forms. The secondary consists of those hypochondriacal states arising in association with depressive illness, schizophrenic disorders, and organic cerebral disease. An example of the dangers of missing the secondary nature of some hypochondriacal disorders can be illustrated by the following case.

Case 4

A 75-year-old man, with a mild post-traumatic arthritis of his ankle joint began to complain of pains all over his body, especially over his bones and in many other joints. Nothing very specific could be found and he was reassured, although without avail. He drove his attending physicians to distraction. Finally, after the finding of a slightly raised serum acid phosphatase level, and following a rectal examination, disseminated prostatic carcinoma was diagnosed and terminal palliative heroin was prescribed.

At this stage he was referred, by a more senior colleague, to a psychiatrist. The patient gave a definite history of feeling sad, worse in the mornings, with poor concentration and a lack of drive. He was waking early, experiencing suicidal thoughts and felt hopeless about the future. He was wholly preoccupied with the agonizing pain that passed all over his body. Relatives confirmed that this man was not usually hypochondriacal, although always rather rigid and a perfectionist. They also recalled that he had seemed somewhat subdued and 'down' before he began to complain of his pains.

After several days treatment for withdrawal of heroin he was given electroconvulsive therapy and made a rapid and uncomplicated recovery. When questioned afterwards about the pain in his ankle he said that it was certainly there but did not trouble him and he could ignore it. All other pains had gone.

This patient illustrates three valuable lessons: first, hypochondriacal symptoms can markedly overlie a more subtle depressive illness; second, insistent and unremitting complaints can lead doctors to desperate and ill-founded measures in order to be able to do something...anything!; and third, that where the depression has such delusional intensity then electroconvulsive therapy is often the treatment of choice.

Patients with primary hypochondriasis can also be divided into three groups:

(1) those with bodily preoccupations;
(2) those with disease phobia;
(3) those experiencing disease conviction.

The first condition is self-explanatory, but the other two merit further explanation. Disease phobia is the fear of contracting a particular disease, but disease conviction is the profound belief that the patient harbours some specific condition, sometimes held with delusional intensity (Pilowsky 1967).

The importance of hypochondriasis as part of normal ageing is taken for granted by most laymen and many doctors. The Duke University studies (Busse and Pfeiffer 1969) carried out on community-resident volunteers emphasize the prominence of hypochondriasis, but perhaps insufficient allowance was made for the special nature of their method for selecting the sample.

In a random sample of community residents in Newcastle-upon-Tyne, 300 subjects from 65 to 80 years of age and without psychosis or dementia, were interviewed to detect the prevalence of hypochondriasis, the results of which are shown in Table 31.2 (Bergmann 1970).

These figures suggest that hypochondriasis is rare in normal older people, whereas moderate or severe states mainly occur in those with longstanding neurosis or personality disorders. In order to identify primary hypochondriasis in old age, an enquiry into lifelong or longstanding hypochondriacal traits is therefore necessary. It is safe to assume that if hypochondriasis appears to arise in old age then a vigorous search should be made for another psychiatric disorder as the primary condition. Hypochondriasis in old age carries a significantly increased risk of suicide (d'Alarcon 1964). Occult physical ill health may also manifest itself in a hypochondriacal form.

The management of hypochondriasis is difficult. The following suggestions combine the author's views with those of Pilowsky (1983) and

Table 31.2 Prevalence of hypochondriasis in a random sample of 65- to 80-year-old community residents

	None (%)	Mild (%)	Moderate/severe (%)
Normals	93	7	<1
Recent neurosis	67	26	7
Chronic neurosis and personality disorder	64	19	17

Taken from Bergmann 1970 with permission.

with the more specifically gerontological approach of Busse and Pfeiffer (1969).

1. All hypochondriacal patients should receive a thorough physical examination in the first instance.
2. Patients should be seen regularly, and in the initial part of the interview be allowed to air their physical concerns.
3. The doctor should be alert to the emergence of underlying worries and causes of grief, and encourage their ventilation at the expense of physical symptoms.
4. Appointments should be time-limited on a prearranged basis and manipulation of these arrangements should be resisted.
5. Always check for an underlying depression—and then check again!

Borderline personality disorder in later life

Among the younger patients the criteria contained in the DSM-IV include identity disturbance, impulsivity, self-mutilation, risk-taking, and substance abuse. However, it is difficult to identify such a picture in later life.

Perry (1993) conducted a review of follow-up studies ranging in duration from 2 to 16 years. In the longest follow-up, 9% of subjects had committed suicide and 42% appeared to have recovered. The other 49% continued to merit the diagnosis of borderline personality disorder. The Links *et al.* (1999) study was for a 7-year period, but very similar results were obtained. Again about 6% of the sample were dead, mainly following suicidal acts. A large number, nearly 30%, refused to participate. Just under half the subjects continued to merit the diagnosis of borderline personality disorder. It is, therefore, difficult to identify elderly patients still suffering from borderline personality disorder.

Rosowsky and Gurian (1991) claimed to identify troublesome and disturbed residents in nursing-home settings, whom they considered to be suffering from borderline personality disorder:

> Identity disturbance in old age may be evidenced by an inability to formulate future plans or pursue goal directed activities. Anorexia maybe a substitute for more obvious forms of self mutilation, and elderly patients with severe personality disorders may disrupt nursing homes and other service delivery systems.

It is difficult to seek any point of resemblance to borderline personality in earlier life. However, the suggestion that various types of personality disorder may be found in elderly people who prove to be troublesome in residential care and community settings, could provide a valuable base for research in future. The troublesome older person, with no evidence of a dementing illness or of major psychiatric illnesses, might provide a worthwhile target for research into the later life manifestations of personality disorder.

Personality traits and the experience of distress in later life

Using the data from the 300 respondents seen in Newcastle-upon-Tyne (Bergmann 1971), the relationship could be examined between various types of personality traits and events in earlier life, social factors, physical disability, current complaints and symptoms. A retrospective life review was carried out on all respondents using a standardized semi-structured interview schedule in order to evaluate the various types of personality traits. On the basis of clinical judgement, subjects could be assigned to various personality groups, the four most common being:

(1) the anxiety prone,
(2) the insecure and rigid,
(3) the paranoid and hostile, and
(4) the inadequate.

Significant correlations are shown in Table 31.3. It can be seen that, although all the personality types described here manifest problems in earlier life, those with anxiety-prone and insecure traits suffer from more complaints and symptoms than do the paranoid and inadequate groups. The anxiety-prone personality also seems to furnish the strongest predisposition towards late-onset neurosis, most often of a depressive type (Bergmann 1971).

Table 31.3 The relationship between personality traits and other factors

	Anxiety prone	Insecure and rigid	Paranoid and hostile	Inadequate
Early and experiences and personal history	Early marriage[a] Marital disharmony[a]	Poor relationship with Parents[b] Loss of parents < 15 years Psychiattic disorder as a child[a] Low in birth order[a]	Poor relationship with Parents Childhood neurotic traits Marital disharmony[a]	Marital disharmony[a]
Social facors		Few children alive[a]	Poor work record[a]	Poor work record[c] Poor club attendence < 60 years[a]
Physical disability	Poor mobility[a]			Main system gastrointestinal[b] Age[a]
Complaints	Poor sleep[b] Sees own health as poor[b] Hypochondriasis[a]	Poor sleep[a] Loneliness[a]	Hypochondriasis[b]	
Symptoms	Psychic tension[c] Lifelong worrier[c] Autonomic overactivity[c] Depressive symptomsc	Obsessional[c] Autonomi[c] overactivity[c] Psychic tension[c] Phobic[b]	Historical[a] Depressive symptoms[a]	Depression[a]

[a] $p < 0.05$ [b] $p < 0.01$; [c] $p < 0.001$

Looking at the correlations with variables that have a bearing on experience in childhood, the insecure personalities seem to have more experience of early childhood trauma. Thus, the hypothesis could be put forward that the anxiety-prone personalities arise from a more genetic and biological origin, whilst insecure traits result more from the impact of their early environment. Slater and Shields (1969) in twin studies of anxiety, suggest a link between genetic factors and the predisposition to anxiety.

Paranoid personality traits in later life may not be as maladaptive as they appear to be in earlier years. The vicissitudes of old age, poverty, loss, and isolation can often be combated by the hostile extra punitive attitude of such people; psychiatrists seeing only the end of the spectrum where adjustment and coping mechanisms fail. Verwoerdt (1981) stated that such personalities, 'may have counterphobic features and an inclination to use defences of the high energy variety, mastery through attack; projection with subsequent attempts to move aggressively against the externalized threat'. Such a type of adjustment was evident in a proportion of random sample subjects seen by the author (Bergmann 1978).

One example of this type of personality is given below.

Case 5

A 66-year-old lady, lived with a dull, inadequate husband whom she ruled with a rod of iron. She was bizarrely dressed in voluminous ill-fitting trousers showing a large expanse of pink knickers, and talking volubly. She suffered from moderately severe ischaemic heart disease and lived in a small cluttered and decaying house. She expressed many dislikes and hatreds, of ethnic minorities of all types, and with great pride told a story of when she hit a neighbour until she made his face bleed. Nevertheless, she owned her house, had two student lodgers, was very alert, competent, and kept very good financial control of her affairs. She maintained a quarrelsome relationship with general practitioners and hospital specialists preferring, successfully, to dictate to them her own treatment. Her earlier life resembled in many ways that of the chronic neurotic group, but the difference appeared to be that she fought back with great energy and drive, winning most of her battles.

Inadequate personalities, with their longstanding failures—occupational, social, and in achieving permanent relationships, often fitted in rather better in later life. They took up the submissive roles and were able in many ways to gratify their caregivers by their compliance and by letting themselves be patronized.

In conclusion, when assessing personality traits in older people, psychiatrists must ask whether they suffer from the effects of their personality, or at the least do others suffer to the point where their endurance is exhausted and the patient may come to harm? If the answer is in the affirmative, then perhaps some intervention may be justified.

Coping with major psychiatric disorder—the effect of comorbid personality disorder

Major depressive disorder

Fogel and Westlake (1990) reviewing Axis II diagnoses in 2322 psychiatric inpatients with an Axis I diagnosis of depression found there was a lower rate of Axis II diagnoses of personality disorder in those patients over the age of 64 compared to younger patients, the prevalence being 11.2% and 17.1%, respectively. There was, however, an excess of compulsive personality disorders in the older group, which comprised 45% of older patients with an Axis II disorder.

The question arises: to what degree are the personality disorders found in the course of a depressive illness part of the depressive state or pre-existing personality traits? Abrams *et al.* (1987) compared recovered depressive patients with matched controls. Employing a standardized personality disorder examination (PDE), they found that patient groups had a higher trait score and concluded that the patient group experienced a higher lifetime personality dysfunction. A later study (Abrams *et al.* 1994) compared the dimensional personality score before and after treatment and between patients with early- and late-onset depression. 'Schizotypal', 'dependent', 'obsessive–compulsive' and 'passive-aggressive' trait scores reduced significantly after treatment, while other traits did not. The mean dimensional personality trait scores were higher for the early-onset depressive group.

Having examined the relationship of personality disorder in later life and depressive illness the question then arises as to what the effect is of personality disorder on the clinical course of depression in later life? Vine and Steingart (1994) examined older patients with depression treated in a day hospital. Abnormal personality traits were assessed before and after treatment and found in 33% and 36% of the sample, respectively. They concluded that the presence of personality disorder, especially histrionic, borderline, narcissistic, and antisocial traits adversely affected the outcome. Poor response to crisis intervention (Andreoli *et al.* 1993) and also to treatment with desipramine (Peselow *et al.* 1992) has been observed in the presence of personality disorder in older patients with depressive illness.

It has long been a belief by practising psychiatrists that the presence of personality disorder adversely affects the treatment of depressive illness. Gradman *et al.* (1999) consider this question thoroughly. Their review of the literature includes nine surveys which all show the adverse effects of personality disorder on the treatment of depressive illness. They report a second controlled-outcome study of the treatment of depression, employing a number of modalities including drug treatments and cognitive–behavioural therapy. For a sub-sample of older patients they included a rating scale, the MCMI to assess the presence of personality disorder. These patients had also completed the Beck Depression Inventory and the Hamilton Rating Scale for Depression. The conclusion of Gradman and colleagues was that older, significantly depressed outpatients with personality disorder were less likely to respond well to treatments compared to those with similar depressive diagnoses but without Axis II pathology.

Anxiety disorder

Anxiety disorder is a longstanding and persistent neurotic problem. It is of interest to examine how much this is associated with types of personality disorder and how older subjects compare to younger ones.

A recent study has addressed these issues (Coolidge *et al.* 2000) by examining community-resident volunteers, comprising: a younger group of students, and an older one consisting of family members and recruits from local seniors' centres. The measure of anxiety was the Brief Symptom Inventory, a self-report measure consisting of 53 items. Personality disorder was measured by a 225-item questionnaire developed by the principal author and based on the DSM-IV criteria for personality disorder. Coping mechanisms were also measured using a standardized scale.

The study showed that generalized anxiety states appeared to be no more common in older adults than in younger persons, and that the types of personality disorder more common in the older anxious group were the obsessive–compulsive, schizoid, and avoidant personality disorders. It was also found that the coping strategies of anxious older adults were different from those of the non-anxious older adults. It appeared that anxious older adults relied on more dysfunctional coping strategies such as mental and behavioural disengagement. A final conclusion was that anxious younger people suffered from personality disorders, which were far more florid than those of the older sample.

Personality disorder adversely affects many psychiatric illnesses. The effect is on recovery from the illness and also on the coping mechanisms required to deal with the adverse circumstances that so many older people suffer from during the course of their later lives.

Dysthymic disorder

Personality disorder seems to affect the prognosis of depressive illnesses and their response to treatment. Dysthymic personalities (Akiskal 1983) survive into old age and such people, when they succumb to a depressive illness, may require urgent treatment. After the treatment they may show little more than a recovery of their 'vital' functions, but still complain unabatedly and manifest a gloomy view of life.

Conversely, it is too easy for a psychiatrist treating an unresponsive patient to invoke the effect of personality, rather than the inefficacy of medical care.

Blazer and Williams (1980) found a prevalence of dysphoria, depressive symptoms without depressive illness, of 4.5%, but at least some of this group may have been suffering from a dysthymic disorder of longer duration. An enquiry from relatives or an informant, who have known the patient for a long time, may on the one hand reveal periods of good functioning and a positive attitude in earlier life, or on the other a lifelong gloomy, negative, and anhedonic picture.

Dysthymic disorder is a persistent and chronic condition. It is not necessarily a disease of old age but often persists into the senium. The personality disorders most closely associated were examined by Devanand *et al.* (2000). Obsessive–compulsive disorders were the most commonly observed traits (17.1%), while avoidant personality traits were also frequently seen (11.8%). Nevertheless, personality disorder was less frequently seen in older patients with dysthymia than in younger patients with dysthymic disorder. The associated personality disorders of elderly patients with dysthymic disorder resembles that observed in patients with major depressive disorder. This finding may suggest that, in old age, dysthymic disorder is more closely related to the major depressive disorders.

In younger adults a different pattern of associated personality disorder is found. Antisocial, borderline, histrionic, and narcissistic types of personality disorder occur more commonly.

The influence of personality traits on organic psychiatric disorders

It is evident to clinicians that the psychiatric state of any patient with dementia is influenced substantially by personality factors. Taking two patients with only moderate dementia, they may have very different prognoses with regard to survival in the community because of their differing personality traits. One patient may be hostile, angry, denying his need for help, and rejecting all offers of support. Another, no less demented, may be pleasant, acknowledge the help of others with gratitude, and make friendly and pleasant relationships with formal and informal carers. Premature institutionalization faces the former and the successful maintenance of a place in the community rewards the latter.

The scientific study of personality disorder presenting within a dementing illness raises methodological difficulties. An important question, in the first instance, is whether personality disorder can be evaluated in the presence of dementia. Behavioural disturbances, deviations of sexuality, and psychotic and affective symptoms are all found alongside the cognitive deficits in dementia (Burns and Levy 1992). The interaction of more subtle personality traits is readily obscured by such florid features of the illness. However, attempts to overcome these difficulties have been tackled using standardized questionnaires with relatives and other close friends. Strauss *et al.* (1993), employing two informants, demonstrated acceptable reliability and distinguished between current personality states and traits preceding the dementing illness. The personality changes arising with the progress of the dementia of the Alzheimer type could also be identified by informants (Siegler and Costa 1985). These changes included increased neuroticism, less extroversion, and less conscientiousness.

Do personality problems get worse with increasing dementia and do they hasten the progression of a dementing illness? Rubin *et al.* (1984) addressed this question. They studied a group of mildly demented patients and normal controls over a 50-month period. They made an assessment of three aspects of behaviour, which they considered indicative of different personality traits: passive, agitated, and self-centred. Personality ratings were not standardized but taken from a simple clinical questionnaire. The progression of the dementing illness was measured by the Clinical Dementia Rating (CDR) (Hughes *et al.* 1982). More behavioural deterioration followed the progression of the dementia. However, patients with mild dementia and behavioural problems deteriorated no more rapidly than those who had mild dementia without behavioural problems. This work is important not so much for its result but because it indicates the need for more reliable and valid measures of personality.

Petrie *et al.* (1989) indicated that progression of behavioural changes was a complex matter. They compared patients with 'senile dementia of the Alzheimer's type' (SDAT) and matched controls and followed both groups over a 3-year period. They found considerable heterogeneity in response patterns:

- initial change with little further change on progression;
- ongoing change with progression;
- no change;
- regression of previously psychopathological features.

And they were able to characterize reliably the premorbid profiles on a number of occasions.

Aitken *et al.* (1999) adopted a novel approach to the study of personality change in dementia. Their rating scale is based on a personality inventory used to measure the psychological sequelae of severe blunt head injuries. The study reports major changes ranging from positive personality characteristics to their negative counterparts. For example, the characteristic of being 'energetic' has at its other end the characteristic of being ' lifeless'.

The questionnaire is based on responses given by informants concerning the patient's personality before and after the onset of dementia. The authors found a large negative change in the personality characteristics after the onset of dementia: 70% of the sample had negative changes on all dimensions of personality measured. They also examined differences in personality change between vascular dementia and Alzheimer-type dementia. The total sum of the change in personality traits as a consequence of the dementia was more severe for vascular than for Alzheimer-type dementia. As far as physical factors were concerned, the presence of extrapyramidal signs was the strongest independent predictor of personality change.

Although this study does not correspond to others, which in the main employ questionnaires derived from DSM-III-R and DSM-IV, and the reliability and repeatability of the questionnaire may not have been established in the usual way, nevertheless it combines reliable psychiatric diagnoses of dementia and neuropsychiatric and physical assessment with the ratings of personality. That combination of an informant-based questionnaire, valid for the DSM categories of personality disorder, together with appropriate neuropsychiatric data and physical health measurements, would be of help in advancing our understanding of the interaction of personality changes and dementia. The agreement between categorical diagnoses and informant interviews gathered from relatives of patients with dementia has not been very reliable. However, dimensional ratings of personality produce a greater level of agreement (Molinari *et al.* 1998).

Family relationships and personality disorder

Can maladaptive traits be identified and demonstrated to have some effect?

There are considerable methodological difficulties in demonstrating any effects of personality with even a degree of scientific objectivity. A preliminary and tentative approach was reported by Bergmann *et al.* (1984). This was a retrospective case-record study of 60 patients seen for the first time in a day-hospital setting.

As well as physical dependency and cognitive impairment, various aspects of the elderly person's personality and interaction were assessed. These included a 'submissiveness–dominance' rating (SD), a 'negative–positive communication' rating (NPC) and an 'autonomy–dependence' rating (AD). Inter-rater reliabilities were satisfactory and a 3-month global outcome rating was made, having regard to physical, social, and psychiatric factors. The outcome rating also gave satisfactory reliability measures. Overall, those patients who communicated most positively with praise and thanks and approval in their dealings with their carers, i.e. a positive NPC rating, had the best 3-month outcome on the global rating. Taking only those patients with dementia, then submissive patients did better than dominant ones. These findings indicate, perhaps somewhat indirectly, the importance of aspects of personality function in the welfare of older and demented people. The need for a prospective study with more valid and objective measures of personality is evident and might lead to more effective counselling and training of carers. For instance, could a case be made for assertiveness training for the carers of at least some demented people? Could some behavioural programme be set up to reward positive communication? Better research in this field could have both theoretical and practical advantages.

Various maladaptive personality traits can be identified in patients with dementia. Only some of the common patterns will be outlined.

Denial and pseudo-independence

Patients showing this reaction pattern often come to the notice of the clinician through a failure to cope. They may present with poor nutrition, a neglected household, failing self-care, and poor personal hygiene. The patient may have reasonable preservation of cognitive function, but any attempt to suggest help or enlist more support is met with a blank wall of denial.

The patient may say, 'I go out shopping every day…my memory is fine…I have no difficulty with my money…I am making really good meals…I don't know why my daughter worries so much about me.' In reality, the patient may be crippled, live up four flights of stairs, with no food in the larder, and the gas cut off for non-payment of bills, while money is found under blankets and mattresses. Only a crisis with temporary or permanent removal to institutional care may resolve the situation.

Paranoid reactions

Paranoid reactions are commonly found in demented patients and may be the presenting feature of an organic state. The patient may misinterpret some noise and explain that burglars are in her flat. Objects may be lost and accusations of theft follow. Visits by strangers or even relatives may become the focus of a persecutory plot. Such reactions also have an adaptive function since they offer the hope that when the external threats have been subdued, then a favourable outcome can still be expected, however long the battle.

Withdrawal-restriction of contacts and reduction of activities

In many ways this reaction is an adaptive one, in that the patient reduces the chances of failure to cope with the environment and the resulting anxiety. Only simple and well-known activities are carried out and the patient may refuse to go out on trips, or leave the house. Conflicts often arise from the well-meaning attempts of friends to give variety and stimulation to the patient's life. Anger, abuse, and sometimes aggression may arise and the relative may end up feeling hurt and rejected. Counselling and advice may help to prevent a breakdown of relationships.

The treatment of personality disorder in later life

The arguments that have centred on the issue of whether personality disorder is treatable also apply in old age. However, the more limited treatment aims in later life might make interventions more rewarding.

Pharmacological treatment

There is no information, which embodies valid, controlled, double-blind trials for the treatment of personality disorder in later life. Empirically, various psychotropic agents have been employed. These include antidepressants, tranquillizers, and mood stabilizers. The basis for choosing a particular agent is to target the predominant symptom. However, the scales are heavily weighted even against such an approach. Among the most important negative factors are the absence of a therapeutic relationship in many cases, poor compliance with medication, and sometimes abuse of medication.

Soloff (1997) has advanced a theoretical approach, which might offer a fruitful way forward in future and could make use of functional imaging. Instead of taking blanket diagnoses of personality disorder, he suggests that concepts incorporating neurobehavioural findings from animal studies might be more helpful. The dimensions to which he refers include concepts such as impulsivity, harm-avoidance, novelty-seeking, and reward-dependence. He proposes that many of these concepts are already associated with neurotransmitter pathways, and that various ways forward in the investigation of these relationships may be explored, including the activation of the HPA (hypothalamic–pituitary– adrenal axis) and the measurement of specific responses. He also suggests that in the case of personality disorder, pharmacotherapy has too often been directed at acute-state symptoms rather than the latent trait vulnerabilities.

Psychotherapeutic treatments

Cognitive–behavioural therapies

Goisman (1999) reviews the position of cognitive–behavioural therapy with older patients suffering from personality disorders. The emphasis should be on the 'here and now', on presenting problems, and immediate behavioural difficulties. He suggests that target symptoms within the syndromes, represented by the diagnosis of personality disorder, should be the focus of therapeutic aims. Examples of such symptoms and behaviours would be impulsiveness, acting out, substance abuse, and suicidal behaviour.

Special adaptations to suit older patients might include the slowing of the pace of therapy, the use of multiple sensory modes to present material, and, where necessary, a didactic approach. The possibility of including aids to memory should also be considered. Therapy should be of short duration and be problem- and goal-oriented.

Dynamic therapies (see also Chapter 16)

Reports of dynamic therapies for older patients with personality disorder are largely descriptive rather than evaluative (Abrams 1994). In his review he emphasizes the need to consider dynamic therapy for personality disorder in later life in conjunction with the other modalities already mentioned. These would include the treatment of Axis I disorders and symptomatic pharmacotherapy.

The difference in handling the transference with older patients is also of importance. Whereas with younger patients the focus is on childhood events and relationships with parents, with older patients, suffering from personality disorders, the experiences of later life and the 'here and now' relationship with the therapist assume a greater prominence. Abrams (1994) states that, 'there is a need to focus on the patient's present reality.'

It is important to consider what issues are especially relevant to people in later life (Bergmann 1983) rather than to try and fit the therapeutic framework, within which older people are treated, into the Procrustean Bed of classical psychoanalysis. These issues will be briefly reviewed:

1. *Grief, mourning, and loss.* Dynamic grief work and the issues of restitution and refocusing of the cathectic bonds are still highly relevant with older people. However, loss is far more extensive than simply bereavement. Such losses include the loss of physical powers and capacities, especially those that have contributed to the older persons self-esteem, the loss of status, and the losses that accompany a reduced income. These are just some of the broader issues which may have to be explored.
2. *Life review.* (See Butler 1968.) There is often a need to review the meaning of one's life at its latter end, an issue which at times can profitably be taken up by a therapist. A historical approach may well be useful in this task.
3. *Learned helplessness.* (See Seligman 1975.) In old age many situations occur where elderly persons are left helpless, and whatever action they take they cannot influence their environment; nor can they exert any power or influence over their fate. In these cases therapeutic interventions have to come from many sources. The most important is a change of attitude by all the people who care for and treat elderly people. The need to be involved in decisions concerning their lives is an important therapeutic counter to the feeling of helplessness. Cognitive and behavioural treatments will also be of value in changing the patient's feelings of despair and helplessness. Finally, attention should be drawn to providing a safe place where patients can discharge their feelings of rage and anger, which usually have to be choked down. Goldfarb, as long ago as 1967, recognized the need for a patient to feel able to influence and even to some extent to manipulate the therapist. Such an attitude runs counter to all accepted dynamic approaches to younger patients. However, a good case can be made for adopting and modifying the approach to older patients.

Conclusions

The diagnosis of major psychiatric illness (Axis I disorders) is of great importance. Many illnesses are now amenable to treatment and estimates of prognosis, morbidity, and mortality can help to improve the planning of psychiatric services.

Nevertheless, it is undeniable that older people with the same diagnosis can be found in very different settings. Personality disorder, personality change, and maladaptive lifelong personality traits may well account for a substantial proportion of this variation. To understand the nature of personality disorders in old age and develop better ways of management and the delivery of treatment will be one of the important future tasks for old age psychiatry.

References

Abrams, R. C. (1994). Management. In *Principles and practice of geriatric psychiatry* (ed. J. R. M. Copeland,

M. T. Abouh-Saleh, and D. G. Blazer), pp. 783–90. Wiley, Chichester.

Abrams, R. C. and Horowitz, S. V. (1996). Personality disorder after age 50: a meta-analysis. *Journal of Personality Disorder*, **10**, 271–81.

Abrams, R. C., Alexopoulos, G. S., and Young, R. (1987). Geriatric Depression and DSM-III-R Personality Disorder Criteria. *Journal of the American Geriatrics Society*, **35**, 383–6.

Abrams, R. C., Rosendahl, E., Card, C., and Alexopoulos, G. S. (1994). Personality disorder correlates of late and early onset depression. *Journal of the American Geriatrics Society*, **42**, 727–31.

Abrams, R. C., Spielman, L. A., Alexopoulos, G. S., and Klausner, E. (1998). Personality disorder symptoms and functioning in elderly depressed patients. *American Journal of Geriatric Psychiatry*, **6**, 24 –30.

Aitken, L., Simpson, S. and Burns, A. (1999). Personality change in dementia. *International Psychogeriatics*, **11**, 263–71.

Akiskal, H. S. (1983). Dysthymic disorder: psychopathology of proposed chronic depressive subtypes. *American Journal of Psychiatry*, **140**, 11–20.

Ames, A. and Molinari, V. (1994). Prevalence of personality disorder in community-living residents. *Journal of Geriatric Psychiatry and Neurology*, **7**, July–September, 189–94.

Andreoli, A., Frances, A., Gex-Fabry, M., Aapro, N., Gerin, P., and Dazord, A. (1993). Crisis intervention in depressed patients with and without DSM-III-R personality disorders. *Journal of Nervous and Mental Disease*, **181**, 732–7.

Aviram, A., Silverberg, D. S., and Carel, R. S. (1987). Hypertension in European immigrants to Israel: the possible effects of the Holocaust. *Israeli Journal of Medical Science*, **23**, 257–63.

Bergmann, K. (1970). M.D. Thesis. Sheffield University.

Bergmann, K. (1971). The neuroses of old age. In *Recent developments in psychogeriatrics*, Vol. 6 (ed. D. W. K. Kay and A. Walk), pp. 39–50. *British Journal of Psychiatry*, Special Publications, London.

Bergmann, K. (1978). Neurosis and personality disorder in old age. In *Studies in geriatric psychiatry* (ed. A. D. Isaacs and F. Post), pp. 41–76. Wiley, Chichester.

Bergmann, K. (1983). Psychotherapy in the elderly. In *Handbook of Psychiatry* 4 (ed. G. F. M. Russell and L. Hersov), pp. 110–12. Cambridge University Press, Cambridge.

Bergmann, K., Manchee, V., and Woods, R. T. (1984). Effect of family relationships on psychogeriatric patients. *Journal of the Royal Society of Medicine*, **77**, 840–4.

Blazer, D. and Williams, C. (1980). Epidemiology of dysphoria and depression in an elderly population. *American Journal of Psychiatry*, **137**, 439–44.

Burns, A. and Levy, R. (1992). Clinical diversity in late onset Alzheimer's disease. *Maudsley Monograph number 34*, Oxford University Press, Oxford.

Busse, E. W. and Pfeiffer, E. (1969). *Behaviour and adaptation in later life. Functional psychiatric disorder in old age: hypochondriasis*, pp. 203–9. Little, Brown and Company, Boston.

Butler, R. N. (1968). Towards a psychiatry of the life cycle: implications of sociopsychologic studies of the aging process for the psychotherapeutic situation. In *Ageing in modern society* (ed. A. Simon and L. J. Epstein), pp. 233–48. Psychiatric Research Reports of the American Psychiatric Association, Washington, DC.

Carmil, D. and Carel, R. S. (1986). Emotional distress and satisfaction in life among Holocaust survivors: a community study of survivors and controls. *Psychological Medicine*, **16**, 141–9.

Ciompi, L. (1969). Follow up studies on the evolution of former neurotic and depressive states in old age: clinical and psychodynamic aspects. *Journal of Geriatric Psychiatry*, **3**, 99–106.

Clarke, A. N. G., Mankikar, G. D., and Gray, I. (1975). Diogenes syndrome: a clinical study of gross self neglect in old age. *Lancet*, **i**, 366–73.

Coolidge, F. L., Segal, D. L., Hook, J. N., and Stewart, S. (2000). Personality disorders and coping among older anxious adults. *Journal of Anxiety Disorders*, **14**, 157–72.

Costa, P. T., McCrae, R. R., and Arenberg, D. (1983). Recent research on personality and aging. In *Longitudinal studies of adult psychological development* (ed. K. W. Schaie), pp. 222–65. Guilford Press, New York.

Cummings, E. and Henry, W. (1961). *Growing old: the process of disengagement*. Basic Books, New York.

Cummings, J. L., Petry, S., Dian, L., Shapira, J., and Hill, M. A. (1990). Organic personality disorder in dementia syndromes: an inventory approach. *Journal of Neuropsychiatry and Clinical Neuroscience*, **2**, 261–7.

D'Alarcon, R. (1964). Hypochondriasis and depression in the aged. *Gerontologia Clinica (Basel)*, **6**, 266–77.

Devanand, D. P., Turret, N., Moody, B. J., Fitzsimons, L., Peyser, S., Mickle, K., *et al.* (2000) Personality disorders in elderly patients with dysthymic disorder. *American Journal of Geriatric Psychiatry*, **8**, 188–195.

Erikson, E. (1959). The healthy personality. In *Psychological Issues*, Vol. 1. International University Press, New York.

Ernst, K. (1959). Die Prognose der Neurosen. *Monograph Neurologie, Psychiatrie*, No. 85. Springer, Berlin.

Essen-Moller, E. (1956). Individual traits and morbidity in a Swedish rural population. *Acta Psychiatrica Scandinavica*, Suppl. 100.

Fogel, B. S. and Westlake, R. (1990). Personality disorder and diagnoses and age in in-patients with major depression. *Journal of Clinical Psychiatry*, **51**, 232–5.

Gao, S., Dolan, N., Hall, K. S., and Hendrie, H. C. (2000). The association of demographic factors and physical illness with personality change in a community sample of elderly African Americans. *American Journal of Geriatric Psychiatry*, **8**, 209–43.

Goisman, R. M. (1999). Cognitive–behavioral therapy, personality disorders, and the elderly: clinical and theoretical considerations. In *Personality disorders in older adults* (ed. E. Rosowsksky, R. C. Abrams, and R. A. Zweig), pp. 215–28. Lawrence Erlbaum, New Jersey.

Goldfarb, A. I. (1967). The psychodynamics of dependency and the search for aid. In *The dependencies of old people* (ed. Karsh). Occasional papers in gerontology No. 6, 1–16. Institute of Gerontology the University of Michigan, Wayne State University, MI,

Golomb, M., Fava, M., Abraham, M., and Rosenbaum, J. F. (1995). The relationship between age and personality in depressed outpatients. *Journal of Nervous and Mental Disease*, **183**, 43–4.

Gradman, T. J., Thompson, L. W., and Gallagher-Thompson, D. (1999). Personality disorder and treatment outcome. In *Personality disorders in older adults* (ed. E. Rosowsksky, R. C. Abrams, and R. A. Zweig), pp. 69–94. Lawrence Erlbaum, New Jersey.

Hagnell, O. Ojesjo, L. and Rorsmann, B. (1994). Prevalence of mental disorders, personality traits and mental complaints in the Lundby study. A point prevalence study of the 1957 Lundby cohort of 2612 inhabitants of a geographically defined area who were re-examined in 1972 regardless of domicile. *Scandinavian Journal of Social Medicine*. Suppl. **50**, 1–77.

Havighurst, R. J. (1963). Successful aging. In *Processes of aging*, Vol. 1 (ed. W. C. Tibbetts and W. Donahue), pp. 161–72. Longmans Green, New York.

Havighurst, R. J., Neugarten, B. L., and Tobin, S. S. (1968). Disengagement and patterns of aging. In *Middle age and aging* (ed. B. L. Neugarten). University of Chicago Press, Chicago, IL.

Himmelfarb, S. and Murrell, S. A. (1984). The prevalence and correlates of anxiety symptoms in older adults. *Journal of Psychology*, **116**, 159–67.

Hueston, W. J., Werth, J., and Mainous, A. G. (1999). Personality disorder traits: prevalence and its effects on health in primary care patients. *International Journal of Psychiatry in Medicine*. **29**, 63–74.

Hughes, C. P., Berg, L., Danziger, W. L., Coben, L. A., and Marshall, R. (1982). A new clinical scale for the staging of dementia. *British Journal of Psychiatry*, **140**, 558–65.

Kastrup, M. (1985). Characteristics of a nationwide cohort of psychiatric patients—with special reference to the elderly and chronically admitted. *Acta Psychiatrica Scandinavica*, **71**(Suppl. 319), 107–15.

Kay, D. W. K., Beamish, P., and Roth, M. (1964). Old age and mental disorder in Newcastle upon Tyne. *British Journal of Psychiatry*, **110**, 146–58.

Kunic, M. E., Mulsant, B. H., Rifai, A. H., Sweet, R. A., Pasternak, R., and Zubenko, G. S. (1994). Diagnostic rate of comorbid personality disorder in elderly psychiatric inpatients. *American Journal of Psychiatry.* **151**, 603–5.

Lehr, U. (1986). Aging as fate and challenger: the influence of social, biological and psychological factors. In *Mental health in the elderly* (ed. H. Hafner, G. Moschel, and N. Sartorius), pp. 57–67. Springer-Verlag, Berlin.

Leon, G. R., Gillum, B., Gillum, R., and Gouze, M. (1979). Personality and change over a 30 year period—middle age to old age. *Journal of Consulting Clinical Psychology*, **47**, 517–24.

Links, P. S., Heslegrave, R., and Van Reekum, R. (1999). Impulsivity: core aspect of borderline personality disorder. *Journal of Personality Disorders*, **13**, 1–9.

Lowenthal, M. F. (1964). Social and mental illness in old age. *American Social Revue*, **29**, 54–70.

Lowenthal, M. F. and Boler, D. (1965). Voluntary vs involuntary social withdrawal. *Journal of Gerontology*, **20**, 363–71.

Macmillan, D. and Shaw, P. (1966). Senile breakdown of personal and environmental standards of cleanliness. *British Medical Journal*, **ii**, 1032–7.

Molinari, V., and Marmion, J. (1993). Personality disorders in geropsychiatry outpatients. *Psychological Reports*, **73**, 256–8.

Moliari, V., Kunic, M. E., Mulsant, B., and Rifai, A. H. (1998). The relationship between patient, informant social worker and consensus diagnosis of personality disorder in elderly depressed inpatients. *American Journal of Geriatric Psychiatry*, **6**, 36–44.

Myers, J. K, Weissman, M. M., Tischler, G. L., Holzer, C. E., Leaf, P. J., Orvaschel, H., *et al.* (1984). Six-month prevalence of psychiatric disorders in three communities. *Archives of General Psychiatry*. **41**, 959–67.

Neugarten, B. L. (1977). Personality and aging. In *Handbook of the psychology of aging* (ed. J. E. Birren and K. W. Schaie), pp. 626–49. Van Nostrand and Reinhold, New York.

Orrell, M., Sahakian, B. J., and Bergmann, K. (1989). Self-neglect and frontal lobe dysfunction. *British Journal of Psychiatry*, **155**, 101–5.

Perry, J. C. (1993). Longitudinal studies of personality disorders. *Journal of Personality Disorders,* Suppl. Spring, 63–85.

Peselow, E. D., Fieve, R. R., and DiFiglia, C. (1992). Personality traits and response to imipramine. *Journal of Affective Disorders*, **24**, 209–16.

Petrie, S., Cummings, J. L., Hill, M. A., and Shapira, J. (1989). Personality alterations in dementia of the Alzheimer type: a three year follow-up study. *Journal of Geriatric Psychiatry and Neurology*, **2**, 203–7.

Pilowsky. I. (1967). Dimensions of hypochondriasis. *British Journal of Psychiatry*, **113**, 89–93.

Pilowsky, I. (1978). A general classification of abnormal illness behaviour. *British Journal of Medical Psychology*, **51**, 131–7.

Pilowsky, I. (1983). Hypochondriasis. In *Handbook of psychiatry*, 4, The neuroses and personality disorder (ed. G. F. M. Russell and L. A. Hersov), pp. 319–25. Cambridge University Press, Cambridge.

Pollit, J. (1957), The natural history of obsessional states. *British Medical Journal*, **i**, 194–8.

Rosokowsky, E. and Gurian, B. (1991). Borderline personality disorders in later life. *International Psychogeriatrics*, **3**, 39–52.

Rubin, E. H., Morris, J. C., and Berg, L. (1984). The progression of personality change in senile dementia of the Alzheimer's type. *Journal of the American Geriatrics Society*, **35**, 721–5.

Saunders, P. A., Copeland, J. R., Dewey, M. E., Gilmore, C., Larkin, B. A., Phaterpekar, H., *et al.* (1993). The prevalence of dementia, depression and neurosis in later life: the Liverpool MRC-ALPHA Study. *International Journal of Epidemiology*, **22**, 839–47.

Savage, R. D., Gaber, L. B., Britton, P. G., Bolton, N., and Cooper, A. (1977). *Personality and adjustment in ageing*. Academic Press, London.

Schaie, K. W. and Parham, I. M. (1976). Stability of adult personality traits: fact or fable. *Journal of Personality and Social Psychology*, **34**, 146–58.

Seligman, M. E. P. (1975). *On depression development and death*. Freeman, San Francico, CA.

Siegler, I. C. and Costa, P. T. (1985). Biological influence on behaviour. In *Handbook of the psychology of aging* (ed. J. E. Birren and K. W. Schaie), pp. 95–166. Van Nostrand and Reinhold, New York.

Siegler, I. C., Dawson, D. V., and Welsh, K. A. (1994). Caregiver ratings of personality change in Alzheimer's disease patients: A replication. *Psychology and Aging*, **9**, 464–6.

Simon, A. (1980). The neuroses, personality disorders, alcoholism, drug use and misuse and crime in the aged. In *Handbook of mental health and aging* (ed. J. E. Birren and R. B. Sloane), p. 654. Prentice Hall, Englewood Cliffs, N J.

Slater, E. and Shields, J. (1969). Genetical aspects of anxiety. *British Journal of Psychiatry*, Special Publication **3**, 62–71.

Soloff, P. (1997). Psychobiologic perspectives on treatment of personality disorder. *Journal of Personality Disorders*, **11**, 336–44.

Strauss, M. E., Pasupathi, M., and Chatterjee, A. (1993). Concordance between observers on descriptions of personality change in Alzheimer's disease. *Psychology and Aging*, **8**, 475–80.

Tennant, C., Goulston, K., and Dent, O. (1986). Australian prisoners of war of the Japanese: post-war psychiatric hospitalization and psychiatric morbidity. *Australia and New Zealand Journal of Psychiatry*, **20**, 334–40.

Thomae, H. (1976). *Patterns of aging—findings from the Bonn Longitudinal Study of Aging*. Karger, Basel.

Townsend, P. (1957). *The family life of old people*. Routledge, London.

Verwoerdt, A. (1981). *Clinical geropsychiatry* (2nd edn), p. 94. Williams and Wilkins, Baltimore, MD.

Vine, R. G. and Steingart, A. B. (1994). Personality disorder in the elderly depressed. *Canadian Journal of Psychiatry*, **39**, 392–8.

Williams, W., Weiss, T. W., Edens, A., Hjohnson, M., and Thornby, J. L. (1998). Hospital utilization and personality characteristics of veterans with psychiatric problems. *Psychiatric Services*, **49**, 370–5.

32 Late-onset schizophrenia and very late-onset schizophrenia-like psychosis

Robert Howard

Historical development of diagnostic concepts

Paraphrenia to late paraphrenia

The classification of schizophrenia-like and paranoid disorders in the elderly has a long and somewhat confusing history, which can largely be blamed for the currently uncertain nosological position of such patients. To Kraepelin (1894) *dementia praecox* was fundamentally a disorder of emotion and volition; *paraphrenia* was characterized by hallucinations and delusions without deterioration or disturbance of affective response; and *paranoia* involved the insidious development of a permanent delusional system which resulted from internal causes and was accompanied by perfect preservation of orderly thinking, acting, and will. However, by the eighth edition of his textbook in 1913, Kraepelin was expressing serious doubts about the assumptions on which his conception of dementia praecox had been based. In some cases a complete and lasting recovery was seen and the relationship between onset and early adult life was not absolute. Indeed, Bleuler (1911) had introduced the term 'schizophrenia' to get away from the concept of the disorder as an adolescent mental deterioration. The notion of paraphrenia as a distinct entity was further discredited following Mayer's (1921) follow-up of Kraepelin's 78 original cases. At least 40% of his patients had developed clear signs of dementia praecox within a few years and only 36% could still be classified as paraphrenic. Many of the paraphrenics had positive family histories of schizophrenia, and the presenting clinical picture of those patients who remained 'true' paraphrenics did not differ from those who were later to develop signs of schizophrenia. Some 31 years later in 1952, Roth and Morrisey resurrected both terminology and controversy with their choice of the term 'late paraphrenia' to describe patients who they believed had schizophrenia, but with an onset delayed until after the age of 55 or 60 years. The term was intended to be descriptive; to distinguish the illness from the chronic schizophrenic patients seen in psychiatric institutions at the time, and to emphasize the clinical similarities with the illness described by Kraepelin. Their choice of the term was perhaps unfortunate because two particular points of misconception often seem to arise in relation to it; and it is vital now to set these straight. Late paraphrenia was never intended to mean the same thing as paraphrenia and Kraepelin certainly did not emphasize late age of onset as a feature of the illness.

Late schizophrenia

Both Kraepelin (1913) and Bleuler (1911) observed that there was a relatively rare group of schizophrenics who had an onset of illness in late middle or old age and who, on clinical grounds, closely resembled those who had an onset in early adult life. Utilizing a very narrow conception of dementia praecox and specifically excluding cases of paraphrenia, Kraepelin (1913) reported that only 5.6% of 1054 patients had an onset after the age of 40 years. If the age of onset was set at 60 years or greater, only 0.2% of patients could be included.

Manfred Bleuler (1943) carried out the first specific and systematic examination of late-onset patients and defined late schizophrenia as follows:

1. Onset after the age of 40.
2. Symptomatology that does not differ from that of schizophrenia occurring early in life (or if it does differ it should not do so in a clear or radical way).
3. It should not be possible to attribute the illness to a neuropathological disorder because of the presence of an amnestic syndrome or associated signs of organic brain disease.

Bleuler found that between 15% and 17% of two large series of schizophrenic patients had an onset after the age of 40. Of such late-onset cases, only 4% had become ill for the first time after the age of 60. Later authors confirmed that while onset of schizophrenia after the age of 40 was unusual, onset after 60 should be considered even rarer. From 264 elderly schizophrenic patients admitted in Edinburgh in 1957, only 7 had an illness that had begun after the age of 60 (Fish 1958). Using very broad criteria for the diagnosis of schizophrenia (including schizoaffective, paraphrenic, and other non-organic non-affective psychoses) and studying 470 first contacts from the Camberwell Register, Howard *et al.* (1993*a*) found 29% of cases to have been over 44 years of age at onset.

Kraepelin and E. Bleuler both considered late-onset cases to have much in common with more typically early-onset schizophrenia, a view supported by M. Bleuler's report (1943) of only very mild phenomenological variance from early-onset cases. His 126 late-onset cases were, however, symptomatically milder, had less affective flattening and were less likely to have formal thought disorder than patients with a younger onset. Fish (1960) reported that the clinical picture presented by 23 onset-after-40 patients did not differ importantly from patients who were young at onset, but believed that with increasing age at onset schizophrenia took on a more 'paraphrenic' form.

Late paraphrenia

Kay and Roth (1961) studied a group of 39 female and 3 male patients given a diagnosis of late paraphrenia in Graylingwell Hospital between 1951 and 1955. All but six of these cases were followed-up for 5 years. The cases notes of 48 female and 9 male late paraphrenics admitted to a hospital in Stockholm between 1931 and 1940 were also collected and these cases followed until death or until 1956. Over 40% of the Graylingwell late paraphrenics were living alone, compared with 12% of affective patients and 16% of those with organic psychoses who were of comparable ages. Late paraphrenics were also socially isolated. Although the frequency of visual impairment at presentation (15%) was no higher than in comparison groups with other diagnoses, some impairment of hearing was present in 40% of late paraphrenics and this was considered severe in 15%. Deafness was only present in 7% of affective patients. Focal cerebral disease was identified in only 8% of late paraphrenic patients at presentation. Primary delusions, feelings of mental or physical influence, and hallucinations were all prominent and the prognosis for recovery was poor. Kay and Roth concluded that, at least descriptively, late paraphrenia was a form of schizophrenia, but that its aetiology might be multifactorial. This is a view at variance with that of most current workers in the field (Howard *et al.* 2000) and at least one distinguished schizophrenia researcher (Andreasen 1999).

From a detailed analysis of 1250 first admissions to a hospital in Gothenburg, Sjoegren (1964) identified 202 elderly individuals who conformed to the French concept of paraphrenia (Magnan 1893): well-organized and persistent paranoid delusions with hallucinations occurring in clear consciousness. Sjoegren argued cogently that together with constitutional factors, ageing itself produces effects (feelings of isolation and loneliness, social and economic insecurity, and heightened vulnerability) which contribute to the development of paranoid reactions.

Felix Post (1966) collected a sample of 93 patients to whom he gave the non-controversial and self-explanatory label 'persistent persecutory states' and made a point of including cases regardless of coexisting organic brain change. Within this broad category he recognized three clinical subtypes: a schizophrenic syndrome (34 of 93 patients), a schizophreniform syndrome (37 patients), and a paranoid hallucinosis group (22 patients). Post regarded those patients with the schizophrenic syndrome as having a delayed form of the illness with only partial expression. Post's patients were treated with phenothiazines and he was able to demonstrate that the condition was responsive to antipsychotic medication. Success or failure of treatment were related to the adequacy of phenothiazine treatment and its long-term maintenance.

From a series of 45 female and 2 male late paraphrenics (identified using the same criteria as Kay and Roth), admitted to St Francis' Hospital in Hayward's Heath between 1958 and 1964, Herbert and Jacobson (1967) confirmed many of Kay and Roth's (1961) observations. In addition, they found an unexpectedly high prevalence of schizophrenia among the mothers (4.4%) and siblings (13.3%) of patients.

Late paraphrenia as a heterogeneous disorder or disorders

With the exception of Grahame (1984), and perhaps Roth and Kay in their most recent paper (1999), who have suggested that late paraphrenia should be regarded purely as the manifestation of schizophrenia in old age, most workers writing since the late 1960s have considered these patients to be a heterogeneous group. This view was initially proposed by Post (1966) who considered that only about a third of his patients had schizophrenia. In a 10-year, case-note, follow-up of 47 patients with paranoid psychosis from the Camberwell Register, Holden (1987) revealed heterogeneity in terms of the contribution of organic and affective factors. Even after excluding 10 patients who probably represented misdiagnosed cases of affective and organic psychoses at the time of initial contact, Holden was able to recognize a further 'organic group' of 13 late paraphrenics who had progressed to a diagnosable dementia during 3 years of follow-up. His conclusions as to what his follow-up revealed about the heterogeneous nature of patients with late-life paranoid syndromes were neatly summarized in the title of his paper: 'Late paraphrenia or the paraphrenias'.

ICD-10 and DSM-IV: the end for late paraphrenia

Diagnostic guidelines published by authoritative organizations such as the World Health Organization (WHO) and the American Psychiatric Association (APA) reflect the views of many contemporary clinicians who were consulted at the draft and field trial stages. Inclusion or exclusion of a particular diagnosis in published diagnostic schemes thus reflects the current credence given to the nosological validity of that diagnosis, plus an indication of its general usefulness in clinical practice.

Late paraphrenia, included within ICD-9 (WHO 1984), has not survived as a separate codeable diagnosis into ICD-10 (WHO 1992). There are three possible diagnostic categories available to old age psychiatrists for the accommodation of patients previously diagnosed late paraphrenic. These are schizophrenia, delusional disorder, and other persistent delusional disorders. It seems likely that most cases will be coded under schizophrenia (F20.-) (Quintal *et al.* 1991; Howard *et al.* 1994*a*), although the category of delusional disorder (F22.0) is suggested as a replacement for 'paraphrenia (late)' in the diagnostic guidelines. Distinction between cases of schizophrenia and delusional disorder within ICD-10 is very much dependent on the quality of auditory hallucinations experienced by patients and is subject to some unhelpful ageism. The guidelines for delusional disorder (F22.0) in ICD-10 state that; 'Clear and persistent auditory hallucinations (voices)...are incompatible with this diagnosis' (WHO 1992). Rather confusingly for old age psychiatrists, these same guidelines for a diagnosis of delusional disorder further suggest however, that: '...occasional or transitory auditory hallucinations, particularly in elderly patients, do not rule out this diagnosis, provided that they are not typically schizophrenic and form only a small part of the overall clinical picture'. To add further to diagnostic delirium, the guidelines also include the suggestion that: 'Disorders in which delusions are accompanied by persistent hallucinatory voices or by schizophrenic symptoms that are insufficient to meet criteria for schizophrenia...' should be coded under the category other persistent delusional disorders (F22.8). Since the majority of late paraphrenic patients who hear distinct hallucinatory voices also have a rich variety of schizophrenic core symptoms, very few will be diagnosed as 'other persistent delusional disorders'.

The inclusion within DSM-III-R (APA 1987) of a separate category of late-onset schizophrenia for cases with an illness onset after the age of 44 years seems largely to have been a reaction to the unsatisfactory and arbitrary upper age limit for onset that had hitherto prevailed for a diagnosis of schizophrenia. DSM-IV (APA 1993) contains no separate category for late-onset schizophrenia and this presumably reflects the general North American view of a direct continuity between cases of schizophrenia whatever their age at onset.

The author's personal view is that late paraphrenia has proved (at least in European psychiatry) to be a clinically useful diagnosis, the adoption of which helped to advance the recognition and study of late-onset psychoses. Because of its possibly heterogeneous nature, the lack of clarity regarding its relationship with schizophrenia, and its failure to achieve international recognition, the survival of late paraphrenia has always been threatened and perhaps we should not mourn it.

Terminology and classification for the future

The important questions now are: have ICD-10 and DSM-IV been fair to abandon any facility for coding late-onset within schizophrenia and the delusional disorders, and do we need diagnostic categories that distinguish the functional psychoses with onset in later life from schizophrenia? In the previous edition of this textbook, Raymond Levy and myself argued for a slight modification of ICD-10 and DSM-IV diagnostic coding to record late age at onset. On reflection, such minor tinkering with classificatory systems, which we believed had rather missed the point with this group of patients, seemed inadequate and unlikely to gain acceptance with international colleagues. This provided the spur to establish an international consensus on diagnosis and terminology (Howard *et al.* 2000), which may form the basis for consideration of these patients within future revisions of DSM and ICD. When the Late-onset Schizophrenia International Consensus Group met in 1998, they agreed that the available evidence from the areas of epidemiology, phenomenology, and pathophysiology supported heterogeneity within schizophrenia with increasing age at onset up to the age of 60 years. Schizophrenia-like psychosis with onset after the age of 60 years (i.e. what we used to call late paraphrenia) was considered to be distinct from schizophrenia. The consensus group recommended that cases with onset between 40 and 59 years be termed late-onset schizophrenia and that the group with onset after 60 years should be called very late-onset schizophrenia-like psychosis (VLOSLP). The latter term is long-winded and unmemorable, but at least is unambiguous and had the unprecedented support of both European and North American old age psychiatrists. In spite of his antipathy for the term, the author is sufficiently pragmatic to accept that for reasons outlined above many old age psychiatrists will wish to keep 'late paraphrenia.' *From this point in this chapter the term* 'late paraphrenia' *will however be used only for patients already described as such in the literature.*

Clinical features

Schizophrenic symptoms

Although Bleuler (1943) believed that it was impossible to separate early- and late-onset patients on clinical grounds, he acknowledged that a later onset was accompanied by less affective flattening and a more benign course. Formal thought disorder is seen in only about 5% of cases of DSM-III-R late-onset schizophrenia (Pearlson *et al.* 1989) and could not be elicited from any of 101 late paraphrenics (Howard *et al.* 1994*a*). First-rank symptoms of Schneider are seen, but are less prevalent in later onset cases. Thought-insertion, block, and withdrawal seem to be particularly uncommon (Grahame *et al.* 1984; Pearlson *et al.* 1989; Howard *et al.* 1994*a*) and negative symptoms are unusual (Almeida *et al.* 1995*a*).

Delusions

Persecutory delusions usually dominate the presentation, although in a series of 101 late paraphrenics, delusions of reference (76%), control (25%), grandiose ability (12%), and of a hypochondriacal nature (11%) were also present (Howard *et al.* 1994*a*). Partition delusions are found in about two-thirds of cases. They are the belief that people, animals, materials, or radiation can pass through a structure that would normally constitute a barrier to such passage. This barrier is generally the door, ceiling, walls, or floor of a patient's home and the source of intrusion is frequently a neighbouring residence (Herbert and Jacobson 1967; Pearlson *et al.* 1989; Howard *et al.* 1992*a*).

Affective symptoms

The coexistence of affective features in late-onset schizophrenia is well recognized clinically, but there have been no controlled studies comparing such features in early- and late-onset cases. Atypical, schizoaffective and cycloid psychoses are all characterized by affective features, tend to arise later in life, and affect women more than men (Cutting *et al.* 1978; Levitt and Tsuang 1988). Among late paraphrenic patients, Post (1966) reported depressive admixtures in 60% of cases, while Holden (1987) considered that 10 of his 24 'functional' late paraphrenic patients had affective or schizoaffective illnesses. These patients also had a better outcome in terms both of institutionalization and 10-year survival compared with paranoid patients. Such observations have led to the suggestion that some later onset schizophrenics or late paraphrenics may have variants of primary affective disorder (Murray *et al.* 1992).

Cognitive deficits

Kay and Roth (1961) recognized that a degree of overlap between functional and organic psychoses in senescence existed and pointed out that, particularly in the elderly, it was misleading to consider psychiatric illness in isolation from other symptoms: '...we are most prone to encounter depressive psychosis after an attack of pneumonia, manic episodes after surgical operations, paranoid disorders with and without physical illness in old people with a mild memory defect'.

Post (1966) did not exclude patients with associated organic impairment from his study and found proven organic cerebral change in 16 of his 93 cases of persistent persecutory states. He concluded that simple paranoid and schizophrenia-like syndromes could commonly complicate early dementia but that, in such cases, disorders of memory and concentration could clearly be seen to have preceded the emergence of persecutory symptoms.

Attempts to identify and characterize the patterns of cognitive impairment associated with these conditions began with Hopkins and Roth (1953) who administered the vocabulary subtest from the Wechsler–Bellevue Scale, a shortened form of the Raven's Progressive Matrices, and a general test of orientation and information, to patients with a variety of diagnoses. They reported that 12 late paraphrenic patients performed as well as a group of elderly depressives and better than patients with dementia on all three tests.

Naguib and Levy (1987) evaluated 43 late paraphrenics (having already excluded subjects with a diagnosable dementia) with the Mental Test Score, Digit Copying Test, and the Digit Symbol Substitution Test. Patients performed less well than age-matched controls on both the MTS and DCT.

Miller and co-workers (1991) have published comprehensive neuropsychological assessments of patients with what they term 'late life psychosis'. These patients performed less well than age-matched controls on the Mini-Mental State Examination (MMSE), the Wechsler Adult Intelligence Scale-Revised, the Wisconsin Card Sorting Test, Logical Memory and Visual Reproduction subtests from the Wechsler Memory Scale, a test of verbal fluency, and the Warrington Recognition Memory Test. Patients were, however, not well matched with controls for educational attainment and premorbid intelligence and some of the patients clearly had affective psychoses and dementia syndromes (Miller *et al.* 1992), so that it is probably not fair to equate them with late paraphrenics or late-onset schizophrenics.

Almeida (1995*a*) carried out a very detailed neuropsychological examination of 40 patients with late paraphrenia in South London. Using cluster analysis of the results he identified two groups of patients The first was a 'functional' group characterized by impairment restricted to executive functions, in particular a computerized test assessing extra- and intradimensional attention set shift ability and a test of planning. Such patients had a high prevalence and severity of positive psychotic symptoms and lower scores on a scale of neurological abnormalities. A second 'organic' group of late paraphrenics showed widespread impairment of cognitive functions, together with a lower frequency of positive psychotic symptoms and a high prevalence of abnormalities on neurological examination (Almeida *et al.* 1995*b*).

Stability of cognitive deficit

In his 10-year, case-note, follow-up study, Holden (1987) considered a group of late paraphrenics who progressed to a frank dementia in the first 3 years to have 'organic' late paraphrenia. Such patients had lower scores on cognitive testing on entry to the follow-up period, a reduced female-to-male ratio, and were less likely to have first-rank symptoms than 'functional' late paraphrenics. None of the organic patients showed a full symptomatic recovery and, perhaps not surprisingly, the functional patients had a superior 10-year survival. Holden's organic group almost certainly represented patients with dementia whose non-cognitive symptoms had led their physicians to make a diagnosis of paranoid psychosis. Strikingly, only 8% of his functional group of late paraphrenics developed dementia during the follow-up period, so that the risk of cognitive decline in these patients would appear to have been no higher than in the elderly general population.

The sole published attempt to follow cognitive performance prospectively was reported by Hymas and colleagues (1989) who retested Naguib and Levy's (1987) late paraphrenics after a mean of 3.7 years. Out of the original 43 patients, 31 had survived the follow-up and only 2 of these (and 1 out of 17 surviving controls) had evidence of a global deterioration that the authors considered amounted to a dementia. This favourable cognitive prognostic result needs to be interpreted in the light of the brevity of the follow-up and the observation that one-third of the late paraphrenics, but only 1 control, showed a decline of more than 4 points on the Mental Test Score during this period. It is probably safest to conclude from these studies that patients with misdiagnosed dementia will (not surprisingly) reveal their true condition after a few months, but that functional patients often have mild cognitive impairment at presentation and will continue to experience a gentle decline in performance (Almeida 1999).

Aetiology

Family studies

Reviewing the literature on family history in schizophrenia, Gottesman and Shields (1982) reported that the overall risk of schizophrenia in the relatives of an affected proband is about 10%, compared with a risk of around 1% for the general population.

Kendler *et al.* (1987) concluded that there was no consistent relationship between age at onset and familial risk for schizophrenia, but data from patients with an onset in old age were not included in this analysis. The literature on familiality in late-onset schizophrenia and related psychoses of late life is sparse and inconclusive, partly due to variations in illness definition and age at onset, but principally because of the difficulties inherent in conducting family studies in patients who often have very few surviving first-degree relatives. The results of those few studies, specifically of late-onset psychoses, reviewed by Castle and Howard (1992), suggest a trend for increasing age at the onset of psychosis to be associated with a reduced risk of schizophrenia in first-degree relatives. Thus studies involving subjects with illness onset after the age of 40 or 45 years have reported rates of schizophrenia in relatives of between 4.4% and 19.4% (Bleuler 1943; Huber *et al.* 1975; Pearlson *et al.* 1989), while those with onsets delayed to 50 or 60 years have yielded rates of between 1.0% and 7.3% (Funding 1961; Post 1966; Herbert and Jacobson 1967). More recently, two studies of patients with late onset psychosis—one study with onset after the age of 50 (Brodaty *et al.* 1999) and the other study with onset after 60 years (Howard *et al.* 1997) have reported no increase in the prevalence of schizophrenia among relatives of patients compared to those of healthy comparison subjects. In a controlled family study involving data from 269 first-degree relatives of patients with onset after 60 and 272 relatives of healthy elderly subjects, the estimated lifetime risk for schizophrenia with an onset range of 15 to 90 years was 2.3% for the relatives of cases and 2.2% for the relatives of controls (Howard *et al.* 1997).

Genetic markers

Two attempts to link late paraphrenia to genetic markers for potentially related neuropsychiatric disorders have been unsuccessful. Mohsen Naguib and co-workers (1987) investigated the association between late paraphrenia and HLA type and failed to confirm an association with the HLA-A9 genotype which had been reported for paranoid schizophrenia. We have been unable to establish an association between late paraphrenia and one of the alleles of apolipoprotein E (ApoE). The *APOE ε4* allele frequency among a group of 46 late paraphrenic patients was 0.043 (Howard *et al.* 1995*b*), compared with reports of 0.141 in normal elderly controls (Saunders *et al.* 1993) and 0.382 in populations of patients with Alzheimer's disease (Saunders *et al.* 1993).

Brain imaging

Structural

Computed tomography (CT)

The first CT study specifically to examine patients with schizophrenic symptoms with an onset in late life was performed by Miller *et al.* (1986). They scanned five female patients, whose age at onset of symptoms ranged from 58 to 81 years; three of the patients had extensive cortical and subcortical infarcts and one had normal-pressure hydrocephalus. The scan appearances were so abnormal that the authors entitled their paper 'Late life paraphrenia: an organic delusional syndrome'. It has to be said that selection of patients with exclusion of those with a history or clinical signs of neurological disease or dementia has not confirmed this conclusion for the majority of cases.

Rabins *et al.* (1987) determined ventricle-to-brain ratios (VBRs) with CT in 29 patients whose onset of illness had been after the age of 44 years. Mean VBR was 13.3% in patients and 8.6% in a group of 23 age-matched controls. Naguib and Levy (1987) prospectively identified and CT-scanned 45 cases of late paraphrenia and reported an increase in VBR measurements that was strikingly similar to that of Rabins *et al.*'s late-onset schizophrenics. Mean VBR in patients was 13.09% compared to 9.75% in controls. Since larger values of VBR were not associated with illness duration or any measured cognitive parameters, Naguib and Levy suggested that the observed structural abnormality may have preceded the appearance of psychosis. A more recent examination of the scans of these patients demonstrated more frontal cortical atrophy in those patients who had not experienced Schneiderian first-rank symptoms (Howard *et al.* 1992*b*).

Förstl and co-workers (1994) have reported the results of quantitative CT measurements of the third and lateral ventricles, sylvian and anterior fissures in 14 patients with 'late paranoid psychosis' (onset after 50 years), 14 patients with Alzheimer's disease (AD), and 14 'undemented controls'. All the measurements from the paranoid patients yielded values that were intermediate between the controls and AD patients. For example, VBR was 1.83% in controls, 12.22% in paranoid psychosis, and 16.9% in AD patients. Length of illness came close to being significantly inversely correlated with the areas of the third ($r = -0.46$) and lateral ($r = -0.43$) ventricles. Paranoid psychosis patients who had first-rank symptoms had significantly smaller VBR values than those who did not (10.6% compared to 14.7%).

Exclusion from CT studies of patients with obvious neurological signs or a history of stroke, alcohol abuse, or dementia has shown that structural abnormalities other than in large ventricles of patients with late paraphrenia are probably no more common than in healthy aged controls. Despite adhering to such exclusions however, Flint *et al.* (1991) found unsuspected cerebral infarction on the scans of 5 out of 16 of their late paraphrenic patients. Most of these infarcts were subcortical or frontal, and they were more likely to occur in patients who had delusions but no hallucinations. The results of this study need to be interpreted with some caution, since only 16 of a collected sample of patients had actually undergone CT scanning: it is of course possible that these represented the more 'organic' cases, or at least those thought most likely to have some underlying structural abnormality.

Magnetic resonance imaging (MRI)

The superiority of MRI over CT, both in terms of grey/white matter resolution and visualization of deep white matter, is established. The results of some MRI studies of changes in periventricular and deep white matter in patients with paranoid psychosis however, must again be viewed with some caution—few have assessed abnormalities in the white matter in any kind of standardized manner, and appropriate control populations, matched for cerebrovascular risk factors, are rarely used. Miller and colleagues (1989, 1991, 1992) have reported the results of structural MRI investigations in patients with what they have termed 'late life psychosis'. They have reported that 42% of non-demented patients with an onset of psychosis after the age of 45 (mean age at scanning 60.1 years) had white matter abnormalities on MRI, compared to only 8% of a healthy age-matched control group. The appearance of large patchy white matter lesions (WMLs) was six times more likely in the temporal lobe, and four times more common in the frontal lobes, of patients than controls (Miller *et al.* 1991). These authors hypothesized that, although insufficient to give rise to focal neurological signs, WMLs might produce dysfunction in the overlying frontal and temporal cortex and that this could contribute to psychotic symptomatology. They acknowledged that since WMLs in the occipital lobes could also be implicated, it might not be possible to pinpoint an isolated anatomical white matter lesion that predisposed to psychosis. When comparisons were made between those patients who had structural brain abnormalities on MRI (10 patients) with those who did not (7), there were no significant differences on age, educational level, IQ, or performance on a wide battery of neuropsychological tests. Measurements of VBR indicated a non-significant increase in patients (10.6%) compared to controls (8.8%). The DSM-III-R (APA 1987) diagnoses of the 24 patients at entry to this study were schizophrenic disorder (late-onset type) (10), delusional disorder (7), schizophreniform psychosis (2), and psychosis not otherwise specified (5), but at least 12 were shown to have organic cerebral conditions. Our own studies of white matter signal hyperintensities among patients with late paraphrenia from whom we have tried to exclude organic cases have suggested they may be no more common in such patients than in healthy community-living elderly controls (Howard *et al.* 1995*a*), a finding replicated in a sample of late-onset schizophrenia patients in the United States (Symonds *et al.* 1997).

Pearlson *et al.* (1993) have reported the results of a volumetric MRI study of late-onset schizophrenic patients based on a sample of 11 individuals with an illness onset after the age of 55 years. Third ventricle volume was significantly greater in late-onset schizophrenics (mean value 561 mm^3) than in an age-matched control group (mean 386 mm^3). VBR estimations were higher among the late-onset schizophrenics (mean 9.0) than controls (mean 7.1), but this difference did not reach accepted levels of statistical significance. Mean percentage cerebrospinal fluid (CSF) volume, compared to whole brain, was 11.8% in normal controls and 15.5% in late-onset schizophrenics, but this difference was not statistically significant.

We have reported the results of volumetric MRI studies based on the scans of 47 patients with late paraphrenia, 31 of whom satisfied ICD-10 criteria for a diagnosis of schizophrenia and 16 for delusional disorder. While total brain volume was not reduced in the patients compared with 35 elderly community-living controls, lateral and third ventricle volumes were increased. Among the subgroup of late paraphrenics with schizophrenia, lateral ventricle volumes were 6.6% higher on the right and 12.1% higher on the left than control values, while in patients with delusional disorder the volumes were increased by 74.6% and 93.5%, respectively (Howard *et al.* 1994*b*). Delusional disorder patients 63.64 cm^3 had smaller left temporal lobe 68.10 cm^3 volumes than 69.09 cm^3 schizophrenic and control subjects, but this difference failed to reach accepted levels of statistical significance after the effects of multiple comparisons had been taken into account (Howard *et al.* 1995*c*). Measurements of the frontal lobes, hippocampus, parahippocampus, thalamus, and basal ganglia structures failed to demonstrate further differences between patient and control subjects. These negative results are in accord with a recent North American volumetric study examining the thalamus in late-onset schizophrenia. Corey-Bloom *et al.* (1995) compared MRI scans of the brains of 16 late-onset and 14 early-onset schizophrenic patients and of 28 normal elderly controls. All subjects were over the age of 45 years. Patients with late-onset schizophrenia had significantly larger lateral ventricles than normal comparison subjects and significantly larger thalamic volumes than the patients with early-onset schizophrenia.

Functional

Regional cerebral blood flow studies

With single photon emission tomography (SPET) of the brain it is possible to measure and image regional cerebral blood flow in a relatively non-invasive manner. In patients with vascular dementia, SPET demonstrates multifocal perfusion deficits (Myers *et al.* 1988), whilst in Alzheimer's disease symmetrical bilateral posterior temporoparietal hypoperfusion is seen (Johnson *et al.* 1987; Miller *et al.* 1990). In Pick's disease, bifrontal and anterior bitemporal hypoperfusion occurs (Risberg 1987). Some studies of patients with schizophrenia who have had onset in early adult life show global cortical hypoperfusion or hypometabolism (Gur *et al.* 1985; Mathew *et al.* 1988), while others demonstrate frontal hypoperfusion (Berman *et al.* 1988; Weinberger *et al.* 1988).

There have been few studies of blood flow in patients with a late-onset, schizophrenia-like illness or in patients with early dementia and paranoid symptomatology. Miller *et al.* (1992) studied 18 DSM-III-R (APA 1987) late-onset schizophrenics with SPET using [^{99}Tc]hexamethyl propyleneamine oxime (HMPAO) which gives a high-resolution (approx. 7 mm) qualitative image of relative cerebral perfusion. Regional cerebral blood flow was described in right and left frontal, parietal, temporal, occipital, thalamic, and basal ganglia regions. Hypoperfusion was defined as a blood flow less than 66% of maximal cerebral uptake. Of the 18 schizophrenic patients in the study, 11 (61%) had MRI evidence of either WMLs or multiple strokes, 9 of whom had focal or multifocal deficits on SPET suggesting vascular injury. Normal SPET perfusion scans were seen in 5 patients; 1 had an Alzheimer's disease-type pattern; and 12 had a pattern suggesting multi-infarct dementia. Only 4 out of 30 normal controls had abnormal SPET scans. In the light of previous suggestions that temporal and frontal dysfunction may be important in the pathogenesis of psychosis (e.g. Cummings 1985), Miller *et al.* (1992) further evaluated regional temporal, parietal, and frontal perfusion in these patients and their controls. Some 13 of 18 late-life psychosis patients, compared with 7 of 30 control subjects, had unilateral or bilateral temporal hypoperfusion ($p < 0.003$); 7 of 18 patients and 4 of 30 controls had frontal hypoperfusion ($p < 0.002$); and 15 of 18 (83%) late-life psychosis patients, compared to 27% of controls, had either frontal or temporal hypoperfusion. These results support the view of this group of workers who emphasize the contribution of vascular structural brain abnormalities in the aetiology of late-onset schizophrenia-like psychoses.

Dopamine D_2 receptors

Pearlson *et al.* (1993) have reported the results of a positron emission tomography (PET) study in late-onset schizophrenia. Subjects were 10 female and 3 male never-medicated patients who met DSM-III-R diagnostic criteria for schizophrenia and had an illness onset after the age of 55 years. Mean age at scanning was 74 years. Control subjects were recruited by local newspaper advertisement and from hospital staff members. Two PET scans were obtained for each subject to estimate caudate D_2-receptor density (B_{max}) (Wong *et al.* 1986*a–c*). The first scan was performed before any neuroleptic exposure. At 4 hours prior to the second scan, a single dose of 7.5 mg unlabelled oral haloperidol was administered to reveal binding under conditions in which the D_2 receptor was almost completely blocked. Measured D_2-receptor density was elevated among the late-onset schizophrenics compared to the values for control subjects. Our own examination of striatal D_2-receptor binding with SPET in six never-medicated patients who also satisfied DSM-III-R criteria for late-onset schizophrenia (Howard *et al.* 1993*b*) did not demonstrate an increase in D_2-receptor binding compared to age-matched control subjects. Therefore, functional imaging has not yet convincingly demonstrated the presence of abnormalities in the number or function of dopamine D_2 receptors in patients with late paraphrenia or late-onset schizophrenia who have not received antipsychotic medication

Sex ratio

The female preponderance of individuals who have an onset of schizophrenia or a schizophrenia-like psychosis in middle or old age is a consistent finding. Among late-onset schizophrenics (onset after 40–50 years) females have been reported to constitute 66% (Bleuler 1943), 72% (Klages 1961), 82% (Gabriel 1978), 85% (Marneros and Deister 1984), or 87% (Pearlson *et al.* 1989) of patients. In studies of patients with an illness onset at 60 years or over, the female preponderance is even greater: 75% (Sternberg 1972), 86% (Howard *et al.* 1994*a*), 88% (Kay and Roth 1961), or 91% (Herbert and Jacobson 1967).

Two reports have indicated the presence of a subgroup of female schizophrenia patients with later illness onset who typically do not have a positive family history of schizophrenia (Shimizu and Kurachi 1989; Gorwood *et al.* 1995). Typically, a later illness onset, particularly in females, is associated with a milder symptom profile and better outcome, better premorbid social adjustment, and a lower prevalence of structural brain abnormalities than in (mostly male) patients with an early illness onset. This has led to the suggestion that sex differences in schizophrenia may reflect different psychiatric disorders. Hence, Castle and Murray (1991) have suggested that early-onset, typically male schizophrenia is essentially a heritable neurodevelopmental disorder, while late-onset schizophrenia in females may have aetiologically more in common with affective psychosis than with the illness seen in males.

Sensory deficits

Deafness has been experimentally (Zimbardo *et al.* 1981) and clinically (Moore 1981) associated with the development of paranoid symptoms. Deficits of moderate to severe degree affect 40% of patients with late paraphrenia (Kay and Roth 1961; Herbert and Jacobson 1967) and are more prevalent than in elderly depressed patients or normal controls (Post 1966; Naguib and Levy 1987). Deafness associated with late-life psychosis is more usually conductive than degenerative (Cooper *et al.* 1974) and generally of early onset, long duration, bilateral, and profound (Cooper 1976; Cooper and Curry 1976). Corbin and Eastwood (1976) suggested that deafness may reinforce a pre-existing tendency to social isolation, withdrawal, and suspiciousness. Further, auditory hallucinations are the psychopathological phenomenon most consistently associated with deafness (Keshavan *et al.* 1992). There are several reports of improvement in psychotic symptoms after the fitting of a hearing aid (Eastwood *et al.* 1981; Khan *et al.* 1988; Almeida *et al.* 1993), although it has to be said that clinical practice suggests that this is not usually the case.

Visual impairment, most commonly a consequence of cataract or macular degeneration, is also commoner in elderly paranoid psychosis patients than those with affective disorder, and there is a higher coincidence of visual and hearing impairment in paranoid than affective patients (Cooper and Porter 1976). An association between visual impairment and the presence of visual hallucinations (Howard *et al.* 1994*a*) echoes Keshavan's findings with deafness.

Premorbid personality

A consistent theme in descriptions of patients who develop paranoid psychoses late in life is the presence of abnormal personality traits; most often schizoid or paranoid personality types (Kay and Roth 1961; Post 1966; Kay *et al.* 1976). Although these patients are known to experience relationship difficulties, reflected by their low rates of marriage and the apparently reduced numbers of children born to those who do marry (Kay and Roth 1961; Herbert and Jacobson 1967), this contrasts with their premorbid educational and occupational adjustment which is often good (Pearlson and Rabins 1988). Hence, abnormalities in personality function in these patients have a characteristic specificity. Kay and Roth (1961) reported paranoid and schizoid personality traits (characterized by jealousy, suspiciousness, emotional coldness, arrogance, egocentricity, and extreme solitariness) in 45% of patients. A further 30% were described as explosive, sensitive, or belonging to religious minority groups. Late paraphrenics were also more likely to be living alone (40%) than patients of the same age with affective disorders (12%) or organic psychoses (16%). Acknowledging that premorbid personality abnormality seemed almost universal in late paraphrenia, Kay and Roth (1961) identified a subgroup comprising 20% of their sample who were characterized by severely abnormal premorbid personalities, who developed paranoid delusions, but did not hallucinate. Such patients had longstanding abnormalities of personality of a kind that interfered with relationships, a high age of first admission (generally over 75 years), and delusions that were almost always confined to ideas of theft, ill-treatment, or poisoning by people in everyday contact with the patient. The onset of psychosis was often hard to date in such individuals, since relatives tended to regard symptoms as an extension and caricature of the usual personality.

Felix Post (1966) believed that the personalities of patients with persistent persecutory states could frequently be recognized as having been paranoid in early life. From 87 patients for whom he had information about their premorbid personality function, 35 had what he termed 'paranoid traits', in that they had been quarrelsome, sensitive, suspicious, or generally hostile. He described other patients as having been odd, eccentric, histrionic, or pretentious, and in only 26 cases was he able to conclude that the premorbid personality had been free of significant abnormality.

Premorbid personality in late and mid-life paranoid psychoses and the quality of premorbid relationships within families and with friends were assessed retrospectively by Kay *et al.* (1976). This study is an important one because, through the use of structured patient and informant interviews, it represented a first effort to overcome some of the problems inherent in any retrospective attempt at defining premorbid personality. From a consecutive series of first admissions to a psychiatric hospital the authors selected 54 cases of paranoid and 57 of affective psychosis who were over the age of 50. Patients and close relatives or friends were independently given a semi-structured clinical interview, designed to cover a wide range of paranoid traits. The paranoid patients were rated more highly, both by themselves and informants, on items that suggested they had greater difficulty in establishing and maintaining satisfactory relationships premorbidly. They had also been significantly more shy, reserved, touchy, and suspicious and less able to display sympathy or emotion. Through principal components analysis of the results, the authors derived a 'prepsychotic schizoid personality factor'; consisting of unsociability, reticence, suspiciousness, and hostility.

Retterstol (1966) has argued that since personality deviations in paranoid patients are recognizable at a very early age, factors in the childhood and adolescence of patients are important in determining a predisposition to paranoid psychosis later in life. Key experiences in the later development of paranoid psychoses are proposed to be those which provoke feelings of insecurity or which damage the self-image of an individual whose personality is already overtly sensitive. Gurian *et al.* (1992) have also provided evidence for the importance of childhood experiences in the development of paranoid psychosis in late life. Among nine Israeli patients with delusional disorder, these authors found a high prevalence of 'war refugees'. These were individuals who had survived the Armenian or Nazi Holocausts or been forced to leave their native country. The authors proposed an association between the presence of extremely life-threatening experiences in childhood, a failure to produce progeny, and the development of paranoid delusional symptoms in late life in response to a stressful situation such as widowhood. Just how early the threatening experience needs to be is not clear. Cervantes *et al.* (1989) found the risk of developing a paranoid psychosis to be doubled in immigrants from Mexico and Central America who were escaping war or political unrest compared with those who had moved for economic reasons. Thus, the period during which a personality may be rendered sensitive to the later development of paranoid psychosis by exposure to trauma is presumably not limited to early childhood.

Exactly how important abnormalities in personality functioning are in the aetiology and onset of late-life paranoid psychoses is unclear. Whilst there is evidence linking social trauma in childhood or early adult life to the later development of psychosis, it is perhaps more plausible to view the abnormal premorbid personality as an early marker of impending psychosis, rather than to regard the psychosis as an outcome of earlier personality dysfunction.

Management/treatment

Establishing a therapeutic relationship

Although these patients are often described as hostile, and relationships with neighbours, GP, and the local police have frequently been affected by their psychotic symptoms by the time psychiatric referral is considered, the author's experience is that they are often also extremely lonely. Without entering into any kind of collusion, it is always possible at least to take the time to listen to the patient's account of her persecution, and not difficult to express sympathy for the distress she is experiencing. Sometimes a brief admission to hospital or the establishment of regular visits by the community psychiatric nurse (CPN) can be rendered acceptable as an attempt to 'get to the bottom' of whatever is going on. Once a relationship of trust and support has been established, patients will often accept medication and visits from members of the psychiatric team without really ever developing insight into their condition. Telling the patient directly that he or she has a mental illness is probably the quickest way to join a list of perceived persecutors, and hence use of the Mental Health Act should be reserved until all else has failed. Even though this may mean that the patient does not receive antipsychotic medication, the provision and maintenance of a relationship of trust with a member of staff who can absorb complaints about, for example, a patient's neighbours will do more to reduce distress than will an enforced prescription. Relatives and friends should be advised to encourage the patient to reserve discussion of such complaints to the time that the CPN visits, if this is possible. Of course, there is no single strategy which is best for all patients. For most patients, interventions delivered to their own homes (CPN or volunteer visits, home helps, and meals-on-wheels) seem to be most acceptable; and although some will respond well to the activities and company provided by a day hospital or centre, many will decline to attend. The potential role of psychological treatments in the management of psychotic symptoms in younger patients is becoming clearer, but elderly psychotic patients are not routinely considered for these, which is unfortunate and unfair (Aguera-Ortiz and Reneses-Prieto 1999).

Rehousing

Since these patients are often persistent and able complainers and may have highly restricted and encapsulated delusional systems, their complaints about neighbours or the home environment are sometimes taken at face value by social services' staff. It is therefore not uncommon to discover that, by the time of the first psychiatric referral, a patient has been rehoused at least once in the preceding months. As a general rule, even if it results in a brief reduction of complaints from the sufferer, provision of new accommodation is followed within a few weeks by a re-emergence of symptoms. The obvious distress this causes is sufficient reason always to advise patients and social workers against such moves, unless they are being considered for non-delusional reasons or following successful treatment of psychosis.

Antipsychotic medication

There are good reasons to suspect that a smaller number of late- than early-onset patients with schizophrenia or schizophrenia-like psychoses show a complete response to antipsychotic medication. For example, Rabins and colleagues (1984) found no, or only a partial, response to neuroleptics in 43% of schizophrenic patients with an onset after 44 years of age, while Pearlson *et al.* (1989) reported that 54% of their patients fell into this category. In reports of patients with late paraphrenia, the comparable rates range from 49% (Post 1966) to 75% (Kay and Roth 1961). The general conclusion from such studies is that while drugs relieve some target symptoms, the overall treatment response to medication is modest (Branchey *et al.* 1978; Raskind and Risse 1986).

It would be useful to know which illness parameters are associated with a poor response to medication. Pearlson *et al.* (1989) found a poor response to neuroleptics to be associated with the (rare) presence of thought disorder and with schizoid premorbid personality traits. The presence of first-rank symptoms, a family history of schizophrenia, and gender had no effect on treatment response. In a late paraphrenic patient group, Holden (1987) found auditory hallucinations and affective features to predict a favourable response. This may of course simply reflect a better natural history in such patients.

Among a group of 64 late paraphrenic patients prescribed neuroleptic medication for at least 3 months, 42.2% showed no response, 31.3% a partial response, and 26.6% a full response to treatment (Howard and Levy 1992). Compliance with medication, receiving depot rather than oral medication, and support by a CPN if the patient was an outpatient all had a positive effect on treatment response. Patients prescribed depot medication received on average a lower daily dose in chlorpromazine equivalents than those prescribed oral medication. Hence use of depot, rather than the oral route, is associated with a better response rate (a significantly higher proportion of patients treated with a depot formulation had improved symptoms) despite the administration of smaller amounts of medication.

Novel antipsychotic medications

Because of its anticholinergic activity and relatively weak blockade of striatal dopamine D_2 receptors, low-dose clozapine seemed a very promising drug for the treatment of those elderly psychotic patients with individual sensitivity to extrapyramidal symptoms caused by typical neuroleptics (Jeste *et al.* 1993). Clozapine has anticholinergic, hypotensive, and sedating effects and has been shown to impair memory function even in young patients (Goldberg and Weinberger 1994). Despite a couple of early positive case reports (Oberholzer *et al.* 1992) it has not found favour with those of us who regularly prescribe for older patients.

Risperidone is a benzisoxazole derivative with an extremely strong binding affinity for serotonin 5-HT_2 receptors, a strong affinity for dopamine D_2 receptors, and a high affinity for a_1- and a_2-adrenergic and histamine H_1 receptors (Cohen 1994; Livingstone 1994). Of all the atypicals, clinical experience with risperidone in this patient group is most extensive. Early reports with this drug suggested that activity at 5-HT_2 receptors appeared to be important in the treatment of complex visual hallucinations (Sadzot *et al.* 1989; Howard *et al.* 1994*b*), which had been traditionally regarded as treatment-resistant (Post 1965; Howard and Levy 1994). Risperidone has efficacy in the treatment of hallucinations and delusions in elderly patients at low doses (typically 0.5–2 mg per day (Heylen *et al.* 1988; Howard *et al.* 1994*b*). When compared with treatment with traditional neuroleptics in open-label studies, risperidone has been shown to improve cognitive function (Jeste *et al.* 1999) and to result in a significantly lower cumulative incidence of tardive dyskinesia (Jeste *et al.* 1998, 2000). Since the risk of developing extrapyramidal symptoms, hypotension, and somnolence increases with higher doses, prescription of more than 2 mg per day should be avoided if possible. Also, since patients with dementia with Lewy bodies may present with hallucinations and delusions before cognitive deficit is apparent, caution should always be exercised in the prescription of any antipsychotic medication.

Olanzapine has a similar receptor binding profile to clozapine but doesn't appear to cause the anticholinergic and sedating problems seen with the latter agent, probably because it has antipsychotic activity at much lower doses. A starting dose of 2.5 mg per day is generally well tolerated and can be increased to 10 mg per day if no adverse events appear. Anecdotal evidence suggests that olanzapine is less likely to cause extrapyramidal symptoms than risperidone, but more likely to produce sedation and weight gain. However, this has not been subjected to testing by controlled trial, and the choice as to which of these two atypicals is prescribed will depend very much on individual experience.

Guidelines for prescribing

There is no real evidence that any particular drug is more effective than another in this group of patients. The choice of drug for each individual patient should thus be based on considerations of concomitant physical illness and other treatments received, together with the specific side-effect profile of the drug (Tran-Johnson *et al.* 1994). While there is an argument that all patients should be commenced on depot (Raskind and Risse 1986), treatment will usually be commenced at a low dose of an oral preparation and it is easy to argue that this should be one of the atypicals because of the reduced risk of early and delayed emergent side-effects. Patients who do not respond to oral treatment (whether due to poor compliance or genuine treatment-resistance) can be treated with a depot preparation. Successful treatment of patients with a depot preparation can often be achieved using very modest doses. For example, the mean prescribed dose of a depot agent in Howard's and Levy's (1992) study was 14.4 mg of flupentixol decanoate or 9 mg of fluphenazine decanoate every 2 weeks. In those patients who continue to experience psychotic symptoms after receiving a depot preparation for several weeks, the dose can be increased by 10% every 2–3 weeks until a response is seen or side-effects emerge. There is no reason why patients in the community should not be maintained on a depot preparation for several years, so long as (*and this is very important*) they are monitored through examination by the prescriber for the presence of extrapyramidal side-effects at least once every 3 months, in addition to regular reports from the nurse who gives the injection. Over the next few years we can expect to see the development of depot preparations of the atypicals. Indeed, trials of depot risperidone are in progress at the time of writing. If these trials prove successful I have little doubt that this will represent the optimal way of delivering antipsychotic treatment to these patients.

Conclusions

The history of schizophrenia and schizophrenia-like psychoses that have onset in later life is a long one, but it is only in the last three decades that any real attempts have been made to study patients with these conditions and understand how they might relate to psychoses arising earlier in the life cycle. The aetiological roles of premorbid personality functioning and degenerative and genetic factors are still not elucidated fully, although most recent brain imaging studies indicate that gross degenerative changes are not present. If compliance with neuroleptic medication can be established and maintained, the prognosis for symptomatic improvement is good.

References

Aguera-Ortiz, L. and Reneses-Prieto, B. (1999). The place of non-biological treatments. In *Late-onset schizophrenia* (ed. R. Howard, P. V. Rabins, and D. J. Castle), pp. 233–60. Wrightson Biomedical, Petersfield.

Almeida, O. (1999). The neuropsychology of schizophrenia in late life. In *Late-onset schizophrenia* (ed. R. Howard, P. V. Rabins, and D. J. Castle), pp. 181–90. Wrightson Biomedical, Petersfield.

Almeida, O., Forstl, H., Howard, R., and David, A. S. (1993). Unilateral auditory hallucinations. *British Journal of Psychiatry*, **162**, 262–4.

Almeida, O., Howard, R., Levy, R., and David, A. (1995*a*). Psychotic states arising in late life (late paraphrenia). Psychopathology and nosology. *British Journal of Psychiatry*, **166**, 205–14.

Almeida, O., Howard, R., Levy, R., and David, A., and Morris, R. (1995*b*). Clinical and cognitive diversity of psychotic states arising in late life (late paraphrenia). *Psychological Medicine*, **25**, 699–714.

American Psychiatric Association. (1987). *Diagnostic and statistical manual of mental disorders—third edition revised*. APA, Washington, DC.

American Psychiatric Association. (1993). *Diagnostic and statistical manual of mental disorders—fourth edition*. APA, Washington, DC.

Andreasen, N. C. (1999). I don't believe in late-onset schizophrenia. In *Late-onset schizophrenia* (ed. R. Howard, P. V. Rabins, and D. J. Castle), pp. 111–26. Wrightson Biomedical. Petersfield.

Berman, K. F., Illowsky, B. P., and Weinberger, D. R. (1988). Physiological dysfunction of dorsolateral prefrontal cortex in schizophrenia. *Archives of General Psychiatry*, **45**, 616–22.

Bleuler, E. P. (1911). *Dementia praecox or the group of schizophrenias*. Deuticke. Leipzig.

Bleuler, M. (1943). Die spatschizophrenen krankheitsbilder. *Fortschritte der Neurologie Psychiatrie*, **15**, 259–90.

Branchey, M. H., Lee, J. H., Amin, R. and Simpson, G. M. (1978). High- and low-potency neuroleptics in elderly psychiatric patients. *Journal of the American Medical Association*, **239**, 1860–2

Brodaty, H., Sachdev, P., Rose, N., Rylands, K., and Prenter, L. (1999). Schizophrenia with onset after age 50 years. 1. Phenomenology and risk factors. *British Journal of Psychiatry*, **175**, 410–15.

Castle, D. J. and Howard, R. (1992). What do we know about the aetiology of late-onset schizophrenia? *European Psychiatry*, **7**, 99–108.

Castle, D. J. and Murray, R. M. (1991). The neurodevelopmental basis of sex differences in schizophrenia. *Psychological Medicine*, **21**, 565–75.

Cervantes, R. C., Salgado-Snyder, V. N., and Padilla, A. M. (1989). Post-traumatic stress in immigrants from Central America and Mexico. *Hospital and Community Psychiatry*, **40**, 615–19.

Cohen, L. J. (1994). Risperidone. *Pharmacotherapy*, **14**, 253–65.

Cooper, A. F. (1976). Deafness and psychiatric illness. *British Journal of Psychiatry*, **129**, 216–26.

Cooper, A. F. and Curry, A. R. (1976). The pathology of deafness in the paranoid and affective psychoses of later life. *Journal of Psychosomatic Research*, **20**, 107–14.

Cooper, A. F. and Porter, R. (1976). Visual acuity and ocular pathology in the paranoid and affective psychoses of later life. *Journal of Psychosomatic Research*, **20**, 107–14.

Cooper, A. F., Curry, A. R., Kay, D. W. K., Garside, R. F., and Roth, M. (1974). Hearing loss in paranoid and affective psychoses of the elderly. *Lancet*, **ii**, 851–4.

Corbin, S. and Eastwood, M. R. (1976). Sensory deficits and mental disorders of old age: Causal or coincidental associations? *Psychological Medicine*, **16**, 251–6.

Corey-Bloom, J., Jernigan, T., Archibald, S., Harris M. J., and Jeste D. V. (1995). Quantitative magnetic resonance imaging of the brain in late-life schizophrenia. *American Journal of Psychiatry*, **152**, 447–9.

Cummings, J. (1985). Organic delusions: phenomenology, anatomical correlations and review. *British Journal of Psychiatry*, **146**, 184–97.

Cutting, J. C., Clare, A. W., and Mann, A. H. (1978). Cycloid psychosis: investigation of the diagnostic concept. *Psychological Medicine*, **8**, 637–48.

Eastwood, M. R., Corbin, S., and Reed, M. (1981). Hearing impairment and paraphrenia. *Journal of Otolaryngology*, **10**, 306–8.

Fish, F. (1958). A clinical investigation of chronic schizophrenia. *British Journal of Psychiatry*, **104**, 34–54.

Fish, F. (1960). Senile schizophrenia. *Journal of Mental Science*, **106**, 938–46.

Flint, A., Rifat, S., and Eastwood, M. (1991). Late-onset paranoia: distinct from paraphrenia? *International Journal of Geriatric Psychiatry*, **6**, 103–9.

Forstl, H., Dalgalarrondo, P., Riecher-Rossler, A., Lotz, M., Geiger-Kabisch C., and Hentschel, F. (1994). Organic factors and the clinical features of late paranoid psychosis: a comparison with Alzheimer's disease and normal ageing. *Acta Psychiatrica Scandinavica*, **89**, 335–40.

Funding, T. (1961). Genetics of paranoid psychoses in late life. *Acta Psychiatrica Scandinavica*, **37**, 267–82.

Gabriel, E. (1978). *Die Langfristige Entwicklung der Spatschizophrenien*. Karger. Basel.

Goldberg, T. E. and Weinberger, D. R. (1994). The effects of clozapine on neurocognition: an overview. *Journal of Clinical Psychiatry*, **55**(Suppl. B), 88–90.

Gorwood, P., Leboyer, M., Jay, M., Payan C., and Feingold, J. (1995). Gender and age at onset in schizophrenia: Impact of family history. *American Journal of Psychiatry*, **152**, 208–12.

Gottesman, I. I. and Shields, J. (1982). *Schizophrenia, the epigenetic puzzle*. Cambridge University Press, Cambridge.

Grahame, P. S. (1984). Schizophrenia in old age (late paraphrenia). *British Journal of Psychiatry*, **145**, 493–5.

Gur, R. E., Gur, R. C., Skolnik B. E., Caroff, S., Obrist, W. D., Resnick S., *et al.* (1985). Brain function in psychiatric disorders: III. Regional cerebral blood flow in unmedicated schizophrenics. *Archives of General Psychiatry*, **42**, 329–34.

Gurian, B. S., Wexler, D., and Baker, E. H. (1992). Late-life paranoia: possible associations with early trauma and infertility. *International Journal of Geriatric Psychiatry*, **7**, 277–84.

Herbert, M. E. and Jacobson, S. (1967). Late paraphrenia. *British Journal of Psychiatry*, **113**, 461–7.

Heylen, S. L., Gelders, Y. G., and Vanden Bussche, G. (1988). Risperidone (R 64 766) in the treatment of behavioural symptoms in psychogeriatric patients: pilot clinical investigation. *Presented at International Symposium of Psychogeriatrics*, Laussane, Switzerland, April 28th.

Holden, N. (1987). Late paraphrenia or the paraphrenias: a descriptive study with a 10-year follow-up. *British Journal of Psychiatry*, **150**, 635–9.

Hopkins, B. and Roth, M. (1953). Psychological test performance in patients over 60. Paraphrenia, arterio-sclerotic psychosis and acute confusion. *Journal of Mental Science*, **99**, 451–63.

Howard, R. and Levy, R. (1992). Which factors affect treatment response in late paraphrenia? *International Journal of Geriatric Psychiatry*, **7**, 667–72.

Howard, R. and Levy, R. (1994). Charles Bonnet syndrome plus: complex visual hallucinations of Charles Bonnet type in late paraphrenia. *International Journal of Geriatric Psychiatry*, **9**, 399–404.

Howard, R., Castle, D., O'Brien, J., Almeida, O., and Levy, R. (1992*a*). Permeable walls, floors, ceilings and doors. Partition delusions in late paraphrenia. *International Journal of Geriatric Psychiatry*, **7**, 719–24.

Howard, R., Forstl, H., Naguib, M., Burns, A., and Levy, R. (1992*b*). First-rank symptoms in late paraphrenia: cortical structural correlates. *British Journal of Psychiatry*, **160**, 108–9.

Howard, R., Castle, D., Wessely, S., and Murray, R. (1993*a*). A comparative study of 470 cases of early and late-onset schizophrenia. *British Journal of Psychiatry*, **163**, 353–7.

Howard, R., Cluckie, A., and Levy, R. (1993*b*). Striatal D_2 receptor binding in late paraphrenia. *Lancet*, **342**, 562.

Howard, R., Almeida, O., and Levy, R. (1994*a*). Phenomenology, demography and diagnosis in late paraphrenia. *Psychological Medicine*, **24**, 397–410.

Howard, R., Almeida, O., Levy, R., Graves, M., and Graves, P. (1994*b*). Quantitative magnetic resonance imaging in delusional disorder and late-onset schizophrenia. *British Journal of Psychiatry*, **165**, 474–80.

Howard, R., Cox, T., Mullen, R., Almeida, O., and Levy, R. (1995*a*). White matter signal hyperintensities in the brains of patients with late paraphrenia and the normal community-living elderly. *Biological Psychiatry*, **38**, 86–91.

Howard, R., Dennehey, J., Lovestone, S., Birkett, J., Sham, P., Powell, J., *et al.* (1995*b*). Apolipoprotein E genotype and late paraphrenia. *International Journal of Geriatric Psychiatry*, **10**, 147–80.

Howard, R., Mellers, J., Petty, R., Bonner, D., Menon, R., Graves, M., *et al.* (1995*c*). Magnetic resonance imaging of the temporal and frontal lobes, hippocampus, parahippocampal and superior temporal gyri in late paraphrenia. *Psychological Medicine*, **25**, 495–503.

Howard, R., Graham, C., Sham, P., Dennehey, J., Castle, D. J., Levy, R., *et al.* (1997). A controlled family study of late-onset non-affective psychosis (late paraphrenia). *British Journal of Psychiatry*, **170**, 511–14.

Howard, R., Rabins, P. V., Seeman, M. V., Jeste, D. V., and the International Late-Onset Schizophrenia Group (2000). Late-onset schizophrenia and very-late-onset schizophrenia-like psychosis: an international consensus. *American Journal of Psychiatry*, **157**, 172–8.

Huber, G., Gross, G., and Schuttler, R. (1975). Spat schizophrenie. *Archiv fur Psychiatrie und Nervenkrankheiten*, **22**, 53–66.

Hymas, N., Naguib, M., and Levy, R. (1989). Late paraphrenia: a follow-up study. *International Journal of Geriatric Psychiatry*, **4**, 23–9.

Jeste, D. V., Lacro, J. P., Gilbert, P. L., Kline, J., and Kline, N. (1993). Treatment of late-life schizophrenia with neuroleptics. *Schizophrenia Bulletin,*, **19**, 817–30.

Jeste, D. V., Lohr, J. B., Eastham, J. H., Rockwell, E., and Caligiuri, M. P. (1998). Adverse effects of long-term use of neuroleptics: human and animal studies. *Journal of Psychiatric Research*, **32**, 201–14.

Jeste, D. V., Lacro, J. P., Palmer, B., Rockwell, E., Harris, M. J., and Caligiuri, M. P. (1999). Incidence of tardive dyskinesia in early stages of neuroleptic treatment for older patients. *American Journal of Psychiatry*, **156**, 309–11.

Jeste, D. V., Okamoto, A., Napolitano, J., Kane. J. M., and Matinez, R. A. (2000). Low incidence of persistent tardive dyskinesia in elderly patients with dementia treated with risperidone. *American Journal of Psychiatry*, **157**, 1150–5.

Johnson, K. A., Mueller, S. T., Walshe, T. M., English, R. J., and Holman, B. L. (1987). Cerebral perfusion imaging in Alzheimer's disease. Use of single photon emission computed tomography and iofetamine hydrochloride. *Archives of Neurology*, **44**, 165–8.

Kay, D. W. K. and Roth, M. (1961). Environmental and hereditary factors in the schizophrenias of old age ('late paraphrenia') and their bearing on the general problem of causation in schizophrenia. *Journal of Mental Science*, **107**, 649–86.

Kay, D. W. K., Cooper, A. F., Garside, R. F., and Roth, M. (1976). The differentiation of paranoid from affective psychoses by patients' premorbid characteristics. *British Journal of Psychiatry*, **129**, 207–15.

Kendler, K. S., Tsuang, M. T., and Hays, P. (1987). Age at onset in schizophrenia: a familial perspective. *Archives of General Psychiatry*, **44**, 881–90.

Keshavan, M. S., David, A. S., Steingard, S., and Lishman, W. A. (1992). Musical hallucinations: a review and synthesis. *Neuropsychiatry, Neuropsychology and Behavioural Neurology*, **5**, 211–23.

Khan, A. M., Clark, T., and Oyebode, F. (1988). Unilateral auditory hallucinations. *British Journal of Psychiatry*, **152**, 297–8.

Klages, W. (1961). *Die Spatschizophrenie*. Enke, Stuttgart.

Kraepelin, E. (1894). Die abgrenzung der paranoia. *Allgemeine Zeitschrift fuer Psychiatrie*, **50**, 1080–1.

Kraepelin, E. (1913). *Psychiatrie, ein Lehrbuch fur Studierende und Artze*. Barth, Leipzig.

Levitt, J. J. and Tsuang, M. T. (1988). The heterogeneity of schizoaffective disorder: implications for treatment. *American Journal of Psychiatry*, **145**, 926–36.

Livingstone, M. G. (1994). Risperidone. Lancet, **343**, 457–60.

Magnan, V. (1893). *Lecons cliniques sur les maladies mentales*. Bureaux de Progres Medical. Paris.

Marneros, A. and Deister, A. (1984). The psychopathology of 'late schizophrenia'. *Psychopathology*, **17**, 264–74.

Mathew, R. J., Wilson, W. H., Tant, S. R., Robinson, L., and Prakash, R. (1988). Abnormal resting regional cerebral blood flow patterns and their correlates in schizophrenia. *Archives of General Psychiatry*, **45**, 542–9.

Mayer, W. (1921). Uber paraphrene psychosen. *Zeitschrift fur die Gesamte Neurologie und Psychiatrie*, **71**, 187–206.

Miller, B., Benson, F., Cummings, J. L., and Neshkes, R. (1986). Late paraphrenia: an organic delusional syndrome. *Journal of Clinical Psychiatry*, **47**, 204–7.

Miller, B. L., Lesser, I. M., Boone, K., Goldberg, M., Hill, E., Miller, M. H., *et al.* (1989). Brain white-matter lesions and psychosis. *British Journal of Psychiatry*, **155**, 73–8.

Miller, B. L., Mena, I., Daly, J., Giombetti, R. J., Goldberg, M. A., Lesser, I., *et al.* (1990). Temporal-parietal hypoperfusion with SPECT in conditions other than Alzheimer's disease. *Dementia*, **1**, 41–5.

Miller, B. L., Lesser, I. M., Boone, K., Hill, E., Mehringer, C., and Wong, K. (1991). Brain lesions and cognitive function in late-life psychosis. *British Journal of Psychiatry*, **158**, 76–82.

Miller, B. L., Lesser, I. M., Mena, I., Villanueva-Meyer, J., Hill-Gutierrez, E., Boone, K., *et al.* (1992). Regional cerebral blood flow in late-life-onset psychosis. *Neuropsychiatry, Neuropsychology and Behavioural Neurology*, **5**, 132–7.

Moore, N. C. (1981). Is paranoid illness associated with sensory deficits in the elderly? *Journal of Psychosomatic Research*, **25**, 69–74.

Murray, R. M., O'Callaghan, E., Castle, D. J., and Lewis, S. W. (1992). A neurodevelopmental approach to the classification of schizophrenia. *Schizophrenia Bulletin*, **18**, 319–32.

Myers, J. S., Rogers, R. L., Judd, B. W., Mortel, K. F., and Sims, P. (1988). Cognition and cerebral blood flow fluctuate together in multi-infarct dementia. Stroke, **19**, 163–9.

Naguib, M. and Levy, R. (1987). Late paraphrenia: neuropsychological impairment and structural brain abnormalities on computed tomography. *International Journal of Geriatric Psychiatry*, **2**, 83–90.

Naguib, M., McGuffin, P., Levy, R., Festenstein, H., and Alonso, A. (1987). Genetic markers in late paraphrenia: a study of HLA antigens. *British Journal of Psychiatry*, **150**, 124–7.

Oberholzer, A. F., Hendriksen, C., Monsch, A. U., Heierli, B., and Stahelin, H. B. (1992). Safety and effectiveness of low-dose clozapine in psychogeriatric patients: a preliminary study. *International Psychogeriatrics*, **4**, 187–95.

Pearlson, G. D. and Rabins, P. V. (1988). The late onset psychoses: possible risk factors. *Psychiatric Clinics of North America*, **11**, 15–32.

Pearlson, G. D., Kreger, L., Rabins, P., Chase, G. A., Cohen, B., Wirth, J., *et al.* (1989). A chart review study of late-onset and early-onset schizophrenia. *American Journal of Psychiatry*, **146**, 1568–74.

Pearlson, G. D., Tune, L. E., Wong, D. F., Aylward, E., Barta, P., Powers, R. E., *et al.* (1993). Quantitative D_2 dopamine receptor PET and structural MRI changes in late-onset schizophrenia. *Schizophrenia Bulletin*, **19**, 783–95.

Post, F. (1965). *The clinical psychiatry of late life*. Pergamon, Oxford.

Post, F. (1966). *Persistent persecutory states of the elderly*. Pergamon, Oxford.

Quintal, M., Day-Cody D., and Levy R. (1991). Late paraphrenia and ICD-10. *International Journal of Geriatric Psychiatry*, **6**, 111–16.

Rabins, P. V., Pauker, S., and Thomas, J. (1984). Can schizophrenia begin after age 44? *Comprehensive Psychiatry*, **25**, 290–3.

Rabins, P. V., Pearlson, G., Jayaram, G., Steele, C., and Tune, L. (1987). Ventricle-to-brain ratio in late-onset schizophrenia. *American Journal of Psychiatry*, **144**, 1216–18.

Raskind, M. A. and Risse, S. C. (1986). Antipsychotic drugs and the elderly. *Journal of Clinical Psychiatry*, **47**, (Suppl.), 17–22.

Retterstol, N. (1966). *Paranoid and paranoiac psychoses. A personal follow-up investigation with special reference to aetiological, clinical and prognostic aspects. Oslo Universitetsforlaget*. Thomas, Springfield, IL.

Risberg, J. (1987). Frontal lobe degeneration of non-Alzheimer type. III. Regional cerebral blood flow. *Archives of Gerontoloy and Geriatrics*, **6**, 225–33.

Roth, M. and Kay, D. W. K. (1999). Late paraphrenia: a variant of schizophrenia manifest in late life or an organic clinical syndrome? A review of recent evidence. *International Journal of Geriatric Psychiatry*, **13**, 775–84.

Roth, M. and Morrisey, J. (1952). Problems in the diagnosis and classification of mental disorders in old age. *Journal of Mental Science*, **98**, 66–80.

Sadzot, B., Baraban, J. M., Glennon, R. A., Lyon, R. A., Leonhardt, S., Jan, C-R., *et al.* (1989). Hallucinogenic drug interactions at human brain 5-HT2 receptors: implications for treating LSD-induced hallucinogenesis. *Psychopharmacology*, **98**, 495–9.

Saunders, A., Strittmater, W., Schmechel, D., St George-Hyslop, P., Pericak-Vance, M., Joo, S., *et al.* (1993). Association of apolipoprotein E allele e4 with late-onset familial and sporadic Alzheimer's disease. *Neurology*, **43**, 1467–72.

Shimizu, A. and Kurachi, M. (1989). Do women without a family history of schizophrenia have a later onset of schizophrenia? *Japanese Journal of Psychiatry and Neurology*, **43**, 133–6.

Sjoegren, H. (1964). Paraphrenic, melancholic and psychoneurotic states in the pre-senile and senile periods of life. *Acta Psychiatrica Scandinavica*, Supplement 176.

Sternberg, E. (1972). Neuere forschungsergebnisse bei spatschizophrenen psychosen. *Fortschritte der Neurologie Psychiatrie*, **40**, 631–46.

Symonds, L. L., Olichney, J. M., Jernigan, T. L., Corey-Bloom, J., Healy, J. F., and Jeste, D. V. (1997). Lack of clinically significant gross structural abnormalities in MRIs of older patients with schizophrenia and related psychoses. *Journal of Neuropsychiatry and Clinical Neuroscience*, **9**, 251–8.

Tran-Johnson, T. K., Harris, M. J., and Jeste, D. V. (1994). Pharmacological treatment of schizophrenia and delusional disorder of late life. In *Principles and practice of geriatric psychiatry* (ed. J. R. M. Copeland, M. T. Abou-Saleh, and D. G. Blazer), pp. 685–92. Wiley, New York.

Weinberger, D. R., Berman, K. F., and Illowsky, B. P. (1988). Physiological dysfunction of dorsolateral prefrontal cortex in schizophrenia. *Archives of General Psychiatry*, **45**, 609–15.

WHO (World Health Organization). (1984). *9th revision of the International classification of diseases: mental disorders*. WHO, Geneva.

WHO (World Health Organization). (1992). *The ICD-10 classification of mental and behavioural disorders*. WHO, Geneva.

Wong, D. F., Gjedde, J., and Wagner, H. N. (1986*a*). Quantification of neuroreceptors in the living human brain. 1. Irreversible binding of ligands. *Journal of Cerebral Blood Flow and Metabolism*, **6**, 137–46.

Wong, D. F., Gjedde, J., Wagner, H. N., Dannals, R. F., Douglas, K. H., Links, J. M., *et al.* (1986*b*). Quantification of neuroreceptors in the living human brain. 2. Assessment of receptor density and affinity using inhibition studies. *Journal of Cerebral Blood Flow and Metabolism*, **6**, 147–53.

Wong, D. F., Wagner, H. N., Tune, L. E., Dannals, R. F., Pearlson, G. D., Links J. M., *et al.* (1986*c*). Positron emission tomography reveals elevated D_2 dopamine receptors in drug-naive schizophrenics. *Science*, **234**, 1558–63.

Zimbardo, P. G., Anderson, S. M., and Kabat, L. G. (1981). Induced hearing deficit generates experimental paranoia. *Science*, **212**, 1529–31.

33 Graduates

Patrick Campbell and Hema Ananth

Introduction

'Graduates' is a term that was originally applied to people who entered mental hospitals as non-elderly patients and stayed on in the institution, 'graduating' to elderly status. Arie and Jolley (1982) introduced the term for people (about 20% of the UK mental hospital population, they said) who were defined by the 1972 planning guidelines for the elderly mentally ill (DHSS 1972) as 'Patients who entered hospitals for the mentally ill before modern methods of treatment were available and have grown old in them after many years there'. The guidelines had given a succinct summary of what was thought to be needed for them: 'Number diminishing. New accommodation not needed, but improved conditions'.

At that time, many other psychiatrists and policy-makers would have agreed with Arie and Jolley's prediction that 'most are likely to live out their lives in hospital', a forecast which seemed both realistic and humane. Now, however, most mental hospitals in England have closed or are to close in line with government policy (Jenkins 1994), and those graduates able to survive long enough have been, or will be, rehoused elsewhere, perhaps included in reprovision plans mainly aimed at patients with Alzheimer's disease, or moved to a variety of community settings, or transferred to other hospitals.

There is no term yet for people with mental illness enduring into old age who are not long-term hospital residents but whose needs will require continuing attention in the community. The term 'graduates' now needs to encompass them too.

Hospital closure plans have brought this under-championed group of patients more to the fore. *Forget me not*, the Audit Commission's (2000) review of services for older people with mental health problems, includes a very brief mention, noting, rather clumsily, that: 'A small number of people who developed severe and enduring mental health problems when young, such as schizophrenia, are growing older...Many are physically frail and need considerable support'. Others, recognizing more emphatically the significance of the conjunction of hospital closures and an ageing population, call for greater recognition of the needs of this neglected group (e.g. Abdul-Hamid *et al.* 1998; Rodriguez-Ferrera and Vassilas 1998, Palmer *et al.* 1999*b*). In the USA, deinstitutionalization advanced earlier and faster, impelled by social and fiscal reformers temporarily united by a rare 'coalescence of ideologies' (Bachrach 1997): the Committee on Aging of the Group for the Advancement of Psychiatry has now recognized a 'crisis' with respect to the understanding of the nature and treatment of schizophrenia in older persons, and critical gaps in service provision (Cohen *et al.* 2000). Cost considerations (Knapp 1997) may encourage greater political recognition. A study in the USA showed that costs for the most elderly patients with schizophrenia are similar to those for the youngest, and higher than for those of intermediate age (Cuffel *et al.* 1996).

The last decade has seen a welcome proliferation of research into the nature of the disabilities of graduate patients: old assumptions that they are simply 'institutionalized' people who missed the boat of modern treatment are no longer good enough. Now that graduates are recognized as more than an embarrassing reminder of the under-visited back wards of old mental hospitals and of failures and limitations of treatment, they can be seen to share with their counterparts outside hospital a continuing significance for psychiatry. This goes far beyond the still-pressing territorial question of whether they should be cared for by psychiatrists for general adult mental illness, or by psychiatrists for the elderly, or go on being at risk of being relatively ignored by both. Quite apart from the immediate clinical priorities of finding better ways to meet the needs of graduate patients and their carers, the possibility exists that research into the nature of mental illness as its sufferers approach, or reach, the end of their lives may yield fundamental discoveries about its pathogenesis and the validity, or otherwise, of diagnostic categorization.

The problems of characterization: the historical perspective

Questions about who mental hospital graduates are, and why they remained so long in hospital, touch on important uncertainties: about the causes and natural history of mental illness and of schizophrenia in particular, rates of mortality and onset of Alzheimer's disease and other physical illnesses and handicaps in mentally ill people, rates of potential recruitment by attainment of 'new long-stay' status, the consequences of institutional care, the effectiveness and hazards of treatments, variations in local policies for discharge and resettlement, and social and medical attitudes towards elderly people with mental disorder. Since the age of 60 or 65 is commonly taken as a cut-off point in research studies of patients with adult-onset mental illness, and studies in psychiatry of the elderly have tended to concentrate on illnesses with an onset or first presentation in old age, these questions are hard to answer.

Surveys of mental hospital populations formerly provided the main avenue by which knowledge about graduates reached the medical literature. Clinical experience of graduate patients as individuals is seldom documented, and the richness of their diversity receives scant justice. For Pitt (1982), elderly chronic schizophrenics are a 'hardy, eccentric group who need very little care until they become physically infirm with age. They have become well adjusted to life in a mental hospital and are often useful in carrying out ward chores'. From Glenside Hospital (Ford *et al.* 1987) the view sounded less sanguine: there the long-stay 'remnant', mostly over age 55, male, and suffering from schizophrenia, were found to have poor social functioning and few outside contacts. 'These severely handicapped people continue to live in impoverished ward environments with only minimal staff. They also suffer personal poverty, no longer being able to supplement their income from industrial therapy; they survive on a basic allowance which scarcely provides a packet of cigarettes a day'. Mayer-Gross, Slater and Roth (1954) wrote of the chronic patient with schizophrenia who had 'come to an arrangement with his illness' and observed that 'Judged by their physique many schizophrenics look much younger than their years, especially if they live a sheltered life in hospital'. 'Nevertheless', they added, retaining the statement even in the 1969 edition of their textbook, 'on the average they die comparatively early, from tuberculosis or some other intercurrent illness'.

Today, causes of death are unlikely to include tuberculosis, but how much else has changed? Are elderly hospital graduates hardy survivors or underprivileged and specially handicapped victims, or, in varying degree, both at once? Seeking an answer in the literature by extrapolating the results of studies on non-elderly long-stay patients is tempting when specific studies on many aspects of the graduate population are still so few, but may be misleading.

Statistics

Counting the numbers of mental hospital graduates is not without its problems, since age and length of stay or duration of illness are commonly not taken into account when enumerating the graduate group within a hospital or other specified population, and terms like 'old long-stay' may have a variety of meanings. 'Old' in this sense is usually contrasted with 'new', and refers to the duration of the current admission rather than to the patient's chronological age. Referring to patients who were 'old' long-stay in this sense, the DHSS (1975) stated in *Better services for the mentally ill*, 'They are not easy to define in numerical terms'. At the time of the census of mental hospitals in 1971 there were 104 638 occupied beds in mental illness hospitals in England, of which 75 923 were occupied by patients who had been in hospital for more than one year; 57% of this group had been in hospital for more than 10 years, and 39% (0.65 per 1000 population) more than 20 years.

By 1986 elderly patients constituted nearly two-thirds of resident hospital patients (DHSS 1988). Of 60 280 people resident in mental illness beds at the end of 1986, 34 340 were aged over 65 years; 21 500 had been resident for more than a year and 11 300 for more than 5 years. In the previous decade, there had been a fall of 15.7% in the numbers of resident elderly people compared to a 40% fall in younger patients. Therefore at the start of the 1990s, surviving mental hospitals were 'increasingly dominated by their population of elderly patients' (Benbow and Jolley 1992). In the USA in 1955 there were 560 000 people in state mental hospitals, a figure that fell to 77 000 for a larger population; this represented a fall from 339 to 31 per 100 000, with the latter constituting possibly only 3% of people with schizophrenia (Bachrach 1997). The transfer of elderly hospital residents to other institutions such as large nursing homes occurred on so great a scale as to earn the new word of 'transinstitutionalization', but elderly patients still constituted over 20% of the census of American state hospitals (Moak 1990). In Italy, 25 000 people were reported (Crepet 1990) to be the 'asylum residue' in the mental hospitals banned by Law 180 of 1978; Jones and Poletti (1986) noted that those residents admitted before 1980 were regarded simply as the victims of institutional oppression. In Spain, a decisive policy of closing psychiatric hospitals in Andalusia has seen the Institute of Social Services taking many aged adults from psychiatric long-stay wards into its institutions (Torres-Gonzalez 1995).

Hitherto, studies of the prevalence of graduate-type people in community populations have been very limited and not specially targeted. An attempt in South Camden (Campbell *et al.* 1990) to identify all patients with schizophrenia known to health, social, and voluntary services on a single day revealed a very high prevalence of schizophrenia in this inner-city area of 55 000 people. Of the 530 total identified 20% were in hospital. 65 people were identified with schizophrenia and age over 65, of whom 23% were in hospital. 12 of the 65 had a secondary diagnosis of senile dementia (Taylor 1990, personal communication). Studies of the prevalence of schizophrenia in a rural site in Scotland compared with two urban areas in South London by McCreadie *et al.* (1997*b*) showed similar figures for White males and females over the age of 60 (18–19% and 24–26%, respectively of the cases identified), with much lower figures for non-White (0% in Scotland, 6–8% in London). In an age- and sex-stratified sample of 5222 people aged 65 or over taken from general practitioner lists in Liverpool, Copeland *et al.* (1998) found a prevalence of DSM-III-R schizophrenia of 0.12% and of delusional disorder 0.04%. No cases of schizophrenia were found in a similar study in Dublin by Kirby *et al.* (1997).

The rising proportion of elderly graduates

Even a century ago, the increasing proportion of elderly people in asylums was causing concern to the Commissioners in Lunacy, whose report on Friern Hospital in 1894 noted that more than 10% of the hospital population were aged 65 and over (Hunter and Macalpine 1974). In the period before closure, that proportion had risen greatly. At Knowle, for instance, Shawcross *et al.* (1987) reported that 30% of the long-stay patients not cared for by psychogeriatricians were aged over 65 years. In two mental hospitals in Leicester, Levene *et al.* (1985) found that more than half (59%) of the 26% of patients who had been inpatients for more than 10 years were aged over 65, with 31% of this group aged 75 or over, and 7% aged 85 or more. Clifford *et al.* (1991) surveyed five hospitals and, within them, all those patients without a diagnosis of senile dementia who had been in hospital for over a year. The population (numbering 1308, with a slight predominance of females) was predominantly elderly, with an average age of 64.5 years and an average length of stay of 24.5 years—70% had a diagnosis of schizophrenia, 40% were aged over 70. In Cane Hill Hospital before it closed in 1992, the mean age of the 246 long-stay patients was 67, and the average length of stay was 26 years (quoted by Leff 1997*a*). In Broadmoor, 8% of patients were aged over 60 years, and most had been admitted in their twenties and thirties (Wong *et al.* 1995, quoted by Yorston 1999).

Rates of decline and recruitment

Surveys of Glenside Hospital in Bristol, between 1960 and 1985 (Ford *et al.* 1987), showed that the rate of decline of the hospital population appeared to be slowing. Nearly one-third of the patients in 1985 had been resident since 1960. Before the era of widespread mental hospital closures, death rather than discharge had accounted for most of the decline in numbers of graduates and other long-stay patients (Wing 1986). Their declining number in UK mental hospitals is illustrated in Jennings *et al.*'s (1989) review of the evidence from eight UK case-registers between the end of 1977 and of 1983. The elderly occupied at least half the beds in all areas, and around a third of beds were occupied by the very-long-stay (5 years and over), of whom the majority were elderly. Case-register statistics suffer from a difficulty in distinguishing between elderly inpatients suffering from diseases of old age and those who become old in hospital. An attempt to separate the two, by examining patients aged under 65 at the start of their admission, showed that at least two-thirds of elderly very-long-stay patients were admitted before their 65th birthday; 90% or more of elderly patients with schizophrenia were admitted before age 65. To interpret such figures, and the wide variation between different areas, demands recognition of the need to adjust for population changes (Der 1989), the local demography, and correlations between the scale of need for hospital beds and indices of social deprivation such as Jarman's (1983), as well as differences in practice and policy (Hirsch 1988). In Scotland, for instance, closure plans developed more gradually, and bed occupancy had been higher than in England (Wing 1986). There, too, great variations were seen, as shown by McCreadie *et al.*'s (1991) survey of long-stay patients (defined as those admitted before the age of 65 and resident for more than 6 years), in psychiatric hospitals serving more than 83% of the Scottish population. Across hospitals, long-stay patients accounted for 19 to 123 per 100 000 population, with an overall rate of 59 per 100 000. Most patients were male, single, and over 60 years of age, and 41% had been in hospital more than 30 years.

Predicting the need for beds

Within the hospital population, predictive studies of which patients were to become graduates are lacking. Findings from a survey at Friern Hospital (1983), a large Victorian asylum in North London which was closed in 1993, showed that the numbers of patients who remained in the hospital from admissions in each half-decade of the half-century prior to 1975 until the census date in 1983 stayed surprisingly constant, apart from a small dip in the war years (Table 33.1). Examination of the age structure of the hospital population showed a median age of 59 for patients with schizophrenia (Fig. 33.1). There was no obvious change in numbers from before or

Table 33.1 Year of current admission to Friern Hospital—52% of patients had stayed less than 4 years; 50 patients had stayed longer than 50 years

Year of admission	Number of patients
Before 1920	5
1920 – 1924	12
1925 – 1929	18
1930 – 1934	26
1935 – 1939	28
1940 – 1944	16
1945 – 1949	25
1950 – 1954	30
1955 – 1959	33
1960 – 1964	37
1965 – 1969	43
1970 – 1974	37
1975 – 1979	138
1980 – 1983	391

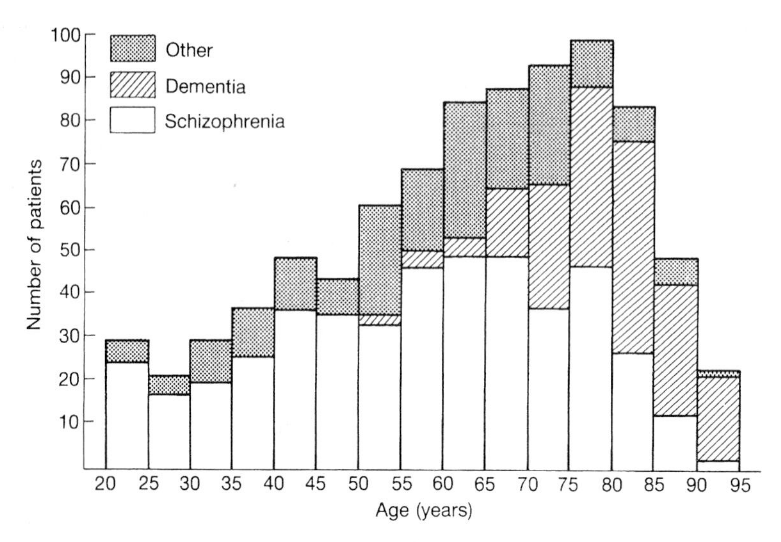

Fig. 33.1 Age structure and diagnosis (Friern Hospital 1983).

after the introduction of modern treatments. The figures show that there was a continuing core of patients, albeit a very small minority of acute admissions, whose illnesses were so disabling that prolonged hospital care continued to be an unavoidable requirement.

The 1970s saw the emerging recognition of a 'new' long-stay population in mental hospitals, suffering from a variety of persistent severe disabilities, most commonly schizophrenia, affective illness, and organic disorders (Bewley *et al.* 1981). Mann and Cree (1976) surveyed 15 mental hospitals in England and Wales to study patients under the age of 65 who had stayed for 1 to 3 years. Over 50% of the study sample were aged over 45 and only 17% had been admitted for the first time; one-quarter of them had spent more than 5 years in a mental hospital before the present admission. The authors suggested that 34% needed further hospital care; their estimate of need had already been quoted in *Better services for the mentally ill* (DHSS 1975). This document had stressed that the guidelines it gave for the bed needs in the new service 'are in addition to the beds—gradually declining in numbers—which will be required for many years to meet the needs of the 'old' long-stay patients...who are already in the mental illness hospitals'. A study in Scotland (McCreadie *et al.* 1985) of 14 hospitals serving 56% of the Scottish population found that only 20% of the 'new long-stay' patients aged 18–64 had been discharged 2 years later. 'Many of the new chronics will become old chronics', concluded the authors. In Clifford *et al.*'s (1991) survey of five hospitals, one in three of the patients who had stayed for more than a year had been in hospital for less than 10 years, showing that patients were still accumulating in these hospitals.

In 1992, a national audit of new long-stay patients was undertaken on a cohort of patients in England and Wales, with some also from Scotland and Northern Ireland, by the Royal College of Psychiatrists Research Unit (Lelliott *et al.* 1994). This was a major enterprise designed to provide guidance for policy-makers, purchasers, and clinicians about service structure, service delivery, and clinical practice. Psychiatrists from 59 services participated, and patients were included if, on the census day, they were aged 18–64 at the time of admission and had been occupying a hospital bed for between 6 months and 3 years. A cohort of 431 patients resident in hospital for between 1 and 3 years was directly comparable to another cohort studied 20 years earlier by Mann and Cree (1976). Compared to the 1972 sample, the 1992 cohort had a higher proportion of men, single people, those with a diagnosis of schizophrenia, those admitted formally, and fewer first admissions. The most striking differences were that the 1992 cohort was much more likely to be detained (29% vs. 9%) at the time of admission and to have had multiple admissions. Overall, the cohort was heterogeneous, with the younger patients (aged between 18 and 34) predominantly single males, often with a history of violence or criminality; 35% were formally detained. The older group (aged 55–67) included a larger proportion of women who were married or had been married. They had fewer positive symptoms but poorer physical health, and were thought to have been at risk of physical neglect if discharged. This age/gender distribution, with the younger new long-stay patients predominantly male, and the older, female, had been consistently noted (e.g. in Mann and Cree 1976; Clifford *et al.* 1991). Combining prevalence data led Kavanagh *et al.* (1995) to estimate that of the 13% of patients with schizophrenia who were hospital inpatients, about two-thirds were long-stay.

Against a background of falling rates for long-stay inpatients, Holloway *et al.* (1999) found that a 1995 cohort from a deprived inner-city catchment area were more symptomatic than the 1993 cohort, more commonly detained, and more often from an ethnic minority. Only 9% remained inpatients for the entire 4-year follow-up.

Predicting needs for services

In the postclosure era, the prediction of future need should be based on epidemiological work in community populations as a whole, but such knowledge is generally lacking. The concept of the 'undischargeable' patient in a hospital bed must give way to a notion of people in a defined population with a range of needs associated with continuing high dependence on services, as explored by Wykes (1983) in Camberwell. From this perspective, the long-term highly dependent patient, other than people with Alzheimer's disease, will most commonly suffer from schizophrenia, but nearly half the total will have other disorders such as short-cycle manic depressive psychoses, chronic depression, or severe chronic neuroses. Personality disorders and alcohol abuse are common complications. Many patients have multiple disabilities, such as epilepsy, learning disabilities, brain damage, sensory deficits, and neurological disorders and physical illness (Wing 1986). The impact of recreational drug use can be expected to affect the future pattern of psychotic and other disorders in older people. Differential take-up of services by ethnic minorities, and the advancing age of the Afro-Caribbean urban population with a heightened prevalence of schizophrenia will require particular attention.

But our question here must be more specific. How many of these patients will graduate to elderly status and still need services? How many people are there now, who are at present not in hospital but are approaching old age—in the care, perhaps, of elderly siblings or very elderly parents—who will no longer be supportable outside institutional care when their carers become incapacitated or die? The patients of the new postclosure era are likely to be very different from those who spent many years in hospital and were, as Lamb (1993), observing from the USA, describes it, 'institutionalized into passivity'. A comparison of a rural population of people with schizophrenia surveyed in 1981 and again in 1996 in an area with good service provision (Kelly *et al.* 1998), shows the price that may be paid for the greater freedom of treatment in the community rather than hospital: the patients in the more recent cohort were more severely ill, as measured by mental state assessment, and there were more adverse effects of drugs. There was no change in social adjustment.

Psychiatric diagnosis

In recent times, the great majority of graduate patients in mental hospitals have suffered from schizophrenia. The diagnosis of affective psychosis is far behind in second place, followed by small numbers of other diagnoses including learning disability, personality disorders, and organic disorders other than Alzheimer's disease at the time of admission. Some have supervening dementia. Cunningham Owens and Johnstone's

(1980) survey of all the patients in Shenley Hospital provides illustrative figures: 524 of 635 patients resident for at least a year were diagnosed as having schizophrenia by Feighner (1972) criteria, with males slightly outnumbering women; 47 fulfilled St Louis criteria for primary affective disorder, with a preponderance of women. At Glenside (Ford *et al.* 1987) 76% of patients resident for 5 years or more had schizophrenia, compared to 5% with dementia. By 1990 (Eastley and Lucas 1992), the proportion of patients with schizophrenia at Glenside had fallen to 65% and with dementia had risen to 10%, reflecting the death of many old long-stay patients with schizophrenia and the greater longevity of patients with dementia. At Friern (1983), the comparable population had 74% schizophrenia, 7% primary senile dementia, and 5% primary affective disorder.

Reports of these surveys, as is so often the case, do not provide figures for the graduate population as such. A common finding is the relative predominance of men in the long-stay population (e.g. Ford *et al.* 1987; Leff 1991; McCreadie *et al.* 1991). This may be consistent with evidence of a relatively better prognosis for schizophrenia in women (Angermeyer *et al.* 1989; Harrison *et al.* 1996), but this gender difference tends to be more marked in short-term, rather than very long-term outcome (Yassa *et al.* 1991; Lewis 1992). The generally greater longevity of women should tend to reduce or reverse this predominance in the graduates over 65.

Hospital surveys reveal other minor but significant diagnostic subgroups among hospital graduates, such as patients with learning disability, who may formerly have received care in mental handicap hospitals. A similar variety of diagnoses has been recorded among the 'new long-stay'. Mann and Cree (1976) found remarkably few differences between the 15 hospitals they studied—schizophrenia, at 44.4%, was less common, and affective disorders, at 15.8%, more common than in graduate hospital populations.

How younger people with psychiatric illnesses other than schizophrenia progress into old age appears to have been little studied in recent years, though excess mortality is well recognized (Lloyd *et al.* 1996). Nor is it easy to find discussion in the psychogeriatric literature of the significance of the psychiatric history prior to old age. Reviews of natural history and chronicity in affective disorder (e.g. Scott 1988) have emphasized the frequent occurrence of a chronic course for depression, particularly in women. A past history of depression is said to be a risk factor for depression in later life (e.g. Evans and Mottram 2000), and it is commonly stated that in recurrent affective disorder the episodes of illness become longer and the intervals between episodes of unipolar or bipolar relapse become shorter with increasing age, but these familiar clinical axioms do not appear to have been examined by recent research. The extent to which early-onset depression may be a risk factor for the later development of dementia is still uncertain, and the question may become confused with the different issue of how often depression is a prodromal symptom of incipient dementia (See Chapter 27). A Swedish population study by Pálsson *et al.* (1999) of a sample of 85-year-olds showed an increased risk of dementia where there was a history of early-onset major depression (before age 65) but not for later-onset depression. Other studies do not provide a clear consensus. A history of major psychiatric illness long preceding, and apparently unrelated to, the onset of dementia was found by Cooper and Holmes (1998) in 12.5% of 559 people with dementia entered on the Camberwell dementia case register, compared to 3.4% who had a history of psychiatric illness before the age of 70 in a matched control group, a highly significant difference with an odds ratio of 3.6. The significance of white matter abnormalities on magnetic resonance imaging (MRI), if detectable before the age of 65, for subsequent outcome in the older age group where such lesions appear to be associated with poorer cognitive performance (Kramer-Ginsberg *et al.* 1999) and for outcome of depression (O'Brien *et al.* 1998), is still uncertain.

The disabilities of graduate patients

A very wide range of disabilities is found in the graduate population in mental hospitals. At one extreme are physically fit and active elderly people, who remained in hospital primarily because they had nowhere else to go or because of their determined opposition to discharge. At the other are people so helplessly disabled as to need total nursing care, whose disability may have been attributed, rightly or wrongly, to supervening Alzheimer's disease. Neither the duration of stay in hospital nor graduate status alone provide a sound basis for planning appropriate care in other environments.

Cognitive impairments in graduate patients

Does functional mental illness damage intellectual ability, and if it does, what is the nature of the cognitive deficit, and is it progressive? The past decade has seen a remarkable proliferation of research into these questions. Repeated demonstration of cognitive impairment with onset at a relatively early age in a proportion of patients with schizophrenia (reported, for example, by Taylor and Abrams 1984) was often dismissed on ideological grounds as explicable by psychological factors of motivated withdrawal, environmental factors of institutional care, or purported invalidity of test results.

Kraepelin (1920), towards the end of his career, acknowledged the many factors which might cause schizophrenic symptoms, but none the less employed the phrases 'destruction of conscious volition' and 'irreversible dementing cortical disturbances' to characterize dementia praecox, even in an era when the progressive restriction of the term 'dementia' to cognitive deterioration was well established (Berrios 1990) and Bleuler's introduction of a more 'psychological' approach to schizophrenia was well known. But Mayer-Gross, Slater, and Roth (1954–69), in all editions of their textbook, continued to aver that: 'If dementia is used...as meaning impairment of intelligence, in contrast to impairment of personality, schizophrenia does not lead to dementia', and that: 'Potentially his [the schizophrenic's] formal intelligence is preserved and so is his knowledge'. They did, however, concede that this statement: 'while certainly adequate for the great majority of chronic schizophrenics', might not be sufficient for all, since: 'Some, who are often compared to burned-out ruins, come very close to the picture of organic dementia'.

Nowadays, however, poor performance on psychological tests is regarded as evidence of 'genuine' cognitive impairment in the majority of non-elderly patients with schizophrenia, correlating with 'real-life' functional disability and outcome (Klapow *et al.* 1997; Harvey *et al.* 1998). O'Carroll (2000) provides a valuable review of the field. His summary of recent research findings includes the following conclusions: significant cognitive impairment is common in schizophrenia, affecting up to 75% of patients; a wide range of cognitive functions are affected, particularly memory, attention, motor skills, executive function, and intelligence; the cognitive impairment often pre-dates the illness onset; it is an intrinsic part of the illness and is observed in young, drug-naïve patients; efforts to explain the core features of schizophrenia as a consequence of specific neuropsychological abnormalities have been disappointing; cognitive impairment is related to social and functional outcome.

The wide range of impairments on cognitive testing, affecting all domains measured by standard clinical tests, emerges from a meta-analysis by Heinrichs and Zakzanis (1998) of 204 studies comparing schizophrenic patients with controls. Two studies demonstrating onset before overt illness are particularly remarkable. From among the 5362 individuals taken as a random sample of births in England, Scotland, and Wales during one week in 1946 for inclusion in the Medical Research Council's National Survey of Health and Development, some 30 patients developed schizophrenia between the ages of 16 and 43. These patients were found to have had low educational test scores at ages 8, 11, and 15 years, with earlier developmental delays in walking, more speech problems, and poorer social skills (Jones *et al.* 1994). Low intelligence and poor performance on verbal tasks and a mechanical knowledge test were identified as risk factors for the later development of schizophrenia in a study of 50 000 men conscripted into the Swedish Army between 1969 and 1970, of whom 195 were later admitted to hospital with schizophrenia (David *et al.* 1997).

The functional consequence of neurocognitive deficits in schizophrenia is a growing field of research interest, which has been reviewed by Green *et al.* (2000). They propose that concepts such as learning potential and social cognition can act as mediating mechanisms through which basic neurocognitive processes are related to skill acquisition and functional outcome. Earlier interest in the possibility that patterns of test results may indicate particular kinds of brain localization of the underlying pathology, an approach which has yielded no clear consensus, is now regarded by O'Carroll (2000) as 'old fashioned', having been based on tests largely devised to identify specific brain damage in an era before high-resolution brain imaging was possible. Schizophrenia does not appear to be associated with a characteristic 'signature' pointing to lateralized or differential cognitive impairment (Blanchard and Neale 1994). The possibility still exists, however, that different clusters of cognitive impairments (such as the five identified by Heinrichs and Awad (1993) in a factor-analytic study of four cognitive tests in 104 patients with chronic schizophrenia) could reduce and clarify some of the heterogeneity of schizophrenia's clinical presentation and outcome.

Of particular relevance to graduate patients are the questions as to whether the cognitive impairment so often associated with schizophrenia becomes worse over time, perhaps aggravated by extraneous factors such as institutional and drug treatment, and whether it leads to an enhanced susceptibility to Alzheimer's disease. The clinical experience is that outcomes are very diverse: although some patients show a progressive worsening of cognitive performance, perhaps leading to the picture of dementia, others do not. A review by Rund (1998) of 15 studies with a follow-up period of at least a year concludes that after the onset of schizophrenia, cognitive deficits are relatively stable over long periods. Such evidence is interpreted as suggesting that schizophrenia is not a degenerative process but a static encephalopathy. A distinction between the cognitive impairments associated with schizophrenia and with Alzheimer's disease has been drawn from cross-sectional studies which have included elderly patients with schizophrenia. Heaton *et al.* (1994), for instance, compared normal controls, ambulatory patients with Alzheimer's disease, and three groups of patients with schizophrenia (early onset-young, early onset-old, and late onset) on a battery of tests and concluded that the neuropsychological impairment is unrelated to current age, age at onset, or duration of illness. The three schizophrenic groups were similar to one another on test performance, but different from normal controls or patients with Alzheimer's disease. A study by McGurk *et al.* (2000) of 168 elderly patients with schizophrenia, followed up on average 15 months later, confirmed and extended earlier studies that cognitive impairments are predictive, both cross-sectionally and longitudinally, of adaptive life skills. Negative symptoms, but not positive symptoms, were correlated with impaired adaptive skills. Positive correlation of cognitive decline with age and/or duration of illness is noted in some studies (e.g. Cuesta *et al.* 1998; Seno *et al.* 1998) but not in others (e.g. Mockler *et al.* 1997). The majority of 31 elderly patients with schizophrenia (aged 60–76 years) studied by Heinik *et al.* (1997) scored below the normal range in the clock-drawing test of the Cambridge Cognitive Examination (Roth *et al.* 1998), and the impairment correlated with the duration of illness. Relative preservation of reading ability has been noted in several studies (e.g. Nelson *et al.* 1990; Harvey *et al.* 2000), thereby providing a stable measure of premorbid intelligence (Morrison *et al.* 2000).

The diversity of functional outcome in schizophrenia seems to be increased in elderly patients (Friedman *et al.* 1999), with marked cognitive decline occurring in some patients that can be correlated with poor functional outcome. Cognitive and functional decline over a 30-month period in a subset of geriatric patients with schizophrenia could be detected in a study of 326 patients by Harvey *et al.* (1999). The decline could not be attributed to a progressive degenerative dementing disease. Some 30% of patients with baseline scores in the less impaired range showed worsening of their scores to moderate or more severe impairment; however,

7% of the sample with lower baseline scores appeared to improve. Transatlantic comparison of patients with schizophrenia aged over 70 studied by Harvey *et al.* in New York and the Team for Assessment of Psychiatric Services, TAPS (Leff 1991) in London, (Harvey *et al.* 1997*a*), showed a similar severity of cognitive impairment and correlation with adaptive functioning but differences in three out of four measures of the latter, suggesting that cognitive impairment was a common feature in poor-outcome patients with schizophrenia, irrespective of the system of care, while adaptive functioning might be more responsive to environmental factors.

An interesting clinical pointer to severe cognitive deficit is the phenomenon of disorientation for personal age. Stevens *et al.* (1978) had found this to some degree in 25% of chronically ill schizophrenic patients. Several subjects had shown marked cognitive decline during the first few years of illness. At Shenley, Buhrich *et al.* (1988) found that 22 of 510 patients identified their age as being within 5 years of their first admission to mental hospital; a striking example of age-disorientation which was correlated with severe cognitive defects but found not to be related to premorbid IQ or past physical treatments. In a study by Harvey *et al.* (1995) which examined age-related changes in cognitive functioning in 393 patients with schizophrenia, ranging from 25 to 95 years of age, all test items changed with age linearly over time: with aspects of orientation, concentration, and delayed recall most impaired in younger patients; and naming and sentence repetition most preserved in the oldest patients. Patients with age-disorientation had more severe cognitive impairments at each age, and the age-related changes in global impairment were more severe in these patients. Age-disorientation proved extremely stable in a 1-year follow-up study. The same authors (Lombardi *et al.* 1996) found that age-disorientation—defined as the mis-stating of age by 5 years or more—was also evident in about 20% of a sample of geriatric patients with chronic mood disorders, and that these patients performed worse on the Mini-Mental State Examination (MMSE; Folstein *et al.* 1975) than those without. In a Canadian study of 110 patients with chronic illness, age-disorientation was found in 12 (28%) of the 43 patients who were institutionalized with schizophrenia (and 5 of the 12 had MMSE scores in the dementia range); but it was not observed in other patients with schizophrenia who were not institutionalized, nor in those with other psychoses, whether or not they were institutionalized (Gabriel 1997). The phenomenon was observed in only 6% of patients with schizophrenia in the long-stay wards of three Dutch mental hospitals by Selten and Cath (1995), who suggested it could result from an interaction between serious illness and poor psychosocial treatment. This view is opposed by Manschreck *et al.* (2000) who found that social withdrawal did not differentiate between age-disoriented patients, who constituted 30% of their sample, and matched controls. The age-disoriented patients were more severely impaired on various measures, including severity of symptoms and mental state performance.

The current surge of interest in the cognitive disorders of schizophrenia gives prominence to further questions about their potential mutability, including their possible aggravation by antipsychotic drug therapy, and their potential treatability by psychological and/or pharmacological means. Green and Neuchterlein (1999), for example, claim that: 'with a growing confidence that some neurocognitive deficits in schizophrenia can be modified, questions that seemed irrelevant only a few years ago are now fundamental.' The review by Sharma (1999) provides helpful guidance to the existing literature and complex methodological issues relating to typical and atypical antipsychotic drugs, from which emerges some evidence that atypical antipsychotics, especially clozapine, may sometimes improve some aspects of cognitive performance. The occurrence of severe neurocognitive deficits in patients never treated with antipsychotics (e.g. McCreadie *et al.* 1997*a*) indicates that although antipsychotic drugs may be contributory, they are not the cause of the cognitive impairments. This is the firm conclusion drawn by O'Carroll (2000), whose review also includes a helpful critique of 'cognitive rehabilitation' and its promise for the future. Studies in which the performance on particular tests can be improved by special coaching and inducements (e.g. Wexler *et al.* 1997) may not lead to gains in functional ability. Wykes *et al.* (1999), however, showed the possibility of a more generalized improvement on cognitive tests, and improved self-esteem, in a randomized controlled trial of a very intensive, individual 'cognitive remediation' package. Some improvement in cognition was also observed in the control group who received intensive occupational therapy.

Evidence for different syndromes within schizophrenia

The recent interest in cognitive impairment in schizophrenia as an intrinsic and early development in the evolution of the illness, extends earlier work which explored the possibility of characterizing different pathophysiologies and aetiologies in schizophrenia through analysis of clinical symptoms. The seminal pioneering studies of Wing and Brown (1970) had emphasized two clinical syndromes, one primarily characterized by social withdrawal and relatively stable over time, the other by productive psychotic symptoms and greater fluctuation. Recalling the evolution of these studies, Wing (1989) stated that for more than 30 years he had seen the relationship between psychological deficit (cognitive defect, negative syndrome) and the productive (florid, positive) symptoms as lying at the heart of the mystery of schizophrenia. In the 1950s it was easy to demonstrate a syndrome whose central characteristic, statistically, was social withdrawal, highly correlated with which were slowness, underactivity, poverty of speech, lack of interests, and poor self-care. The total sum was stable over quite long periods. Also associated, but less stable and subject to much greater fluctuation over time, was a syndrome termed 'socially embarrassing behaviour', composed of four elements: overactivity; talking to self; posturing and mannerisms; and threatening or violent behaviour. Further research into the possibility of identifying different syndromes within schizophrenia was further stimulated by Crow's hypotheses (1980, 1989) that two syndromes, type I and type II, represent independent dimensions of pathology in schizophrenia—with type II (characterized by negative symptoms such as flattened affect and poverty of speech) reflecting structural brain abnormality, which is also clinically manifest as cognitive deficit and abnormal involuntary movements. The concept of the negative syndrome was broadened by Andreasen (1982; Andreasen and Olsen 1982) who introduced the widely used Scale for Assessment of Negative Symptoms (SANS) comprising five subscales: blunted affect; alogia; avolition; anhedonia; and attentional impairment. A further distinction between primary and secondary negative symptoms, the latter resulting perhaps from social deprivation, depression, or drug side-effects, was drawn by Carpenter *et al.* (1985).

More recent work (reviewed by Liddle, Carpenter, and Crow 1994) examined the correlations of negative symptoms, which may be particularly striking in some graduate patients, perhaps accounting in large measure for the difficulty of achieving rehabilitation and resettlement. Semple *et al.* (1999), for instance, report an inverse relationship between interpersonal competence and negative symptoms in elderly patients compared to age-matched controls. Despite inconsistency of terminology and categorization of symptoms and other methodological problems, research has in general suggested the independence of positive and negative symptoms and intercorrelations between negative symptoms, cognitive impairments, and tardive dyskinesia, in support of the Crow model, and shown that negative symptoms can be reliably differentiated from depression (Kibel *et al.* 1993). Further elaboration of the Crow model to recognize three or more syndromes may be appropriate. A factor analysis of scale items on the SANS led Liddle (1987) to propose three syndromes, named as: psychomotor poverty (closely resembling, in Liddle's view, Crow's narrowly defined negative syndrome); disorganization (incorporating formal thought disorder); and reality distortion (various delusions and hallucinations). The three-dimensional model was found by Sauer *et al.* (1999) to be appropriate in 131 elderly patients with schizophrenia; negative and disorganized syndromes showed different correlations with neuropsychological and motor phenomena. Other attempts have been made to correlate the three syndromes with different patterns of performance on neurocognitive tests (e.g. Berman *et al.* 1997; Norman *et al.* 1997; Baxter and Liddle 1998). A quantified EEG study by Harris *et al.* (1999) favoured the three-syndrome model over the two-syndrome. A small MRI study by Chua *et al.* (1997) showed correlations between specific grey matter volumes and the psychomotor poverty and disorganization syndromes. Liddle (1987) acknowledges that the syndromes do not encompass all the symptoms of schizophrenia, and that incorporation of two further identifiable syndromes, of depression and psychomotor excitement, lead to a five-syndrome model. Cardno *et al.* (1996) suggest the 'positive' factor subdivides into paranoid symptoms, first-rank delusions and first-rank hallucinations. Another factor-analytic study by Lindenmayer *et al.* (1994) identified five factors as negative, positive, excitement, cognitive, and depression/anxiety domains. A Japanese study by Hori *et al.* (1999), using factor-analysis of items on the Manchester Scale, concludes that the classification of symptoms changes with increasing duration of illness. Negative symptoms appear to be more stable than positive over time, the latter showing a greater tendency to fluctuation, even in elderly patients (Putnam *et al.* 1996). Mojtabai (1999) reviewed 22 studies to examine the association of duration of illness with the structure of illness, and concluded that the structure of symptoms evolves over time, following a consistent pattern. In the early stages of illness, negative and positive symptoms form cohesive dimensions, but with time the dimensions become less cohesive and the boundaries less clear.

Further evidence of the heterogeneity of schizophrenia is provided by the more favourable outcome in developing countries, demonstrated, for example, by the WHO study (Jablensky *et al.* 1992). The possibility that schizophrenia with late onset after the age of 45 may be different from early-onset cases is discussed in Chapter 32. Schizoaffective disorder, also, has proved difficult to distinguish from schizophrenia (Evans *et al.* 1999*a*).

The search for structural brain abnormality

Progress in brain imaging techniques has confirmed the evidence of structural brain abnormalities in schizophrenia in both non-elderly and elderly patients, but earlier hopes that these could be correlated with illness severity, diagnostic subtype, or other clinical features of the illness have generally not been sustained. A study by Johnstone *et al.* (1990), for instance, showed that increased ventricular size in inpatients with schizophrenia was significantly associated with impaired social behaviour and with movement disorder, and was particularly evident in patients with early-onset illness. This suggests that at least some of the structural changes in schizophrenia may occur at a time when the brain is still developing, and that age of onset is an important determinant of social and intellectual impairment. Andreasen *et al.* (1990), however, in a study which provided a critical reappraisal of their earlier work, found that enlarged ventricles were not a statistically significant correlate of the 'negative' clinical subtype. They therefore had to conclude that the hypothesis of a type of schizophrenia due to early neurological injury had not been confirmed by computed tomography. A meta-analysis by Van Horn and McManus (1992) of 39 studies of ventricular:brain ratio (VBR) as a measure of ventricular size in schizophrenia concluded that, while there was an indisputable difference in VBR between patients with schizophrenia and controls, the difference was smaller than had formerly been thought and, although of theoretical interest as regards aetiology, it was probably too small to be of practical significance in diagnosis or the differentiation of subtypes. Davis *et al.* (1998) report a computed tomographic (CT) study repeated at an interval averaging 5 years, which indicated that progressive ventricular enlargement may be a feature of a subtype of patients with severe deficits in self-care, here defined as 'Kraepelinian'.

Brain imaging with MRI and single photon emission computed tomography (SPECT) did not provide a statistically significant differentiation of treatment-responsive and -unresponsive patients in a study by Lawrie *et al.* (1995), though the two groups were significantly differentiated by neuropsychological tests. In a review of 40 studies of volumetric MRI in schizophrenia, Lawrie and Abukmeil (1998) conclude that median percentage volume differences reveal that several brain structures are reduced in schizophrenia to a greater extent than expected from overall reductions in brain volume (found in all studies, to some small degree)—evident in both temporal lobes and the amygdala/hippocampal complex, with possible reductions in the parahippocampal and superior temporal gyri and the thalamus. Increases in the lateral ventricles were greatest in the body and occipital horns. Segmentation studies suggest that grey matter is reduced but that white matter volumes may be increased in men. Temporolimbic volume reductions in schizophrenia on MRI found by Gur *et al.* (2000) showed differences between the sexes in the amygdala and superior temporal gyrus, but hippocampal grey matter volume was reduced in both sexes for the hippocampus and temporal pole. The abnormalities were evident in patients with first-episode illness, and correlated more strongly with cognitive performance than symptom severity. Increased cerebellar vermis volume and a trend for more hemispheric volume asymmetry in patients with schizophrenia on MRI has been reported (Levitt *et al.* 1999) following interest in the possible role of the cerebellum in higher cognitive functions. Structural MRI data from 110 studies are reviewed by McCarley *et al.* (1999). Notable among the conclusions is the report that frontal lobe abnormalities were less consistently found than evidence for functional frontal lobe dysfunction might suggest; 55% of studies described volume reduction. Most of the data were consistent with a developmental model, but growing evidence was compatible, also, with progressive, neurodegenerative features, suggesting a 'two-hit' model of schizophrenia. Affective disorders do not show similar features.

Functional brain-imaging techniques, such as fMRI (functional MRI), PET, SPECT and MRS (magnetic resonance spectroscopy) (Buckley and Friedman 2000), offer hope of further clarification. For example, a PET study showed that 'hypofrontality' in schizophrenia, indicated by reduced prefrontal blood flow and relative failure of activation of the left dorsolateral prefrontal cortex on the performance of cognitive tasks, may be symptom-related and remit with improvement (Spence *et al.* 1998).

Another perspective on the possibility of demonstrating structural brain abnormalities in patients with schizophrenia has come from neuropathological studies of postmortem brains, which received renewed interest through technological advances (e.g. Pakkenberg 1987; Kleinman *et al.* 1988). Bruton *et al.* (1990) reported impressive findings from a prospective study of the brains of 56 patients with schizophrenia matched for age and sex with normal controls. Brains of patients who had had schizophrenia showed significantly reduced brain weight and length and increased ventricular size, and also contained more non-specific focal pathology and fibrillary gliosis. Female patients with schizophrenia had lived longer than men. The report by Crow *et al.* (1989) of a postmortem study showing ventricular enlargement to be greater in the left temporal horn than in the right has stimulated further research into the possibility that the pathology of schizophrenia is asymmetrical, with lateralized brain deficits underlying, perhaps, a failure of hemispheric dominance for language, as postulated by Crow (1998). Significant left-sided reduction in the superior temporal gyrus, differentially related to age of onset in males and females, is reported in a postmortem study of 29 patients with schizophrenia and 27 controls by Highley *et al.* (1999), who review other studies both supporting and conflicting with their findings. Reduced volumes in the parahippocampal and fusiform gyri on the left side, with reversed asymmetry compared to normal subjects, and gender differences, are reported by the same group (McDonald *et al.* 2000).

Another focus of interest has been the question of whether Alzheimer disease pathology is more frequent in postmortem brains of schizophrenic patients, and whether there is a distinctive pathology underlying severe cognitive deficits in older patients with schizophrenia. Several recent studies (e.g. Dwork *et al.* 1998; Murphy *et al.*, 1998; Niizato *et al.* 1998; Purohit *et al.* 1998) and a meta-analysis by Baldessarini *et al.* (1997) of 10 studies indicate that Alzheimer-type pathology is not more frequent in the population with schizophrenia than in the general population (and may even be less), nor is there an increased frequency associated with antipsychotic drug treatment. These findings reverse earlier studies, based on archival material, which suggested such increases. Neither neuronal degeneration nor loss correlate with cognitive impairment in elderly patients with schizophrenia.

Social disabilities and the effects of institutional care

In the period preceding widespread hospital closures several common features of social disability could be discerned among the more disabled non-demented patients who had been in hospital for a very long time, as reviewed by Wing and Furlong (1986). The chief common feature was a record of contact with services stretching back long before the index admission. Very few had roots in an outside community, had had recent employment, were married or in touch with a spouse, or had a home to go to, though most had relatives somewhere. In many cases, social disablement had remained severe and intractable despite the fact that assessment and care had been as good as possible. The authors identify five major factors, commonly interacting, which often complicate treatment or set limits to the degree of independence which can be achieved, namely: (1) risk of harm to self or others; (2) unpredictability of behaviour and liability of relapse; (3) poor motivation and capacity for self-management or performance of social roles; (4) lack of insight; and (5) low public acceptability.

A key reference point for studies of social disability in schizophrenia and its relation to institutional care is the Three Hospitals study by Wing and Brown (1970), which showed how measures of social withdrawal correlated with a lack of social stimulation, as indicated by measures of, for example, time spent doing nothing. Wing (1989) provided a summary of the evolution of this very influential work. An earlier study, reported in 1962, of the long-stay populations of two hospitals had shown that social withdrawal scores were correlated with length of stay, as were ignorance of elementary facts about the outside world, absence of plans for the future, and the wish to stay in hospital. In the later 8-year study of three hospitals greatly differing in their delivery of care (Wing and Brown 1970), no evidence emerged of any general tendency to deterioration. The four main conclusions were that a core deficit in many patients is impervious to social influence and constitutes a threat of deterioration if the social environment becomes understimulating, that it is amplified by conditions of social poverty, and that it can possibly be reversed by socially enriching the environment; effort, however, needs to be sustained, and this need continues if the patient is discharged. Recognition of the risks of overvigorous stimulation in precipitating acute relapse, and the influence of life events, led to research on what later came to be called 'high expressed emotion' (Brown *et al.* 1962; Vaughn and Leff 1976).

Vital as these studies have been in the recent corpus of psychiatric knowledge and opinion in the UK, they beg several questions when we consider the predicament of elderly graduate patients, particularly as regards the narratives of their lives, the natural history of their illnesses and disabilities, their prognosis, and the possible response to therapeutic endeavours or resettlement in alternative environments. Wing and Brown (1970) remark that age seemed to have surprisingly little significance throughout the analysis of findings. A selection criterion for the patients studied had been that they were under 60 (and female), but no separate analysis is provided for patients who were 65 or older when the final survey (which had shown in two of the three hospitals a falling-off of the improvements noted at the four-year follow-up) was undertaken after 8 years.

The association between social poverty and clinical poverty found in Wing and Brown's study was re-examined in a fourth hospital (Horton) 30 years later by Curson *et al.* (1992), and was found to be much weaker than in the original study. Reluctance to be discharged was not related to length of stay. In a commentary on the study, Wing (1992) noted that the proportion of patients in the more severe impairment categories in the study by Curson *et al.* was markedly lower than in

1960, and that there was little variation within which to test their hypothesis The much improved social milieu at Horton could be expected to provide a milieu in which negative impairments were reduced to their basic biological levels, beyond which little amplification could be expected because of the environment.

Three processes of change over time are commonly spoken of when referring to elderly graduates. Two of these, namely the effects of institutional care and ageing, are seen as progressively disabling, and the word 'frail' starts being added as an epithet for all elderly patients, though it is quite inappropriate for some. The third, the alleged 'burning-out' of schizophrenia, should perhaps work in the opposite direction. Direct observation of elderly patients in a mental hospital provides evidence of such diversity of outcome that no general tendency distinctive of this group of people is apparent. Wing and Brown (1970), commenting on their three-hospital study, expected that: 'If social improvements had not been taking place at the hospitals the tendency would have been for the patients to become more withdrawn and reticent, simply with the passing of the years. That such deterioration was mainly prevented, and that so large a proportion as one-fifth of the patients actually improved, is a considerable achievement'.

The question of deterioration

Cross-sectional studies of people in hospitals show increasing degrees of dependency among the older residents with the longest lengths of stay, and such findings are liable to be interpreted as evidence of progressive deterioration or damage from institutional care as described by Martin (1955), Barton (1959), and Goffman (1961). Indeed, proponents of antimedical ideologies have claimed that the disabilities of graduate and other long-stay patients are to be understood more as the result of progressive effects of 'institutionalization' than as anything else. The impact of such opinions on mental health policies and their dangerously negative impact on attitudes towards the prospects for patients with schizophrenia (powerfully criticized by Abrahamson, 1993) makes it important to explore how much such indices of apparently increasing disability reflect individual changes attributable to duration of stay, ageing, or deterioration due to illness processes. The influence on cross-sectional findings of selective mortality and discharge of less disabled or better motivated people should not be overlooked.

Questions as to whether, and how often, schizophrenia carries with it an intrinsic tendency to 'deterioration' are still debated. If it does, when and at what rate does it occur, and how much impairment is super-added as a result of institutional care? Is there a 'ceiling' effect so that the effects of the illness or institutionalization or both together attain their greatest degree early in the course of the illness or of hospital stay, so that beyond a certain point disability cannot show much worsening?

Many patients afflicted by schizophrenia continue to suffer a very poor outcome. Reviewing 10 outcome studies, from Kraepelin's of 1913 to Huber *et al.*'s of 1979, Cutting (1986) observed that bad outcome after a first admission for schizophrenia had fallen from 83% in the 1900s to under 26% in the 1970s. The outlook becomes worse after subsequent admissions. The five most powerful overall predictors of poor outcome were social isolation, long duration of episode, a past history of psychiatric treatment, being unmarried, and a history of behavioural symptoms in childhood. In the Cologne studies reported by Marneros *et al.* (1992), 148 patients with schizophrenia were included in a cohort studied after an average of more than 25 years from the index episode of illness. Of these, 24.3% had lived in a mental hospital permanently for more than 3 years; 41% were able to care for themselves and meet the needs of dependent family members; and only 7% had achieved full remission.

However, too much emphasis on the possibly deteriorating course of schizophrenia can lead to a misleadingly pessimistic and fatalistic attitude, which overlooks the wide heterogeneity of outcome and the many patients for whom improvement is possible. Harding *et al.* (1987) in Vermont followed 269 very chronic subjects over an average of 32 years and found that one-half to two-thirds of all cohort subsamples had achieved significant improvement or recovery. Commenting on this and other very-long-term studies, the authors (Harding *et al.* 1992) see the data as demonstrating the existence of a more flexible and dynamic process than one envisaged by a deterioration model, in which the patient is not just a passive actor but a more active participant than has been appreciated. They see the illness as being more of a prolonged one than a chronic one, in which the focus shifts back from the disorder to the person. In attempting to understand the picture of chronicity, it has been difficult to separate out the residual effects of the disorder, the effects of institutionalism, the adoption of the patient role, the lack of rehabilitation, reduced economic opportunities, reduced social status, the side-effects of medication and the role of lack of staff expectations, self-fulfilling prophecies, and the lack of hope. The patients in Harding *et al.*'s study were particularly notable for appearing to demonstrate the possibility of late recovery. As many as 68% of the survivors were reported to show no further symptoms and signs of schizophrenia, and good global functioning was found in 60%. They were, however, patients specially selected for an active rehabilitation programme, and it is important not to equate them with those patients housed in the back wards of hospitals of recent times (Harrison and Mason 1993). The limitations of these and other 'outcome' studies, arising from sampling biases and other methodological deficits, should be emphasized, particularly in order to avoid underallocating resources to the treatment of schizophrenia (Schwartz *et al.* 1992)

In 1983 a discussion on schizophrenic deterioration in the *British Journal of Psychiatry* (Cutting *et al.* 1983) illustrated viewpoints current at that time. M. Bleuler had observed that 10% of patients sink into such a severe state of deterioration that they need permanent nursing care, a proportion unaffected by modern treatments. Ciompi emphasized that the importance of psychosocial factors was at least equal to, if not greater than, organic factors. In his long-term follow-up study (Ciompi 1980) of a sample of 1642 patients diagnosed schizophrenic on first admission, 6% showed a catastrophic course, with acute onset leading directly to severe end-state, and 42% had unfavourable outcomes. Despite the mean age of 74 at follow-up more than half were still working. Treatment had made no effect on outcome. The later half of life often appeared to exert a 'levelling, smoothing and calming influence' on schizophrenia. Statistically, the further a person advanced into old age, the more probable was a favourable course of illness. Mortality had been heavy. A total of 289 patients were followed up after an average interval of 36.9 years, about a quarter of whom spent more than 20 years in hospital. Abrahamson reported findings of a survey which had included particular attention to graduate patients. His survey of 300 chronic patients at Goodmayes showed the expected highly significant correlation between the length of stay and social withdrawal, as found by Wing and Brown (1970), but Abrahamson noted that this might result from studying different cohorts with different individual deterioration. Scores varied a lot in the first two decades of hospital stay, and it was not until the end of the third decade that scores increased markedly and persistently to establish the overall correlation between length of stay and social withdrawal. Taking the case-notes of three samples of individual patients with different degrees of disability, Abrahamson found surprising degrees of long-term consistency. Levels of disability at the time of the survey were strikingly similar to those recorded at or shortly after the index admission, even when this had taken place four or five decades earlier. In less than 10% was the final state worse than the initial, and even here, deterioration had been confined to the first third of their admission. Improvement, which had occurred in about 25% of patients, had developed predominantly in the middle or last third of their admission. The pattern was thus the reverse of that predicted by either a progressive or threshold model.

If there is an early 'critical period' in the development of schizophrenia followed by a relatively stable plateau, and treatment resistance becomes established in the earliest years of the illness, vigorous treatment efforts need to be focused on the early stages (Birchwood *et al.* 1997). The possibility that earlier and more effective treatments with medication, cognitive therapy, and improved social management can improve the longer term outcome of schizophrenia is an area of active debate.

The persistence and evolution of schizophrenic symptoms

The occurrence and frequency of the phenomenon of 'burning-out' in schizophrenia, described as an amelioration of symptoms at ages above 55 by Bridge *et al.* (1978) who reviewed outcome studies, are still disputed. Differences of perspective influence the way 'outcome' studies are viewed. Breier *et al.* (1992), for instance, appear optimistic in suggesting that after an early phase of deterioration and a middle one of stabilization, there is a third phase of illness consisting of an 'improving course for many patients'. Evidence of 'burning out' was not found in the TAPS baseline studies among hospital residents (Leff 1991) which demonstrated a continuing high prevalence of florid psychotic symptoms. A 13-year follow-up study of 67 patients with ICD-9 schizophrenia identified in Nottingham in 1978–80, who were assessed at onset and at 1, 2, and 13 years (Mason *et al.* 1996), showed that the amount of time spent in psychotic episodes and in hospital is greatest in the first year of follow-up, but stable thereafter. There was a small deterioration in social adjustment between 2 and 13 years. The data did not support a concept of progressive deterioration, nor of progressive amelioration, and there was no 'late recovery'.

The relative effects of illness severity and duration, age, and duration of institutional care are hard to disentangle. Cunningham Owens and Johnstone's study at Shenley (1980) showed increasing disability with age and duration of stay; assessed abnormalities correlated, too, with features of the illness at its worst and with past academic record, but not with previous physical treatment. Positive symptoms did not correlate with any other assessed abnormality, and the persistence of very florid schizophrenic symptoms after many years in hospital was not uncommon. A comparison (Johnstone *et al.* 1981) with a sample of patients discharged 5–9 years previously showed no significant differences between the two groups for positive schizophrenic symptoms and current behavioural performance, nor for negative features when age and duration of illness were corrected for. A reduction in positive and disorganized symptoms with increasing age but no age effect for formal thought disorder or negative symptoms (which were worse in men) was reported in a cross-sectional study by Schultz *et al.* (1997). Increasing severity of negative symptoms with age and the amelioration of some positive symptoms were found by Gur *et al.* (1996) in a study that included very elderly patients. Women had less negative symptoms than men, a difference evident until the eighth decade. Thought disorder may have separate components which change differently with time, poverty of speech becoming more common and severe but disconnection problems becoming less evident (Harvey *et al.* 1997*b*).

An illustration of the declining prevalence of some positive features of schizophrenia among longer stay hospital inpatients is provided by the Friern survey (1983). A comparison of mental state items for patients with schizophrenia in different categories of duration of stay (1–5 years, 5–10 years, and over 10 years) showed a progressive decrease in the frequency of delusions (63% to 36%), and liability to marked exacerbations of illness (63 to 48%), a progressive increase in negative symptoms (from 61% to 73%), and little change in hallucinations (40% to 36%). Most striking was the increasing social isolation of the longest stay, with 54% having no outside contact, only 19% having regular visitors, and 41% knowing of no family members.

Wing and Brown (1970) suggest that the lowered prevalence of positive symptoms in long-stay patients is more likely to be due to protection from the strains of everyday life than the effects of medication or the natural history of schizophrenia. Great variability of symptoms, even among negative features, was shown by Johnstone *et al.* (1987) in a 4-year follow-up of 92 patients (mean age 58.7 years) on medium-dependency wards, and they observed neither obvious deterioration nor improvement. Unaccountably, retardation got significantly better, but poverty of speech tended to increase. In general, negative features were more stable, but none were irreversible. Levene *et al.*'s (1985) study in Leicestershire found that those elderly patients who had been in hospital for more than 10 years were less incapacitated, both socially and physically, than their shorter stay counterparts, though they clearly exhibited much higher levels of incapacity than younger patients. 41% of the elderly long-stay group had low scores on social withdrawal. Among long-stay residents with schizophrenia surveyed at Horton Hospital by Milne *et al.* (1993), advancing age was found to be significantly related to decline in social activity and reduction in speech.

A re-examination of the results for the Friern Hospital survey of 1985 examined dependency ratings (Reedhead 1985) among all patients resident there for more than a year, who were either aged 75 or over either/or suffering from dementia. These ratings, which took in five scales and were scored and combined into high-, medium-, and low-dependency categories, showed that even graduate patients who had stayed in hospital for more than 20 years and were over 75 years of age scored less on ratings of physical and social disability than patients with dementia who were between the ages of 65 and 75.

Not surprisingly, elderly patients with schizophrenia who are studied in community settings tend to have less severe symptoms than their counterparts remaining in hospital, who tend to be more cognitively impaired (Harvey *et al.* 1998; Evans *et al.* 1999*b*). In the South Camden survey (Campbell *et al.* 1990) elderly patients in the community before hospital closure were found to have lower scores on Krawiecka *et al.* (1977) scale ratings of depression, hallucinations, poverty of speech, and flattened affect. In contrast, they had better ratings on most Social Behaviour Schedule (Wykes and Sturt 1986) items and for physical illness and incontinence than those in hospital, but they scored higher on self-assessed loneliness. Ratings were similar in both groups for delusions, anxiety, and retardation (Taylor 1990, personal communication). In a study of patients with schizophrenia living in the community and aged over 55 years, Cohen *et al.* (1996) found probable pervasive depression in 44%. They reported that six variables were strong predictors, namely the presence of positive symptoms, physical limitations interfering with activities, younger age, diminished linkage of members of the social network, lower income, and a smaller proportion of social network members providing sustenance.

Physical illness and disability

The high prevalence of physical disability and handicap among long-stay residents is liable to be overlooked when planning for alternative accommodation. It increases with age, but is not confined to elderly patients or those with the longest duration of stay. In the Friern (1983) survey, for instance, physical illness requiring systemic medication was noted in 25% of schizophrenic patients resident over 10 years, but was also noted in 20% of those resident for between 1 and 5 years. The presence of significant physical handicap was recorded in 17% and 14% of these groups, respectively. In a study of the 168 old long-stay patients at Crichton Royal Hospital, Stewart (1991) found only 20% apparently free of physical ill-health—80% were aged over 60 years; 24% were unable to walk unaided; 17% had significant hearing problems; and 8% were partially or totally blind. Neurological disorders were the most prevalent, with physical illness, including epilepsy in 9%, and tardive dyskinesia in 6%. Cardiovascular problems were present in 25%, gastrointestinal in 14%, endocrine in 11%, and genitourinary in 10%; 4% had been treated for a tumour in the past year or had a known inoperable growth.

Concomitant physical illness is also likely to be an important aspect of the disabilities of graduate patients in the community, but may go undetected. In a study of long-term users of psychiatric services aged under 65 (Brugha *et al.* 1989) more than half of those aged 50 or over had a physical health problem, and this age group accounted for half of all who were regarded as having an unmet need. The importance of medical comorbidity, especially in older patients with schizophrenia, is reviewed by Jeste *et al.* (1996). Excessive morbidity and hospitalization for somatic disease was reported by Dalmau *et al.* (1997) in a controlled study of 775 patients with schizophrenia. In a national sample of veterans discharged from US Veterans'

Administration (VA) hospitals, a diagnosis of schizophrenia predicted a decreased use of medical services, indicating a need for better integration of medical and psychiatric services (Druss and Rosenheck 1997).

Neurological disorders

The presence of neurological abnormalities in patients with schizophrenia was described in detail by E. Bleuler (1950), who remarked, for instance, on his experience of making the diagnosis sometimes simply by seeing the patient's gait. More recently there has been renewed interest in the 'soft' neurological signs of schizophrenia (e.g. King *et al.* 1991). Rogers (1985) studied the 100 patients in Friern who had the earliest recorded dates of admission. Their mean age was 71.5, and the mean duration of their current admission 42.8 years; 92 had had diagnoses of schizophrenia. Fewer than half were receiving antipsychotic drugs, and 21 had received none in the past 15 years. In 98 of the patients, motor disorders had been recorded (and in 71 in at least five of the ten categories examined), before neuroleptic medication became available. Motor abnormalities had been noted at first admission in 88 patients. The motor disorders found, as consistently reported in earlier studies of mental hospital patients, included disorders of posture and tone, motor performance, inappropriate activity, abnormal movements, automatic movements, and disorders of speech production. Although variable in individual patients at different times, the disorders had been a constant feature of this group of patients at all stages in their illness, and could not be attributed merely to hospitalization, physical treatment, or undiagnosed neurological illness. Functional MRI has shown some evidence of associated dysfunction in the sensorimotor cortex and supplementary motor area (e.g. Schröder *et al.* 1995). Boks *et al.* (2000) reviewed 17 studies, comparing the prevalence of 30 neurological signs in patients with schizophrenia, affective disorders, and healthy controls. Lack of extinction, dysdiadochokinesia, and poor tandem walk, finger–thumb opposition, and articulation were significantly more common in schizophrenia than affective disorders. Some signs, however, were common in both, with several, including poor stereognosis and rhythm tapping, even commoner in mood disorders than schizophrenia. Impaired motor coordination seemed most specific to schizophrenia. A review by Wolff and O'Driscoll (1999) concludes that about 20% of neuroleptic-naïve patients with schizophrenia have increased rates of parkinsonism and neurological soft signs, and an increased rate has been reported in first-degree relatives.

The involuntary movements of tardive dyskinesia are now widely recognized as an association with dopamine-blocking antipsychotic drugs, which may still be under-recognized in long-stay patients (Macpherson and Collis 1991). Debate continues as to how much the vulnerability to this disorder may be an intrinsic part of the schizophrenic disease process. Liddle *et al.* (1993) found that both orofacial and trunk and limb dyskinesias were significantly associated with negative symptoms, but that only the former showed a significant increase in prevalence with increasing age, suggesting a synergistic interaction between the pathological process underlying negative symptoms and age-related neuronal changes. In patients with schizophrenia never treated with neuroleptics, McCreadie *et al.* (1997*a*) found no association between dyskinesia and poorer memory, but the latter was associated with negative symptoms. The possibility of an overlap in neurological substrate between cognitive changes, negative symptomatology, tardive dyskinesia, and parkinsonism has been further explored in elderly patients (e.g. Chen *et al.* 1996; Byne *et al.* 1998, 2000; Palmer *et al.* 1999*a*). No single concept of pathophysiology has been identified. Fenton (2000) has reviewed 14 studies of the spontaneous occurrence of tardive dyskinesia in neuroleptic-naïve patients with schizophrenia, and reports a rate of about 4% in first-episode patients, rising with age to 40% in those aged 60 or over.

Incontinence

Incontinence of urine, and less often of faeces, is a very common problem in long-stay patients, often underinvestigated, yet of vital importance to the carers. Levene *et al.* (1985) found that more than 50% of patients aged over 65 in two mental hospitals were incontinent of urine at least once a week. In a sample of 49 graduates aged over 65 at Cane Hill Hospital, of whom 82% had schizophrenia, Holloway *et al.* (1994) found nearly half (46%) were incontinent of urine or faeces once or more a week. At Friern (1983) 32% of patients with schizophrenia and a duration of stay over 10 years were incontinent of urine, compared to 22% of those with durations of between 1 and 5 years. In addition, 25% of them were incontinent of faeces, compared to less than 10% of those with a 1–5 year stay. These remarkable figures prompted more detailed studies, including medical and urodynamic investigations. Carrick *et al.* (1988) confirmed that over a third of the hospital population had regular problems of incontinence, and nearly two-thirds of these were also faecally incontinent. The mean age of patients investigated was 74.3 years, and less than half had senile dementia. A complex variety of problems emerged as likely to be contributory, most notably physical disability, inefficient bladder emptying, and colonic faecal stasis. Demented patients were more frequently and heavily incontinent than patients with other (mostly schizophrenic) diagnoses, were more prone to constipation, and were harder to manage. Only very careful individual assessments and specially tailored programmes for treatment seemed likely to bring any useful benefit. Urodynamic studies by Bonney *et al.* (1997) showed bladder detrusor hyperreflexia in some patients with schizophrenia: the authors propose that bladder dysfunction and incontinence are previously unrecognized neurobiological correlates for schizophrenia. A 5-year follow-up of long-stay patients discharged from hospital in the TAPS project showed that some patients regained continence after leaving hospital (Leff and Trieman 2000).

Other physical problems

Besides the expected range of physical diseases—particularly cardiovascular and respiratory diseases associated with heavy cigarette smoking—diabetes, bone fractures, sensory deficits of eyesight and hearing, epilepsy, static organic defects from brain injury, problems of dental care, and foot ailments are among the many disorders likely to require assessment and expert help. Many graduate patients have been edentulous for years and cannot accept dentures, which are quickly lost or claimed to be unwearable, or insist they are content with a few stumps of teeth. Conjunctivitis may be a recurring problem, particularly in faecally incontinent patients who rub their eyes. Longstanding constipation may be caused or aggravated by antipsychotic drugs, and be resistant to aperients and enemas, which may leave the rectum empty but the colon still loaded with faeces.

Epidemiological evidence of both positive and negative statistical associations between schizophrenia and other illnesses is reviewed by Jablensky (1988). Increased risk has been found, for instance, for arteriosclerotic heart disease and myxoedema. Rheumatoid arthritis appears to be rare, a negative association confirmed in many studies reviewed by Oken and Schulzer (1999), who conclude the rate could be as low as about 10% of the rate in the general population. Efforts to account for this led them to propose a hypothesis concerning the platelet-activating factor system and to consider the glutamatergic dysfunction hypothesis of schizophrenia, with possible implications for pharmacotherapy. A WHO record-linkage study found reduced risk of all cancers, especially lung cancer in both sexes (reported in some other studies, and very surprising in view of the frequency of heavy smoking), in patients with schizophrenia in Denmark, but other studies in Nagasaki and Honolulu did not give similar results (Gulbinat *et al.* 1992). A pronounced increase in breast cancer was found in Nagasaki and some increase in Japanese women in Honolulu. No significant increase could be inferred from the Danish data. Cancer mortality in schizophrenia is further reviewed by Saku *et al.* (1995) and Brown (1997).

Mortality

It has long been recognized that schizophrenia is associated with increased mortality. In the earlier accounts of mental hospital statistics, tuberculosis and other physical illness resulting from poor conditions account for most of the excess. Higher than normal mortality in long-stay patients under the age of 65 was reported by Mayer-Gross, Slater, and Roth (1969), who quoted Sjogren's study of 1948 which indicated that life-expectancy for patients with schizophrenia in and outside hospital was about three-quarters of the normal. In the follow-up study of 532 people discharged from Shenley Hospital over a 10-year period, patients of both sexes with schizophrenia suffered a twofold increase in mortality compared to the general population (Anderson *et al.* 1991); the principal causes of death were suicide and 'accidents' in both sexes, and cardiovascular disorder, especially myocardial infarction and cerebrovascular accidents, in women. The topic is reviewed by Brown (1997) who provides a meta-analysis of published studies involving cohorts since 1952. The overall excess mortality was indicated by a standardized mortality rate (SMR) of 151, with a significantly greater excess among males than females, but no gender difference in natural-cause mortality. Suicide, the largest single cause of the excess deaths, accounted for 12% of all deaths in the analysis and about 28% of the excess deaths. Natural deaths account for about 59% of the excess mortality. The SMR appears to decrease exponentially with age, largely due to the high rate of suicide in the young, and the natural-cause SMR probably also falls with age, though more gradually. Overall, the excess mortality appears similar to that associated with chronic physical diseases such as diabetes, but it is lower than that of organic mental disease. Published studies show considerable variation in results. Although aggregate SMR figures from more recent studies are lower than those of asylum cohorts, Brown concludes that the evidence is not sufficient to indicate whether this is a real change. High figures for suicide are reported in a cohort of nearly 8000 patients from the Salford case register, followed for up to 18 years (Baxter and Appleby 1999). Suicide risk was increased more than tenfold in schizophrenia, affective disorder, and personality disorder. The risk was highest at younger ages but remained increased throughout life. Lifetime risks of suicide in schizophrenia, affective disorder, and alcoholism, commonly quoted as 10, 15, and 15% respectively, may be lower and in the region of 4, 6, and 7%, according to Inskip *et al.* (1998). Their analysis of published studies shows how rates may be overestimated if cohorts are not followed to extinction and if extrapolation is made on the basis of the higher excess mortality seen soon after onset of the illness, as is particularly the case with schizophrenia.

A question of recent concern is whether moving elderly graduate patients from familiar hospital surroundings to other environments is likely to increase mortality. Such fears are not confirmed by the TAPS Project in a 5-year follow-up of people discharged from two hospitals (Trieman *et al.* 1999), but some earlier studies, mainly from the USA, had shown alarming increases in mortality following relocation (Morriss *et al.* 1988). The preparation, sensitivity, and care with which relocation is undertaken are likely to be crucial. A 5-year follow-up of the 49 graduate patients surveyed by Holloway *et al.* (1994), who left a closing mental hospital, found 45% had died. The figure was lower than the 70% mortality predicted from a projection based on age-specific mortality rates for mental hospital survivors, but higher than the 33% mortality predicted from general population mortality rates.

Approaches to care

The individual dimension

An adequate description of treatment and care for individual graduate patients would encompass a consideration of good practices in adult psychiatry and psychiatric rehabilitation (Shepherd 1988), as well as the psychiatric, physical, and social care of elderly people with a very wide range of strengths and disabilities. A few points, however, may be emphasized here, with the reservation that the concept of 'good practice' must beg many questions, and may fragment into controversy about particular approaches to individual problems where no better yardstick is available. It is a realm where exhortation is much easier than practice, where evaluation of care practices has seldom been attempted (Lavender 1987) and where general ideological strategies, such as that proposed by some of the more extreme advocates of 'normalization' (Wolfensberger 1972), may be speciously attractive. Quite often it may be difficult to weigh conflicting values in trying to work for what is best for patients as individuals or groups. It may be appropriate to seek answers not so much in the isolated details of care practice (which may seldom present such clear-cut consequences as, say, the occurrence of pressure-sores) but in the overall humanity and individual responsiveness of the care programme as a whole, which will be harder to measure or change. In hospital, and now also in community homes, an important requirement is to try to overcome rigidity and pessimism in the attitudes liable to be found among some nursing and medical staff and other care attendants, which are not just due to shortage of time and other resources: they reflect the negative aura which may surround elderly long-term patients, who are liable to be seen, particularly in settings which also provide for younger people, as offering little therapeutic reward. Evidence of such disinterest may be abundant in hospital wards: disorganized medical case-notes without recent summaries or entries, other than by duty doctors called for physical emergencies; the lack of any clear diagnostic formulation, list of problems, or individual care-plan; prescription charts that have been unchanged for months or even years; lack of up-to-date knowledge about the patient's family and any social contacts; absence of ready-to-hand information about the patient's past life and interests; lack of recent attention to daily activities, use of finances, clothing and other personal possessions, eyesight, hearing, dental care and chiropody; and other signs of physical neglect such as absence of regular physical reviews or follow-up of physical abnormalities found in previous investigations. Problems of incontinence or other disabilities and problem behaviours may have been accepted for years by staff without medical investigation, systematic attempts at treatment, or even modern incontinence garments. Care practices stressing attention to routine and cleanliness may become excessively rigid and restrictive, denying opportunities for personal choice and motivation. All too often it seems as if the individuality and humanity of the patient become progressively lost sight of, leaving only a 'known chronic schizophrenic' whose needs are condensed into a brief account of major problem behaviours. Records are liable to be lost or incomplete when patients are transferred to new accommodation.

Even more than in the case of acute patients, the need is for ingenuity and painstaking effort to try to identify islands of normal or potentially improvable function that can foster communication and mental and physical activity. The primacy of the patient's subjective experience can easily be lost (Strauss 1994), and the experienced quality of life may be quite different from an objectively measured standard of living. Skantze *et al.* (1992), for example, found that in a Swedish sample of people with chronic schizophrenia, complaints about 'inner experience', mental health, contacts, leisure, and work were common despite a reasonable standard of living. Patients' perception of their needs may be different from those of their carers. For example, 17% of 23 elderly graduates surveyed in the Nunhead and Norwood PriSM community surveys in South London reported thoughts of harming themselves, compared to only 5% reported by staff (Abdul-Hamid *et al.* 1999). The organization of advocacy services, as promised now by the *National Plan* (DoH 2000) for the NHS, may help to articulate what patients want and what they have a right to expect. As Williams and Wilkinson (1995) emphasize, the patients' perspective must be understood in greater detail, if mental health services are to become more people-centred and closer to the people they serve. Slade *et al.* (1999) insist that: 'The patient's perspective on their difficulties (especially their unmet needs) must be central to mental health care', an obligation which should be heeded in providing for graduates as much as for younger patients.

Some elderly graduates may enjoy attending workshops even when they are long past ordinary retirement age. Others will greatly benefit from the active input of appropriately motivated occupational therapists, and of other therapists in art, music, reminiscence, and communication skills, who have discovered the enjoyment of working with older patients. Some patients have a rich store of knowledge about their past life, and in this regard their graduate status deserves appreciation. Outings, holidays, and other social and recreational events should be organized, and funds and transport will need to be sought for such purposes. Cultural and religious values should be explored and attended to. Sexual needs, despite much evidence of older people's capacity for sexual enjoyment, are seldom assessed.

A positive benefit of the move to hospital closure has been the way staff with a different, non-hospital perspective have drawn renewed attention to the extreme social poverty of many individual patients' lives in hospital, and to the dangers of excessive regimentation or understimulation and apathy. These staff have sought to engage patients in everyday domestic and recreational activities, with greater responsibility for self-care, shopping and cooking, handling money, making contact with relatives, and travel. Some patients can be seen to respond to these new endeavours with an enthusiasm and an improvement in behaviour and functioning never believed possible in hospital; others remain largely unengageable, but their resistance may fluctuate and should not be assumed to be permanent or irreversible. Input needs to be sustained, or, as Wing and Brown (1970) highlighted, progress can be quickly lost.

Placing graduate patients in wards or community settings for people with Alzheimer's disease carries a double danger: the patient is likely to be understimulated and become more helpless, apathetic, and liable to incontinence; plans for reprovision may underestimate the severity of need if the graduate person's place is eventually taken by a patient with the greater disabilities of Alzheimer's disease. However, elderly patients can be vulnerable to abuse, exploitation, or aggression when living on wards or in houses which also accommodate younger patients who are more physically robust and mobile.

Medication

A common finding in patients who have spent many years in mental hospitals, particularly in situations where staff turnover is rapid, is that they continue to receive substantial amounts of psychotropic medication. This is often prescribed in a great variety of forms and dosage over the years, without anybody being able to say for sure what good, if any, it does them and why they are being prescribed a particular dosage or combination of drugs. In a small study of long-stay residents at Park Prewitt hospital, many of whom were elderly, Allen and Pugh-Williams (1992) found only 62% had had their drugs reviewed in the past year, mostly following some change in behaviour. Surveys of prescribing psychotropic drugs for people with chronic mental illness in hospital or the community have highlighted the frequency of polypharmacy and other questionable prescribing practices (e.g. Muijen and Silverstone 1987; Holloway 1988). Trends towards prescribing higher doses of antipsychotic medication in the treatment of schizophrenia have been noted in recent years. In two audits of prescribing at Horton Hospital in 1991 and 1993, Warner *et al.* (1995) found in both that nearly half the patients were being prescribed doses which, when converted to chlorpromazine equivalents, were in excess of the British National Formulary guidelines for chlorpromazine. Possible excessive mortality associated with polypharmacy emerges in a study by Waddington *et al.* (1998).

In practice, some elderly patients will benefit from cautious reduction or withdrawal of antipsychotic drugs (as studied by Harris *et al.* 1997): the drugs may dampen initiative, cause excessive sedation, stiffness or akathisia, and aggravate weight gain, constipation, and possibly sleep disturbance (Staedt *et al.* 2000). It may be difficult to be sure if such a trial (which may precipitate or aggravate tardive dyskinesia) is justifiable if there has been a history of previous relapse into florid symptomatology when drugs were previously discontinued; it may be similarly difficult to be sure if the patient might benefit from an increase in dosage or the exhibition or withdrawal of antimuscarinic agents or other medication. Antimuscarinic drugs can cause side-effects such as dry mouth, blurred vision, and constipation: they may also cause memory deficits which can be of clinical significance (Siris 1993) and may aggravate the symptoms of tardive dyskinesia.

It may be helpful, within the overall primacy of avoiding unwarranted risk to the patient, to try to make the prescribing of medication a continuing systematic exploration of different hypotheses about possible benefits or absence of benefit. However, the long time-scale needed and the patient's tendency to show fluctuations of mental state and behaviour independent of treatment approaches may make evaluation difficult. Preparation of a graphic life-chart of medication received, doses, and noted effects can be a useful first step. The common routine prescription of antimuscarinic drugs, laxatives, enemas, analgesics, and hypnotics should be reviewed.

The special risks of prescribing for elderly patients are reviewed elsewhere in this volume. Although negative symptoms of schizophrenia tend to be less responsive to antipsychotic medication than positive symptoms, there is evidence that the newer atypical antipsychotic agents may be effective in treating both positive and negative symptoms (Chan *et al.* 1999; Jeste *et al.* 1999), with less severe extrapyramidal effects, less liability to cause tardive dyskinesia, and possibly even a beneficial effect on cognitive impairment. Effective treatments for negative symptoms could be particularly valuable for graduate patients (Schultz *et al.* 1997). Accounts of experience with clozapine, olanzapine, and risperidone (e.g. Sajatovic *et al.* 1998; Madhusoodanan *et al.* 1999) in elderly patients are now accumulating, though randomized controlled trials are awaited. A report of the monitoring of 12 760 clozapine recipients in the UK and Ireland (Munro *et al.* 1999) includes mention of 263 patients aged between 65 and 75 years of age and 74 patients aged 75 or over. The risk of agranulocytosis increased with age (at least until 65), the hazard rising 53% for each 10-year increase in age. This has been noted previously. Barak *et al.* (1999) found 133 elderly patients without medical comorbidity reported in the literature to have received clozapine: mean dosage of clozapine was 134 mg daily, and the drug appeared to have been safe, tolerated, and effective. Oral drugs are likely to be more acceptable than depot injections (Desai *et al.* 1999). Patients with severe manic-depressive disorders may benefit from active therapy of resistant illness, and full doses may be needed. The risk of precipitating lithium toxicity even when blood levels are within the therapeutic range should not be forgotten.

Managing the environment

A useful maxim in all work with chronically disabled people is that even if, for the present, the patient's behaviour and disabilities cannot be improved very much, it is still possible to work towards an improved quality of life by improving the physical and social environment. Attention to the needs of the carers is a vital element of the latter. Privacy, opportunities for having personal clothing and other possessions, and provision of quiet and more sociable areas, domestic-scale kitchens, access to open spaces, shops and recreational facilities, conveniently placed toilets with well-marked access routes, and aids to reality-orientation are basic necessities still often lacking.

But how is one to decide what is best needed for patients who have grown accustomed to their present accommodation and are reluctant to leave? Where possible the patient's cooperation should be enlisted in planning a future which has personal value and meaning for that person, as illustrated and exhorted by, for example, Thomas *et al.* (1990). Much will depend on the availability of different local options. Abrahamson's work at Goodmayes demonstrated well how patients can be engaged, even after very many years in hospital, in making appropriate choices for their future, particularly when they are enabled to understand what different options actually mean (Abrahamson *et al.* 1989).

Planning for services

Attempts to communicate medical and nursing knowledge about requirements for care to non-medical people planning services for graduates may be severely hampered by a lack of understanding of the different aspects of requirement, which may vary from the predominantly medical, such as the need for treatment of physical illness or supervision of medication, to the primarily social. The concept of 'dependency' may blur or even exclude from consideration important distinctions between different kinds of disability and problem behaviours. It is important to examine specific aspects of graduates' preferences, capacities, and functioning. Bachrach (1978), a trenchant observer of deinstitutionalization in the USA, urged that: 'Emphasis must be moved away from programs and places towards the patients themselves'. Since then, there has been greater recognition of the cogency of the views of service users and their carers. Planning should be based on assessments of individual and local need, as demanded by the 1990 NHS and Community Care Act and reiterated by many others, including the Audit Commission (2000) in relation to elderly people. The development of CANE, the Camberwell Assessment of Need for the Elderly (Reynolds *et al.* 2000), may provide a valuable tool. Comprising 26 items, it records staff, carer, and patient views, and has been found to be easily used without professional training by a wide range of staff. Baker and Hall's (1984) REHAB scale and Clifford's (1986) Community Placement Questionnaire (CPQ) have been extensively used in planning for hospital closure. Although both scales show high levels of agreement on some measures, they did not identify the same individuals as being potentially hard to place in a study by Nelson *et al.* (1992). The CPQ includes staff opinions as to the specific requirements of patients with regard to a range of community facilities and may be more useful in service planning, but it is unlikely that any single measure can be relied upon to identify people who will be hard to place in the community. The MRC Needs for Care Assessment (Brewin *et al.* 1987) has also been used with long-stay inpatients by Pryce *et al.* (1993) in a study of patients of whom many were elderly, two-thirds had a clinical diagnosis of schizophrenia and almost half showed evidence of cognitive impairment; the mean length of illness was 26 years and most had multiple problems. Although few unmet needs for treatment were found, there were extensive unmet needs for social skills assessment, especially on a ward destined for closure, whose staffing levels had declined.

The use of computerized systems to record individual needs, care-plans, and outcome measures, though widely advocated, is still in its infancy. Much is hoped for from the forthcoming minimum data set (Glover 2000). The Health of the Nation Outcome Scale developed for the elderly (HoNOS 65+, Burns *et al.* 1999) offers promise as a simple means of monitoring progress.

Residential options

It is important to avoid confusing requirements for a high level of nursing care and supervision with requirements for continued stay in hospital, if there is a real opportunity to plan for alternative and better environments in which adequate care can be provided. The distinction is not made in most published estimates of how many patients could be discharged from hospital. At Claybury, for instance, Carson *et al.* (1989) found a particularly disabled and elderly population, with 63% of patients on longer stay wards rated as 'severely handicapped' on the REHAB scale and only 15% as showing 'potential for discharge'. The wide range of residential services which may be needed to provide an appropriately graduated series of options is helpfully discussed by Wing and Furlong (1986).

A variety of schemes may be proposed for elderly graduates, including transfer to other hospitals, settlement in old people's homes, purpose-built or -converted group homes, more intensively staffed homes, or private nursing homes. New community houses for chronically disabled ex-hospital patients may lack any plans or provisions for residents as they become older, and their staff may face anxious dilemmas as to whether residents should move on to the more institutional care provided by nursing homes, or back into hospital if behaviour, mobility, or incontinence deteriorate. The provision of shared bedrooms, a relic of the old barrack-room mentality of the hospital culture and a way of cutting down on requirements for space, was common in the early rush to closure of hospitals, justified on the basis that old comrades would want to stick together. Attitudes have been changing in favour of single bedrooms as the predictable inflexibility of shared arrangements has become evident. Promises of 'homes for life', so enthusiastically given when achievement of hospital closure was the priority aim, have at times had to be quickly ignored by a new generation of service managers faced with the mounting costs of community provision, particularly for ageing residents whose needs for care can no longer be met in a hostel environment planned for younger people. Large disparities may exist in the personal remuneration of residents in different types of care setting and may become a disincentive to move. Relocation to more distant accommodation may present difficult questions about who will be responsible for continuing medical supervision.

New administrative structures and priorities

The changing UK framework of policy for mental-health care of the elderly is described elsewhere in this volume (see Chapter 20). It can be hoped that the forthcoming National Service Framework for the mental health of the elderly will provide some recognition of the special needs of graduate patients. As policy demands for a high-quality service become more explicit, professionals may be faced with a widening gap between aspiration and achievable practice, finding services increasingly fragmented and incoherent (Haddad and Knapp 2000). The importance of the general practitioner's role is stressed again by the Audit Commission (2000), but their report also highlights the wide variation in attitudes and training of GPs in dealing with mental illness. The positive possibilities in relation to schizophrenia are enthusiastically advocated by King and Nazareth (1996). Guidelines for good practice are outlined by Burns and Kendrick (1997).

Wide variations between districts in their expenditure on mental health—by a factor of seven—was previously noted by the Audit Commission (Renshaw 1994), and spending does not appear to be closely correlated with need. Fragmentation of professionals and services, inflexible budgets, poor availability of information to clinical managers and purchasers, and training inadequately addressing the needs of people in the community, particularly those with longer term needs, are among other points noted. Some guidance for purchasers was offered by the Department of Health's *Handbook on the mental health of older people* (DoH 1997), which recognizes GPs' central role in coordinating services for the patients' physical and mental health needs.

A swing in emphasis for all services in favour of those with more severe and enduring mental illness has been demanded, with greater attention to outreach services, crisis intervention, and care management by unified health and social service teams, but evidence of their effectiveness for graduate patients has yet to emerge. With caseloads in Inner London averaging 37 clients per community psychiatric nurse (CPN) (MILMIS Project Group 1995), demands for Supervision Registers (Holloway 1994) and closer follow-up of at-risk patients, and increased administrative work associated with the still patchily implemented Care Programme Approach (Bindman *et al.* 1999; Schneider *et al.* 1999), it is unlikely that the needs of many graduate patients who lack family support can be adequately met outside some sort of institutional care.

Studying the consequences of hospital closures

The closing of a mental hospital and its replacement by community facilities is 'a vast natural experiment, which is going on nationally and internationally' (Leff 1991). Concern has been voiced that the people who were supposed to benefit most from the closure of the large institutions may have fared the worst (Grove 1994). The lack of prospective studies of the consequences of closing down a mental hospital and reproviding for all its long-stay residents in community facilities is highlighted by a review of mental hospital closure programmes by O'Driscoll (1993). The TAPS study of the closure of Friern and Claybury hospitals provides a valuable exception, with positive results for most people resettled out of hospital (Leff 1991; Leff *et al.* 2000). Other European studies provide further evidence of elderly patients doing well in new community environments after relocation from hospital (e.g. Donnelly *et al.* 1997; Borge *et al.* 1999). Encouraging results which suggest that reprovision benefits elderly long-term residents with functional illness come from Trieman *et al.*'s (1996) report, part of the TAPS project, on 130 functionally ill, long-stay patients whose outcome was studied over 3 years from baseline assessments—71 were still alive, equally distributed between hospital and community facilities. The behaviour of the patients who left hospital was stable and even improved slightly over time, while those who remained became more disturbed. Those remaining in hospital markedly deteriorated in their cognitive function, but those who left declined to a much lesser extent.

Lack of planning foresight in providing a specialist nursing home for the elderly functionally mentally ill was noted by Holloway *et al.* (1994). They found that for surviving graduate patients resettled from Cane Hill hospital and surveyed over a 5-year interval, most patients' needs, as assessed by a quality-of-life profile, were adequately met within their new settings; however, severe deficits and unmet needs were found in the areas of structured activities, leisure, and companionship. The majority were moved outside the catchment area, mainly to residential and nursing home facilities, but only a few (14%) expressed a desire to return to hospital. The authors noted that significant numbers of elderly graduates had been moved into hostels designed for people with severe psychiatric problems: the services were now struggling with the needs for physical care.

The burden of care

High levels of psychological morbidity have been extensively reported in the carers of patients with Alzheimer's disease (see Chapter 21), and benefit to carers and patients from cognitive-behavioural family intervention has been reported (Marriott *et al.* 2000). The profound impact of severe functional illness on families and other informal carers is also recognized (Fadden *et al.* 1987), with effects severe enough to qualify as evidence for minor psychiatric 'caseness' (e.g. in 45% of the carers of former long-stay patients studied by McGilloway *et al.* 1997), especially in women. The burden does not lessen with time (Brown and Birtwistle 1998). Formal acknowledgement of the needs and rights of carers has become more explicit in recent policy documents, including the National Service Framework for Mental Health for the non-elderly (NHS Executive 1999). Greater attention to the role of paid carers has highlighted the urgent need for appropriate training and career development (Leff 1997*b*).

General adult psychiatrist or psychiatrist for the elderly?

Moves to resettle graduate mental hospital patients in the community, combined with the growing development of specialist psychiatric services for the elderly, have raised questions about how dividing lines should be drawn between the responsibilities of psychiatrists for 'general adult' mental illness and psychiatrists for the elderly in the care of these patients. There appears to be no formula which can substitute for good local cooperation and agreement between consultants and their associated teams, and no basis for service policies, often directed more towards exclusion than acceptance, which are not motivated by desire to meet individual patients' needs in the best way possible. A general service which disowns its patients as they attain their 65th birthday deserves no more respect than a service for the elderly that excludes people from their rights to help, which may best serve their needs, simply because they have a history of mental disorder preceding the age of seniority.

The growth of substantial links between psychiatrists for the elderly and GPs, with the majority of teams having community psychiatric nurses working in GP surgeries and community teams, as enumerated in the surveys reported by Banerjee *et al.* (1993) and by Wattis *et al.* (1999), should be an encouraging basis for a more focused approach to the needs of graduates.

In 1982, the Health Advisory Service's report *The rising tide* noted that 'the chronically mentally ill in old age are not yet included in most services [for old age], mainly because of the size of the problem and the way they are so deeply embedded in general psychiatry'. Guidelines from the Royal College of Psychiatrists (1987) for consultant posts in the psychiatry of old age (which Rodger and Wattis (1995) found poorly observed in a small audit of job descriptions) insist that: 'There should be a clear statement on the local policy of allocation of responsibility for the population aged over 65. In particular this should refer to the arrangements and criteria which are to be used for the transfer of patients from the "general adult" service to the "old age" service'. A 1985/6 survey of consultants in old age psychiatry (Royal Colleges 1989) found that 82% of respondents with five or more sessions in old age psychiatry said they took responsibility for all mental illness in a given catchment area and age group (usually over 65), compared to 75% in a previous survey in 1980. Of the remainder, half looked after those patients with organic brain disorders only. A further survey in 1996 of UK psychiatrists working in old age psychiatry, with a response rate of just 51%, is reported by Wattis *et al.* (1999). In just over a fifth of cases, general psychiatrists provided some services to old people, restricted to functional illness in three-quarters. Nearly two-thirds of respondents took over psychiatric responsibility for patients growing old in the community. but only just over a third for those growing old in hospital. For functional disorders nearly all services had an age cut-off, mainly at 65 years (range 60–75 years). A postal survey by Green *et al.* (1997), answered by 145 consultants in old age psychiatry in England, Scotland, and Wales, highlighted the lack of coherent planning and policy for graduate patients, with responses describing some successful innovative schemes but also situations where the graduates were slotted inappropriately into existing facilities. Interagency cooperation was not easy to achieve. A majority of respondents felt that individual need should dictate which service, the general adult or the elderly, should be responsible, but it was acknowledged to be a contentious issue. On the subject of graduate patients the earlier joint report of the two Royal Colleges (1989) commented: '...it is customary for chronic institutionalized patients who reach advanced age to remain under the care of their original services unless there are clear nursing reasons for transfer. The drive towards community and group home care for chronically mentally ill people will, however, increase the demand on psychogeriatric services in the future and necessitate provision for such people if community support breaks down'. If that is to be the case, those services will need to have the physical and human resources and commitment to do the job. As knowledge develops about the efficacy of newer medical, psychological, and social interventions in schizophrenia and other long-term mental illness, and about the practical kinds of help that can be offered to carers as well as sufferers, there must be a danger that graduate patients and their carers will suffer no less from inequalities in care provision in the community than they formerly did in mental hospitals. At a time of heightened aspirations for the improvement of services for the elderly, and a new round of administrative mergers and reorganization, graduates are still at risk of moving from a shamefully low status within one sector of psychiatry to a no-more exalted status within another.

References

Abdul-Hamid, W., Holloway, F., and Silverman, M. (1998). The needs of elderly chronic mentally ill—unanswered questions. *Aging and Mental Health*, **2**, 167–70.

Abdul-Hamid, W., Johnson, S., Thornicroft, G., Holloway, F., and Silverman, M. (1999). The needs of elderly graduates. *International Journal of Geriatric Psychiatry*, **14**, 984–5.

Abrahamson, D. (1993). Institutionalisation and the long-term course of schizophrenia. *British Journal of Psychiatry*, **162**, 533–8.

Abrahamson, D., Swatton, J., and Wills, W. (1989). Do long-stay patients want to leave hospital? *Health Trends*, **21**, 17–19.

Allen, D. and Pugh-Williams, S. (1992). General medical care of long-stay psychiatric patients: a pilot study. *Psychiatric Bulletin*, **16**, 332–7.

Anderson, C., Connelly, J., Johnstone, E. C., and Owens, D. G. C. (1991). Disabilities and circumstances of schizophrenic patients—a follow-up study: V. Cause of death. *British Journal of Psychiatry*, **159**(Suppl. 13), 30–3.

Andreasen, N. C. (1982). Negative symptoms in schizophrenia: definition and reliability. *Archives of General Psychiatry*, **39**, 784–8.

Andreasen, N. C. and Olsen, S. (1982). Negative v. positive schizophrenia: definition and validation. *Archives of General Psychiatry*, **39**, 789–94.

Andreasen, N. C., Flaum, M., Swayze II, V. W., Tyrrell, G., and Arndt, S. (1990). Positive and negative symptoms in schizophrenia: a critical reappraisal. *Archives of General Psychiatry*, **47**, 615–21.

Angermeyer, M. C., Goldstein, J. M., and Kuehn, L. (1989). Gender differences in schizophrenia: rehospitalisation and community survival. *Psychological Medicine*, **19**, 365–82.

Arie, T. and Jolley, D. J. (1982). Making services work: organisation and style of psychogeriatric services. In *The psychiatry of late life* (ed. R. Levy and F. Post), pp. 222–51. Blackwell, Oxford.

Audit Commission (2000). *Forget me not: mental health services for older people*. Audit Commission Publications, Abingdon.

Bachrach, L. L. (1978). A conceptual approach to deinstitutionalisation. *Hospital and Community Psychiatry*, **29**, 573–8.

Bachrach, L. L. (1997). Lessons from the American experience in providing community-based services. In *Care in the Community: illusion or reality?* (ed. J. Leff), pp. 21–36. Wiley, Chichester.

Baker, R. and Hall, J. N. (1984). *REHAB: Rehabilitation Evaluation Hall and Baker: user's manual*. Vine Publishing, Aberdeen.

Baldessarini, R. J., Hegarty, J. D., Bird, E. D., and Benes, F. M. (1997). Meta-analysis of postmortem studies of Alzheimer's disease-like neuropathology in schizophrenia. *American Journal of Psychiatry*, **154**, 861–3.

Banerjee, S., Lindesay, J., and Murphy, E. (1993). Psychogeriatricians and general practitioners: a national survey. *Psychiatric Bulletin*, **17**, 592–4.

Barak, Y., Wittenberg, N., Naor, S., Kutzuk, D., and Weizman, A. (1999). Clozapine in elderly psychiatric patients: tolerability, safety and efficacy. *Comprehensive Psychiatry*, **40**, 320–5.

Barton, R. (1959). *Institutional neurosis*. John Wright, Bristol.

Baxter, D. and Appleby, L. (1999). Case register study of suicide risk in mental disorders. *British Journal of Psychiatry*, **175**, 322–6.

Baxter, R. D. and Liddle, P. F. (1998). Neuropsychological deficits associated with schizophrenic syndromes. *Schizophrenia Research*, **30**, 239–49.

Benbow, S. M. and Jolley, D. J. (1992). A cause for concern—changing the fabric of psychogeriatric care. *Psychiatric Bulletin*, **16**, 533–5.

Berman, I., Viegner, B., Merson, A., Allan, E., Pappas, D., and Green, A. I. (1997). Differential relationships between positive and negative symptoms and neuropsychological deficits in schizophrenia. *Schizophrenia Research*, **25**, 1–10.

Berrios, G. (1990). Memory and the cognitive paradigm of dementia during the 19th century: a conceptual history. In *Lectures on the history of psychiatry: the Squibb series* (ed. R. M. Murray and T. Turner), pp. 194 –211. Gaskell, London.

Bewley, T. H., Bland, M., Mechen, D., and Walch, E. (1981). 'New chronic' patients. *British Medical Journal*, **283**, 1161–4.

Bindman, J., Beck, A., Glover, G., Thornicroft, G., Knapp, M., Leese, M., *et al*. (1999). Evaluating mental health policy in England. Care Programme Approach and supervision registers. *British Journal of Psychiatry*, **175**, 327–30.

Birchwood, M., McGorry, P., and Jackson, H. (1997). Early intervention in schizophrenia. *British Journal of Psychiatry*, **170**, 2–5.

Blanchard, J. J. and Neale, J. M. (1994). The neuropsychological signature of schizophrenia: generalised or differential deficit? *American Journal of Psychiatry*, **151**, 40–8.

Bleuler, E. (1950). *Dementia praecox or the group of schizophrenias* (trans. J. Zinkin). International Universities Press, New York.

Boks, M. P., Russo, S., Knegtering, R., and van den Bosch, R. J. (2000). The specificity of neurological signs in schizophrenia: a review. *Schizophrenia Research*, **43**, 109–16.

Bonney, W. W., Gupta, S., Hunter, D. R., and Arndt, S. (1997). Bladder dysfunction in schizophrenia. *Schizophrenia Research*, **25**, 243–9.

Borge, L., Martinsen, E. W., Ruud, T., Watne, O., and Friis, S. (1999). Quality of life, loneliness, and social contact among long-term psychiatric patients. *Psychiatric Services*, **50**, 81–4.

Breier, A., Schreiber, J. L., Dywer, J., and Pickar, D. (1992). Course of illness and predictors of outcome in chronic schizophrenia; implications for pathophysiology. *British Journal of Psychiatry*, **161**(Suppl. 18), 38–43.

Brewin, C., Wing, J., Manger, S. P., and MacCarthy, B. (1987). Principles and practice of measuring needs in the long-term mentally ill: the MRC Needs for Care Assessment. *Psychological Medicine*, **17**, 971–81.

Bridge, T. P., Cannon, H. E., and Wyatt, R. J. (1978). Burned-out schizophrenia: evidence for age effects on schizophrenic symptomatology. *Journal of Gerontology*, **33**, 835–9.

Brown, G. W., Monck, E., Carstairs, G. M., and Wing, J. K. (1962). Influence of family life on the course of psychiatric illness. *British Journal of Preventive and Social Medicine*, **16**, 55–68.

Brown, S. (1997). Excess mortality of schizophrenia: a meta-analysis. *British Journal of Psychiatry*, **171**, 502–8.

Brown, S. and Birtwistle, J. (1998). People with schizophrenia and their families: fifteen-year outcome. *British Journal of Psychiatry*, **173**, 139–44.

Brugha, T. S., Wing, J. K., and Smith, B. L. (1989). Physical health of the long-term mentally ill in the community: is there unmet need? *British Journal of Psychiatry*, **155**, 777–81.

Bruton, C. J., Crow, T. J., Frith, C. D., Johnstone, E. C., Owens, D. G. C., and Roberts, G. W. (1990). Schizophrenia and the brain: a prospective clinico-neuropathological study. *Psychological Medicine*, **20**, 285- 304.

Buckley, P. F. and Friedman, L. (2000). Magnetic resonance spectroscopy: bridging the neurochemistry and neuroanatomy of schizophrenia. *British Journal of Psychiatry*, **176**, 203–5.

Buhrich, N., Crow, T. J., Johnstone, E. C., and Owens, D. G. C. (1988). Age-disorientation in chronic schizophrenia is not associated with pre-morbid intellectual impairment or past physical treatment. *British Journal of Psychiatry*, **152**, 466–9.

Burns, A., Beevor, A., Lelliott, P., Wing, J., Blakey, A., Orrell, M., *et al.* (1999). Health of the Nation Outcome Scales for elderly people (HoNOS 65+). *British Journal of Psychiatry*, **174**, 424–7.

Burns, T. and Kendrick, T. (1997). The primary care of patients with schizophrenia: a search for good practice. *British Journal of General Practice*, **47**, 515–20.

Byne, W., White, L., Parrella, M., Adams, R., Harvey, P. D., and Davis K. L. (1998). Tardive dyskinesia in a chronically institutionalised population of elderly schizophrenic patients: prevalence and association with cognitive impairment. *International Journal of Geriatric Psychiatry*, **13**, 473–9.

Byne, W., Stamu, C., White, L., Parrella, M., Harvey, P. D., and Davis, K. L. (2000). Prevalence and correlates of parkinsonism in an institutionalised population of geriatric patients with chronic schizophrenia. *International Journal of Geriatric Psychiatry*, **15**, 7–13.

Campbell, P. G., Taylor, J., Pantelis C., and Harvey, C. (1990). Studies of schizophrenia in a large mental hospital proposed for closure, and in two halves of an inner London borough served by the hospital. In *International perspectives in schizophrenia research* (ed. M. Weller), pp. 185–202. John Libbey, London.

Cardno, A. G., Jones, L. A., Murphy, K. C., Asherson, P., Scott, L. C., Williams, J., *et al.* (1996). Factor analysis of schizophrenic symptoms using the OPCRIT checklist. *Schizophrenia Research*, **22**, 233–9.

Carpenter, W. T., Heinrichs, D. W., and Alphs, L. D. (1985). Treatment of negative symptoms. *Schizophrenia Bulletin*, **11**, 440–52.

Carrick, J., Ramchurn, L., and Malone-Lee, D. (1988). Urinary incontinence in a large psychiatric hospital. *Health Trends*, **20**, 118–19.

Carson, J., Shaw, L., and Wills, W. (1989). Which patients first: a study from the closure of a large psychiatric hospital. *Health Trends*, **21**, 117–20.

Chan, Y. C., Pariser, S. F., and Neufeld, G. (1999). Atypical antipsychotics in older adults. *Pharmacotherapy*, **19**, 811–22.

Chen, E. Y. H., Lam, L. C. W., Chen, R. Y. L., and Nguyen, D. G. H. (1996). Negative symptoms, neurological signs and neuropsychological impairments in 204 Hong Kong Chinese patients with schizophrenia. *British Journal of Psychiatry*, **168**, 227–33.

Chua, S. E., Wright, I. C., Poline, J.-B., Liddle, P. F., Murray, R. M., Frackowiack, R. S. J., *et al.* (1997). Grey matter correlates of syndromes in schizophrenia. A semi-automated analysis of structural magnetic resonance images. *British Journal of Psychiatry*, **170**, 406–10.

Ciompi, L. (1980). The natural history of schizophrenia in the long term. *British Journal of Psychiatry*, **136**, 413–20.

Clifford, P. I. (1986). *The Community Placement Questionnaire*. National Unit for Psychiatric Research and Development, London.

Clifford, P., Charman, A., Webb, Y., and Best, S. (1991). Planning for community care: long-stay populations of hospitals scheduled for rundown or closure. *British Journal of Psychiatry*, **158**, 190–6.

Cohen, C. I., Talavera, N., and Hartung, R. (1996). Depression among aging persons with schizophrenia who live in the community. *Psychiatric Services*, **47**, 601–7.

Cohen, C. I., Cohen, G. D., Blank, K., Gaitz, C., Katz, I. R., Leuchter, A., *et al.* (2000). Schizophrenia and older adults. An overview: directions for research and policy. *American Journal of Geriatric Psychiatry*, **8**, 19–28.

Cooper, B. and Holmes, C. (1998). Previous psychiatric history as a risk-factor for late-life dementia: a population-based case-control study. *Age and Ageing*, **27**, 181–8.

Copeland, J. R., Dewey, M. E., Scott, A., Gilmore, C., Larkin, B. A., Cleave, N., *et al.* (1998). Schizophrenia and delusional disorder in older age: community prevalence. *Schizophrenia Bulletin*, **24**, 153–61.

Crepet, P. (1990). A transition period in psychiatric care in Italy ten years after the reform. *British Journal of Psychiatry*, **156**, 27–36.

Crow, T. J. (1980). Molecular pathology of schizophrenia: more than one disease process? *British Medical Journal*, **280**, 66–8.

Crow, T. J. (1989). A current view of the type I syndrome: age of onset, intellectual impairment, and the meaning of structural changes in the brain. *British Journal of Psychiatry*, **155**(Suppl. 7), 15–20.

Crow, T. J. (1998). Nuclear schizophrenic symptoms as a window on the relationship between thought and speech. *British Journal of Psychiatry*, **173**, 303–9.

Crow, T. J., Ball, J., Bloom, S. R., Brown, R., Bruton, C. J., Colter, N., *et al.* (1989). Schizophrenia as an anomaly of development of cerebral asymmetry. A postmortem study and a proposal concerning the genetic basis of the disease. *Archives of General Psychiatry*, **46**, 1145–50.

Cuesta, M. J., Peralta, V., and Zarzuela, A. (1998). Illness duration and neuropsychological impairments in schizophrenia. *Schizophrenia Research*, **33**, 141–50.

Cuffel, B. J., Jeste, D. V., Halpain, M., Pratt, C., Tarke, H., and Patterson, T. L. (1996). Treatment costs and use of community mental health services for schizophrenia by age cohorts. *American Journal of Psychiatry*, **153**, 870–6.

Cunningham Owens, D. G. and Johnstone, E. C. (1980). The disabilities of chronic schizophrenia. *British Journal of Psychiatry*, **136**, 384–95.

Curson, D. A., Pantelis, C., Ward, J., and Barnes, T. R. E. (1992). Institutionalism and schizophrenia 30 years on: clinical poverty and the social environment in three British mental hospitals in 1960 compared with a fourth in 1990. *British Journal of Psychiatry*, **160**, 230–41.

Cutting, J. (1986). Outcome of schizophrenia: overview. In *Contemporary issues in schizophrenia* (eds. A. Kerr and P. Snaith), pp. 433–44. Gaskell, London.

Cutting, J., Bleuler, M., Ciompi, L., Crow, T. J., Abrahamson D., and Tantam, D. (1983). Discussion: schizophrenic deterioration. *British Journal of Psychiatry*, **143**, 77–84.

Dalmau, A., Bergman, B., and Brismar, B. (1997). Somatic morbidity in schizophrenia—a case control study. *Public Health*, **111**, 393–7.

David, A. S., Malmberg, A., Brandt, L., Allebeck, P., and Lewis, G. (1997). IQ and risk for schizophrenia: a population-based cohort study. *Psychological Medicine*, **27**, 1311–23.

Davis, K. L., Buchsbaum, M. S., Shihabuddin, L., Spiegel-Cohen, J., Metzger, M., Frecska, E., *et al.* (1998). Ventricular enlargement in poor-outcome schizophrenia. *Biological Psychiatry*, **43**, 783–93.

Der, G. (1989). The effects of population changes on long-stay inpatient rates. In *Health services planning and research; contributions from psychiatric case registers* (ed. J. K. Wing) pp. 53–7. Gaskell, London.

Desai, N. M., Huq, Z., Martin, S. D., and McDonald, G. (1999). Switching from depot antipsychotics to risperidone: results of a study of chronic schizophrenia. The Schizophrenia Treatment and Assessment Group. *Advances in Therapy*, **16**, 78–88.

DHSS (1972). *Services for mental illness related to old age.* Department of Health and Social Security. Circular HM (72)71. HMSO, London.

DHSS (1975). *Better services for the mentally ill.* HMSO, London.

DHSS (1988). *Mental health statistics for England.* Government Statistical Service, London.

DoH (Department of Health). (1997). *Handbook on the mental health of older people.* Department of Health, London.

DoH (2000). *The National Plan. A plan for investment. A plan for reform.* Department of Health, London.

Donnelly, M., McGilloway, S., Mays, N., Perry, S., and Lavery, C. (1997). A 3- to 6-year follow-up of former long-stay psychiatric patients in Northern Ireland. *Social Psychiatry and Psychiatric Epidemiology*, **32**, 451–8.

Druss, B. G. and Rosenheck, R. A. (1997). Use of medical services by veterans with mental disorders. *Psychosomatics*, **38**, 451–8.

Dwork, A. J., Susser, E. S., Keilp, J., Waniek, C., Liu, D., Kaufman, M., *et al.* (1998). Senile degeneration and cognitive impairment in chronic schizophrenia. *American Journal of Psychiatry*, **155**, 1536–43.

Eastley, R. J. and Lucas, P. (1992). Thirty years on: the Glenside Hospital Surveys 1960–1990. *Psychiatric Bulletin*, **16**, 542–4.

Evans, J. D., Heaton, R. K., Paulsen, J. S., McAdams, L. A., Heaton, S. C., and Jeste, D. V. (1999*a*). Schizoaffective disorder: a form of schizophrenia or affective disorder? *Journal of Clinical Psychiatry*, **60**, 874–82.

Evans, J. D., Negron, A. E., Palmer, B. W., Paulsen, J. S., Heaton, R. K., and Jeste, D. V. (1999*b*). Cognitive deficits and psychopathology in institutionalized versus community-dwelling elderly schizophrenia patients. *Journal of Geriatric Psychiatry and Neurology*, **12**, 11–15.

Evans, M. and Mottram P. (2000). Diagnosis of depression in elderly patients. *Advances in Psychiatric Treatment*, **6**, 49–56.

Fadden, G., Bebbington, P., and Kuipers, L. (1987). The burden of care: the impact of functional psychosis on the patient's family. *British Journal of Psychiatry*, **150**, 285–92.

Feighner, J. P., Robins, E., Guze, S., Woodruff, R. A., Winokur, G., and Munoz, R. (1972). Diagnostic criteria for use in psychiatric research. *Archives of General Psychiatry*, **26**, 57–62.

Fenton, W. S. (2000). Prevalence of spontaneous dyskinesia in schizophrenia. *Journal of Clinical Psychiatry*, **61** (Suppl. 4), 10–14.

Folstein, M. F., Folstein, S. E., and McHugh, P. R. (1975). 'Mini- Mental State': a practical method for grading the cognitive state of patients for the clinician. *Journal of Psychiatric Research*, **12**, 189–98.

Ford, M., Goddard, C., and Lansdall-Welfare, R. (1987). The dismantling of the mental hospital? Glenside hospital surveys 1960–1985. *British Journal of Psychiatry*, **151**, 479–85.

Friedman, J. I., Harvey, P. D., Kemether, E., Byne, W., and Davis, K. L. (1999). Cognitive and functional changes with aging in schizophrenia. *Biological Psychiatry*, **46**, 921–8.

Friern Hospital (1983). *Inpatient survey 1983.* Friern Hospital Medical Committee.

Friern Hospital (1985). *The 1985 Friern Hospital survey: a guide for district planning.* Friern Hospital Medical Committee.

Gabriel, A. (1997). Disorientation in chronic psychiatric patients. *Canadian Journal of Psychiatry*, **42**, 864–8.

Glover, G. (2000). The minimum data set. At last—information! *Psychiatric Bulletin*, **24**, 163–4.

Goffman, E. (1961). *Asylums; essays on the social situation of mental patients and other inmates.* Penguin, Harmondsworth.

Green, M. F. and Nuechterlein, K. H. (1999). Should schizophrenia be treated as a neurocognitive disorder? *Schizophrenia Bulletin*, **25**, 309–19.

Green, M. F., Kern, R. S., Braff, D. L., and Mintz, J. (2000). Neurocognitive deficits and functional outcome in schizophrenia: are we measuring the 'right stuff'? *Schizophrenia Bulletin*, **26**, 119–36.

Green, S., Girling, D. M., Lough, S., Ng, A. M. N., and Whitcher, S. K. (1997). Service provision for elderly people with long-term functional illness. *Psychiatric Bulletin*, **21**, 353–7.

Grove, B. (1994). Reform of mental health care in Europe: progress and change in the last decade. *British Journal of Psychiatry*, **165**, 431–3.

Gulbinat, W., Dupont, A., Jablensky, A., Jensen, O. M., Marsella, A., Nakane, Y., *et al.* (1992). Cancer incidence of schizophrenic patients: results of record linkage studies in three countries. *British Journal of Psychiatry*, **161**(Suppl. 18), 75–85.

Gur, R. E., Petty, R. G., Turetsky, B. I., and Gur, R. C. (1996). Schizophrenia throughout life: sex differences in severity and profile of symptoms. *Schizophrenia Research*, **21**, 1–12.

Gur, R. E., Turetsky, B. I., Cowell, P. E., Finkelman, C., Maany, V., Grossman, R. I., *et al.* (2000). Temporolimbic volume reductions in schizophrenia. *Archives of General Psychiatry*, **57**, 769–75.

Haddad, P. and Knapp, M. (2000). Health professionals' views of services for schizophrenia—fragmentation and inequality. *Psychiatric Bulletin*, **24**, 47–50.

Harding, C. M., Brooks, G. W., Ashikaga, T., Strauss, J. S., and Breier, A. (1987). The Vermont longitudinal study of persons with severe mental illness: I. Methodology, study sample and overall status 32 years later. *American Journal of Psychiatry*, **144**, 718–26. and II. Long-term outcome of subjects who retrospectively met DSM-III criteria for schizophrenia. *American Journal of Psychiatry*, **144**, 727–35.

Harding, C. M., Zubin, J., and Strauss, J. S. (1992). Chronicity in schizophrenia: revisited. *British Journal of Psychiatry*, **161**(Suppl. 18), 27–37.

Harris, A. W., Williams, L., Gordon, E., Bahramali, H., and Slewa-Younan, S. (1999). Different psychopathological models and quantified EEG in schizophrenia. *Psychological Medicine*, **29**, 1175–81.

Harris, M. J., Heaton, R. K., Schalz, A., Bailey, A., and Patterson, T. L. (1997). Neuroleptic dose reduction in older psychotic patients. *Schizophrenia Research*, **27**, 241–8.

Harrison, G. and Mason, P. (1993). Schizophrenia—falling incidence and better outcome? *British Journal of Psychiatry*, **163**, 535–41.

Harrison, G., Croudace, T., Mason, P., Glazebrook, C., and Medley, I. (1996). Predicting the long-term outcome of schizophrenia. *Psychological Medicine*, **26**, 697–705.

Harvey, P. D., Lombardi, J., Kincaid, M. M., Parrella, M., White, L., Powchik, P., *et al.* (1995). Cognitive functioning in chronically hospitalised schizophrenic patients: age-related changes and age-disorientation as a predictor of impairment. *Schizophrenia Research*. **17**, 15–24.

Harvey, P. D., Leff, J., Trieman, N., Anderson, J., and Davidson, M. (1997*a*). Cognitive impairment in geriatric chronic schizophrenic patients: a cross-national study in New York and London. *International Journal of Geriatric Psychiatry*, **12**, 1001–7.

Harvey, P. D., Lombardi, J., Leibman, M., Parrella, M., White, L., Powchik, P., *et al.* (1997*b*). Age-related differences in formal thought disorder in chronically hospitalized schizophrenic patients: a cross-sectional study across nine decades. *American Journal of Psychiatry*, **154**, 205–10.

Harvey, P. D., Howanitz, E., Parrella, M., White, L., Davidson. M., Mohs, R. C., *et al.* (1998). Symptoms, cognitive functioning, and adaptive skills in geriatric patients with lifelong schizophrenia: a comparison across treatment sites. *American Journal of Psychiatry*, **155**, 1080–6.

Harvey, P. D., Silverman, J. M., Mohs, R. C., Parrella, M., White, L., Powchik, P., *et al.* (1999). Cognitive decline in late-life schizophrenia: a longitudinal study of geriatric chronically hospitalised patients. *Biological Psychiatry*, **45**, 32–40.

Harvey, P. D., Moriarty, P. J., Friedman, J. I., White, L., Parella, M., Mohs, R. C., *et al.* (2000). Differential preservation of cognitive functions in geriatric patients with lifelong chronic schizophrenia: less impairment in reading compared with other skill areas. *Biological Psychiatry*, **47**, 962–8.

Health Advisory Service (1982). *The rising tide: developing services for mental illness in old age.* Health Advisory Service, London.

Heaton, R., Paulsen, J. S., McAdams, L. A., Kuck, J., Zisook, S., Braff, D., *et al.* (1994). Neuropsychological deficits in schizophrenics. Relationship to age, chronicity, and dementia. *Archives of General Psychiatry*, **51**, 469–76.

Heinik, J., Vainer-Benaiah, Z., Lahav, D., and Drummer, D. (1997). Clock-drawing test in elderly schizophrenia patients. *International Journal of Geriatric Psychiatry*, **6**, 653–5.

Heinrichs, R. W. and Awad, A. G. (1993). Neurocognitive subtypes in chronic schizophrenia. *Schizophrenia Research*, **9**, 49–58.

Heinrichs, R. W. and Zakzanis, K. K. (1998). Neurocognitive deficit in schizophrenia: a quantitative review of the evidence. *Neuropsychology*, **12**, 426–45.

Highley, J. R., McDonald, B., Walker, M. A., Esiri, M. M., and Crow, T. J. (1999). Schizophrenia and temporal lobe asymmetry: a postmortem stereological study of tissue volume. *British Journal of Psychiatry*, **175**, 127–34.

Hirsch, S. R. (Chairman) (1988). *Psychiatric beds and resources: factors influencing bed use and service planning: report of a working party of the section for Social and Community psychiatry of the Royal College of Psychiatrists.* Gaskell, London.

Holloway, F. (1988). Prescribing for the long-term mentally ill: a study of treatment practices. *British Journal of Psychiatry*, **152**, 511–15.

Holloway, F. (1994). Supervision registers: recent government policy and legislation. *Psychiatric Bulletin*, **188**, 593–4.

Holloway, F., Rutherford, J., Carson, J., and Dunn, L. (1994). 'Elderly graduates' and a hospital closure programme. *Psychiatric Bulletin*, **18**, 534–7.

Holloway, F., Wykes, T., Petch, E., and Lewis-Cole, K. (1999). The new long-stay in an inner-city service: a tale of two cohorts. *International Journal of Social Psychiatry*, **45**, 93–103.

Hori, A., Tsunashima, K., Watanabe, K., Takekawa, Y., Ishihara, I., Terada, T., *et al.* (1999). Symptom classification of schizophrenia changes with the duration of illness. *Acta Psychiatrica Scandinavica*, **99**, 447–52.

Huber, G., Gross, G., and Scheuttler, R. (1979). *Schizophrenie. Eine verlaufs- und sozial-psychiatrische Langzeitstudie*. Berlin, Springer.

Hunter, R. and Macalpine, I. (1974). *Psychiatry for the poor: 1851 Colney Hatch Asylum: Friern Hospital 1973*. Dawsons of Pall Mall, London.

Inskip, H. M., Harris, E. C., and Barraclough, B. (1998). Lifetime risk of suicide for affective disorder, alcoholism and schizophrenia. *British Journal of Psychiatry*, **172**, 35–7.

Jablensky, A. (1988). Epidemiology of schizophrenia. In *Schizophrenia: the major issues* (ed. P. Bebbington and P. McGuffin), pp. 19–35. Heinemann (and the Mental Health Foundation), Oxford.

Jablensky, A., Sartorius, N., Ernberg, G., Anker, M., Korten, A., Cooper, J. E., *et al.* (1992). Schizophrenia: manifestations, incidence and course in different cultures. A World Health Organisation ten-country study. *Psychological Medicine* (Monograph Suppl. 20).

Jarman, B. (1983). Identification of underprivileged areas. *British Medical Journal*, **286**, 1705–9.

Jenkins, R. (1994). The health of the nation: recent government policy and legislation. *Psychiatric Bulletin*, **18**, 324–7.

Jennings, C., Der, G., Robinson, C., Rose, S., de Alarcon, J., Hunter, D., *et al.* (1989). Inpatient statistics from eight psychiatric case-registers 1977–83. In *Health services research and planning: contributions from psychiatric case registers* (ed. J. K. Wing), pp. 13–58. Gaskell, London.

Jeste, D. V., Gladsjo, J. A., Lindamer, L. A., and Lacro, J. P. (1996). Medical co-morbidity in schizophrenia. *Schizophrenia Bulletin*, **22**, 413–30.

Jeste, D. V., Rockwell, E., Harris, M. J., Lohr, J. B., and Lacro, J. (1999). Conventional vs. newer antipsychotics in elderly patients. *American Journal of Geriatric Psychiatry*, **7**, 70–6.

Johnstone, E. C., Cunningham Owens, D. G., Gold, A., Crow, T. J., and Macmillan, J. F. (1981). Institutionalisation and the defects of schizophrenia. *British Journal of Psychiatry*, **139**, 195–203.

Johnstone, E. C., Owens, D. G. C., Frith, C. D., and Crow, T. J. (1987). The relative stability of positive and negative features in chronic schizophrenia. *British Journal of Psychiatry*, **150**, 60–4.

Johnstone, E. C., Owens, D. G. C., Bydder, D. M., Colter, N., Crow, T. J., and Frith, C. D. (1990). The spectrum of structural brain changes in schizophrenia: age of onset as a predictor of cognitive and clinical impairments and their cerebral correlates. *Psychological Medicine*, **19**, 91–103.

Jones, K. and Poletti, A. (1986). The 'Italian Experience' reconsidered. *British Journal of Psychiatry*, **148**, 144–50.

Jones, P., Rodgers, B., Murray, R., and Marmot, M. (1994). Child development risk factors for adult schizophrenia in the British 1946 birth cohort. *Lancet*, **344**, 1398–402.

Kavanagh, S., Opit, L., Knapp, M., and Beecham, J. (1995). Schizophrenia: shifting the balance of care. *Social Psychiatry and Psychiatric Epidemiology*, **30**, 206–12.

Kelly, C., McCreadie, R. G., MacEwan, T., and Carey, S. (1998). Nithsdale Schizophrenia Surveys 17. Fifteen year review. *British Journal of Psychiatry*, **172**, 513–17.

Kibel, D. A., Lafont, I., and Liddle, P. F. (1993). The composition of the negative syndrome of chronic schizophrenia. *British Journal of Psychiatry*, **162**, 744–50.

King, D. J., Wilson, A., Cooper, S. J., and Waddington, J. L. (1991). The clinical correlates of neurological soft signs in chronic schizophrenia. *British Journal of Psychiatry*, **158**, 770–5.

King, M. and Nazareth, I. (1996). Community care of patients with schizophrenia: the role of the primary care health team. *British Journal of General Practice*, **46**, 231–7.

Kirby, M., Bruce, I., Radic, A., Coakley, D., and Lawlor, B. A. (1997). Mental disorders among the community-dwelling elderly in Dublin. *British Journal of Psychiatry*, **171**, 369–72.

Klapow, J. C., Evans, J., Patterson, T. L., Heaton, R. K., Koch, W. L., and Jeste, D. V. (1997). Direct assessment of functional status in older patients with schizophrenia. *American Journal of Psychiatry*, **154**, 1022–4.

Kleinman, J. E., Casanova, M. F., and Jaskiw, G. E. (1988). The neuropathology of schizophrenia. *Schizophrenia Bulletin*, **14**, 209–16.

Knapp, M. (1997). Costs of schizophrenia. *British Journal of Psychiatry*, **171**, 509–18.

Kraepelin, E. (1920). Die Ersheinungensformen des Irreseins. *Z. ges Neurol. Psychiat.*, **62**, 1–29. [Patterns of mental disorder. In *Themes and variations in European psychiatry* (ed. S. R. Hirsch and M. Shepherd), pp. 7–30. John Wright, Bristol, 1974. (trans. H. Marshall)#]

Kramer-Ginsberg, E., Greenwald, B. S., Krishnan, K. R., Christiansen, B., Hu, J., Ashtari, M., *et al.* (1999). Neuropsychological functioning and MRI signal hyperintensities in geriatric depression. *American Journal of Psychiatry*, **156**, 438–44.

Krawiecka, M., Goldberg, D., and Vaughan, M. (1977). Standardised psychiatric assessment scale for chronic psychotic patients. *Acta Psychiatrica Scandinavica*, **55**, 299–308.

Lamb, H. R. (1993). Lessons learned from deinstitutionalisation in the US. *British Journal of Psychiatry*, **162**, 587–92.

Lavender, A. (1987). Improving the quality of care on psychiatric hospital rehabilitation wards: a controlled evaluation. *British Journal of Psychiatry*, **150**, 476–81.

Lawrie, S. M. and Abukmeil, S. S. (1998). Brain abnormality in schizophrenia. A systematic and quantitative review of volumetric magnetic resonance imaging studies. *British Journal of Psychiatry*, **172**, 110–20.

Lawrie, S. M., Ingle, G. T., Santosh, C. G., Rogers, A. C., Rimmington, J. E., Naidu, K. P., *et al.* (1995). Magnetic resonance imaging and single photon emission tomography in treatment-responsive and treatment-resistant schizophrenia. *British Journal of Psychiatry*, **167**, 202–10.

Leff, J. P. (1991). Evaluation of the closure of mental hospitals. In *The closure of mental hospitals* (ed. P. Hall and I. F. Brockington), pp. 25–32. Gaskell for The Royal College of Psychiatrists, London.

Leff, J. (1997*a*). The future of community care. In *Care in the community: illusion or reality?* (ed. J. Leff), p. 204. Wiley, Chichester.

Leff, J. (1997*b*). The downside of reprovision. In *Care in the community: illusion or reality?* (ed. J. Leff), pp. 167–74. Wiley, Chichester.

Leff, J. and Trieman, N. (2000). Long-stay patients discharged from psychiatric hospitals. Social and clinical outcomes after five years in the community. The TAPS Project 46. *British Journal of Psychiatry*, **176**, 217–23.

Leff, J., Trieman, N., Knapp, M., and Hallam. A. (2000). The TAPS project. A report of 13 years of research, 1985–1998. *Psychiatric Bulletin*, **24**, 165–8.

Lelliott, P., Wing, J., and Clifford, P. (1994). A national audit of new long-stay psychiatric patients. I: method and description of the cohort. *British Journal of Psychiatry*, **165**, 160–9.

Levene, L. S., Donaldson, L. J., and Brandon, S. (1985). How likely is it that a District Health Authority can close its large mental hospitals? *British Journal of Psychiatry*, **147**, 150–5.

Levitt, J. J., McCarley, R. W., Nestor, P. G., Petrescu, C., Donnino, R., Hirayasu, Y., *et al.* (1999). Quantitative volumetric MRI study of the cerebellum and vermis in schizophrenia: clinical and cognitive correlates. *American Journal of Psychiatry*, **156**, 1105–7.

Lewis, S. (1992). Sex and schizophrenia: vive la difference. *British Journal of Psychiatry*, **161**, 445–50.

Liddle, P. F. (1987). The symptoms of chronic schizophrenia: a re-examination of the positive-negative dichotomy. *British Journal of Psychiatry*, **151**, 145–51.

Liddle, P. F., Barnes, T. R. E., Speller, J., and Kibel, D. (1993). Negative symptoms as a risk factor for tardive dyskinesia in schizophrenia. *British Journal of Psychiatry*, **163**, 776–80.

Liddle, P., Carpenter, W. T., and Crow, T. (1994). Syndromes of schizophrenia: classic literature. *British Journal of Psychiatry*, **165**, 721–7.

Lindenmayer, J. P., Bernstein-Hyman, R., and Grochowski, S. (1994). Five-factor model of schizophrenia. Initial validation. *Journal of Nervous and Mental Disease*, **182**, 631–8.

Lloyd, K. R., Jenkins, R., and Mann, A. (1996). Long-term outcome of patients with neurotic illness in general practice. *British Medical Journal*, **313**, 26–8.

Lombardi, J., Harvey, P. D., White, L., Parrella, M., Powchik, P., and Davidson, M. (1996). Age-disorientation in chronically hospitalised patients with mood disorders. *Psychiatry Research*, **60**, 87–90.

McCarley, R. W., Wible, C. G., Frumin, M., Hirayasu, Y., Levitt, J. J., Fischer, I. A., *et al.* (1999). MRI anatomy of schizophrenia. *Biological Psychiatry*, **45**, 1099–119.

McCreadie, R. G., Latha, S., Thara, R., Padmavathi, R., and Ayankaran, J. R. (1997*a*). Poor memory, negative symptoms and abnormal movements in never-treated Indian patients with schizophrenia. *British Journal of Psychiatry*, **171**, 360–3.

McCreadie, R. G., Leese, M., Tilak-Singh, D., Lofyus L., MacEwan, T., and Thornicroft, G. (1997*b*). Nithsdale, Nunhead and Norwood: similarities and differences in prevalence of schizophrenia and utilisation of services in rural and urban areas. *British Journal of Psychiatry*, **170**, 31–6.

McCreadie, R. G., Robinson, A. D. T., and Wilson, A. O. A. (1985). The Scottish survey of new chronic inpatients: 2 year follow-up. *British Journal of Psychiatry*, **147**, 637–40.

McCreadie, R. G., Stewart, M., Robertson, L., and Dingwall, J. M. (1991). The Scottish survey of old long-stay inpatients. *British Journal of Psychiatry*, **158**, 398–402.

McDonald, B., Highley, J. R., Walker, M. A., Herron, B. M., Cooper, S. J., Esiri, M. M., *et al.* (2000). Anomalous asymmetry of fusiform and parahippocampal gyrus gray matter in schizophrenia: a postmortem study. *American Journal of Psychiatry*, **157**, 40–7.

McGilloway, S., Donnelly, M., and Mays, N. (1997). The experience of caring for former long-stay psychiatric patients. *British Journal of Clinical Psychology*, **36**, 149–51.

McGurk, S. R., Moriarty, P. J., Harvey, P. D., Parrella, M., White, L., and Davis, K. L. (2000). The longitudinal relationship of clinical symptoms, cognitive functioning, and adaptive life in geriatric schizophrenia. *Schizophrenia Research*, **42**, 47–55.

Macpherson, R. and Collis, R. (1991). Failure to recognise tardive dyskinesia in the long-stay population. *Psychiatric Bulletin*, **15**, 725–6.

Madhusoodanan, S., Brecher, M., Brenner, R., Kasckow, J., Kunik, M., Negron, A. E., *et al.* (1999). Risperidone in the treatment of elderly patients with psychotic disorders. *American Journal of Geriatric Psychiatry*, **7**, 132–8.

Mann, S. and Cree, W. (1976). 'New' long-stay psychiatric patients: a national survey of fifteen mental hospitals in England and Wales 1972/3. *Psychological Medicine*, **6**, 603–16.

Manshreck, T. C., Maher, B. A., Winzig, L., Candela, S. F., Beaudette, S., and Boshes, R. (2000). Age-disorientation in schizophrenia: an indicator of progressive and severe psychopathology, not institutional isolation. *Journal of Neuropsychiatry and Clinical Neurosciences*, **12**, 350–8.

Marneros, A., Deister, A., and Rohde, A. (1992). Comparison of long-term outcome of schizophrenic, affective and schizoaffective disorders. *British Journal of Psychiatry*, **161**(Suppl. 18), 44–51.

Marriott, A., Donaldson, C., Tarrier, N., and Burns, A. (2000). Effectiveness of cognitive-behavioural family intervention in reducing the burden of carers of patients with Alzheimer's disease. *British Journal of Psychiatry*, **176**, 557–62.

Martin, D. (1955). Institutionalisation. *Lancet*, **ii**, 1188–90.

Mason, P., Harrison, G., Glazebrook, C., Medley, I., and Croudace, T. (1996). The course of schizophrenia over 13 years. A report from the International Study on Schizophrenia (ISoS) coordinated by the World Health Organisation. *British Journal of Psychiatry*, **169**, 580–6.

Mayer-Gross, W., Slater, E. and Roth, M. (1954). *Clinical Psychiatry*. 3rd edn (1969) by E. Slater and M. Roth. Baillière, Tindall and Cassell, London.

Milne, S., Curson, D., Wilkie, A., and Pantelis, C. (1993). Social morbidity of a long-stay mental hospital population with chronic schizophrenia. *Psychiatric Bulletin*, **17**, 647–9.

MILMIS Project Group (1995). Monitoring inner London mental illness services. *Psychiatric Bulletin*, **19**, 276–80.

Moak, G. S. (1990). Discharge and retention of psychogeriatric long-stay patients in a state mental hospital. *Hospital and Community Psychiatry*, **41**, 445–7.

Mockler, D., Riordan J., and Sharma, T. (1997). Memory and intellectual deficits do not decline with age in schizophrenia. *Schizophrenia Research*, **26**, 1–7.

Mojtabai, R. (1999). Duration of illness and structure of symptoms in schizophrenia. *Psychological Medicine*, **29**, 915–24.

Morrison, G., Sharkey, V., Allardyce, J., Kelly, R. C., and McCreadie R. G. (2000). Nithsdale schizophrenia surveys 21: a longitudinal study of National Audit Reading Test stability. *Psychological Medicine*, **30**, 717–20.

Morriss, R. K., Bowie, P. C. W., and Spencer, P. V. (1988). The mortality of long-stay patients following interhospital relocation. *British Journal of Psychiatry*, **152**, 705–6.

Muijen, M. and Silverstone, T. (1987). A comparative hospital survey of psychotropic drug prescribing. *British Journal of Psychiatry*, **150**, 501–4.

Munro, J., O'Sullivan, D., Andrews, C., Arana, A., Mortimer, A., and Kerwin, R. (1999). Active monitoring of 12,670 clozapine recipients in the UK and Ireland: beyond pharmacovigilance. *British Journal of Psychiatry*, **175**, 576–80.

Murphy, G. M., Lim, K. O., Wieneke, M., Ellis, W. G., Forno, L. S., Hoff, A. L., *et al.* (1998). No neuropathologic evidence for an increased frequency of Alzheimer's disease among elderly schizophrenics. *Biological Psychiatry*, **43**, 205–9.

Nelson, H. E., Pantelis, C., Carruthers, K., Speller, J., Baxendale, S. and Barnes, T. R. E. (1990). Cognitive functioning and symptomatology in chronic schizophrenia. *Psychological Medicine*, **20**, 357–65.

Nelson, H. E., Milne, S., Weatherley, L., and Clifford, P. (1992). Predicting requirements for community care. *Psychiatric Bulletin*, **16**, 17–18.

NHS Executive (1999). National Service Framework for Mental Health. Modern standards and service models. Department of Health, London.

Niizato, K., Arai, T., Kuroki, N., Kase, K., Iritani, S., and Ikeda, K. (1998). Autopsy study of Alzheimer's disease brain pathology in schizophrenia. *Schizophrenia Research*, **31**, 177–84.

Norman, R. M. G., Malla, A. K., Morrison-Stewart, S. L., Helmes, E., Williamson, P. C., Thomas, J., *et al.*(1997). Neuropsychological correlates of syndromes in schizophrenia. *British Journal of Psychiatry*, **170**, 134–9.

O'Brien, J., Ames, D., Chiu, E., Schweitzer, I., Desmond, P., and Tress, B. (1998). Severe deep white matter lesions and outcome in elderly patients with major depressive disorder: a follow up study. *British Medical Journal*, **317**, 982–4.

O'Carroll, R. (2000). Cognitive impairment in schizophrenia. *Advances in Psychiatric Treatment*, **6**, 161–8.

O'Driscoll, C. (1993). The TAPS Project. 7: Mental hospital closure—a literature review of outcome studies and evaluative techniques. *British Journal of Psychiatry*, **162** (Suppl. 19), 7–17.

Oken, R. J. and Schulzer, M. (1999). At issue: schizophrenia and rheumatoid arthritis: the negative association revisited. *Schizophrenia Bulletin*, **25**, 625–38.

Pakkenberg, B. (1987). Postmortem study of chronic schizophrenic brains. *British Journal of Psychiatry*, **151**, 744–52.

Palmer, B. W., Heaton, R. K., and Jeste, D. V. (1999*a*). Extrapyramidal symptoms and neuropsychological deficits in schizophrenia. *Biological Psychiatry*, **45**, 791–4.

Palmer, B. W., Heaton, S. C., and Jeste, D. V. (1999*b*). Older patients with schizophrenia: challenges in the coming decades. *Psychiatric Services*, **50**, 1178–83.

Pálsson, S., Aevarsson, Ó., and Skoog, I. (1999). Depression, cerebral atrophy, cognitive performance and incidence of dementia. Population study of 85-year-olds. *British Journal of Psychiatry*, **174**, 249–53.

Pitt, B. (1982). *Psychogeriatrics: an introduction to the psychiatry of old age* (2nd edn). Churchill Livingstone, Edinburgh.

Pryce, I. G., Griffiths, R. D., Gentry, R. M., Hughes, I. C. T., Montague, L. R., Watkins, S. E., *et al.* (1993). How important is the assessment of social skills in current long-stay patients? An evaluation of clinical response to needs for assessment, treatment, and care in a long-stay psychiatric inpatient population. *British Journal of Psychiatry*, **162**, 498–502.

Purohit, D. P., Perl, D. P., Haroutunian, V., Powchik, P., Davidson, M., and Davis K. L. (1998). Alzheimer disease and related neurodegenerative diseases in elderly patients with schizophrenia: a postmortem neuropathologic study of 100 cases. *Archives of General Psychiatry*, **55**, 205–11.

Putnam, K. M., Harvey, P. D., Parrella, M., White, L., Kincaid, M., Powchik, P., *et al.* (1996). Symptom stability in geriatric chronic schizophrenic inpatients: a one-year follow-up study. *Biological Psychiatry*, **39**, 92–9.

Reedhead, C. (1985). *Rating scales of dependency*. Hackney Community Psychiatry Research Unit, London.

Renshaw, J. (1994). The Audit Commission's review of mental health services. *Psychiatric Bulletin*, **18**, 421–2.

Reynolds, T., Thornicroft, G., Abas, M, Woods, B., Hoe, J., Leese, M., *et al.* (2000). Camberwell Assessment of Need for the Elderly (CANE). *British Journal of Psychiatry*, **176**, 444–52.

Rodger, C. R. and Wattis, J. P. (1995). Job descriptions for consultant posts in psychiatry of old age. *Psychiatric Bulletin*, **19**, 96–8.

Rodriguez-Ferrera, S. and Vassilas, C. A. (1998). Older people with schizophrenia: providing services for a neglected group. It's the quality of the environment that matters, not where it is. *British Medical Journal*, **317**, 293–4. [Editorial]

Rogers, D. (1985). The motor disorders of severe psychiatric illness: a conflict of paradigms. *British Journal of Psychiatry*, **147**, 221–32.

Roth, M., Huppert, F. A., Tym, E., and Mountjoy, C. Q. (1998) *CAMDEX—the Cambridge examination for mental disorders of the elderly*. Cambridge University Press, Cambridge.

Royal Colleges (1989). *Elderly people with mental illness: specialist services and medical training*. A joint report by the Royal College of Physicians of London and Royal College of Psychiatrists, London.

Royal College of Psychiatrists (1987). Guidelines for regional advisers on consultant posts in the psychiatry of old age. *Bulletin of the Royal College of Psychiatrists*, **11**, 240–2.

Rund, B. R. (1998). A review of longitudinal studies of cognitive functions in schizophrenia patients. *Schizophrenia Bulletin*, **24**, 425–35.

Sajatovic, M., Perez, D., Brescan, D., and Ramirez, L. F. (1998). Olanzapine therapy in elderly patients with schizophrenia. *Psychopharmacological Bulletin*, **34**, 819–23.

Saku, M., Tokudome, S., Ikeda, M., Kono, S., Makimoto, K., Uchimura, H., *et al.* (1995). Mortality in psychiatric patients, with a specific focus on cancer mortality associated with schizophrenia. *International Journal of Epidemiology*, **24**, 366–72.

Sauer, H., Hornstein, C., Richter, P., Mortimer, A., and Hirsch, S. R. (1999). Symptom dimensions in old-age schizophrenics. Relationship to neuropsychological and motor abnormalities. *Schizophrenia Research*, **39**, 31–8.

Schneider, J., Carpenter, J., and Brandon, T. (1999). Operation and organisation of services for people with severe mental illness in the UK. A survey of the Care Programme Approach. *British Journal of Psychiatry*, **175**, 422–5.

Schröder, J., Wenz, F., Schad, L. R., Baudendistel, K., and Knopp, M. V. (1995). Sensorimotor cortex and supplementary motor area changes in schizophrenia: a study with functional magnetic resonance imaging. *British Journal of Psychiatry*, **167**, 197–201.

Schultz, S. K., Miller, D. D., Oliver, S. E., Arndt, S., Flaum, M., and Andreasen, N. C. (1997). The life course of schizophrenia: age and symptom dimensions. *Schizophrenia Research*, **23**, 15–23.

Schwartz, F., Terkelsen, K. G., and Smith, T. E. (1992). Long-term outcomes in schizophrenia. *Archives of General Psychiatry*, **49**, 502–3.

Scott, J. (1988). Chronic depression. *British Journal of Psychiatry*, **153**, 287–97.

Selten, J. P. and Cath, D. C. (1995). Low prevalence of age-disorientation in Dutch long-stay patients. *Schizophrenia Research*, **14**, 141–3.

Semple, S. J., Patterson, T. L., Shaw, W. S., Grant, I., Moscona, S., and Jeste, D. V. (1999). Self-perceived interpersonal competence in older schizophrenic patients: the role of patient characteristics and psychosocial factors. *Acta Psychiatrica Scandinavica*, **100**, 126–35.

Seno, H., Shibata, M., Fujimoto, A., Koga, K., Kanno, H., and Ishino, H. (1998). Evaluation of Mini Mental State Examination and Brief Psychiatric Rating Scale on aged schizophrenic patients. *Psychiatry and Clinical Neurosciences*, **52**, 567–70.

Sharma, T. (1999). Cognitive effects of conventional and atypical antipsychotics in schizophrenia. *British Journal of Psychiatry*, **174** (Suppl. 38), 44–51.

Shawcross, C. R., Davies, H., and Taylor, S. (1987). The effect of community care on long-stay patients at Knowle Hospital. *Bulletin of the Royal College of Psychiatrists*, **11**, 414–16.

Shepherd, G. (1988). Practical aspects of the management of negative symptoms. *International Journal of Mental Health*, **16**, 75–97.

Siris, S. G. (1993). Adjunctive medication in the maintenance treatment of schizophrenia and its conceptual implications. *British Journal of Psychiatry*, **163**(Suppl. 22), 66–78.

Skantze, K., Malm, U., Dencker, S. J., May, P. R., and Corrigan, P. (1992). Comparison of quality of life with standard of living in schizophrenic out-patients. *British Journal of Psychiatry*, **161**, 797–801.

Slade, M., Leese, M., Taylor, R., and Thornicroft, G. (1999). The association between needs and quality of life in an epidemiologically representative sample of people with psychosis. *Acta Psychiatrica Scandinavica*, **100**, 149–57.

Spence, S. A., Hirsch, S. R., Brooks, D. J., and Grasby, P. M. (1998). Prefrontal cortex activity in people with schizophrenia and control subjects. Evidence from positron emission tomography for remission of 'hypofrontality' with recovery from acute schizophrenia. *British Journal of Psychiatry*, **172**, 316–23.

Staedt, J., Dewes, D., Danos, P., and Stoope G. (2000). Can chronic neuroleptic treatment promote sleep disturbances in elderly schizophrenic patients? *International Journal of Geriatric Psychiatry*, **15**, 170–6.

Stevens, M., Crow, T. J., Bowman, M., and Coles, E. C. (1978). Age-disorientation in chronic schizophrenia: a constant prevalence of 25% in a mental hospital population? *British Journal of Psychiatry*, **133**, 130–6.

Stewart, M. (1991). The physical health of old long-stay inpatients in one psychiatric hospital. *Psychiatric Bulletin*, **15**, 404–6.

Strauss, J. S. (1994). The person with schizophrenia as a person. II: approaches to the subjective and complex. *British Journal of Psychiatry*, **164** (Suppl. 23), 103–7.

Taylor, M. A. and Abrams, R. (1984). Cognitive impairment in schizophrenia. *American Journal of Psychiatry*, **141**, 196–201.

Thomas, D., Holt, V., Illingworth, M., Maddocks, N., and Robinson, E. (1990). Designing services with people who are elderly. In *Community care; people leaving long-stay hospitals* (ed. S. Sharkey and S. Barna), pp. 51–72. Routledge, London.

Torres-Gonzalez, F. (1995). Mental health care in Spain. *Psychiatric Bulletin*, **19**, 254–7.

Trieman, N., Wills, W., and Leff, J. (1996). TAPS project 28: does reprovision benefit elderly long-stay mental patients? *Schizophrenia Research*, **21**, 199–208.

Trieman, N., Leff, J., and Glover, G. (1999). The TAPS Project 45: the fate of long-stay psychiatric patients resettled in the community. *British Medical Journal*, **319**, 13–16.

Van Horn, J. D. and McManus, I. C. (1992). Ventricular enlargement in schizophrenia: a meta-analysis of studies of the ventricle: brain ratio (VBR). *British Journal of Psychiatry*, **160**, 687–97.

Vaughn, C. E. and Leff, J. P. (1976). The influence of family and social factors on the course of psychiatric illness. *British Journal of Psychiatry*, **129**, 125–37.

Waddington, J. L., Youssef, H. A., and Kinsella, A. (1998). Mortality in schizophrenia: antipsychotic polypharmacy and absence of adjunctive anticholinergics over the course of a 10-year prospective study. *British Journal of Psychiatry*, **173**, 325–9.

Warner, J. P., Slade, R., and Barnes, T. R. E. (1995). Change in neuroleptic prescribing practice. *Psychiatric Bulletin*, **19**, 237–9.

Wattis, J., MacDonald, A., and Newton P. (1999). Old age psychiatry: a speciality in transition. *Psychiatric Bulletin*, **23**, 331–5.

Wexler, B. E., Hawkins K. A., Rounsaville, B., Anderson, M., Sernyak, M. J., and Green M. F. (1997). Normal neurocognitive performance after extended practice in patients with schizophrenia. *Schizophrenia Research*, **26**, 173–80.

Williams, B. and Wilkinson, G. (1995). Patient satisfaction in mental health care: evaluating an evaluative method. *British Journal of Psychiatry*, **166**, 559–62.

Wing, J. K. (1986). The cycle of planning and evaluation. In *The provision of mental health services in Britain: the way ahead* (ed. G. Wilkinson and H. Freeman), pp. 35–48, Gaskell, London.

Wing, J. K. (1989). The concept of negative symptoms. *British Journal of Psychiatry*, **155**(Suppl. 7), 10–14.

Wing, J. K. (1992). Comment on institutionalisation and schizophrenia. *British Journal of Psychiatry*, **160**, 241–3.

Wing, J. K. and Brown, G. W. (1970). *Institutionalism and schizophrenia*. Cambridge University Press, London.

Wing, J. K. and Furlong, R. (1986). A haven for the severely disabled within the context of a comprehensive psychiatric community service. *British Journal of Psychiatry*, **149**, 449–57.

Wolfensberger, W. (1972). *The principle of normalisation in human services*. National Institute of Mental Retardation, Toronto.

Wolff, A. L. and O'Driscoll, G. A. (1999). Motor deficits and schizophrenia: the evidence from neuroleptic-naïve patients and populations at risk. *Journal of Psychiatry and Neurosciences*, **24**, 304–14.

Wykes, T. (1983). A follow-up of 'new' long-stay patients in Camberwell 1977–82. *Psychological Medicine*, **12**, 177–90.

Wykes, T. and Sturt, E. (1986). The measurement of social behaviour in psychiatric patients: an assessment of the reliability and validity of the SBS schedule. *British Journal of Psychiatry,* **148**, 1–11.

Wykes, T., Reeder, C., Corner, J., Williams, C., and Everitt, B. (1999). The effects of neurocognitive remediation on executive processing in patients with schizophrenia. *Schizophrenia Bulletin*, **25**, 291–307.

Yassa, R., Uhr, S., and Jeste, D. V. (1991). Gender differences in chronic schizophrenia. In *The elderly with chronic mental illness* (ed. E. Light and B. D. Lebowitz), pp. 16–30. Springer, New York.

Yorston, G. (1999). Aged and dangerous. Old-age forensic psychiatry. *British Journal of Psychiatry*, **174**, 193–5.

34 Substance abuse in the elderly

Roland M. Atkinson

Introduction

Recognition of substance abuse in the elderly

Recent literature demonstrates that alcohol and drug dependence constitute a public health problem of moderate proportion in the elderly. Still, clinicians have been slow to recognize these problems, in part because of the erroneous view, espoused in several papers during the 1960s, that these disorders were seldom to be seen after middle age. It was believed that lifelong alcoholics and drug addicts either died prematurely or recovered spontaneously, and that late-onset addiction was rare. Trained to this view, clinicians do not expect to encounter these disorders in elderly persons. Compounding this problem is the fact that symptoms of substance abuse in older persons may mimic findings of other medical and behavioural disorders, leading to misdiagnosis.

Another complex phenomenon is the underreporting of problems to and by clinicians. Contributing to this are: older patients' faulty recall of even recent consumption; the reluctance of elderly individuals and their families to disclose such problems because of shame, or the belief that alcohol or drugs are the last remaining comfort; lack of third parties (employers, courts, spouse) who often discover younger substance abusers; therapeutic pessimism; and faulty methods of documentation in medical records. These factors, together with differences in demographics and health care referral and delivery patterns, probably account for the variability in reported prevalence of elderly substance abuse, and for the fact that these problems tend to remain hidden from broader social and medical scrutiny.

General terms and concepts in the field of substance abuse

Several terms are defined in Table 34.1 as they will be used in this chapter. A general 'substance abuse model', embracing alcohol, licit and illicit psychoactive drugs, is supported by recent research suggesting common biobehavioural bases for these disorders. The concept of 'drug use behaviour' emphasizes use patterns that may apply to any substance, implying that characteristics of the user and the social context of use are often as important as the pharmacological properties of the drug in the development of clinical disorders. The resulting risk-use continuum (Table 34.2) further suggests that categorical diagnostic distinctions (e.g. between 'alcoholic' and 'social drinker') can be arbitrary. Changes in a person's pattern of use, in either direction along the continuum, can occur over time. An individual may use one substance differently than another substance, or switch from one to another. The development and promulgation, beginning in 1980, of explicit criteria for the diagnosis of substance use disorders has aided epidemiological and clinical research. Two currently used sets of criteria for substance dependence, the fundamental behavioural disorder underlying most substance abuse problems, are listed in Table 34.3. While similar, these criteria differ sufficiently that agreement between them on case classification is far from perfect (k = 0.67) (Caetano and Tam 1995). Several general sources are given in the reference list for the reader desiring further clinical information on substance abuse.

Table 34.1 Definitions of some terms used in the substance abuse field

Term	Definition
Psychoactive	Any chemical—alcohol, therapeutic agent, industrial compound, or illicit drug—with important effects on the central nervous system.
Substance	A psychoactive that typically is associated with a substance use disorder. The term includes alcohol, opioids, sedative-hypnotics, and antianxiety agents of the barbiturate and benzodiazepine types, psychomotor stimulants, especially amphetamines and cocaine, tobacco products, and certain over-the-counter psychoactives. The terms *chemical* and *drug* in this context are synonymous with substance (e.g. 'chemical dependence', 'drug abuse').
Standard drink	A standard drink of beverage alcohol is equivalent to a 12 fl. oz. (US; 355 ml) domestic beer (alcohol content about 4%), a 5 fl. oz. (US; 148 ml) glass of table wine (about 12% alcohol), or a mixed drink containing 1 to 1.5 fl. oz (US; 29–40 ml) hard liquor (about 40% alcohol).
Use	Appropriate medical or social consumption of a psychoactive in a manner that minimizes the potential for dependence or abuse.
Heavy use	Use of a substance in greater quantity than the usual norms, but without obvious negative social, behavioural, or health consequences. Heavy alcohol or tobacco users may be dependent upon the substance. *At-risk* or *risky* drinkers refer to heavy consumers of alcohol, usually at rates of ≥ 15–21 drinks/week for men, ≥ 10–14 for women, or binges in which ≥ 4–6 drinks are consumed on a single drinking occasion. Safe drinking levels for elderly persons are recommended by the US National Institute on Alcohol Abuse and Alcoholism not to exceed 7 drinks/week or 2 drinks on a single drinking occasion.
Misuse	Use of a prescribed drug in a manner other than directed. The term can mean overuse, underuse, improper dose sequencing, lending, or borrowing another's medication, with or without harmful consequences.
Problem use	Use of a substance in a manner that induces negative social, behavioural, or health consequences. A 'problem' may or may not meet criteria for substance dependence or abuse, although many do. Alcohol 'problems' or drug 'problems' are categories often used by epidemiologists in community prevalence surveys.
Abuse	Of a substance is defined in DSM-IV (American Psychiatric Association 1994) as a maladaptive pattern of substance use leading to clinically significant impairment or distress, as manifested by one or more of the following, occurring within a 12-month period: (1) recurrent substance use resulting in failure to fulfill major role obligations at work or home; (2) recurrent substance use in physically hazardous situations; (3) recurrent substance-related legal problems; (4) continued substance use despite having persistent or recurrent social or interpersonal problems caused or exacerbated by the effects of a substance (pp. 182–3).
Harmful use	(ICD-10—World Health Organization 1992) approximates abuse in definition. Both imply milder severity of substance involvement than in substance dependence.
Dependence	Upon a substance is defined by explicit diagnostic criteria, such as those listed in DSM-IV or ICD-10 (see Table 34.2). Serious and persistent involvement in the heavy use of the substance is the rule. These approaches set aside the older distinction between *physical dependence* and *psychological dependence*, which are now viewed as differing manifestations of similar disorders. The terms *alcoholism* and *addiction* are usually used as synonyms for dependence on alcohol and other drugs, respectively.
Substance use disorder	A clinical condition in which substance abuse or substance dependence can be diagnosed.
Substance abuse, chemical dependence, and addictions	These terms are often used to refer to the entire professional/scientific field.

Table 34.2 A continuum of drug use behaviour[a]

Experimental	Social-recreational	Circumstantial-situational	Intensified	Compulsive
Low		Continuum of use frequency and risks[b]		High
Descriptions:				
No more than 10–15 trials	Stable	Use related to: Recurring situation(e.g. social anxiety, sexual inhibition)	Daily or frequent sporadic use	Daily or frequent use
	Social			High dose
Social			Low dose	
	Patterned (drug supply and equipment for use kept on hand)			Deterioration of social, vocational, and health functioning
Non-patterned (fortuitous)		Symptom (e.g. recurrent insomnia, pain)	Outwardly normal functioning	
Normative in youth		Life stress	Life activities beginning to orbit around drug-related elements	
	Internalized 'norms' or rules for safe use	Abuse or dependence can occur		Life orbits around drug use
				Dependence present
			Dependence likely	

[a]Adapted from United States National Commission on Marihuana and Drug Abuse 1973.
[b]Risks are social, vocational, and health. For illicit drugs, the risks of overdose and criminal arrest are present all along the continuum.

Epidemiology

Risk factors

Risk factors for substance use disorders in the elderly are listed in Table 34.4. Predisposing factors are similar at all ages. Factors that may increase substance exposure and consumption level and thus set the stage for abuse or dependence in some individuals, include: demographics (e.g. gender and ethnicity); chronic illnesses for which controlled substances are often prescribed on a regular basis; institutionalization in long-term care settings; and several psychological and social factors, especially negative affects associated with loss and loneliness (Dupree and Schonfeld 1998). Gerontologists have often attributed late-life substance use problems to major loss and other life stress, but this relationship is in fact quite enigmatic. Although clinically one often sees cases in which major stress accompanies increased alcohol or drug use, it is not easy at times to determine whether a particular life event is a consequence or a cause of substance abuse. Factors that increase or prolong the effects of substances with age (i.e. pharmacokinetic and pharmacodynamic factors) may increase their dependence liability, although studies proving such an effect with regard to alcohol, benzodiazepines, or opioid analgesics are so far lacking (Ozdemir *et al.* 1996). Regular alcohol or psychoactive drug use can also increase functional impairment caused by a variety of illnesses that are more common in old age, e.g. cognitive, cardiovascular, pulmonary, gastrointestinal, and metabolic disorders. Clinical complications can arise from adverse drug–drug interactions between psychoactive substances and other prescribed medications (Adams 1995; Korrapati and Vestal 1995). At the same time, some elders may overuse alcohol or sedatives as medication to abate arthritic pain or insomnia. These alterations in biological sensitivity to drugs, comorbid medical illness, and medication interactions can lead to biomedical problems in the elderly at substance consumption rates that would have caused little or no difficulty earlier in life.

Table 34.3 DSM-IV versus ICD-10 criteria for substance dependence

DSM-IV criteria*	ICD-10 criteria*
1. Tolerance, as defined by either of the following: (a) need for markedly increased amounts of the substance to achieve intoxication or desired effect; or (b) markedly diminished effect with continued use of the same amount of the substance.	1. Strong desire or sense of compulsion to take the substance.
2. Withdrawal, as manifested by either of the following: (a) characteristic withdrawal syndrome for the substance; or (b) the same (or a closely related) substance is taken to relieve avoiding withdrawal symptoms.	2. Difficulties in controlling substance-taking behavior in terms of its onset, termination or levels of use.
3. The substance is often taken in larger amounts or over a longer period than was intended.	3. A physiological withdrawal state when substance use has ceased or been reduced, as evidenced by: the characteristic withdrawal syndrome for the substance; or use of the same (or a closely related) substance with the intention of relieving or avoid withdrawal symptoms.
4. There is a persistent desire or unsuccessful efforts to cut down or control substance use.	4. Evidence of tolerance, such that increased doses of the psychoactive substance are required in order to achieve effects originally produced by lower doses (clear examples of this are found in alcohol- and opiate-dependent individuals who may take daily doses sufficient to incapacitate or kill nontolerant users).
5. A great deal of time is spent in activities necessary to obtain the substance (e.g. visiting multiple doctors or driving long distances), use the substance (e.g. chain smoking), or recover from its effects.	5. Progressive neglect of alternative pleasures or interests because of psychoactive substance use, Increased amount of time necessary to obtain or take the substance, or to recover from its effects.
6. Important social, occupational, or recreational activities are given up or reduced because of substance use	6. Persisting with substance use despite clear evidence of overtly harmful consequences, such as harm to the liver through excessive drinking, depressive mood states consequent to periods of heavy substance use, or drug-related impairment of cognitive functioning; efforts should be made to determine that the user was actually, or could be expected to be, aware of the nature and extent of the harm.
7. Substance use is continued despite knowledge of having a persistent or recurrent physical or psychological problem that is likely to have been caused or exacerbated by the substance (e.g. current cocaine use despite recognition of cocaine-induced depression, or continued drinking despite a peptic ulcer made worse by alcohol consumption).	

*DSM-IV, *Diagnostic and statistical manual of mental disorders*, 4th edn (American Psychiatric Association, 1994, p. 181).
ICD-10, *International classification of diseases*, 10th edn (World Health Organization, 1992, pp. 75–6). For either system, at least 3 of the listed criteria must be met in the same 12-month period to make the diagnosis of dependence on a substance.

Table 34.4 Risk factors for substance abuse in the elderly

Predisposing factors
Family history (alcohol)
Previous substance abuse
Previous pattern of substance consumption (individual and cohort effects)
Personality traits (sedative-hypnotics, anxiolytics)
Factors that may increase substance exposure and consumption level
Gender (men—alcohol, illicit drugs; women—sedative-hypnotics, anxiolytics)
Chronic illness associated with pain (opioid analgesics), insomnia (hypnotic drugs), or anxiety (anxiolytics)
Long-term prescribing (sedative-hypnotics, anxiolytics)
Caregiver overuse of 'as needed' medication (institutionalized elderly)
Life stress, loss, social isolation
Negative affects (depression, grief, demoralization, anger) (alcohol)
Family collusion and drinking partners (alcohol)
Discretionary time, money (alcohol)
Factors that may increase the effects and abuse potential of substances
Age-associated drug sensitivity (pharmacokinetic, pharmacodynamic factors)
Chronic medical illnesses
Other medications (alcohol–drug, drug–drug interactions)

Comparative prevalence of geriatric substance use disorders

Tobacco, alcohol, and prescribed sedative–hypnotic drugs account for most of the substance dependence problems seen in the elderly. As in younger age groups, cigarette smoking is the most common substance abuse problem in the elderly. In every survey reporting both alcohol and prescription drug cases, alcohol abuse cases exceed drug abuse cases by a significant margin.

Principles of diagnosis and treatment

Assessment of geriatric substance use disorders

General approaches

Denial of substance abuse is common in affected persons of all ages. Reasons for this include substance-induced amnesia for intoxication episodes, shame about reliance on alcohol or drugs, pessimism about recovery, and, of course, the desire to continue use. For these reasons, careful rapport building through repeated contacts, enquiry with relatives, caregivers and others in the social network, reviews of medical and pharmacy records, and home visitation are especially useful case assessment methods. An instrument intended to guide home assessment by visiting nurses and social caseworkers is presented in Table 34.5. Based on clinical experience and published case reports, this outline was devised to assist a prevention/intervention project focusing on elderly substance abusers within a diversified suburban community mental health programme in Oregon. The DSM-IV and ICD-10 dependence criteria (Table 34.3) offer a reasonable framework for acquiring information in order to establish a clinical diagnosis.

Special examinations

Physical and laboratory findings can help to establish a diagnosis of alcohol dependence, but offer little in typical drug cases. Toxicological examinations of urine, blood, and breath samples for suspected substances may be the most useful findings to corroborate the history. Neuropsychological evaluation and brain imaging (computed axial scanning, magnetic resonance imaging (MRI)) may help to identify complicating brain disorders, although primary dementias and dementias secondary to alcohol or drug abuse may produce similar initial cognitive or morphological deficits. In so far as substance-induced

Table 34.5 Senior substance abuse assessment tool: Clackamas County Mental Health Services, Oregon (for in-home assessment by case-workers (unpublished, abridged))

A. *Descriptive account*
1. Medications (including prescription drugs, over-the-counter drugs, home remedies, alcohol)
2. Health problem list
3. Hospitalizations (note especially those for falls or mental health problems)
4. Observations of environment (organization, cleanliness, odours) and the elderly person (grooming, weight, skin colour, swelling, bruises, burns)

B. *Observations check-list*
1. Environmental clues to substance abuse
   - Alcohol odour
   - Squalid surroundings
   - Cigarette burns on furniture
   - 'Nesting' (TV, other paraphernalia arranged so the person spends long periods in one seat)
   - Concern expressed by significant others
   - Complaints about behaviour from neighbours
2. Physical problems
   - Eyes yellow or bloodshot
   - Sallow skin
   - Red nose
   - Oedema
   - Diarrhoea
   - Incontinence
   - Malnutrition
   - Anorexia
   - Injuries
   - Bruises at furniture level
   - Falls to the side (rib fractures)
   - Gastritis
   - Gout
   - Hypertension
   - Indigestion
   - Hypothermia
   - Tremors
3. Emotional status
   - Depression
   - Loneliness
   - Anxiety
   - Frequent mood swings
   - Lack of motivation
   - Irritability
   - Helplessness
4. Behavioural observations
   - Self-neglect
   - Social isolation
   - Resists help
   - Unusual or erratic behaviour
   - Strong negative response to questions about alcohol (drugs)
   - Chronic insomnia or change in sleep pattern
   - Slurred speech or unsteady gait
5. Thinking processes
   - Confusion
   - Disorientation
   - Suicidal ideation
   - Impaired abstract reasoning
   - Memory loss
   - Slowed thought process

defects either remain static or actually improve with prolonged abstinence (Golombok *et al.* 1988; Salzman *et al.* 1992; Oslin *et al.* 1998), serial psychometric testing and brain imaging may be useful in differential diagnosis.

Clinical features

Signs and symptoms of substance use disorders

In old age these can be subtle, atypical, or mimic symptoms of other geriatric illness. In mild or circumscribed cases among community-dwelling elderly people, episodic alcohol abuse or low-dose benzodiazepine dependence may not produce physical signs or complaints, and may easily be concealed from others. Moderate alcohol dependence may have a circumscribed clinical presentation of increasingly uncontrolled hypertension or diabetes mellitus, while moderate benzodiazepine or alcohol dependence may present with the complaint of daytime drowsiness or forgetfulness. In more severe cases, substance abuse can produce delirium or dementia, which the clinician may falsely attribute to other causes. Other serious but non-specific presenting signs and symptoms, for example poor grooming, depression, erratic changes of mood or behaviour, malnutrition, bladder and bowel incontinence, muscle weakness or frank myopathy, gait disorders, recurring falls, burns, or head trauma, may be caused by unsuspected alcohol or drug abuse.

Features often associated with alcohol or sedative dependence

These include heavy tobacco use, chronic pain syndromes or insomnia, persistent family discord, a course of inexplicable 'ups and downs', a pattern of doing well in hospital but poorly at home, and patient defensiveness when queried about substance use. When such factors are noted, the clinician needs to be alert to the possibility of underlying substance dependence.

Treatment and case management

The goals of substance abuse treatment in the elderly are threefold: stabilization and reduction of substance consumption; treatment of coexisting problems; and arrangement of appropriate psychological and social interventions to reduce relapse risks. Reducing consumption may be simple and straightforward in mild dependence, especially if the older person is highly cooperative. In other cases it may be very complicated and hazardous, requiring hospital care or a protracted outpatient course of treatment, in cases of longstanding, high-dose dependence. Treatment of coexisting problems can be a crucial step, especially when chronic pain, chronic insomnia, or a mood disorder has been a major factor sustaining the substance dependence, or when serious medical complications of substance abuse are present. Psychosocial interventions range from informal plans (e.g. arranging for increased visits by loved ones, or enrolment in a senior citizens' activity programme or day centre), to formal interventions (e.g. admission to a senior citizens' substance abuse programme, or to residential care).

Alcohol use disorders

Prevalence

Even though alcohol use and alcohol problems decline with age, they still constitute a significant public health problem. Recent community surveys show that alcohol use in the US is most prevalent in the 25–45-year age group. Furthermore, it declines stepwise in older age cohorts, so that 12-month prevalence levels of 46% are reached for persons aged 55 and older who report any alcohol use (Ruchlin 1997), and 30% for those who report having consumed at least 12 drinks in the past 12 months (Grant 1997). Rates of any recent alcohol use continue to decline after age 55, to 25% of persons age 85 and older (Ruchlin 1997). Rates for heavy and problem alcohol use by older adults vary widely depending upon the population sampled and definitions of use (Atkinson 1990). Community prevalence rates of alcohol use disorders indicate that about 2–3% of elderly men and under 1% of elderly women in the US suffer from these disorders (Helzer *et al.* 1991; Grant 1997). Because older adults with alcohol problems also have high rates of comorbid medical disorders, they are represented much more commonly in clinical settings. Surveys of elderly clinical cohorts, showing rates of current alcohol problems from 4% to 23%, are summarized in Table 34.6.

Older men are twice as likely to be using alcohol as older women, and are two to six times more likely than women to be problem drinkers. These patterns hold true across diverse ethnic and racial groups. Once alcohol dependence develops it is more likely to persist in older men than in women. Several factors contribute to the decline in drinking and drinking problems with age, including premature deaths of early-onset alcoholics, moderation or cessation of drinking with age by surviving alcoholics and social drinkers, and cohort effects. The epidemiology of alcohol use and abuse in older adults is reviewed in greater detail elsewhere (Atkinson 2000).

Early- versus late-onset alcohol problems

Retrospective studies of community-dwelling elderly people have noted subsets who report increasing their alcohol consumption in later life, either for the first time or following a fluctuating pattern established earlier. More recent household

Table 34.6 Prevalence of active alcohol problems among older adults in US clinical settings

Setting (Reference)	Age cut-off for sample	Sample size	Gender	Frequency of active alcoholism (%)
General medical outpatient clinic, Omaha NE (Jones *et al.* 1993)	≥ 65	154	both	4
Acute medical inpatient wards, San Diego CA (Schuckit *et al.* 1980)	≥ 65	222	men	6
Community geriatric outreach mental health team, Seattle WA (Reifler *et al.* 1982)	≥ 60	2309	both	9
Primary care medical clinic, Indianapolis IN (Callahan and Tierney 1995)	≥ 60	3954	both	11
Emergency department visitors, Chapel Hill NC (Adams *et al.* 1992)	≥ 65	205	both	14
Nursing-home admissions, Portland, OR (Joseph *et al.* 1995)	> 50*	117	both*	18
Geriatric psychiatry residential treatment unit, Tampa FL (Speer and Bates 1992)	≥ 55	128	both	23

*Mean age 69 years; SD 8.6; 97% of sample male

surveys and clinical reports demonstrate that an onset of initial drinking problems at age 50 or older is not uncommon. However, people with early-onset alcoholism who achieved prolonged abstinence in middle life but later relapsed can be mistaken for late-onset cases (Atkinson 1994). The notion that late-onset alcohol dependence usually occurs secondary to a mood or organic mental disorder has not been upheld by recent systematic studies. Many persons with late-onset alcohol problems were social drinkers (Neve *et al.* 1997) or heavy or reactive drinkers (Schutte *et al.* 1998) in the past. Late-onset alcohol problems are typically milder and more circumscribed than those beginning earlier in life. Compared with early-onset cases, late-onset problem drinkers also tend to have less alcoholism among relatives, less psychopathology, and higher socioeconomic status—a larger proportion of late-onset problem drinkers are women (Atkinson 1994; Liberto and Oslin 1995). While there is clinical evidence to support the view that late-onset drinking problems often begin in reaction to life stress (e.g. Finlayson *et al.* 1988), it is not true that this group exhibits more reactive drinking than early-onset alcoholics. Compared with alcoholism of long duration, late-onset problems tend to resolve more often without formal treatment (Moos *et al.* 1991). However, there is little evidence to suggest that late-onset patients respond more favourably to treatment than early-onset patients.

Therapeutic use and health maintenance value of alcohol

Use for socialization, appetite, and sleep

Several careful studies (reviewed in Atkinson and Kofoed 1984) demonstrated that modest amounts of alcohol can enhance patient socialization and morale, and thus the use of small amounts of beverage alcohol has been advocated as a social adjuvant in elder residential-care facilities. However, residents who have cardiovascular or cognitive disorders, or who receive benzodiazepines, should not use alcohol. Clinicians who advise outpatients to use alcohol as a social adjuvant should recall that controls existed in the residential studies to regulate the quantity consumed and to assure its use within a social context. Iatrogenic alcohol use disorders are not unknown. Similar cautions apply in advising older patients to use alcohol to enhance their appetite or induce sleep. In fact, sleep is progressively disturbed by habitual bedtime alcohol use (Hartford and Samorajski 1982).

Safe drinking levels

Generally recommended safe ceiling levels for healthy elders are no more than 14 standard drinks per week or 3 drinks per drinking occasion for older men, and 7 drinks per week or 2 drinks per drinking occasion for women. Older women sustain substantially higher blood alcohol levels after a standard alcohol load than men (Lucey *et al.* 1999).

Protective value of alcohol against coronary heart disease and other disorders

An intriguing epidemiological finding is the association of regular—but moderate—alcohol use (up to two standard drinks/day) with a lower morbidity and mortality from coronary heart disease, especially in men, when compared to that in heavy alcohol users and abstainers. This 'U'- or 'J'-shaped relationship appears to be quite robust. Why should teetotallers have a higher morbidity and mortality than moderate drinkers? The abstainer group is heterogeneous and includes former alcoholics and those perhaps predisposed to cardiac disease, but other factors seem to be implicated. Further study is needed to determine the respective contributions of an alcohol-induced rise in high-density lipoproteins (Srivastava *et al.* 1994), antioxidant effects of beverage alcohol (Artaud-Wild *et al.* 1993; Soleas *et al.* 1997), and other alcohol-associated biological mechanisms (Davidson 1989) in the moderate drinkers, as well as the contribution of adverse health events and less adaptive coping skills more commonly noted in the abstainers (Mertens *et al.* 1996).

A more general apparent protective effect of moderate drinking on mortality from all causes has also been demonstrated in several studies (e.g.

Colditz *et al.* 1985; Mertens *et al.* 1996; Thun *et al.* 1997), even taking into account those diseases for which increasing alcohol consumption is clearly associated with higher mortality. In one study of 490 000 persons aged 35 to 70, moderate drinking reduced the overall mortality by about 20%, although much of this general effect on mortality may be related to cardiovascular disease (Thun *et al.* 1997). Recent reports have indicated that a moderate alcohol intake (especially red table wine) may have a beneficial effect on cognitive status and a possible protective effect against the development of age-related retinal macular degeneration (reviewed in Atkinson 2000), but these findings require further study.

Reactive drinking

Old age alcohol problems, especially those of late onset, are often depicted in gerontology literature as a consequence of late-life losses and other stresses of ageing, but the stress-reactive hypothesis for problem drinking in old age has been difficult to validate (Finney and Moos 1984). People with increasing alcohol problems in association with major losses are, however, not uncommonly encountered in clinical practice. Once a pattern of excessive alcohol use has been established, evanescent negative-affect states (e.g. depression, sadness, boredom, anger, tension) may trigger repeated drinking episodes (Dupree and Schonfeld 1998). Patients with longstanding alcohol use disorders may be especially vulnerable to increased or recurrent late-life alcohol problems in conjunction with stress (see Cases 1 and 2 below).

Clinical features of alcohol use disorders

Primary features

There is no evidence that the elderly differ from other age groups in the primary manifestations of their alcohol dependence (Table 34.3). Circumscribed abuse or harmful use (for example, complication of a pre-existing medical disorder or drinking and driving, without evidence of other problems—see Case 4 below) is common in late-onset cases.

Associated features and complications

Alcohol intoxication may occur at lower dose levels in older persons, because of increased biological sensitivity. Several characteristic laboratory abnormalities accompanying many cases of alcohol dependence are listed in Table 34.7. While there is no evidence that alcohol withdrawal disorders (the tremulous syndrome, hallucinosis, seizures, and delirium tremens) occur at different rates in the elderly, alcohol withdrawal is more difficult to treat in this group of people and may be associated with greater mortality (Liskow *et al.* 1989; Brower *et al.* 1994). Older alcoholic patients are at high risk for the development of multiple medical problems (for extensive reviews see Gambert and Katsoyannis 1995; Smith 1995). Alcohol-related liver disease, when present, carries a poor prognosis if drinking continues (Woodhouse and James 1985). A number of cancers (mouth, oesophagus, pharynx, larynx, liver, colorectal), hypoglycaemia, hyperuricaemia, hypertriglyceridaemia, osteoporosis, anaemias, congestive heart failure, aspiration pneumonia, and accidental injuries can also be caused or aggravated by alcohol dependence. Breast cancer in one large recent survey was 1.3 times more common in women who currently drink than in non-drinkers (Thun *et al.* 1997). Moreover, the control of hypertension and diabetes mellitus is compromised by excessive drinking.

Behavioural complications

Mild to moderate depressive symptoms are present in more than half of all alcoholics entering treatment, regardless of their age (Atkinson 1999). In the majority of cases, such depressive symptoms appear to be alcohol-induced (in many cases even meeting the criteria for major depression), since scores on depression measures usually fall to normal levels without specific antidepressant treatment after 2 to 4 weeks' sobriety (Case 1 below) (Brown *et al.* 1995). Affective disorders are diagnosed much less often than simple depressed mood (see Table 34.10). Alcohol problems are found in a variable proportion of older suicides, the reported range being 7% to 30% or more; interestingly, the

Table 34.7 Frequency of laboratory abnormalities in elderly and younger inpatients with alcoholism[a]

	Results[c]			
	Patients ≥ 65 years[d]		Younger patients[d]	
Blood tests[b]	Number tested	Percent abnormal	Number tested	Percent abnormal
MCH increased	213	71	123	57**
AST increased	214	56	123	42*
GGT increased	123	55	101	48
MCV increased	213	44	124	17**
Glucose increased	206	32	124	36
Uric acid increased	201	21	123	<1**
Albumin decreased	186	17	115	3**
Alkaline phosphatase increased	213	11	123	15
Triglycerides increased	191	16	122	19
Phosphorus increased	198	9	124	11

[a]Adapted from Hurt *et al.* 1988.
[b]MCH, mean corpuscular hemoglobin; AST, aspartate aminotransferase; GGT, gamma-glutamyltransferase; MCV, mean corpuscular volume.
[c]Number, number of patients tested in each age group; percent, percent of patients tested in the age group who had an abnormal value.
[d]Older patients: $n = 216$; mean age 69.6 years; age range 65 to 83 years. Younger patients: $n = 125$; mean age 44.3 years; age range 19 to 64 years.
**$p < 0.01$ using Wilcoxon two-sample rank sum test to compare age groups for proportion having an abnormal value; *$p < 0.05$; for others, $p > 0.3$.

association of alcoholism with suicide may be stronger in late middle-aged men than in old age or women (Conwell *et al.* 1990). Social impairment ranges from being mild to very severe—presenting in extreme cases as 'senile squalor' or 'Diogenes' syndrome' (MacMillan and Shaw 1966; Kafetz and Cox 1982; Wrigley and Cooney 1992; Cooney and Hamid 1995).

Ageing and alcohol neurotoxicity

Alcohol use and cognition in non-alcoholics

The neurotoxicity of alcohol increases with age (reviewed in detail in Atkinson 2000), with pharmacokinetics playing a role in its development. For instance, a non-alcoholic man in his sixties may have a peak blood alcohol level 20% higher than a man in his thirties after a standard alcohol load, and for women this difference is even greater (Lucey *et al.* 1999). But even when one controls for blood alcohol level, performance is more impaired with age after a standard alcohol load, indicating an increasing neuropharmacodynamic effect of alcohol with age. This has been demonstrated on measures of subjective intoxication experience, memory, performance on divided attention tasks, and body sway and hand dexterity, after single alcohol doses. Cognitive performance also tends to be impaired in older social drinkers tested in the sober state, but only at relatively high consumption levels (e.g. above 21 drinks/week) (Parsons and Nixon 1998). Regional cerebral blood flow is reduced in otherwise healthy elderly volunteers, proportional to their reported alcohol consumption level (Meyer *et al.* 1984).

Varieties of cognitive loss in alcoholics

Following prolonged drinking, alcoholics often show cognitive impairment, which tends to be both more extensive and protracted with age (reviewed in more detail in Atkinson 2000). Such lingering deficits, demonstrable for weeks to months after the last drinking bout, and resulting in psychosocial dysfunction, can occur in up to 9% of mixed-age abstinent alcoholic patients. Older abstinent alcoholics continue to show a gradual resolution of memory and other deficits over periods ranging from several months to as long as 5 years after discontinuing alcohol. Current nosologies have not offered very satisfactory categories for these slowly resolving disorders, with the result that unofficial terms are coined instead, for example 'reversible alcoholic cognitive deterioration' (Lishman 1997).

There are also many cases in which neurological deficits appear to be irreversible. Some of these persisting, alcoholism-related CNS disorders take distinctive forms, such as the alcohol amnestic disorder (Wernicke–Korsakoff syndrome), cerebellar cortical degeneration, and rarer entities like central pontine myelinosis and dementia associated with demyelination of the corpus callosum (Marchiafava–Bignami disease). These disorders not only have fairly specific clinical manifestations but also special neuropathological features that distinguish them from other types of dementia.

Is there an 'alcoholic dementia?'

In contrast, the question of whether prolonged, excessive alcohol consumption can cause a diffuse dementia ('alcoholic dementia', or 'alcohol-induced persisting dementia') remains controversial almost 50 years after Courville (1955) first proposed such a disorder (reviewed in Smith and Atkinson 1995). On the one hand, it has been asserted that alcohol is as important a cause of dementia as vascular disease (Lishman 1990), while others counter that, in a heavy drinking society, alcoholism and dementia can often be coincident without any causal connection (Ryan and Butters 1986; Victor *et al.* 1989). A lack of distinctive clinical markers and specific gross neuropathology have complicated the study of alcoholic dementia, and in current nosologies the diagnosis of alcohol-induced persisting dementia tends to be made by exclusion. Viewed in this light, the tendency of dementia researchers to confine their study of alcohol-related dementias to the Wernicke–Korsakoff and rarer syndromes mentioned above, often simply excluding persons with a history of heavy alcohol use from more general studies of dementia, is understandable. Early surveys suggested that only a small proportion of dementia cases were associated with prior alcoholism (2–3% in US and 7% in UK community surveys, 1–15% in clinical cohorts, most under 10%), reinforcing the tendency of researchers to disregard this elusive category. These surveys typically suffered, however, from inadequate information about patients' alcohol use and their neurological and neuropsychological status. Three more recent clinical studies of older demented cohorts (Table 34.8), based on systematic information, demonstrate that prior heavy alcohol exposure is more common (22–24% of cases) than earlier reports had indicated, especially in men. These reports also demonstrate that routine clinical records seriously under-represent alcoholism and heavy drinking in the histories of demented cohorts. Even these careful studies are flawed, however, in two important respects: they are retrospective and uncontrolled.

Recent research on dementia in mixed-age alcoholic populations

In mixed-age groups of alcoholic patients without an amnestic disorder, alcohol neurotoxicity is

Table 34.8 Dementia and prior heavy alcohol exposure: retrospective studies

Author: setting (*n*)	Criteria	Men (%)	Women (%)	Total (%)
King (1986): Dementia clinic, Baltimore (65)	DSM-III alcohol use disorder, or heavy alcohol consumption	29	17	22
Smith and Atkinson (1994): Dementia clinic, Portland (120)	Heavy alcohol consumption (3-4 drinks/day)	22	–	22
Carlen *et al.*1994: Long-term care facilities, Ontario (130)	Alcoholism, medical records and current questionnaires	37	12	24

suggested by a number of deficits in neuropsychological performance (Ryan and Butters 1986; Parsons and Nixon 1993; Parsons 1994) and by evidence from brain imaging studies of atrophy of the cerebral cortex, corpus callosum, anterior hippocampus, diencephalon, caudate nucleus, and parts of the limbic system, including the mesial temporal lobe and thalamus (studies reviewed in Atkinson 2000). Age, rather than duration of alcoholism, tends to be the most critical factor in the manifestation of both the cognitive performance and imaging findings. Cortical changes reflect a loss of both grey and white matter, occur in older alcoholic individuals beginning about the fifth decade, and are over and above the changes associated with normal ageing (Jernigan *et al.* 1991; Pfefferbaum *et al.* 1992, 1997). These losses are especially evident in frontal areas (Kril *et al.* 1997; Pfefferbaum *et al.* 1997). Frontal cortical deficits have also been demonstrated in positron emission tomographic (PET) studies in older alcoholics (Gilman *et al.* 1990; Adams *et al.* 1993), as well as in studies of regional cerebral blood flow and event-related potentials.

There is also evidence that the imaged frontal cortical defects are related to impairment in neuropsychological performance: indeed, the pattern of test performance deficits in patients with chronic alcoholism has, in recent years, prompted the 'frontal lobe hypothesis' (Oscar-Berman and Hutner 1993). According to this view, the vulnerability of the frontal lobes to alcohol accounts for many of the persistent neuropsychological deficits in patients with chronic alcoholism, including problem-solving, abstraction, organization, judgement, and working memory (studies reviewed in Kril *et al.* 1997; Pfefferbaum *et al.* 1997). On the other hand, widespread damage throughout the brain is also indicated by recent research, and other models besides the frontal lobe hypothesis can explain a number of performance deficits in persons with chronic alcoholism who do not have an amnestic disorder (Evert and Oscar-Berman 1995). For example, deficits in visual–spatial–motor skills may instead be associated with tissue loss in the anterior parietal cortex (Pfefferbaum *et al.* 1997) or with ventricular dilatation, rather than cortical atrophy (DiSclafani *et al.* 1995). Furthermore, there is ample evidence of tissue loss in deeper diencephalic and limbic structures in non-amnestic patients (Jernigan *et al.* 1991), which might be the primary basis for cerebral dysfunction and even cortical tissue loss (in accord with the 'continuity theory' that attributes all neurological lesions in alcoholics to the same fundamental subcortical processes).

Histopathological findings in older persons with alcoholism include neuron loss and damage (Samorajski *et al.* 1984) and reduced dendritic connections (Ryan and Butters 1986). Several studies point in particular to changes in the frontal cortex in chronic alcoholics (e.g. neuron loss, shrinkage of the neuronal soma, and loss or shrinkage of large pyramidal cells from the superior frontal cortex) (Harper and Kril 1989, 1990; Kril and Harper 1989). Such changes also occur with normal ageing, suggesting that an age-related decline in brain structural integrity, especially in the frontal lobes, reduces the margin of safety and leaves the brains of old, relative to young, persons more susceptible to alcohol neurotoxicity (Pfefferbaum *et al.* 1997).

Alcohol as a risk factor for dementia

Whether there is a distinctive alcoholic dementia may be the wrong question to ask—or at least not the only question—nor, necessarily, the most important question. Alcohol could be a risk factor, like hypertension, that increases a person's vulnerability to dementia. That is, rather than typically producing a distinctive dementia, alcohol, operating as one influence among several, could contribute to Alzheimer's, vascular, or other forms of dementia. Alcohol exposure directly (i.e. neurotoxic effects of ethanol or its metabolic products) or indirectly (e.g. through reducing the bioavailability of dietary thiamine) impairs CNS function and structure in a variety of ways. Furthermore, alcoholics are known to be at high risk for repeated head trauma and infectious diseases, which could predispose them to dementia. Heavy drinking is also associated with the aggravation of hypertension and various other cardiovascular diseases, and thus could contribute indirectly to a vascular presentation of dementia (Fisman *et al.* 1996). This notion is consistent with preliminary clinical data from our programme (Atkinson 1997) and with data from the Liverpool longitudinal study of community-dwelling elderly people, showing that men aged 65 and older who were previously heavy drinkers were 4.6 times more likely to have a current diagnosis of any form of dementia than non-heavy drinking men (Saunders *et al.* 1991). Although these data sets are small, the hypothesis and findings to date suggest a clinical research approach worth pursuing, i.e. including alcohol in multifactorial studies of the aetiology of dementia. If it proves true that alcohol is a common causal factor in many cases of dementia, at least in men, it will be important for clinicians to consider alcohol more carefully in routine dementia assessments.

Differential diagnosis of dementia in alcoholics and heavy drinkers

Current diagnostic criteria for alcohol-induced persisting dementia are given in Table 34.9(a), but they presume an aetiological connection between past alcohol use and present dementia that is often impossible for clinicians to specify with confidence. Some recent efforts have been made to improve the differential diagnosis by specifying additional provisional features that appear to be regularly associated with dementia in alcoholics and heavy drinkers (Osuntokun *et al.* 1994; Oslin *et al.* 1998). Features favouring alcohol-related dementia include: a history of prolonged heavy alcohol use; the presence of peripheral polyneuropathy and/or gait ataxia; sparing of naming (i.e. absence of dysnomia); evidence, after a period of abstinence, of stabilization or improvement in cognitive functioning or reversal of cerebral atrophy seen on MRI; and several other characteristics that are also summarized in Table 34.9(b). This approach to differential diagnosis, if affirmed by prospective studies, may help distinguish more precisely between alcohol-associated dementia, Alzheimer's dementia, and mixed cases. Case 3 below illustrates a number of the features emphasized here.

Comparative prevalence of comorbid psychiatric disorders in ageing alcoholics

Among substance-related comorbidities, active tobacco dependence—principally from cigarette smoking—is highly prevalent in elderly alcoholics (about 50–70%), active dependence on prescribed sedatives, anxiolytics, and opioid analgesics varies (2–14%) depending on the cohort studied, and recent illicit drug abuse is very uncommon in ageing alcoholics. Non substance-related psychiatric comorbidities in clinical datasets vary even more, depending upon the cohort and setting where studied. Data from three recent reports are summarized in Table 34.10, which shows that mood, cognitive, and anxiety disorders are the most common comorbid psychiatric conditions in this age group. Determining in a particular case whether depression or cognitive deficits are secondary to recent alcohol use or represent a true comorbid disorder may be difficult within the usual time constraints of inpatient care or consultation; and mixed pictures do occur (e.g. comorbid depression aggravated by alcohol effects on mood) (Atkinson and Misra 2001).

Course of problem drinking in old age

Based on retrospective reports, the span from the onset of the first alcohol problem to the date of entry into current treatment can be as long as 50 years. Over this course, drinking may have been steady, progressive, or variable; in some cases, sober periods of 10 years or more occur between problem-drinking episodes. In one small prospective study, Schuckit and his colleagues (1980) conducted careful clinical assessments and then followed older alcoholic and non-alcoholic patients in their late sixties and early seventies for 3 years, finding relapses and remissions in several cases, as well as the onset of new problem drinking in 5% of controls. In a much larger prospective 4-year repeated telephone survey of over 1600 community-dwelling, late middle-aged drinkers and non-drinkers, 37% initially reported one or more current alcohol problems (Moos *et al.* 1991). Resolution of current problems within the next year occurred in 29% of the problem

Table 34.9(a) DSM-IV diagnostic criteria for alcohol-induced persisting dementia*

A The development of multiple deficits manifested by both:
- (1) memory impairment (impaired ability to learn new information or to recall previously learned information); and
- (2) one or more of the following cognitive disturbances:
  - (a) aphasia (language disturbance);
  - (b) apraxia (impaired ability to carry out motor activities despite intact motor function);
  - (c) agnosia (failure to recognize or identify objects despite intact sensory function); and/or
  - (d) disturbance in executive functioning (i.e. planning, organization, sequencing, abstracting).

B. The cognitive deficits in criteria A1 and A2 each cause significant impairment in social or occupational functioning and represent a significant decline from a previous level of functioning.

C. The deficits do not occur exclusively during the course of a delirium and persist beyond the usual duration of alcohol intoxication or withdrawal.

D. There is evidence from the history, physical examination, or laboratory findings that the deficits are etiologically related to the persisting effects of alcohol use.

*From American Psychiatric Association 1994

Table 34.9(b) Features that may distinguish between alcohol-related and Alzheimer's dementias*

Features	Alcohol-induced persisting dementia	Alzeheimer's dementia
Meets criteria for dementia	+	+
Cortical atrophy on MRI	+	+
Long history of heavy drinking	+	–
Ataxia may be present	+	–
Peripheral polyneuropathy may be present	+	–
Cerebellar atrophy may be present on MRI	+	–
Abstinence halts cognitive decline	+	–
Cortical atrophy can be reversed	+	–
Anomia/dysnomia prominent	–	+
Cognitive decline continues despite abstinence	–	+
CSF 'tau' protein may be elevated	–	+

*Symbols '+' and '–' mean that the finding is more (+) or less (–) likely to be associated with this form of dementia; MRI, magnetic resonance imaging of the brain; CSF, cerebrospinal fluid.

Based on Morikawa *et al.* 1999; Oslin *et al.* 1998; Smith and Atkinson 1995

Table 34.10 Psychiatric comorbidity (%) in older adults with alcohol use disorders

Comorbid Disorder	Atkinson *et al.* 2001 OP, A, ≥ age 55, DSM-IV, n = 101[a]	Finlayson *et al.* 1988 IP, A, ≥ age 65, DSM-III, n = 216[a]	Blow *et al.* 1992 OP, MH, age 60–69, DSM-III, n = 3986[a]	Blow *et al.* 1992 OP, MH, ≥ age 70, DSM-III, n = 543*a*
Any other disorder (one or more)	55	about 50*b*	48	55
Mood disorder	24	12	21	21
(Major depression)	(15)	(8)	(9)	(12)
(Bipolar disorder)	(4)	(2)	(5)	(4)
(Dysthymic disorder)	(5)	(1)	(8)	(5)
Dementia and cognitive disorders	13	25	9	18
Anxiety disorder	5	< 1	10	10
Post-traumatic stress disorder	8	0	4	2
Schizophrenia	2	0	9	8
Personality disorder	not reported	3	6	4

[a]Setting: IP = inpatient; OP = outpatient; A = alcohol treatment program; MH = mental health or psychiatric treatment program. All studies were from a single setting except for Blow *et al.*, which was pooled data from 172 VA facilities.
[b]Not reported in paper; personal communication from senior author, 1994.

drinkers. Early-onset problem drinkers remitted less often (24%) and tended to solve their problems by seeking professional help, while persons with recent-onset problems remitted more often (41%) and tended to resolve their problems without professional help. Gains made at one year were sustained at the fourth year resurvey in 70% of the remitted problem group (Schutte *et al.* 1994). Among non-problem drinkers at baseline, 8% developed one or more alcohol-related problems in the next year. Predictors of new problem drinking included a history of heavy drinking and increased drinking when under stress or feeling depressed (Schutte *et al.* 1998). There is evidence that social drinkers tend to modify their consumption downward with age, while problem drinkers are more likely to choose to abstain. The rate of problem drinking after age 85 is negligible. Mortality rates are very high when active drinking continues in the face of frank dementia or active alcohol-related liver disease.

Diagnosis, intervention, and management

Screening and diagnosis

Screening for alcohol problems should be part of the initial evaluation of all new geriatric patients. A standard screening measure such as the 'CAGE' questionnaire may be useful in some settings (Table 34.11(a)). This simple set of non-pejorative questions has been validated several times on elderly samples. However, it is important to recognize that as many as 60% of community-dwelling 'at-risk' older drinkers are CAGE-negative (Adams *et al.* 1996). Thus it is important to ascertain current alcohol consumption in addition to asking about drinking problems, taking care to translate the patient's definition of 'a drink' into standard units (see Table 34.1). Another questionnaire, the 24-item geriatric version of the Michigan Alcoholism Screening Test (MAST-G), has been validated for use with hospitalized elderly patients (Table 34.11(b)) (Blow 1991; Joseph *et al.* 1995). It is a more cumbersome instrument than the CAGE and may be most useful in postscreening follow-up. Positive findings at screening indicate those cases requiring a more thorough evaluation of current drinking problems, patient and family interviews, domiciliary visits, discussion with other caregivers, and physical and laboratory examinations.

Intervention

Once the diagnosis is established it is important to present the information thoroughly and objectively to the patient and spouse, or other close relative or caregiver, as a basis for urging an appropriate course of action. It is helpful to reassure the patient and family that older persons with drinking problems actually have tended to fare as well as or better than younger persons in a variety of treatment settings (Atkinson 1995).

Management of mild, circumscribed abuse

In mild cases and, especially, in 'at-risk' drinkers who do not yet have major alcohol-related problems, success can be achieved sometimes simply by offering advice to cut down or abstain, accompanied by informal social interventions as needed. This form of 'brief intervention' has been demonstrated to be effective in reducing alcohol consumption in two US studies of older heavy drinkers in medical practice rolls (Blow 1999; Fleming *et al.* 1999).

Management of more serious abuse or dependence

The person with more pervasive alcoholism should enter an outpatient alcoholism treatment programme, preferably one that offers specialized services for ageing patients (Center for Substance Abuse Treatment 1998). Successful programmes have been set up within mental health centres (Dupree *et al.* 1984) and general substance abuse programmes (Atkinson *et al.* 1998). Alcoholics Anonymous (AA) may also be a useful alternative (see Case 2 below), particularly when age-specific groups are available. Family involvement in treatment improves adherence and outcome. Ambulatory, gradual detoxification is often achieved without resort to medications or hospital admission. Use of the deterrent drug disulfiram can be hazardous, but naltrexone appears to be safe in

Table 34.11 Screening instruments for alcohol problems in older adults

Table 34.11(a) CAGE measure (Ewing 1984)

1. Have you ever felt you ought to **C**ut down on your drinking?
2. Have people **A**nnoyed you by criticizing your drinking?
3. Have you ever felt bad or **G**uilty about your drinking?
4. Have you ever had a drink first thing in the morning to steady your nerves or get rid of a hangover (**E**ye-opener)?

KEY: 2 or more answered positive suggests alcoholism or problem drinking (current or past).

Table 34.ll(b) Michigan Alcoholism Screening Test-Geriatric version (Blow 1991)

1. After drinking have you ever noticed an increase in your heart rate or beating in your chest?
2. When talking with others, do you ever underestimate how much you actually drink?
3. Does alcohol make you sleepy so that you often fall asleep in your chair?
4. After a few drinks, have you sometimes not eaten or been able to skip a meal because you didn't feel hungry?
5. Does having a few drinks help decrease your shakiness or tremors?
6. Does alcohol sometimes make it hard for you to remember parts of the day or night?
7. Do you have rules for yourself that you won't drink before a certain time of day?
8. Have you lost interest in hobbies or activities you used to enjoy?
9. When you wake up in the morning, do you ever have trouble remembering part of the night before?
10. Does having a drink help you sleep?
11. Do you hide your alcohol bottles from family members?
12. After a social gathering, have you ever felt embarrassed because you drank too much?
13. Have you ever been concerned that drinking might be harmful to your health?
14. Do you like to end an evening with a nightcap?
15. Did you find your drinking increased after someone close to you died?
16. In general, would you prefer to have a few drinks at home rather than go out to social events?
17. Are you drinking more now than in the past?
18. Do you usually take a drink to relax or calm your nerves?
19. Do you drink to take your mind off your problems?
20. Have you ever increased your drinking after experiencing a loss in your life?
21. Do you sometimes drive when you have had too much to drink?
22. Has a doctor or nurse ever said they were worried or concerned about your drinking?
23. Have you ever made rules to manage your drinking?
24. When you feel lonely does having a drink help?

KEY: 5 or more 'yes' responses is indicative of an alcohol problem (current or past).

geriatric cases and has shown some promise for reducing the extent of drinking lapses (Oslin *et al.* 1997*a,b*). Reports are lacking on the safety and efficacy of acamprosate in elderly persons, but it could prove equal to naltrexone in reducing craving and severe drinking lapses in this population. In studies of mixed-age patients, antidepressant drugs—tricyclics and selective serotonin-reuptake inhibitors—appear to affect favourably the course of drinking in alcoholics with current comorbid depression (Litten and Allen 1998; Atkinson 1999), but there is little evidence that these agents deter drinking in non-depressed patients.

Management of severe dependence

The most serious cases should be referred to an alcoholism inpatient treatment unit, which is also indicated when outpatient efforts fail. If severe medical or psychiatric complications are present, or major withdrawal is anticipated or already occurring, initial treatment on an acute medical or general psychiatric inpatient unit is warranted. Intractable heavy drinking in the face of dementia or other coexisting major mental disorder may force placement in residential care, where, unfortunately, alcoholic patients are not always welcomed. In a few US locales, 'alcohol-free' foster homes and other residential facilities have been established, staffed by personnel trained to care for recovering alcoholics in an accepting manner.

Other approaches

Social group methods for outpatient alcoholism rehabilitation are indicated for most persons not handicapped by severe dementia, chronic psychosis, or severe personality disorder. However, in age-heterogeneous AA or clinical treatment groups, elderly persons may be offended by the profanity and disclosure of past antisocial behaviour by younger members. Elders are more likely to engage successfully if the group is composed of age peers and led in a low-keyed, emotionally supportive manner (Atkinson *et al.* 1998). Peer-bonding and shared reminiscing in such groups are probably important factors in retention (see Cases 1 and 4 below). Frank discussion of personal and family problems often follows several months of more superficial discourse. Cognitive–behavioural psychotherapeutic and educational methods, using very specific, manual-assisted techniques, have also been shown to be very useful with older adult alcoholics (Dupree *et al.* 1984; Dupree and Schonfeld 1998). Demented or chronically psychotic patients are best managed in a psychiatric day treatment or home visitation programme. Some others with personality disorders and major mental illness can best be managed individually in a psychiatric outpatient clinic, preferably in conjunction with an alcoholism group (see Case 2 below).

Monitoring alcohol and drug use

In outpatient settings it is desirable to monitor substance use in recovering elderly problem drinkers. Such monitoring must be conducted in the spirit of assisting rather than intruding. Patients, relatives, and fellow group members (who may establish social ties outside the meetings) should regularly be queried and encouraged to offer information on drinking 'slips' spontaneously. Randomly conducted, unannounced breath and urine examinations cannot, of course, be expected to catch many instances of drinking relapse or surreptitious psychoactive drug use. Such testing is recommended because of the strong 'message' it conveys to patients that the staff are striving to be as thorough as possible in monitoring efforts. Often older alcoholics in treatment who resume drinking are apt to stay away from group meetings. In this circumstance, a home visit by the group leader may clarify whether a drinking relapse has occurred.

Case studies

Case 1

Early-onset, 'familial' alcohol dependence: (DB) A 65-year-old retired stockbroker was referred to a geriatric substance abuse programme by the general psychiatry unit after rapid resolution of acute depressive symptoms and suicidal thoughts without specific treatment. His lifelong daily drinking had resulted in 'blackouts' at age 13, military court martial for drunken disorderly conduct at 18, and, in later adulthood, falls resulting in injury, business failures, and a divorce. He had never been treated for alcoholism. Several paternal uncles, all four siblings, and an adult son are alcoholic, but there is no family history of depression. After retirement at age 63, he drank more 'from boredom' and still more after his second wife left him for another man. Despondent over this loss, he thought of suicide and sought psychiatric treatment. He reported an active 47 packet-year cigarette smoking habit (a packet-year is the average number of packets (20 cigarettes each) smoked per day multiplied by the number of years of the smoking habit). He had a self-limited, untreated depressive episode at age 39 following an alcohol-related business failure.

He was physically fit, and, after resolution of initial depressed mood, his mental status showed only mildly variable affect. MCV and MCH on the blood count were elevated, without anaemia. After engaging successfully in a supportive social therapy group for older problem drinkers, he remained abstinent over the next year and stabilized his social circumstances. Depression did not reoccur, and his former subjective complaint of forgetfulness also waned. After a year of sobriety his Mini-Mental State score was 26/30.

Comment: In this case a middle-class man with longstanding alcoholism was vulnerable to increased drinking problems when faced with life stressors in his sixties. Although depressive symptoms were probably induced by a combination of losses, alcohol effects and perhaps a predisposition to mood disorder, the sequence of events suggests primary alcohol dependence with secondary depression. Abstinence from alcohol and peer social support, rather than antidepressant treatment, have determined his favourable course.

Case 2

Early-onset alcohol dependence with comorbid affective disorder: (IC) A 69-year-old recently divorced woman was admitted to the medical service after being found unconscious at home. Her blood alcohol level was 332 mg/100 ml. She gradually regained consciousness and had an uncomplicated recovery with supportive medical care. She had drunk table wine regularly throughout adulthood, up to a gallon (US, equivalent to about 28 standard drinks) per week, consuming more when confronted by stress, anxiety, or depressive symptoms. Consumption had escalated even further in the past few months after she was divorced by her husband of 46 years. Always dependent upon others, she feared she could not look after herself and said she drank more to assuage her fear and despair, until she 'lost control.' She had, over the last 15 years, also solicited and overused prescribed benzodiazepines and codeine-containing analgesic compounds for a variety of minor emotional and physical complaints. She had not smoked cigarettes. She had received various antidepressant medications over the past several years, but had not been hospitalized for psychiatric problems. Her family history was negative for alcoholism and mood disorder.

Physical assessment showed obesity and first-degree heart block. Chronic atypical chest pain was minimally responsive to angina treatments. Mental status was not remarkable after recovery from alcohol-induced coma, which was judged not to be a suicidal act. She joined and sustained involvement in AA, and has remained abstinent from alcohol for nearly 5 years. She was gradually weaned from longstanding daily low doses of clorazepate and triazolam as well.

However, after 2 years she still had not adapted to living alone and developed symptoms of major depression. She was admitted to a general psychiatry inpatient unit where she responded to doxepin. Thereafter she was maintained on antidepressants and, during regular supportive individual psychotherapy, was encouraged to live more independently. After 3 years she has not had a depressive relapse, was able to attend her granddaughter's wedding 1000 miles away, and recently journeyed from the US on a vacation trip to France.

Comment: It is not clear in this woman's history whether alcohol dependence or depressive episodes occurred first. But it is apparent that, unlike the situation in the first case, a major depressive episode arose after a lengthy period of abstinence. Alcohol excess could not be implicated in the aetiology of this episode, and specific antidepressant treatment was necessary. Her positive engagement in AA attests to the usefulness of this path to recovery for some elderly alcoholics.

Case 3

Early-onset alcohol dependence with probable alcohol-related dementia: (EB) A 77-year-old retired cook was admitted to hospital following an alcohol withdrawal seizure that occurred shortly after he entered a local alcohol detoxification centre where he was well known. He had consumed alcohol to the point of intoxication nearly every day for the past 50 years, had had multiple arrests over many years for drunken driving and public intoxication, and in recent years lived in a single room-occupancy hotel in a poor section of the inner city and drank a pint (US) to a fifth of whiskey (equivalent to 16 to 25 standard drinks) daily. He used no other drugs but had a greater than 100 packet-year cigarette smoking history, though he had cut down recently to 4–6 cigarettes daily. On admission he was drowsy but rousable, disoriented except to person, and unable to participate in other cognitive testing. Extraocular movements were intact, and there was no nystagmus or gaze preference. His only other medical problem was degenerative joint disease. His blood alcohol level was still 125 mg/100 ml, there were mild abnormalities in liver function tests, and the MCH was elevated. Awake EEG showed intermittent slowing consistent with a toxic or metabolic abnormality or diffuse structural disease, and a CT examination of the head showed global atrophy both above and below the tentorium, without focal lesions. A week later, following successful resolution of his alcohol withdrawal and doses of intramuscular thiamine, he achieved a Mini-Mental State score of 18/30, with deficits in attention, orientation, memory, and construction.

Cognitive deficits persisted during the patient's subsequent 9-month stay in a locked, alcohol-free nursing home, in spite of adequate nutritional repletion. He was then referred to the dementia clinic, where his Mini-Mental State score was 21/30. Performance on other tests showed marked impairment of attention, short-term memory, similarities, and visuoconstructional skills as well as mild impairment in language repetition, judgement, and calculation. Language comprehension and naming were intact. Neurological examination showed marked impairment of tandem gait and a positive Romberg test. There was symmetrical bilateral loss of proprioception and vibratory sensation in his feet. Deep tendon reflexes were absent except for a trace response at the knees. Extraocular movements were intact.

Comment: This man's situation illustrates the phenomena commonly seen in cases where alcohol appears to be a major factor in dementia: namely, persisting, widespread cognitive impairment, without the dense amnesia seen in Wernicke–Korsakoff cases or dysnomia as commonly seen in Alzheimer's dementia; associated peripheral neurological findings of polyneuropathy and ataxia; brain imaging evidence of diffuse cortical atrophy; a history of heavy, prolonged consumption of alcohol; and no evidence of further cognitive decline—a stable course or perhaps even slight improvement—with abstention from alcohol.

Case 4

Late-onset, circumscribed alcohol abuse: (GB) A 73-year-old, divorced, retired electrician was referred to a geriatric substance abuse programme by the district court after his third drink-driving arrest in the past 3 years. For many years he drank daily with his friends in taverns, but denied any alcohol-related problems until his ex-wife died 4 years ago. Shortly thereafter he moved to a new, semi-rural locale which proved disappointing. He was uncertain whether his customary alcohol intake, typically six beers (6 standard drinks) daily with occasional wine or whiskey as well, might have increased. In any event he was arrested on three occasions for driving erratically after leaving his favourite tavern (blood alcohol level on each occasion was higher than the legal limit of 80 mg/100 ml). He quit his five packet/day cigarette habit at age 48, and had had no other substance use problem. He had never been treated, and the family history was negative, for alcoholism. A son's heroin addiction, however, had been another source of recent worry. He complained of forgetfulness, but the psychiatric history was otherwise negative.

Physical evaluation showed degenerative osteoarthritis of several joints, open-angle glaucoma, and essential hypertension, all in reasonable control. On mental status he had slight trouble finding words and his thinking was somewhat tangential. After 10 months in a supportive social therapy group for older problem drinkers, he had moved close to the hospital, remained sober, and claimed that his memory and sense of well-being had both improved. His arthritis, however, troubles him more now that he is sober. His Mini-Mental State score after 10 months was 25/30.

Comment: It is possible that unsteady driving by this gentleman was the consequence of both increased alcohol consumption following life stressors and increased biological (cerebellar) sensitivity to alcohol effects with age. In a US metropolitan setting in which people rely on public transport, it is unlikely that this man's drinking would have come to clinical attention. Yet it is clear in retrospect that his well-being and memory were suffering as consequences of his daily drinking. Elderly alcoholics often complain that musculoskeletal pain is more bothersome without alcohol, and this can be a threat to abstinence.

Sedative-hypnotic drug use disorders

Prevalence of use, misuse, and dependence

Young adult abusers of benzodiazepines consume such drugs outside of medical supervision, use them for euphoriant effects, escalate the dose over time, and continue use despite adverse consequences. Such behaviours are very uncommon in older people. However, long-term prescribing of these agents can produce physical dependence with characteristic 'discontinuance symptoms' when the drug is stopped, and chronic toxicity from long-term exposure to these agents is more likely in old age.

Benzodiazepine use by community-dwelling elderly people

This class of sedative-hypnotics has achieved dominance over the past 30 years because of the relative safety and efficacy of these agents in the treatment of insomnia and anxiety. Although the number of benzodiazepine prescriptions peaked in the mid-1970s and has since been in decline worldwide, use of these drugs in the elderly has not changed appreciably in recent years, even though the individual agents change. Surveys of community-dwelling elderly people suggest that 5% to 15% are currently prescribed benzodiazepines. Similar surveys also suggest, though, that most older persons use these agents as directed. When misuse occurs, it tends to be in the direction of underuse.

Long-term benzodiazepine use and the development of dependence

It is now well established that regular, daily therapeutic doses of any benzodiazepine, if prolonged beyond 4 to 12 months, depending upon the pharmacokinetics of the particular drug, can result in the development of physical dependence *without* dose escalation (Higgitt 1988; American Psychiatric Association 1990). There is little tolerance to the anxiolytic and antipanic effects of diazepam, alprazolam, or other drugs in this class. Tolerance to their hypnotic effects, on the other hand, is well documented, so that addiction to increasingly high doses is also possible, especially in persons who take a benzodiazepine over a protracted period for chronic insomnia.

Clinical surveys have long indicated that the elderly are more likely to receive benzodiazepines for prolonged periods than younger persons. Indeed, the most likely long-term benzodiazepine user is the elderly female (Ancill and Carlyle 1993). The most recently reported prescription surveys show continuing evidence of this pattern (e.g. Isacson *et al.* 1992; Thomson and Smith 1995; Simon *et al.* 1996). Although receipt of a prescription does not necessarily mean that the patient uses the drug every day, these findings demonstrate that many elderly patients are, at the very least, placed at risk for developing benzodiazepine dependence by the manner in which these drugs are prescribed.

The prevalence of drug dependence of all types in persons age 65 and older reported in community epidemiological surveys is very low, but such data almost certainly do not reflect low-dose benzodiazepine dependence, which is typically unrecognized by the patient and poorly measured by the dependence criteria.

Institutional benzodiazepine use

Wide concern has been expressed that in nursing homes and residential-care facilities older patients may be particularly likely to be dosed with excessive sedatives to control behaviour. While a few surveys indicate higher rates of benzodiazepine use in these settings than in community-dwelling elderly, details such as duration of treatment are often lacking. The practice of open-ended dispensing of nightly benzodiazepines for sleep is certainly to be discouraged. Most cases of benzodiazepine-induced or aggravated cognitive impairment and ataxia are seen in this circumstance. Recent efforts to rationalize and curb the use of these agents and other psychoactives in nursing homes have produced mixed results. A reduced use of benzodiazepines has been demonstrated in some settings (e.g. Avorn *et al.* 1992; Gilbert *et al.* 1993; Schmidt *et al.* 1998), but in others, perhaps because of improved recognition of anxiety disorders or reduction in use of neuroleptics, benzodiazepine use has in fact *increased* in the past few years (Borson and Doane 1997; Lasser and Sunderland 1998).

Risk factors for benzodiazepine dependence

Pharmacological factors

Besides duration of treatment, other variables influencing the likelihood of dependence are higher drug dose level, shorter pharmacokinetic elimination half-life, and higher milligram potency of the agent (American Psychiatric Association 1990).

Patient factors

These include prior or concurrent alcoholism or sedative-drug dependence, chronic insomnia (rather than anxiety) as the target symptom for which the drug is prescribed, and coexisting chronic painful physical illness or personality disorder.

Clinical features and complications

Low-dose benzodiazepine dependence

When initiating benzodiazepine treatment or stepping up the dose, there is a transitional period until a new plasma steady-state drug level is achieved, during which toxic effects may occur transiently, consisting of one or more of the following symptoms: sedation, ataxia, and increased reaction time. Age-related pharmacokinetic and pharmacodynamic changes render the elderly especially susceptible to these effects, and the duration until steady state is more protracted with age, as well. Varying degrees of chronic toxicity may build up, especially in the elderly, once steady state is achieved at a maintenance dose level that is continued long-term; but in many cases low doses for long periods will cause few if any obvious physical or behavioural sequelae, as long as the drug is taken regularly. Persistence of the patient in assuring a steady supply of the agent is perhaps the most noteworthy behavioural feature in long-term dependence (see Case 5 below), and some persons may withhold information about the extent of their use or sources.

Complications: chronic toxicity

Chronic toxicity has subtle manifestations at low doses, and becomes more obvious when dose escalation follows the development of tolerance. In an older person, even at therapeutic dose levels, toxicity may be manifest by persistent ataxia leading to falls, depressed mood which can be mistaken for an affective disorder, oversedation, memory impairment and other cognitive dysfunction, and possibly frank dementia (American Psychiatric Association 1990). Memory impairment typically is the consequence of drug disruption of memory consolidation (transfer of newly learned information from short- to long-term memory) (Barbee 1993). While the effect size may be small, because of baseline deficits in recall in the elderly, the additional impairment produced by benzodiazepines can represent a more severe compromise than the same dose given to younger persons (Woods and Winger 1995). Benzodiazepines can also induce anterograde amnesia. One recent large US health maintenance organization study of persons over age 65 demonstrated that any benzodiazepine use was associated significantly with impairment in functional status, independent of comorbid medical disorders (Ried *et al.* 1998).

Mechanisms underlying age-associated changes in response to benzodiazepines

As a person ages, alterations occur in the volume of distribution, elimination half-life, and clearance of metabolized benzodiazepines, producing higher steady-state plasma drug concentrations (Greenblatt *et al.* 1991*a,b*; Ozdemir *et al.* 1996). However, even when old and young patients have comparable plasma drug concentrations, the elderly develop more sedation, psychomotor impairment, and memory problems (Bertz *et al.* 1997; Greenblatt *et al.* 1991*a,b*), suggesting an increased neuropharmacodynamic effect with age. Basic mechanisms accounting for an age-associated increased sensitivity to benzodiazepines have not been determined, but may involve postreceptor mechanisms in GABAergic neurons and second messenger systems (Ozdemir *et al.* 1996).

Complications associated with comorbid disorders

Benzodiazepines may contribute to respiratory insufficiency in patients with pulmonary disorders (see Case 6 below), increased falls and incoordination in patients with cerebellar disease or compromised vascular supply to the posterior fossa, or deteriorating status in demented or depressed patients. These agents potentiate the effects of alcohol and opioids. Cimetidine and propanolol interfere with the metabolism of benzodiazepines and can raise their blood levels, but the clinical importance of these effects appears to be small.

Discontinuance symptoms

Following abrupt termination of benzodiazepines after long-term use, clinically significant discontinuance symptoms occur in as many as 90% of patients who have been taking low daily doses (these symptoms are summarized in Table 34.12). Often symptoms can be quite distressing and sometimes very serious. Symptoms occurring after cessation of long-term benzodiazepines often represent a mixture of 'rebound', 'reoccurrence', and true withdrawal symptoms (American Psychiatric Association 1990). Rebound symptoms are identical to those for which the drug was originally prescribed, but they reoccur rapidly, are more severe or intense than in the past, and resolve in a few days. Reoccurrence symptoms are also identical to the original symptoms, but they reappear gradually, never exceed their original intensity, and persist. They represent a return to the chronic symptom pattern that had been suppressed by drug therapy. Some symptoms, like restlessness or irritability, are common and can represent any of the three types of discontinuance phenomena, depending upon the history, intensity, and time course. Other symptoms, like psychosis, seizures, or delirium (see Case 6 below), are uncommon and almost always represent true withdrawal phenomena, defined as new or novel symptoms for that patient, with early- or late-onset, but typically lasting only 2–4 weeks. True withdrawal phenomena have been reported to occur in 20–50% of mixed-age chronic benzodiazepine users after discontinuation (Roy-Byrne and Hommer 1988; Schweizer *et al.* 1990). There is limited evidence that older adults tolerate tapered drug withdrawal as well as or better than younger adults (Schweizer *et al.* 1989).

Diagnosis, outcome, and management

Diagnosing dependence and withdrawal

Benzodiazepine dependence and withdrawal may be initially overlooked in hospitalized elderly patients who do not or cannot disclose their daily use of these agents, and the deteriorating course that ensues may be misdiagnosed as myocardial infarction, hypertensive crisis, or infection (Whitcup and Miller 1987). Delirium may be a more common presentation of withdrawal in older patients and be misattributed to other causes (Foy *et al.* 1995). Among outpatients, many cases of dependence on benzodiazepines are evident only when one takes note of a longstanding prescription. Low-dose dependence is not proven, however, merely by the record of longstanding prescriptions. One patient may not take the agent regularly, while another may also be surreptitiously consuming supplies garnered from multiple sources. Benzodiazepine toxicity and possible dependence should always be considered when patients have poorly explained sedation, ataxia, depression, or cognitive impairment. A search for undisclosed prescription bottles should be conducted, with the aid of relatives and home visitation, and a urine examination for benzodiazepines should be obtained, when there is strong suspicion of surreptitious benzodiazepine use.

Table 34.12 Benzodiazepine discontinuance symptoms*

Specific symptoms by frequency		
Frequent	Common	Uncommon**
Anxiety	Flu-like symptoms (nausea, coryza, lethargy, diaphoresis)	Delirium
Insomnia	Sensitivity to sound, touch, or light	Seizures
Restlessness	Aches and pains	Persistent tinnitus
Agitation	Blurred vision	Depersonalization
Irritability	Depression	Derealization
Muscle tension	Nightmares	Paranoid delusions
	Hyper-reflexia	Hallucinations
	Ataxia	Psychosis
	Autonomic hyperactivity	

*Adapted with permission from American Psychiatric Association 1990
**Typically when present these represent true withdrawal symptoms

Drug discontinuation in the dependent patient

Gradual discontinuation of the drug is indicated, at least in those dependent patients who suffer from chronic toxicity or other complications, or who have developed tolerance with dose escalation above the therapeutic range (Higgitt *et al.* 1985; American Psychiatric Association 1990). One's goal is to proceed slowly enough in decremental reductions to avoid major withdrawal problems and minimize other discontinuance symptoms. Some patients, especially those who have developed lengthy, high-dose habits, may require many months' tapering to avert serious discontinuance symptoms. As the dose reaches lower levels, the size and frequency of decrements may have to be reduced even further, especially for high-potency, short half-life drugs like alprazolam. One must, in the end, tailor the reduction schedule to meet individual needs, although a period of 1–4 months is often sufficient. It is no small feat to persuade some elderly persons to give up benzodiazepines, and various intervention strategies may be needed. In some cases one may have to settle for a reduction to very low drug doses rather than complete discontinuation.

Adjunctive measures in managing drug discontinuation

Several drug substitutes, including propanolol, clonidine, carbamazepine, buspirone, and barbiturates, have been studied, but none clearly merits widespread use (American Psychiatric Association 1990; Roy-Byrne and Ballenger 1993). Psychological therapies (Golombok and Higgitt 1993) and self-help groups (Tattersall 1993) can be useful adjuncts for persons withdrawing from benzodiazepine dependence.

Outcome of medically supervised benzodiazepine withdrawal

Despite evidence that old age is not associated with more severe withdrawal, studies of mixed-age patient groups show that older persons have a poorer outcome following therapeutic attempts to discontinue benzodiazepines after longstanding use (studies reviewed in Atkinson 2000). Older age was associated with both difficulty completing withdrawal protocols and an increased likelihood of relapse to benzodiazepine use despite completion of a cessation programme. The mean age of subjects in these follow-up studies was 40–50 years, but the numbers of elderly persons were small. Risk factors for relapse in such studies of mixed-aged patients, besides older age, include casual efforts to discontinue (as opposed to participation in a formal protocol), personality pathology, dependence on agents with short half-lives, higher drug doses, higher caffeine intake, and continued psychiatric symptomatology (Atkinson 2000).

For long-term benzodiazepine users who do succeed in discontinuing use of these agents, several studies indicate the possibility of at least some improvement in cognitive functioning (Golombok *et al.* 1988; Salzman *et al.* 1992; Tonne *et al.* 1995), and, in addition, improvement, or at least no deterioration, in symptoms of anxiety, depression, or insomnia (e.g. Schweizer *et al.* 1990; Salzman *et al.* 1992). One study of 76 patients (mean age 62) successfully withdrawn from chronic benzodiazepine use found that medical and mental health visits fell from 25.4 per year before detoxification to 4.4 per year afterward (Burke *et al.* 1995). But other studies suggest that the majority of patients who successfully withdraw from benzodiazepines will continue to experience significant anxiety, depression, and insomnia, and thus remain at risk for a return to use of these agents (Atkinson 2000).

Managing long-term benzodiazepine use

Ideally, benzodiazepines should be used over short periods (weeks to a few months) for acute episodes of anxiety or insomnia. One encounters patients, however, who might continue to benefit from long-term treatment. Deciding when to prescribe long-term can be quite difficult, requiring consideration of the patient's relief from morbid anxiety symptoms balanced against the hazards of chronic toxicity and physical dependence (Ancill and

Carlyle 1993). Long-term, low-dose therapy may be justified especially in patients whose anxiety responds better to a benzodiazepine than to alternative therapies, and who are reliable, have no history of alcoholism or drug addiction, and can be well supervised medically (American Psychiatric Association 1990). In these circumstances, however, the physician should anticipate the likelihood of inducing physical dependence and seek the informed consent of patient and family in deciding how to proceed. Moreover, as in the case of the epileptic or diabetic patient, steps should be taken to protect the patient from inadvertent abrupt drug withdrawal (see Case 6 below), e.g. by clearly documenting the status of the patient as a long-term benzodiazepine user in the medical record and by educating patient and family never to stop the drug abruptly.

Case studies

Case 5

Uncomplicated low-dose benzodiazepine dependence presenting as a mixture of reoccurrence and rebound symptoms after drug discontinuation: (MA) An 82-year-old widow, living independently, asked a private consultant internist to prescribe diazepam for sleep and nerves. Her practitioner had previously prescribed this medication, 5 mg at night, to help with insomnia, one of several side-effects she had developed during a phase of excessive thyroxine treatment for hypothyroidism 2 years earlier, and she had continued to use it nearly daily. Her doctor had recently refused to renew the prescription, saying that he feared she might become dependent upon diazepam, although she had not increased the dose. She subsequently developed early-night insomnia and awakenings later in the night for the next several weeks, as well as an increase in her longstanding symptoms of nervousness and worry. She had had no other substance use habits or problems.

Aside from well-controlled hypothyroidism and ocular (lenticular) cataracts, her physical health was excellent. She was well groomed and poised, with normal mental status. The consultant declined to prescribe for her but did discuss the situation with her practitioner, who reinstituted night-time diazepam, 5 mg, temporarily. Her symptoms improved. Her physician then more carefully explained the possibility of low-dose dependence, and she agreed to gradually taper off the drug. Some 4 months later she was sleeping reasonably well, having been without diazepam for 3 months.

Comment: This woman's increased nervousness represented a reoccurrence of the chronic mild anxiety that had long pre-dated, but was temporarily suppressed by, diazepam use. The insomnia more likely was a 'rebound' symptom. If some sleep benefit from the drug occurred during the 2 years prior, it probably resulted indirectly from the antianxiety effects of the diazepam, hence the lack of tolerance and dose build-up, a not uncommon situation in older persons with anxiety and insomnia accompanying chronic medical illness.

Case 6

Benzodiazepine dependence presenting as withdrawal delirium after discontinuation: (WJ) A 72-year-old, divorced, chronically disabled, former labourer was admitted to the medical service with a 2-week history of shortness of breath. He was lethargic and cyanotic. His acute respiratory insufficiency was found to have been caused by acute pneumonia and congestive heart failure, superimposed on chronic obstructive pulmonary disease and ischaemic cardiomyopathy. He responded to appropriate treatment, becoming alert, breathing easily, and displaying good skin colour within 48 hours. On the third hospital day, however, he became progressively delirious despite normalizing blood gases and improved cardiac function. He responded slightly but briefly to small intramuscular doses of lorazepam but not at all to droperidol.

Relatives disclosed that he was a chronic alcoholic who lived upstairs above a tavern, where he spent his days and evenings. He had also taken prescribed diazepam, 10 to 20 mg daily, for at least 7 years. Some 3 months earlier, during a 6-day medical hospitalization for cardiac evaluation, he showed no withdrawal symptoms, but, significantly, he was maintained on diazepam, 5 mg four times daily, during that hospital stay. In the few weeks before the present admission, he reportedly had taken about 30% more than the prescribed diazepam doses (perhaps 25 to 30 mg daily), and his urine at admission was positive for benzodiazepines. He had not, however, been given diazepam during this admission.

When evaluated by a consulting psychiatrist on the fourth hospital day, he displayed a variable level of consciousness and verbal responsiveness, moderate motor agitation, negativism, and disorientation to place and time. Oral diazepam doses were begun, 5 mg every 8 hours. Within 48 hours his delirium had generally cleared, and he was discharged to outpatient status 6 days later.

Comment: Unexpected delirium is not uncommon when patients dependent upon alcohol or a prescribed drug enter hospital and do not have the substance continued. Since this man had consumed both alcohol and diazepam before admission, and the onset of his delirium after 3 days is consistent with withdrawal from either, one cannot be certain which agent (or perhaps both) to implicate. His straightforward response to modest diazepam replacement doses does, however, tend to suggest that diazepam withdrawal was responsible for his second bout of delirium.

Pre-existing substance dependence predisposes a person to the development of low-dose physical dependence on benzodiazepines. Coexisting alcohol and prescription drug dependence constitutes the most common form of polydrug dependence seen in older people. The combination undoubtedly contributed to this man's episode of acute respiratory insufficiency. The presence of active alcoholism, lack of clear-cut benefits from diazepam, as well as its misuse, prompted the recommendation that this patient have his diazepam doses tapered over several months and then discontinued.

Tobacco and other drug use disorders

Tobacco (nicotine) dependence

Although older adults are less likely to smoke than younger adults, tobacco dependence is the most common of all substance use disorders in the elderly. It is entirely obvious, thus taking no special effort to establish the diagnosis, and arguably accounts for far more medical disability and mortality in the elderly than abuse of all other substances combined. Because of its low behavioural toxicity, however, tobacco dependence has held little interest for psychiatrists. Compulsive tobacco use is rooted, none the less, in an abnormal behaviour pattern that merits the attention of mental health professionals.

Prevalence

US community survey data for 1994 showed that among persons age 65 and older, 13% of men and 11% of women were regular daily cigarette smokers (National Center for Health Statistics 1996).

Diagnosis

Nicotine dependence is characterized by the pursuit of pleasurable effects from nicotine use, a compulsive pattern of use despite knowledge of the health hazards, withdrawal symptoms, tolerance, and craving and relapse with abstinence. Some of the usual criteria for substance dependence (Table 34.3) are not very satisfactory because low behavioural toxicity and easy access to cheap tobacco products make several of these criteria irrelevant. When moderate to heavy daily use of tobacco is discontinued, smokers experience a variety of unpleasant mood and physical symptoms that begin within hours of abstinence. Psychological symptoms include irritability, anxiety, depression, and craving. Physiological symptoms include low energy, concentration difficulties, headache, increased appetite, and non-specific somatic complaints. There is little investigation into age-related changes in the prevalence or severity of these withdrawal symptoms.

Adverse health consequences

If the pleasures of smoking are immediate, the complications are long delayed. Indeed, 75% of the years of potential life lost because of premature smoking-attributable deaths in the US are estimated to occur in the period from age 65 on (US Public Health Service 1988). Smoking doubles the risk of death from combined causes in persons aged 35–70 (Thun *et al.* 1997). Major health problems associated with tobacco dependence are well known, and include: various cancers; heart, peripheral, and cerebrovascular disease; chronic obstructive lung disease; peptic ulcer; osteoporosis; burns; reduced body weight; impaired sense of taste and smell; loss of mobility; and poorer physical functioning (studies reviewed in Atkinson 2000). Smoking also interferes with the metabolism of many drugs (Dawson and Vestal 1984).

Smoking cessation by the elderly

It is not certain whether older smokers are more or less successful than younger persons in quitting, but it is clear that most successful quitters achieve this goal spontaneously, without participating in a specialized treatment programme. Successful quitters often cite health concerns, death of loved ones who smoked, or a physician's advice as motivating factors. Of those continuing to smoke, many say they want to quit and up to half have tried recently. Nevertheless, currently smoking elders may be less likely than younger smokers to believe in the health hazards of smoking and more likely to view smoking as a positive habit to enhance coping, reduce stress, and control weight (Orleans *et al.* 1994a). Older smokers report the same reasons as younger smokers for return to smoking after quitting: irritability, weight gain, fear of weight gain, friction with family members, and inability to concentrate.

Among smoking cessation methods, some, like rapid smoking aversion therapy or medicinal nicotine substitutes (polacrilex gum, transdermal patches), may be contraindicated in older patients with coronary artery disease, cardiac arrhythmias, hypertension, or diabetes mellitus. Brief intervention in primary care medical settings and self-help guides can, when appropriately tailored to elderly individuals, produce 6-month to 1-year quit rates as high as 20%, compared to spontaneous quit rates of 5–10% (Morgan *et al.* 1996; Rimer and Orleans 1994). Transdermal nicotine patch therapy has yielded a 6-month quit rate of 29% in one naturalistic study of elderly smokers (Orleans *et al.* 1994*b*). Bupropion has been demonstrated to favourably affect smoking cessation in several careful studies of mixed-age, non-depressed smokers (Hurt *et al.* 1997; Jorenby *et al.* 1999), doubling the 12-month quit rate of placebo controls. Bupropion appears to be equal in effects to nicotine replacement methods (Hughes *et al.* 1999). Unfortunately the use of this drug specifically in ageing smokers has not received attention. Quit rates by any method seem to be influenced favourably by more frequent contact with supervising personnel, although elderly patients voice a preference for minimal contact approaches, which, for economic reasons, should in most cases be tried first.

After stopping tobacco use, elderly persons experience greater longevity, reduced morbidity and mortality from myocardial infarction, reduced risk of death from smoking-related cancers and chronic obstructive lung disease, and improvement in pulmonary function and hip bone mineral density, compared to their contemporaries who continue smoking. The reduced risk of death becomes evident within 1–2 years after quitting, and approaches that of never-smokers after 15–20 years of abstinence (LaCroix and Omenn 1992).

Does smoking protect against dementia?

Beginning in the early 1980s, more than 30 studies have now examined whether smoking is associated with lower rates of Alzheimer's dementia (AD) and dementia in general, but most are not reliable since they tend to be relatively small, retrospective, cross-sectional, case-control surveys of prevalent cases (Doll *et al.* 2000). In one review, 4 of 17 such studies demonstrated a protective effect of regular smoking against AD (Lee 1994). Confounding variables, such as differential mortality (Ott *et al.* 1998; Wang *et al.* 1999), and smoking-related non-dementing illnesses that increase the proportion of smokers among control cases (Doll *et al.* 2000) have often made results of such studies difficult to interpret. More recent, prospective, population-based studies of incident cases are consistent in demonstrating that current regular smoking either has little or no association with AD or overall dementia rates (Broe *et al.* 1998; Wang *et al.* 1999; Doll *et al.* 2000) or is associated with a greater, not lesser, risk of AD and dementias (Ott *et al.* 1998; Merchant *et al.* 2000).

Still, new reports of a protective effect of smoking in AD based on prevalent case series continue to appear (Hillier and Salib 1997; Tyas *et al.* 2000). Two additional findings may stimulate continuing interest in this theme. There is evidence that nicotine inhibits amyloid formation (Salomon *et al.* 1996), and that senile plaque formation is less prominent in the brains of patients with AD who were smokers than in the brains of non-smoking AD case controls (Ulrich *et al.* 1997). There is also evidence from the prospective studies cited above that the risk of AD is lower in smokers who possess the *APOE* (apolipoprotein E) $\varepsilon 4$ allele than in those who lack this allele (Van Duijn *et al.* 1995; Ott *et al.* 1998; Merchant *et al.* 2000).

Other drug dependence

Illicit drug use disorders

Abuse of illicit drugs by the elderly is very uncommon, being found as a rule only in ageing criminals and long-term heroin addicts. A recent, sporadically observed phenomenon is the abuse of illicit substances by older persons susceptible to influence by younger loved ones who are themselves drug abusers. Use of illegal drugs may impair social functioning and expose the user to legal and health risks. Clinical disorders vary by drug class (opioids, stimulants, sedative-hypnotics of the barbiturate type, marijuana, and hallucinogens).

Opioid addiction

This is the best studied form of illicit drug abuse in older persons. Typical addicts are men who have survived their addiction for many years, led socially isolated lives, and been secretive about drug use. They have tended to avoid law enforcement agents, and often continue to support their drug habits through legal employment into their sixties (see Case 7 below). They tend to practise scrupulous hygiene with needles and syringes, and may substitute 'cleaner' drugs like hydromorphone for heroin when available. They enter methadone maintenance as they become too old to 'hustle,' and the methadone clinic may become their main social network. Some older addicts tolerate methadone poorly. Few, however, accept or do well in drug-free treatment.

Case 7

Early-onset heroin addiction: (CD) A 63-year-old, separated, food service worker sought treatment in a geriatric substance abuse programme because he feared relapse into heroin addiction. He first smoked heroin at age 30 aboard ship when he was a merchant seaman, escalated to sniffing heroin and sporadic intravenous dosing, and was a daily intravenous heroin addict almost continuously from age 32 until the present, except for periods of imprisonment for drug addiction (ages 33–37 years, 37–46, and 47–48). He constantly varied the dose based on finances and drug availability, taking as little as one dose a day to avoid withdrawal. He tried methadone maintenance briefly twice, but dropped out because he did not get high on methadone and also feared, paradoxically, that methadone would suppress pain-signalling medical problems. Recent separation from his spouse, loss of contact with his son who was sent to live with other relatives in Germany, and financial problems, were associated with fairly steady heroin dosing for the past 6 months. He also began to smoke freebase ('crack') cocaine sporadically 2 years ago, a habit acquired from a girlfriend. He has not been arrested since age 47 and has worked steadily. He reports a 41 packet-year cigarette habit, but denies alcohol or other drug excess. There is no maternal family history of substance abuse, but he has no information about his father's family. He underwent brief residential detoxification before applying for follow-up outpatient treatment.

Physical assessment showed only mild essential hypertension. Mental status was normal except for shyness. His Mini-Mental State score was 27/30. He was accepted for treatment in a supportive social therapy group on a trial basis when he refused to re-enter methadone maintenance. A urine drug screen was positive for cocaine the week he began treatment. He continued to show evidence of heroin and/or cocaine in several subsequent tests. He was discharged from the programme after 2 months for habitual non-compliance and referred to methadone maintenance.

Comment: Social group treatment alone is usually not an adequate approach for heroin addicts, unlike older alcoholics. US methadone maintenance programmes report increasing numbers of ageing addicts whose heroin use began in their twenties and thirties.

Prescription opioid analgesic dependence

Dependence on prescribed opioid analgesics occurs less commonly than benzodiazepine dependence and tends to be longstanding (beginning typically before old age) and associated with chronic pain disorders and high levels of psychopathology (Finlayson and Davis 1994). Whether opioid dependence liability changes with age is uncertain (Ozdemir *et al.* 1996).

Over-the-counter (OTC) drugs

Use of psychoactive OTCs by the elderly is common. There is a potential for medical and behavioural problems from habitual overuse of the many available products containing antihistamines, anticholinergics, caffeine, aspirin, or the newer non-steroidal anti-inflammatory agents (Kofoed 1985). Anticholinergics may affect cognition. Chronic salicylate toxicity increases with age and may produce a dementia-like syndrome associated with tinnitus and irritability (Grigor *et al.* 1987; Bailey and Jones 1989). No data exist about the true extent of OTC dependence and complications.

Polysubstance abuse

Mixed-substance problems in the elderly are not uncommon, and usually take the form of coexisting dependence on alcohol and either prescribed sedatives (see Case 6 above) or opioid analgesics (Finlayson *et al.* 1988; Finlayson and Davis 1994). Use of multiple illicit drugs is limited to ageing criminals and longstanding opioid addicts (see Case 7 above). There is little specific information on the treatment of prescription opioid, OTC, or polysubstance problems in the elderly.

Prevention of elderly substance abuse

Alcohol and drug dependence in the elderly can be reduced. Prevention should begin with public and private institutions sponsoring better preretirement planning for employees' future roles and constructive uses of time, including substance use education. Retirement communities, and senior citizens' organizations and periodicals, can promote smoking cessation and moderation of alcohol use.

Health providers and social caseworkers can provide advice and education on the adverse health and behavioural effects of alcohol and tobacco, and programmes for smoking cessation and alcohol use reduction can be made more easily accessible. Medical practitioners need continuing education on conservative prescribing of psychoactive drugs and on screening for the early recognition of alcohol and benzodiazepine dependence. Improved institutional milieus for the ageing population must stress alternatives to sedation for behavioural control.

Acknowledgement

The author thanks Dr Rob Olsen and Dr David M. Smith for providing two of the case studies.

Further reading

Begleiter, H. and Kissin, B. (ed.) (1996). *The pharmacology of alcohol and alcohol dependence.* Oxford University Press, New York.

Donovan, D. M. and Marlatt, G. A. (ed.) (1988). *Assessment of addictive behaviors.* Guilford, New York.

Edwards, G., Marshall, E. J., and Cook, C. C. H. (1997). *The treatment of drinking problems: a guide for the helping professions* (3rd edn). Cambridge University Press, London.

Lader, M., Edwards, G., and Drummond, D. C. (ed.) (1993). *The nature of alcohol and drug related problems.* Oxford University Press, Oxford.

Lowinson, J. H., Ruiz, P., Millman, R. B., and Langrod, J. G. (ed.) (1997). *Substance abuse: a comprehensive textbook* (3rd edn). Williams and Wilkins, Baltimore, MD.

Schuckit, M. A. (2000). *Drug and alcohol abuse* (5th edn). Kluwer Academic/Plenum, New York.

References

Adams, K. M., Gilman, S., Koeppe, R. A., Kluin, K. J., Brunberg, J. A., Dede, D., *et al.* (1993). Neuropsychological deficits are correlated with frontal hypometabolism in positron emission tomography studies of older alcoholic patients. *Alcoholism (NY)*, **17**, 205–10.

Adams, W. L. (1995). Interactions between alcohol and other drugs. *International Journal of the Addictions*, **30**, 1903–23.

Adams, W. L., Magruder-Habib, K., Trued, S., and Broome, H. L. (1992). Alcohol abuse in elderly emergency department patients. *Journal of the American Geriatrics Society*, **40**, 1236–40.

Adams, W. L., Barry, K. L., and Fleming, M. F. (1996). Screening for problem drinking in older primary care patients. *Journal of the American Medical Association*, **276**, 1964–7.

American Psychiatric Association (1990). *Benzodiazepine dependence, toxicity, and abuse*. American Psychiatric Press, Washington, DC.

American Psychiatric Association (1994). *Diagnostic and statistical manual of mental disorders* (4th edn). American Psychiatric Press, Washington, DC.

Ancill, R. J. and Carlyle, W. W. (1993). Benzodiazepine use and dependency in the elderly: Striking a balance. In *Benzodiazepine dependence* (ed. C. Hallstrom), pp. 238–51. Oxford University Press, Oxford.

Artaud-Wild, S. M., Connor, S. L., Sexton, G., and Connor, W. E. (1993). Differences in coronary mortality can be explained by differences in cholesterol and saturated fat intakes in 40 countries but not in France and Finland. *Circulation*, **88**, 2771–9.

Atkinson, R. M. (1990). Aging and alcohol use disorders: diagnostic issues in the elderly. *International Psychogeriatrics*, **2**, 55–72.

Atkinson, R. M. (1994). Late-onset problem drinking in older adults. *International Journal of Geriatric Psychiatry*, **9**, 321–6.

Atkinson, R. M. (1995). Treatment programs for aging alcoholics. In *Alcohol and aging* (ed. T. P. Beresford and E. S. L. Gomberg), pp. 186–210. Oxford University Press, New York.

Atkinson, R. M. (1997). Alcohol and drug abuse in the elderly. In *Psychiatry in the elderly* (2nd edn) (ed. R. Jacoby and C. Oppenheimer), pp. 661–86. Oxford University Press, Oxford.

Atkinson, R. M. (1999). Depression, alcoholism and ageing: a brief review. *International Journal of Geriatric Psychiatry*, **14**, 905–10.

Atkinson, R. M. (2000). Substance abuse. In *Textbook of geriatric neuropsychiatry* (2nd edn) (ed. C. E. Coffey and J. L. Cummings), pp. 367–400. American Psychiatric Press, Washington, DC.

Atkinson, R. M. and Kofoed, L. L. (1984). Alcohol and drug abuse. In *Geriatric medicine*, Vol. 2 (ed. C. K. Cassell and J. R. Walsh), pp. 219–35. Springer-Verlag, New York.

Atkinson, R. M. and Misra, S. (2001). Mental disorders and symptoms in older alcoholics: solving the puzzles of psychiatric comorbidity. In *Treating alcohol and drug abuse in the elderly* (ed. A. M. Gurnack and N. Osgood. Springer-Verlag, New York. (In press.)

Atkinson, R. M., Turner, J. A., and Tolson, R. L. (1998). Treatment of older adult problem drinkers: lessons learned from 'The Class of '45.' *Journal of Mental Health and Aging*, **4**, 197–214.

Atkinson, R. M., Ryan, S. C., and Turner, J. A. (2001). Variation among aging alcoholic patients in treatment. *American Journal of Geriatric Psychiatry*, **9**, 275–82.

Avorn, J., Soumerai, S. B., Everitt, D. E., Ross-Degnan, D., Beers, M. H., Sherman, D., *et al.* (1992). A randomized trial of a program to reduce the use of psychoactive drugs in nursing homes. *New England Journal of Medicine*, **327**, 168–73.

Bailey, R. B. and Jones, S. R. (1989). Chronic salicylate intoxication: A common cause of morbidity in the elderly. *Journal of the American Geriatrics Society*, **37**, 556–61.

Barbee, J. G. (1993) Memory, benzodiazepines, and anxiety: integration of theoretical and clinical perspectives. *Journal of Clinical Psychiatry*, **54**(10, suppl.) 86–97.

Bertz, R. J., Kroboth, P. D., Kroboth, F. J., Reynolds, I. J., Salek, F., Wright, C. E., *et al.* (1997). Alprazolam in young and elderly men: sensitivity and tolerance to psychomotor, sedative and memory effects. *Journal of Pharmacology and Experimental Therapeutics*, **281**, 1317–29.

Blow, F. (1991). Michigan Alcoholism Screening Test—Geriatric Version (MAST-G). University of Michigan Alcohol Research Center, Ann Arbor, Michigan.

Blow, F. C., Cook, C. A. L., Booth, B. M., Falcon, S. P., and Friedman, M. J. (1992). Age-related psychiatric comorbidities and level of functioning in alcoholic veterans seeking outpatient treatment. *Hospital and Community Psychiatry*, **43**, 990–5.

Blow, F. C. (1999). The effectiveness of an elder-specific brief alcohol intervention for older hazardous drinkers. *The Gerontologist*, **39** (Special issue 1), 569.

Borson, S. and Doane, K. (1997). The impact of OBRA-87 on psychotropic drug prescribing in skilled nursing facilities. *Psychiatric Services*, **48**, 1289–96.

Broe, G. A., Creasey, H., Jorm, A. F., Bennett, H. P., Casey, B., Waite, L. M., *et al.* (1998). Health habits and risk of cognitive impairment and dementia in old age: A prospective study on the effects of exercise. *Australia and New Zealand Journal of Public Health*, **22**, 621–3.

Brower, K. J., Mudd, S., Blow, F. C., Young, J. P., and Hill, E. M. (1994). Severity and treatment of alcohol withdrawal in elderly versus younger patients. *Alcoholism (NY)*, **18**, 196–201.

Brown, S. A., Inaba, R. K., Gillin, J. C., Schuckit, M. A., Stewart, M. A., and Irwin, M. R. (1995). Alcoholism and affective disorder: clinical course of depressive symptoms. *American Journal of Psychiatry*, **152**, 45–52.

Burke, K. C., Meek, W. J., Krych, R., Nisbet, R., *et al.* (1995). Medical services used by patients before and after detoxification from benzodiazepine dependence. *Psychiatric Services*, **46**, 157–60.

Caetano, R. and Tam, T. W. (1995). Prevalence and correlates of DSM-IV and ICD-10 alcohol dependence: 1990 US national alcohol survey. *Alcohol and Alcoholism*, **30**, 177–86.

Callahan, C. M. and Tierney, W. M. (1995). Health services use and mortality among older primary care patients with alcoholism. *Journal of the American Geriatrics Society*, **43**, 1378–83.

Carlen, P. L., McAndrews, M. P., Weiss, R. T., Dongier, M., Hill, J.-M., Menzano, E., *et al.* (1994). Alcohol-related dementia in the institutionalized elderly. *Alcoholism (NY)*, **18**, 1330–4.

Center for Substance Abuse Treatment (1998). *Substance abuse among older adults: treatment improvement protocol #26*. US Department of Health and Human Services, Public Health Service, Substance Abuse and Mental Health Services Administration, Rockville, Maryland, DHHS Publ. No. (SMA) 98–3179. (A copy of this guide may be obtained at no charge by calling the National Clearinghouse for Alcohol and Drug Information at 1–800–729–6686.)

Colditz, G. A., Branch, L. G., Lipnick, R. J., Willet, W. C., Rosner, B., Posner, B., *et al.* (1985). Moderate alcohol and decreased cardiovascular mortality in an elderly cohort. *American Heart Journal*, **109**, 886–9.

Conwell, Y., Rotenberg, M, and Caine, E. D. (1990). Completed suicide at age 50 and over. *Journal of the American Geriatrics Society*, **38**, 640–4.

Cooney, C. and Hamid, W. (1995). Review: Diogenes syndrome. *Age and Ageing*, **24**, 451–3.

Courville, C. B. (1955). *The effects of alcohol on the nervous system of man.* San Lucas Press, Los Angeles.

Davidson, D. M. (1989). Cardiovascular effects of alcohol. *Western Journal of Medicine*, **151**, 430–9.

Dawson, G. W. and Vestal, R. E. (1984). Smoking, age, and drug metabolism. In *Smoking and aging* (ed. R. Bosse and C. L. Rose), pp. 131–56. Lexington Books, Lexington, MA.

DiSclafani, V., Ezekial, F., Meyerhoff, D. J., MacKay, S., Dillon, W. P., Weiner, M. W., *et al.* (1995). Brain atrophy and cognitive function in older abstinent alcoholic men. *Alcoholism (NY)*, **19**, 1121–6.

Doll, R., Peto, R., Boreham, J., and Sutherland, I. (2000). Smoking and dementia in male British doctors: A prospective study. *British Medical Journal*, **320**, 1097–102.

Dupree, L. W. and Schonfeld, L. (1998). Cognitive-behavioral and self-management treatment of older problem drinkers. *Journal of Mental Health and Aging*, **4**, 215–32.

Dupree, L. W., Broskowski, H., and Schonfeld, L. (1984). The Gerontology Alcohol Project: a behavioral treatment program for elderly alcohol abusers. *The Gerontologist*, **24**, 510–16.

Evert, D. L. and Oscar-Berman, M. (1995). Alcohol-related cognitive impairments: an overview of how alcoholism may affect the workings of the brain. *Alcohol Health and Research World*, **19**, 89–96.

Ewing, J. A. (1984). Detecting alcoholism: the CAGE questionnaire. *Journal of the American Medical Association*, **252**, 1905–7.

Finlayson, R. E. and Davis, Jr, L. J. (1994). Prescription drug dependence in the elderly population: demographic and clinical features of 100 inpatients. *Mayo Clinic Proceedings*, **69**, 1137–45.

Finlayson, R. E., Hurt, R. D., Davis, L. J., and Morse, R. M. (1988). Alcoholism in elderly persons: a study of the psychiatric and psychosocial features of 216 inpatients. *Mayo Clinic Proceedings*, **63**, 761–8.

Finney, J. W. and Moos, R. H. (1984). Life stressors and problem drinking among older persons. In *Recent developments in alcoholism*, Vol. 2 (ed. M. Galanter), pp. 267–88. Plenum, New York.

Fisman, M., Ramsay, D., and Weiser, M. (1996). Dementia in the elderly alcoholic—a retrospective clinico-pathological study. *International Journal of Geriatric Psychiatry*, **11**, 209–18.

Fleming, M. F., Barry, K. L., Adams, W. L., and Stauffacher, E. A. (1999). Brief physician advice for alcohol problems in older adults: a randomized community-based trial. *American Journal of Family Practice*, **48**, 378–84.

Foy, A., O'Connell, D., Henry, D., Kelly, J., Cocking, S., and Halliday, J. (1995). Benzodiazepine use as a cause of cognitive impairment in elderly hospital inpatients. *Journals of Gerontology*, **50A**, M99–106.

Gambert, S. R. and Katsoyannis, K. K. (1995). Alcohol-related medical disorders of older heavy drinkers. In *Alcohol and aging* (ed. T. P. Beresford and E. S. L. Gomberg), pp. 70–81. Oxford University Press, New York.

Gilbert, A., Innes, J. M., Owen, N., and Sansom, L. (1993). Trial of an intervention to reduce chronic benzodiazepine use among residents of aged-care accommodation. *Australia and New Zealand Journal of Medicine*, **23**, 343–7.

Gilman, S., Adams, K., Koeppe, R. A., *et al.* (1990). Cerebellar and frontal hypometabolism in alcoholic cerebellar degeneration studied with positron emission tomography. *Annals of Neurology*, **28**, 775–85.

Golombok, S. and Higgitt, A. (1993). Psychological treatments for benzodiazepine dependence. In *Benzodiazepine dependence* (ed. C. Hallstrom), pp. 296–309. Oxford University Press, Oxford.

Golombok, S., Moodley, P. J., and Lader, M. (1988). Cognitive impairment in long-term benzodiazepine users. *Psychological Medicine*, **18**, 365–74.

Grant, B. F. (1997). Prevalence and correlates of alcohol use and DSM-IV alcohol dependence in the United States: results of the National Longitudinal Alcohol Epidemiologic Survey. *Journal of Studies on Alcohol*, **58**, 464–73.

Greenblatt, D. J., Harmatz, J. S., and Shader, R. I. (1991*a*). Clinical pharmacokinetics of anxiolytics and hypnotics in the elderly: therapeutic considerations (Part I). *Clinical Pharmacokinetics*, **21**, 165–77.

Greenblatt, D. J., Harmatz, J. S., and Shader, R. I. (1991*b*). Clinical pharmacokinetics of anxiolytics and hypnotics in the elderly: therapeutic considerations (Part II). *Clinical Pharmacokinetics*, **21**, 262–73.

Grigor, R. R., Spitz, P. W., and Furst, D. E. (1987). Salicylate toxicity in elderly patients with rheumatoid arthritis. *Journal of Rheumatology*, **14**, 60–6.

Harper, C. and Kril, J. (1989). Patterns of neuronal loss in the cerebral cortex in chronic alcoholic patients. *Journal of the Neurological Sciences*, **92**, 81–9.

Harper, C. G. and Kril, J. J. (1990). Neuropathology of alcoholism. *Alcohol and Alcoholism*, **25**, 207–16.

Hartford, J. T. and Samorajski, T. (1982). Alcoholism in the geriatric population. *Journal of the American Geriatrics Society*, **30**, 18–24.

Helzer, J. E., Burnam, A., and McEvoy, L. T. (1991). Alcohol abuse and dependence. I*n Psychiatric disorders in America. The Epidemiologic Catchment Area Study* (ed. L. N. Robins and D. A. Regier), pp. 81–115. The Free Press, New York.

Higgitt, A. C. (1988). Indications for benzodiazepine prescriptions in the elderly. *International Journal of Geriatric Psychiatry*, **3**, 239–43.

Higgitt, A. C., Lader, M. H., and Fonagy, P. (1985). Clinical management of benzodiazepine dependence. *British Medical Journal*, **291**, 688–90.

Hillier, V. and Salib, E. (1997). A case-control study of smoking and Alzheimer's disease. *International Journal of Geriatric Psychiatry*, **12**, 295–300.

Hughes, J. R., Goldstein, M. G., Hurt, R. D., and Shiffman, S. (1999). Recent advances in the pharmacotherapy of smoking. *Journal of the American Medical Association*, **281**, 72–6.

Hurt, R. D., Finlayson, R. E., Morse, R. M., and Davis, L. J. (1988). Alcoholism in elderly persons: medical aspects and prognosis of 216 inpatients. *Mayo Clinic Proceedings*, **63**, 753–60.

Hurt, R. D., Sachs, D. P. L., Glover, E. D., Offord, K. P., Johnston, J. A., Dale, L. C., *et al.* (1997). A comparison of sustained-release bupropion and placebo for smoking cessation. *New England Journal of Medicine* **337**, 1195–202.

Isacson, D., Carsjo, K., Bergman, U., *et al.* (1992). Long-term use of benzodiazepines in a Swedish community: an eight-year follow-up. *Journal of Clinical Epidemiology*, **45**, 429–36.

Jernigan, T. L., Butters, N., DiTraglia, G., Schafer, K., Smith, T., Irwin, M., *et al.* (1991). Reduced cerebral grey matter observed in alcoholics using magnetic resonance imaging. *Alcoholism (NY)*, **15**, 418–27.

Jones, T. V., Lindsey, B. A., Yount, P., and Soltys, R. (1993). Alcoholism screening questionnaires: are they valid in elderly medical outpatients. *Journal of General Internal Medicine*, **8**, 674–8.

Jorenby, D. E., Leischow, S. J., Nides, M. A., Rennard, S. I., Johnston, J. A., Hughes, A. R., *et al.* (1999) A controlled trial of sustained-release bupropion, a nicotine patch, or both for smoking cessation. *New England Journal of Medicine*, **340**, 685–91.

Joseph, C. L., Ganzini, L., and Atkinson, R. M. (1995). Screening for alcohol use disorders in the nursing home. *Journal of the American Geriatrics Society*, **43**, 368–73.

Kafetz, K. and Cox, M. (1982). Alcohol excess and the senile squalor syndrome. *Journal of the American Geriatrics Society*, **30**, 706.

King, M. B. (1986). Alcohol abuse and dementia. *International Journal of Geriatric Psychiatry*, **1**, 31–6.

Kofoed, L. L. (1985). OTC drug overuse in the elderly: what to watch for. *Geriatrics*, **55**, 55–60.

Korrapati, M. R. and Vestal, R. E. (1995). Alcohol and medications in the elderly: complex interactions. In *Alcohol and aging* (ed. T. P. Beresford and E. S. L. Gomberg), pp. 42–55. Oxford University Press, New York.

Kril, J. J. and Harper, C. G. (1989). Neuronal counts from four cortical regions of the alcoholic brain. *Acta Neuropathologica*, **79**, 200–4.

Kril, J. J., Halliday, G. M., Svoboda, M. D., and Cartwright, H. (1997). The cerebral cortex is damaged in chronic alcoholics. *Neuroscience*, **79**, 983–98.

LaCroix, A. Z. and Omenn, G. S. (1992). Older adults and smoking. *Clinics of Geriatric Medicine*, **8**, 69–87.

Lasser, R. A. and Sunderland, T. (1998). Newer psychotropic medication use in nursing home residents. *Journal of the American Geriatrics Society*, **46**, 202–7.

Lee, P. N. (1994). Smoking and Alzheimer's disease: a review of the epidemiological evidence. *Neuroepidemiology*, **13**, 131–44.

Liberto, J. G. and Oslin, D. W. (1995). Early versus late-onset of alcoholism in the elderly. *International Journal of the Addictions*, **30**, 1799–818.

Lishman, W. A. (1990). Alcohol and the brain. *British Journal of Psychiatry*, **156**, 635–44.

Lishman, W. A. (1997). *Organic psychiatry: the psychological consequences of cerebral disorder*. Blackwell, Oxford.

Liskow, B. I., Rinck, C., Campbell, J., and DeSouza, C. (1989). Alcohol withdrawal in the elderly. *Journal of Studies on Alcohol*, **50**, 414–21.

Litten, R. Z. and Allen, J. P. (1998). Pharmacologic treatment of alcoholics with collateral depression: issues and future directions. *Psychopharmacological Bulletin*, **34**, 107–10.

Lucey, M. R., Hill, E. M., Young, J. P., Demo-Dananberg, L., and Beresford, T. P. (1999). The influences of age and sex on blood ethanol concentrations in healthy humans. *Journal of Studies on Alcohol*, **60**, 103–10.

MacMillan, D. and Shaw, P. (1966). Senile breakdown in standards of personal and environmental cleanliness. *British Medical Journal*, **2**, 1032–7.

Merchant, C., Tang, M. X., Albert, S., Manly, J., Stern, Y., and Mayeux, R. (2000). The influence of smoking on the risk of Alzheimer's disease. *Neurology*, **54**, 777–8.

Mertens, J. R., Moos, R. H., and Brennan, P. L. (1996). Alcohol consumption, life context, and coping predict mortality among late-middle-aged drinkers. *Alcoholism (NY)*, **20**, 313–19.

Meyer, J. S., Largen, Jr, J. W., Shaw, T., Mortel, K. F., and Rogers, R. (1984). Interaction of normal aging, senile dementia, multi-infarct dementia, and alcoholism in the elderly. In *Alcoholism in the elderly. Social and biomedical issues* (ed. J. T. Hartford and T. Samorajski), pp. 227–51. Raven, New York.

Moos, R. H., Brennan, P. L., and Moos, B. S. (1991). Short-term processes of remission and nonremission among late-life problem drinkers. *Alcoholism (NY)*, **15**, 948–55.

Morgan, G. D., Noll, E. L., Orleans, C. T., Rimer, B. K., Amfoh, K., and Bonney, G. (1996). Reaching midlife and older smokers: tailored interventions for routine medical care. *Preventive Medicine*, **25**, 346–54.

Morikawa, Y.-I., Arai, H., Matsushita, S., Kato, M., Higuchi, S., Miura, M., *et al.* (1999). Cerebrospinal fluid tau protein levels in demented and nondemented alcoholics. *Alcoholism (NY)*, **23**, 575–7.

National Center for Health Statistics (1996). Cigarette smoking among adults—United States, 1994. *Morbidity and Mortality Weekly Reports*, **45**, 588–90.

Neve, R. J. M., Lemmens, P. H., and Drop, M. J. (1997). Drinking careers of older male alcoholics in treatment as compared to younger alcoholics and to older social drinkers. *Journal of Studies on Alcohol*, **58**, 303–11.

Orleans, C. T., Jepson, C., Resch, N., and Rimer, B. K. (1994*a*). Quitting motives and barriers among older smokers. *Cancer*, **74**, 2055–61.

Orleans, C. T., Resch, N., Noll, E., Keintz, M. K., Rimer, B. K., Brown, T. V., *et al.* (1994*b*). Use of transdermal nicotine in a state-level prescription plan for the elderly. *Journal of the American Medical Association*, **271**, 601–7.

Oscar-Berman, M. and Hutner, N. (1993). Frontal lobe changes after chronic alcohol ingestion. In *Alcohol-induced brain damage*. National Institute on Alcohol Abuse and Alcoholism Research monograph No. 22 (ed. W. A. Hunt and S. J. Nixon), pp. 121–56. US Government Printing Office, Rockville, Maryland.

Oslin, D., Liberto, J. G., O'Brien, J., and Krois, S. (1997*a*). The tolerability of naltrexone in treating older, alcohol dependent patients. *American Journal of Addictions*, **6**, 266–70.

Oslin, D., Liberto, J. G., O'Brien, J., Krois, S., and Norbeck, J. (1997*b*). Naltrexone as an adjunctive treatment for older patients with alcohol dependence. *American Journal of Geriatric Psychiatry*, **5**, 324–32.

Oslin, D., Atkinson, R. M., Smith, D. M., and Hendrie, H. (1998). Alcohol related dementia: proposed clinical criteria. *International Journal of Geriatric Psychiatry*, **13**, 203–12.

Osuntokun, B. O., Hendrie, H. C., Fisher, K., McMahon, D., and Brittain, H. (1994). The diagnosis of dementia associated with alcoholism: a preliminary report of a new approach. *West African Journal of Medicine*, **13**, 160–3.

Ott, A., Slooter, A. J. C., Hofman, A., van Harskamp, F., Witteman, J. C. M., Van Broeckhoven, C., *et al.* (1998). Smoking and risk of dementia and Alzheimer's disease in a population-based cohort study: The Rotterdam Study. *Lancet*, **351**, 1840–3.

Ozdemir, V., Fourie, J., Busto, U., and Naranjo, C. A. (1996). Pharmacokinetic changes in the elderly: do they contribute to drug abuse and dependence? *Clinical Pharmacokinetics*, **31**, 372–85.

Parsons, O. A. (1994). Determinants of cognitive deficits in alcoholics: the search continues. *The Clinical Neuropsychologist*, **8**, 39–58.

Parsons, O. A. and Nixon, S. J. (1993). Neurobehavioral sequelae of alcoholism. *Behavioral Neurology*, **11**, 205–18.

Parsons, O. A. and Nixon, S. J. (1998). Cognitive functioning in sober social drinkers: a review of the research since 1986. *Journal of Studies on Alcohol*, **59**, 180–90.

Pfefferbaum, A., Lim, K. O., Zipursky, R. B., *et al.* (1992). Brain gray and white matter volume loss accelerates with aging in chronic alcoholics: a quantitative MRI study. *Alcoholism (NY)*, **16**, 1078–89.

Pfefferbaum, A., Sullivan, E. V., Mathalon, D. H., and Lim, K. O. (1997). Frontal lobe volume loss observed with magnetic resonance imaging in older chronic alcoholics. *Alcoholism (NY)*, **21**, 521–9.

Reifler, B. V., Kethley, A., O'Neill, P., Hanley, R., Lewis, S., and Stenchever, D. (1982). Five-year experience of a community outreach program for the elderly. *American Journal of Psychiatry*, **139**, 220–3.

Ried, L. D., Johnson, R. E., and Gettman, D. A. (1998). Benzodiazepine exposure and functional status in older people. *Journal of the American Geriatrics Society*, **46**, 71–6.

Rimer, B. K. and Orleans, C. T. (1994). Tailoring smoking cessation for older adults. *Cancer*, **74**, 2051–4.

Roy-Byrne, P. P. and Ballenger, J. C. (1993). Pharmacological treatments for benzodiazepine dependence. In *Benzodiazepine dependence* (ed. C. Hallstrom), pp. 310–22. Oxford University Press, Oxford.

Roy-Byrne, P. P. and Hommer, D. (1988). Benzodiazepine withdrawal: overview and implications for treatment of anxiety. *American Journal of Medicine*, **84**, 1041–52.

Ruchlin, H. S. (1997). Prevalence and correlates of alcohol use among older adults. *Preventive Medicine*, **26**, 651–7.

Ryan, C. and Butters, N. (1986). The neuropsychology of alcoholism. In *The neuropsychology handbook* (ed. D. Wedding, A. Horton, and J. Webster), pp. 376–409. Springer, New York.

Salomon, A., Jao, S-C., Marcinowski, K., *et al.* (1996). Nicotine inhibits amyloid formation by the beta peptide. *Biochemistry*, **35**, 13568–78.

Salzman, C., Fisher, J., Nobel, K., Glassman, R., Wolfson, A., and Kelley, M. (1992). Cognitive improvement following benzodiazepine discontinuation in elderly nursing home residents. *International Journal of Geriatric Psychiatry*, **7**, 89–93.

Samorajski, T., Persson, K., Bissell, C., Brizzee, L., Lancaster, F., and Brizzee, K. R. (1984). Biology of alcoholism and aging in rodents: brain and liver. In *Alcoholism in the elderly. Social and biomedical issues* (ed. J. T. Hartford and T. Samorajski), pp. 43–63. Raven, New York.

Saunders, P. A., Copeland, J. R. M., Dewey, M. E., Davidson, I. A., McWilliam, C., Sharma, V., *et al.* (1991). Heavy drinking as a risk factor for depression and dementia in elderly men. *British Journal of Psychiatry*, **159**, 213–16.

Schmidt, I., Claesson, C. B., Westerholm, B., Nilsson, L. G., and Svarstad, B. L. (1998). The impact of regular multidisciplinary team interventions on psychotropic prescribing in Swedish nursing homes. *Journal of the American Geriatrics Society*, **46**, 77–82.

Schuckit, M. A., Atkinson, J. H., Miller, P. L., and Berman, J. (1980). A three year follow-up of elderly alcoholics. *Journal of Clinical Psychiatry*, **41**, 412–16.

Schutte, K. K., Brennan, P. L., and Moos, R. H. (1994). Remission of late-life drinking problems: a 4-year follow-up. *Alcoholism (NY)*, **18**, 835–44.

Schutte, K. K., Brennan, P. L., and Moos, R. H. (1998). Predicting the development of late-life late-onset drinking problems: a 7-year prospective study. *Alcoholism (NY)*, **22**, 1349–58.

Schweizer, E., Case, W. G., and Rickels, K. (1989). Benzodiazepine dependence and withdrawal in elderly patients. *American Journal of Psychiatry*, **146**, 529–31.

Schweizer, E., Rickels, K., Case, W. G., and Greenblatt, D. B. (1990). Long-term therapeutic use of benzodiazepines, II: Effects of gradual taper. *Archives of General Psychiatry*, **47**, 908–15.

Simon, G. E., VanKorff, M., Barlow, W., Pabiniak, C., and Wagner, E. (1996). Predictors of chronic benzodiazepine use in a health maintenance organization sample. *Journal of Clinical Epidemiology*, **49**, 1067–73.

Smith, D. M. and Atkinson, R. M. (1994). Alcohol and dementia: neurological and neuropsychological features of 59 patients in a dementia registry. In *Textbook of geriatric neuropsychiatry* (ed. C. E. Coffey and J. L. Cummings), p. 306 (discussion) and p. 307 (Table 15-7). American Psychiatric Press, Washington, DC.

Smith, D. M. and Atkinson, R. M. (1995). Alcoholism and dementia in the elderly. *International Journal of the Addictions*, **30**, 1843–69.

Smith, J. W. (1995). Medical manifestations of alcoholism in the elderly. *International Journal of the Addictions*, **30**, 1749–98.

Soleas, G. J., Diamandis, E. P., and Goldberg, D. M. (1997). Resveratrol: a molecule whose time has come? And gone? *Clinical Biochemistry*, **30**, 91–113.

Speer, D. C. and Bates, K. (1992). Comorbid mental and substance disorders among older psychiatric patients. *Journal of the American Geriatrics Society*, **40**, 886–90.

Srivastava, L. M., Vasisht, S., Agarwal, D. P., and Goedde, H. W. (1994). Relation between alcohol intake, lipoproteins and coronary artery disease: the interest continues. *Alcohol and Alcoholism*, **29**, 11–24.

Tattersall, M. (1993). Self-help groups and benzodiazepine dependence. In *Benzodiazepine dependence* (ed. C. Hallstrom), pp. 323–36. Oxford University Press, Oxford.

Thomson, M. and Smith, W. A. (1995). Prescribing benzodiazepines for noninstitutionalized elderly. *Canadian Family Physician*, **41**, 792–8.

Thun, M. J., Peto, R., Lopez, A. D., Monaco, J. H., Henley, S. J., Heath, Jr., C. W., *et al.* (1997). Alcohol consumption and mortality among middle-aged and elderly US adults. *New England Journal of Medicine*, **337**, 1705–14.

Tonne, U., Hiltunen, A. J., Vikander, B., Engelbrektsson, K., Bergman, H., Bergman, I., *et al.* (1995). Neuropsychological changes during steady-state drug use, withdrawal and abstinence in primary benzodiazepine-dependent patients. *Acta Psychiatrica Scandinavica*, **91**, 299–304.

Tyas, S. L., Koval, J. J., and Pederson, L. L. (2000). Does an interaction between smoking and drinking influence the risk of Alzheimer's disease? Results from three Canadian data sets. *Statistics in Medicine*, **19**, 1685–96.

Ulrich, J., Johannson-Locher, G., Seiler, W. O., and Stahelin, H. B. (1997). Does smoking protect from Alzheimer's disease? Alzheimer-type changes in 301 unselected brains from patients with known smoking history. *Acta Neuropathologica*, **94**, 450–4.

US National Commission on Marihuana and Drug Abuse (1973). *Drug use in America: problem in perspective*, pp. 93–8. US Government Printing Office, Washington, DC.

US Public Health Service (1988). State-specific estimates of smoking-attributable mortality and years of potential life lost—United States, 1985. *Morbidity and Mortality Weekly Report*, **37**, 689–93.

Van Duijn, C. M., Havekes, L. M., Van Broeckhoven, C., *et al.* (1995). Apolipoprotein E genotype and association between smoking and early-onset Alzheimer's disease. *British Medical Journal*, **310**, 627–31.

Victor, M., Adams, R. D., and Collins, G. H. (1989). *The Wernicke–Korsakoff syndrome and related neurologic disorders due to alcoholism and malnutrition* (Contemporary neurology series, Vol. 3). F.A. Davis, Philadelphia.

Wang, H. X., Fratiglioni, L., Frisoni, G. B., Viitanen, M., and Winblad, B. (1999). Smoking and the occurrence of Alzheimer's disease: cross-sectional and longitudinal data in a population-based study. *American Journal of Epidemiology*, **149**, 640–4.

Whitcup, S. M. and Miller, F. (1987). Unrecognized drug dependence in psychiatrically hospitalized elderly patients. *Journal of the American Geriatrics Society*, **35**, 297–301.

Woodhouse, K. W. and James, O. F. W. (1985). Alcoholic liver disease in the elderly: presentation and outcome. *Age and ageing*, **14**, 113–18.

Woods, J. H. and Winger, G. (1995). Current benzodiazepine issues. *Psychopharmacology*, **118**, 107–15.

World Health Organization (1992). *The ICD-10 classification of mental and behavioural disorders*. World Health Organization, Geneva.

Wrigley, M. and Cooney, C. (1992). Diogenes syndrome. *Irish Journal of Psychological Medicine*, **9**, 37–41.

V | *Sexuality, ethics, and medico-legal issues*

35 Sexuality in old age

Catherine Oppenheimer

The teenage grand-daughter of an 83-year-old lady found her studying an information leaflet about AIDS that had just been put through the letterbox. The girl said reassuringly, 'I don't think you need to worry about that, Granny'. With gentle reproof, the old lady replied, 'What do *you* know about my sex life?'

Both public understanding and scientific interest in the sexuality of old age have matured considerably in the last few decades. The growth of the literature devoted to this topic is striking in itself: in the number of articles published, in the variety of journals available, and in the range of professionalism of the studies undertaken. Nurses in particular have been leaders in important areas of research, and sociology and feminism have made their contribution. Sexuality in old age can no longer be regarded as a neglected subject, nor is discussion of it now so dominated by issues of illness, loss, and aberration; though none of these should be neglected either.

Among the most dramatic changes in the field, of course, has been the development of treatments for erectile impotence that involve only medication by mouth, in place of the rather daunting methods of local treatment that were available previously. General practitioners and specialists in urology and andrology are now the key professionals in this area; and psychiatry has less to contribute—except perhaps where problems with the physical act of intercourse are only part of a more complex individual or emotional difficulty for the couple concerned.

Other areas in which important progress has been made (which will be discussed in greater detail later in this chapter) are: the scope and variety of surveys into sexual interest and activity in old age (see p. 840); observational studies of sexuality in institutional care (see p. 852); investigations into the impact of dementia on marital relationships, and particularly on the spouses of the person affected (see p. 850); consideration of ethical issues, and specifically of competence to participate voluntarily in a sexual relationship (see pp. 851–2); and the development of a clearer understanding of appropriate interventions where sexual problems arise—including educational and other supportive approaches, both to informal carers and to staff in institutions (see pp. 854–8).

Other routes into the literature are provided by textbooks (such as Schiavi's (1999) excellent work on ageing and male sexuality) and many of the articles cited elsewhere in this chapter (e.g. Drench and Losee (1996), Mattiasson and Hemberg (1998), Routasalo and Isola (1996), Gladstone (1995), and Ghusn (1995).

Attitudes to sexuality

Earlier literature (Golde and Kogon 1959; La Torre and Kear 1977) document negative attitudes to sexuality in old age: particularly among younger people, but also among older people.

A common finding in these earlier studies was the poor self-image of older people: they saw themselves as less attractive than younger people, and less entitled to the enjoyment of sexual pleasure (Cameron 1970; Wasow and Loeb 1979; White and Catania 1982). Their attitudes were conservative, they were poorly informed, and they felt uncomfortable in discussing sex with an interviewer (e.g. Persson 1980). Other studies, however, emphasized the eagerness of older people to learn more, and their interest in participating in research in this field (Hite 1976; Wasow and Loeb 1979).

More recent work suggests that some positive changes have occurred: Gibson *et al.* (1999), comparing the attitudes of residents (of a Veterans' facility in Canada), their spouses, and the staff; Walker and Ephross (1999), in a helpful and detailed survey of knowledge and attitudes in 68 homes; Loehr *et al.* (1997), describing a focus group with older Canadian women; and Minichiello *et al.* (1996) in a population survey in Australia, all point out the greater openness and willingness to engage in discussions on sexuality by the participants in their studies.

By contrast, Davey Smith *et al.* (1997) found that inclusion of questions on sexuality in their epidemiological study in Wales was threatening recruitment to the study, so they later removed those questions. Hillman and Stricker (1996) in an interesting survey of 241 college students, demonstrated how positively the students' knowledge and attitudes were affected by their having a good relationship with a grandparent: without such a relationship, however, knowledge itself did not translate into a positive attitude. Walker *et al.* (1998) carried out a survey of knowledge and attitudes in eight long-term care facilities in California, comparing the older residents with the care staff, and suggested that, overall, the staff had more tolerant attitudes than the residents. However, some of the detailed findings belie this, for example with regard to homosexuality and to the availability of erotic magazines in the home, where the residents were more liberal in their opinions.

In summary, our collective understanding of sexuality in old age has advanced some way from a narrow focus on sexual performance and age-related physiological changes. Sexuality, in the old as well as the young, encompasses far more than this (West 1975; Thompson *et al.* 1990). It includes all the physical intimacies comfortably nested in the familiarity of a settled couple: the happiness of having your back scratched for you, being hugged, warming your toes on another's feet in bed, not bothering whether the bathroom door is locked; and the relaxed acceptance of altered physical appearance, because of the unbreakable links of memory back to the time when the attraction and the relationship first began. Likewise it includes the appreciative eye, the alert awareness of sexual potential in every new encounter, and the romance and excitement inherent in the consciousness of being admired. Sexuality is linked with a proud sense of identity, with the ability to value oneself in giving and receiving, with having a place in someone else's life, and with being on friendly terms with one's own body.

One might argue that this gives too wide a meaning to 'sexuality'. But in fact the meaning attributed to an action will depend on who is doing the attributing: what is innocent for me may be erotic for you. The district nurse, secure in her own sexual relationship with her husband and in the love of her children, may mean nothing more than kindly attention as she bathes the widower, who lost the only person really close to him some 15 years ago. But her actions may carry much greater emotional meaning for him, and he may respond accordingly.

The care offered to older people is often more intimate and (happily) often more freely affectionate than to patients or residents of other ages; yet the carers are more likely to be untrained, and may be working on their own. The unspoken sexuality implicit in caring relationships needs to be understood and accepted (Webb 1987). Otherwise its overt expression is the more shocking and confusing when it does break through.

Physical touching of older people by their carers is a complex and essential area of study, relating as it does to respect for the privacy of the older person, the ability of the carer to give comfort or conversely to communicate reserve and distance, and all the ethical and emotional issues arising from these. The topic is well discussed especially in the nursing literature (e.g. Genevay 1975; Langland and Panicucci 1982; Mattiasson and Hemberg 1998; Kaplan 1996). Routasalo and Isola (1996) give a thorough and sensitive account of the issues, based on structured interviews with 30 nurses and 25 older patients from long-term wards in Finland, backed by an extensive literature review. Autton (1989) offers a comprehensive review of touch which is not confined to old age.

The ethics of non-sexual touching in psychotherapeutic relationships are considered by Bancroft (1984) who also discusses the value of taboo, in allowing certain freedoms within its boundary: we shall return later to this idea.

Not only are older people more likely to trigger stereotyped attitudes to their sexuality, they are also more vulnerable to damage by those attitudes. Young and independent people can choose to ignore what other people think. Some older people may also have enough independence to do so, but a significant proportion are not so lucky. At some point they have to live their lives in public—within a younger family, in a residential home or a hospital ward, or with help coming into their home from outside. Then the pressure on them to behave according to the norms set by the *providers* of help may be too strong to allow them to live their sexuality as they want. A poignant example of this vulnerability arose when an elderly transsexual patient, living a wholly female social life, needed an emergency prostatectomy. The surgical team had immense difficulty in accepting her chosen gender identity while giving her the physical care she needed. Bauer (1999), in a detailed interview study with five caregivers, highlights the different ways in which privacy is lost by residents in long-term care, and the failure of staff and administration to appreciate the importance of this deprivation.

It is not only the attitudes of the young to the old that matter, but also how old people themselves feel about each others' sexuality (e.g. Silverstone and Wynter 1975; Snyder and Spreitzer 1976). In a residential home the greatest problem faced by staff may be the attitudes of residents towards one of their number of whose behaviour they disapprove. But there may also be differences between staff over social rules, and moral beliefs, perceived conflict between the needs of the individual and of the institution, and personal feelings (of embarrassment, revulsion, or frustration), which will be stressful and confusing. (LaTorre and Kear 1977; Szasz 1983). It is then difficult for the staff to respond in any coherent or helpful way to problems that arise, and their difficulties are compounded if the institution is one in which open discussion of sexual matters is impossible. This is why institutional and educational approaches may be the most effective response to a 'sexual problem' expressed through the behaviour of one individual resident. Such an approach may begin with a meeting with staff—and the query most likely to come up in discussion will be 'but is it *normal*?'

Normal sexuality in old age—methodological issues

The collection of objective data on sexual behaviour began with Kinsey and his colleagues (Kinsey *et al.* 1948 1953), and useful information from the data gathered then still emerged decades later (Christenson and Gagnon 1965; Christenson and Johnson 1973). Later Masters and Johnson (1966), by the direct observation of volunteers in the laboratory, obtained information on the sexual physiology of aged men and women which has never yet, in its detail or objectivity, been surpassed. (However, both Kinsey and Masters and Johnson drew their conclusions from a comparatively small number of elderly subjects.) Since then, a growing number of studies has focused specifically on the elderly. The best of these studies have helped to identify important methodological difficulties in this field, which should be considered before the findings of the studies can be discussed.

Cohort effects

Any study examining the effects of ageing on a particular phenomenon, which takes a cross-section of the population at a given point in time and then compares people in one age-group with those in another, is confounding ageing and cohort effects. The older people in the sample may differ from the younger, not because of their age but because of the era they were born into. George and Weiler (1981) discuss this issue very thoroughly in relation to studies of sexual behaviour in older people. Studies of sexuality are particularly vulnerable to the cohort effect (Traupmann 1984); for example, Christenson and Johnson's study (1973), which looked at never-married women in their sixties and seventies, yielded data on this age-group that are still worth quoting now—although the women who were studied were born in the 1890s, and therefore belong to a cohort 50 years older than the 60- and 70-year-olds of today. (Compare their findings with those of Bretschneider and McKoy 1988.)

Problems with sampling

The early studies (Kinsey 1948 1953; Masters and Johnson 1966; first wave of the Duke University studies (Verwoerdt *et al.* 1969*a,b*)#) were carried out with volunteers, and most later studies have followed this example or have drawn their subjects from attenders at clinics (e.g. Weizman and Hart 1987). A few studies have been based on representative community samples (e.g. Persson 1980; Feldman *et al.* 1994), but they are rare. The constraints of cost, willingness of potential subjects to participate, and willingness of *others* (families, administrators of old-age homes, and so on) to permit the participation of elderly people (Wasow and Loeb 1979) usually end in biasing the sample of responders in some way. Systematic investigation of the sexual behaviour of people who are not competent to consent to being interviewed is practically non-existent (but see Ehrenfeld *et al.* 1997). Even with volunteer subjects, some topics are less likely to be studied than others: elderly people have been found (Sander 1976; Wasow and Loeb 1979) to be particularly reluctant to talk about masturbation. Young interviewers find it difficult to mention the subject of sexuality to older people: for example Pfeiffer (1977) observed that for this reason data on sexual activity were obtained from only 4 of the 14 unmarried elderly women in his sample. The setting from which the sample is drawn is likely to affect the findings: Todarello and Boscia (1985) showed marked differences in measures of sexual activity between people living at home and in institutions. The reliability of older people's memories for their early sexual history was discussed by Martin (1981), who concluded that reliability was high. The effect of different survey methods (such as self-administered questionnaire versus unstructured interview, for example) has been mentioned by some authors but not studied systematically (Monteiro *et al.* 1987 and Malatesta 1988 noted that older people preferred to answer their questionnaire in a small group setting, with ample opportunity for discussion; so also did Loehr *et al.* (1997)). Cultural influences on sexual behaviour and attitudes may have a role in determining differences between the elderly citizens of different countries, but it is not possible at present to draw any conclusions about these.

Individual versus grouped data

The Duke University studies vividly demonstrated (George and Weiler 1981) the value of longitudinal as compared to cross-sectional data, not only in separating out ageing and cohort effects, but also in identifying individual patterns of behaviour and their stability over time: patterns that would otherwise have been concealed within group averages. Thus although on average it is true to say that sexual activity declines between the ages of 55 and 70, for some individuals the opposite occurs, and their activity increases over that period of their lives (see below). Some studies do not differentiate between age-groups, or between those currently married or not. People within a given age-group will differ in their current level of sexual interest and activity, and in the sexual histories that shaped the attitudes and habits of their present age.

Sexuality in its wide (affectional) and narrow (coital) senses

Most studies are primarily concerned with coital sex; some include masturbation, sexual fantasy, and dreams (e.g. Martin 1981; Todarello and Boscia 1985); but few cover the wider aspects of sexuality. Some enquire into the length and happiness of relationships and the pleasure derived from sexuality in the past. However, many studies tacitly assume that coital sexual activity equates with enjoyable sex: it is not necessarily so for everybody, particularly not for women in the era under study. Non-coital, affectionate aspects of the relationships between sexual partners (actual or potential) have been little examined so far (West 1975); the study by Persson (1980) of a sample of 70-year-old Swedish men and women is an exception.

Stable heterosexual relationships between physically fit people as the implied norm—and those outside the norm.

Relatively little has been written about the lives of homosexual people of either sex as they grow older (Dressel and Avant 1983). Dorfman *et al.* (1995) compared a group of homosexual elders with their heterosexual counterparts in California. Admittedly this was a selected group (urban, middle-class, and well educated). They found that the homosexual group had built their social networks more around friendships than family relationships (the women more so than the men); these networks were fruitful and supportive, and the subjects were neither more lonely nor more depressed than heterosexual elders. Wojciechowski (1998), in a review of the literature on older lesbians, confirmed these findings; but also highlighted the vulnerability of couples who have not been publicly recognized to interference by others in decisions about their care, in bereavement, and in their property rights (see also p. 853). Slusher *et al.* (1996) give a good description of a support group for older gay and lesbian people and of the issues raised by the group.

The sexuality of single people living isolated lives is also neglected in the literature (but see Christenson and Johnson 1973; Stephens 1974; Corby and Zarit 1983).

Lastly, the issue of sexuality in the setting of illness is relatively unexplored. Physical illness is known to be one of the commonest sources of interference in the sexual lives of older people, and frequently signals the end of sexual intercourse in the partnership (especially where it is the male who is ill). An end to intercourse does not necessarily mean the end to all sexuality in the relationship, however: some couples are able to make a happy and successful adaptation to the handicap (e.g. see Traupmann 1984), though others sadly do not (Neuhaus and Neuhas 1982; Kral 1984; Helgason *et al.* 1996*b*; Buzzelli *et al.* 1997; Korpelainen *et al.* 1999). No studies appear to have been carried out on the *process* of adjusting a sexual relationship to the common illnesses of old age, such as stroke and Parkinson's disease, with the exception of dementia (p. 850).

What does 'normality' mean?

What is quoted as 'normal' may depend on the point that the speaker is trying to make. If it is assumed that no-one over the age of 60 can enjoy sex, then the assumption is refuted by demonstrating that a few people enjoy sex up to the age of 80, showing there is no absolute physiological or psychological bar to sexual activity in old age. If the reasoning then shifts to asking: 'If people over 60 *can* enjoy sex, why isn't everyone doing so?', then more detailed answers are needed. For example, it may be that a proportion of people in each age-band is failing to enjoy the opportunities for sexual activity that they would like for themselves (e.g. White 1982 found that 17% of his sample of people in their eighties would have liked to be sexually active, although currently they had no opportunity).

It is now accepted that 'normality' covers a very wide range of individual variation (e.g. see Martin 1981); that professionals need to respect the individuality of each person, rather than measuring them against some imaginary norm; and that the available data can be used to liberate both old and young from misleading notions of what is normal (and therefore allowable), and to give them permission to follow their feelings about what is right and pleasant for them and those they love (also see Kaplan 1996).

Normal sexuality in old age—findings

Taking account of these methodological points, we can now turn to what is known about sexuality in old age, concentrating more on themes emerging from the literature than on numerical findings that are specific to the context of each study. More detailed information can be found through the following reviews: Berezin (1969); Pfeiffer (1977); Friedeman (1978); Comfort (1980*b*); Corby and Solnick (1980); Ludeman (1981); Weg (1983); Schiavi (1990, 1999).

Data from the longitudinal study of healthy community volunteers, carried out by the Duke University Center for the Study of Aging and Human Development (Newman and Nichols

1960; Verwoerdt *et al.* 1969*a,b*; Pfeiffer and Davis 1972; George and Weiler 1981) showed that some 60% of married subjects (in this sample) aged 60–69, nearly the same proportion of those aged 70–74, and 25% of those aged 75 and over were sexually active. Even in extreme old age sexual activity did not disappear: one-fifth of the men in their eighties and nineties reported intercourse once a month or less. (By comparison, one-third of men in this age group in Todarello and Boscia's study (1985) reported 'occasional coitus').

Some important determinants of sexual activity were identified: age, gender (men were more sexually active than women of the same age), married status (a more important influence on sexual activity in women than men), own physical health (more important for men), and health of the partner (more important for women). Sexual interest was ascertained separately from sexual activity: in all age groups interest was commoner than activity, and though it became less common in the older age groups, this age effect was less marked than for sexual activity. The discrepancy between interest and activity was greater for women than for men, but at all ages the prevalence of sexual interest was less in women than in men.

The median age for stopping intercourse was 68 for men, 60 for women (but this included both married and widowed subjects). Within any age-group some individuals were more active and others less so. If they were divided into groups according to their *current* level of activity then they were found to differ in their sexual histories (those active in old age were always more interested in sex); and to differ in their future course (their level of sexual activity tended to remain stable over time and they mostly fell into the same groups when reclassified several years later) (George and Weiler 1981). Thus the modal pattern is to maintain a relatively stable level of sexual activity throughout a lifetime up to the age of around 70 or older; for some individuals, however, activity will decrease, and for others it will increase for a while.

Women showed the same stability of sexual activity over time, but (in the samples studied) a lower level on average than in men of the same age. Persistence of sexual interest and activity into old age is in women less closely related to the age of onset of sexual activity; it seems to be influenced more by social factors (e.g. Todarello and Boscia 1985) and by the degree to which their sexual experience was orgasmic (Christenson and Gagnon 1965). In other words, women who had enjoyed sex continued to be sexually active for longer than those who had not. This happy coincidence of scientific finding with common sense is supported by single-case accounts of women (Hite 1976) whose levels of sexual activity and interest were low throughout their first sexual relationship (usually in marriage), but dramatically increased in late life when they embarked on a new and more satisfactory relationship.

In considering the findings of the Duke University studies, it is important to remember that they refer to a sample of people born at the end of the nineteenth century or earlier, whereas a similar sample recruited today would contain people born in the 1930s and later, in a very different social climate. It is interesting to compare the findings of a more recent study (Bretschneider and McKoy 1988), also in California, of elderly people (aged 80 and over) in residential homes. This was a cross-sectional, volunteer study; only a third of the people approached gave answers to the questionnaire, but within that group 65% of the men and 30% of the women reported that they still had intercourse at least sometimes. Touching and caressing were more frequent, reported by 82% of the men and 64% of the women.

Later surveys have complemented the earlier findings discussed here. Some are based on samples from the general (aged) population, for example: Johnson (1996)—questionnaire survey of 164 community-resident volunteers; Dello Buono *et al.* (1998*b*)—335 people aged 65–106 recruited through their GPs in Padua, Italy, part of an international study conducted by the World Health Organization; Minichiello *et al.* (1996)—844 older people drawn randomly from the electoral role in Australia, part of a general health survey; Helgason *et al.* (1996*a*)—questionnaire survey of 319 men, an age-stratified community sample in Sweden; Davey Smith *et al.* (1997)—a 20-year follow-up study of 2512 men in Wales, an 'add-on' to a study of cardiovascular mortality.

Other studies have targeted specific groups: Matthias *et al.* (1997)—1216 community recipients of Medicare in California; Dello Buono (1998*a*)—38 centenarians, as a subgroup of the study mentioned above; Bortz and Wallace (1999)—1002 members of the 50+ Fitness Association, a selected group of physically active and highly motivated Americans; Ehrenfeld *et al.* (1997)—a study of nursing observations of 160 patients with dementia in long-term care in Israel; Archibald (1998)—a survey of sexuality and dementia in 23 social service residential-care homes in England, using managers' reports.

Many of the findings from these studies echo those of the earlier ones. Age, physical fitness, gender, and mental health are important factors in influencing sexual interest and activity. (For example, Dello Buono found their centenarians to be much less interested in sex than the younger-old members of the sample). Across the board, about two-thirds of older people are interested in sex, while one-third are sexually active; however about two-thirds of those who are sexually inactive are content to be so. Men tended to be more interested in sexual intercourse, women more in affection and loving touch, while neither rated oral sex very highly (Johnson 1996). Padoani *et al.* (2000) dissected out the influence of cognitive status on sexual activity in the Italian study and showed a relationship between higher scores on quality-of-life scales, maintenance of sexual activity, and cognitive status. In their view, 'rather than being a determining factor in sexual behaviour, cognitive integrity seems to play an important role in preserving an adequate ability to overcome the cultural, psychological and physical hurdles which hinder complete expression of sexual life.' Implicitly or explicitly, the same conclusion surfaces in many other studies of dementia and sexuality in old age.

The Duke University investigators asked their subjects in whom the level of sexual activity had *declined* to suggest why this occurred. Men tended to give as their reasons the onset of illness and the loss of a partner. Their sexual interest tended to persist even where activity had declined. For women, the chief reasons given for a decline in sexual activity were: loss of the partner, illness of the partner, and illness in themselves. Loss of a partner is both commoner and more of a handicap for women, in that women survive longer then men, and tend to be younger than their husbands, so that there are many more widows than widowers. On average, a woman can expect to survive her spouse by about 6 years (Bancroft 1989). Remarriage is less common for women than for men, both because there are fewer potential partners of the same or older ages, and because social pressures tend to discourage a partnership between an older woman and a younger man. Sexual relationships outside marriage are also probably harder for women to establish than for men. Some authors have suggested that the natural solution to this demographic imbalance would be for women at this age to establish homosexual relationships with each other (Ludeman 1981), but the available evidence suggests that it is rare for women to change their sexual orientation and preferences in late life.

Solitary sexual activity (both for people in established relationships and for people on their own) in the form of masturbation has proved more difficult to study, because elderly people (of both sexes) are reluctant to discuss it either in general or with reference to themselves. The strongly negative attitude to masturbation current during the early years of elderly people makes it more likely that those who do masturbate will deny it, so that the available data may be an underestimate of the number of people who find satisfaction in this form of sexual expression. One of the respondents in the Hite report (1976) clearly expresses the complex feelings that may accompany this simple sexual act: 'Masturbation has been important to me because I cannot seek sex outside of marriage, rotten as it is. So, masturbation is a release, but I do not practice it intensely because of religious and parental taboos left over from childhood...I enjoy masturbation 'during', but later feel guilty and then try to rationalize'. Corby and Solnick (1980) report a Danish study giving the prevalence of masturbation in men as 43% at age 70–75, dropping to 21% at age 80–95; Weizman and Hart (1987) in a study of healthy married men aged 60–71 reported a prevalence of 41%. Christenson and

Gagnon 1965 reported a prevalence of 25% in married women aged 65, and zero in married women aged 70, whereas 33% of the *previously* married women aged 65 masturbated, and 25% of those aged 70. Catania and White (1982) discuss the determinants of masturbation (in a study of interviews with volunteers). In Bretschneider and McKoy's (1988) study, 72% of men and 40% of women reported that they masturbated at least sometimes, but (as in other studies) many of the subjects simply avoided the question.

Less is known about the non-genital aspects of the sexual life of elderly people. Malatesta *et al.* (1988), in a study of widows (volunteers, aged 40–89, excluding those engaged in a relationship or living in an institution), enquired into the self-perceived *obstacles* to meeting sexual needs, the degree of *unhappiness* attributed to loss of a sexual companion, and the alternative activities that might *satisfy* their 'affectional and sexual needs'. Older widows were less conscious of obstacles (such as believing themselves unattractive); were less unhappy than younger widows about the loss of physical aspects of their relationship, but just as unhappy about the loss of companionship; and more likely to choose activities such as 'being with grandchildren' rather than 'going out on a date' or 'touching your body for sexual feelings' as alternative ways of meeting their affectional needs. The authors commented on the sexual pleasure derived by the older widows from having their hair done and wearing lingerie, and suggested that such activities should be taken seriously in therapy and education directed towards older widows. In Bretschneider and McKoy's (1988) study, 88% of the men and 71% of the women fantasized or daydreamed (at least once a year) 'about being close, affectionate and intimate with the opposite sex'.

Sexual physiology in old age

Detailed reviews of this topic are available elsewhere (e.g. Corby and Solnick 1980; Schiavi 1999), and only an outline will be given here, concentrating on the physiological events of sexual response, rather than on hormonal influences on sexuality.

Physiological changes in the female

Masters and Johnson (1966, 1970) analysed sexual response in four phases: excitement (arousal), plateau, orgasm, and resolution; and identified changes with age in all of these, primarily in the intensity of the muscular and vasocongestive events that are involved in sexual function. During the *arousal* phase in women, the increased blood flow to the pelvic organs takes place with lesser intensity in old age, so that vasocongestion of the vaginal wall, and vaginal lubrication are both reduced. This effect is particularly marked when oestrogen lack has caused thinning and shrinkage of the vaginal tissues, which also tends to reduce the expansile capacity of the vagina. These atrophic changes are more severe in women who have not been engaged in sexual intercourse: conversely, regular intercourse or masturbation tends to protect genital tissue from these hormonally associated changes. The sensitivity of the clitoris to sexual stimulation is unimpaired, but where the pelvic tissues have undergone atrophy they are more liable to trauma from physical stimulation, in which case the sensations will be of irritation or pain rather than sexual arousal. The phase of *orgasm* undergoes relatively little change with ageing. The number of uterine and vaginal contractions occurring during orgasm tends to be less, but the sensation is reported to be unaltered, and those women who experience multiple orgasms retain that capacity as they age. Sometimes the uterine contractions are spasmodic rather than rhythmical, and are experienced as painful: the authors relate this particularly to the oestrogen-deprived state. The phase of *resolution* is more rapid than in youth.

Physiological changes in the male

In the *arousal* phase in older men, erections are slower to develop, and require more direct tactile stimulation than in younger ages, where psychic stimulation plays a proportionately greater role. The erections are usually less intense: they are less firm, less elevated, and persist for a shorter time. Often the penis, though sufficiently erect to allow intromission, does not become fully stiff until the moment of ejaculation. Nocturnal erections and emissions are less frequent. (But this reduced frequency does not predict less satisfactory intercourse: Schiavi 1990.) The scrotal and testicular changes associated with arousal are also less intense. In the *plateau* phase, the 'point of ejaculatory inevitability' is less distinct than at a younger age, and it is possible for the older male to prolong the enjoyment of the plateau phase for much longer before experiencing the need to ejaculate. In the phase of *orgasm*, ejaculation takes place with fewer contractions and with a lesser volume of ejaculate, less forcefully expressed, but the intensity of the sensation of orgasm is not necessarily altered, and is a source of as much pleasure as in youth. Enjoyable intercourse without orgasm is common (and is linked to the phenomenon of 'less pressure to ejaculate' noted above). The *resolution* following arousal is more rapid in older men, and the refractory period that follows (during which renewed arousal cannot be achieved) is markedly longer than in youth. Older men may have a refractory period of 24 hours or more after orgasm, compared to the few minutes found in adolescence: but if ejaculation has not taken place then re-arousal can occur much sooner.

The effect of these physiological changes on the quality of a sexual relationship appears to depend very much on the attitudes of the partners, and on the freedom with which they can communicate with each other about their sexuality (e.g. see Sander 1976). Kaplan (1989) makes a sharp distinction between pathological effects on sexual physiology and the effects of normal ageing on male erectile function. She terms the latter *presbyrectia,* highlighting four aspects of clinical importance: erections are softer, need more stimulation, last for a shorter time, and are more vulnerable to anxiety or stress. The ability of a couple to adjust to these normal age-related changes is crucial for the survival of their sexual relationship. The gradual nature of the changes allows people who are secure and flexible to adapt their style of lovemaking—an adaptation that is seen by many as a gain rather than a loss. In the eyes of these couples, sex becomes less hasty and pressurized, more equally shared between the two: women take on a more active role in foreplay, men become more able to enjoy the romantic accompaniments of lovemaking (Kaplan 1981, 1989; Robinson 1983; Traupmann 1984). One of the respondents in the Hite Report (1976) wrote: 'It's a matter of growth and development, from a simplistic yes-or-no view of sex to much greater complexity, variety, subtlety, fluidity... many of us come rather late to the recognition of her or his unique and intricate sexual personality'.

Sexual problems

An informal questionnaire survey among colleagues in a variety of disciplines (unpublished) requested information on the problems they encountered concerning sexuality in old age. The replies indicated that the professional groups who had been made most aware, during the course of their work, of the sexuality of their patients were district nurses and community psychiatric nurses, field social workers, and care staff in residential homes. There were interesting differences in the nature of the problems identified by different professional groups: for example general practitioners most often cited impotence in elderly men (and, to a lesser extent, vaginal dryness in women), while staff of residential and nursing homes commonly identified the problem of sexual behaviour occurring in an inappropriate social context. (One respondent who had experience both as a nurse and as a residential careworker commented that in the former role she had been asked about physical problems concerning sexuality, while in the latter role people tended to ask her about emotional problems.)

The literature on sexual problems in old age reflects a similar diversity of perspective, and coverage of the field is patchy. At one extreme are the studies of older individuals who choose to seek help for something that they recognize as a source of distress to them individually or in their relationships (e.g. Hirst and Watson 1996). In this, they differ little from younger people who seek help for their sexual problems. At the other extreme are the studies of institutions or staff who have some responsibility for the behaviour, including sexual behaviour, of people in their care; where the people concerned have not sought and may not wish for any help in this area. In between lies a range of difficulties and a variety of levels of personal distress. We shall cover this area under the following headings: taking a sexual history; the effects of physical illness and medication on sexuality; relationship problems arising within established couples; dementia occurring in one partner in the relationship; sexuality in public settings; the sexuality of elderly people on their own; and individual elderly people and their professional carers.

Taking a sexual history

Sexual problems do not always declare themselves in advance to professionals, so that they can prepare their thoughts and arrange their attitudes to meet the challenge with composure. Patients can unexpectedly reveal a difficulty, in contexts devoted to other purposes, and professionals need to feel able to respond comfortably to them no matter how the problem has presented.

The principles of taking a sexual history are not altered by the age of the patient: Hawton (1985) gives an excellent account of these. They include:

(1) establishing a language that is comfortable for both the interviewer and interviewed, and in which clear information can be exchanged;
(2) using open questions to map out the area to be discussed, and closed questions to establish exact details;
(3) clarifying the problem by asking for a description of a specific occasion on which it occurred;
(4) taking a longitudinal view—the history from childhood, family attitudes, the sources of sexual information, through all relationships, and especially the early history of the present relationship;
(5) seeking information about the good periods of the relationship, and what the partners valued in each other then;
(6) interviewing both partners in a relationship wherever possible, both separately and together;
(7) heeding the importance of the medical and psychiatric history: illnesses, operations, and medication, both prescribed and non-prescribed;
(8) formulating the problem in terms of predisposing, precipitating, and maintaining factors; presenting the formulation to the patient (or couple), and ensuring they understand it and find it acceptable.

This description assumes that there has been an open acknowledgement of a sexual problem, that it has come to the attention of someone capable of helping with it, and that both the professional and the patient are willing to work at the problem together. This might be the situation, for example, when an elderly man consults his own doctor about his fear that he is becoming impotent. A clinic for sexual disorders may receive most of its referrals of older people in this way (e.g. Hirst and Watson 1996).

But the starting point can be less clear-cut than this. Two situations may illustrate this. A traditional gynaecological consultation takes place in circumstances that are clearly contrived to distance genital anatomy and physiology as far as possible from love and eroticism. The relaxation of taboo that licences the stranger to see and touch the sexual organs of the woman is made possible only by the strong boundary taboo set round it—a boundary that tacitly discourages talk of sexuality. In a similar fashion, nursing routines have tacit rules that separate the physical intimacies of washing a patient from the emotional intimacy that might otherwise be associated with that act (Burnside 1975). (In the survey among staff, mentioned earlier, a district nurse wrote: 'I have found that it is important to be very academic about doing things which involve a person's private parts, to the point of seeming cold, in order to protect myself from attention I did not want'.) Just as constrained, but in the opposite sense, is the counselling interview—in which profound feelings of love, grief, dependence, or abandonment can be accepted and discussed, but where the client may feel quite unable to talk about physical intimacy despite its equal emotional significance.

Trespassing outside the customary boundaries of a consultation provokes embarrassment; but often much of the embarrassment comes from the doctor. In fact, when given the opportunity, people are generally more ready to discuss a sexual difficulty than professionals assume (West 1975), and are willing to enter into detail when the first tentative statement receives a serious response. A community psychiatric nurse commented on her patients' eagerness to talk about sexual issues: 'The majority of functional clients and dementia carers bring it up, and...can't wait to be given permission to talk...they volunteer a vast amount of information and feelings.' Another wrote: '...when they do raise the subject they have a great need to express feelings...admissions of needs, regrets and frustrations both past and present'. (There are also important and specific cultural issues here that must be taken into account: see Qureshi 1989.)

Case 1

A 69-year-old woman had been seen by successive doctors in the psychiatric outpatient clinic for many years, for surveillance of her manic-depressive illness. She mentioned in passing that her sexual relationship with her husband had recently declined. On a bad day the doctor might have let the remark pass, with the subliminal thought 'probably normal for her age', but he was feeling energetic and had recently been reading about sexuality, so he asked if she would like to tell him more about her difficulty. He learned that, throughout her marriage, she had not enjoyed the oral sex that her husband liked, but rather than tell him so (because 'it might upset him') she had found it easier lately simply to discourage his sexual advances. Although this successfully avoided oral sex, it created new problems because she missed the comfort of their former physical closeness, and her husband began to withdraw from her emotionally. There was a happy outcome to the doctor's energy: the discussion of her difficulty with an outsider helped the patient to talk to her husband, and they found a more comfortable compromise between their different preferences.

Too many elderly people have found that a hesitant allusion to a sexual difficulty in a consultation has been met by a stunned silence or an embarrassed diversion of conversation. Too many doctors, in all specialties, feel uncomfortable and inadequately prepared for such an exploratory remark. In fact the doctor only needs to say: 'I'm glad you came to see me: can you tell me more about this?', and to listen with interest and sympathy. He may then find that simply telling the story has given the patient much relief, or he may discover within the story the ideas for its solution. If not, it is very appropriate then to say that he needs to consider the problem further, or ask for advice, and to arrange another appointment. The effect of that is very different from an initial response which conveys the message: 'That is not something I wish to discuss'. Beyond this, suitable training in psychosexual medicine is available and can greatly enhance the doctor's usefulness to patients with sexual difficulties (Mathers *et al.* 1994).

Effects of physical illness and medication on sexuality

One of the commonest reasons given by elderly people for ending sexual activity is the onset of physical illness, which may operate through a number of different mechanisms. Physical illness may generate unfounded anxieties about the *risks* of sexual activity (as in heart disease or stroke); it may make intercourse *difficult*, exhausting, or painful (as in respiratory disease or arthritis); or it may impair *responsiveness* of the sexual organs (as in diabetes or peripheral vascular disease). Physical illness may undermine *self-confidence* and the feeling of attractiveness (as in mutilating operations such as mastectomy or colostomy), and it may have a direct effect in reducing sexual *desire* (perhaps in Parkinson's disease and Alzheimer's disease (Zeiss *et al.* 1990), and certainly in depressive illness).

One systematic study (Feldman *et al.* 1994) of a sexual problem was part of a community-based survey in Massachusetts of 1709 randomly sampled healthy men aged between 40 and 70, and which examined the phenomenon of impotence. The authors chose a broad perspective on this problem: potency 'was addressed as a subjective state', using a self-administered questionnaire which included questions on the subjects' satisfaction with their sex life and with their relationship with their partner, on their partners' satisfaction with them, and on the frequency of sexual activity with their partner. Answers to these questions were combined with those to questions on erectile function itself to give a composite measure of potency at three levels: minimal, moderate, and complete impotence. (The validity of this composite measure was tested by comparison with a 'calibration sample' of men directly assessed at a urology clinic.)

The prevalence of 'impotence' assessed in this way was strongly related to age. For example, in men aged 40, 5% were completely impotent, while 15% were so at the age of 70. Moderate impotence occurred in 17% of 40-year-olds, and 34% of 70-year olds.

The relationship of impotence to a variety of medical risk factors was also examined. The most important effects were seen with heart disease, hypertension, diabetes, medication associated with these diseases, a low level of high-density lipoprotein, and psychological measures of anger, depression, and low dominance. Smoking intensified the effects of cardiovascular risk; and (in this study) alcohol intake had a minor effect and obesity had none.

Stroke

There are two valuable studies to cite here. Buzzelli and colleagues (1997) interviewed patients and their spouses a year after their stroke and found a decline in the frequency of intercourse (compared to the time before the stroke). They also found that the spouses' fear of causing harm, or feelings of being put off by the stroke, were more important factors in this decline than any physical disability resulting from the stroke itself. Korpelainen and colleagues (1999) surveyed 192 patients and 94 of their spouses who were participating in poststroke adjustment courses. They found a marked decrease in libido (both in the patients and their partners) and a general decrease in satisfaction, possibly linked with the difficulty that both spouses and partners felt in discussing the issues between themselves, including their fear of impotence. The authors highlighted a need for poststroke counselling to encompass these issues.

Incontinence

Roe and May (1999) interviewed a number of people (of all ages) identified by the nurse visiting them at home as having adjusted particularly well or particularly badly to their incontinence, and to the use of catheters and other incontinence devices. They quote vivid case examples to make their argument that the urethra and sexuality are closely linked, and that nurses offering care in this area must understand both the practical details and the emotional implications. Atkinson(1997) in a single case study reinforces this point.

Prostate disease

Folklore predicts impotence after prostatectomy, but the risk of this depends on the surgical technique and on the illness (benign hypertrophy or prostatic cancer) that required the operation (Catalona *et al.* 1993). In a case-note audit of transurethral prostatectomy, Thorpe *et al.* (1994) found that 12% of patients who were previously sexually active had major erectile problems after surgery, and 24% had ejaculatory dysfunction. Interestingly, 10% of the sample reported an improvement of sexual function that had been impaired preoperatively, including 9% who regained erectile capacity. Prostatectomy will reduce the volume of ejaculate and may cause retrograde ejaculation into the bladder, so that the experience of ejaculating may be different (Neuhaus and Neuhaus 1982; Schover and Jensen 1988).

As a non-surgical treatment for benign prostatic hyperplasia, finasteride has been reported (Gormley *et al.* 1992) to cause a loss of libido in 6%, a reduced volume of ejaculate in 4.4%, and erectile impotence in 5% of men taking 1 mg. daily.

A notable study in this area is that of Helgason *et al.* (1996*b*). This was a questionnaire survey of 430 men with cancer of the prostate and 435 controls (randomly selected and age-matched). The authors found diminished sexual activity in the patients and considerable distress related to this. More importantly, they asked their subjects to indicate their personal trade-offs between longevity and loss of potency (since this trade-off should of course be considered by men who are making a decision about surgery for prostate cancer). The authors found a remarkable range of strongly held individual views, both within the patient group and the controls. For example 19% of men in the control group said that they would not be willing to risk their sexual function even if it was proved that the treatment prolonged life, given that they had an 80% chance of being alive after 10 years without any curative treatment. On the other hand, 38% of men would choose treatment irrespective of eventual effects on their sexual function. Of the men who had actually had prostate cancer, 63% said they were willing to trade-off the possibility of a longer life for an intact sexual function. Practically, the findings of this study are important to surgeons and oncologists in counselling their patients; methodologically they are significant in showing how individual variation and personal choice can and should be a legitimate part of an orthodox scientific investigation.

A further aspect of physical illness that needs to be considered in its own right is the effect of *medication*. The list of drugs that can interfere with sexual function is very long (Parkinson and Bateman 1994): among them should be noted antidepressants (Baier and Philipp 1994; Mir and Taylor 1998), antipsychotics, antihypertensive medication, thiazide diuretics, and benzodiazepines (Kellett 1989). Much less commonly, medication can enhance (or overstimulate) sexual function: this has been described with L-dopa (Brown *et al.* 1978), and with trazodone (Scher *et al.* 1983; Purcell and Ghurya 1995).

Relationship problems arising within established couples

Problems arising within the sexual relationship of an elderly couple may have emotional or physical origins, or both. The general principles of the framework now well established for the sexual counselling of younger couples (Masters and Johnson 1970; Kaplan 1981; Hawton 1985; Bancroft 1989) are equally appropriate for the problems of older people, so we shall concentrate on aspects particular to old age.

Bretschneider and McCoy (1988) asked their respondents who had a regular sexual partner what problems they experienced: those most frequently cited (by both men and women) were fear of poor performance, inability to achieve or maintain an erection, vaginal dryness and pain, and lack of opportunities for sexual encounters. Sexual dysfunction in older couples may arise simply from a lack of information about the normal age-related changes in sexual physiology. A slower onset of arousal, or a reduced need to ejaculate, may be interpreted by the man as the onset of impotence, or by the woman as a sign of declining interest in her; and their fearful or offended reactions can then aggravate the difficulty (Masters and Johnson (1970), Sander (1976), and Kaplan (1989) give good examples). There may be additional fears of unattractiveness or loss of fitness, or jealousy of younger potential rivals. (A large disparity in age may be an important factor: a couple aged 50 and 30 may feel comfortably matched, but 30 years later the 80-year-old may have a very different perspective on life from the 60-year-old spouse.)

Frequently, physical and psychological factors will interact, and old anxieties or conflicts may emerge in the new context. In a man who already feels insecure and pessimistic about his sexual function, one failed attempt to ejaculate in the same way as before may be enough to trigger a psychogenic impotence, with performance anxiety creating a self-fulfilling prophecy. Convinced that he will fail in intercourse, he may avoid occasions for making love (with all its wider connotations), and for showing physical affection in any other way, for fear of being expected to go further. The less he is able to talk to his wife about his fear and his reasons for avoiding intercourse, the greater the risk of this outcome.

In a similar way, if illness has reduced the capacity to respond to stimulation, and this is something the couple cannot understand or discuss, then they cannot compensate for it. In a relationship where the assumption was that the man always takes the major role in lovemaking, the wife may be quite unused to stroking her husband's penis as part of their preparation for intercourse, and so she cannot help him if this is what he needs (for example, see Gustavii 1983).

Illness can affect a sexual relationship in more subtle ways: if one partner is looking after the other, disabled partner, then the mutuality of the relationship is under threat. The ill partner may lose the self-esteem which reassures him that he is still contributing to the relationship; or the caring partner may think it unkind and selfish to make demands on the sexual responsiveness of the one who is ill (e.g. Litz *et al.* 1990). Even simple actions can have far-reaching effects, such as when the couple decide they should sleep apart so as to give the ill partner a better night's rest.

Much will depend on how the couple understood their sexual relationship previously. If they saw it as a self-interested need experienced by one of them, which the other would kindly or dutifully fulfil, they may have difficulty maintaining it under adverse circumstances. If withdrawal from sexual contact was used by either partner to signal anger in the relationship, then an unexpected difficulty in one of them may also be interpreted—mistakenly in this case—as a punitive action. But if they saw their sexuality as an important element of the bond between them, to which either of them could give extra care whenever it was in danger of weakening, then their chances of coping well with the effects of disability are much better. Examples of successful adaptation are quoted by Traupmann (1984) from the survey by Brecher (1984). One such quotation reads: 'In my late sixties, I began to find sexual intercourse physically tiring—especially holding my body off the bed...Then I discovered how to plant one hip firmly on the mattress to support my weight, and to enter my partner sideways. This proved to have many advantages, including the ease with which I could stroke her clitoris and she could stimulate my penis with her fingers...Sex takes longer these days—and now that it is less fatiguing, it is more enjoyable.'

The effects of dementia occurring in one partner in a sexual relationship

It is important to note that although the illness itself is a tragedy, the effects on sexuality need not always be bad. For many couples in this situation, the physical relationship can remain a source of comfort and mutual support, long after other forms of communication have narrowed down to the unequal exchange between a carer and the recipient of care. (A touching aspect of this is the determination of some couples to go on sharing a double bed, even when mobility difficulties or incontinence create major practical problems.)

Sadly, it is more common for dementia to impair the sexual component—like so many other elements—in a relationship. This is sympathetically discussed by Mace and Rabins (1981) and by Litz *et al.* (1990).It is not unusual for the dementing partner still to feel sexual interest, but to be unaware that the quality of the relationship has changed. The change may have come about because the demented person has become childlike, or uncouth, or inconsiderately demanding, or because of erectile problems (Zeiss *et al.* 1990). The carer-partner may find it difficult to respond, if he or she is struggling with a mixture of feelings that includes compassion and affection for the sake of the past, but no longer any sexual attraction for a partner who has lost the subtle skills of courtship. It is harder still if the feelings include irritation or disgust, and can become intolerable if the relationship that existed before the illness was already on the margin of survival.

Case 2

The wife of a man with a dementing illness felt unable to resist his demands for sexual contact, distressing as they were to her. Throughout their marriage he had been violent at times towards her, and with good reason she was now scared that he would be unable to understand or accept a refusal from her, and would assault her again. The ambivalence of her feelings towards him, which had earlier prevented her from leaving this violent relationship, continued to complicate her attempts (and the attempts of the social worker involved with her) to deal with the problem (see also Chapter 37).

In a longitudinal study of 97 patients with dementia living (at entry to the study) at home with a carer, sexual problems were noted by the carer at some point during the illness in 27 subjects (Hope, personal communication of unpublished findings). The three main categories of problem were 'inappropriate talking', 'exposure', and 'inappropriate behaviour'. In many cases the problem was transient, but in a few it persisted for months or even years. The severity and frequency of problems was very variable, and the carer's perception might influence what was counted as a problem. (For instance, examples of 'inappropriate behaviour' ranged from 'wants to sit beside other patients and put his hand on their knee' to 'grabs women's breasts' or regular masturbation.)

An important study in this area is that of Wright (1998) who conducted a 5-year follow-up of two groups of couples, one in which one partner had a dementing illness, and a control group where neither partner was ill. At baseline the partners in the two groups reported the same levels of affection and sexual activity, but over the 5 years, while reported affection remained steady for the control spouses, it declined in the spouses in the dementia group—except, interestingly, when the person with dementia had been admitted to institutional care, after which affection in the spouse recovered significantly. Fewer couples with a partner with dementia maintained sexual activity (27% at 5 years after onset of the dementia) compared to control spouses (of whom 82% were sexually active at the same period). However, in those partnerships with dementia where sexual activity was maintained, the mean frequency of sexual contact was higher than in controls, and demands for frequent contact were reported by 50% of their caregivers. Sexual activity in these couples was also related to the spouses' physical health and freedom from depression, but not to the cognitive state of the ill partner.

Gladstone (1995) surveyed 87 married people living in institutions and 74 spouses living in the community whose partner was in institutional care. The interviews were analysed by Gladstone into categories according to the respondents' perception of changes to their marriages resulting from institutionalization; these were discussed in terms of the psychological need to preserve a sense of continuity, whether through 'external continuity' (for example, continuing to provide practical help in small ways), or 'internal continuity' (by maintaining self-perception and memories of the past). Haddad and Benbow (1998) give a comprehensive review of sexual problems associated with dementia.

Sexuality in public settings

In the informal survey of professional staff cited earlier, the commonest problem identified was that of sexual behaviour in public. 'A male resident with his hand in a female resident's underclothing, touching her, in a lounge with other residents sitting there.' 'Public fondling. The apparent lack of sensitivity to the presence of other residents.' 'Suggestiveness in front of other residents which is embarrassing. It's difficult to know what to say, to take it as a joke or take offence.' Szasz's (1983) study of the attitudes of staff in a large extended care unit showed that they identified a similar range of unwanted sexual behaviours, which he categorized as 'sex talk', 'sexual acts', and 'implied sexual behaviour' (such as openly reading pornography). Interestingly, staff observed that patients were consistent in the type of sexual behaviour they adopted; and the only behaviour that staff regarded as acceptable was hugging, and kissing on the cheek. Archibald (1998), from a postal questionnaire answered by managers of residential homes, reported that the sexual issues they most frequently encountered were 'men and women holding hands; male residents attempting to touch staff; masturbation; and male residents (with no cognitive problems) attempting to establish relationships with female residents who were cognitively impaired'.

The discomfort caused to care staff by the open display of sexuality can interact with discomfort from another source: worries about the legitimacy of a relationship. A married couple may be encouraged to keep their sexual intimacies to their bedroom, but residents with no socially sanctioned tie will generate much more anxiety and conflict among the staff, unsure whether to encourage a more private expression of the couple's sexual feeling, or to try and put a stop to it altogether (e.g. see Loeb and Wasow 1975; Silverstone and Wynter 1975). Lichtenberg (1997) in a helpful survey of the literature, and Lichtenberg and Strzepek (1990) discuss the ethical issues in such situations, clarifying the conflict between supporting autonomous decision-making and protecting from abuse. The notion of competence is central to their analysis, and they offer a helpful framework for understanding this concept where participation in relationships is concerned. The three elements of competence they describe are: awareness of the relationship (for which memory is required); ability to avoid exploitation (in which the capacity to decline unwanted contact is crucial); and awareness of risks (which involves the ability to foresee the consequences of ending the relationship). Two case studies illuminate their analysis. Richardson and Lazur (1995) and Ghusn (1995) also offer thorough and helpful reviews of this area.

Ehrenfeld *et al.* (1999) report an observational study of sexual behaviour in eight old people's homes. Nurses participating in this study, using standardized checklists and reporting forms, collected data on the behaviour of 48 patients. In their analysis the authors distinguish three categories of sexual behaviour: love and caring; romance; and eroticism (the rarest form of behaviour in this sample). They offer illustrative examples, and an interesting in-depth discussion of the ethical and emotional issues.

The families of elderly residents can play an important role, for good or ill, in determining how much freedom the residents have to enter into relationships. A residential social worker wrote: 'I have found that when two consenting adults develop and consummate a relationship in a residential setting, the relationship comes under great pressure to stop from many areas. Often family, other residents, staff, find reasons for trying to end the relationship.'

Case 3

An elderly lady with dementia who was cared for at home by her husband, came regularly for respite care to a psychogeriatric unit. She responded happily to the advances of a resident in the unit (who was also demented); but the nursing staff found it impossible to agree among themselves how decisively they should, for the sake of her husband, intervene and curb her interest.

Similarly, staff and residents of a home find it hard to deal with the sexuality implicit in the behaviour of residents who wander at night and climb into another resident's bed. This is not to deny that it is extremely alarming for an elderly person in a home to wake suddenly and find a stranger in their room: but the drama invested in such incidents seems to owe as much to sexual fears as to fear of any other danger.

One aspect of sexuality that can cause particular tension in communal settings is homosexuality. Whereas staff may take an affectionate interest in the development of a heterosexual relationship between two of their residents, and a marriage in an old people's home is usually a source of general rejoicing, the corresponding development of a homosexual relationship provokes anxiety, conflict, and sometimes hostility and outrage (e.g. Kassel 1983). A social worker in our survey quoted the case of an elderly lesbian woman 'who went into other accommodation following the death of her partner after a long relationship. She has just started a relationship with another resident but they feel they have to keep it secret'.

Perhaps the behaviour that arouses the strongest feelings is masturbation in public, and community and residential staff are equally concerned by it. A community nurse noted how he was asked frequently for advice 'on what they [care staff] perceive as inappropriate masturbation and ways that I can stop them [residents] doing it. They often seem surprised when I suggest that it is *where* they are doing it that is inappropriate and not the act itself' (also see Comfort 1980*a*; Kassel 1983).

One environment particularly devoid of privacy for the expression of sexual affection, even between acknowledged partners, is the hospital ward. Comfort (1980*a*) has written eloquently about the deprivation imposed on elderly couples when one of them is admitted to hospital: a deprivation particularly tragic if the illness is terminal, and the opportunity for the final physical expression of comfort and leave-taking is lost.

The sexuality of elderly people on their own

For people who have been in a relationship ended by the death of the partner, this is part of the larger issue of bereavement. It is important for those who counsel in bereavement not to shy away from the physical aspects of the loss, or to forget that a vital aspect of personal identity has been lost when a sexual relationship is ended by death. The grief of the loss is compounded when the relationship was not a publicly acknowledged one (for example a homosexual or an extra-marital relationship). Then the partner may be deprived of any recognition as a mourner, as well, perhaps, as having earlier been excluded from major decisions affecting their lover's life (such as a move into residential care, or decisions on the treatment of intercurrent illness near the time of death). A social worker wrote in reply to our survey: 'If we do have homosexual people in our homes it is likely that they will have been bereaved. If they do not feel safe to discuss their sexuality they will not be able to grieve openly in the same way as widows and widowers—and yet they may have lost a life partner in the same way'. These points are vividly illustrated by Stuart (1994), the carer in such a relationship.

For some elderly people, bereavement is lifelong; for others, it is the beginning of a new way of living, and a release from tiresome responsibilities (e.g. Thompson *et al.* 1990). Some would like to establish a new sexual relationship: the chances of finding a new marriage partner are much greater for men than women, but many older women would not contemplate a sexual relationship outside marriage (Snyder and Spreitzer 1976). Others feel differently. One widow quoted in Hammond (1987) wrote: 'I'm 81, and when my husband was alive I thought sex was the most fun in the world, but now that I'm a widow, it's kind of hard to find someone to play with'. Expressing the same idea in a different way, one of the women quoted in the Hite report (1976) wrote: 'I am answering your questionnaire because I feel there are not enough statistics about women septuagenarians (I am seventy-eight), not enough understanding of the widow's situation. At my age and without responsibilities I do not want matrimony but I have a continuing sex drive which keeps me looking fifteen to twenty years younger than my chronological age. Also I had heart surgery two years ago, which has completely rejuvenated me. I want to live to the fullest extent of my capabilities.' One difficulty that may arise in new relationships at this age stems from sexual anxiety or expectations that either partner may have of themselves or of the other. One form of this is so-called 'widower's impotency' (Comfort 1980*b*). Sadly, some re-marriages may lead to new problems, including sexual abuse (Ron and Lowenstein 1999).

Older people who have always chosen to live alone will have different needs, and will often be better adjusted to their situation than are those who come to a solitary life after bereavement. They have been little studied (see Christenson and Johnson 1973 for women, no comparable study for men, Corby and Zarit 1983 for an overview).

Individual elderly people and their professional carers

Care staff (in any profession) may encounter sexual advances at any level of subtlety from the elderly people they care for. These advances may range from tentative invitations to wordless physical actions, and may evoke a conflicting mixture of feelings in the carer (Griffiths 1988). Mostly the carers do not wish to upset the elderly person (sometimes they are afraid of provoking a violent response to rejection), nor do they want to appear encouraging. Their embarrassment includes a fear that they may be overreacting, and a recognition that the subtle understatements used in ordinary social life will not help them here. Caught unprepared, the carer may respond with laughter or a teasing response to hide her embarrassment, or may try to ignore the event and act as though it has not happened. Either of these responses risk being understood as encouragement (or at best, ambiguity) by the elderly person. If he (or she) then tries the same advance on another occasion, before long he will acquire the label of 'a behaviour problem'. But the carer who is at ease with the issue of sexuality is much more likely to give a clear response: to indicate straightforwardly that the person's need has been understood but cannot be responded to in the way that he wants, while preserving affection and respect on both sides of the relationship (see also

Mattiason and Hemberg 1998; Routasalo and Isola 1996).

Management of sexual problems

Information

Most writers on sexuality in old age, from Masters and Johnson (1970) onwards, have emphasized the necessity of disseminating accurate information about normal sexual physiology and about the acceptability of sexual feelings and behaviour in later life, so as to dispel harmful attitudes and preconceptions. The publication of books easily accessible to the general public (Felstein 1978; Hammond 1987; Greengross and Greengross 1989), and programmes on radio and television are important vehicles for this process. The education of professionals, whether in health or social services, is also vital. A theme that repeatedly occurs in the literature on intervention is the value of educational programmes in allowing carers to understand the issues and their own reactions better, to allow unfounded fears to be relieved, to share dilemmas, and to think together about solutions. Walker and Ephross (1999) offer a model outline of the content of such a programme. Mayers and McBride (1998) describe a 3-hour workshop for care staff in geriatric long-term care homes, followed up by questionnaires to assess the usefulness of the workshop. Participants found it valuable and enjoyable. Sadly, however, the untrained caregivers found it hard to get away from their work, and so it was mainly senior staff who attended. This is a problem often encountered in Britain by psychogeriatricians and community psychiatric nurses (CPNs) who try to set up teaching programmes in nursing and residential homes; and it re-emphasizes the crucial importance of a real and practical commitment to education by the managers of homes. White and Catania (1982) describe the effects of a formal educational programme set up in an old people's home (targeted on the residents, their families, and the care staff); a fourfold increase in sexual activity was reported by the study group of residents, following the programme. Webb (1987) describes the effect of an enlightened senior nurse on the attitudes of a group of gynaecological nurses. The Dementia Services Development Centre has produced materials on sexuality and dementia (book and video) for staff education—see the address at the end of this chapter.

Attitudes

Better information contributes to the process of changing attitudes, but opportunities may also need to be created in which the new information can be shared, so that people can feel safe to modify or abandon their former attitudes. It is quite wrong to assume that people who have difficulty in publicly discussing sexual behaviour are inhibited because of discomfort in their own sexual relationships. The persistence of social taboos on public talk about sex is quite enough to account for inhibition in such discussions, and the false assumption can be a serious barrier to fruitful discussion. If the staff of an old people's home are invited to a meeting to discuss sexual problems in their residents, they may be afraid to discuss their thoughts in case they reveal to their seniors or to a visiting professional some personal hang-up or inexperience of which they are unaware; and they may need to be reassured on this point before any other discussion can take place.

Respondents to our survey reported that they were frequently called on for advice and information in helping care staff or relatives to deal with sexual issues. A central part of this educational process lies in encouraging the carers to express feelings, attitudes, and assumptions, so that they can be discussed and possibly modified. For example, a social worker wrote: 'Relatives ask for advice on how to stop an active sex life of parents or a parent and the new partner. Sometimes care staff find aged consenting couples distasteful and ask social workers to halt it.' A head of home wrote: 'Care staff have on occasions asked for guidelines if a resident is found masturbating. Advised to leave resident alone if in own bedroom, if in lounge etc. to report to senior member of staff on duty. Explained it is quite healthy for sexual activity in elderly people'. A member of a home's care staff wrote: 'Attitudes of staff [concern me]. They can find this situation humorous or disgusting rather than concentrating on client's needs for an active fulfilling physical relationship. And possibly denying the rights of clients'. A psychologist wrote: 'Carers...are on occasion provoking the behaviour they complain of, by badinage, teasing...trying to forbid all expressions of sexuality rather than find ways of defining acceptable outlets'. Szasz (1983) discusses similar issues.

Prevention of problems

The sexual difficulties that can arise after an illness or operation, or as a consequence of medication, might be prevented if better-informed nurses and doctors discussed with their patients beforehand any sexual implications of their condition. Lawton and Hacker (1989) reported that, among the women referred to their clinic for gynaecological cancers, at least a third of the women over the age of 70 who had radical surgery were still sexually active; and they emphasized the importance of preoperative counselling that encompasses the sexuality of elderly patients. Thorpe *et al.* (1994) found that in only 30% of their sample (of men undergoing prostatectomy) was there a record of preoperative counselling about the possibility of retrograde ejaculation following surgery. Moreover, men over 70 were significantly less likely to have been advised on the sexual consequences of their operation than the younger men in the study. Korpelainen *et al.* (1999) discuss the importance of counselling after stroke.

Simple counselling for sexual problems

Many sexual difficulties, especially those arising in untroubled relationships and related to physical illness, can be helped by relatively simple advice. For example, couples limited by painful joints from enjoying sexual intercourse may be encouraged to try different positions, pillows for support of hips and limbs, different timing for their analgesic medication, or taking a warm bath before intercourse to relax painful muscles. Vaginal dryness and atrophy may need lubricants and hormonal treatment.

Often patients do not need specific medical treatment or advice, but with a little help can find their own solutions. Gustavii (1983) quotes a telling example: 'A rural district nurse arrived at the home of a 70-year-old man to change his catheter. He asked whether she was married. When she replied that she was not, he did not reveal why he had asked. The explanation came 1 year later, when her vacation substitute was asked the same question. She replied that she was married. On hearing this response, the man dared to ask her to leave the catheter out for a few hours so that he could have sexual intercourse with his wife. Naturally, his request was granted, and now the regular nurse follows this routine'. A 72-year-old woman with an 80-year-old husband quoted by Traupmann (1984) wrote: 'My husband's joints are painful—so that limits his activity, but his mind and disposition are fine so I am lucky...He has not had a full erection for at least eight years...but he is such a delightful, delicious caresser that he can give me an orgasm without [intercourse]. He does not crave this activity as often as I do but the quality is worth waiting for. In any case, I can piece out with masturbation'. Some couples less confident in their sexuality might need to share the problem with an understanding outsider, and to receive 'permission' to experiment, before they could arrive at this couple's solution.

Prescription of new medication is not often helpful with sexual problems, though it is always important to review the medication the patient is taking for other reasons. (For example, anti-parkinsonian medication can sometimes provoke unwanted sexual behaviour.) Occasionally antidepressant treatment may be indicated, where the problem seems to be part of a mood disorder: but many classes of antidepressants depress sexual function, though moclobemide seems to be free of this side-effect (Baier and Philipp 1994). Medication to suppress sexual activity in dementia is discussed later (p. 857).

The literature on sexuality and disability (not confined to older people) is a good source of practical advice (Heslinga 1974; Schover and Jensen 1988); information is also available from SPOD—the address is given at the end of this chapter.

Psychosexual counselling in non-specialist settings.

Counselling depends first of all on a clear understanding of the problem. Though this appears obvious, in fact the history given by the patient will be coloured by his perception of what is wrong, while the perception *itself* may be the source of the difficulty. For example, a general practitioner consulted by an elderly man because of impotence may think first of organic causes, echoing the patient's own assumptions, and both may miss the possibility that factors in his relationships and in his thinking are contributory. However, the habit of taking a systematic sexual history (see p. 846 in this chapter) and of always asking to see the partner will help to ensure that the contributions of early sexual experience, mistaken assumptions, anxious pessimism, and the responses of the wife to her husband are not neglected, and these may offer hopeful opportunities for intervention (Hawton 1988). The sexual history needs to be supplemented by a medical and psychiatric history (especially alert to the possibility of depression and alcoholism) and a review of medication, followed by a thorough physical examination. The importance of interviewing the spouse should be explained, and arrangements made for seeing each partner individually, followed by time with the couple together. At this joint meeting, a careful and unhurried explanation is given to the couple, concerning the nature of the problem, the likely reasons why it arose, the factors that may be perpetuating it, and the ways in which it can be helped. This explanation needs to be thought through a little beforehand, so that it can be presented in a way that does not lay blame on either partner, leaving room for positive steps to be taken. Even where nothing else is possible, there is usually scope for helping communication and understanding between the partners. The explanation (formulation) is followed by time and encouragement for the couple to ask questions, through which the doctor assures himself that they have both understood what he has said. Further details on counselling are beyond the scope of this chapter, and the interested reader is referred to Kaplan (1981) and Hawton (1985) as a helpful starting point, and to Runciman (1975), Felstein (1978), Teri and Reifler (1986), Kaplan (1989), Litz *et al.* (1990), and Pinfold (1994) for informal accounts of such counselling in the elderly.

Specialist advice

By and large, such advice falls into two categories: specialist psychosexual counselling, and specialist urogenital advice.

Where the psychological and relationship issues contributing to a sexual problem are too time-consuming or complex for the general practitioner or other member of the primary care team to deal with, help may be sought from Relate (formerly the Marriage Guidance Council), or (in some areas) from psychosexual clinics provided through the local psychiatric service. The Association of Sexual and Marital Therapists (see the end of this chapter) holds a list of therapists; and the Institute of Psychosexual Medicine organizes training for doctors interested in this field (Mathers 1994).

Enormous advances in the understanding and treatment of organic difficulties in sexual function, especially the organic element in impotence, have taken place in the last few years (Krane *et al.* 1989; Gregoire and Pryor 1993; Kirby 1994). A wide variety of treatments is available, foremost among them being sildenafil as a convenient and safe (with appropriate precautions) oral treatment for impotence. Older methods are still available when required, including intracavernosal self-injection of papaverine, prostaglandin E_1, and other vasoactive compounds; hormonal treatment; external devices; and implantable prostheses. The patient and his problem need careful assessment in a specialist clinic, and the choice of treatment will be based on that assessment. Although only a minority of elderly people may require such a referral, it is no longer necessary either for doctors or patients to see impotence as an insoluble problem.

Interventions to modify 'inappropriate' sexual behaviour, particularly in dementia

Harris and Wier (1998) survey the literature on sexual behaviour in dementia. They point out that a decrease in sexual interest and activity is far more common than hypersexuality, that behavioural and educational methods of management are to be preferred but are under-researched, and that carers rarely report their concerns to professionals though they have few strategies for coping with problems themselves.

Often the first reaction of worried relatives or staff in the face of sexual behaviour that they find aberrant or distressing, is to seek a medical solution: surely, they think, some medication could solve the problem. There are indeed occasions when medication may be necessary and effective. Lothstein *et al.* (1997) summarize their experience with 39 patients referred over 5 years to a geriatric outpatient clinic with a variety of severe problems in sexual behaviour (including incest, child abuse, sexual aggression), many in the setting of longstanding cognitive impairment. On the basis of their experience, they recommend first-line treatment with selective serotonin-reuptake inhibitors (SSRIs) and, if unsuccessful, the use of antiandrogens or oestrogen patches. They review the indications and contraindications to these treatments, and give a comprehensive survey of the relevant literature. Kuhn *et al.* (1998) report a single case where (after a variety of other interventions) medroxyprogesterone acetate (Provera), in association with nursing interventions, was effective in modifying the hypersexual behaviour of a male patient with Alzheimer's disease, whose inappropriate behaviour was causing considerable problems in the long-stay facility where he had been admitted, and was threatening his placement there.

Major tranquillizers are sometimes used to control inappropriate sexual actions, but they may be ineffective unless given at doses that cause unacceptable levels of sedation. Nadal and Allgulander (1993) report the successful use of cyproterone acetate (an antiandrogen) in a woman with Pick's disease and intractable masturbation, in whom antipsychotic and antidepressant medication had been ineffective. It is noteworthy that the patient agreed to the treatment (her husband consented to it); and that the beneficial effect of the drug was slow in onset and persisted when the drug was withdrawn after 5 months.

However, before turning to medication which can have undesirable side-effects, it is generally better to look for non-drug interventions. Sometimes these have been very ingenious: there is a charming report by Fielo and Warren (1997), of a case in which nursing students helped to modify the behaviour of a 95-year-old man who was regularly inviting prostitutes to his flat. He was thought to be putting himself at risk, both of robbery and of sexually transmitted disease, but careful thought was given to balancing this risk against respect for his autonomous personal choices. Tunstull and Henry (1996) give an unusually practical and candid account of interventions undertaken in a nursing home to devise ways in which the sexual feelings of the residents could be creatively expressed; education of staff in supporting this approach and in developing skills in limit-setting was an important part of the programme. Ragno (1996) also details creative solutions to engaging the interest of residents, and emphasizes the valuable role that activities organizers and creative therapists can play in making sure that gender-appropriate activities are available to residents.

For such approaches in institutional care to work, it is obviously important for the leaders in the homes, and their management, to give them their support. Ehrenfeld *et al.* (1997) describe a committee set up by a number of chief nurses jointly to consider problem cases; the emphasis in their discussions was on achieving a proper balance between the individual residents' needs and their safety and dignity (which was usually the concern of their carers). Doyle *et al.* (1999), in a sensitive account of the approach of a Catholic nursing home in Ontario to sexual issues among their residents, describe the team approach to the cases where a resident who lacks capacity has begun to enter into a relationship with another. They also discuss unwanted behaviour towards other residents and towards members of staff, and the guidelines developed to help staff to respond to these appropriately. Philo *et al.* (1996) describe a useful 'decision tree' for guiding the management of inappropriate sexual behaviour in institutional care, based on efforts to understand any underlying unmet needs that are being expressed through the sexual behaviour.

Problems should not have the last word. One should end rather with a recognition of the beauty and importance of sexuality in old age. The quotation comes from an interview Weg (1983) with a 74-year-old woman:

> Sex isn't as powerful a need as when you're young, but the whole feeling is there; it's as nice as it ever was. He puts his arms around you, kisses you, and it comes to you—satisfaction and orgasm—just like it always did...don't let anybody tell you different.

Acknowledgement

The help of colleagues who participated in our survey; and of Helen Sarah Tyndel for her excellent research assistance, is acknowledged with gratitude.

Useful addresses

Association of Sexual and Marital Therapists, PO Box 62, Sheffield S10 3TS.

Dementia Services Development Centre, University of Stirling, Stirling FK9 4LA. Telephone 01786 467 740. Fax 01786 466 846.

SPOD (Sexual Problems of the Disabled), 286, Camden Road, London N7 0BJ. Telephone 20 7607 8851.

References

Archibald, C. (1998). Sexuality, dementia and residential care: managers report and response. *Health and Social Care in the Community* 6, 95–101.

Atkinson, K. (1997). Incorporating sexual health into catheter care. *Professional Nurse*, **13**, 146–8.

Autton, N. (1989). *Touch: an exploration*. Darton, Longman and Todd, London.

Baier, D. and Philipp, M. (1994). Effects of antidepressants on sexual function. *Fortschritte der Neurologie. Psychiatrie*, **62**, 14–21.

Bancroft, J. (1984). Ethical aspects of sexuality and sex therapy. In *Psychiatric ethics* (ed. S. Bloch and P. Chodoff), pp. 160–84. Oxford University Press, Oxford.

Bancroft, J. (1989). *Human sexuality and its problems* (2nd edn), pp. 282–98. Churchill Livingstone, Edinburgh.

Bauer, M. (1999). Their only privacy is between their sheets. *Journal of Gerontological Nursing* **25**, 27–41.

Berezin, M. A. (1969). Sex and old age. A review of the literature. *Journal of Geriatric Psychiatry*, **2**, 131–49.

Bortz, W. M. and Wallace, D. H. (1999). Physical fitness, aging, and sexuality. *Western Journal of Medicine*. **170**, 167–9.

Brecher, E. and the Editors of Consumers Union. (1984). *Love, sex and aging*. Little, Brown. Boston, MA.

Bretschneider, J. G. and McKoy, N. L. (1988). Sexual interest and behaviour in healthy 80- to 102-year-olds. *Archives of Sexual Behaviour*, **17**, 109–29.

Brown, E., Brown, G. M., Kofman, O., *et al.* (1978). Sexual function and effect in parkinsonian men treated with L-dopa. *American Journal of Psychiatry*, **135**, 1552–5.

Burnside, I. M. (1975). Sexuality and the older adult: implications for nursing. In *Sexuality and aging* (ed. I. M. Burnside), pp. 26–34. University of Southern California Press, Los Angeles.

Buzzelli, S., Di Francesco, L., Giaquinto, S., and Nolfe, G. (1997). Psychological and medical aspects of sexuality following stroke. *Sexuality and Disability*, **15**, 261–70.

Cameron, P. (1970). The generation gap: beliefs about sexuality and self-reported sexuality, *Developmental Psychology*, **3**, 272.

Catalona, W. J. and Basler, J. W. (1993). Return of erections and urinary continence following nerve sparing radical retropubic prostatectomy. *Journal of Urology*, **150**, 905–7.

Catania, J. A. and White, C. B. (1982). Sexuality in an aged sample: cognitive determinants of masturbation. *Archives of Sexual Behaviour*, **11**, 237–45.

Christenson, C. V. and Gagnon, J. H. (1965). Sexual behaviour in a group of older women. *Journal of Gerontology*, **20**, 351–6.

Christenson, C. V. and Johnson, A. B. (1973). Sexual patterns in a group of older never-married women. *Journal of Geriatric Psychiatry*, **7**, 80–9.

Comfort, A. (1980*a*). *Practice of geriatric psychiatry*, pp. 84–6. Elsevier. New York.

Comfort, A. (1980*b*). Sexuality in later life. In *Handbook of mental health and aging* (ed. J. E. Birren and R. B. Sloane), pp. 885–92. Prentice-Hall, Eaglewood Cliffs, NJ.

Corby, N. and Solnick, R. L. (1980). Psychosocial and physiological influences in sexuality in the older adult. In *Handbook of mental health and aging* (ed. J. E. Birren and R. B. Sloane), pp. 893–921. Prentice-Hall, Eaglewood Cliffs, NJ.

Corby, N. and Zarit, J. M. (1983). Old and alone: the unmarried in later life. In *Sexuality in the later years: roles and behavior* (ed. R. B. Weg), pp. 131–45. Academic Press, New York.

Davey Smith, G., Frankel, S., and Yarnell, J. (1997). Sex and death: are they related? Findings from the Caerphilly Cohort Study. *British Medical Journal*, **315**, 1641–4.

Dello Buono, M., Urciuoli, O., and De Leo, D. (1998*a*). Quality of life and longevity: a study of centenarians. *Age and ageing*, **27**, 207–16.

Dello Buono, M., Zaghi, P. C., Padoani, W., Scocco, P., Urciuoli, O., Pauro, P., *et al.* (1998*b*). Sexual feelings and sexual life in an Italian sample of 335 elderly 65 to 106-year-olds. *Archives of Gerontology and Geriatrics*, (Suppl. 6), 155–62.

Dorfman, R., Walters, K., Burke, P., Hardin, L., Karanik, T., Raphael, J. and Silverstein, E. (1995), Old, sad and alone: the myth of the aging homosexual. *Journal of Gerontological Social Work*, **24**(1/2), 29–44.

Doyle, D., Bisson, D., Janes, N., Lynch, H., and Martin, C. (1999). Human sexuality in long-term care. *The Canadian Nurse*, **95**, 26–9.

Drench, M. E. and Losee, R. H. (1996). Sexuality and sexual capacities of elderly people. *Rehabilitation Nursing*, **21**, 118–23.

Dressel, P. L. and Avant, W. R. (1983). Range of alternatives. In *Sexuality in the later years: roles and behavior* (ed. R. B. Weg), pp. 185–207. Academic Press, New York.

Ehrenfeld, M., Tabak, N., Bronner, G., and Bergman, R. (1997). Ethical dilemmas concerning sexuality of elderly patients suffering from dementia. *International Journal of Nursing Practice,* **3**, 255–9.

Ehrenfeld, M., Bronner, G., Tabak, N., Alpert, R., and Bergman, R. (1999). Sexuality among institutionalized elderly patients with dementia. *Nursing Ethics*, **6**, 144–9.

Feldman, H. A., Goldstein, I., Hatzichristou, D. G., Krane, R. J., and McKinlay, J. B. (1994). Impotence and its medical and psychosocial correlates: results of the Massachusetts male aging study. *Journal of Urology*, **151**, 54–61.

Felstein, I. (1970). *Sex in later life*. Penguin, Harmondsworth.

Fielo, S. B. and Warren, S. A. (1997). Sexual expression in a very old man: a nursing approach to care. *Geriatric Nursing*, **18**, 61–4.

Friedeman, J. S. (1978). Factors influencing sexual expression in aging persons: a review of the literature. *Journal of Psychiatric Nursing and Mental Health Services*, **16**, 34–47

Genevay, B. (1975). Age is killing us softly,... when we deny the part of us which is sexual. In *Sexuality and aging* (ed. I. M. Burnside), pp. 67–75. University of Southern California Press, Los Angeles.

George, L. K. and Weiler, S. J. (1981). Sexuality in middle and late life. *Archives of general psychiatry*, **38**, 919–23.

Ghusn, H. (1995). Sexuality in institutionalised patients. *Physical Medicine and Rehabilitation*, **9**, 475–86.

Gibson, M. C., Bol, N., Woodbury, M. G., Beaton, C., and Janke, C. (1999). Comparison of caregivers', residents', and community-dwelling spouses' opinions about expressing sexuality in an institutionalised setting. *Journal of Gerontological Nursing*, **25**, 30–9.

Gladstone, J. W. (1995). The marital perceptions of elderly persons living or having a spouse living in a long-term care institution in Canada. *The Gerontologist*, **35**, 52–60.

Golde, P. and Kogan, N. (1959). A sentence completion test for assessing attitudes toward old people. *Journal of Gerontology*, **14**, 355–63.

Gormley, G. J., Stoner, E., Bruskewitz, R. C., Imperato-McGinley, J., Walsh, P. G., McConnell, J. D., *et al.* for the Finasteride Study Group. (1992). The effect of finasteride in men with benign prostatic hyperplasia. *New England Journal of Medicine*, **327**, 1185–91.

Greengross, W. and Greengross, S. (1989). *Living loving and ageing: sexual and personal relationships in later life* Age Concern England, Mitcham, Surrey,

Gregoire, A. and Pryor, J. P. (ed.) (1993). *Impotence: an integrated approach to clinical practice*. Churchill Livingstone, Edinburgh.

Griffiths, E. (1988). No sex please, we're over 60. *Nursing Times*, **84**, 34–5.

Gustavii, B. (1983). A view from Sweden. In *Sexuality in the later years: roles and behaviour* (ed. R. B. Weg), pp. 271–5. Academic Press, New York.

Haddad, P. M. and Benbow, S. M., (1993). Sexual problems associated with dementia: part 1. Problems and their consequences, and part 2. Aetiology, assessment and treatment. *International Journal of Geriatric Psychiatry*, **8**, 547–51 and 631–7.

Hammond, D. B. (1987). *My parents never had sex: myths and facts of sexual aging* Prometheus Books, Buffalo, NY.

Harris, L. and Wier, M. (1998). Inappropriate sexual behaviour in dementia: a review of the treatment literature. *Sexuality and Disability*, **16**, 205–17.

Hawton, K. (1985). *Sex therapy: a practical guide.* Oxford Medical Publications, Oxford University Press, Oxford.

Hawton, K. (1988). Erectile dysfunction and premature ejaculation. *British Journal of Hospital Medicine*, **40**, 428–36.

Helgason, A. R., Adolfsson, J., Dickman, P., Arver, S., Fredrikson, M., Göthberg, M., *et al.* (1996*a*). Sexual desire, erection, orgasm and ejaculatory functions and their importance to elderly Swedish men: a population-based study, *Age and Ageing*, **25**, 285–91.

Helgason, A. R., Adolfsson, J., Dickman, P., Fredrikson, M., Arver, S., and Steineck, G. (1996*b*). Waning sexual function—the most important disease-specific distress for patients with prostate cancer. *British Journal of Cancer*, **73**, 1417–21.

Heslinga, K. (1974). *Not made of stone. The sexual problems of handicapped people.* Stafleu's Scientific, Leyden and Charles Thomas, IL.

Hillman, J. L. and Stricker, G. (1996). Predictions of college students' knowledge of and attitudes toward elderly sexuality: the relevance of grandparental contact. *Educational Gerontology*, **22**, 539–55.

Hirst, J. F. and Watson, J. P. (1996). Referrals aged 60+ to an innercity psychosexual dysfunction clinic. *Sexual and Marital Therapy*, **11**, 131–46.

Hite, S. (1976). *The Hite report: a nationwide study of female sexuality*. Dell, New York.

Johnson, G. K. (1996). Older adults and sexuality: a multidimensional perspective. *Journal of Gerontological Nursing*, **22**, 6–15. *Also* correspondence following the article: *Journal of Gerontological Nursing*, **23**, 52–5.

Kaplan, H. S. (1981). *The new sex therapy: active treatment of sexual dysfunctions*. Pelican Books, Penguin Books, Harmondsworth, Middlesex.

Kaplan, H. S. (1989). The concept of presbyrectia. *International Journal of Impotence Research*, **1**, 59–65.

Kaplan, L. (1996). Sexual and institutional issues when one spouse resides in the community and the other lives in a nursing home. *Sexuality and Disability*, **14**, 281–93.

Kassel, V. (1983). Long-term care institutions. In *Sexuality in the later years: roles and behaviour* (ed. R. B. Weg), pp. 167–84. Academic Press, New York.

Kellett, J. M. (1989). Sex and the elderly. *British Medical Journal*, **299**, 934.

Kinsey, A. C., Pomeroy, W. B., and Martin, C. E. (1948). *Sexual behaviour in the human male*. WB Saunders, Philadelphia.

Kinsey, A. C., Pomeroy, W. B., Martin, C. E., and Gebhard, P. H. (1953). *Sexual behaviour in the human female*. W. B Saunders, Philadelphia.

Kirby, R. S. (1994). Impotence: diagnosis and management of male erectile dysfunction. *British Medical Journal*, **308**, 957–61.

Korpelainen, J. T., Nieminen, P., and Myllyla, V. V. (1999). Sexual functioning among stroke patients and their spouses. *Stroke*, **30**, 715–19.

Kral, V. A. (1984). Sexual problems in old age. In *Handbook of studies on psychiatry and old age* (ed. D. W. Kay and G. D. Burrows), pp. 329–36. Elsevier,

Krane, R. J., Goldstein, I., and Saenz de Tejada, I. (1989). Impotence. *New England Journal of Medicine*, **321**, 1648–59.

Kuhn, D. R., Greiner, D., and Arseneau, L. (1998). Addressing hypersexuality in Alzheimer's disease. *Journal of Gerontological Nursing*, **24**, 44–50.

Langland, R. M. and Panicucci, C. L. (1982). Effects of touch on communication with elderly confused clients. *Journal of Gerontological Nursing*, **8**, 152–5.

LaTorre, R. A. and Kear, K. (1977). Attitudes towards sex in the aged. *Archives of Sexual Behaviour*, **6**, 203–13.

Lawton, F. G. and Hacker, N. F. (1989). Sex and the elderly. *British Medical Journal*, **299**, 1279. [Letter]

Lichtenberg, P. A. (1997). Clinical perspectives on sexual issues in nursing homes. *Topics in Geriatric Rehabilitation*, **12**, 1–10.

Lichtenberg, P. A. and Strzepek, D. M. (1990). Assessments of institutionalized dementia patients' competencies to participate in intimate relationships. *The Gerontologist*, **30**, 117–20.

Litz, B. T., Zeiss, A. M., and Davies, H. D. (1990). Sexual concerns of male spouses of female Alzheimer's disease patients. *The Gerontologist*, **30**, 113–16.

Loeb, M. B. and Wasow, M. (1975). Sexuality in nursing homes. In *Sexuality and aging* (ed. I. M. Burnside), pp. 35–41. University of Southern California Press, Los Angeles.

Loehr, J., Verma, S., and Seguin, R. (1997). Issues of sexuality in older women. *Journal of Women's Health*, **6**, 451–7.

Lothstein, L. M., Fogg-Waberski, J., and Reynolds, P. (1997). Risk management and treatment of sexual disinhibition in geriatric patients. *Connecticut Medicine*, **61**, 609–18.

Ludeman, K. (1981). The sexuality of the older person: review of the literature. *The Gerontologist*, **21**, 203–8

Mace, N. L. and Rabins, P. V. (1981). *The 36-hour day. A family guide to caring for persons with Alzheimer's disease, related dementing illnesses, and memory loss in later life*, pp. 100–2, 168–70, 217–18. Johns Hopkins University Press, Baltimore, MD.

Malatesta, V. J., Chambless, D. L., Pollack, M., and Cantor, A. (1988). Widowhood, sexuality and aging: a life span analysis. *Journal of Sex And Marital Therapy*, **14**, 49–62.

Martin, C. E. (1981). Factors affecting sexual function in 60–79-year-old married males. *Archives of Sexual Behavior*, **10**, 399–420.

Masters, W. H. and Johnson, V. E. (1966). *Human sexual response*. Little, Brown, Boston.

Masters, W. H. and Johnson, V. E. (1970). *Human sexual inadequacy*. Little, Brown, Boston.

Mathers, N., Bramley, M., Draper, K., Snead, S., and Tobert, A. (1994). Assessment of training in sexual medicine. *British Medical Journal*, **308**, 969–72.

Matthias, R. E., Lubben, J. E., Atchison, K. A., and Schweitzer, S. O. (1997). Sexual activity and satisfaction among very old adults: results from a community-dwelling Medicare population survey. *The Gerontologist*, **37**, 6–14.

Mattiasson, A. C. and Hemberg, M. (1998). Intimacy—meeting needs and respecting privacy in the care of elderly people: what is a good moral attitude on the part of the nurse/carer? *Nursing Ethics*, **5**, 527–34.

Mayers, K. S. and McBride, D. (1998). Sexuality training for caretakers of geriatric residents in longterm care facilities. *Sexuality and Disability*, **16**, 227–36.

Minichiello, V., Plummer, D., and Seal, A. (1996). The 'asexual' older person? Australian Evidence. *Venereology*, **9**, 180–8.

Mir, S. and Taylor, D. (1998). Sexual adverse effects with new antidepressants. *Psychiatric Bulletin*, **22**, 438–41.

Monteiro, W. O., Noshirvani, H. F., Marks, I. M., and Lelliott, P. J. (1987). Anorgasmia from clomipramine in obsessive-compulsive disorder: a controlled trial. *British Journal of Psychiatry*, **151**, 107–12.

Nadal, M. and Allgulander, S. (1993). Normalization of sexual behaviour in a female with dementia after treatment with cyproterone. *International Journal of Geriatric Psychiatry*, **8**, 265–7.

Neuhaus, R. H. and Neuhaus, R. H. (1982). Sexuality and aging. In *Successful aging*, pp. 71–82. Wiley, New York.

Newman, G. and Nichols, C. R. (1960). Sexual activities and attitudes in older persons. *Journal of the American Medical Association*, **173**, 33–5.

Padoani, W., Dello Buono, M., Marietta, P., Scocco, P., Zaghi, P. C., and De Leo, D. (2000). Influence of cognitive status on the sexual life of 352 elderly Italians aged 65–105 years. *Gerontology*, **46**, 258–65.

Parkinson, M. and Bateman, N. (1994). Disorders of sexual function caused by drugs. *Prescribers' Journal*, **34**, 183–90.

Persson, G. (1980). Sexuality in a 70-year old urban population. *Journal of Psychosomatic Research*, **24**, 335–42.

Pfeiffer, E. (1977). Sexual behaviour in old age. In *Behaviour and adaptation in late life* (ed. E. W. Busse and E. Pfeiffer), pp. 130–41. Little, Brown, Boston.

Pfeiffer, E. and Davis, G. C. (1972). Determinants of sexual behavior in middle and old age. *Journal of the American Geriatrics Society*, **20**, 151–8.

Philo, S. W., Richie, M. F., and Kaas, M. J. (1996). Inappropriate sexual behaviour. *Journal of Gerontological Nursing*, **22**, 17–22.

Pinfold, S. M. (1994). The joys of ageing. *Care of the Elderly*, **April**, 140–4.

Purcell, P. and Ghurye, R. (1995). Trazodone and spontaneous orgasms in an elderly postmenopausal woman: a case report. *Journal of Clinical Psychopharmacology*, **15**, 293–5.

Qureshi, B. (1989). *Transcultural medicine*. Kluwer, Lancaster.

Ragno, J. G. (1996). Successful redirection of the sexually disruptive resident. *Activities, Adaptation and Aging*, **21**, 37–41.

Richardson, J. P. and Lazur, A. (1995). Sexuality in the nursing home patient. *American Family Physician*, **51**, 121–4.

Robinson, P. K. (1983). The sociological perspective. In *Sexuality in the later years: roles and behaviour* (ed. R. B. Weg), pp. 81–103. Academic Press, New York.

Roe, B. and May, C. (1999). Incontinence and sexuality: findings from a qualitative perspective. *Journal of Advanced Nursing*, **30**, 573–9.

Ron, P. and Lowenstein, A. (1999). Loneliness and unmet needs of intimacy and sexuality—their effect on the phenomenon of spousal abuse in second marriages of the widowed elderly. *Journal of Divorce and Remarriage*, **31**(3/4), 69–89.

Routasalo, P. and Isola, A. (1996). The right to touch and be touched. *Nursing Ethics*, **3**, 165–76.

Runciman, A. (l975). Problems older clients present in counseling about sexuality. In *Sexuality and aging* (ed. I. M. Burnside), pp. 54–66. University of Southern California Press, Los Angeles.

Sander, F. (1976). Aspects of sexual counseling with the aged. *Social casework*, **57**, 504–10.

Scher, M., Krieger, J. N., and Juergens, S. (1983). Trazodone and priapism. *American Journal of Psychiatry*, **140**, 1362–3.

Schiavi, R. C. (1990). Sexuality and aging in men. *Annual Review of Sex Research*, **1**, 227–49.

Schiavi, R. C. (1999). *Aging and male sexuality*. Cambridge University Press, Cambridge.

Schover, L. R. and Jensen, S. B. (1988). *Sexuality and chronic illness: a comprehensive approach*. Guilford Press, New York.

Silverstone, B. and Wynter, L. (1975). The effects of introducing a heterosexual living space. *The Gerontologist*, **15**, 83–7.

Slusher, M. P., Mayer, C. J., and Dunkle, R. E. (1996). Gays and Lesbians Older and Wiser (GLOW): a support group for older gay people. *The Gerontologist*, **36**, 118–23.

Snyder, E. E. and Spreitzer, E. (1976). Attitudes of the aged toward nontraditional sexual behavior. *Archives of Sexual Behavior*, **5**, 249–54.

Stephens, J. (1974). Romance in the SRO. Relationships of elderly men and women in a slum hotel. *The Gerontologist*, **14**. 279–82.

'Stuart'. (1994). Between the anger and the tears. *Alzheimer's Disease Society Newsletter*, **November**, p. 3.

Szasz, G. (1983). Sexual incidents in an extended care unit for aged men. *Journal of the American Geriatrics Society*, **31**, 407–11.

Teri, L. and Reifler, B. V. (1986). Sexual issues of patients with Alzheimer's disease. *Medical Aspects of Human Sexuality*, **2**, 86–91.

Thompson, P., Itzin, C., and Abendstern, M. (1990). *I don't feel old. The experience of later life*. Oxford University Press, Oxford.

Thorpe, A. C., Cleary, R., Coles, J., Reynolds, J., Vernon, S., and Neal, D. E. (1994). Written consent about sexual function in men undergoing transurethral prostatectomy. *British Journal of Urology*, **74**, 479–84.

Todarello, O. and Boscia, F. M. (1985). Sexuality in aging: a study of a group of 300 elderly men and women. *Journal of Endocrinological Investigation*, **8**(Suppl. 2), 123–30.

Traupmann, J. (1984). Does sexuality fade over time? A look at the question and the answer. In *Geriatric Psychiatry*, Vol. 17 (ed. D. Blau and R. Kahana), pp. 149–59. International Universities Press,

Turnstull, P. and Henry, M. E. (1996). Approaches to resident sexuality. *Journal of Gerontological Nursing*, **22**, 37–42.

Verwoerdt, A., Pfeiffer, E., and Wang, H-S. (1969*a*). Sexual behavior in senescence. Changes in sexual activity and interest of aging men and women. *Journal of Geriatric Psychiatry*, **24**, 163–80.

Verwoerdt, A., Pfeiffer, E., and Wang, H-S. (1969*b*). Sexual behavior in senescence. II. patterns of sexual activity and interest. *Geriatrics*, **24**, 137–54

Walker, B. L. and Ephross, P. H. (1999). Knowledge and attitudes toward sexuality of a group of elderly. *Journal of Gerontological Social Work*, **31**(1/2), 85–107.

Walker, B. L., Osgood, N. J., Richardson, J. P., and Ephross, P. H. (1998). Staff and elderly knowledge and attitudes towards elderly sexuality. *Educational Gerontology*, **24**, 471–89.

Wasow, M. and Loeb, M. B. (1979). Sexuality in nursing homes. *Journal of the American Geriatrics Society*, **27**, 73–9.

Webb, C. (1987). Nurses' knowledge and attitudes about sexuality: report of a study, *Nurse Education Today*, **7**, 209–14.

Weg, R. B. (1983). The physiological perspective. In *Sexuality in the later years; roles and behaviour* (ed. R. B. Weg), pp. 39–80. Academic Press, New York.

Weizman, R. and Hart, J. (1987). Sexual behaviour in healthy married elderly men. *Archives of Sexual Behavior*, **16**, 39–44.

West, N. D. (1975). Sex in geriatrics—myth or miracle? *Journal of the American Geriatrics Society*, **23**, 551–2.

White, C. B. (1982). Sexual interest, attitudes, knowledge, and sexual history in relation to sexual behavior in the institutionalized aged. *Archives of Sexual Behavior*, **11**, 11–21.

White, C. B. and Catania, J. A. (1982). Psychoeducational intervention for sexuality with the aged, family members of the aged, and people who work with the aged. *International Journal of Aging and Human Development*, **15**, 121–38.

Wojciechowski, C. (1998). Issues in caring for older lesbians. *Journal of Gerontological Nursing*, **24**, 28–33.

Wright, L. K. (1998). Affection and sexuality in the presence of Alzheimer's disease: a longitudinal study. *Sexuality and Disability*, **16**, 167–79.

Zeiss, A. M., Davies, H. D., Wood, M., and Tinklenberg, J. R. (1990). The incidence and correlates of erectile problems in patients with Alzheimer's disease. *Archives of Sexual Behavior*, **19**, 325–31.

36 Ethics and the psychiatry of old age

Julian C. Hughes

Introduction

Plumbing and philosophy are both activities that arise because elaborate cultures like ours have, beneath their surface, a fairly complex system which is usually unnoticed, but which sometimes goes wrong. In both cases, this can have serious consequences. (Midgley 1996)

In the practice of old age psychiatry the need for attention to the ethical plumbing should be obvious. There are the big issues, such as genetic testing, the rationing of expensive drugs, advance directives, and physician-assisted suicide. But it is important to see, too, that ethical issues are involved in ordinary day-to-day practice.

The first patient to be seen in a community outpatient clinic is mildly manic. Should she be managed at home or in the hospital? This is a clinical question, but embedded within it are matters of value. The wishes of the patient and her family are relevant to the decision and these wishes will reflect their values. The second person in the clinic has been fully investigated and the diagnosis is probable Alzheimer's disease. Should the patient be told? Or the family? Or both? The third person has an alcohol problem and is deteriorating physically. He denies the problem and refuses all help, but seems depressed. At what point should he be admitted under compulsion for further assessment? Or does he have a right to drink himself to death? In short, clinical problems are fraught with ethical issues. So much so, indeed, that Fulford (1987) raised the question concerning whether medicine should be regarded as a branch of ethics. Taking the ethical perspective more clearly brings into view the notion of the patient-as-a-person rather than, say, the notion of the patient-as-a-machine.

Clinical problems require practical know-how. This clinical know-how is multifarious, but it requires a sound ethical basis. This chapter deals with the practical business of ethical plumbing in old age psychiatry. As Midgley goes on to suggest, given how the plumbing system has evolved, it is difficult now to get a clear overview, let alone to start afresh. My aim is to see why things are as they are in particular areas. Further insights into ethical reasoning can be gained from Gillon (1986). Alternative treatment of ethical issues in old age psychiatry can be found in Oppenheimer (1999); or, with respect to dementia, in Jones (1997). Ethical guidelines relating to Alzheimer's disease have appeared in the US (Post and Whitehouse 1995) and in Canada (Fisk *et al.* 1998). For a sustained and significant discussion of many of the ethical issues raised in connection with Alzheimer's disease the reader should consult Post (2000).

Approaches to philosophical medical ethics

As Table 36.1 shows, there are many different approaches to theorizing in ethics. In the course of this chapter I shall highlight where I feel some of these approaches have relevance. But since my approach is firmly rooted in the business of old age psychiatry, I prefer to put aside particular ethical theories and approach the issues from the perspective of the *person*. Medical ethics is a matter both of conceptual analysis (philosophical plumbing) and of practice. I shall consider a number of issues relevant to practice, but my

Table 36.1 Theories and approaches to ethical issues

Absolutism	The view that certain actions are *always* wrong or *always* obligatory, whatever their consequences.
Casuistry	Arguing case by case, in the light of basic moral instincts, but with regard to the important differences between cases.
Communicative ethics	The correct answer to an ethical dilemma requires a commitment to free and open communication on the part of individuals and institutions.
Consequentialism	The rightness or wrongness of an action depends on its consequences.
Deontological ethics	Certain actions must be done as a duty (*deon*) regardless (to *some* extent) of their consequences.
Feminist ethics	Taking into account experiences and values more typical of women than of men, feminism stresses the importance of interdependent relationships in which caring for others is implicit in a person's moral life.
The Four Principles	Beneficence: doing good; Non-maleficence: avoiding harm; Autonomy: allowing self-rule; Justice: distributing goods fairly.
Intuitionism	What is right can be directly seen (or intuited) by the mind or conscience.
Narrative ethics	The rightness (or wrongness) of an action will become apparent in the context of a detailed story.
Natural Law ethics	A moral theory favoured by the Catholic religious tradition: reason can determine basic human goods, constitutive of human flourishing, which ought to guide action.
Prescriptivism	Moral terms are used primarily to guide action, to tell people what to do.
Religious ethics	What is right or wrong depends upon religious traditions (e.g. *Halakah* in the Jewish tradition; *Sharia'* in the Islamic tradition) or precepts.
Situation ethics	In ethical dilemmas in medicine, issues must be decided on the basis of the actual situation: different decisions reflect different situations.
Utilitarianism	A form of consequentialism which takes the maximization of pleasure (and the minimization of pain) as the measure of a good action.
Virtue ethics	What counts in ethics is the habitual disposition of the person: an action is good if it reflects a virtuous character.

Note: For further details and theories the reader should consult the sources of this table: Gillon and Lloyd (1994) and Honderich (1995). Communicative ethics is discussed in Moody (1992).

approach to these issues, via the perspective of the person, requires that I consider, albeit briefly, what being a person entails.

The person as a situated embodied agent

The notion of 'the person' is by no means unproblematic. Generally speaking, when the notion of personhood raises its head in ethical discourse, it is usually intended as a way of marking someone as a being worthy of a certain sort of dignity and respect. Of course, there are all sorts of problems in defining what a person is and in establishing whether there is any crucial distinction between human persons and other animals. These philosophical arguments are beyond my remit.

There has been, however, much attention paid to the problem of personal identity and, in particular, to the views of Parfit (1984) who has stressed, following Locke (1690), that personal identity is maintained by there being appropriate psychological continuity and connectedness.

This position has been used in medical ethics to discuss issues relevant to old age psychiatry. For instance, if psychological continuity and connectedness are lost in dementia, because failing memory means that a psychological state now cannot be connected to the psychological states of yesterday, then (it is argued) there is not enough psychological continuity to claim that the person today is the same as the person yesterday. The theories of Locke and Parfit concerning the person, however, are not the only ones in town. An alternative thought is that the notion of a person is uncircumscribable, but will be characterized by those possibilities which lie open to human beings (Wiggins 1987). For, whether or not other beings warrant similar characterization, our current conception of the person is tied tightly to our understanding of the *human* person, with all that this entails (Wilkes 1988).

One way of shedding light upon what it is to be a human person is to consider persons as *situated-embodied-agents*. Whilst this concept does not deny the importance of a person's psychological life, it also emphasizes the significance of the human *body* for the human person and the extent to which the person is *situated*, or embedded, in a context of human social relations, culture, and history. In this way, the situated-embodied-agent view of the person broadens the view of Locke and Parfit. Adopting this perspective of the person will have been worthwhile if it enriches our understanding of ethical issues relating to old age psychiatry.

What is clear in the present climate of dementia care is that the person is centre-stage. Undoubtedly, the emphasis on the personhood of people with dementia owes an enormous debt to the work of the late Tom Kitwood. Kitwood (1997) defines personhood as: 'a standing or status that is bestowed upon one human being, by others, in the context of relationship and social being'. He goes on to say, 'It implies recognition, respect and trust'. His talk of an 'ethic of the context' implies the importance of a person's situatedness (Kitwood 1998).

In the pages that follow, therefore, I shall approach ethical issues from the perspective of the person and I shall characterize the person broadly as a situated-embodied-agent.

The person as an agent

Autonomy versus paternalism

One of the key ethical tensions in medical practice is that between the need to recognize the person as an autonomous agent and the inclination to act paternalistically for the benefit of patients. Autonomy is one of the four principles of medical ethics (Beauchamp and Childress 1994) and many regard it as fundamental to liberal ethical theories which emphasize the right of individuals to self-determination. Beneficence, that is the requirement that medical practitioners should do good, need not be in conflict with the notion of autonomy, but easily can be.

Case 1

Mr A. has some cognitive impairment and lives alone in the community. He is using excessive alcohol on occasions. He regards it as his right to drink when he wants to. It gives him pleasure and he lacks the insight to see the potential for harm.

If we respect Mr A.'s autonomy, he will remain in the community drinking excessively from time to time and placing himself at more or less risk. The paternalistic action, in an attempt to be beneficent, would be to take him into hospital under compulsion. Reference to the principles of autonomy and beneficence here helps to clarify the ethical dilemma, but does not solve it. Other approaches might help to elucidate why this person acts (as an agent) in the way that he does. Perhaps we can gain an understanding of Mr A. as an agent that will help to inform (ethically) the decisions we might be forced to make concerning his care.

For instance, narrative ethics encourages us to view people in the context of their stories. Making sense of a particular aspect of someone's life requires an understanding of that life as a whole. Maybe the tendency to abuse alcohol episodically is linked to intrusive memories of earlier trauma. The narrative view, understanding Mr A.'s actions as part of an overall history, again does not in itself solve the ethical dilemma, but it increases our understanding and thereby makes it more likely that we will act for the good. Our well-meant, paternalistic inclination to make him safe might, perhaps, be supplanted now by the aim of providing treatment to ameliorate the effects of the earlier trauma. And part of that might involve supporting him at home. The risks will still remain, but the hope is that Mr A.'s distress and tendency to abuse alcohol will be lessened.

Capacity and consent: the case of antidementia drugs

If the tension between autonomy and paternalism is central to many issues in medical ethics, lack of capacity is typically the source of ethical dilemmas in caring for people with dementia. Under British law, in the case of adults, only the person him or herself can consent to treatment. Consent, which must be uncoerced, involves capacity, which in turn involves understanding. The reason for this is precisely that we recognize persons as agents. To inflict unwanted treatment upon someone undermines his or her agency and personhood. The difficulties involved in doing what is right are clearly shown when we think of the new antidementia drugs. For one thing, although competence can be operationalized (Chapter 40), at its core the notion of consent involves an evaluative and contextualized judgement (Hughes 2000*a*).

Case 2

Mrs B. has a mild Alzheimer's type of dementia. Although she minimizes her problems, she accepts the suggestion that she is forgetful. She responds positively to the news that there are drugs available which can help with memory.

How much more does Mrs B. need to understand before we can say that she has given valid consent? There are a number of pertinent points. First, capacity to consent is always specific to a particular action or treatment. But then, is Mrs B. simply required to consent to take a tablet that might help her memory or should the consent be more thoroughly informed? If Mrs B. had previously studied neurochemistry, she might (arguably) need to understand a good deal about the medication; but perhaps not if her education were minimal.

A second pertinent point is whether the level of capacity required should be inversely proportional to the importance of the treatment. So, if the treatment is exceedingly important, the level of capacity need not be so high. Whereas, if the treatment is merely optional, the level of capacity should be much higher. In the case of antidementia drugs, however, the importance or otherwise of the treatment is again relative to the individual. It would depend on what was and is important to the person.

The third point, recognized in British law for instance, is that an adult is presumed to have capacity. In effect, this point restates the importance of recognizing that persons are agents. Our inclination, therefore, should be to presume that a person (by virtue of being a person) has the capacity to make decisions and act. Thus, recognizing someone's personhood must involve attempting to make it easy for them to act. This will require effective communication, which in turn suggests the need for patience, time, a willingness to explain in simple terms (even if the person was once a neurochemist!), and to re-explain, along with empathic understanding. It might also mean setting a less stringent criterion for full understanding or memory when a person with dementia needs to make a decision, so as to enable them to make their own choice, precisely in order to recognize the person as a person. In this way the person's autonomy is respected. Autonomy, then, is rooted in what is constitutive of persons, namely that they are agents and should accordingly, as Kant decreed, be treated as ends in themselves (Kant 1785).

The use of the currently available antidementia drugs, however, raises other issues with relevance to alternative principles, which are also derivable from Kant's argument that rational agents should adopt the Golden Rule and 'do as they would be done by' (Scruton 1982). First, in accordance with the principle of beneficence, do these drugs actually do good? The improvement in cognitive performance is, in itself, a good. The evidence that cholinesterase inhibitors affect non-cognitive features of dementia too, such as hallucinations and agitation, is also of benefit (Burns *et al.* 1999). Second, however, do they (in keeping with the principle of non-maleficence) cause no harm? The side-effects of the current drugs are largely transient and mild, but what of the possibility that they might prolong a person's distress by prolonging the awareness of decline (Post and Whitehouse 1998*a*)? Third, the principle of justice should make us consider the fair use of resources. Some have suggested that spending large sums of money on expensive drugs for some people with dementia might divert funds and (just as importantly) our attention from more basic forms of care (Whitehouse 1996).

Ethical issues, therefore, concerning the use of antidementia drugs can be discussed from the point of view of the person as an agent. As rational agents, according to Kant, we ought to derive certain principles to guide our actions. But underlying the principles is a concern to respect persons, which we do by acting ourselves in accordance with the dictates of rational agency.

Telling the truth

That we should be truthful with patients, their families, and carers, as well as with colleagues, seems unproblematically certain. However, total honesty in any relationship can be hurtful; at least, it might do no good. It is the same in clinical practice.

Case 3

Mr C. develops late paraphrenia. He has no previous history of mental illness, but becomes convinced that the people next door are spying on him and plotting against him as part of a huge conspiracy. He is so perturbed he calls the police.

To tell Mr C. that his delusions *are* delusional is unlikely to be useful. To acknowledge the reality of his experiences *for him* is both honest and useful as a way of building trust, since it acknowledges his own world in which he regards himself as a competent agent. To deny the reality that Mr C. experiences is to undermine his standing as an agent in the world. To accept that he has such experiences and to offer assistance (by providing him with a safe haven or drugs to ease the experience), maintains his personhood without dishonesty.

One of the ways, again linked to consent, in which the advent of antidementia drugs has challenged clinical practice, is that there is a greater need to discuss the diagnosis with our patients. Once again there is a need to tell the truth. Pinner (2000) provides a useful summary of research in this area and concludes that the questions are *when* and *how* we should tell the diagnosis truthfully, not *whether* we should. In a survey of the relations of people with Alzheimer's disease, 83% did not wish their relative to be told, while 71% said they would like to be told themselves if they developed the condition (Maguire *et al.* 1996). This can be interpreted in terms of agency. As agents we wish to know things that concern us; but, somewhat worryingly, we deny such agency to people with dementia. The reasons given for not wishing people with dementia to know their diagnosis tend to be consequentialist: people with dementia will not understand or will be frightened; the information will cause stress and worry because of the poor prognosis. The arguments in favour of telling the diagnosis tend to emphasize the autonomy of the agent: the person can make plans, sort out their financial affairs, accept help and advice far more easily. It can also be argued that the person has a *right* to know, to which there is the correlative *duty* on the part of the doctor to tell the person the diagnosis.

Despite a growing interest in the issue of telling the diagnosis, as in many other areas of dementia research, the perspective of the patient has (so far) been largely ignored (Cotrell and Schulz 1993). In Smith *et al.* (1998), when carers were asked how helpful the diagnosis had been *to the patient*, a mean rating score of 7 was given (where 1 indicated that being told the diagnosis was bad or unhelpful and 10 indicated it was good or helpful). The range (from the 56 respondents) was from 1 to

10. One carer reported that the patient had been pleased to know that there was a physical explanation for his condition. Many felt the diagnosis was made too late to have been much use. There were also cases in which the diagnosis seemed to be unhelpful and might have contributed to hopelessness and depression. Similarly, Husband (2000) reports a study in which knowledge of the diagnosis of dementia led to behaviour likely to result in low self-esteem, self-stigmatization, and impaired quality of life. Telling the diagnosis, therefore, necessitates support.

In Marzanski (2000), people with dementia were asked what they would like to know. The majority (21/30) wished to know what was wrong with them or wished to have more information if they already knew; 10 wished to know the diagnosis, but in 4 cases the participants could not specify exactly what it was they wanted to know. In this study 30% did not wish to know what was wrong with them or did not wish to receive any further information about their illness. Some of these people lacked insight and did not accept that there were any problems. But at least one simply said, 'I have enough troubles'. Pinner (2000) states it is not a question of *whether* to tell the truth; but Marzanski (2000) adds that whether the person with dementia *wishes to know* is the question that needs asking. The individual person as an agent may or may not wish to know. The clinicoethical imperative for the doctor is to be honest, but to discern the person's wishes and needs.

Advance directives

One way in which a person's wishes can be known is if they are recorded in advance. The advance directive (or 'Living Will') enables the person to exercise control—to act as an agent—over decisions that might be made concerning his or her medical treatment in the future (Hope 1992, 1996). In effect, advance directives are usually advance *refusals*, since a person cannot demand a particular treatment, but can stipulate that certain treatments should *not* be used under certain circumstances if he or she should become incompetent. Nevertheless, advance directives may authorize that life-prolonging measures be maintained (Mason *et al.* 1999). The point of the advance directive, then, is to encourage autonomy even for the person who is no longer able to exercise the agency that autonomy promotes.

Whilst this seems laudable, numerous concerns have been raised regarding the use of advance directives. Can they be specific enough for the circumstances of clinical practice? Who will define the terms that might be used, such as 'severe' or 'advanced'? How can we be certain that a person has not altered his or her view? Would it be possible to determine later that the person was non-coerced and informed at the time of making the directive, and can we be certain that the person correctly anticipated what it would be like to have had, say, a stroke? Will people be capable of appreciating the complexities of possible future decisions and might not medical advances render earlier directives irrelevant or, at least, uninformed?

Undoubtedly such questions reflect areas of real difficulty. But similar difficulties must arise in connection with testamentary capacity and Wills, so we might anticipate that good clinical practice, combined with a sensible, workable, legal framework will lead to solutions. Instead, it seems more worthwhile to consider here the underlying ethical rationale for advance directives. If advance directives add to the potential for agency amongst patients, they will enhance our conception of the patient-as-a-person.

As a preliminary, it appears practicable to use advance directives, even in early dementia. First, there are ways of assessing capacity to complete an advance directive (Fazel *et al.* 1999). Second, it does *not* appear that asking people with early dementia questions about hypothetical future severe illnesses is upsetting and it may indeed be helpful (Finucane *et al.* 1993). Certainly, a person's understanding of the issues involved in, for example, enteral tube feeding can be improved (Krynski *et al.* 1994). Moreover, when 76 medical inpatients in London hospitals were asked about advance directives, 82% had not heard of them, but 74% expressed an interest in writing such a 'Living Will'—most commonly in order that their views would be known, but also to lessen the burden on their families (Schiff *et al.* 2000). In this study, at least 90% said they would refuse surgery, artificial feeding, ventilation, and cardiopulmonary resuscitation at the end of a terminal illness, whilst over 80% would refuse subcutaneous or intravenous fluids or antibiotics at such a time. Amongst 78% of the participants, the single condition most feared was advanced dementia: these patients would choose 'comfort only' care in advanced dementia, compared, for example, to 53% who would choose 'comfort only' if they had double incontinence. Whilst this indicates that people may have particular preconceptions of certain states, which may or may not be justified, it also shows a desire to express a view, to exercise agency and control over their lives. Furthermore, there is evidence that advance directives make decision-making easier for doctors, more uniform, and more in keeping with the previously expressed wishes of patients (Waddell *et al.* 1997).

Still, whilst the enhancement of patient autonomy seems a straightforward advantage of advance directives, they raise profound questions concerning personhood. Based on the view of Parfit (1984), that personal identity is a matter of psychological continuity and connectedness, Glover (1988) suggests:

> the psychological unity of a life is not all-or-none. Memories or intentions can fade or disappear. I can be linked psychologically to other stages of my life to a greater or lesser degree. If I am hit in old age by senile dementia, perhaps nearly all my present self will have faded out.

Thus it might be that a man before and after dementia is a different person (Hope 1995). Or it could even be suggested that in severe dementia, since there is no psychological continuity at all, there is no person and the advance directive made by the earlier person is irrelevant (Buchanan 1988).

Over against this view, Dworkin (1986) commends an 'integrity-based theory of autonomy', which:

> focuses not on individual decisions one by one, but the place of each decision in a general program or picture of life the agent is creating and constructing, a conception of character and achievement that must be allowed its own distinctive integrity.

Hence we should respect the 'precedent autonomy' of advance directives, even when this contradicts our inclination to treat the chest infection of the otherwise seemingly contented person with dementia:

> If I decide, when I am competent, that it would be best for me not to remain alive in a seriously and permanently demented state, then a fiduciary could contradict me only by exercising an unacceptable form of moral paternalism. (Dworkin 1993)

By considering advance directives as an expression of preferences and by regarding preferences as dispositions to act, Savulescu and Dickenson (1998*a*) offer an alternative view. They commend a person's present dispositional preferences as commanding more respect than past preferences. When pressed, they agree that past preferences might still carry some weight in dementia, but they feel that there needs to be a corrective towards present preferences (Savulescu and Dickenson 1998*b*). Otherwise people will feel that an advance directive, made in the past, might disadvantage them in the present. Underlying these thoughts is a commitment to the notion of the person as an agent and the tension is between past and present agency.

In different ways, Dresser (1998) and Brock (1998) have drawn attention to the moral, cultural and legal norms, and values that surround such decisions. Elsewhere it has been argued that, whilst liberal theory, with its emphasis on autonomy, supports the use of advance directives, it is enhanced by feminist critiques which stress the importance of personal relationships in advance-care planning (Ikonomidis and Singer 1999). We have already noted that, when asked, people cite the reduction of the burden on the family as a reason for completing an advance directive. So the conflict between past and present agency will necessarily be worked out in a situated context: the context of family, community, and culture. In the United Kingdom this was recognized in a government paper on decision-making for incapacitated people:

> the advance statement is not...to be seen in isolation, but against a background of doctor–patient dialogue and the involvement of other carers who may be able

to give an insight as to what the patient would want in the particular circumstances of the case. (Lord Chancellor's Department 1997)

Advanced directives will not dissolve all problems, but they do focus our attention on agency and consequently on the status of the patient as a person. But persons are not just agents, they are situated agents, and for the most part they are primarily situated in the context of a family.

The person in the family

Confidentiality

Case 4
Mr D. is an 82-year-old widower who lives on his own with only a modicum of outside support. Over the course of 4 months, and following the death of his sister and a bout of influenza, his standards of self-care decline. The GP prescribes an antidepressant, but there is no improvement and Mr D. is referred to a specialist. He is seen within a week. The old age psychiatrist then receives a phone call from Mr D.'s son stating that he should have been present when his father was seen. The son also asks for the psychiatrist's opinion regarding his father.

Most families, even when they live at a distance, show concern for their relations. Physicians have a duty to respect confidentiality (Joseph and Onek 1999); but there is a natural inclination to involve other family members when looking after the elderly. At least in the case of the competent elderly, there is no reason for confidential medical information to be shared without their specific consent. The old age psychiatrist who saw Mr D. might already have realized that Mr D. would have preferred his son to be present during their meeting and might already have undertaken to discuss matters with the son. But, if this is not the case, the psychiatrist must consult with Mr D. before breaking confidentiality.

When someone lacks capacity, however, the case is not so clear. In dementia it is commonplace to discuss patients with relatives, neighbours, and carers. In the usual situation, a patient is seen at home with the family around. Whilst it cannot be presumed that the patient wishes family or carers to be involved, it is often difficult either to gain sufficient history or to make a workable treatment plan without the full involvement of the family. In these cases, the person is not just situated in the family as a matter of fact, she may be utterly dependent upon them. But dependency might arise from other mental illnesses too, such as from depression or anxiety. The mistake, however, is to presume that dependency is a necessary concomitant of old age.

Case 5
Mrs E. is an elderly widow with mild dementia who is admitted by the physicians with a chest infection. As she improves physically it becomes obvious that she is depressed. She ascribes her depression, in part, to her feelings of helplessness in the face of her overbearing daughter-in-law, herself a doctor, who is now dominating Mrs E.'s life. The daughter-in-law seems genuinely concerned for Mrs E., who (she feels), can no longer cope at home.

In this case it is important that confidences are maintained. Mrs E. needs to regain some sense of agency, but the relationship with the son and daughter-in-law must not be put in jeopardy. In other words, confidentiality must be respected (and Mrs E. allowed space in which to act), but the importance of the family (in which Mrs E. is situated) is a fact that has to be understood. A true appreciation of Mrs E.'s situated agency, an understanding of her as a person, will affect the planning of her discharge, which might include social support to lessen her dependence on her daughter-in-law, but might also involve family therapy.

Ethical issues for carers

Given that the person is usually situated in the context of a family (although there are occasionally non-familial main carers), it is inevitable that ethical issues arise within this context. Ethical issues from the perspective of the main carers (as opposed to issues arising for professional carers) have scarcely been studied. In a relatively large study (Pratt *et al.* 1987), of the 216 respondents to an open question about other issues that might lead to a better understanding of caregiving, 54% raised ethical concerns. Some 42% of the responses related to the responsibility of giving care within the family. Issues centred on problems to do with sharing the care and the moral responsibility to give care based on notions of reciprocity ('she looked after us, now we must look after her') and vulnerability. Conflicts with other obligations were obvious (in 29%), as were issues around finance and standards of care. Three carers described how important it was for them to have been able to discuss the wishes of the person with dementia, either before they became ill, or at the time of diagnosis.

In a qualitative case report, Butterworth (1995) presented the account of a daughter who had been caring for her mother for 15 years. The issues raised were: the need for more information, including the need for a diagnosis; the importance of the relationship with the GP; the cost of caring and the need for more funding; a need for support, for good respite care, and better training of professional carers.

It becomes clear that carers face a wide range of ethical issues, many of which have an everyday character. It is also clear that carers' issues bring into focus a whole variety of approaches to ethical problems. In one case caring is a deontological matter, to do with doing one's duty; in another case caring is more like a habitual disposition, a virtue. Elsewhere, according to a feminist interpretation, caring is a matter of nurturing, as the carer was once nurtured. Or, the onus of caring is justified in religious terms: the burden of caring must be offered up. It is a testing of the spirit through which the carer might grow (Klein 1989). What is common to these different approaches, however, is the situatedness of the person with dementia in a nexus of relationships which tends to be familial. The ethical decisions, which have to be made, are inevitably made within this relational context.

Treatment decisions: surrogates, end-of-life, and artificial feeding

What is certain is that the decisions are not easy. Deciding when to treat and how vigorously is a matter which often involves families. In itself this is an acknowledgement of the fact recognized in practice, if not strictly speaking in law, that part of my personhood quintessentially involves others. These significant others are naturally turned to when I can no longer make decisions for myself. Of course, families are not the only significant others involved in the care of elderly people. Care staff in residential homes, for instance, can form close bonds with the people they look after. In addition, sometimes old people facing death have none other than the hospital team to make decisions for them. Doctors and nurses then, necessarily, stand proxy for the family and provide the context within which someone's personhood must be preserved (Murphy 1984). In part, the need for surrogate decision-makers arises because of the new possibilities offered by technology in medicine. An example of this, which is now encroaching on practice in old age psychiatry, is feeding by percutaneous endoscopic gastrostomy (PEG).

Where the person is incompetent to make decisions about treatment, the alternatives are: to act in their best interests, proxy decision-making, substituted judgements, or advance directives (Hope and Oppenheimer 1997). Things are not, however, always straightforward. Arras (1988) demonstrates the problem of using either the substituted judgement or the best interests' criteria to decide on whether it is appropriate to place a gastrostomy tube in the severely demented 85-year-old Mrs Smith, who has continually pulled out her nasogastric (NGT) tube, but who has life-threatening dysphagia. Arras shows that arriving at a substituted judgement from either her previously expressed values or from her current aversive behaviour is problematic. Determining her best interests seems to depend on the particular definition of the good being used. Instead, Arras commends a procedural solution: in grey areas we should rely on the decision of 'a trustworthy surrogate' unless there is 'a clear violation of best interests'. But while respecting the views of Arras, this just seems to raise the same practical ethical questions concerning best interests and trustworthiness.

The thought that the family, the normal source of 'a trustworthy surrogate', should decide is tempting (Rabins and Mace 1986). It fits in with the notion that the person is a situated agent, since the family provides the normal context for this situatedness. There are concerns, however, about an immediate appeal to the family, which are little to do with the worry that families are avaricious. Most families are, on the contrary, benign. If their decisions sometimes reflect a degree of self-interest (which might include the need to assuage feelings of understandable, but perhaps unwarranted, guilt), the decisions of medical staff are prone, at least, to other influences (e.g. the pressure on beds, the difficulties of certain interventions, or the cost). But beyond these worries is the concern that, in UK law, the family cannot make a proxy decision. This is likely to change, given the proposal for a Continuing Power of Attorney, which allows the person to nominate someone to make decisions, not just about property and finance (as in an Enduring Power of Attorney), but also regarding personal and health care matters (Lord Chancellor's Department 1999). Yet there is still a further concern which stems from conceptual ambiguities concerning the person. We shall arrive at the ambiguities by way of empirical research.

When 36 relatives of patients with Alzheimer's and 34 physicians from various specialties were asked about surrogate decision-making (Silberfeld *et al.* 1996), the physicians made more frequent use of records of patients' wishes and relied more on objective tests. In addition, they tended to talk with the patient and with colleagues more frequently. Families coped by relying on their subjective overall impression. These families were less inclined than the physicians to refer to advance directives. The physicians, it seemed, were attempting, in accordance with contemporary trends, to make a best estimate of what the patient would have wanted in the circumstances. Families found decision-making more burdensome than the physicians. The study concludes that physicians need to engage with families in making these difficult decisions, to guide and support them.

In another study (Moe and Schroll 1997), competent and incompetent residents from nursing homes, relations, and staff members were compared in their responses to questions about a hypothetical case. The greatest degree of disagreement existed between relatives of incompetent residents and staff members concerning whether hospital referral and attempts at curative treatment were required, rather than just palliation. Relations were significantly more likely to seek curative treatments. Meanwhile it appeared that most elderly people welcomed the chance to discuss treatments such as resuscitation, intubation, and tube-feeding, even though it also appears that many physicians fail to discuss these difficult issues with patients (Golin *et al.* 2000).

These studies suggest the potential for disagreement between families, professional carers, and physicians. But they also point us in the direction of a process (van der Steen *et al.* 2000). It is a process which starts by trying to ascertain the wishes of the patient, even in dementia. It then moves us towards significant others (family or friends), professional carers, and physicians. The process should involve measures to settle disputes between surrogates and must recognize uncertainty and the need for public education (AGS Ethics Committee 1996). Centre-stage is the person, situated in the context of family, carers, culture, and law.

This is all well and good, but is there yet agreement on what is actually *right* in these circumstances? This is a matter of values, but it is worth noting that empirical research can continue to shed light on these issues. For instance, Hurley *et al.* (1996) demonstrated that, in comparison with aggressive medical treatment of infections in Alzheimer's disease, palliative care was less invasive, did not accelerate progression of the disease and conserved resources. But talk of what is right or wrong brings us back to the conceptual difficulties we mentioned earlier. For in question are the wishes of the demented Mrs Smith (Arras 1988). The procedural solution ('a trustworthy surrogate') seemed too simple. The process suggested above, necessitated by the seeming likelihood of disagreement, is more thorough since it involves broader enquiry (which should include Mrs Smith) and more open negotiation.

But the problem remains the impenetrable wishes of Mrs Smith.

One of the distinctions informing the discussion concerning Mrs Smith is that between her biographical and biological life. Arras (1988) suggests that in severe dementia, whilst Mrs Smith exists biologically, her biography is over. The real meaning of her life is at an end. Interestingly, many of those who take a narrative view, whom we might guess would have sympathy with talk of biography, seem to reject this:

> Being able to experience episodes of our lives as whole and meaningful stories is an important aspect of our narrative competence. The demented person gradually loses this competence. The care giver then has an important task helping her or him experience wholeness and meaning. (Norberg 1994)

In other words, the story of a person's life can still be told by others. But the biological–biographical split is fuelled both by the notion that a person's self is a matter of self-awareness and by the psychological continuity and connectedness view of Parfit (1984). Hence,

> an individual's ability to remember past experiences is crucial to his or her personal identity. The fact that a patient with severe dementia has a body and brain is not enough to establish that the patient is the same person as they were before...What makes people the same persons that they were...is that they perceive a narrative chain linking their many memories, goals, and beliefs...Indeed, without the long term and short term memory to develop new connections they are not persons at all. (Doyal and Wilsher 1994)

So, conceptual ambiguities, which have practical relevance, surround the notion of the person. The distinction between biology and biography suggests either that personhood involves both of these two facets, or that personhood is located either predominantly in biology, or predominantly in biography. It is worth noting in passing that there are, both in practice (Howell 1984) and in philosophy (Williams 1973), arguments that stress the importance of the body for the person. The characterization I am using stresses *embodied* agency. Even if we simply focus on biography, however, questions are raised. Does this persist into advanced dementia? Is biography maintained by others? Should present biography (Dresser 1995) or past biography (Newton 1999) hold sway? These arguments are illuminating and important because they help to focus our attention on different aspects of personhood. But there seems no way to judge between these principled stances. What then becomes important is actually what we do. In a sense there is no further justification (Hughes 1995). The *process* by which we decide becomes all-important.

Our philosophical ponderings have provided grounds for broadening the process. We shall have to have regard to the person's previously stated wishes, as well as to present preferences, which the person must be encouraged to express. In addition, the views of those others, professional and non-professional, who are now engaged with the patient must be heard. Negotiation and communication within this engaged context become critically important in defining the outcome and its validity. This is the communicative ethics of Moody (1992), which is based 'on shared discourse among persons who respect the position of others in the communication process itself'. Moody continues: 'the problem is to define and promote the concrete conditions that promote such communication in all stages of life, including old age'. In fact, the communicative process, which I am advocating, is a description of how a person's best interests should be determined (see Lord Chancellor's Department 1999, and Hughes 2000*a*).

There is, however, something of a hermeneutic circle here, for if the process of good practice, with respect to the person, involves broad consultation, one interpretation is that this is because involvement with others is an essential part of what we understand by being 'a person'. It is not, as Post (1990) suggests, that buried within someone with severe dementia is a continuing biography, which we must presume. Rather we accept that others are involved in a person's biography (Kitwood 1993). In any case, there is increasing empirical and ethical support for the view that the self is *not* in fact deeply hidden, even in severe dementia. Instead, many authors stress the importance of listening to the voice of the person with dementia, even when communication makes this difficult (Sabat and Harré 1994, Callaghan 1995, Lyman 1998). The solution, therefore, to the problem generated by the impenetrable wishes of Mrs Smith is not that those inner wishes are suddenly made overt. It is rather that, within the situated context of Mrs Smith as a person, the distinction between inner wishes and outer desires breaks down (Hughes 2000*b*). Mrs Smith's *inner* wishes are *outer*, partly because of things she once said and partly because of what she now says or does. Her 'inner' wishes are likely to have some resonance with the wishes of those close to her who know her well. They are likely to be determined by *overt* facts concerning her values and her present medical condition. And all of this can be determined, *outwardly*, by thorough, open communication and negotiation between all those involved. What is important is the process of communication. The aim of this communication is to bring into the open those facts—both past and present (Berghmans 1997)—which allow us to make a decision concerning what is right, not on the basis of serendipity, but on the basis of her status as a situated-embodied-agent.

Artificial feeding again, futility, ordinary and extraordinary means

Case 6

Mrs F. is in a nursing home for people with severe dementia. She has been dependent on nursing staff for all activities of daily living for several years. She has not been able to communicate for some while and she has become immobile. She has gradually been losing weight. She requires feeding, but the amounts she eats have been lessening. A swallowing assessment by the speech therapist and advice from the dietitian have led to changes in her feeding, but finally she makes no effort to eat food, even when it is placed in her mouth.

Case 7

Mr G. also has marked dementia, but has lived happily in a residential home for some years. He has been able to attend to some of his personal needs. He is able to communicate, and the only difficulty has been his tendency occasionally to wander and to shout at other residents and visitors if they disturb his routine. He becomes acutely unwell and requires hospital admission. He develops an unexplained dysphagia, which is still being investigated. The immediate problem, however, is that he cannot swallow. He will not tolerate a nasogastric tube.

The possibility of PEG feeding is a technological advance, but it brings with it difficult decisions concerning when and when not to treat. If we presume that Mrs F. and Mr G. have no advance directives and have never clearly stated a preference concerning how they should be treated, the sort of broad, communicative process we have discussed above must take place. As well as Mrs F. and Mr G., it should involve family carers, but the views of the nursing and care staff in the homes will be vital too (Jansson *et al.* 1995; Goodhall 1997). This process brings the possibility of disagreement, perhaps because of the fear of litigation, or because of a tradition of paternalism or strongly held views about the sanctity of life (Rosin and Sonnenblick 1998; Garanis-Papadatos and Katas 1999).

Disagreements about PEG feeding also reflect different intuitions concerning the nature of feeding. The key legal decisions in England and the United States concerned Tony Bland and Nancy Cruzan, respectively, both of whom were in a persistent vegetative state (PVS). The implications of these cases are wide-ranging (see Mason *et al.* 1999 for details), but they establish that artificial feeding should be regarded as a *treatment* which could, therefore, under certain circumstances be withheld in the interests of the patient. This legal view, however, goes against the intuition that feeding is an aspect of basic care and nurture. It offends the intuition that if we stop feeding we are starving the person to death.

As in most debates in medical ethics, it is worth establishing the facts. Finucane *et al.* (1999) conclude their evidence-based review of the literature on tube-feeding people with advanced dementia by stating that they found, 'no direct data to support tube-feeding of demented patients with eating difficulties for any of the commonly cited indications'. Their review found no good evidence that tube-feeding prevented aspiration pneumonia, prolonged survival, reduced the risk of pressure sores or infection, or improved function or comfort. In addition, they found numerous adverse effects for both NGT and PEG feeding, which range from local irritation to potentially fatal complications. On the basis of this type of evidence, Gillick (2000) argues that artificial feeding is inappropriate in advanced dementia. On this view, Mrs F.'s difficulty with eating signals the severity of her dementia. She has entered the final stage of her disease and her treatment should be palliative.

One way to put this would be to say that PEG feeding for Mrs F. would be futile. The notion of futility has become important in medical ethics (Gillon 1997). In qualitative terms, medical futility has been defined thus:

> if a patient lacks the capacity to appreciate the benefit of a treatment, or if the treatment fails to release a patient from total dependence on intensive medical care, that treatment should be regarded as futile. (Schneiderman and Jecker 1995)

There are at least two problems with this definition. First, it would seem to discount all non-palliative treatments for people with moderate to severe dementia. Mr G.'s treatment, according to this definition, is futile in the same way as Mrs F's. Callaghan (1995) warns against equating people with dementia, even in the later stages, with people in a persistent vegetative state. People with dementia, it can be argued, over against those in PVS, continue to exhibit agency. (As *embodied* agents they also experience pain and suffering, but it is the situated nature of their agency that marks them out specifically as human persons.) This allows a rational basis for treating depression in people with advanced dementia. Anorexia might, after all, be a symptom of depression. But, on the definition above, treatment is futile. This cannot be so if it relieves a distressing condition. Second, the notion of futility emphasizes facts—which we have noted to be important—but not values.

The process of deciding these difficult cases must be based on communication and negotiation in the best interests of the patient (Lennard-Jones 1999). Even if the notion of futility has a role, the communication must be sensitive (Weber and Campbell 1996) and must involve appropriate support for all those involved, particularly the family (Mezey *et al.* 1996). Rather than futility, this process emphasizes the situatedness of the person with dementia. The person is situated in a historical and familial context. But the context also involves laws and traditions. These will, inescapably, affect the communication and negotiation. Certain traditions emphasize certain values. Still, there is at least the possibility that open discussion might alter the perception of how these values are applicable in a particular case.

For instance, Roman Catholic moral philosophy has made use of a distinction between 'ordinary' and 'extraordinary' means. This distinction suggests we are *bound* to take ordinary measures to sustain life, but we are *not* bound to take extraordinary measures. The difficulty, however, is to define these terms. Feeding by NGT now seems 'ordinary' in medical practice. Is PEG feeding? Well, 'the distinction between ordinary and extraordinary means draws its sense from a framework of assumptions' (Linacre Centre Papers 1979). So we are impelled to consider context. The fundamental assumption, according to this tradition, is that human life is a 'basic good'. This assumption however, is not used irrespective of circumstances. Hence,

> certainly there is a moral obligation to care for oneself and to allow oneself to be cared for, but this duty must take account of concrete circumstances. It needs to be determined whether the means of treatment available are objectively proportionate to the prospects for improvement. To forego extraordinary or disproportionate means is not the equivalent of suicide or euthanasia; it rather expresses acceptance of the human condition in the face of death. (John Paul II 1995)

The process of communication, therefore, to decide whether to use PEG feeding for Mrs F. and Mr G., is itself situated and relies on embedded assumptions and values as well as upon facts. Even within a tradition which stresses the 'sanctity of life' it should be possible, with care, to negotiate a position which recognizes human life as a good, but also accepts the inevitability of death. Whilst Mrs F., whose death is now imminent, requires palliative care (and hence PEG feeding would be extraordinary), arguably

Mr G.(whose dysphagia is unexplained and forms no part of his expected decline) should be given PEG feeding to keep him alive. Thus, the same treatment (PEG feeding) is ordinary in one circumstance and extraordinary in another. Similarly, it might be argued, artificial nutrition (by whatever means) is nurturing and a means of expressing basic human care in one case, but is medical treatment (as the law suggests) in another case. (There are three similar approaches to ethical problems which might be relevant here, and which I have briefly defined in Table 36.1, namely casuistry, situation ethics, and communicative ethics.) The important point is that different cases must be dealt with differently: PVS is not the same as dementia and dementia is different in different individuals. So it is the situated context of the person within the family and the broader community which determines how the process of decision-making will go. Furthermore, this situated context involves both facts and values.

Genetics

The astonishing advances in our understanding of the genetic basis of diseases (see Chapter 7) has raised many issues and questions. I have tried to summarize these in Table 36.2. As this demonstrates, the ethical issues related to genetics are worthy of much greater attention than can be given here (Post and Whitehouse 1998*b*). Indeed, it is likely that unforeseen ethical issues will arise as the practical usefulness of genetic advances increases. It is also clear from Table 36.2 that the issues relate not only to us as individual agents, but also to us as persons situated in a familial and societal context.

At least in the case of autosomal dominant inheritance, as seen in some forms of early-onset Alzheimer's disease, we have the experience of Huntington's disease on which to draw. Genetic counselling, both before and after testing, is now regarded as central to good practice (Nuffield Council on Bioethics 1993). Although there is a risk that testing positive for a disease such as Huntington's might cause depression, risk factors can be delineated and support given (Codori *et al.* 1997). Burgess (1994) found the most significant changes following testing seemed to be in relation to other family members. 'Survivor guilt' was experienced by those with decreased risk of the disease. Because of the potential impact on the family, there are clearly arguments in favour of involving other family members in decisions concerning testing (Eaton 1999). The consequences of testing are likely to contribute to our sense of whether such tests are right or wrong. A broadly utilitarian approach, therefore, might be adopted towards many of the issues raised in Table 36.2.

Although the ethical issues concerning autosomal dominant conditions are difficult enough, calculating how to maximize utility or happiness (or minimize pain and suffering) is even more problematic where susceptibility genes are concerned. Because the predictive value of tests for genetic alleles such as *APO e4* is low, and because of the continuing importance of non-genetic factors in late-onset Alzheimer's disease, authoritative bodies in both the US (Post *et al.* 1997) and the UK (Nuffield Council on Bioethics 1998) have advised against the introduction of genetic testing in disorders with multiple causes. This reasoning will be relevant to other mental disorders with multifactorial aetiology too. Nevertheless, testing in some families with autosomal dominant early-onset Alzheimer's disease might be warranted after full discussion within the family.

Moving beyond the family, there are of course others who might benefit from genetic information. Although insurance companies, as well as employers generally, can be regarded as potentially malevolent users of genetic information, this need not be the case (Cook 1999). Even so, whilst we might be able to identify prudential and moral reasons for knowing some of our personal genetic information, it has been argued that,

> As long as people whose genes deviate from those of the average individual are likely to face suspicion and discrimination, societies cannot legitimately force people to know about their hereditary composition. (Takala and Gylling 2000)

Table 36.2 Ethical issues raised by the advances in genetics

- Benefits and risks (including the risk of emotional harm and stigma) of genetic testing to individuals
- Effects of testing on other family members
- The rights of other family members
- Need to involve families in discussions concerning testing
- Need for sophisticated genetic counselling
- Need for valid consent and the difficulties involved in conveying information about risk to enable valid consent to be given
- Accessibility of testing
- Need for, and bounds of, confidentiality (in health, in research, amongst employers and insurers)
- General need for ethical guidelines for genetic research and practise
- Need to keep genetic information gleaned from research away from participants, carers, or treating physicians, except in exceptional circumstances and only with appropriate counselling
- Control of uses made of genetic material by researchers beyond the uses for which consent gained
- Possibility that a genetic test might reveal increased risks in conditions other than that under investigation
- Need for genetic research to be scientifically sound and, therefore, the need for competent and sufficiently experienced local research ethics committees
- Legitimacy of claims by others on genetic information
- Need to respect the wishes and rights of those who are now incompetent, or dead, but who might be able to supply samples for genetic analysis
- Ownership of DNA sequences
- Concerns over the cloning of human tissue
- Prospect of genetic information imposing an ethical burden on people to alter their lifestyles, occupations, or reproductive choices
- Protection of public from inappropriate advertising and marketing of genetic tests
- Need for public education

Sources: Burgess (1994); Farmer *et al.* (2000); Lovestone *et al.* (1996); McConnell *et al.* (1999); Nuffield Council on Bioethics (1998).

The move beyond the family should also make us alert to issues broader than those raised by consequentialist ethics. We need to consider the social and historical meaning of conditions such as Alzheimer's disease (McConnell *et al.* 1999). We might wish to consider also the place of suffering in our lives (Cassel 1998). Post (1994*a*) asks:

> is it wrong to assume that suffering is the necessary result of every genetic defect, or that lives with degrees of physical suffering cannot be creative and meaningful?

He points out too that contingency is at the heart of human experience and, similarly, he suggests that people with dementia challenge in a useful way our notions of human perfection and normality. Nevertheless, Post (1999) clearly accepts the ethical imperative to make scientific progress to delay or prevent Alzheimer's dementia. The broader societal perspective on genetics, which inevitably raises the spectre of eugenics, makes clear that scientific progress occurs not solely in the physicochemical realm, but also in the space of values. Medical practice, for the same reason, is a matter of ethics as much as a matter of science (Fulford 1989). But the values in which medical practice are embedded should also impel us to further research:

> despite...the baggage of its history, psychiatry should not be treated differently from any other branch of medicine with respect to genetic research. To do so is a form of discrimination against those who suffer from psychiatric disorders, and could possibly prevent the benefits deriving from genetic research. (Farmer *et al.* 2000)

The person embedded in the community

People belong to families, but they are also embedded in communities. A community tends to operate in accordance with certain norms. In this section the theme will be the tension that can arise between the actions of individual agents and the norms of communities. Sometimes how a person lives is a concern to other members of the community. Sometimes the actions of others will need to be controlled within the community. If, for instance, the person wanders inappropriately, or drives a car erratically, other members of the community will have concerns and might positively object. The old age psychiatrist quickly becomes involved in these situations when it is an elderly person upsetting the community. In which case, however, does it not seem as if old age psychiatry is akin to community policing? And if this is so, then surely Szasz (2000) is correct in his assertion that psychiatry is, in effect, a branch of the law? I shall, first, consider the arguments concerning some specific conflicts that can arise in the community and, then, return to look at the underlying philosophical plumbing.

Community care

Case 8

Mr H. has been on the medical ward for 3 weeks having been admitted with 'acute on chronic' confusion, caused by a chest infection, which has now been treated. His memory problems and disorientation persist. He has a mild dementia. He wishes to return home, where he lives alone. His family say that he will be all right at home, but an occupational therapy (OT) assessment shows him to be lacking in most basic skills. He tends to wander on the ward and he is occasionally incontinent of urine (perhaps because of disorientation). The district nurse reports that before his admission he had been neglecting his self-care and the home had become quite squalid.

The case of Mr H. is not unusual. I suspect that most old age psychiatrists called to advise would favour Mr H. being discharged home with suitable arrangements being made for increased community care. But we only need to change a few details in the story and the decision becomes more difficult. What if the family do not support him going home? What if his dementia were moderate? What if there were a clear history that he used to wander at night when at home? Even in Mr H.'s 'straightforward' case, discharge from hospital can raise ethical issues for the whole clinical team (Cummings and Cockerham 1997). In terms of principles, there is a conflict between autonomy and beneficence. Strang *et al.* (1998) put the point thus: 'Respect for personal freedom and the desire to help and protect vulnerable people frequently appear to demand opposite interventions'. Their response is to suggest that we need valid and reliable ways to assess the capacity to make such decisions. An alternative, which would have some appeal in the current political climate, would be to insist on an appropriate 'risk assessment'.

Both of these suggestions, however, even if they have the value of attempting to bring some sort of objectivity to the decision, might miss the central ethical dilemma. Even if Mr H. fails the assessment of his capacity to make the decision about where he should live, and even if the risk assessment shows him to be at significant risk, he is likely still to want to go home. What is at stake is Mr H.'s freedom. Clinical assessments, even using standardized, well-validated instruments, do not in this sort of circumstance eradicate the extent to which values are embedded in the decisions that have to be made.

Intuitionism (see Table 36.1) is an ethical theory with almost no supporters nowadays (Hudson 1967). For if we say our intuition is that it is right to treat all infections in people with dementia, there are quite likely to be many people with an alternative intuition! Intuitionism does not supply a way around this disagreement. Similarly, the current trend in medical practice is against intuition. It would be no good saying, for instance, that my *intuition* is that you will survive surgery; you will want to know the facts and figures. And yet, is there not something to be said for the suggestion that our unease about *simply* saying that Mr H. must be in care is a matter of *conscience*? Perhaps we have an intuition that we should give him a chance. The substantial point is that intuitions might lead us to moral precepts, to statements about what is right or wrong with which all (right thinking) people will agree.

This might seem a vain hope, but let us for a second presume it is not. What will then be important is *the way in which* rightness and wrongness are worked out in practice. The question will be *how* intuitions and conscience are shaped and allowed to influence our decisions. The shaping of conscience is a matter far beyond my scope, but the moral intuitions of doctors will have something to do with medical education, which emphasizes the importance of medical ethics in the medical curriculum. How intuitions are allowed to influence our practical decisions, however, *is* a matter with which this chapter has been concerned. Once more, the *process* of making a decision is all-important. It is a process that must make room for an appreciation of values, not just facts, and allow for the possibility of conflicting values which will necessitate (literally) *careful* negotiation with an openness to the possibility of different weights being given to competing moral precepts.

Perhaps the thought that, under these circumstances, Mr H. should be discharged to his home reflects a deep-seated intuition in favour of respecting autonomy. This intuition surely underlies the humane sentiments expressed by Winner (1999):

> Empowering frail old people who wish to leave hospital requires clinicians to be liberal and permissive in the best sense of these much-abused words, to find practical ways of loosening constraints and giving vulnerable people the benefit of any doubt...A good clinical service is one that has a small but definite incidence of discharges that go wrong: a paternalistic service that never risks sending a doubtful prospect home should only seem desirable to the uninformed.

Yet it remains the case that these decisions are difficult for clinicians and can cause ethical unease (or pangs of conscience?). In a qualitative study involving physicians looking after elderly people in the community, Kaufman (1995) revealed three sources to the dilemmas experienced by physicians. The first source of stress was the assessment of risk and deciding 'how, when, and to what degree' to intervene 'in the lives of frail old people who want to retain their autonomy and continue to live at home'. Second, deciding how far to try to force modifications of behaviour was a difficulty. The behaviour concerned ranged from compliance with medication, to changes in the consumption of addictive substances, to the reduction of squalor and the acceptance of home care services. Physicians wondered what was 'correct' or 'ethical' in these circumstances. Third, there were concerns about the whole issue of placement into long-term care. In discussing these issues, Kaufman (1995) points out that an important feature of medical decision-making is that 'it is both influenced by and embedded in broader social practices and cultural values'.

The nuances of this social and cultural embedding are brought out in a paper by Collopy (1988), in which he discusses the notion of autonomy in long-term care. Collopy defines autonomy in such a way as to ensure that 'the autonomous person is not a lone, isolated, atomistic agent making decisions without ties to other people, social institutions, and traditions of thought and action'. He shows that autonomy,

> is an internally problematic concept, bristling with distinctions and polarities that can be ethically perplexing even in settings where professionals are committed to client self-determination.

For instance, there is a distinction between a *decisional* element to autonomy (having preferences and being able to make decisions) and an *executional* element (actually being able to implement such decisions). Mr H. has the autonomy to decide he wishes to live at home, but he lacks the autonomy to put this into effect. Talk of respecting his autonomy is in danger of conflating such polarities. He might, as a further example, express his autonomy by 'authentic' choices, which are consonant with his character, or by 'inauthentic' choices, which are seriously out of character. Bringing out the *authentic* element to autonomy stresses the need to consider a person's lifelong values and the individual's situatedness in a history, as well as in a social and cultural context. The conclusion of Collopy's analysis is that the multiplicity of elements involved in the notion of autonomy shows 'the range and fertile dynamics of self-determination'. Hence,

> Fixation on a particular aspect or interpretation of autonomy can lead...to a narrow constraining or a tyrannical enlargement of this value.

So decisions relating to community care are fraught with ethical difficulties. There is little doubt that there will always be factual matters to consider (such as the severity of Mr H.'s dementia), but interventions in the lives of elderly people, as in the lives of younger people, are either wanted or unwanted. And, if unwanted, they need to be justified, as a matter of conscience, but also in line with the values that permeate the person's embeddedness in the community.

Behaviour control

Various types of behaviour might appear at different times during the course of a person's dementia (Hope *et al.* 1999). Some of these behaviours are upsetting and some involve definite risks. Difficult decisions have to be made about how far to intervene. Once again, facts and values are involved. Dodds (1996) argues that there is little literature to suggest that mechanical restraints are effective, whilst at the same time there is evidence that they might do harm. These empirical data are linked to the philosophical argument that autonomy should be respected and, therefore, the onus should be on people who consider using restraints to justify their actions. This does not really do justice to the complexities of the notion of autonomy. Nor does it show much consideration for the other values involved in these difficult situations. For instance, Dawkins (1998), from the perspective of a nurse, considers the various principles that might be relevant to using restraint in the elderly, but then emphasizes caring as a virtue:

> The ethics of care maintains that many human relationships involve persons who are vulnerable, dependent, ill, and frail, and that the desirable moral response is attached attentiveness to needs, not detached respect for rights.

Dawkins (1998) also points towards a process that begins by specifying the norms that are relevant and proceeds to balance the competing norms as a way of deciding in a particular case what is best. The process should also involve the acquisition of facts. The contextual nature of the decision is clear; but so too is the possibility that notions such as 'autonomy' can be used glibly.

Behaviour can be controlled by drugs, as well as by mechanical restraint. Factual evidence, for instance that neuroleptics may be associated with more rapid cognitive decline in dementia (McShane *et al.* 1997), has led to an awareness of potential harm. In America, the Omnibus Budget Reconciliation Act of 1987 enforced restrictions on the prescription of neuroleptics in Medicare- and Medicaid-certified nursing homes. Research seems to be confirming that there are non-pharmacological ways of managing difficult behaviours (Gormley and Howard 1999). Interestingly, much of this research proceeds by regarding the person with dementia as a situated agent: in other words, interventions take into account the whole context and history of the person. This sort of approach seems instantly more ethical.

On the other hand, there are occasions when neuroleptic medication might be the best alternative.

Case 9

Mr J. has a moderately severe dementia and lives with his brother, who knows that he would always have wanted to stay at home. But Mr J. is tending to get up at night and wander. This is wearing out his brother, who is not getting enough sleep. Furthermore, when his brother remonstrates with him at night, Mr J. becomes physically aggressive. Mr J.'s brother has come to rely on thioridazine (a neuroleptic), which both sedates and calms Mr J. He recognizes that he might be causing some harm to Mr J., but alternative medications have not worked so well.

Caregiver stress and dangerousness are recognized circumstances in which it might be appropriate to use neuroleptics (Post 1994*b*; Gormley and Howard 1999). But it should also be recognized that there are contexts in which main carers in the community might also use *physical* restraint—by locking doors to prevent wandering or by positioning furniture so that a spouse cannot attempt to get out of bed unaided—and the judgement concerning the ethics of these manoeuvres would again have to be open to particular facts and embedded values.

Driving and wandering

A basic agentive competence is the ability to go places. Losing the ability to drive can be both a major psychological blow and a huge practical difficulty (Freedman and Freedman 1996). It may well be the job of the old age psychiatrist to advise on this issue. In one sense, the decision should be made on empirical grounds and there is, in fact, a good deal of effort being put into attempts to delineate when it is that a person with cognitive impairment is no longer safe to drive (Dubinsky *et al.* 2000) (Chapter 42). The issue is, however, one that also involves wider societal norms. For the issue is precisely to decide how much risk we are prepared to tolerate on our roads. Since we tolerate a certain amount of risk from young male drivers and (at least in the UK) from people driving with low levels of alcohol in their blood, there are good grounds for arguing that a mild degree of cognitive impairment should not preclude driving (Dubinsky *et al.* 2000). Even so, stopping anyone from driving is a restriction of their liberty. Concern for the individual agent's rights, therefore, should perhaps encourage us to seek laws that differentiate between the capacities of different cognitively impaired people.

Case 10a

Mr K. has very mild cognitive impairment. He continues to drive and his wife depends on him to get her to the shops. Mrs K. always accompanies her husband in the car. They had a worrying incident recently when they attempted to drive at night in the rain on an unfamiliar route. Mr K. became very anxious and disoriented. His wife had to coax him along slowly, aware that he was causing irritation to other drivers.

Should Mr K. have his licence revoked? Or would a better option be for him to have regular driving tests and, for now, to be restricted to driving in a limited area, in daylight, only in good weather, only when accompanied by his wife, outside the 'rush hour', and avoiding motorways (Shua-Haim and Gross 1996)?

Mr K. may eventually have to stop driving, but at least his (and Mrs K.'s) independence has been maintained for longer. How he is actually prevented from driving will depend on the circumstances, but attempts should be made to be honest with him. If he does not agree to stop, confidentiality will have to be broken eventually, but best practice suggests that this should be discussed with him. This is, again, a matter of acknowledging his agency. Nevertheless, such a discussion needs to be sensitive to the extent to which his sense of agency might depend on his perception of himself as a competent driver. It might be better, therefore, for the discussion to be hypothetical and tentative, to reflect the ethos of the caring doctor rather than that of the community police officer.

Case 10b

Mr K. now has a moderate dementia. Since he was stopped from driving he has taken to walking every afternoon. One afternoon he goes out to watch his grandson play football, but he goes to the wrong pitch and he then gets lost coming home. He sometimes leaves the house without telling his wife and on one occasion this was after dark.

Mr K.'s driving put him and others in the community at risk. His wandering places only him at risk (at present), but it is a considerable concern to his family and friends. About 40% of people with dementia get lost outside the home and this leads to greater caution on the part of their main carers, who often lock doors to prevent wandering (McShane *et al.* 1998*a*). The worry about wandering may hasten the person's admission to long-term care. In one way or another, therefore, confinement is the response of the community to wandering. The duty to care, whether on the part of the professional or the family member, outweighs the duty to respect the person's liberty. Philosophical scrutiny in this area, therefore, shows the person embedded in a field of facts and values, where the estimation of duties and moral intuitions will depend upon particularities rather than broad principles.

In the future it might be that Mr K.'s tendency to wander and get lost might be lessened by technological advances. Electronic tags can sound an alarm when a boundary is crossed and electronic tracking devices can help to locate people with an appropriate electronic transmitter.

McShane *et al.* (1994) argue that, whilst a tag that sets off an alarm (perhaps when a person tries to leave a residential home) is a restriction of liberty, this might be 'a price worth paying for the safety of the person and others'. Meanwhile, in the right circumstances, a tracking device might 'enhance the liberty and safety of people' such as Mr K.

Interestingly, however, this latter view was changed to some extent by a later survey of carers concerning the use of tracking devices (McShane *et al.* 1998*b*). For, in fact, very few carers said they would give patients more freedom if they had such a device. Those who actually had experience of using a tracking device had not given the person they cared for more freedom. 'A more relevant ethical justification was that the device had the capacity to reduce the length of time that someone was lost, thereby lessening the chances that they would sustain or cause an accident' (McShane *et al.* 1998*b*). Additionally, using these devices focuses attention on the needs of the person with dementia and thereby contributes to the person's overall assessment.

Against the advocacy of electronic tracking, some might argue that these devices infringe a person's privacy. McShane *et al.* (1994) state this will only be the case if the person is trying to hide. But there *might* be such cases, albeit in rather particular circumstances, and too readily to accept the use of electronic tagging and tracking devices could be to ride roughshod over a person's basic human rights. In any case, medical involvement in the use of tagging and tracking devices brings us back to Szasz (2000) and the suggestion that psychiatry is really a branch of the law.

Old age psychiatry and community policing

Sometimes people make a distinction between the 'social-work-side' and the 'biological-physician-side' of being an old age psychiatrist. One way to counter Szasz's (1960) seminal paper, which suggests that mental illness is a myth (because illnesses must have a physical basis and mental illnesses do not), is to focus on the biological aspects of old age psychiatry. Ignoring the social nature of much normal clinical practice, however, is difficult. And it is in this social context, in the community in which the person is embedded, that ethical issues arise. Mr A. with alcoholic dependence and dementia, Mr C. with late paraphrenia, and the wandering Mr K. might all need to be detained under mental health legislation against their wishes, or might otherwise need to be coerced into accepting certain sorts of care or treatment. It is because of the social embeddedness of persons that they are treated one way rather than another, and that old age psychiatrists inevitably act, on occasions, on behalf of the community with respect to the persons under their care.

The truth is that clinical practice, just as it involves facts and values, is also biological and social at one and the same time. It is psychological, ethical, spiritual, and legal too. Indeed, any facet of being a person, a situated-embodied-agent, will be relevant to clinical practice. Others have argued against Szasz (see Megone 2000), but in one respect, at least, I agree with him.

Precisely because the person is embedded in a community, because the person's mental illnesses (whether 'organic' or 'functional') will have an effect in the community, and because the old age psychiatrist will sometimes have to take action to limit these effects, old age psychiatry is indeed, 'in effect, a branch of the law' (Szasz 2000). It is also 'coercive' at times; and it may 'incarcerate' people because of 'misbehaviour'. Ignoring the use of emotive language, I argue that these social and ethical functions of old age psychiatry are not just necessary manifestations of social control which are delegated to psychiatrists, but rather they are a manifestation of good clinical practice. The embedded nature of the elderly person with a mental illness means that it is not possible to understand (have any empathy with) his or her situation without regard to the context of the family and the wider community. Moreover, the old age psychiatrist is a part of the broader community and inevitably acts on its behalf.

The key question is whether, in discharging our biological, psychological, social, and legal functions, old age psychiatrists are acting ethically. But there is no doubt that old age psychiatrists perform all of these functions. We *must* do in order to look after people with mental illnesses. Whether we act ethically or not is itself worked out in a historical, cultural, and social context. Here, as we have seen, there may be disagreements in terms of values and intuitions, but the process of deciding what is right involves being engaged in open communication and negotiation. Our engagement as doctors in this context is an important factor. We are not simply disengaged agents of the state. Although we are embedded in the community, our engagement, *as* clinicians, is with the person who is ill. It is through this engagement that we shall work out, not only what is wrong with them and what to do about it, but what it is right to do in this particular case. Both clinically and ethically, the important things are trust and respect. Szasz has highlighted the extent to which clinical practice must involve civil practices; he has perhaps ignored the extent to which this applies to the whole of medicine. But medicine, including old age psychiatry, is enriched by an appreciation of the extent to which it is embedded, in a social and ethical context of civil practices.

> Civil practices are each of them ways of dispensing a single commodity: respect. This word sums up all that is bestowed on someone as he is made the beneficiary of non-violence, non-fraudulence, truth-telling, promise-keeping and benevolence. On the other side, to be the beneficiary of such treatment, to count as an appropriate object of respect, is in a social, if not a metaphysical, sense of the term, to be a person. (Pettit 1980)

The person and the polis

The person is situated in a wider context still; not just the context of family and community, but of the whole society, the body politic (*the polis*). In this section I shall consider three large fields relevant to old age psychiatry: ethical issues relevant to research, rationing and ageism, and the morality of decisions at the end of life.

Research

The possibility of unethical research is real. For instance, the 1930s saw the start of the inhumanity of Nazi research (Müller-Hill 1991) and the end of the twentieth century witnessed an increasing awareness of research fraud (Farthing 1998). The political response to the Nazi atrocities in the field of human research led to the Nuremberg Code in 1947 and the Helsinki Declaration in 1964 (revised 1983) (BMJ 1996). In recent years, again as a reflection of the political nature of research, a number of ethical guidelines for research with people with dementia have been suggested (High *et al.* 1994; Post *et al.* 1995; AGS Ethics Committee 1998; Brodaty *et al.* 1999). A central ethical difficulty in research in dementia, reflected in these guidelines, is the inability to gain valid consent.

A person might have the capacity to consent to participate in research early in the course of a dementia, but probably not later. As always, capacity is specific to a decision, so it will depend on the complexity of the particular research. In this regard research raises the same problems as does the treatment of people who lack capacity to give consent. For instance, strictly speaking, consent must persist throughout the research, even as cognitive function declines. But when consent has been assessed in dementia research, it has been found distinctly lacking (Agarwal *et al.* 1996). Even harder to deal with, however, is the issue of *non-therapeutic* research. For here we cannot appeal to 'best interests', since (by its nature) the research will be of no benefit to the person concerned. We are still left with the options of proxy decision-making, substituted judgements, or advance directives.

Relying on proxies or surrogates to give consent in dementia research can be difficult for the practical reason that they may be hard to find, either because they do not exist, or because they are themselves unable to engage in the process of giving informed consent (Baskin *et al.* 1998). Furthermore, even if proxies are often motivated by altruism (Lynöe *et al.* 1998), there is evidence they do not know the views of the people they stand proxy for anyway; instead, they tend to be more protective than the people themselves would be (Muncie *et al.* 1997). This might have the effect of preventing or impeding important research.

The conflicting motivation behind attempts to lay down guidelines for research in dementia has been both that vulnerable potential participants need protection *and* that the severity of the illness necessitates and warrants a massive research effort. Thus we see the encroachment of the *polis* in to the research arena: even if the research does not benefit you, there are good utilitarian reasons why you should be used even in the absence of your consent, since the research will benefit society as a whole. This may or may not sound alarming, depending on the good that is expected to come from the research and the potential for harm to those who participate. But this apparently reasonable utilitarian stance comes up against the Kantian imperative that people should never be used solely as means, but only as ends in themselves (Kant 1785). In dementia research, this will allow some leeway for therapeutic research, but it still poses difficulties for non-therapeutic research, where the person is (on the face of it) being used solely as a means to an end.

Whereas the idea of substituted judgements concerning consent to participate in research seems very problematic (it is often difficult enough to establish clearly the incompetent person's previously expressed wishes on resuscitation, let alone on whether they would wish to participate in a neuroimaging study using radioisotopes!), at first blush, advance directives might provide a solution, even in non-therapeutic research. If all the usual caveats are in place (the advance directive must have been written when the person was competent, etc., and be relevant to the research now being considered), an advance directive allows the person to exercise agency in a situation that might occur in the future. The researcher then has evidence of (at least) precedent valid consent.

As in our earlier discussion, however, the ethical standing of advance directives needs to be carefully considered. This will be particularly the case in non-therapeutic research involving more than minimal risks and/or burdens to the participant (Berghmans 1998). An advance directive can add to the surety of a decision, but is unlikely to be sufficient on its own, since (if for no other reason) it will require interpretation by others at a particular time and place. None the less, as with substituted judgements, there are practical problems with advance directives for research. For one thing, they are hardly ever in existence. So there remains a gap between the ethical 'gold standard' of an advance directive properly interpreted and applied, with full consultation amongst family and other carers, and the practical needs of researchers to recruit participants for their studies.

Within this gap, Sachs (1994) has endorsed the use of 'a rather informal, even somewhat amorphous, advance consent process'. This would be akin to the process I described in connection with treatment decisions, again with an emphasis on the quality of the discourse (Post *et al.* 1994). The aim would be to establish a person's wishes on the basis of what they and those close to them have said, with attention being paid not simply, in a legalistic fashion, to the requirements of valid consent, but also to the values and preferences (both past and present) expressed by the person concerned. Although such a process would take time, since it would involve written records of the consensus achieved as a result of detailed conversations with all concerned, it would (arguably) satisfy the demands of both utilitarian and deontological (Kantian) ethics. It should be possible to recruit participants with dementia, who cannot give informed consent, even for non-therapeutic studies. Yet the researchers will have met their duty to avoid using people *solely* as means, since the person will have been involved beyond the minimal requirement of assent. This possibility is predicated on the notion of the person as a situated-embodied-agent. It recognizes the reality of the person as someone located in a history, a value system, and social context. Of course, some research will still be precluded, but that is an inescapable feature of the inclination to respect persons *as such*. It is also an indication, perhaps, that unbridled utilitarianism is a threat to the integrity of persons.

An emerging problem in treatment research in dementia concerns the use of placebos. The effectiveness of the cholinesterase inhibitors means that there is now a standard against which new treatments should be measured (Kawas *et al.* 1999). Whilst this clearly applies to cognitive function, the situation is not so clear for other symptoms in dementia. Cholinesterase inhibitors have been found effective, for instance, in non-cognitive symptoms in dementia (McKeith *et al.* 2000), but so too have some of the newer atypical antipsychotic medications (de Deyn and Katz 2000). Selecting appropriate controls, therefore, for drug trials in dementia is not simply a research problem, but an ethical one.

This brings us back to the involvement of the *polis* (the body politic). Research carries on in the broad context of society and the person's participation in research has to be judged with this broad perspective in view. This entails, amongst other things, that the *polis* must exert some control over research. In the UK this function is vested in local and multicentre research ethics committees. But the responsibilities of such committees and whether they are equipped to deal with them are matters of continuing debate (Blunt *et al.* 1998; Williamson *et al.* 2000).

The situatedness of the person in a society, which is inevitably political, cuts in different directions. It means that the person with dementia is not just an individual, but is an engaged individual. The person's autonomous agency must be respected and respect for this agency, when the person cannot articulate it, will involve those others who contribute to the individual's personhood. In addition, however, given that research is important for society, there is *some* weight to be attached to the thought that individuals, as part of that society, should be given at least the opportunity to contribute to the advancement of its store of knowledge (Berghmans and ter Meulen 1995). Similarly, the researcher (as an individual agent) pursues his or her own interests (such as the need to make a living and seek advancement) in pursuing research and seeking research grants (Morris 1994). At the same time, however, the researcher must be cognizant of both the needs and values of the research participants with whom he or she has engaged, as well as the norms and laws that govern research. In this social and historical context, the researcher (and research ethics committees) should have regard, 'not only to the content of research, but also to the process' (Kitwood 1995).

There are two further (and somewhat contradictory) thoughts which emerge from reflection on the moral and political nature of medical research. This is an example of the complexity of the underlying 'philosophical plumbing'. First, most clearly in the case of non-therapeutic research, the aim is to increase our knowledge. It could be argued that, whether or not this knowledge has practical benefits, it is in itself a good. Aristotle, for instance, who was a research scientist as well as a philosopher, regarded the desire for knowledge as a part of human nature (Barnes 1982). In which case, we should all share a commitment to scientific research. But this, perhaps, depends upon what it is about knowledge that is important and, thus, whether a particular piece of scientific research is worthwhile as judged by what is good for human beings, or what it is for human beings, as such, to flourish. The second thought takes us back to the importance of the individual agent in the *polis*. For even if it is generally accepted that scientific knowledge is important, the scientific understanding of the world (especially perhaps if this understanding tends to be reductionist concerning values) need not be one to which the individual subscribes. There must, therefore, be the option for individuals to contract out. In this regard, Berghmans (1998) quotes Jonas (1989):

> Let us not forget that progress is an optional goal, not an unconditional commitment, and that its tempo in particular, compulsive as it may become, has nothing sacred about it.

Rationing and ageism

This section considers issues relating to justice and the distribution of resources. In any given polity health care resources are inevitably finite, whilst the demand for better health care invariably outstrips the supply. The upshot is that health care is a matter of economics. The ethical concern is that the *polis*, in deciding how to distribute health resources, should do so in a just manner. This instantly raises, for my purposes, the question: what constitutes a just distribution of health care resources to the elderly? Implicit in this question is an acceptance of the need for rationing.

For a more detailed discussion of theories of rationing than I intend to give, the reader should consult Hope and Oppenheimer (1997). My comments are merely an addendum to that discussion, using the perspective of the person as a situated-embodied-agent.

At the end of the 1980s, a number of philosophers, on various grounds, accepted that it was not unjust for health care resources to be allocated in favour of the young rather than the old. Daniels (1988), for instance, used his 'prudential life-span account' to argue that, since we will all be old, it is not unfair for us to limit spending, say on renal dialysis, to those below a certain age. This is unlike discrimination on the basis of sex or race because usually we also expect to be old, but not to change sex or race. Callahan (1987), who talks of a 'natural life span' of about 80 years, argues that after this time the elderly should only receive palliative care, rather than attempts being made to increase the length of their lives. The suggestion is that elderly people should accept this natural life span as a matter of wisdom and not seek further resources. Veatch (1988) argues that younger people deserve more resources because they have lived less of their lives and are, therefore, worse off than older people.

One problem with Daniels's argument is that different cohorts of elderly *are* treated differently. The social welfare system (as it operates in the UK) is based on the 'principle of intergenerational transfers' (Johnson 1999). There is an implicit contract between generations according to which the current workforce agrees to transfer resources to the former generation of workers and their dependants. The expectation is that the future workforce, some as-yet-unborn, will do the same for the current workers. This creates a problem, because in the future the retired workforce will be much bigger and so, short of depriving themselves, the then-workforce will either have to be more productive, or the retired population will have to put up with less by way of state social welfare than the current elderly population. At some point there will be a cohort that is depriving itself to maintain an elderly population, with no prospect of being similarly supported in its old age. If different cohorts are treated differently, prudent distribution of resources within a life-span becomes more difficult. It is a moot point whether the intergenerational contract will then hold. At some stage a political decision might determine that certain sorts of support are no longer available for older people. Whether or not this is an injustice will depend upon the other decisions that are being made within the *polis*. It is the nexus of decisions in the political sphere that will help to determine the moral shape of the *polis* as a whole.

Arguments about a just distribution of resources, therefore, inevitably involve the *polis*. It has been argued that the isolated and the demented have a basic requirement for meaningful relationships (Howe and Lettieri 1999). Yet it is not at all obvious that the *polis* would necessarily undertake to meet such a need. For instance, at the time of writing, the UK is in the midst of a passionate debate concerning the long-term care of the elderly (Heath 2000). Whilst personal care must still be paid for, the government has committed itself to meeting the costs of nursing care for nursing home residents. In this debate, Stern (2000) suggests that the funding of long-term care is 'not a healthcare issue at all but a wholly political one'; whilst Arie (2000) feels it necessary to speak up for 'frail and dependent old people' and argue against 'taxation by mode of dying'. Inevitably, it seems, old age psychiatrists and their patients are situated in a political context.

Within this context, it might seem reasonable that scarce resources should be rationed in favour of the young over against the elderly. Age, it seems, is a reasonable basis upon which to make a choice, all other things being equal. The use of quality adjusted life years (QALYs) seems to support this view. Rather than rehearse the arguments concerning QALYs (see Hope and Oppenheimer 1997) (see also Chapter 8), I shall just note that whether or not they explicitly discriminate against the old, it can be argued that they do so *in fact*, because it will mostly be the case that the older person can expect fewer QALYs than the younger person (Harris 1987).

Here, the situatedness of the person in the *polis* is relevant. Despite the *a priori* reasonableness of a policy that uses age as a basis for discrimination, it is unreasonable inasmuch as it undermines the standing of persons in society. As in the case of sexism and racism, what is wrong with ageism is that it negatively evaluates those aspects of a life (in this case, the person's age, the *sine qua non* of the person's history) that are an essential part of who they are. The discrimination, the '-ism', therefore *dis*-values the person *qua* person. Hence, Lesser (1999) argues that an illness can provide grounds for treating people differently (and the illness might be a consequence of age), but age itself is irrelevant.

QALYs and policies that support the distribution of resources preferentially away from the old, undervalue the history, values, culture, experience, and agency that help to define older people as persons. Old age itself becomes devalued and, thereby, the quality of the older person's life is further jeopardized (Leaman 1999). It might be, of course, that at a certain age, or in certain circumstances, the elderly person would encourage the spending of resources on someone younger. But this then is a choice and not a prejudice. It will be based on facts and values of importance to the person.

What is central here is the idea that ageism (regarding age as a good ground for discrimination), even if justifiable in individual cases, should not be accepted as public policy. As Harris (1987) argues, the requirement that the State uphold the civil rights of citizens and deal justly between them,

> means that a society, through its public institutions, is not entitled to discriminate between individuals in ways that mean life or death for them on grounds which count the lives or fundamental interests of some as worth less than those of others.

The decisions which might be reasonable in my case should not be accepted as generally applicable if this means that some people will be discriminated against as persons. A just distribution of health care resources to the elderly must recognize the respect due to persons *as such* and, since this involves respecting the person's age, it undermines the legitimacy of ageist policies.

Thus, the distribution of health resources is inherently a matter of politics. Politics, however, is grounded, as economics is grounded, in the individual decisions of people. Just as the person is situated in the *polis*, so the *polis* is constituted by persons. In deciding these matters, then, not only facts, but also personal values, will play a part. Decisions about the allocation of resources to older people will require conversations 'about the elements of a valuable life, and about the other social goods which ought to be protected or promoted through health policy' (Cribb 1999). Old age psychiatrists and others who work with older people have a role to play in the discourse that shapes policy. Such discourse should be free of ageism as an accepted political principle and open to the possibility of a type of moral growth that will enhance and not enfeeble personhood.

Euthanasia and ending life

The issues of euthanasia, physician-assisted suicide, and rational suicide hover at the periphery in the practice of medicine, in debates in clinical ethics, and in the media. Occasionally a report from The Netherlands, a legal case, or a patient brings the issues into full view. In concluding this chapter I can only gesture at some of the arguments, but I hope that here (as elsewhere in the chapter) the reader will find directions to more sustained accounts of these important issues.

Case 11

Mr L. suffers chronic pain from osteoarthritis. He has been a heavy smoker and he develops ischaemia of the foot. He requires an amputation, but the wound heals badly and the amputation has to be extended to below the knee. He also has chronic obstructive pulmonary disease. He develops a series of chest and urinary tract infections. He develops obvious depressive symptoms and he states that he will no longer accept antibiotics. He hopes in this way that he will die. He is treated with an antidepressant, but his negative cognitions do not improve. The expectation is that he will soon develop a further infection, such is his debilitated state.

It is fairly clear that Mr L. has a depressive disorder, but he also has understandable reasons for feeling that life is no longer worth living. It might be decided that his depression should be treated more vigorously. But what if he continues to say that he will not accept further antibiotic medication? Will there come a stage at which it might have to be accepted that his wish to die is 'rational', in the sense that it is *not* motivated by his depressive illness?

Mr L. is not actually saying that he wishes to kill himself. Indeed he is accepting treatment of his depression. But he raises the same concerns as someone who wishes, apparently on 'rational' grounds, to commit suicide. Burgess and Hawton (1998) discuss the case of Dr Chabot in The Netherlands, who assisted Mrs Bosscher in her suicide. Dr Chabot had found no evidence of a 'depression that would have responded to drugs' and her wish to die was regarded as rational in the face of her unhappiness caused by the death of her two sons. Dr Chabot reported the case, in accordance with the Dutch rules, and the case was referred to the local court. Having been dismissed by lower courts, since it was regarded as a test case of psychiatric euthanasia, it went to the Dutch Supreme Court. Dr Chabot was found guilty of unlawful assisted suicide, but only because he had failed to follow the exact guidelines of the Dutch Royal Medical Association. He was not punished and continued to practise medicine.

The case demonstrates that, in the context of Dutch law regarding euthanasia, suffering need not be physical and a person does not need to be terminally ill. From their own case histories Burgess and Hawton (1998) conclude that suicidal wishes sometimes do not seem to arise from treatable mental illnesses. They also conclude that, since suicide seems to be a 'natural and not uncommon outcome of depression and schizophrenia', suicidal patients with serious untreatable mental illnesses 'could be considered to have a potentially terminal illness, and euthanasia in these cases could be seen as akin to euthanasia in cases of terminal physical illness'.

None of their cases was an elderly patient, but the issues raised by Burgess and Hawton are not infrequently seen in the elderly. It is not that elderly patients frequently ask to be killed, although some express the wish that they were dead. But it is sometimes the case that their suffering, either mental or physical, is great enough to give them what appear to be good grounds for wishing to die. Psychiatric training tends to encourage the view that suicidal thoughts (even in the absence of plans and intentions) are a symptom of depression; and old age psychiatrists are determined that depression in the elderly should be treated. But it seems correct to say 'that to choose to die, or to lose the will to live, becomes rational or irrational in virtue of what motivates it' (Matthews 1998). For this reason the concept of 'rational' in the context of suicide must be in inverted commas. The point is not the 'rationality', but the motivation and whether this has authentic grounds, rooted not in mental illness but in the person's true, uncoerced, agentive concerns and values. A psychiatric illness might well make the motivation irrational, but this need not invariably be so. Mr L. demonstrates the difficulty in knowing when pursuing psychiatric treatment is futile. Inasmuch as his wish to die is motivated by 'rational' grounds, he presents the challenge that will face physicians and psychiatrists in the UK should physician-assisted suicide become legal.

Those who argue in favour of voluntary euthanasia can claim that allowing self-determination secures the person's best interests (Nowell-Smith 1994) and preserves the person's dignity (Fairbairn 1999). Those who argue against voluntary euthanasia can claim that it involves intentionally killing innocent people and (similarly) offends a notion of basic human dignity (Gormally 1994). The issues have been more thoroughly pursued in *Euthanasia examined* (Keown 1995), which includes a sustained debate between Harris and Finnis.

Harris (1995) argues:

> Euthanasia should be permitted, not because everyone should accept that it is a right, nor because to fail to do so violates a defensible conception of the sanctity of life, but simply because to deny a person control of what, on any analysis, must be one of the most important decisions of life, is a form of tyranny, which

like all acts of tyranny is an ultimate denial of respect for persons.

Alternatively, against euthanasia, Finnis (1995) argues:

> [A] being that once has human (and thus personal) life will remain a human person while that life (the dynamic principle for that being's integrated organic functioning) remains—i.e. until death. Where one's brain...has been so damaged as to impair or even destroy one's capacity for intellectual acts, one is...[a] damaged human person...In sustaining human bodily life, in however impaired a condition, one is sustaining the person whose life it is. In refusing to choose to violate it, one respects the person in the most fundamental and indispensable way.'

Rather than pursue the details of this particular debate here, I should rather note the central importance attached to the notion of a person. What is, perhaps, missing from this debate is the broader conception of the person as a situated-embodied-agent. This broader view of the person might influence the debate in two areas: first, concerning the notion of intention; second, with respect to the idea of human dignity.

The notion of intention often enters the debate in connection with the doctrine of double effect (Doyal 1999; Gillon 1999). This doctrine suggests a distinction between *intending* a bad outcome and *foreseeing* a bad outcome. If, in giving an injection, my intention is to kill the patient, then I have done wrong. But if my intention is to relieve the patient's pain, then even if I foresee that the injection will shorten the patient's life, I have not done wrong, because I have not intended to kill the patient. Many doctors accept this doctrine as clear and helpful in clinical practice. But many philosophers and ethicists have found it problematic (Glover 1977). A major problem is that *intending something* is regarded as an inner activity, something that occurs in the mind. In which case, a person can say that he or she intended almost anything. The notion of intention as an inner activity is the bend in the philosophical plumbing I wish to scrutinize briefly.

What if 'intending something' is not regarded as simply an inner activity? What if the concept of an intention must have some outer manifestation in order for it to retain its sense? When I intend something, there must be some link with certain things in the (outer) human world in order for the concept of intention to have any meaning in that world. Without elaborating the point, it can be seen that the concept of intention relies on certain features of the world being as they are; which is to say that the concept is embedded in a human linguistic context, and is enmeshed with the notion of the person as a situated-embodied-agent. Our intentions are not just private things, they are (at least in principle) subject to public scrutiny. Thus, having given a standard dose of morphine by injection, my claim that I intended to relieve the person's pain is justified. But, having given a large injection of potassium chloride, my claim that I did not intend the patient to die, but only to relieve the pain, is not justified. This has nothing to do with what it was that I said to myself as I gave the injection. It is to do with the potentially visible practices that intending something must involve.

So, if the divide between 'inner' and 'outer' is largely porous, the doctrine of double effect will be supportable, but only because human actions are embedded in circumstances which contribute to any determination of their rightness or wrongness. It is the 'outer' circumstances that characterize actions as either justifiable or unjustifiable killing. Intentions are crucially important. But they cannot be regarded as solely 'inner' acts, disengaged from the situated context of the human agent.

Concerning human dignity, there is an acceptance by the Royal Dutch Medical Association that 'it can be justified for a doctor to assist in the suicide of a patient who is in the early stages of dementia because this patient fears the prospect of an inevitable loss of human dignity or *ontluistering*' (Berghmans 1999). Meanwhile, the Dutch Association of Nursing Home Physicians, whilst accepting that life can be terminated in exceptional cases of unbearable human suffering, does not accept that the notion of *ontluistering* is relevant. For, 'the now demented patient cannot experience the *ontluistering* that the previously competent former self of the patient has expressed as a condition for life termination' (Berghmans 1999).

Berghmans (1999) proceeds to raise some conceptual questions about the notion of loss of human dignity or *ontluistering*. How can we know what this state, which we regard ahead of time as undignified, is actually like to experience? Is *ontluistering* simply a subjective matter? Is there no intersubjectivity involved? And, if it is partly objective, what are its characteristics? The notion that human persons are situated-embodied-agents immediately brings in intersubjectivity and objectivity, and makes it possible that the physical and emotional environment will contribute to whether or not there is *ontluistering*. Kitwood (1997), after all, spoke of the possibility of a 'malignant social environment' in dementia care.

If this is the case, then the broad notion of the person as a situated being suggests that human dignity is at least in part a function of the environment and reflects the idea that personhood is partly maintained by others. It might be, therefore, that the need for euthanasia and physician-assisted suicide, as a response to *ontluistering*, would become unnecessary. This would reflect the idea that personhood is partly maintained by others. The thought that what is really required is better care for people with dementia, rather than euthanasia, reflects the thought that what is required for people with terminal illnesses is good-quality terminal care. This has led to the suggestion that in severe dementia there is an imperative for the development of hospice-type care (Sachs 1995; Roth 1996; Post 1997).

The *polis* is, therefore, relevant to end-of-life decisions. Not only will it make the laws, which should aim to encourage respect for persons, it will also provide the forum in which what best constitutes such respect must be worked out. And one worry about promoting suicide as a way of dealing with some of the infirmities of the elderly is that, in so doing, we might erode the value that should be attached to human life as such and, in particular, make the elderly feel undervalued as people (Post 1990). Hence,

> When faced with a problem that may seem insoluble, it will often emerge that the real issue concerns communication and relationships...Closer attention to the humane art that is medicine, rather than the technical discipline it threatens to become...would almost certainly avoid many of these problems...Therefore we would argue that compassionate, restrained care and the judicious use of those resources that have a proven beneficial role in terms of pain relief, comfort and dignity are the best response to the needs of people with tragic and terminal diseases. (Campbell *et al.* 1997)

Conclusion: the person in the world

In this chapter I have made use of the notion of the person as a situated-embodied-agent to discuss a number of ethical issues in old age psychiatry. The discussion has often demonstrated the importance of both facts and values in everyday clinical decisions. The notion that we, whether as patients or as health-care workers, are situated in our histories, which link with the histories of others and which are embedded in broader familial, societal, cultural, and spiritual contexts, helps to emphasize the importance of communication and the process by which ethically difficult decisions and disputes should be handled.

The discussion raises issues for medical ethics too. Philosophy should lead us to look more clearly, or perhaps from a different perspective, at the conceptual plumbing that underlies our thoughts and actions. But medical ethics also relies on accurate facts. There is, therefore, an empirical side to it (Hope 1999). Moreover, many of the values with which it deals will be embedded in discourse and narrative. Medical ethics should then rely, to some extent, not only on quantitative but also on qualitative studies. This will involve ethnographic approaches as a way of elucidating the values that operate within our situated contexts (Robertson 1996). Increasingly, whilst not forgetting our own values, it will be the values of patients themselves which must be heard. Part of our responsibility, as ethical practitioners, will be to facilitate the expression of those values.

In this chapter I have placed the person in the pivotal position. Philosophical reflection can increase our understanding of personhood, but one of the things that contributes to the excitement of clinical practice is the potential it has to broaden our grasp of human nature and of what it is to be a person in the world.

Acknowledgement

I am extremely grateful to Professor Tony Hope who made detailed comments on a draft of this chapter. He has encouraged me to clarify the argument in parts and to avoid some pitfalls. His generous help has improved the chapter; the remaining faults are my own.

References

Agarwal, M. R., Ferran, J., Ost, K., and Wilson, K. C. M. (1996). Ethics of 'informed consent' in dementia research—the debate continues. *International Journal of Geriatric Psychiatry*, **11**, 801–6.

AGS (American Geriatrics Society) Ethics Committee (1996). Making treatment decisions for incapacitated older adults without advance directives. *Journal of the American Geriatrics Society*, **44**, 986–7.

AGS (American Geriatrics Society) Ethics Committee (1998). Informed consent for research on human subjects with dementia. *Journal of the American Geriatrics Society*, **46**, 1308–10.

Arie, T. (2000). Funding long term care for older people. *British Medical Journal*, **321**, 238. [Letter]

Arras, J. D. (1988). The severely demented, minimally functional patient: an ethical analysis. *Journal of the American Geriatrics Society*, **36**, 938–44.

Barnes, J. (1982). *Aristotle*. Oxford University Press, Oxford.

Baskin, S. A., Morris, J., Ahronheim, J. C., Meier, D. E., and Morrison, R. S. (1998). Barriers to obtaining consent in dementia research: implications for surrogate decision-making. *Journal of the American Geriatrics Society*, **46**, 287–90.

Beauchamp, T. L. and Childress, J. F. (1994). *Principles of biomedical ethics* (4th edn). Oxford University Press, Oxford.

Berghmans, R. L. P. (1997). Ethical hazards of the substituted judgement test in decision making concerning the end of life of dementia patients. *International Journal of Geriatric Psychiatry*, **12**, 283–7.

Berghmans, R. L. P. (1998). Advance directives for non-therapeutic dementia research: some ethical and policy considerations. *Journal of Medical Ethics*, **24**, 32–7.

Berghmans, R. L. P. (1999). Ethics of end-of-life decisions in cases of dementia: views of the Royal Dutch Medical Association with some critical comments. *Alzheimer Disease and Associated Disorders*, **13**, 91–5.

Berghmans, R. L. P. and ter Meulen, R. H. J. (1995). Ethical issues in research with dementia patients. *International Journal of Geriatric Psychiatry*, **10**, 647–51.

Blunt, J., Savulescu, J., and Watson, A. J. M. (1998). Meeting the challenges facing research ethics committees: some practical suggestions. *British Medical Journal*, **316**, 58–61.

BMJ (*British Medical Journal*) (1996). The Nuremberg Code (1947); Declaration of Helsinki (1964). *British Medical Journal*, **313**, 1448–9.

Brock, D. W. (1998). Commentary on 'The time frame of preferences, dispositions, and the validity of advance directives for the mentally ill'. *Philosophy, Psychiatry, & Psychology*, **5**, 251–3.

Brodaty, H., Dresser, R., Eisner, M., Erkunjuntti, T., Gauthier, S., Graham, N., *et al.* (1999). Consensus statement: Alzheimer's Disease International and International Working Group for Harmonization of Dementia Drug Guidelines for research involving human subjects with dementia. *Alzheimer Disease and Associated Disorders*, **13**, 71–9.

Buchanan, A. (1988). Advance directives and the personal identity problem. *Philosophy and Public Affairs*, **17**, 277–302.

Burgess, M. M. (1994). Ethical issues in genetic testing for Alzheimer's disease: lessons from Huntington's disease. *Alzheimer Disease and Associated Disorders*, **8**, 71–8.

Burgess, S. and Hawton, K. (1998). Suicide, euthanasia, and the psychiatrist. *Philosophy, Psychiatry, & Psychology*, **5**, 113–26.

Burns, A., Russell, E., and Page, S. (1999). New drugs for Alzheimer's disease. *British Journal of Psychiatry*, **174**, 476–9.

Butterworth, M. (1995). Dementia: the family caregiver's perspective. *Journal of Mental Health*, **4**, 125–32.

Callahan, D. (1987). *Setting limits: medical goals in an aging society*. Simon and Schuster, New York.

Callahan, D. (1995). Terminating life-sustaining treatment of the demented. *Hastings Center Report*, **25**, 25–31.

Campbell, A., Charlesworth, M., Gillett, G., and Jones, G. (1997). *Medical ethics*. Oxford University Press, Auckland.

Cassel, C. K. (1998). Genetic testing and Alzheimer disease: ethical issues for providers and families. *Alzheimer Disease and Associated Disorders*, **12**, S16–S20.

Codori, A.-M., Slavney, P. R., Young, C., Miglioretti, D. L., and Brandt, J. (1997). Predictors of psychological adjustment to genetic testing for Huntington's disease. *Health Psychology*, **16**, 36–50.

Collopy, B. J. (1988). Autonomy in long term care: some crucial distinctions. *Gerontologist*, **28**(Suppl.), 10–17.

Cook, E. D. (1999). Genetics and the British insurance industry. *Journal of Medical Ethics*, **25**, 157–62.

Cotrell, V. and Schulz, R. (1993). The perspective of the patient with Alzheimer's disease: a neglected dimension of dementia research. *Gerontologist*, **33**, 205–11.

Cribb, A. (1999). The felicific calculus strikes back. In *Ageing, autonomy and resources* (ed. A. Harry Lesser), pp. 188–200. Ashgate, Aldershot.

Cummings, S. M. and Cockerham, C. (1997). Ethical dilemmas in discharge planning for patients with Alzheimer's disease. *Health* and *Social Work*, **22**, 101–8.

Daniels, N. (1988). *Am I my parents' keeper? An essay on justice between the young and the old*. Oxford University Press, Oxford.

Dawkins, V. H. (1998). Restraints and the elderly with mental illness: ethical issues and moral reasoning. *Journal of Psychosocial Nursing*, **36**, 22–7.

De Deyn, P. P. and Katz, I. R. (2000). Control of aggression and agitation in patients with dementia: efficacy and safety of risperidone. *International Journal of Geriatric Psychiatry*, **15**, S14–S23.

Dodds, S. (1996). Exercising restraint: autonomy, welfare and elderly patients. *Journal of Medical Ethics*, **22**, 160–3.

Doyal, L. (1999). When doctors might kill their patients. The moral character of clinicians or the best interests of patients? *British Medical Journal*, **318**, 1432–3.

Doyal, L. and Wilsher, D. (1994). Withholding and withdrawing life sustaining treatment from elderly people: towards formal guidelines. *British Medical Journal*, **308**, 1689–92.

Dresser, R. (1995). Dworkin on dementia: elegant theory, questionable policy. *Hastings Center Report*, **25**, 32–8.

Dresser, R. (1998). Commentary on 'The time frame of preferences, dispositions, and the validity of advance directives for the mentally ill'. *Philosophy, Psychiatry, & Psychology*, **5**, 247–9.

Dubinsky, R. M., Stein, A. C., and Lyons, K. (2000). Practice parameter: risk of driving and Alzheimer's disease (an evidence-based review). *Neurology*, **54**, 2205–11.

Dworkin, R. (1986). Autonomy and the demented self. *Millbank Quarterly*, **64**, 4–16.

Dworkin, R. (1993). *Life's dominion. An argument about abortion and euthanasia.* Harper Collins, London.

Eaton, M. L. (1999). Surrogate decision making for genetic testing for Alzheimer disease. *Genetic Testing*, **3**, 93–7.

Fairbairn, G. (1999). Ending lives: age, autonomy and the quality of life. In *Ageing, autonomy and resources* (ed. A. Harry Lesser), pp. 88–115. Ashgate, Aldershot.

Farmer, A. E., Owen, M. J., and McGuffin, P. (2000). Bioethics and genetic research in psychiatry. *British Journal of Psychiatry*, **176**, 105–8.

Farthing, M. J. G. (1998). Coping with fraud. *Lancet*, **SIV**, 11.

Fazel, S., Hope, T., and Jacoby, R. (1999). Assessment of competence to complete advance directives: validation of a patient centred approach. *British Medical Journal*, **318**, 493–7.

Finnis, J. (1995). A philosophical case against euthanasia. In *Euthanasia examined: ethical, clinical and legal perspectives* (ed. J. Keown), pp. 23–35. Cambridge University Press, Cambridge.

Finucane, T. E., Beamer, B. A., Roca, R. P., and Kawas, C. H. (1993). Establishing advance directives with demented patients: a pilot study. *Journal of Clinical Ethics*, **4**, 51–4.

Finucane, T. E., Christmas, C., and Travis, K. (1999). Tube feeding in patients with advanced dementia. *Journal of the American Medical Association*, **282**, 1365–70.

Fisk, J. D., Sadovnick, A. D., Cohen, C. A., Gauthier, S., Dossetor, J., Eberhart, A., *et al.* (1998). Ethical guidelines of the Alzheimer Society of Canada. *Canadian Journal of Neurological Sciences*, **25**, 242–8.

Freedman, M. L. and Freedman, D. L. (1996). Should Alzheimers disease patients be allowed to drive? A medical, legal, and ethical dilemma. *Journal of the American Geriatrics Society*, **44**, 876–7.

Fulford, K. W. M. (1987). Is medicine a branch of ethics? In *Persons and personality. A contemporary inquiry* (ed. A. Peacocke and G. Gillett), pp. 130–49. Blackwell, Oxford.

Fulford, K. W. M. (1989). *Moral theory and medical practice.* Cambridge University Press, Cambridge.

Garanis-Papadatos, T. and Katas, A. (1999). The milk and the honey: ethics of artificial nutrition and hydration of the elderly on the other side of Europe. *Journal of Medical Ethics*, **25**, 447–50.

Gillick, M. R. (2000). Rethinking the role of tube feeding in patients with advanced dementia. *New England Journal of Medicine*, **342**, 206–10.

Gillon, R. (1986). *Philosophical medical ethics.* Wiley, Chichester.

Gillon, R. (1997). 'Futility'—too ambiguous and pejorative a term? *Journal of Medical Ethics*, **23**, 339–40.

Gillon, R. (1999). When doctors might kill their patients. Foreseeing is not necessarily the same as intending. *British Medical Journal*, **318**, 1431–2.

Gillon, R. and Lloyd, A. (ed.) (1994). *Principles of health care ethics.* Wiley, Chichester.

Glover, J. (1977). *Causing death and saving lives.* Penguin, Harmondsworth.

Glover, J. (1988). *I: The philosophy and psychology of personal identity.* Penguin, Harmondsworth.

Golin, C. E., Wenger, N. S., Liu, H., Dawson, N. V. Teno, J. M., Desbiens, N. A., *et al.* (2000). A prospective study of patient–physician communication about resuscitation. *Journal of the American Geriatrics Society*, **48**, S52–S60.

Goodhall, L. (1997). Tube feeding dilemmas: can artificial nutrition and hydration be legally or ethically withheld or withdrawn? *Journal of Advanced Nursing*, **25**, 217–22.

Gormally, L. (1994). Against voluntary euthanasia. In *Principles of health care ethics* (ed. R. Gillon and A. Lloyd), pp. 763–74. Wiley, Chichester.

Gormley, N. and Howard, R. (1999). Should neuroleptics be used in the management of nursing home residents with dementia? *International Journal of Geriatric Psychiatry*, **14**, 509–11.

Harris, J. (1987). QALYfying the value of life. *Journal of Medical Ethics*, **13**, 117–23.

Harris, J. (1995). Euthanasia and the value of life. In *Euthanasia examined: ethical, clinical and legal perspectives* (ed. J. Keown), pp. 6–22. Cambridge University Press, Cambridge.

Heath, I. (2000). Dereliction of duty in an ageist society. *British Medical Journal*, **320**, 1422.

High, D. M., Whitehouse, P. J., Post, S. G., and Berg, L. (1994). Guidelines for addressing ethical and legal issues in Alzheimer disease research: a position paper. *Alzheimer Disease and Associated Disorders*, **8**(Suppl. 4), 66–74.

Honderich, T. (1995). *The Oxford companion to philosophy.* Oxford University Press, Oxford.

Hope, T. (1992). Advance directives about medical treatment. *British Medical Journal*, **304**, 398.

Hope, T. (1995). Personal identity and psychiatric illness. In *Philosophy, psychology and psychiatry* (ed. A. P. Griffiths), pp. 131–43. Cambridge University Press, Cambridge.

Hope, T. (1996). Advance directives. *Journal of Medical Ethics*, **22**, 67–8.

Hope, T. (1999). Empirical medical ethics. *Journal of Medical Ethics*, **25**, 219–20.

Hope, T. and Oppenheimer, C. (1997). Ethics and the psychiatry of old age. In *Psychiatry in the elderly* (2nd edn), (ed. R. Jacoby and C. Oppenheimer), pp. 709–35. Oxford University Press, Oxford.

Hope, T., Keene, J., Fairburn, C. G., Jacoby, R., and McShane, R. (1999). Natural history of behavioural changes and psychiatric symptoms in Alzheimer's disease: a longitudinal study. *British Journal of Psychiatry*, **174**, 39–44.

Howe, E. G. and Lettieri, C. J. (1999). Health care rationing in the aged. Ethical and clinical perspectives. *Drugs and Aging*, **15**, 37–47.

Howell, M. (1984). Caretakers' views on responsibilities for the care of the demented elderly. *Journal of the American Geriatrics Society*, **32**, 657–60.

Hudson, W. D. (1967). *Ethical intuitionism*. Macmillan, London.

Hughes, J. (1995). Ultimate justification: Wittgenstein and medical ethics. *Journal of Medical Ethics*, **21**, 25–30.

Hughes, J. C. (2000*a*). Ethics and the anti-dementia drugs. *International Journal of Geriatric Psychiatry*, **15**, 538–43.

Hughes, J. C. (2000*b*). Response to Case 6.2—Ida Harbottle. In *In two minds: a casebook of psychiatric ethics* (ed. D. Dickenson and K. W. M. Fulford), pp. 195–6. Oxford University Press, Oxford.

Hurley, A. C., Volicer, B. J., and Volicer, L. (1996). Effect of fever-management strategy on the progression of dementia of the Alzheimer type. *Alzheimer Disease and Associated Disorders*, **10**, 5–10.

Husband, H. J. (2000). Diagnostic disclosure in dementia: an opportunity for intervention? *International Journal of Geriatric Psychiatry*, **15**, 544–7.

Ikonomidis, S. and Singer, P. A. (1999). Autonomy, liberalism and advance care planning. *Journal of Medical Ethics*, **25**, 522–7.

Jansson, L., Norberg, A., Sandman, P.-O., and Åström, G. (1995). When the severely ill elderly patient refuses food. Ethical reasoning among nurses. *International Journal of Nursing Studies*, **32**, 68–78.

John Paul II (1995). *Evangelium vitae*. Libreria Editrice Vaticana, Vatican City.

Johnson, P. (1999). Population ageing, social security, and the distribution of economic resources. In *Ageing, autonomy and resources* (ed. A. Harry Lesser), pp. 142–60. Ashgate, Aldershot.

Jonas, H. (1989). Philosophical reflections on experimenting with human subjects. In *Contemporary issues in bioethics* (3rd edn) (ed. T. L. Beauchamp and L. R. Walters), pp. 432–40. Wadsworth, Belmont, CA.

Jones, R. G. (1997). Ethical and legal issues in the care of demented people. *Reviews in Clinical Gerontology*, **7**, 147–62.

Joseph, D. I. and Onek, J. (1999). Confidentiality in psychiatry. In *Psychiatric ethics* (3rd edn) (ed. S. Bloch, P. Chodoff, and S. A. Green), pp. 105–40. Oxford University Press, Oxford.

Kant, I. (1785). *Foundations of the metaphysic of morals*. Published as *The moral law* (trans. H. J. Paton, 1948). Hutchinson, London.

Kaufman, S. R. (1995). Decision making, responsibility, and advocacy in geriatric medicine: physician dilemmas with elderly in the community. *Gerontologist*, **35**, 481–8.

Kawas, C. H., Clark, C. M., Farlow, M. R., Knopman, D. S., Marson, D., Morris, J. C., *et al.* (1999). Clinical trials in Alzheimer disease: debate on the use of placebo controls. *Alzheimer Disease and Associated Disorders*, **13**, 124–9.

Keown, J. (ed.) (1995). *Euthanasia examined: ethical, clinical and legal perspectives*. Cambridge University Press, Cambridge.

Kitwood, T. (1993). Towards a theory of dementia care: the interpersonal process. *Ageing and Society*, **13**, 51–67.

Kitwood, T. (1995). Exploring the ethics of dementia research: a response to Berghmans and ter Meulen: a psychosocial perspective. *International Journal of Geriatric Psychiatry*, **10**, 655–7.

Kitwood, T. (1997). *Dementia reconsidered. The person comes first*. Open University Press, Buckingham.

Kitwood, T. (1998). Toward a theory of dementia care: ethics and interaction. *Journal of Clinical Ethics*, **9**, 23–34.

Klein, S. (1989). Caregiver burden and moral development. *IMAGE: Journal of Nursing Scholarship*, **21**, 94–7.

Krynski, M. D., Tymchuk, A. J., and Ouslander, J. G. (1994). How informed can consent be? New light on comprehension among elderly people making decisions about tube feeding. *Gerontologist*, **34**, 36–43.

Leaman, O. (1999). Justifying ageism. In *Ageing, autonomy and resources* (ed. A. Harry Lesser), pp. 180–7. Ashgate, Aldershot.

Lennard-Jones, J. E. (1999). Giving or withholding fluid and nutrients: ethical and legal aspects. *Journal of the Royal College of Physicians of London*, **33**, 39–45.

Lesser, H. (1999). Justice and the principle of triage. In *Ageing, autonomy and resources* (ed. A. Harry Lesser), pp. 201–11. Ashgate, Aldershot.

Linacre Centre Papers (1979). *Prolongation of life. Paper 3: Ordinary and extraordinary means of prolonging life*. The Linacre Centre, London.

Locke, J. (1690). *An essay concerning human understanding* (ed. A. D. Woozley, 1964). William Collins/Fount Paperbacks, Glasgow.

Lord Chancellor's Department (1997). *Who decides? Making decisions on behalf of mentally incapacitated adults*. HMSO, London.

Lord Chancellor's Department (1999). *Making decisions*. HMSO, London.

Lovestone, S., Wilcock, G., Rossor, M., Cayton, H., and Ragan, I. (1996). Apolipoprotein E. genotyping in Alzheimer's disease. *Lancet*, **347**, 1775–6.

Lyman, K. A. (1998). Living with Alzheimer's disease: the creation of meaning among persons with dementia. *Journal of Clinical Ethics*, **9**, 49–57.

Lynöe, N., Sandlund, M., and Jacobsson, L. (1998). When others decide: reasons for allowing patients with Alzheimer's disease to participate in nontherapeutic research. *International Psychogeriatrics*, **10**, 435–6.

McConnell, L. M., Koenig, B. A., Greely, H. T., and Raffin, T. A. (1999). Genetic testing and Alzheimer disease: recommendations of the Stanford Program in Genomics, Ethics, and Society. *Genetic Testing*, **3**, 3–12.

McKeith, I. G., Grace, J. B., Walker, Z., Byrne, E. J., Wilkinson, D., Stevens, T., *et al.* (2000). Rivastigmine in the treatment of dementia with Lewy bodies: preliminary findings from an open trial. *International Journal of Geriatric Psychiatry*, **15**, 387–92.

McShane, R., Hope, T., and Wilkinson, J. (1994). Tracking patients who wander: ethics and technology. *Lancet*, **343**, 1274.

McShane, R., Keene, J., Gedling, K., Fairburn, C., Jacoby, R., and Hope, T. (1997). Do neuroleptic drugs hasten cognitive decline in dementia? Prospective study with necropsy follow up. *British Medical Journal*, **314**, 266–70.

McShane, R., Gedling, K., Keene, J., Fairburn, C., Jacoby, R., and Hope, T. (1998*a*). Getting lost in dementia: a longitudinal study of a behavioral symptom. *International Psychogeriatrics*, **10**, 253–60.

McShane, R., Gedling, K., Kenward, B., Kenward, R., Hope, T., and Jacoby, R. (1998*b*). The feasibility of electronic tracking devices in dementia: a telephone survey and case series. *International Journal of Geriatric Psychiatry*, **13**, 556–63.

Maguire, C. P., Kirby, M., Coen, R., Coakley, D., Lawlor, B. A., and O'Neill, D. (1996). Family members' attitudes toward telling the patient with Alzheimer's disease their diagnosis. *British Medical Journal*, **313**, 529–30.

Marzanski, M. (2000). Would you like to know what is wrong with you? On telling the truth to patients with dementia. *Journal of Medical Ethics*, **26**, 108–13.

Mason, J. K., McCall Smith, R. A., and Laurie G. T. (1999). *Law and medical ethics* (5th edn). Butterworths, London.

Matthews, E. (1998). Choosing death: philosophical observations on suicide and euthanasia. *Philosophy, Psychiatry, & Psychology*, **5**, 107–11.

Megone, C. (2000). Mental illness, human function, and values. *Philosophy, Psychiatry, & Psychology*, **7**, 45–65.

Mezey, M., Kluger, M., Maislin, G., and Mittelman, M. (1996). Life-sustaining treatment decisions by spouses of patients with Alzheimer's disease. *Journal of the American Geriatrics Society*, **44**, 144–50.

Midgley, M. (1996). *Utopias, dolphins and computers*. Routledge, London.

Moe, C. and Schroll, M. (1997). What degree of medical treatment do nursing home residents want in case of life-threatening disease? *Age and Ageing*, **26**, 133–7.

Moody, H. R. (1992). *Ethics in an aging society*. Johns Hopkins University Press, Baltimore, MD.

Morris, J. C. (1994). Conflicts of interest: research and clinical care. *Alzheimer Disease and Associated Disorders*, **8**(Suppl. 4), 49–57.

Müller-Hill, B. (1991). Psychiatry in the Nazi era. In *Psychiatric ethics* (2nd edn) (ed. S. Bloch and P. Chodoff), pp. 461–72. Oxford University Press, Oxford.

Muncie, H. L. Jr., Magaziner, J., Hebel, J. R., and Warren, J. W. (1997). Proxies' decisions about clinical research participation for their charges. *Journal of the American Geriatrics Society*, **45**, 929–33.

Murphy, E. (1984). Ethical dilemmas of brain failure in the elderly. *British Medical Journal*, **288**, 61–2. [Letter]

Newton, M. J. (1999). Precedent autonomy: life-sustaining intervention and the demented patient. *Cambridge Quarterly of Healthcare Ethics*, **8**, 189–99.

Norberg, A. (1994). Ethics in the care of the elderly with dementia. In *Principles of health care ethics* (ed. R. Gillon and A. Lloyd), pp. 721–31. Wiley, Chichester.

Nowell-Smith, P. (1994). In favour of voluntary euthanasia. In *Principles of health care ethics* (ed. R. Gillon and A. Lloyd), pp. 753–62. Wiley, Chichester.

Nuffield Council on Bioethics (1993). *Genetic screening: ethical issues*. Nuffield Council on Bioethics, London.

Nuffield Council on Bioethics (1998). *Mental disorders and genetics: the ethical context*. Nuffield Council on Bioethics, London.

Oppenheimer, C. (1999). Ethics in old age psychiatry. In *Psychiatric ethics* (3rd edn) (ed. S. Bloch, P. Chodoff, and S. A. Green), pp. 317–43. Oxford University Press, Oxford.

Parfit, D. (1984). *Reasons and persons*. Oxford University Press, Oxford.

Pettit, P. (1980). *Judging justice. An introduction to contemporary political philosophy*. Routledge and Kegan Paul, London.

Pinner, G. (2000). Truth-telling and the diagnosis of dementia. *British Journal of Psychiatry*, **176**, 514–15.

Post, S. G. (1990). Severely demented elderly people: a case against senicide. *Journal of the American Geriatrics Society*, **38**, 715–18.

Post, S. G. (1994*a*). Genetics, ethics, and Alzheimer disease. *Journal of the American Geriatrics Society*, **42**, 782–6.

Post, S. G. (1994*b*). Ethics of behavior control: a panel discussion. *Alzheimer Disease and Associated Disorders*, **8**(Suppl. 3), 156–8.

Post, S. G. (1997). Physician-assisted suicide in Alzheimer's disease. *Journal of the American Geriatrics Society*, **45**, 647–51.

Post, S. G. (1999). Future scenarios for the prevention and delay of Alzheimer disease onset in high-risk groups. *American Journal of Preventive Medicine*, **16**, 105–10.

Post, S. G. (2000). *The moral challenge of Alzheimer disease: ethical issues from diagnosis to dying* (2nd edn). Johns Hopkins University Press, Baltimore, MD.

Post, S. G. and Whitehouse, P. J. (1995). Fairhill guidelines on ethics of the care of people with Alzheimer's disease: a clinical summary. *Journal of the American Geriatrics Society*, **43**, 1423–9.

Post, S. G. and Whitehouse, P. J. (1998*a*). Emerging antidementia drugs: a preliminary ethical view. *Journal of the American Geriatrics Society*, **46**, 784–7.

Post, S. G. and Whitehouse, P. J. (1998*b*). *Genetics, ethics, and Alzheimer disease*. Johns Hopkins University Press, Baltimore, MD.

Post, S. G., Ripich, D. N., and Whitehouse, P. J. (1994). Discourse ethics: research, dementia, and communication. *Alzheimer Disease and Associated Disorders*, **8**(Suppl. 4), 58–65.

Post, S. G., Grafström, M., Winblad, B., Homma, A., and Rossor, M. N. (1995). International commentaries on 'Guidelines for addressing ethical and legal issues in Alzheimer disease research'. *Alzheimer Disease and Associated Disorders*, **9**, 188–92.

Post, S. G., Whitehouse, P. J., Binstock, R. H., Bird, T. D., Eckert, S. K., Farrer, L. A., *et al.* (1997). The clinical introduction of genetic testing for Alzheimer disease. An ethical perspective. *Journal of the American Medical Association*, **277**, 832–6.

Pratt, C., Schmall, V., and Wright, S. (1987). Ethical concerns of family caregivers to dementia patients. *Gerontologist*, **27**, 632–8.

Rabins, P. V. and Mace, N. L. (1986). Some ethical issues in dementia care. *Clinical Gerontologist*, **5**, 503–12.

Robertson, D. W. (1996). Ethical theory, ethnography, and differences between doctors and nurses in approaches to patient care. *Journal of Medical Ethics*, **22**, 292–9.

Rosin, A. J. and Sonnenblick, M. (1998). Autonomy and paternalism in geriatric medicine. The Jewish ethical approach to issues of feeding terminally ill patients, and to cardiopulmonary resuscitation. *Journal of Medical Ethics*, **24**, 44–8.

Roth, M. (1996). Euthanasia and related ethical issues in dementias of later life with special reference to Alzheimer's disease. *British Medical Bulletin*, **52**, 263–79.

Sabat, S. R. and Harré, R. (1994). The Alzheimer's disease sufferer as a semiotic subject. *Philosophy, Psychiatry, & Psychology*, **1**, 145–60.

Sachs, G. A. (1994). Advance consent for dementia research. *Alzheimer Disease and Associated Disorders*, **8**(Suppl. 4), 19–27.

Sachs, G. A., Ahronheim, J. C., Rhymes, J. A., Volicer, L., and Lynn, J. (1995). Good care of dying patients: the alternative to physician-assisted suicide and euthanasia. *Journal of the American Geriatrics Society*, **43**, 553–62.

Savulescu, J. and Dickenson, D. (1998*a*). The time frame of preferences, dispositions, and the validity of advance directives for the mentally ill. *Philosophy, Psychiatry, & Psychology*, **5**, 225–46.

Savulescu, J. and Dickenson, D. (1998*b*). Response to the commentaries. *Philosophy, Psychiatry, & Psychology*, **5**, 263–6.

Schiff, R., Rajkumar, C., and Bulpitt, C. (2000). Views of elderly people on living wills: interview study. *British Medical Journal*, **320**, 1640–1.

Schneiderman, L. J. and Jecker, N. S. (1995). *Wrong medicine. Doctors, patients, and futile treatment*. Johns Hopkins University Press, Baltimore, MD.

Scruton, R. (1982). *Kant*. Oxford University Press, Oxford.

Shua-Haim, J. R. and Gross, J. S. (1996). The 'co-pilot' driver syndrome. *Journal of the American Geriatrics Society*, **44**, 815–17.

Silberfeld, M., Grundstein-Amado, R., Stephens, D., and Deber, R. (1996). Family and physicians' views of surrogate decision-making: the roles and how to choose. *International Psychogeriatrics*, **8**, 589–96.

Smith, A., King, E., Hindley, N., Barnetson, L., Barton, J., and Jobst, K. A. (1998). The experience of research participation and the value of diagnosis in dementia: implications for practice. *Journal of Mental Health*, **7**, 309–21.

Stern, D. (2000). Funding long term care for older people. *British Medical Journal*, **321**, 238. [Letter]

Strang, D. G., Molloy, D. W., and Harrison, C. (1998). Capacity to choose place of residence: autonomy vs beneficence? *Journal of Palliative Care*, **14**, 25–9.

Szasz, T. S. (1960). The myth of mental illness. *American Psychologist*, **15**, 113–18.

Szasz, T. (2000). Second commentary on 'Aristotle's function argument'. *Philosophy, Psychiatry, & Psychology*, **7**, 3–16.

Takala, T. and Gylling, H. A. (2000). Who should know about our genetic makeup and why? *Journal of Medical Ethics*, **26**, 171–4.

van der Steen, J. T., Muller, M. T., Ooms, M. E., van der Wal, G., and Ribbe, M. W. (2000). Decisions to treat or not to treat pneumonia in demented psychogeriatric nursing home patients: development of a guideline. *Journal of Medical Ethics*, **26**, 114–20.

Veatch, R. M. (1988). Justice and the economics of terminal illness. *Hastings Center Report*, **18**, 34–40.

Waddell, C., Clarnette, R. M., Smith, M., and Oldham, L. (1997). Advance directives affecting medical treatment choices. *Journal of Palliative Care*, **13**, 5–8.

Weber, L. J. and Campbell, M. L. (1996). Medical futility and life-sustaining treatment decisions. *Journal of Neuroscience Nursing*, **28**, 56–60.

Whitehouse, P. J. (1996). Future prospects for Alzheimer's disease therapy: ethical and policy issues for the international community. *Acta Neurologica Scandinavica*, **165**, 145–9.

Wiggins, D. (1987). The person as object of science, as subject of experience, and as locus of value. In *Persons and personality. A contemporary inquiry* (ed. A. Peacocke and G. Gillett), pp. 56–74. Blackwell, Oxford.

Wilkes, K. V. (1988). *Real people. Personal identity without thought experiments*. Clarendon Press, Oxford.

Williams, B. A. D. (1973). *Problems of the Self*. Cambridge University Press, Cambridge.

Williamson, P., Hutton, J. L., Bliss, J., Blunt, J., Campbell, M. J., and Nicholson, R. (2000). Statistical review by research ethics committees. *Journal of the Royal Statistical Society*, **163**, 5–13.

Winner, S. (1999). Practical problems with the discharge of old people from hospital—a physician's perspective. In *Ageing, autonomy and resources* (ed. A. Harry Lesser), pp. 51–66. Ashgate, Aldershot.

37 Elder maltreatment

Rolf D. Hirsch and Bodo R. Vollhardt

Introduction

Although elder maltreatment is not a new phenomenon, it has only been recognized as a major issue of health policy in the last two decades. As the proportion of old people in the population has been increasing in most countries, this problem has been looming large on an international scale (Council of Europe 1992; Kosberg and Garcia 1995). Whereas child- and spouse-abuse became an issue of concern to society and research in the 1960s and 1970s, the topic of elder maltreatment was only recognized in the 1980s. Moreover, different degrees of attention were paid to this issue in different countries. This late recognition of the problem has been followed by comparatively little research, as noted by Lachs and Pillemer (1995). In a 5-year literature search in *Index Medicus*, only 26 articles on the topic of 'elder abuse' were found by the authors, of which only four contained primary data. In contrast, 248 references were found on child abuse. Limited coverage in the medical literature has been accompanied by limited attention to this topic by the medical profession. Thus, only 2% of all reports received between 1989 and 1993 on elder maltreatment in the US—Michigan, where reporting is mandatory, had been supplied by physicians (Rosenblatt *et al.* 1996). Similar observations were also reported by Lachs *et al.* (1997) during their study on the prevalence of elder maltreatment.

One of the main reasons why physicians are under-represented in reports of elder maltreatment may be their lack of familiarity with the problem. In a nationwide survey of American emergency physicians (Jones *et al.* 1997*a*) only 25% of the respondents indicated they had received training on the topic of elder maltreatment during their residency, whereas 63% and 87% had received training on spouse-abuse and child-abuse, respectively. Furthermore, they did not attend continuing medical education programmes on this topic when they went into specialty practice. It was also found that despite mandatory reporting, applicable state laws were generally not known. Although most emergency physicians had seen at least one case of suspected elder maltreatment in the year before the survey, a report was only filed in 50% of cases. However, inadequate familiarity of physicians with the problem of elder abuse is not confined to the United States, as shown by McCreadie *et al.* (2000) in a survey of British general practitioners. Only 39% of the respondents indicated some familiarity with the issue, and 72% showed interest in additional training and education.

Any situation involving maltreatment of an elderly person is usually complex and multifactorial. Most cases have a prior history, and usually more than one type of maltreatment is involved (for example, physical and psychological abuse). Often, the situation is compounded by passivity and helplessness of all involved, and by unfamiliarity with remedial action. A case in point:

Case 1

Mr K, a 66-year-old gentleman, has been cared for at home by his wife since he suffered a stroke 2 years ago. A mild dementia has also been present since that time. In the past several weeks, Mr K. has developed a third-degree pressure ulcer. The apartment is in disarray and has become increasingly filthy. Homecare has been provided during the last few months and the GP has been making weekly visits to Mr K. who has been suffering pains lately. Subsequently, he has been rather restless, frequently moaning and groaning. His wife has been desperate and has indicated that she can not take the situation any longer.

The presence of a pressure ulcer indicates the possibility of negligent care. This judgement, however, is dependent on an assessment of whether the pressure ulcer could have been prevented and whether timely and adequate treatment was given. Other questions raised by the situation include whether risk factors had been present and whether these had been recognized and adequately attended to. Have preventive routines been used appropriately, such as attention to mobility, sufficient turning, attendance to urinary incontinence? Was it at all appropriate to attempt home care in the setting? Had attention been given to the wife who was overburdened with the situation? The answers to such questions will depend on subjective perceptions and judgements and do not lend themselves easily to an objective decision. The complexity involved may prevent an acknowledgement that a maltreatment situation is present and, consequently, the opportunity to take appropriate remedial action may be missed.

Elder persons who are dependent on care, especially those suffering from additional psychiatric problems, are usually without the means to help themselves when they are maltreated. They may react with disturbing behaviour, which may then be followed by more maltreatment, for example being placed in restraints. The role of the physicians in caring for these patients calls for an awareness of the indicators of maltreatment, familiarity with assessment techniques, as well as knowledge about helpful interventions. These are geared towards the prevention, treatment, and rehabilitation for all parties involved in the maltreatment situation, and less towards a search for perpetrators and their punishment.

Definition and types of maltreatment

The problem of elder maltreatment has been an issue for politicians, researchers, and professionals from social sciences, law, psychology, and from health services alike. Each profession dealing with this problem has tended to produce its own views and definitions; for example, if elder maltreatment is viewed as a crime, the definition of elder maltreatment will then be based on the components *intent, injury, and causation.* Elder maltreatment may also be viewed as a social problem. Viewed in this way, the definition will emphasize the role of cultural perceptions, social norms, and standards. Still other views focus on the consequences of damage for the victim, and hold that elder maltreatment is more than just socially undesirable behaviour. Such views prefer to include motivational aspects, and the role of aggression, into the definition of maltreatment.

The literature has applied different terms for similar phenomena, with different shades of meaning for the same problem, such as:

- *Abuse* refers to acts of commission resulting in pain, injury, or constraint of another person. Subsumed under this term are physical, psychological, sexual, and financial types of damages and infringements.
- *Aggression* emphasizes the intent to inflict harm or damage. This aspect is included in some abuse definitions without specifically referring to aggression.
- *Maltreatment* refers to behaviours harmful by their violation of expectations, established rules, or standards. This term is included in the tenth revision of the *International statistical classification of diseases and related health problems* (ICD-10) of the World Health Organization (WHO 1992).
- *Mistreatment* indicates any kind of harmful, improper, or incorrect treatment, including all types of abuse and neglect.
- *Neglect* refers to acts of omission resulting in a failure to provide basic means for the support of physical and emotional health and for basic functions in activities of daily living (ADL). Subsumed under this term are active (wilful failure) as well as passive acts of neglect (non-wilful failure, out of ignorance or lack of skills).
- *Violence* is mostly used to refer to domestic offensive forceful actions against children and spouses; as well as for public crimes.

Table 37.1 ICD-10 codes for elder maltreatment

T 74.–	**Maltreatment syndromes**
T 74.0	Neglect or abandonment
T 74.1	Physical abuse
T 74.2	Sexual abuse
T 74.3	Psychological abuse
T 74.8	Other maltreatment syndromes
T 74.9	Maltreatment syndrome, unspecified

In this chapter we will predominantly use the term *maltreatment* as a generic term and *abuse* as a special type of maltreatment, in accordance with the nomenclature in ICD-10. A total of six different types of maltreatment are listed in the ICD-10 (see Table 37.1), none being supplied with a definition. Criminal offence against the elderly might also be subsumed under this heading, but since it is covered in Chapter 38 we will not discuss this aspect in this chapter.

A review of 21 studies on elder maltreatment found 34 different definitions (Tatara 1990). It is therefore necessary to begin with a precise definition. There is some general agreement in the literature that elder maltreatment covers acts of commission as well as of omission, both resulting in harmful consequences for an elder person. A working definition for different types of maltreatment is given in Table 37.2. Less agreement has been reached as to the typology of mistreatment, and this is particularly true for the definition of self-neglect as a form of maltreatment. However, such an extension of the maltreatment concept has been viewed as difficult and contradictory (O'Brian *et al.* 1999), since self-neglect has been related to different types of problems in the psychiatric literature. In addition, the topic as addressed is highly dependent on situational factors such as the availability of medical treatments and of caregivers, as well as the psychiatric status of the victim: including the capacity to accept or to refuse needed care.

Definitions of maltreatment have also made reference to the care setting. McCreadie *et al.* (2000) define elder mistreatment as:

> Harmful or distressing behaviour to an older person (aged 65 plus) by someone whom he or she should be able to trust, e.g. a family member or a paid carer.

In the definition of the National Council on Elder Abuse (NCEA 2000), additional reference is made to the location of maltreatment by distinguishing between domestic and institutional types of maltreatment. This distinction is important for US state laws that hold paid caregivers criminally liable, while exonerating informal carers such as family members or friends.

As social scientists have pointed out, maltreatment, rather than being only an interpersonal event, is also influenced by a variety of situational and environmental factors (Galtung 1990). These may include inhumane working conditions, negative societal views on ageing, as well as social acceptance of violence as a part of every day life. Such social and situational aspects need to be considered when trying to define maltreatment, since remedial interventions may be targeted at them. These factors are difficult to assess and work their way by indirect effects. In the nursing home, such factors may include, among others, inadequate staffing, failure to provide supervision for the support of the staff, or daily routines organized for the convenience of staff or the institution rather than the residents. In addition to such structural factors, cultural influences may also have an effect. These may be expressed, for example, in views that the elderly are no longer capable of handling their own affairs. Galtung views maltreatment as an infringement of basic human needs including the need of well-being, of survival, of personal identity, and of personal freedom. In this model, maltreatment is viewed as the result of a direct action by a person, that person in turn being influenced by structural and cultural forces (Fig. 37.1). The former are expressed by processes and procedures (procedural), the latter especially by language, ideology, and belief systems. Cultural factors are considered to be difficult to change and hence invariable, and they are liable to legitimize structural forces.

The triangular model, by emphasizing cultural and structural forces as antecedents for maltreatment, tends to de-emphasize personal aspects such as the personality and motivation of the perpetrator, and may even regard the perpetrator as a victim in some instances. This is a

Table 37.2 Types of elder maltreatment

Type of abuse	Definition	Examples	Medical indications
Physical abuse	Forceful acts inflicting pain, injury, or impairment	Hitting, pushing, shoving, inappropriate use of drugs or restraints; force feeding, physical punishment	Unexplained bruises or lacerations, injuries bilateral or in various stages of healing, broken eyeglasses, signs of having been restrained, serum drug levels indicating overmedication
Sexual abuse	Any kind of forced intimate or sexual contact with a person	Sexual explicit advances such as touching, exposure, assault	Bruises around breasts or genitals, vaginal or rectal bleeding, unexplained venereal disease
Psychological (emotional) abuse	Verbal or non-verbal conduct resulting in anguish or distress	Threats, harassement, intimidation, insults, behaviour expressing disinterest in a person, infantilizing behaviour	A sudden change in behaviour of the elder person including agitation, anxiety, depression, withdrawal, or other unusual behaviour.
Financial exploitation	Unauthorized use of an elder's funds or property for the personal gain of the caretaker	Withdrawal from bank account, stealing money or possessions, pressuring elder for signature on documents	Substandard care despite availability of adequate financial resources, unfilled prescriptions for medication or for rehabilitation aids
Neglect	Failure to provide care for basic needs, optimal function, or medical treatments	Inadequate food, fluids, hygiene, clothing, shelter, personal safety, health care	Dehydration, malnutrition, bed sores, poor hygiene of person and/or of living environment, inadequate medication administration, unsafe home
Violation of personal rights	Ignoring elder's rights or capabilities to make own decisions	Not involving an elder in decision-making, inappropriate handling of guardianship	Forced placement in nursing home, limiting the social contacts of elder.

Compiled from Aravanis *et al.* 1992; Fillit and Picariello 1998; National Council on Elder Abuse 2000.

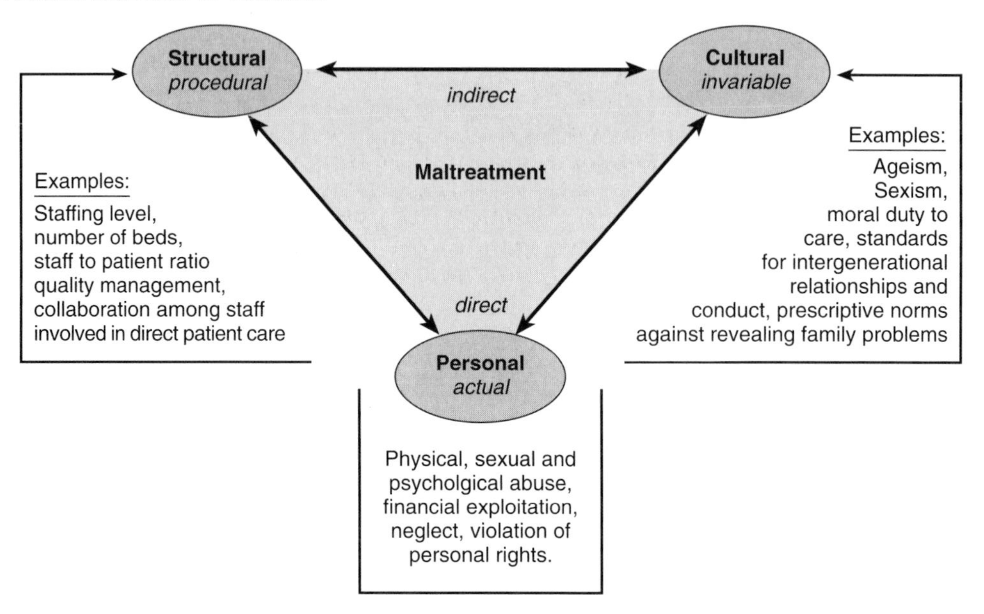

Figure 37.1: The triangular maltreatment model (adapted from Galtung 1990, Hirsch 2000)

stark contrast to the crime model of maltreatment which focuses on the delinquent person, their intent, and culpability. It would, however, be naïve to understand this model as ignoring the personal responsibility of the maltreating person. Rather, this model has pragmatic implications by establishing a frame of reference for remedial interventions based on four tenets:

- the definition of maltreatment as an avoidable infringement of basic human needs. By virtue of its neutrality this definition permits a non-stigmatizing approach to critical situations which require the uncovering and clear presentation of underlying facts in order to allow remedial action;
- the understanding of maltreatment as something that has developed from many sources, each of which may be corrected;
- the need for a multidimensional approach to assessment;
- the avoidance of a dichotomy between victim and perpetrator.

The scope of the problem

Incidence

Mandatory reporting of elder maltreatment to Adult Protective Services (the APS) in the US has provided yearly statistics (collected by the NCEA) on the incidence rates of elder maltreatment in US federal states. According to this administration, the number of reports on elder mistreatment has increased steadily. In 1986 117 000 cases were reported but by 1996 this number had risen to 293 000 cases, corresponding to an increase of 150% in just 10 years (Tatara and Kuzmeskus 1997). However, this number does not necessarily imply that the actual maltreatment of elderly in the general population has increased at that rate. Rather, it may reflect an increased awareness of the problem and/or an improved acceptance of the option to report maltreatment of the elderly.

At present, the best available estimate of the actual incidence rates of elder maltreatment in the

United States has been provided by the National Elder Abuse Incidence Study (NEAIS). This study (NCEA and Westat. Inc. 1998), is based on data collected prospectively on persons representative of the national elder population over the age of 60 not living in institutions. A single definition established by expert consensus was used for case identification. In addition to reports received by the APS agencies, data were collected from specially trained reporters working in community agencies serving senior citizens (sentinel approach). These sentinels were in a position to collect four times as many cases as those officially reported to the APS. Excluding cases of self-neglect, which were also recorded, this study shows an annual incidence of approximately 1.2% of maltreatment cases in the elder population not living in institutions in the United States. This study has done pioneer work in allowing an estimation of the magnitude of unreported cases (the so-called iceberg effect) by showing that for each case of elder maltreatment reported, at least four go unreported.

The reports of elder maltreatment to the APS had a confirmation rate of 49%; in 39% of suspected cases, maltreatment could not be confirmed. Physical abuse had the highest rate of confirmation, 69%, whereas reports on sexual abuse were confirmed in only 7% of the allegations. Most frequently, family members had filed a report (20%), but only one out of five reports was confirmed. Whereas physicians and nursing staff from hospitals had filed 8% of all reports, their confirmation rate was highest, reaching 86%. In almost 90% of confirmed cases, the maltreatment was committed by a member of the family; in order of frequency by adult children (47%), spouses (19%), and other members of the family (24%). The majority of victims were women (67%) in need of care and cognitively impaired. Those over 80 years of age were over-represented. Types of maltreatment included different forms of neglect (54%), physical abuse (15%), financial exploitation (12%), and emotional abuse (8%) (all figures rounded).

Another study from Iowa, where the duty to report is mandatory only for cases involving professional carers, analysed reports made to the APS over a period of 10 years (Jogerst *et al.* 2000). Not included were cases of self-neglect. The confirmation rate of 26.5% was comparatively low. The average yearly incidence rate was 1.27% and was correlated with the local population census and with rates of reported child abuse, among others.

The data from these two studies currently provide the most reliable basis for estimating maltreatment incidence rates in the US. However, methodological constraints, such as subject selection and data collection sensitive to both to under- and over-reporting, limit their generalizability.

Prevalence

Methodological problems with under-reporting, selection bias, and a focus on different aspects on maltreatment are even more prominent in prevalence studies on estimates of elder maltreatment. Such studies have looked at this problem in the community and in domestic, as well as institutional, care-settings for dementia patients.

Community

Prevalence estimates of elder maltreatment in the community range from 1.2% (Kurrle *et al.* 1997) to 10.8% (Hirsch and Brendebach 1999), depending on the method chosen. Most of these estimates are based on self-reports and have been collected retrospectively over different periods. Maltreatment after the age of 65 years was reported by 3.2% of those interviewed by telephone in a study conducted by Pillemer and Finkelhor (1988). Whereas this estimate has been frequently used as an indicator for the prevalence of elder maltreatment in the population at large, this figure, due to a narrow definition and exclusion of some types of maltreatment, has been considered as too conservative, with the true prevalence estimated to be many times greater than the numbers reported. According to the authors, their data point to the role of maltreating spouses and the poor state of health of those maltreated.

With a similar design, studies have been performed in Australia (Kurrle *et al.* 1992),

Canada (Podnieks 1990), England (Ogg and Bennett 1992), Finland (Kivelä *et al.* 1992), Germany (Wetzels *et al.* 1996; Hirsch and Brendebach 1999), and The Netherlands (Comijs *et al.* 1998).

A more standardized procedure has been utilized by Kurrle *et al.* 1997. These authors employed a geriatric assessment that included psychological and social evaluations. Their sample was recruited from an outpatient geriatric programme, where patients presented for medical evaluation. Data on maltreatment were collected retrospectively as well as prospectively. A 1-year prevalence of 1.2% was found. The majority of the victims were care-recipients with physical (67%) or cognitive impairment (37%). In 87% of the cases, maltreatment had been committed at home by family members (spouses in 38%, adult children in 43%). Recorded in order of frequency: psychological and physical abuse, financial exploitation, and neglect were noted. The majority of subjects (65% of all cases) had suffered more than one type of maltreatment.

Estimates on prevalence have also been based on data by the APS agencies. In an epidemiological longitudinal study, Lachs *et al.* (1996) sampled reports for suspected maltreatment from subjects in the cohort. During an 11-year period, 6.4% of the subjects had been reported to the APS agencies, maltreatment was confirmed in 75% of the cases. In order of frequency the types of maltreatment included: self-neglect, neglect, abuse, and financial exploitation.

Domestic care of dementia patients

Table 37.3 gives an overview of empirical studies on maltreatment in the domestic care of dementia patients. This population of persons with impaired communication and severe memory disturbances has been shown to carry a special risk for maltreatment. For this reason, most of the studies have chosen to obtain information on maltreatment by the caregivers. Since one might question the reliability of this kind of information, alternative methods of assessment have employed anonymous questionnaires or covert ratings performed by visiting home services. With appropriate techniques, however, data obtained by personal interview do not contradict the data from studies that have used different methods. Contrary to expectations, caregivers were open to a suggestion for a personal interview and were willing to talk about this problem, in a way that appeared to the investigator to be non-defensive (Pillemer and Moore 1989; Homer and Gilleard 1990; Pillemer and Suitor 1992). All studies reviewed have worked with quantitative methods, have used similar definitions of maltreatment, and collected data with the help of valid measurements. The findings of these studies agree on a number of important points:

- different types of maltreatment are associated with different risk factors;
- reciprocity of maltreatment may be encountered following an established pattern of past spousal relationship;
- psychological abuse is the most frequent form of maltreatment, followed by physical abuse;
- abuse of the caregiver is encountered two to four times as frequently as abuse of the care recipient.

The caregivers were found to be depressed and burdened as a consequence of the caregiving context and the symptoms of dementia. However, not all studies found a clear-cut relationship between abuse and care burden or cognitive impairment. Another important finding of these studies has been a pattern of reactivity for abuse. This replicates earlier findings, obtained with a different method by Hamel *et al.* (1990). Since an abusive pattern established in the premorbid relationship frequently underlies mutual abuse in domestic dementia care, the added release of aggression and behavioural disturbance in dementia (Keene *et al.* 1999; Lyketsos *et al.* 2000) may be expected to increase the risk for abuse in these situations.

Institutional care of dependent elder

Despite public awareness of elder maltreatment in hospitals and nursing homes, heightened from time to time by gruesome reports in the media,

Table 37.3 Maltreatment in domestic dementia-care*

Authors	Methods	Prevalence	Significant findings
Homer and Gilleard 1990	Structured interview and rating scales obtained from 51 Cgs and their 43 Crs, referred for respite care	Overall 6-month prevalence for abuse 45%; including emotional abuse 42%; physical abuse 47%; neglect 12%	Alcoholism and depression scores (Cg); problem-behaviour (Cr), abusive premorbid relationship (Cg and Cr). Mental impairment (Cr) non-significant for maltreament
Paveza *et al.* 1992	Questionnaire and telephone interview obtained from 184 Cgs referred from a multi-site dementia registry	Overall prevalence for violence since dementia diagnosis 17%; 16% directed at Cg; 5% at Cr; 5% in Cd	Depression scores (Cg), living with immediate family but without the spouse (Cr). Cognitive or functional impairment non-significant for maltreatment
Pillemer and Suitor 1992	Structured interview and rating scales obtained from 236 Cgs referred from different dementia screening sites	For unspecified period: 6% of the Cgs had used violence; 25% had been subjected to it; 19% had violent feelings	*Actual violence*: mutual violence (Cd), spouse-status and age (Cg) *Violent feelings:* care-demands, ADL-impairment, behavioural problems (Cr), mutual violence, living together (Cd)
Coyne *et al.* 1993	Postal questionnaires obtained from 342 Cgs picked up from a phone-helpline	Throughout Cd: 12% of Cgs had perpetrated abuse; 33% had been subjected to it	Longer care, more daily care-hours (Cd); functional impairment (Cr), depression scores (Cg)
Cooney *et al.* 1995	Postal questionnaires obtained from 67 Cgs members of a volunteer organization	Overall 1-year prevalence 55%, including: 52% emotional abuse; 12% physical abuse; 12% neglect.	*Physical abuse*: psychological symptoms (Cg), longer caring relationship and mutual abuse, not related: Cr variables *Verbal abuse*: abusive premorbid relationship, mutual abuse (Cd), social isolation (Cg)
Mendonica *et al.* 1996	Ratings by visiting nurses on 82 observed family Cds	Emotional abuse 11%; physical abuse 5%; financial exploitation 5%; various forms of neglect 5%	Physical neglect predicts physical abuse, and psychosocial neglect emotional abuse. Financial exploitation predicts emotional abuse

*Cg stands for Caregiver, Cr for Care-receiver Cd for care-dyad. All numbers are rounded.

little is actually known about the true prevalence of institutional maltreatment. For different reasons research in this area has been difficult. Impairments in memory and communication render interviews with care recipients unreliable, while reporting bias and the need to cover up what might be an offence under penal law make the information obtained from interviews of staff difficult to evaluate. The diversity of organizations and structures in institutions may not be comparable thereby making representative sampling difficult to achieve. Perhaps the only common characteristics of these institutions may be those of a total institution (Goffman 1961) in being governed by administrative regulations, standards, and routines that impinge on the autonomy and privacy of clients. In this setting the boundaries between institutional routines and acts of maltreatment may be difficult to distinguish in a given case. Glendenning (1999) has therefore distinguished institutional or institutionalized maltreatment from individual acts of maltreatment in institutions.

Given these difficulties, indirect indicators may be used to give an estimate of the prevalence of maltreatment in institutions. Suitable indicators for this purpose are the prescribing practices for psychoactive drugs and the use of mechanical restraints. Another approach may be to determine the prevalence of putative indicators for negligent care, such as pressure ulcers.

Nursing homes

Table 37.4 combines findings from two studies that have looked at the prevalence of maltreatment in a sample from different nursing homes in a given area. Different methods of data collection notwithstanding, some conclusions reached by the studies were in agreement. Maltreatment can be related to characteristics of the residents, problems in the interaction between staff and residents, and work satisfaction of the staff. Both studies have also found that resident aggression frequently precedes staff maltreatment and that there may be mutual aggressive interactions between both. Other studies have added further details to this point. With a questionnaire completed anonymously by 126 nursing assistants, Goodridge *et al.* (1996) found a 1-month prevalence of 84% for reported psychological abuse of nursing assistants by residents and a corresponding figure of 58% for physical abuse. Commenting on these findings, Goodridge *et al.* note dryly:

> On average, a nursing assistant in this health care facility may expect to be physically assaulted by residents 9.3 times per month and verbally assaulted 11.3 times per month.

Similar results were obtained by Hagen and Sayers (1995). In a 200-bed facility, these authors found an 8-day prevalence of 182 reported acts of physical aggression by residents against nursing assistants, 6% of which resulted in physical injuries. Most of these incidents occurred during routine nursing care such as dressing and changing (48%), turning and transfer (22%), assisting in meals (8%), and bathing (7%) (all figures rounded).

As Goodridge *et al.* (1996) have shown in their analysis, a situation involving maltreatment of an elder dependent needs to be viewed from the situational context brought about by extreme working conditions and responsibilities unmatched by the level of training. Although nursing assistants or untrained carers take a central role in the care of residents, they receive little appreciation, are underpaid, and are frequently viewed as dispensable at will. While frequently encountering conflict situations with residents, they have usually not received training on interpersonal aspects of nursing care or on conflict-resolving techniques. Therefore resident abuse in institutions needs to be viewed in the context of the institutional structures in the setting. Healthcare Canada (1994, as quoted by Goodridge *et al.* 1996) define systemic abuse as

> harmful situations created, permitted, or facilitated by procedures and processes within institutions including situations where institutions do not provide or structure resources in a manner that allows recognized standards of care to be met.

Table 37.4 Maltreatment in nursing homes

Author	Methods	Prevalence	Significant findings
Pillemer and Moore 1989 Pillemer and Bachman-Prehn 1991	Structured telephone interview of 677 nurses and nursing-aides from different nursing homes	One-year prevalence rates for: *maltreatment observed by staff*: 36% physical abuse,81% psychological abuse *maltreatment committed*: 10% physical and 40% psychological abuse	Abuse associated with less work satisfaction,burn-out symptoms, aggressive behaviour of patients, younger age of care professional, negative attitudes towards patient, staff–patient conflict. Psychological abuse also related to personal life stress of caregiver. No association between and size of facility, staff quality
Schneider 1990	Questionnaires from 205 administrators and nursing staff selected by administrators from different nursing homes	No time period specified *Resident to resident:* psychological aggression often 2–7%, sometimes 6–37%; physical aggression often 1%, sometimes 2–3% *Resident to staff:* psychological aggression often 2–3%, sometimes 8–31%; physical aggression often 0%, sometimes 1% *Staff to resident*: psychological aggression often 1–2%, sometimes 2–11%; physical aggression often 0%, sometimes 6%	Agression related to: *Resident's variables*: cognitive impairment and social competence *Staff variables*: work- and life-satisfaction, stressors *Structural variables*: staffing level, size of facility, census of local town *Milieu variables*: general level of aggression increased in care milieu with number of aggressive acts (violence escalation)

Medical interventions as infringements of basic human needs

Mechanical restraints

The successful implementation of nationwide restraint reduction programmes in nursing homes in the US under the regulations of the Omnibus Budget Reconciliation Act-1987 (OBRA-87) has clearly shown that the restraint practice in use until then had been excessive. From an average of 40%, the rate of restraints has been reduced in US nursing homes to an average of 21% (Williams and Finch 1997). Even this figure may be viewed as excessive when considering restraint rates of 4% in nursing homes in another American study (Neufeld *et al.* 1999). The practice of using restraints has been shown to depend on the geographical location and the staffing level. Improving staffing level and providing special care units to residents suffering from dementia has allowed staff to limit the use of restraints. Whereas considerable reduction in the use of restraints has taken place, there has been no change in the level of resident risk factors (Castle *et al.* 1997).

Despite these successful changes, traditional beliefs continue to influence decision-making about the use of restraints. It is still argued by some that mechanical restraints prevent falls, but in fact restraint use is poorly correlated with standardized fall assessment (Karlson *et al.* 1997). Falls are not prevented by placing residents in restraints, and reducing restraints does not increase the number of falls (Capezuti *et al.* 1996; Neufeld *et al.* 1999). Rather, the risk of falls is increased by the use of mechanical restraints, especially at the point when they are discontinued (Tinetti *et al.* 1992; Arbesman and Wright 1999).

Another frequent reason given for the use of restraint has been to control disturbing behaviour and agitation, particularly in residents suffering from dementia. Experience has shown, however, that restraint use will not control consistently disturbed behaviour but may in fact worsen agitation, and cause anxiety and anguish. It has also been documented that restraints are associated with objective indices for subsequent intellectual decline, immobility, and loss of physical function as well as increased morbidity (Evans and Strumpf 1989). There has also been documentation of lethal complications of restraint use (Parker and Miles 1997). Moreover, it has been shown that the decision to place an elder dependent resident in restraints may not so much reflect the special risk of that person, but features of the institution itself—such as the staff-to-resident ratio, staffing level, geographic location, and restricted reimbursement rates. Another factor relevant for restraint practice is the particular institutional philosophy and the prevailing *myths* (Strumpf and Evans 1991) believed by the staff (Phillips *et al.* 1996; Castle and Fogel 1997). This body of research may be taken as empirical evidence for the relevance of the triangular model proposed by Galtung, considering that mechanical restraints are infringements of basic human needs and that their use:

- may frequently be avoided;
- may depend more on the structure of the care setting rather than on the individual risk profile of the resident;
- may be influenced by cultural attitudes and perceptions.

The current restraint practice in different settings is reflected in point prevalence rates. As reported in the literature, the corresponding figures for geropsychiatric institutions range from 24% to 45% (De Santis *et al.* 1997; Kranzhoff and Hirsch 1997; Karlson *et al.* 1998), from 4% to 22% in nursing homes (Karlson *et al.* 1997; Neufeld *et al.* 1999), and between 17% and 18% in acute geriatric care (Robins *et al.* 1987; Karlson *et al.* 1998). The spread of these figures highlight the role of extraneous factors and a practice of over- and misusing mechanical restraints in current institutional elder care.

Use of psychoactive drugs in nursing homes

The use of psychoactive drugs in nursing homes is common practice: between 17 and 78% of residents will receive at least one prescription of a psychoactive drug (Llorente *et al.* 1998; Schmidt *et al.* 1998). Prescribing practices for drugs have been criticized because of inappropriate choices, hazardous combinations, and failure to discontinue prescriptions at an appropriate time (Board of Directors of the American Association for Geriatric Psychiatry 1992). Such misuse is more prevalent in institutions with less adequate treatment resources (Svarstad and Mount 1991; Riedel-Heller *et al.* 1999). Whereas neuroleptics, hypnotics, and especially benzodiazepines are overused, antidepressants are underused, despite the well-known high prevalence of depression in nursing homes. This prescription practice points to a use of psychoactive drugs that is geared more to the control of non-specific symptoms and less to the specific treatment of a diagnosed psychiatric illness. This disturbing finding may be indicative of inadequate geropsychiatric care in nursing homes. In response to this problem, guidelines have been established by OBRA-87 for the use of psychoactive drugs in US nursing homes, including the requirements for specific indications for drug use, schedules for the reduction and discontinuation of drugs, the employment of non-drug treatment alternatives such as behavioural interventions, and prohibition of as-needed schedules. These regulations have been quite successful in restricting the use of psychoactive drugs, especially when combined with educational programmes. Efforts to reduce psychoactive drug use by offering a visiting consulting service and medical education programmes have been successful in other countries as well, but to a lesser extent than achieved under the OBRA regulations in the US (Schmidt *et al.* 1998; Snowdon 1999).

Putative indicators for neglect: pressure ulcers

Pressure ulcers are generally considered as preventable, and their presence a putative indicator for negligent care. Long ago, Florence Nightingale (1849) considered them 'generally the fault not of the disease but of the nursing'. This traditional view may be justified on the grounds of findings from studies that have established a relationship between pressure ulcers and institutional parameters such as staffing level, number of beds, geographical location, inadequacies in nursing care, in wound treatment, and in medical documentation, as well as a general lack of quality care (Rudman *et al.* 1993; Bergstrom *et al.* 1996; Spector and Fortinsky 1998; Berlowitz *et al.* 1999; Heinemann *et al.* 2000). Despite the availability of standards for risk assessment and preventive measures, these are frequently not used and considerable shortcomings in the prevention and treatment of pressure ulcers may be found in nursing-home care (Bergstrom *et al.* 1996; Heinemann *et al.* 2000). Pressure ulcers have been found more frequently in institutions with other adverse outcomes such as medication errors, a more rapid decline of physical function, and higher levels of disturbing behaviours of residents, typically associated with lower staffing levels and higher staff turnover (Rudman *et al.* 1993; Blegen *et al.* 1998; Ooi *et al.* 1999).

These studies point to the significance of neglect in the institutional care of the elderly. Even though the prevalence and incidence rates reported in the literature may not be fully comparable because different risk profiles in the samples are not adjusted for comparison, the available raw data indicate an incidence for pressure ulcer-stage 2 or above of between 0 and 15%, and up to 38% plus (Bergstrom *et al.* 1996; Rudman *et al.* 1993). The variation in prevalence rates for all stages of pressure ulcers vary from 12% to more than 83% (Spector and Fortinsky 1998; Bours *et al.* 1999). Whereas some of the variation in these figures may actually be accounted for by different risk profiles, these figures nevertheless point to inconsistencies in standards of care, and specifically the lack of quality care in some long-term care institutions. To expect a prevalence of 0%, however, may be unrealistic. This was demonstrated by Hagisawa and Barbenel (1999), who studied pressure ulcer development in a setting with an adequate staffing level and established schedules for routine risk assessment and regular preventive measures. In this setting, annual rates for pressure ulcer development were over 4% (incidence) and over 5% (prevalence).

Causes and consequences

Causal models and risk factors

Prevalence studies have pointed up frequent associations between a maltreatment event and factors in the surrounding situation. These factors have been frequently addressed as risk markers, implying that the likelihood of a maltreatment event is increased in their presence, without the implication of a causal relationship. Diversity and multiplicity of reported risk markers suggest that quite different attendant circumstances may be involved in maltreatment. In an overview of the literature Jones *et al.* (1997*b*) list 19 risk markers for the parties in a maltreatment situation (*victims*, *perpetrators*, and their mutual relationship) as well as 14 factors pertaining to the situational context surrounding the maltreatment event. Reis and Nahmiash (1998) were able to isolate, by discriminant function analysis, 'indicators for abuse' for the person maltreated (including past history of abuse suffered and social isolation) and the person maltreating. The latter include mental health problems and inexperience with caregiving, underdeveloped empathic skills, troubled personal and social relationships, and financial dependence on the care recipient. From the complex tangle of diverse factors, an overview by the NCEA (2000) lists four risk categories: caregiver stress; impairment of dependent elder; cycle of violence; and personal problems of abuser. The relevance of most of these markers in predicting maltreatment has not been well established. In the only published study with a longitudinal prospective design, Lachs *et al.* (1997) found the variables of age, race, poverty, impairments of ADL and cognitive function, as well as the trajectory of cognitive decline, to discriminate the abused from the other subjects in the cohort. Most of the cases were referred for self-neglect to the APS, however, and the authors caution that the sampling may not have been representative.

Cycle of violence

Many studies trying to identify risk markers have been oriented towards existing explanatory models. The first such model was developed in child abuse research. It states that violent behaviour is learned in the family and is then passed on to the next generation. This hypothesis was adapted to elder maltreatment and has led to a number of earlier studies. More recently a large-scale population study has been able to demonstrate an association between elder maltreatment and child abuse in the community at large, but has not analysed this pattern for individual families (Jogerst *et al.* 2000). Maltreatment family dynamics have been found for spousal relationships, in a pattern of mutual abuse turned worse when one spouse became dependent as a consequence of a dementing illness (Homer and Gilleard 1990; Coyne *et al.* 1993). Another lead has been the consistent finding of adult children as the perpetrators of elder maltreatment. There is no study, however, that has looked for a transgenerational transmission of violent behaviour as the cause of maltreatment in these cases. Rather, interpersonal aggression dynamics in elder maltreatment have more often been shown to be reactive, either to aggressive behaviour in the context of a dementing illness, or else in response to caregiver burden. This kind of aggression dynamics is not confined to families but is also prevalent in institutional care, where there may be mutual abuse between residents and staff (Pillemer and Moore 1989; Schneider 1990).

Impairment of dependent elder

Another model has been developed from the observation that elder maltreatment is most prevalent in care dyads. For this paradigm, prospective studies have identified risk markers of functional impairment in physical and cognitive abilities, psychiatric symptoms such as confusion and depression, as well as recent deterioration in cognitive function (Lachs *et al.* 1997; NACEA and Westat Inc.1998). Care dependence has also been shown to be a risk marker in large-scale community studies (Pillemer and Finkelhor 1988; Podniecks 1990). However, findings have been less consistent in this regard in the domestic care of dementia patients. Presumably other factors may increase the risk for maltreatment in this setting including, for example, disturbing behaviour of the care recipient or stress symptoms of the caregiver (Paveza *et al.* 1992; Cooney and Mortimer 1995).

Caregiver stress

Care requirements of the dependent elder will place high emotional, physical, as well financial demands on the caregiver. The resulting burden is a continual challenge to the personal stress-tolerance limits of the carer. Constant pressure by care demands and the necessity to defer one's own needs as well as obligations to family, work, and friends may lead to exhaustion and social isolation as well as to emotional stress symptoms (Coyne *et al.* 1993). Burden notwithstanding, it is frequently not the caregiving context in and of itself, but the added presence of other factors that raise an existing risk situation to a critical level and precipitate maltreatment. Such factors may include specific living arrangements, lack of support for the task of caring, and financial or emotional dependency. Situational trigger events, external stresses, or illness of the caregiver may also acutely raise risk (Jones *et al.* 1997*b*; Kleinschmid 1997). In institutional care, the caregiver's burden is also frequently found to be an antecedent for maltreatment. Of special importance in this regard is the burn-out syndrome of the nursing staff (Pillemer and Moore 1989). In addition, stresses in the personal life of the staff, and institutional factors as well as the situational context have been described (Schneider 1990; Goodridge *et al.* 1996; Glendenning 1999).

Personal problems of the person maltreating

In addition to stress symptoms from the caregiving burden, many studies have uncovered personal problems of the maltreating person, including alcoholism and psychiatric illness. Social isolation, and emotional and material dependence on the care recipient have also been described, as summarized by Jones *et al.* 1997*b* and Kleinschmidt 1997. These factors are interdependent, but, given a cross-sectional study design, it has not been possible to establish whether the factors are antecedents or consequences. Undoubtedly, however, such factors identify persons in trouble who lack the emotional stability to endure the stress of caregiving. Many of the perpetrators are weak and helpless themselves and it may be justified, considering the specifics of a given case, to view the *perpetrator* as a *victim* of attendant circumstances, being unable to take charge of a difficult and overwhelming situation.

A working model for maltreatment

In sum, the literature on risk factors suggests that a one-dimensional approach is not adequate to account for maltreatment. Every maltreatment has its own history and carries along its own risk factors. Drawing on available evidence, Jones *et al.* (1997*b*) have formulated a multidimensional explanatory model, offering a useful tool for educational purposes as well as for professional work with a maltreated elder. However, this model does not account for the structural factors of a maltreatment situation. In our own work we favour a model in which we assume that every caregiver has the individual potential for a maltreatment behaviour in a given situation. The threshold of such behaviour is influenced by personal values and structural factors connected with the caring situation, as well as by the personal characteristics of all people involved in the situation and the kind of relationships among them. The trigger point may be extraneous, such as disturbing behaviour of the elder: e. g. incontinence or communication problems, or acute stress on the caregiver from any source.

Consequences of maltreatment

Field studies from nursing homes have described emotional reactions to maltreatment, especially by neglect (Schneider 1994). These have included depressive symptoms with feelings of helplessness and social withdrawal, suicidal thoughts, and regressive symptoms, but no psychiatric assessment or standardized evaluation has been reported. Single case studies, as reviewed by Wolf

(1997), have indicated the presence of depression, and post-traumatic stress disorder has also been mentioned. A more systematic approach has been taken by Comijs *et al.* 1998, who reported follow-up data on 43 maltreated subjects. Most of these indicated reactions of anger, disappointment, or grief, and one in four reported having reacted with aggressive behaviour in turn. In the study by Hirsch and Brendebach (1999), only 5 of the 44 subjects who reported having suffered maltreatment indicated the absence of any emotional sequelae, whereas all others reported significant emotional distress, including anxiety, feelings of humiliation, and being unable to forget. Only one subject reported an aggressive response in the event. Long-term consequences included avoiding or completely breaking contact with the person maltreating.

In addition to emotional distress reactions, physical effects bearing on mortality have been reported by Lachs *et al.* (1998). During longitudinal follow-up for 9 years, maltreatment as confirmed by the APS was shown to be an independent predictor of early death, all other known mortality risk factors being controlled for.

Assessment

A multi-step procedure is required to understand how a maltreatment situation came about, and to determine what kinds of interventions may be helpful. In any case of suspected maltreatment it is necessary to systematically gather the facts about the situation and about the people involved (Table 37.5). In addition, an evaluation has to be made of whether the maltreated person wants changes made in the situation or is afraid of them, especially when the dreaded consequences of such changes include retaliation or abandonment. In some relationships in which dysfunctional patterns have been entrenched over a long period, there is a great reluctance to accept help from outside.

If it is possible to overcome such barriers, then an evaluation of the people involved and the contextual (structural and cultural) features of the situation is needed. All these aspects are brought into focus by an assessment (Table 37.6). It serves the purpose of uncovering existing maltreatment patterns, finding the points amenable to intervention, and exploring available sources of help. In the majority of cases, antecedents have gone unrecognized for some time. This aspect requires exploration as much as those factors that have precipitated or aggravated the event.

To be able to recognize maltreatment, attention to possible indicators, awareness of 'red flags', and perception of pertinent details is crucial. It is still rare for physicians to recognize the signs of physical abuse, despite distinct indicators and typical clinical presentations (Lachs and Pillemer 1995).

Interventions

Maltreatment may be contagious, and a situation not worked through and resolved will usually be repeated. Usually, professional help is needed to resolve a maltreatment situation and to stabilize the results. Rarely will one intervention suffice to correct a problem; more typically several interventions in collaborative work by several professional groups are required. Physicians, by virtue of the respect and trust they enjoy from the public, have a special role in this task.

Unfortunately many maltreatment situations, by the time they come to light, have been in existence for a long time and have developed into a chronic problem. It may therefore be quite difficult to achieve more than partial success. Some of those afflicted tend to complain but may be reluctant to consider any changes. Others may be unwilling to accept help because of the fear that maltreatment may increase when a third party becomes involved. In such situations, too, mitigation rather than complete change may be all that can be achieved.

Community

Maltreatment in families is a visible manifestation of a destructive pattern in the relationship between family members that has been present for some time. In such families, spouses frequently share a similar background with difficult relationships, including violence, in their families of origin. They are tied together by similar conflicts in their relationship, as well as by weak communication skills. Usually, many signals have been ignored over a long period. Existing ties in the relationships are about to come undone or have already been cut. Violence has become part of the ordinary and has shown up regularly in many different ways. Stress levels have increased and an acute crisis has arisen. Often, one member has escaped or left already, by illness, admission to a hospital or to a nursing home, or by death.

A troubled person seeking help should be encouraged to talk about all their concerns on the initial contact. Prior to any kind of intervention planning it is important to satisfy concerns for safety. The plan must ensure that maltreatment can be brought to a stop immediately. This can mean separation of the parties involved, either by admission to a hospital or referral to social services. Further steps are:

- An attempt needs to be made to arrange for an interview with all involved, alone and together. Such an interview needs to be conducted in a neutral atmosphere. Blame and prejudice need to be avoided, but it may be appropriate for all parties to share their own observations. The focus should be on patterns of maltreatment, and as they relate to patterns of interactions in the family. Strategies for communication skills and conflict-solving techniques, typically absent or underdeveloped in such families, need to be emphasized and potentials for change in the family system pointed out.
- Available local resources that need to be utilized may include counselling services, self-help groups, family support groups, psychosocial services, psychiatric community services, as well as pastoral counselling. The guideline for all such interventions is the basic principle of *help before punishment*.
- If it becomes apparent that social support will not be enough or will be unlikely to succeed in stopping the maltreatment, referral for legal services may be required.

Having an opportunity to talk about their problems and their fears in a private and protected atmosphere may be a significant relief for many families, and grounds for the building of trust, which allows a working alliance to be established, aimed at making and stabilizing necessary changes. Specific interventions following an initial interview depend on the type and intensity of maltreatment, the options agreeable to the parties involved, and their expectations, their value systems, and availability of social support systems. Some examples of possible interventions are listed below:

Level of personal (direct) interventions:

- If there is a psychiatric or medical illness or impairment of one of the parties involved in the maltreatment situation, referral for medical, psychiatric, or rehabilitation services may be necessary.
- For ongoing quarrels and frictions in the spousal relationship, referral for marital counselling or individual therapy may be indicated.
- Conflicts that have arisen from dependency issues require arrangements to be put in place to ensure the right type of distance between the carer and the dependent person (for example, ensuring the carer has their own room, arranging time out from care demands, involving other family members in caregiving tasks), as well as psychotherapeutic interventions to decrease dependency in the relationship.
- For problems involving a violation of personal rights, referral for legal advice may be needed, as well as support from friends, neighbours, or professionals from community services.

Level of structural interventions:

- Referral to community programmes, as indicated, for: senior citizen-assertiveness training and courses on self-defence; local crisis support services, such as telephone helplines and counselling services; or self-help groups.
- Organizing educational programmes for professional service providers on the problem of maltreatment in families and on the types of helpful interventions.
- Getting the topic of elder maltreatment covered by the media. Encourage witnesses of a maltreatment situation to 'blow the whistle',

and to avoid collusion with the perpetrator by inactivity and silence.

Level of cultural interventions:

- Education on violence (questioning beliefs that violence may be unavoidable, offering training in conflict negotiation and conflict resolution, emphasizing non-violent behaviour alternatives).
- Education on ageing (ageist attitudes and how to reduce them, ageing as a normal psycho-physical process, emphasizing the knowledge and wisdom encountered in old age, and competency models of old age).
- Education on how to care for old people (questioning patronizing attitudes towards old people, e.g. how can younger people 'know what's best for old people'?).

Domestic care for the dependent elder

The dependence of an elder person usually means a critical life event for the family. Typically, it has the most severe consequences for daughters and daughters-in-law, since male family members rarely feel obligated to involve themselves directly with the ongoing care. Females in the family usually have to change their lives altogether, and they bear extremes of emotional and physical burden. A critical point is reached when they can no longer maintain their own autonomy because of guilt feelings, unresolved conflicts from their past relationship with the dependent elder, or other conflicts resulting from consequences imposed on their personal lives by caregiving. Such troubled caregivers will tend to drift into social isolation, while at the same time becoming increasingly overburdened. Care burden alone is rarely the cause of a maltreatment. When that has occurred, the caregiver typically has become enmeshed with the person dependent on care in what may be considered a pathological life situation. Outside help has not been acceptable, or even offered, and a climate fostering violent feelings and maltreatment has been in existence for some time. Possible interventions then include

On a personal level:

- Involve other family members in caregiving, optimize the available community services.
- Refer to family support groups (e.g. from the local Alzheimer's society) to share the caregiving experience, to break the sense of isolation, and to learn from other carers' experiences, including, how to cope with the caregiving burden.
- Contact the general practitioner in charge to make him aware of the critical situation and to discuss possible helpful resources with him.

On a structural level:

- Local arrangements for reprieve for caring families (e.g. day care, respite care), counselling services, crisis intervention programmes and help-lines for families involved with care, availability of treatment services.
- Local educational programmes on care techniques and behavioural interventions for families involved in the home care of dementia patients.
- Compensating for the financial disadvantages of family caring, e.g. by counting time spent in care towards social security benefits.
- Financial assistance programmes to allow redesigning living accommodation for care needs.

On a cultural level:

- Awareness programmes (social appreciation of a life limited by dependency and illness, value of domestic care, information about maltreatment of dependent elder in domestic care).

Institutional care

Every institution has its own rules and regulations, its own philosophy reflecting the values and goals of the service. Inherent features of an institution influence the work life of the staff just as much as the life of the clients (residents or patients) being served in that institution. Example for the clients include the availability of a single rooms vs. shared accommodations, convenience of times for meals and basic care, protection of privacy. Coercive measures (restraints, drugs, compulsory admissions) may turn into maltreatment, if not used in the interest of the client's health and in support of their general level of function. Incidents involving pressure ulcers, dehydration, or malnutrition need to be routinely reviewed to rule out maltreatment. Problems between clients and staff involving allegations of maltreatment need to be referred for mandatory review by a neutral committee, composed of different professional groups and administration as well as lay persons from the community.

Interventions in response to maltreatment in institutions may include:

On a personal level:

- Education on types of maltreatment, their manifestations in the institutional setting, as well as corrective interventions, exposing prevailing myths on restraints, staff liability for client falls, etc.
- During team meetings addressing the potential for maltreatment in daily routines, exemplifying maltreatment situations in institutions, analysing sources, and reflecting how to reduce the likelihood of such occurrences.
- Helping staff to examine their own feelings about difficult clients (e.g. recognizing helplessness, resentment, anger, anxiety, and insecurity) and finding ways of not letting such feelings get in the way of caring for such clients.

On a structural level:

- Review care and treatment routines and staff working schedules for their suitability to the needs of clients.
- Implement stress-reduction programmes, increase work satisfaction for staff.
- Implement continuous team supervision, in which the maltreatment potential of work routines or the liability of work routines to bring about maltreatment can be analysed, appropriate changes planned, and the effects of such changes reviewed.
- Improve the environment, with attention to safety, orientation aids and life quality for the clients.

On a cultural level:

- Emphasize the equal status and dignity of both physical and psychiatric illness, of patients both young and old, and of care as well as treatment for old people.
- Achieve a shift in models of care: from a task-oriented model to a model based on human needs and relationships; and from a biomedical to a psychosocial model for the treatment and care of old people.

Society

Maltreatment is a violation of basic human rights. To prevent such violations, democratic constitutions have been brought into existence. For the international community, conventions have been formulated to assert the obligation placed on each state to protect its citizens. Looking at such international conventions it is striking how little consideration has been given to concerns for the elderly. The convention for the political rights of women was formulated in 1952, the declaration of rights for children in 1959, and of mentally retarded persons in 1975. In 1982 an international congress in Vienna convened to deal with the rights of the elderly and formulated recommendations including, among others (United Nations 1983):

> Care is of equal importance to treatment when it comes to diminishing the sequelae of impairments, to strengthen functions left unimpaired, to relieve pains and suffering and to enable the wellbeing and dignity of old people. (From recommendation No. 1.)
>
> The care of dependent elders should not be limited to the effects of illness, but needs to include concerns for overall wellbeing and the interactions of physical, mental, social and ecological factors. Any care to improve the life quality of dependent elders needs to include health care and social care for the family as well. Priority goals of such care are to allow the old person an independent and self determined life as long as possible and not to be excluded from social activities. (From recommendation No. 2.)
>
> Early diagnoses and treatment as well prophylactic measures are needed to forestall illness and impairment in older people. (From recommendation No. 3.)

Table 37.5 Points to clarify when maltreatment is suspected

Why is the report being made now (trigger)?
When and where did the situation take place?
Who is involved/who else was present in the situation?
What are the objective facts?
Is there more than one perpetrator present?
What types of maltreatment are present?
Has this event occurred before?
Is the current situation likely to continue?
Are future occurrences likely?
What personal consequences did the event have?
How does the person reporting feel about the event?
What would the person reporting like to see happen?
Is the report credible?

In arranging for services and care, the participation of the elderly who are served should be promoted. (From recommendation No. 9.)

Any attempt to correct maltreatment is ultimately geared towards preventing the violation of basic human rights or limiting its impact to the extent possible, if prevention cannot be achieved. The international conventions may also be viewed as an attempt to recognize, prevent, and act against elder maltreatment, present on an international scale.

Prevention

One basic requirement for any kind of prevention is effective social condemnation of maltreatment, while providing protection for disadvantaged and weak groups. Current laws for the protection of the elderly are not yet sufficient. The issue of laws against old age discrimination has not been settled. Mandatory reporting has stimulated many valuable efforts for recognizing and preventing elder maltreatment, and at the same time it has also served as a signal that elder maltreatment has an importance equal to that of child abuse and violence against women.

Considering sources of maltreatment and their antecedents, much can be done to prevent or to reduce such events. At the first suspicion of a maltreatment any witness needs to take the situation seriously and to be prepared to take appropriate action, such as involving third parties. General practitioners in particular have an important role in this regard, since they will be among the first to make pertinent observations, to hear about 'family news', to notice stress symptoms or changes in physical and psychological functioning indicative of maltreatment.

In institutions, prevention must be geared towards the staff, their collaboration with one another, and their support from supervisors and administrators. The existence of structures fostering a supportive work environment, the interpersonal climate, and good role models from among their supervisors will contribute to this goal, as much as warmth and support for the clients and the institutional philosophy and human values reflected by it.

Of special importance is continuing professional development for all professionals working with the elderly. Such programmes may help in the self-awareness of one's own violent impulses, to develop a sense for situations where maltreatment may occur, and to understand how to deal with such situations in a helpful and professional way. Little has been written in standard textbooks and professional literature on these topics. It is therefore important for the professional to know where to turn to for discussion and further information. At present, apart from specialist literature on this topic, there are training manuals, structured educational programmes, and other sources for continuous

Table 37.6 Assessment of elder maltreatment

Person afflicted	Maltreatment aspects	Others involved	Contextual factors
Personal characteristics: Identifying data	*Specific details:* Objective signs of abuse or neglect	*Perpetrator:* Identifying data	*Structural factors:* Adequacy of accommodation
Physical examination	Type, frequency, and intensity of maltreatment	Physical and emotional state	Adequacy of care, acceptance for outside services
Mental state examination	Antecedents of current maltreatment situation	Living arrangement, relationship to person maltreated	Financial ressources
ADL- function and physical condition	History of previous maltreatment	Financial or emotional dependence from person maltreated	
Socioeconomic situation	Likelihood of recurrence	Perceived need for changes	
Care and treatment needs, adequacy of services provided			
Living arrangement, relationship to perpetrator			
Motivation for change: Personal view of situation and of need for help and protection	*Interpersonal aspects:* Previous relationship patterns	*Third persons in the situation:* Behaviour in situation (permissive or interventive)	*Cultural factors:* 'Punitive' moral values
Fears of retaliation, of changes in the relationship, of consequences for the perpetrator	Mutual dependence	Fear of perpetrator and of retaliation	Concepts about care needs
Motivation for change and for interventions involved		View of maltreatment situation	Concepts of ageing and of elder needs
Interest in seeing perpetrator punished		Future involvement	

professional education (e.g. Kemshall and Pritchard 1996; Pritchard 1996).

Concluding remarks

The multifaceted presentation of maltreatment in its physical, emotional, social, structural, and cultural dimensions requires a discriminating view for an understanding of the causal web as well as for the recognition of points for interventions. In the family context, it may often be difficult to distinguish between *victim* and *perpetrator*. Usually, maltreatment indicates signs of a destructive relationship pattern, adverse personality characteristics, external stressors, and internal conflicts, as well as social isolation and inadequate support. Therefore, *help before punishment* is the basic principle for interventions. In the institutional context, it is important to consider not only staff maltreatment, but resident aggression as well institutional abuse.

Maltreatment, when encountered, needs to be confronted and alternative ways of handling a situation pursued. Attitudes of denial or of trying to explain it away will encourage more maltreatment. Unfortunately, the need for counselling, support, and services for those afflicted are still not being met. The physician, in the dual role of the patient's advocate and the patient's therapist, has a special responsibility to be aware of maltreatment, to be able to recognize risk factors and the signs of its presence, and to be familiar with the process of assessing for maltreatment and arranging helpful interventions.

References

Aravanis, C., Adelman, R. D., Breckman, R., Fulmer, T. T., Holder, E., Lachs, M., *et al.* (1992). *Diagnostic and treatment guidelines on elder abuse and neglect.* American Medical Association Press, Washington.

Arbesman, R. C. and Wright, C. (1999). Mechanical restraints, rehabilitation therapies, and staffing adequacy as risk factors for falls in an elderly hospitalized population. *Rehabilitation Nursing,* **24**, 122–8.

Bergstrom, N., Braden, B., Kemp, N., Champagne, M., and Ruby E. (1996). Multi-site study of incidence of pressure ulcers and the relationship between risk level, demographic characteristics, diagnoses, and prescription of preventive interventions. *Journal of the American Geriatrics Society,* **44**, 22–30.

Berlowitz, D. R., Anderson, J. J., Brandeis, G. H., Lehner, L. A., Brand, H. K., Ash, A. S. *et al.* (1999). Pressure ulcer development in the VA: characteristics of nursing homes providing best care. *American Journal of Medical Quality,* **14**, 39–44.

Blegen, M. A., Goode, C. J., and Reed, L. (1998). Nurse staffing and patient outcomes. *Nursing Research,,* **47**, 43–50.

Board of Directors of the American Association for Geriatric Psychiatry (1992). Position Statement. Psychotherapeutic Medications in the Nursing Home. *Journal of the American Geriatrics Society,* **40**, 946–9.

Bours, G. J., Halfens, R. J., Lubbers, M., and Haalboom, J. R. (1999). The development of a national registration form to measure the prevalence of pressure ulcers in the Netherlands. *Ostomy Wound Management,* **45**, 28–33, 36–38, 40.

Capezuti, E., Evans, L., Strumpf, N., and Maislin, G. (1996). Physical restraint use and falls in nursing home residents. *Journal of the American Geriatrics Society,* **44**, 627–33.

Castle, N. G., Fogel, B., and Mor, V. (1997). Risk factors for physical restraint use in nursing homes: pre- and post-implementation of the Nursing Home Reform Act. *Gerontologist,* **37**, 737–47.

Comijs, H., Pot, A. M., Smit, H. H., Bouter, L. M., and Jonker, C. (1998). Elder abuse in the community: Prevalence and consequences. *Journal of the American Geriatrics Society,* **46**, 885–8.

Cooney, C. and Mortimer, A. (1995). Elder abuse and dementia—a pilot study. *International Journal of Social Psychiatry,* **41**, 276–83.

Council of Europe. (1992). *Violence against elderly people. Report prepared by the Study Group on Violence against Elderly People.* Council of Europe Press, Strasbourg.

Coyne, A. C., Reichman, W. E., and Berbig, L. J. (1993). The relationship between dementia and elder abuse. *American Journal of Psychiatry,* **150**, 643–6.

DeSantis, J., Engberg, S., and Rogers, J. (1997). Geropsychiatric restraint use. *Journal of the American Geriatrics Society,* **45**, 1515–18.

Evans, L. K. and Strumpf, N. E. (1989). Tying down the elderly. *Journal of the American Geriatrics Society,* **37**, 65–74.

Fillit, H. M. and Picariello, G. (1998). *Practical geriatric assessment.* Greenwich Media, London.

Galtung, J. (1990). Cultural violence. *Journal of Peace Research,* **27**, 291–305.

Glendenning, F. (1999). Elder abuse and neglect in residential settings: the need for inclusiveness in elder abuse research. *Journal of Elder Abuse and Neglect,* **10**, 1–11.

Goffman, E. (1961). *Asylums: essays on the social situations of mental patients and other inmates.* Anchor, Garden City, NY.

Goodridge, D. M., Johnston, P., and Thompson, M. (1996). Conflict and aggression as stressors in the work environment of nursing assistants: implications for institutional elder abuse. *Journal of Elder Abuse and Neglect,* **8**, 49–67.

Hagen, B. F. and Sayers, D. (1995). When caring leaves bruises. *Journal of Gerontological Nursing,* **21**, 7–16.

Hagisawa, S. and Barbenel, J. (1999). The limits of pressure sore prevention. *Journal of The Royal Society of Medicine* **92**, 576–8.

Hamel, M., Gold, P. D., Andres, D., Reis, M., Dastoor, D., Grauer, H., *et al.* (1990). Predictors and consequences of aggressive behavior by community-based dementia patients. *The Gerontologist,* **30**, 206–11.

Heinemann, A., Lockemann, U., Matschke, J., Tsokos, M., and Pueschel, K. (2000). Dekubitus im Umfeld der Sterbephase: Epidemiologische, medizinrechtliche und ethische Aspekte. *Deutsche Medizinische Wochenschrift,* **125**,45–51.

Hirsch, R. D. (2000). Definition und Abgrenzung von Gewalt und Aggression. In *Aggression im Alter* (ed. R. D. Hirsch, J. Bruder, and H. Radebold), pp. 15–43. Bornheim-Sechtem, Chudeck-Druck..

Hirsch, R. D. and Brendebach, C. (1999). Gewalt gegen alte Menschen in der Familie: Untersuchungsergebnisse der Bonner HsM-StudieA. *Zeitschrift für Gerontologie und Geriatrie,* **32**, 449–55.

Homer, A. C. and Gilleard, C. (1990). Abuse of elderly people by their carers. *British Medical Journal,* **301**, 1359–62.

Jogerst, G. J., Dawson, J. D., Hartz, A. J., Ely, J. W., and Schweitzer, L. A. (2000). Community characteristics associated with elder abuse. *Journal of the American Geriatrics Society,* **48**, 513–18.

Jones, J. S., Veenstra, T. R., Seamon, J. P., and Krohmer, J. (1997*a*). Elder mistreatment: national survey of emergency physicians. *Annals of Emergency Medicine,* **30**, 473–9.

Jones, J. S., Holstege, C., and Holstege, H. (1997*b*). Elder abuse and neglect: understanding the causes and potential risk factors. *American Journal of Emergency Medicine,* **15**, 579–83.

Karlson, S., Nyberg, L., and Sandman, P. O. (1997). The use of physical restraints in elder care in relation to fall risk. *Scandinavian Journal of Caring Science,* **11**, 238–42.

Karlson, S., Bucht, G., and Sandman, P. O. (1998). Physical restraints in geriatric care. *Scandinavian Journal of Caring Science*, **12**, 48–56.

Keene, J., Hope, T., Fairburn, C. G., Jacoby, R., Oedling, K., and Ware, C. J. G. (1999). Natural history of aggressive behaviour in dementia. *International Journal of Geriatric Psychiatry,* **14**, 541–8.

Kemshall, H. and Pritchard, J. (1996). *Good practice in risk assessment and risk management.* Kingsley Publishers, London.

Kivelä, S. L., Köngäs-Savaro, P., Kesti, E., Pahkala, K., and Ijäs, M.-L. (1992). Abuse in old age—epidemiological data from Finland. *Journal of Elder Abuse and Neglect,* **4**, 1–8.

Kleinschmidt, K. C. (1997). Elder abuse: a review. *Annals of Emergency Medicine,* **30**, 463–72.

Kosberg, J. I. and Garcia, J. L. (1995). *Elder abuse: International and cross-cultural perspectives.* Haworth Press, New York.

Kranzhoff, E. U. and Hirsch, R. D. (1997). Problemfeld Fixierung in der Gerontopsychiatrie. *Zeitschrift für Gerontologie und Geriatrie,* **30**, 321–6.

Kurrle, S. E., Sadler, P. M., and Cameron, I. D. (1992). Patterns of elder abuse. *Medical Journal of Australia,* **157**, 673–6.

Kurrle, S. E., Sadler, P. M., Lockwood K., and Cameron, I. D. (1997). Elder abuse: prevalence, intervention and outcomes in patients referred to for Aged Care Assesment Teams. *Medical Journal of Australia,***166**, 119–22.

Lachs M. S. and Pillemer, K. (1995). Abuse and neglect of elderly persons. *New England Journal of Medicine,* **332**, 437–43.

Lachs, M. S., Williams, C., O'Brien, S., Hurst L., and Horwitz, R. (1996). Older adults. An 11-year longitudinal study of adult protective service use. *Archives of Internal Medicine*, **156**, 449–53.

Lachs, M. S., Williams, C., O'Brien, M. S., Hurst, L., and Horwitz, R. (1997). Risk factors for reported elder abuse and neglect: a nine-year observational cohort study. *The Gerontologist,* **37**, 469–74.

Lachs, M. S., Williams, C., O'Brien, Pillemer, K. A., and Charlson, M. E. (1998). The mortality of elder mistreatment. *Journal of the American Medical Association*, **280**, 428–32.

Llorente, M. D., Olsen, E. J., Leyva, O., Silverman, M. A., Lewis J. E., and Rivero, J. (1998). Use of antipsychotic drugs in nursing homes: current compliance with OBRA regulations. *Journal of the American Geriatrics Society,* **46** 198–201.

Lyketsos, C. G., Steinberg, M.,Tschanz, J. T., Norton, M. C., Steffens, D. C., and Breitner, J. C. S. (2000). Mental and behavioral disturbance in dementia: findings from the Cache County Study on memory in aging. *American Journal of Psychiatry* **157**, 708–14.

McCreadie, C., Bennett, G., Gilthrope, M. S., Houghton, G., and Tinker, A. (2000). Elder abuse: do general practioners know or care? *Journal of the Royal Society of Medicine,* **93**, 67–71.

Mendonica, J. D., Velamoor, V. R., and Sauve, D. (1996). Key features of maltreatment of the infirm elderly in home settings. *Canadian Journal of Psychiatry,* **41**, 107–13.

(NACEA) National Council on Elder Abuse in collaboration with Westat Inc. (1998). *The National Elder Abuse Incidence Study; Final Report September. Administration on Aging.* Web site www.aoa.gov/abuse/report/Cexecsum.html (visited July 7th 2000).

(NACEA) National Council on Elder Abuse. *The Basics.* NCEA Web site www.gwjapan.com/NCEA/basic/index.html (visited August 26 2000).

Neufeld, R. R., Libow, L., Foley, W. J., Dunbar, J. M., Cohen, C., and Breuer, B. (1999). Restraint reduction reduces serious injuries among nursing home residents. *Journal of the American Geriatrics Society,* **47**, 1202–7.

Nightingale, F. (1849). *Notes on nursing: what it is and is not.* Duckworth Press 1978, Philadelphia.

O'Brian, J. G., Thibault, J. M., Turner, L. C., and Laird-Fick, H. S. (1999). Self-neglect: an overview. *Journal of Elder Abuse and Neglect,* **11**, 1–19.

Ogg, J. and Bennett, G. (1992): Elder abuse in Britain. *British Medical Journal,* **305**, 998–9.

Ooi, W. L., Morris, J. N., Brandeis, G. H., Hossian, M., and Lipsitz, L. A. (1999). Nursing home characteristics and the development of pressure sores and disruptive behaviour. *Age and Ageing,* **28**, 45–52.

Parker, K. and Miles, S. H. (1997). Death Caused by Bedrails. *Journal of the American Geriatrics Society,* **45**, 797–802.

Paveza, G. J., Cohen, D., Eisdorfer, C., Freels, S., Semla, T., Ashford, W., *et al.* (1992). Severe family violence and Alzheimer's disease: prevalence and risk factors. *The Gerontologist,* **32**, 493–7.

Phillips, C. D., Hawes, C., Mor, V., Fries, B. E., Morris, J. N., and Nennstiel, M. E. (1996). Facility and area variation affecting the use of physical restraints in nursing homes. *Medical Care,* **34**, 1149–62.

Pillemer, K. and Finkelhor, D. (1988): The prevalence of elder abuse: a random sample survey. *The Gerontologist,,* **28**, 51–7.

Pillemer, K. and Moore, D. W. (1989). Abuse of patients in nursing homes: findings from a survey of staff. *The Gerontologist,* **29**, 314–20.

Pillemer, K. and Suitor, J. J. (1992).Violence and violent feelings: what causes them among family caregivers? *Journal of Gerontology,* **47**, S165–S172.

Podnieks, E. (1990). *National survey on abuse of the elderly in Canada, The Ryerson Study.* Ryerson Polytechnic Institute, Toronto.

Pritchard, J. (1996). *Working with elder abuse. A training manual for home care, residential and day care staff.* Kingsley Publishers, London.

Reis, M. and Nahmiash, D. (1998). Validation of the Indicators of Abuse (IOA) Screen. *The Gerontologist,* **38**, 471–80.

Riedel-Heller, S. G., Stelzner, G., Schork, A., and Angermeyer, M. C. (1999). Gerontopsychiatrische Kompetenz ist gefragt. *Psychiatrische Praxis,* **26**, 273–6.

Robins, L. J., Boyko, E., Lane, J., and Jahnigen, D. W. (1987). Binding the elderly: a prospective study of the use of mechanical restraints in an acute care hospital. *Journal of the American Geriatrics Society,* **35**, 290–6.

Rosenblatt, D. E., Cho, K.-H., and Durance, P. W. (1996). Reporting mistreatment of older adults. *Journal of the American Geriatrics Society,* **44**, 65–70.

Rudman, D., Mattson, D. E., Alverno, L., Richardson, T. J., and Rudman, I. W. (1993). Comparison of clinical indicators in two nursing homes. *Journal of the American Geriatrics Society,* **41**, 1317–25.

Schmidt, I., Claesson, C. B., Westerholm, B., Nilson, L. G., and Svarstad, B. L. (1998). The impact of regular multidisciplinary team interventions on psychoactive prescribing in Swedish nursing homes. *Journal of the American Geriatrics Society,* **46**, 77–82.

Schneider, H. D. (1990). Bewohner und Personal als Quellen und Ziele von Gewalttätigkeit in Altersheimen. *Zeitschrift für Gerontologie,* **23**, 186–96.

Schneider, H. J. (1994). *Kriminologie der Gewalt.* Hirzel, Stuttgart.

Snowdon, J. (1999). A follow-up survey of psychotropic drug use in Sydney nursing homes. *Medical Journal of Australia,***170**, 299–301.

Spector, W. D. and Fortinsky, R. H. (1998). Pressure ulcer prevalence in Ohio nursing homes: clinical and facility correlates. *Journal of Aging and Health,* **10**, 62–80.

Strumpf, N. E. and Evans, L. K. (1991). The ethical problems of prolonged physical restraint. *Journal of Gerontological Nursing,* **17**, 27–30.

Svarstad, B. L. and Mount, J. K. (1991). Nursing home resources and tranquilizer use among the institutionalized elderly. *Journal of the American Geriatrics Society,* **39**, 869–75.

Tatara, T. (1990). *Elder abuse in the United States: an Issue Paper.* National Aging Resource Center On Elder Abuse, Washington DC. [Quoted by Kleinschmidt 1997]

Tatara, T. and Kuzmeskus, M. A. (1997). *Elder Abuse Information Series.* National Center on Elder Abuse. Web site www. gwjapan.com/NCEA (visited August 26 2000).

Tinetti M., Liu W., and Ginter, S. (1992). Mechanical restraint use and fall related injuries among residents of skilled nursing facilities. *Annals of Internal Medicine,* **116**, 369–74.

United Nations. (1983). *Wiener Internationaler Aktionsplan zur Frage des Alterns. Weltversammlung zur Frage des Alterns,* 26. Juli B 6. August 1992, Vienna, New York.

Wetzels, P. and Greve, W. (1996). Alte Menschen als Opfer innerfamiliärer Gewalt- Ergebnisse einer kriminologischen Dunkelfeldstudie. *Zeitschrift für Gerontologie und Geriatrie,* **29**, 191–200.

Williams, C. C. and Finch, C. E. (1997) Physical restraint: not fit for woman, man, or beast. *Journal of the American Geriatrics Society,* **45**, 773–5.

Wolf, R. S. (1997). Elder abuse and neglect: an update. *Reviews in Clinical Gerontology,* **7**, 177–82.

World Health Organization. (1992). *International statistical classification of diseases and related health problems—10th revision,* Vol. 1. World Health Organization, Geneva.

38 Psychiatric aspects of crime and the elderly

Seena Fazel and Robin Jacoby

The elderly as criminals

Man, 73, on Murder Charge

A man of 73 living in a retirement home has been charged with the murder of an 83-year-old fellow resident, said police last night.

Ralph Barras, a retired soldier, was found with serious head injuries after being hit over the head with a blunt instrument, believed to be a hammer, at the Quintaville Retirement Home in Torquay, Devon. On Tuesday, Mr Barras died in hospital. Police said he had been struck 'a few times'.

The accused man is due to appear before Torquay magistrates this morning.

(*The Daily Telegraph*, August 17th, 2000)

How much crime?

With a growth in the elderly population in Western countries, it would naturally follow that the number of elderly criminals has also been rising. However, estimating how many elderly criminals there are partly depends on the type of statistics gathered. Several factors determine prevalence rates. First, there are varying amounts of unreported and undetected crime. This may impact more on the statistics of the elderly victims of crime than it does on estimates of elderly criminals. But it is possible that many petty offences committed by older persons, such as shoplifting, do not proceed to prosecution or conviction and thus do not appear in statistics. Second, there is no consistent definition of what 'elderly' means in relation to offending, with studies variously including those over 50, 55, 60, or 65 years of age. Third, there are three different indices of crime that may be used: conviction, cautioning, and sentencing. In Britain, when an offence is committed and the police have identified the suspect, they may decide to prosecute or issue a caution; the latter when three conditions are satisfied:

- there is evidence to prosecute;
- the suspect admits the offence;
- the victim agrees to the caution being given.

In England and Wales, there are clear differences in rates of cautioning depending on the age of the suspected offender. The very young are less likely to be prosecuted, and more likely to receive a caution. However, those aged over 60 are as likely to be cautioned as are younger adults (see Table 38.1; caution/convicted rate). However, this was not so 5 years earlier: in 1993, the caution/conviction rate in the over-60s was 2.4. To overcome some of these problems in estimating prevalence, we have opted for the remainder of this chapter to use conviction rates for those of 60 years and older. This has the advantages of allowing comparisons across

Table 38.1 Convictions and cautions by age for men and women in England and Wales, 1998

Age band	10–13	14–59	60+
Convicted	5822	1 434 131	17 613
Cautioned	29 625	254 339	3920
Cautioned/conviction	5.1	0.2	0.2

Source: Home Office 2000—Cm 4649. HMSO, London

different periods and countries, as policies over the threshold for conviction are less likely to vary within and between countries than policies for cautioning and sentencing. 60 years and older is the cut-off used most often in the forensic psychiatry literature.

So what is the impact of the elderly on crime? Overall it is low. Tables 38.2(a) and 38.2(b) show that less than 1% of convictions of men and women were in the over-59s. The other important question is whether the total number of convictions has been increasing. From UK statistics, the evidence points towards a rapid increase in criminal convictions in the elderly.

In 1998, there were 17 613 convictions compared to 2044 in 1993 (Jacoby 1997). Convictions of elderly persons have also been increasing as a proportion of the total number of convictions: in 1993, 0.7% of the total convictions were in the over-59s; in 1998, it had risen to 1.2%. This increase is reflected in the number of incarcerated elderly, which has doubled from 442 in 1993 to 896 in 1998 (Home Office 1999). This partly reflects overall increases in the sentenced prison population in England and Wales, which rose from 37 292 to 49 902 in the same period. However, the proportion of those who were aged over 59 in prison has also doubled in a decade (see Figs 38.1(a) and (b)). A similar trend has been observed in America, where the number of prisoners aged 55 and over grew by over 50% from 1981 to 1991 (Flynn 1992), and where there are about 43 000 sentenced men over 55 in prison (Department of Justice 1997). In Canada, the growth in the population of older offenders in prison is more than ten times that in the population of younger offenders (Uzoaba 1998). The number of receptions of elderly men to prisons in England and Wales has also increased but not as fast the numbers inside prison. This reflects what criminologists call 'punitive bifurcation' whereby those in prison are staying in for longer sentences, while the admission rates are growing less quickly. In 1998, there were 661 receptions of those aged over 59 in prison, compared to 339 in 1993 (Home Office 1999).

What sort of crime?

Armed council tax rebel is a local hero

Villagers rallied yesterday to the support of a pensioner who has held police at bay in an armed siege for four days

The siege...began when George Andrews, 73, turned away bailiffs who arrived on Friday to collect unpaid council tax...

Table 38.2(a) Males found guilty of indictable offences in England and Wales in all courts 1998

Age band	10–20	21–29	30–39	40–49	50–59	60–69	Total
No. of offences	95 088	108 630	60 550	19 409	7102	2170	292 949
% of Total	32.46	37.08	20.67	6.63	2.42	0.74	100

Source: Home Office 2000—Cm 4649. HMSO, London.

Table 38.2(b) Females found guilty of indictable offences in England and Wales in all courts 1998

Age band	10–20	21–29	30–39	40–49	50–59	60–69	Total
No. of offences	13 579	17 573	10 989	3748	1176	256	47 321
% of Total	28.70	37.14	23.22	7.92	2.49	0.54	100

Source: Home Office 2000—Cm 4649. HMSO, London.

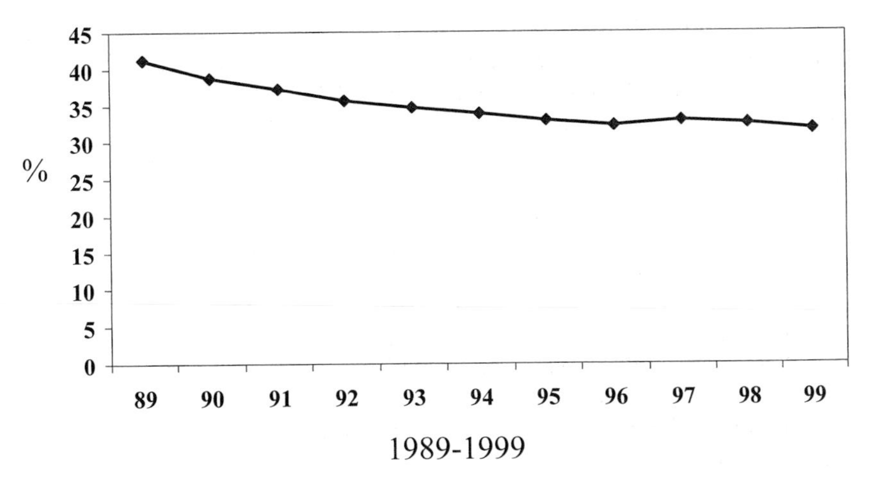

Fig. 38.1(a) Decline in male population aged 15–24 in prison establishments in England and Wales from 1989–99 expressed as a percentage of males of all ages. (Taken with permission from Home Office 2000-Cm 4805. HMSO, London.)

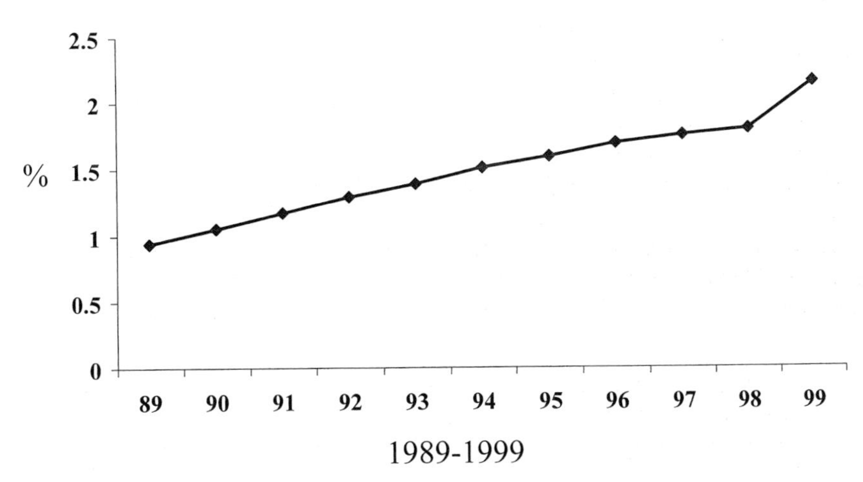

Fig. 38.1(b) Rise in male population aged 60 and over in prison establishments in England and Wales from 1989–99 expressed as a percentage of males of all ages. (Taken with permission from Home Office 2000-Cm 4805. HMSO, London.)

> Edwin Gatehouse, 50, a parish councillor said '...He's doing something a lot of us haven't got the guts to do and that is stand up to the council...'
>
> (*The Times*, August 4th, 1998)

Although the elderly are capable of committing almost any crime, serious offences are rare. To take two examples: of the 904 persons suspected of homicide in England and Wales in 1998, only 34 were persons aged over 59 years, and, of the 673 rapes, 54 were committed by elderly men (Home Office 2000*a*).

In the UK, within their age group, half the convictions of men aged over 59 are for theft and handling, and sexual offences. Compared to younger age groups, elderly men have *proportionately* more convictions for sexual offences and for fraud and forgery. They are less likely to be convicted of violent, drugs-related offences, or

Table 38.3 Patterns of convictions in young and old males as per cent of total offences in their own age group, England and Wales 1998

Age band	10–20	21–29	60–99
Violence against person	11.36	10.39	9.86
Sexual offences	0.79	0.69	20.97
Burglary	15.56	9.32	1.98
Robbery	3.32	1.16	0.14
Theft and handling	37.93	33.09	30.60
Fraud and forgery	2.62	4.90	9.26
Criminal damage	4.05	2.97	1.75
Drugs	10.61	17.73	5.58
Other indictable non-motoring	12.15	16.12	13.82
Indictable motoring	1.62	3.62	6.04

Source: Home Office 2000—Cm 4649. HMSO, London.

Table 38.4 Convictions (men and women) by group of indictable offences in all courts in England and Wales in 1998 as percentage of all convictions for respective offence category

Age band	10–20	21–29	60–99
Violence against person	33.41	33.42	0.62
Sexual offences	16.60	16.77	9.98
Burglary	49.91	33.99	0.14
Robbery	62.65	24.41	0.05
Theft and handling	34.69	35.76	0.63
Fraud and forgery	17.51	36.42	1.20
Criminal damage	38.33	31.83	0.40
Drugs	22.26	44.11	0.28
Other indictable non-motoring	26.94	41.33	0.67
Indictable motoring	17.77	46.74	1.72

Source: Home Office 2000—Cm 4649. HMSO, London.

burglary (see Table 38.3). Table 38.4 shows the percentage of convictions in older men set against those of younger age bands for respective offence categories. It shows that, for all offences apart from sexual ones, older men are convicted for less than 2% of each offence category. The two offences in which the proportion of elderly men convicted for that offence has increased are for sexual offences (~10.0% in 1998 compared to 7.4% in 1993) and convictions for indictable motoring offences (1.7% in 1998 compared to 0.3% in 1993).

Paedophile Free to Live Near Victim

A convicted paedophile who was given a 12-month suspended sentence at Nottingham Crown Court has been allowed to return to his home—next door to his victim. The pensioner who is in ill health, had admitted indecently assaulting a young girl twice and his name and address have been put on the Sex Offenders' Register...

(*The Times*, January 25th, 2001)

Table 38.5 shows the offence categories that attracted sentences of imprisonment for men of all ages in England and Wales. The most striking observation is the large number of sexual offences. Sexual offences as a proportion of all offences committed by a particular age group increase steeply from young to old across all bands. In prisons in England and Wales, about half the elderly male inmates are sex offenders—a proportion that has been growing over the last

Table 38.5 Receptions into prison service establishments of men by age and offence in England and Wales 1999

	All ages	21–24	25–29	30–39	40–49	50–59	over 60
All offences	63635	15905	17133	20596	6772	2505	724
Violence against the person	8926	2159	2356	3126	926	293	66
Sexual offences	2414	139	282	777	538	402	276
Burglary	7294	2517	2352	2005	336	71	13
Robbery	1873	667	546	551	90	16	3
Theft and handling	13813	3983	4099	4261	1087	308	75
Fraud and forgery	2449	285	511	888	458	246	61
Drugs offences	5932	1163	1615	2127	730	241	56
Other offences	19842	4774	5100	6516	2442	861	149
No record	1092	218	272	345	165	67	25

Home Office 2000—Cm 4805. HMSO, London.

decade. In 1993, 43% of the male prison population in England and Wales of over-59s were sex offenders, which figure had risen to 49% by 1998 (Home Office 1998). This large proportion of incarcerated elderly sex offenders is also found in other Western countries. In Canada, for example, half of the male sentenced prison population over 59 are sex offenders (Uzoaba 1998). In the community, elderly sex offenders are also a significant group. One study of men referred to a community treatment programme in England for sex offenders found that 15% were over the age of 60 (Mezey *et al.* 1991).

It is tempting to think that these statistics support the vulgar concept of the *dirty old man*, but the reality is more complex and deserves a closer examination than this glib phrase implies. It is certainly true that old men do commit sexual offences, *but not more frequently than younger men*. Of all sexual offence convictions, currently about 10% are in men over 59 in England and Wales, and about 5% in the US (Department of Justice 1997). Compare this with 18- to 24-year-olds who commit 57% of all sexual offences in the United States, or 21- to 29-year-olds in England and Wales who are responsible for 17% of sexual offences. Nor is it the case that older men commit more sexual offences than any other type of crime. In England and Wales, sex offences constitute 21% of all convictions in the over-59s, which is less than convictions for theft and handling (31%) in the same age group. The fact is that British judges take a more serious view of sexual offences than they do of property offences in older people.

Psychiatric associations

Information on psychiatric associations of crime in the elderly has been collected from different stages of the criminal justice system. The elderly have been the focus of a number of small studies conducted: in police stations; at court; from court liaison referrals; in remand prisons; and in secure hospitals. In addition, there is one larger investigation of elderly convicted prisoners. Findings from these studies will be discussed in the following pages.

Schizophrenia, late-onset schizophrenia, and very late-onset schizophrenia-like psychosis

There is little evidence that schizophrenia or related old age psychoses (see Chapter 32) are linked to offending in the elderly. In support, there are a number of studies of the prevalence of psychotic illness in offender populations. Although *referred* samples of elderly offenders have found rates of schizophrenia as high as 31% (Rosner *et al.* 1991), random samples have reported much lower rates. In a study at a police station in England, 2% of a consecutive sample of men over the age of 60 who were being charged with offences had schizophrenia (Needham-Bennett *et al.* 1996), and another study from Israel found 4% in a sample of 28 consecutive attenders at court (Barak *et al.* 1995). Prison research supports the low prevalence of schizophrenia: of 203 elderly prisoners in England and Wales, 1% had a psychotic illness (Fazel *et al.* 2001).

Very late-onset schizophrenia-like psychosis (late paraphrenia) occurs predominantly in elderly women, who are the group least likely in the entire population (apart from babies and infants) to commit a crime. Of 101 late paraphrenics, none had received convictions for any offences related to their psychotic beliefs (R. Howard, personal communication).

The only evidence in favour of the hypothesis that psychotic illness is related to offending in later life comes from case reports of deluded men and women committing serious crimes. The studies quoted above will exclude those offenders who were directed away from the criminal justice system into hospital. Research designed specifically to avoid this exclusion bias will be necessary to resolve this issue.

The prevalence of schizophrenia in elderly offenders is much lower than the rates of other psychiatric disorders. This may be due to three reasons. The first is the high mortality in younger adults suffering from schizophrenia. Second, elderly men and women are rarely drug abusers, and the emerging evidence from large community-based epidemiological studies is that psychotic disorders lead to an increased risk of offending, particularly when they are combined with illicit drug abuse (Brennan *et al.* 2000). Third, those symptoms in schizophrenia closely correlated with offending, such as delusions or hallucinations that involve perceived threat and override of internal cognitive controls (control/threat-override variety) (Link *et al.* 1998), are less common in those who have suffered from schizophrenia for many years, where the clinical picture is much more likely to be dominated by negative symptoms.

Dementia

The theoretical ground for suggesting a link between dementia and offending is stronger than for other psychiatric disorders. It is possible to envisage that a condition that causes disinhibition could lead to an excess of criminal offending compared with an age-matched population. Support for this comes from studies of aggressive behaviour in patients with dementia in hospital and non-institutional settings, and from prevalence data of dementia at early stages of the criminal justice system.

Reports of violence by hospital inpatients show high rates of aggression in those with dementia—however, these cases are mostly not serious, and typically involve verbal and unarmed aggression. One such study found that the only predictor of aggression in hospital inpatients with dementia was the presence of delusions (Gormley *et al.* 1998). In community settings, where the prevalence of aggression has been found to be 52% in patients with Alzheimer's disease, male gender and the presence of dyspraxia increased the likelihood of assaultative behaviour (Eastley and Wilcock 1997). Frontotemporal dementia has been found to be associated with higher rates of antisocial behaviours compared to patients with Alzheimer's disease (Miller *et al.* 1997).

There are a number of reports at the early stages of the criminal justice system that have found an increased prevalence of dementia in elderly offenders compared to an age-matched population. Retrospective case-note investigations of referrals to forensic services have found 19% with dementia in New York (Rosner *et al.* 1991), and 30% in Israel (Heinik *et al.* 1994). In addition, random samples of elderly male offenders have reported 21% with dementia in a consecutive case series of 28 court attenders (Barak *et al.* 1995); and at a police station, 8% of the 50 men assessed had a diagnosis of dementia (Needham-Bennett *et al.* 1996). In contrast, in a sample of sentenced prisoners, the two cases assigned a diagnosis of dementia had developed the illness whilst in prison (Fazel *et al.* 2001). Two explanations are possible for the discrepancy between the high rates at earlier stages of the criminal justice system and the low rate found in convicted prisoners. The first, and in our opinion the most important, is that demented offenders are diverted away from the criminal justice system. A second explanation is that those with dementia do not possess the cognitive and physical capacity to commit serious crime. There is some support for the first explanation in that the rate of organic brain syndrome was 33% in a sample of 52 elderly patients at secure forensic hospitals (Coid *et al.* 2001), one of the settings to which elderly offenders with overt mental illness would be diverted.

What types of crime are committed by individuals with dementia? There is little research evidence on this and what exists is contradictory. Some reports imply that violent and sexual offences are rare in those with dementia (Knight 1983; Clark and Mezey 1997). Others have found that the elderly who commit homicides are likely to have dementia (Ticehurst *et al.* 1992). In conclusion, it remains unclear to what extent offending in later life is related to dementia. Larger studies of elderly offenders using standardized diagnostic instruments are needed, particularly before diversion to the hospital system has occurred.

Pensioner who killed his wife in 'emotional collapse' freed

A pensioner who killed his senile wife as he told her that he loved her was freed at Sheffield Crown Court yesterday. Anthony Morrison, aged 68, tried to commit suicide after smothering his confused wife.

His life was saved by neighbours and he was admitted to a psychiatric hospital for 6 months...

Morrison was sentenced to two years' probation on condition that he continue to receive psychiatric treatment...

(*The Guardian*, November 19th, 1997)

Affective disorder

The research evidence for the prevalence of affective disorders at different stages of the criminal justice system in elderly offenders is the inverse of that for dementia. Higher than expected rates of affective disorders are found in studies of elderly remand and sentenced prisoners, but lower rates are found at earlier stages of the criminal system. At a police station, Needham-Bennett found 12% had depression, and Barak found that 4% had an affective disorder in a consecutive series of court attenders in Israel (Needham-Bennett *et al.* 1996; Barak, *et al.* 1995, respectively). In contrast, the rates of depressive illness were 30% in a sample of sentenced prisoners in England and Wales (Fazel *et al.* 2001). This compares to a prevalence of depression in age-matched, community-dwelling, elderly men (65–69-year-olds) of about 6% (Saunders *et al.* 1993). The obvious explanation for the increased prevalence in prisoners compared to the community dwellers and those at earlier stages of the criminal system is that the experience of incarceration precipitates depressive illness. Nevertheless, the rates of depression are higher at all stages of the criminal system, suggesting a link between offending and depressive illness in old age. Although epidemiological evidence from younger adults has found conflicting evidence that offending is linked to depression (Tiihonen *et al.* 1997; Brennan *et al.* 2000), it is possible that, in some categories of offending in the elderly, depression may contribute. Shoplifting may represent a defence against the grief associated with a loss or feelings of inferiority: an individual's inability to reconcile themselves to the loss of a spouse or health, work, or independence may lead to an unconscious acting out to obtain symbolic compensation (Moak *et al.* 1988). It is also possible that an elderly person who is depressed will not take steps to avoid detection.

Alcohol abuse

Research examining alcohol-related crime in the elderly is very limited. Some estimates of the prevalence of psychiatric disorders at various levels of the criminal justice system have reported on alcohol abuse, and the findings suggest that rates of alcohol abuse are high. In Taylor's and Parrott's investigation of remand prisoners, 33% of those over 65 had a diagnosis of alcoholism—the highest of any age group (Taylor and Parrott 1988). However, younger adults will have high rates of drug abuse, and it is perhaps more relevant to compare the rates of substance abuse (i.e. alcohol and drugs) rather than alcohol alone to determine the extent to which age-related factors are involved. The lower rate (10%) of alcohol abuse found in convicted prisoners compared to Taylor's and Parrott's remand study is partly attributable to the lack of availability of alcohol in prison. High rates of alcohol abuse are also found at other stages of the criminal justice system. A sample of elderly offenders referred to forensic psychiatric services from court found a rate of 21% (Rosner *et al.* 1991). Another investigation found that 50% of violent offenders referred for psychiatric assessment were alcohol-dependent (Hucker and Ben-Aron 1984). Kratcowski found that in cases of homicide in the elderly, 44% of the offenders and 40% of the victims were under the influence of alcohol (Kratcowski 1990). International comparisons are difficult but suggest a different pattern of offending in the US, where the majority of arrests over the age of 55 in the decade 1964–74 were for alcohol-related offences, mainly drunkenness and drink-driving (Shichor and Kobrin 1978). In the UK, there are currently relatively few convictions for motoring offences committed by elderly people (Table 38.3).

Personality disorder

Zimmer Frame Robber Jailed

An 80-year-old bank robber who uses a Zimmer frame has been jailed for 13 years in Florida. Forest 'Woody' Tucker has been robbing banks since the Thirties. He has escaped from jail 18 times, including, in 1979, from San Quentin, California. Last year he was held after robbing a bank in Jupiter, Florida, of £4000.

(*The Daily Telegraph*, October 23rd, 2000)

Although there are methodological and nosological difficulties in making a diagnosis of personality disorder in the elderly, there are studies which suggest a link between certain personality disorders and elderly offending. The two categories of personality disorder that have been most closely linked to criminal behaviour are antisocial or dyssocial, and paranoid. The evidence for the former comes from large epidemiological studies (Brennan *et al.* 2000; Monahan *et al.* 2000). The suggestion that paranoid personality disorder may be relevant comes from the finding that it is disproportionately represented in prison populations (Singleton *et al.* 1998). In an investigation of elderly convicted prisoners, the rate for antisocial personality disorder was 8% (30% had any personality disorder) (Fazel *et al.* 2001; Table 38.6(a)). In the Office of National Statistics study in England and Wales of psychiatric morbidity in prisoners, 23–26% of the men aged 45–65 were assigned a diagnosis of antisocial personality disorder (see Table 38.6(b)) (Singleton *et al.* 1998). The difference in the rate of antisocial personality disorder between these two studies supports the view that the prevalence has declined by the time old age is reached, and premature death is probably also a factor. One longitudinal investigation found that the mean age of 'settling down' of those with antisocial personality disorder was 40, and that the mean age of death of the one quarter who had died was 52 (Black *et al.* 1995).

Increased prevalence of antisocial personality disorder is also found at other stages of the

Table 38.6(a) Percentages of male prisoners aged >59 years with personality disorder diagnoses

Male sentenced (*n* = 203)	Antisocial PD	5
	Antisocial and other	3
	Other	22
	No PD	70

From the Fazel *et al.* study 2001.

Table 38.6(b) Percentages of male prisoners aged 45–65 with personality disorder diagnoses

Male remand (*n* = 67)	Antisocial PD	8
	Antisocial and other	18
	Other	39
	No PD	36
Male sentenced (*n* = 103)	Antisocial PD	8
	Antisocial and other	15
	Other	30
	No PD	48

From the Office of National Statistics study 1998.

criminal justice system. Of 52 men aged over 59 in English secure psychiatric hospitals 10% had an antisocial personality disorder (Coid *et al.* 2001). At court in Israel, the diagnosis was assigned to 14% of the elderly offenders (Barak *et al.* 1995). These findings are considerably higher than community estimates: in the Epidemiologic Catchment Area study the rate of antisocial personality disorder was 0.2–0.8% in those over 65 (Robins *et al.* 1984). In summary, research in the elderly supports the findings in younger adults that antisocial personality disorder is associated with criminal activity. In relation to other categories of personality disorder, there are too few published data in elderly offenders.

In younger adults, there is a wealth of literature that looks at the personality traits of offenders, using instruments such as the Psychopathy Checklist, the Minnesota Multiphasic Personality Inventory, and the Eysenck Personality Questionnaire. We are not aware of similar research in the elderly. However, there is one study which examined personality traits along DSM-IV dimensions and found that schizoid and obsessive–compulsive traits were particularly associated with sex offending in elderly convicted men (Fazel *et al.* 2002).

'Gentleman burglars' bow as they are jailed

Two gentleman burglars, who wore military ties and blazers to avoid suspicion as they targeted the homes of the wealthy, politely bowed to the judge who jailed them yesterday.
Police now hope the pensioners, John Hughes, 67, and Ian Slack, 65, will keep their promise to give up their criminal careers, which have spanned half a century, and encourage their elderly associates to do the same...

(*The Daily Telegraph*, October 2nd, 1998)

Fitness to plead

Disability in relation to trial or fitness to plead, as it is known in the UK, and competence to stand trial, as it is known in North America, is a generally accepted legal principle originating in English common law in the seventeenth century. In the US, there are an estimated 25 000 examinations per year assessing competence to stand trial, which makes it one of the most frequently requested forensic evaluations. About 7000 defendants every year are thought to be involuntarily committed to public psychiatric hospitals in the US for these evaluations (Steadman and Hartstone 1983). Comparable estimates do not exist in the UK, but it is thought to be far less common. Between 1976–1988, there were a total of 295 established cases of unfitness to plead in English and Welsh courts (Grubin 1991).

No research has specifically looked at elderly individuals' fitness to plead, but it is likely to arise in the context of dementia, and is therefore dealt with in this chapter. The criteria for fitness to plead depend on the jurisdiction, but there are common threads. In the UK, the criteria are the capacity:

- to understand the nature of the charge;
- to understand the meaning of entering a plea;
- to understand the consequence of the plea;
- adequately to instruct lawyers;
- to understand the details of the evidence;
- to understand the court proceedings so as to make a proper defence, for instance by challenging a juror.

In the US, the criteria are based on the ruling of *Dusky* v. *United States* (1960) (Hoge *et al.* 1997), which states that the defendant needs to have 'sufficient present ability to consult with his attorney with a reasonable degree of rational understanding—and whether he has a rational as well as factual understanding of the proceedings against him'. Different American states will have worked out varying specific criteria, but based on this ruling.

Memory impairment, alone, is not grounds for unfitness to plead, and, in difficult cases, a thorough clinical examination looking for cognitive deficits (in addition to memory loss), for example in reasoning and understanding the consequences of decisions, is essential to form an opinion as to the patient's ability to stand trial. A diagnosis of dementia is also not grounds for unfitness to plead, and there may be cases of mild dementia where an individual remains competent, particularly if the clinician uses cognitive aids such as information sheets, and repeats explanations. Our own research has shown that even a diagnosis of dementia on its own is not sufficient to render someone incompetent to write an advance directive (living will) (Fazel *et al.* 1999), which suggests that a general presumption of competence in relation to dementia is required, including in relation to fitness to plead. By the same token, disability in relation to trial must be positively demonstrated.

Research in younger offenders has found that there are some legal and psychiatric correlates of incompetence that may aid in such assessments (James *et al.* 2001). In terms of legal criteria, those concerning the trial, particularly the ability to follow proceedings in court, are better predictors of unfitness to plead than those concerning the charge. Psychiatric correlates of competence have found that there are significant associations between disability in relation to trial and acute psychosis. No associations have been found with depression.

There are no studies specifically of fitness to plead in the elderly. In Grubin's British investigation of 294 cases, 20 were older than 60 years of age (Grubin 1991): 10 suffered from dementia, 9 of whom were over 60 and one who was 57. Other diagnoses in the older people were schizophrenia and other psychotic conditions (9), and personality disorder (1).[1] Outcome was explored, and none of the older subjects was sent to a special security hospital. Only 1 of the 20 older subjects came back to trial, although Grubin judged that almost all of those who were not demented recovered their fitness to plead. This compared with 27% of the younger subjects who eventually came back to trial. At follow-up, of those over 60 years of age, eight had died, three had received absolute discharges, four had their restriction orders lifted, one was still in hospital under restriction, and three had been conditionally discharged from hospital. The fate of one subject was not known.

In summary, older persons in whom there is an issue of fitness to plead are most likely to be psychotic or demented. When demented, they are unlikely to recover the ability to stand trial and usually require hospital treatment that does not have to be of high security. It is also possible that elderly persons who have committed minor offences and are confused at court are found unfit to plead and diverted away from the criminal justice system, which prefers anyway not to bring older people to court if it can be avoided.

The elderly as victims of crime

Scared to Death

Robert Scammell, 22, was jailed for 3½ years at Cardiff Crown Court for frightening a pensioner to death. David Ireland, 68, collapsed and died after he was threatened and his windows smashed at his home near Pontypridd in South Wales. Scammell admitted manslaughter.

(*The Times*, January 25th, 2001)

Broadly speaking there are two types of crime to which the elderly fall victim. The first is maltreatment by relatives or other intimates, which is described in Chapter 37. The second is random ordinary crime such as burglary, robbery, fraud, and violence.

The elderly perceive themselves as being at a higher risk of ordinary crime than other groups in society. The 1996 British Crime Survey of over 10 000 residents living in a variety of areas, from inner city to rural, found that the elderly anywhere felt more unsafe walking alone after dark (Mirrlees-Black *et al.* 1996): 31% of women over 60 years of age felt 'very unsafe', compared to 2% of men aged 16–59. However, these perceptions do not match the actual rates of street crime, as can be seen from Table 38.7. Only 0.5% of elderly women interviewed in the Crime Survey had been mugged, and 0.1% were victims of stranger violence.

Table 38.7 Percentage of individuals victimized once or more (men and women) by age group

Age	16–29	30–59	60+
All contact crimes	13.2	3.9	1.0
Mugging	2.2	0.5	0.4
Stranger violence	4.3	1.2	0.4

From the 1996 British Crime Survey.

Woman, 80, dies after mugging

A youth of 16 was charged with murder after an 80-year-old woman died after being mugged.

Betty Layward died in hospital five hours after her handbag was snatched in Stoke Newington, North London.

(*The Sunday Telegraph*, January 18th, 1998)

As the authors of the previous British Crime Survey point out, these data must be interpreted cautiously. For instance, the elderly are less likely to go out, which puts them at less risk of street crime (and also burglary). Young men aged 16–29 were found to be the most frequent victims of stranger violence (6.5%) but this group is least afraid to put itself at risk; some young men relish the prospect of fighting.

Other notable findings in the Crime Survey were that men and women over 60 were no more likely to worry about burglary or perceive themselves at risk of burglary than younger people. Elderly women felt no more unsafe at home at night alone than younger women, although men were more likely to feel 'very or a bit unsafe' (7%) than younger men (3–4%).

Although many elderly people fear a fatal, predatory attack from a complete stranger, they are not at high risk. In England and Wales in 1998/9, infants under 1 years of age were at the highest risk of being a victim of homicide. Children aged 5–15 faced the lowest risk. Next lowest were children aged 1–4, followed, in equal measure, by those aged 50–69 and those aged 70 and over (see Table 38.8) (Home Office 2000*b*).

Table 38.8 Number of murder victims by age group in England and Wales per million population in each group

	1988	1993	1998/9
Under 1	60	40	71
1–4	12	10	9
5–15	4	2	3
16–29	14	17	20
30–49	13	14	15
50–69	9	7	10
70+	7	7	10
All ages	11	11	13

(Data from Criminal Statistics 2000*b*, Home Office)

Near-blind doctor, 94, begged to keep Lowrys

Two antique dealers took two oil paintings by L. S. Lowry from the home of a partially blind 94-year-old-doctor as he pleaded with them to stop, a jury was told yesterday...

(*The Times*, August 4th, 1998)

Criminal statistics also show that most victims of violence are known to those who kill them. In Britain, 44% of the assaults reported by women were incidents of domestic violence (Mirrlees-Black *et al.* 1996). These data are not broken down by age in the UK, but there are two German studies of elderly victims of homicide (Dankwarth and Püschel 1991; Heinemann and Püschel 1994). They show that about 70% of victims were known to their killers. In both series, where a motive could be established, the most common was financial gain. Other motives include euthanasia, sexual gratification, or delusional mental illness, each in a very small number of cases.

In summary, it can be said that whilst older people do succumb to crimes ranging from the relatively trivial to homicide, their fear of falling victim is greatly out of proportion to the chances of actually becoming one.

Acknowledgements

We are very grateful to Carly Gray and Katie Johnson of the Offenders and Corrections Unit, Research Development and Statistics Directorate of the Home Office for providing the criminal statistics on the elderly for England and Wales.

Notes

1. We have made use of data *not* published in the paper and are grateful to Professor Grubin for making them available to us.

References

Barak, Y., Perry, T., and Elizur, A. (1995). Elderly criminals: a study of first criminal offence in old age. *International Journal of Geriatric Psychiatry*, **10**, 511–16.

Black, D., Baumgard, C., and Bell, S. (1995). A 16- to 45-year follow-up of 71 men with antisocial personality disorder. *Comprehensive Psychiatry*, **36**, 130–40.

Brennan, P., Mednick, S., and Hodgins, S. (2000). Major mental disorders and criminal violence in a Danish birth cohort. *Archives of General Psychiatry*, **57**, 494–500.

Clark, C. and Mezey, G. (1997). Elderly sex offenders against children: a descriptive study of child sex abusers over the age of 65. *Journal of Forensic Psychiatry*, **8**, 357–69.

Coid, J., Fazel, S., and Kahtan, N. (2001). Elderly patients admitted to secure forensic psychiatry services. *Journal of Forensic Psychiatry*. (In press).

Dankwarth, G. and Püschel, K. (1991). Straftaten gegen das Leben—alte Menschen als Opfer und Täter. *Zeitschrift für Gerontologie*, **24**, 266–70.

Department of Justice. (1997). *Profile of US prison inmates*. http://www.ojp.usdoj.gov/bjs/pub/.

Eastley, R. and Wilcock, G. (1997). Prevalence and correlates of aggressive behaviours occurring in patients with Alzheimer's disease. *International Journal of Geriatric Psychiatry*, **12**, 484–7.

Fazel, S., Hope, T., and Jacoby, R. (1999). Dementia, intelligence, and the competence to complete advance directives. *Lancet*, **354**, 48.

Fazel, S., Hope, T., O'Donnell, I., *et al.* (2001). Hidden psychiatric morbidity in elderly prisoners. *British Journal of Pschiatry*. (In press).

Fazel, S., Hope, T., O'Donnell, I., *et al.* (2002). Psychiatric, demographic, and personality characteristics of elderly sex offenders. *Psychological Medicine*. (In press).

Flynn, E. (1992). The graying of America's prison population. *The Prison Journal*, **72**, 77–98.

Gormley, N., Rizwan, M., and Lovestone, S. (1998). Clinical predictors of aggressive behaviour in Alzheimer's disease. *International Journal of Geriatric Psychiatry*, **13**, 109–15.

Grubin, D. (1991). Unfit to plead in England and Wales. *British Journal of Psychiatry*, **258**, 540–8.

Heinemann, A. and Püschel, K. (1994). Tötungsdelikte an alten Menschen. *Zeitschrift für Gerontologie*, **27**, 306–12.

Heinik, J., Kimhi, R., and Hes, J. (1994). Dementia and crime: a forensic psychiatry unit study in Israel. *International Journal of Geriatric Psychiatry*, **9**, 491–4.

Hoge, S. K., Bonnie, R. J., Poythress, N., *et al.* (1997). The MacArthur adjudicative competence study: development and validation of a research instrument. *Law and Human Behavior*, **21**, 141–79.

Home Office. (1998). *Prison Statistics obtained on personal request from Prison Research and Statistics Group, Research, Development and Statistics Directorate*. Home Office, London.

Home Office. (1999). *Prison statistics England and Wales 1998*. HMSO, London.

Home Office. (2000*a*). *Criminal Statistics obtained on personal request from the Offenders and Corrections Unit, Research Development and Statistics Directorate*. Home Office, London.

Home Office. (2000*b*). *Criminal Statistics England and Wales 1998*. HMSO, London.

Hucker, S. and Ben-Aron, M. (1984). Violent elderly offenders—a comparative study. In *Elderly Criminals* (ed. W. Wilbanks and P. Kim), pp. 69–83. Lanham, New York.

Jacoby, R. (1997). Psychiatric aspects of crime and the elderly. In *Psychiatry in the elderly* (2nd edn) (ed. R. Jacoby and C. Oppenheimer), pp. 749–60. Oxford University Press, Oxford.

James, D. V., Duffield, G., Blizard, R., *et al.* (2001). Fitness To Plead: a prospective study of the inter-relationships between expert opinion, legal criteria and specific symptomatology. *Psychological Medicine*, **31**. 139–50.

Knight, B. (1983). Geriatric homicide—or the Darby and Joan syndrome. *Geriatric Medicine*, **13**, 297–300.

Kratcowski, P. (1990). Circumstances surrounding homicides by older offenders. *Criminal Justice and Behavior*, **17**, 420–30.

Link, B. G., Stueve, A., and Phelan, J. (1998). Psychotic symptoms and violent behaviors: Probing the components of 'threat/control-override' symptoms. *Social Psychiatry and Psychiatric Epidemiology*, **33**(Suppl. 1), S55–S60.

Mezey, G., Vizard, E., Hawkes, C., *et al.* (1991). A community treatment programme for convicted child sex offenders: a preliminary report. *Journal of Forensic Psychiatry*, **2**, 11–25.

Miller, B., Darby, A., Benson, D., *et al.* (1997). Aggressive, socially disruptive and antisocial behaviour associated with fronto-temporal dementia. *British Journal of Psychiatry*, **170**, 150–5.

Mirrlees-Black, C., Mayhew, P., and Percy, A. (1996). *The 1996 British Crime Survey (Report 19/96). Research and Statistics Directorate*, Home Office, London.

Moak, G., Zimmer, B., and Stein, E. (1988). Clinical perspective on elderly first-offender shoplifters. *Hospital and Community Psychiatry*, **39**, 648–51.

Monahan, J., Steadman, H. J., Appelbaum, P. S., *et al.* (2000). Developing a clinically useful actuarial tool for assessing violence risk. *British Journal of Psychiatry*, **176**, 312–19.

Needham-Bennett, H., Parrott, J., and Macdonald, A. (1996). Psychiatric disorder and policing the elderly offender. *Criminal Behaviour and Mental Health*, **6**, 241–52.

Robins, L., Helzer, J., Weissman, M., *et al.* (1984). Lifetime prevalence of specific psychiatric disorders in three sites. *Archives of General Psychiatry*, **41**, 949–58.

Rosner, R., Wiederlight, M., Harmon, R., *et al.* (1991). Geriatric offenders examined at a forensic psychiatry clinic. *Journal of Forensic Sciences*, **36**, 1722–31.

Saunders, P., Copeland, J., Dewey, M., *et al.* (1993). The prevalence of dementia, depression and neurosis in later life: the Liverpool MRC-ALPHA study. *International Journal of Epidemiology*, **22**, 838–47.

Shichor, D. and Kobrin, S. (1978). Criminal behavior among the elderly. *The Gerontologist*, **18**, 213–18.

Singleton, N., Meltzer, H., and Gatward, R. (1998). *Psychiatric morbidity among prisoners in England and Wales*. The Stationary Office, London.

Steadman, H. and Hartstone, E. (1983). Defendants incompetent to stand trial. In *Mentally disordered offenders* (ed. J. Monahan and H. Steadman), pp. 37–64. Plenum, New York.

Taylor, P. and Parrott, J. (1988). Elderly offenders: a study of age-related factors among custodially remanded prisoners. *British Journal of Psychiatry*, **152**, 340–6.

Ticehurst, S., Ryan, M., and Hughes, F. (1992). Homicidal behaviour in elderly patients admitted to a psychiatric hospital. *Dementia*, **3**, 86–90.

Tiihonen, J., Isohanni, M., Rasanen, P., *et al.* (1997). Specific major mental disorders and criminality: a 26-year prospective study of the 1966 Northern Finland birth cohort. *American Journal of Psychiatry*, **154**, 840–5.

Uzoaba, J. (1998). *Managing older offenders: where do we stand?* (Report no. 70). Correctional Service of Canada, Ottawa.

39 Testamentary capacity

Harvey D. Posener and Robin Jacoby

....Sed omni
Membrorum damno major dementia, quae nec
Nomina servorum nec vultum agnoscit amici,
Cum quo praeterita coenavit nocte, nec illos
Quos genuit, quos eduxit. Nam codice saevo
Haeredes vetat esse suos: bona tota feruntur
Ad Phialen. Tantum artificis valet halitus oris,
Quod steterat multis in carcere fornicis annis.

But worse than any physical disablement is the dementia that cannot remember servants' names nor recognise the face of a friend with whom he has dined on the previous evening, nor even the children whom he fathered and raised himself. By a cruel testament he forbids his own flesh and blood to be his heirs; all his possessions go to Phiale. So potent was the breath of her mouth that stood on sale at the brothel for many years.

Juvenal, Satire 10, circa 125 AD

Testamentary capacity, or being of sound disposing mind, is the capacity to make a legally valid Will. Thus, whether or not a person has testamentary capacity is a legal and not a medical test.

In England and Wales the execution of Wills (signing them as required in the presence of witnesses) is governed by various Acts of Parliament, such as the Wills Acts (1837, 1861, 1963, and 1968), and in some circumstances the Mental Health Act 1983. As regards testamentary capacity in particular, these statutes are augmented by a large amount of case law. For a clear and concise account of testamentary capacity from the legal standpoint, in which specific cases are referenced, the reader is referred to Volume I, Chapter 4 of the *Seventh edition of Williams on Wills* (Sherrin *et al.* 1995).

The importance of case law in this area is exemplified by the fact that the classic statement of the law still remains the case of *Banks* v. *Goodfellow* which was decided in 1870. The trial concerned the validity of a Will made by John Banks leaving the bulk of his estate to his niece. From the facts it appeared that John Banks had made his Will in 1863. He had been confined as a lunatic for some months in 1841 and from that time he remained subject to a delusion that he was personally molested by a man who had long been dead and that he was pursued by evil spirits whom he believed to be visibly present. These delusions were shown to have existed between 1841 and the date of his death in 1865. His estate was considerable (15 houses). The Court came to the conclusion that Mr Banks's Will *was valid* on the basis that partial unsoundness of mind, which did not actually influence the way in which somebody disposed of their property, did not make a person incapable of validly disposing of his property by a Will.

The then Lord Chief Justice Cockburn stated:

> It is essential...that a testator shall understand the nature of the act and its effects; shall understand the extent of the property of which he is disposing; shall be able to comprehend and appreciate claims to which he ought to give effect; and with a view to the latter object no disorder of mind shall poison his affections, pervert his sense of right and prevent the exercise of his natural faculties – that no insane delusion shall influence his Will in disposing of the property and bring about a disposal of it which, if the mind had been sound, would not have been made.

This still remains the law, and was followed as recently as in the case in 1993 of *Wood* v. *Smith*.

There is nothing in these criteria to prevent a testator from acting in a capricious or frivolous way, or out of mean or even bad motives. As long as testamentary capacity can be established the Will will be valid (*Boughton and Marston* v. *Knight and Others* (1873) Courts of Probate and

Divorce). It may, however, be hard to distinguish between capriciousness and lack of testamentary capacity, and it would probably necessitate an examination of the evidence relating to how the testator behaved throughout his life to come to any valid conclusions.

The criteria for testamentary capacity can therefore be broken down into three distinct elements:

1. The testator must understand the nature of the act and its effects.
2. The testator must be aware of the *extent* of the property being disposed of.
3. The testator must be able to understand the nature and extent of the claims upon him both of those whom he is including in his Will and those whom he is excluding.

The nature of the Act

The Act of making a Will involves understanding that the testator is entering into a document which will take effect upon his death and that the Will will operate in law after his death to determine who receives his estate. That until such time as he dies he can change his Will, although there is some very recent case law which does effectively seem to limit this right. The testator should know:

- whom he has appointed as executors in his Will (if any);
- to whom he has made gifts;
- the extent of those gifts
- and whether those gifts are made outright or conditional upon the occurrence of some event.

In short and at the risk of stating the obvious, but perhaps overlooked at times, the testator should know and understand the contents of his Will. In addition, the testator should understand that the Will will operate to revoke any previous Will that he has made. He should, therefore, be aware as to the differences between his old Will and his new Will and should be aware of the reasons for the changes.

It is clear from a consideration of the above points that, the more complex the Will (and the more complex the estate of the testator), the greater will be the degree of mental capacity required to constitute testamentary capacity in that particular individual (*Park* v. *Park* (1954)).

Extent of the property

It is not necessary for a testator to know the exact value of his estate. However, a testator should understand the extent of the property that is owned solely by him and whether he owns any property jointly with another person, and if so whether upon his death the property will form part of his estate or will simply pass to the surviving joint owner by operation of law. He should be aware of whether there are any assets that will pass outside of his estate as a result of his death. For instance, are there any life policies held upon trust for third parties? Does he have a life interest in a Trust that will now pass to a third party as a result of his death (over which he may or may not have a right to determine who receives the capital and/or income)?

The claims of others

It is worth while setting out again the last part of the test set out in *Banks* v. *Goodfellow*:

> it is essential...that a testator...shall be able to comprehend and appreciate claims to which he ought to give effect; and with a view to the latter object no disorder of mind shall poison his affections, pervert his sense of right or prevent the exercise of his natural faculties – that no insane delusion shall influence his Will in disposing of the property and bring about a disposal of it which, if the mind had been sound, would not have been made.

A testator should be capable of understanding the claims to which he ought to give effect and—if he intends to prefer one beneficiary to another—the reasons why. For example, one potential beneficiary might be financially much better off than another. A testator may have given gifts to one beneficiary during his lifetime but not another. One potential beneficiary's financial needs may be much greater than another, perhaps one potential beneficiary is suffering from either a physical or mental disability which would increase his claim upon the testator's bounty (see example of Mrs C., below). However, as has been stated previously a testator may act capriciously provided that this capriciousness is not caused or influenced by a mental disorder, such as dementia. For example, in the case of *Beal et al.* v. *Henri et al.* (1951) a man disinherited his wife and daughters and left his estate to his mistress. In life he had always been 'eccentric, acted absurdly and foolishly, had wrong headed notions and was extremely difficult to live with. He was also under [a] delusion...' The Court dismissed the claim of his wife and daughters that the Will was invalid, ruling that 'the testator's delusion..., his eccentricity and bad character did not show that he did not appreciate the moral claims on him and did not act in the exercise of his true will in disposing of his property'. In other words his eccentricity and bad character did not in his particular case invalidate his testamentary capacity.

It is obvious from a consideration of the elements of testamentary capacity that are set out above, and from an analysis of what the testator must understand, that the degree of capacity required is relatively high (see *Re Beaney* (1978) *One Weekly Law Reports*)

Impact of delusions on testamentary capacity

As Cockburn CJ indicated in the case of *Banks* v. *Goodfellow*, 'no insane delusion shall influence his Will'. In other words, delusional disorder directly affecting the three criteria for a sound disposing mind, and in particular the third criterion (awareness of those who have a claim on the testator's bounty) can invalidate a Will. Thus, the Will of a man who disinherits his wife and children because of a delusional belief that they are electronically programmed to steal his money for the IRA, would not be valid. However, a valid Will is not invalidated by subsequent mental disorder which impairs testamentary capacity. For instance, a Will made by a healthy person at 55 is not invalidated by very severe dementia at 75.

Nor does insanity *at the time of making a Will* in itself invalidate the Will. In the case of *O'Neil et al.* v. *Royal Trust Co. and McClure et al.* (1946) a woman was bequeathed her husband's estate by him with the request that she in turn bequeath it to his great-nieces. After his death, however, she made a first Will which went against his wishes. Later, she was admitted (for many years) to a private mental hospital with a chronic delusional and hallucinatory psychosis—no diagnosis is stated in the law report but the description strongly suggests paranoid schizophrenia. She was deemed incapable of handling her own financial affairs and legal measures were implemented to manage them on her behalf. Whilst in the mental hospital she made another Will revoking the previous one and fulfilling her husband's request. The Court upheld this last Will because there was no evidence that her delusions or hallucinations had influenced her decision to make the Will or determine its contents. In short she passed the *Banks* v. *Goodfellow* test. Indeed, the case of *Banks* v. *Goodfellow*, discussed above, was directly on the point of delusions and the Court held the Will to be valid.

Dementia

Dementia is the condition *par excellence* which affects testamentary capacity and taxes the expertise of the old age psychiatrist. From a consideration of the points set out above it should be quite clear that the various medical tests for dementia are not directly relevant to the question of testamentary capacity, nor indeed are the criteria for mental disorder under the Mental Health Act 1983. In other words a diagnosis of dementia is not a criterion for testamentary incapacity, nor does having dementia automatically remove the capacity for someone to make a Will. For example, it would certainly be possible for a patient to have moderately severe dementia, as assessed by a score of say 10–20 on the Mini-

Mental State Examination (MMSE) (Folstein *et al.* 1975) and still have testamentary capacity, although it is virtually invariable that those with very severe dementia (MMSE say < 5) are not capable of making a valid Will. To labour the point even more, patients with dementia may be unsure as to the exact date and location, fail the serial subtraction test, and fail to copy the interlocking pentagons accurately and yet pass the *Banks* v. *Goodfellow* test, namely be aware of the nature of the act and the effect of making a Will, be aware of the extent of their property and of the claims of others. Conversely, a patient may not fulfil the criteria for dementia according to the MMSE and yet not have testamentary capacity. For example, he scores 25 but his memory is so poor that he fails to recall that his son has died and that he has grandchildren who might have a claim on his bounty. *In conclusion, the tests for dementia are not the same as those for testamentary capacity.*

Undue Influence

A Will can be declared invalid if it can be proven that the testator was subject to undue influence in making it. Elderly people, especially those suffering from dementia, are clearly vulnerable to undue influence from a variety of sources, not least from relatives or carers. Some professional care agencies do not allow their staff to stay permanently with an elderly client, but rotate them every few weeks, for fear, among other things, that they may try to influence the client into changing a Will or giving them money in some other way. Many old age psychiatrists know of cases where a younger woman (a so-called 'gold-digger') develops a relationship with an elderly mentally frail, wealthy man (sometimes the genders are reversed) which ends in marriage or a new Will in which the man's children are disinherited. However, undue influence is extremely difficult to prove to the standard required by a Court, and it rarely succeeds in a claim against a disputed Will.

Medical opinion

Prospective assessment

Old age psychiatrists and general practitioners are most likely to be asked to give their opinions as to testamentary capacity in cases of presumed or established dementia. A competent solicitor will wish to obtain an opinion any time he acts for an aged client. Opinions are sought both *prospectively and retrospectively*, i.e. before or after a Will has been made—in the latter case usually after the testator's death. Medical practitioners should not certify testamentary capacity prospectively solely on the basis of medical tests. Nor should they certify it when they are not aware of the relevant legal criteria. If a doctor decides to make a statement as to someone's testamentary capacity he should:

- examine the patient specifically in relation to the *Banks* v. *Goodfellow* criteria;

and bearing in mind the points under the various headings previously discussed:

- make contemporaneous notes of the examination;
- and record the reasons for his conclusions.

Case 1

Mrs C. was 90 years of age. She had three daughters, two of whom were married and comfortably off. She lived with the third daughter who was unmarried and had only part-time jobs. She had previously made a Will leaving her considerable estate in equal parts to her three daughters. She asked her solicitor to draw up a new Will leaving everything to her unmarried daughter. The solicitor asked an old age psychiatrist to examine her and give an opinion on her capacity to make a new Will. The psychiatrist found that she had marked memory impairment and scored 21 on the MMSE, i.e. within the accepted range for dementia. However, she very clearly fulfilled the three *Banks* v. *Goodfellow* criteria, and in particular explained (in relation to the third) that her unmarried daughter was in greater need of the money than her sisters, who were not only comfortably off, but had also received financial help in the past. The psychiatrist checked with the solicitor that the woman had given an accurate account of the extent of her property, and he recorded his findings, giving his opinion that she was capable of making a valid Will. The solicitor drew up the Will and asked the psychiatrist to witness its execution. The psychiatrist examined the woman again, immediately before she signed the Will, recorded his findings, and satisfied himself that she had retained testamentary capacity before he formally witnessed her signature. This case has not been tested in Court and is unlikely to be so, which was the whole point of the solicitor's request for the psychiatrist's opinion. However, we believe that an action to contest the Will would not succeed because of the careful evaluation that took place before it was drawn up and executed, and indeed it would be necessary to show that the factual statements made by Mrs C. to the psychiatrist were wrong.

It is impossible to furnish specific rules that could determine whether somebody has testamentary capacity or not. But it is absolutely essential to address the peculiar characteristics of each individual case and to judge from the whole character of the testator whether he does or did have testamentary capacity or not. However, if doctors were to examine patients with specific reference to the three *Banks* v. *Goodfellow* criteria and make careful notes of their findings, the number of disputes arising after the testator's death could be dramatically reduced. Indeed, had a doctor acted as we advise in a case that was later brought before the Court, it would clearly have greatly assisted the judge in reaching a conclusion.

Lucid intervals

As a general rule the testator must be of sound disposing mind both when giving instructions for a Will to be drawn up, and when it is executed. However, it is of course perfectly possible for the mental capacity of a testator to vary from time to time, and indeed in some cases drugs can be used temporarily to increase the mental capacity of a testator, for example naloxone to reverse the effects of opioids. Provided that (for whatever reason) the mental capacity of the testator has increased, whether as a result of a natural cause or of medical treatment so that at the time the Will is executed he does have testamentary capacity, according to the *Banks* v. *Goodfellow* test, then that Will may be valid.

There is a converse position where testamentary capacity can be proved at the time that instructions are given for the preparation of a Will, but during the time that it takes for the Will to be prepared the testator's mental capacity diminishes. For the Will to be valid in these circumstances it is necessary to show that the testator had testamentary capacity both when the instructions to draw up the Will were given *and* when the Will is being executed; and it is necessary for the testator to understand that he is engaged in executing the Will for which he has given instructions. In those circumstances and at the time the Will is executed, it is not necessary for the testator even to remember the instructions that he gave to draw up the Will nor indeed to be capable of understanding them, as long as he does understand that he is executing the Will for which he has given instructions. In the case of *Flynn* v. *Flynn and others* (1982) the testator signed a codicil to his Will when he was gravely ill following a myocardial infarction and only the day before he died. The validity of the codicil was contested on the grounds that he was too ill to have had testamentary capacity when he signed it. The judge dismissed the claim ruling, *inter alia*: that there was ample evidence the codicil had been drawn up on the testator's instructions well before he fell ill; that he clearly had full testamentary capacity when he gave the instructions; and that he knew what he was signing.

Retrospective assessment

Much case law in relation to testamentary capacity arises out of Wills that are contested in Court after the testator's death. A doctor's opinion may be sought either as the testator's former medical attendant (witness as to fact), or as an expert witness. As the former medical attendant, his opinions are admissible in evidence only as to the facts he has observed himself. Since these opinions are based on his case-notes, and because lawyers seek to pick holes in such documents, the value of carefully and legibly recorded observations cannot be overemphasised.

As an expert witness who never examined the testator, a doctor may be asked to study the case records and other relevant documents. If these are put before the Court and *proved in evidence*, the expert witness' opinion is admissible as to the facts therein. He may also give his opinion as to matters of general relevance, for example the clinical features, treatment, and prognosis of conditions such as dementia and delirium. These matters are illustrated below in the case study of Mr A.

Delirium

The testamentary capacity of patients with delirious states also requires some consideration, because litigation may occur when a Will has been made or altered during the patient's terminal illness.

The psychiatrist may be asked, on such occasions, to examine case records, the statements of witnesses, and diagnostic and laboratory reports as the basis for an expert opinion. Regrettably, physicians and surgeons rarely make any record of the patient's mental state. The nursing notes are often much more informative; for example, 'confused and unable to understand what is going on all afternoon—pulled out her drip tube and was continuously restless'. Such observations should be related as far as possible to the relevant time at which instructions for the Will were given or it was signed.

Other factors need to be noted: the mental state before admission to hospital—was there evidence of cerebral vulnerability such as a history of strokes or blackouts in the presence of hypertension? What was the nature of the terminal illness and the likelihood of consequent severe metabolic disturbance; did laboratory investigations indicate electrolyte imbalance, failing renal and hepatic function, severe anaemia or evidence of fulminating infection?

An estimate can be made of the likelihood of severe clouding of consciousness at the probable time, having regard for the clinical findings, for pre-existing cerebral vulnerability—the greater the vulnerability the less the metabolic insult needed to provoke delirium—and for contemporaneous accounts of the mental state. The presence of moderately severe delirium is likely to impair judgement, it can account for persecutory ideas and is likely to make the patient unaware of the facts that are necessary to be of sound disposing mind.

Wills under Part VII of the Mental Health Act 1983

Part VII of the Mental Health Act allows a nominated judge of the Supreme Court to manage the property and affairs of patients who by reason of mental disorder are unable to manage for themselves in this respect. Sections 96 (1) (e) and 97 of Part VII provide for a judge to order an 'authorised person' to execute a will on behalf of a patient. In an important common-sense ruling (quoted by Sherrin *et al.* 1987) the Vice-Chancellor, Sir Robert Megarry, stated that 'the Court will regard the disposition of the estate subjectively from the patient's point of view and will, so to speak sit in his armchair and make for him a will that he or she is likely to have made.' This is clearly a useful and important provision for those with dementia whose estates are large enough and whose dependants would otherwise have difficulties with probate if the patients were to die intestate.

Case 2

Mr A had started his working life as a professional man and later became a successful entrepreneur. He had served in the army.

He had been married twice, his second marriage ending some 7 years before his death. He had two sons by his first marriage. For at least 5 years prior to his death he had cohabited with a Mrs B., whom he did not marry.

As a younger man he was intelligent, quick-witted, and verbally aggressive. He was used to getting his own way and was implacably hostile if opposed. Notwithstanding, he became a man of very considerable means, and he was very careful with his money.

Some 19 years prior to his death his younger brother and partner in his business had died leaving two sons. As a result of Mr A.'s financial manipulations following the death of his brother, these two sons, his nephews, felt deprived by him of their inheritance. They came increasingly to resent this, so that some 13 years later they obliged Mr A. to make irrevocable trusts in their favour for very considerable sums of money, in return for certain favours they had performed for him. The trusts were made with a great deal of acrimony on both sides and relations between Mr A. and his nephews remained, at best, fraught for the rest of his life. Mr A.'s sons were not involved in the pressure brought to bear upon him, but the trusts that he had set up in favour of his sons were not irrevocable and he revoked them shortly afterwards. It would appear that he revoked them as a direct result of the pressure brought to bear upon him by his nephews.

Mr A. had suffered from insulin-dependent diabetes for about 20 years. He was cared for by two specialists until the date of his death. He very rarely saw his GP. Almost certainly as a result of prolonged diabetes Mr A. suffered from cerebrovascular disease and had consulted a neurologist for it. He showed personality changes and memory impairment prior to a series of epileptic convulsions some 2½ years before his death. Shortly after the epileptic convulsions began he had a small stroke with neurological signs of slurred speech, weakness of one hand, and difficulty walking. His speech never normalized prior to his death. Some 18 months before he died he started to have a series of transient ischaemic attacks (TIAs) which continued until his death from a major stroke at the age of 79.

The specialists who treated him for his diabetes noticed a deterioration in his mental state at least 5 years before the date of his death. One of them felt that he had become self-opinionated and dogmatic, childish, irrational, hostile, aggressive, angry, and irritable, especially in relation to people who were close to him, such as his family. He would be rambling on difficult questions, and when this physician was asked by Mr A. formally to certify his testamentary capacity, the doctor declined to do so, having consulted his own solicitor as to the definition of testamentary capacity. The other specialist who treated him for diabetes took a similar view. He noted how Mr A., who had always had a propensity to tell jokes and be a practical joker, started to relate more and more inappropriate jokes at inappropriate times. He also started to show (for him) uncharacteristic behaviour, such as reading a newspaper in the middle of a serious business meeting.

A neurologist had treated Mr A. for 10 years prior to his death, although he had not seen him on more than five occasions. On examination some 2½ years prior to his death, the neurologist stated that Mr A. was having severe mood swings and had difficulty with his short-term memory, although his distant memory remained good. Mr A. was argumentative and illogical in relation to the medical advice given to him. He refused treatment which could avoid a major cerebrovascular accident, and the neurologist noted that he had epilepsy, loss of memory, cerebral atrophy, and that his reasoning and his perception of relationships had changed. He had a tendency to be very irritable with those close to him and suffered from mood swings. The neurologist noted that the stroke which occurred some 2½ years prior to Mr A.'s death had changed his personality and caused a significant amount of damage to his cognitive functions. An MRI scan carried out at that time showed a number of bright signal intensities in the deep cerebral white matter, and the sulci were dilated.

Mr A. had made three Wills since he had started to cohabit with Mrs B. The Wills showed a consistent pattern of increasing bequests to Mrs B. and decreasing bequests to his sons. This culminated in his last Will, some 14 months prior to this death, disinheriting his sons and leaving virtually his entire estate to Mrs B. There was a 7-month gap between this last Will being drafted by a solicitor and its being executed. During this period he had been in the process of creating Trusts in favour of his two sons for a very considerable amount, and which would have restored to them much of what they lost when he had revoked their previous Trusts. However, for reasons which are not clear, these Trusts were never entered into. Shortly before he executed his final Will, Mr A. wrote a letter to the solicitor dealing with the Trusts, in which he instructed him to draft yet another Will leaving an equivalent sum of money to his sons as would have been settled by the Trusts, and the balance to his mistress, Mrs B. The solicitor declined to act (for reasons never stated) and eventually the Will drawn up 7 months previously was executed. Mr A. asked his general practitioner to witness the Will and provide a certificate of testamentary capacity. The general practitioner did this, but never produced contemporaneous clinical notes detailing questions and answers. Nor was he able to set out in detail the questions that he asked Mr A. Furthermore, the few questions that he could remember having asked did not bear directly upon testamentary capacity. He could recall six questions in all. Three of them were invalid simply because he was not in a position to check whether any answer Mr A. gave him was correct or not, namely: what was the last book he had read; what had he done that morning; and what had he done yesterday. Two of the remaining questions would, to some extent, have tested recent memory ability (what had he read in the newspaper; and who was the Prime Minister), although again it should be noted that the general practitioner made no notes to confirm that he asked the questions, nor indeed what the testator's answers were. The final question related to serial subtraction of sevens from a hundred.

Upon Mr A.'s death his two sons challenged his last Will on the grounds that he did not have testamentary capacity. They (the Defendants) obtained a large number of statements from various lay witnesses to show the effects of the cerebrovascular disease including deteriorating short-term memory, increased crudeness of joke telling, rambling, and mood swings. Mr A.'s personal accountant stated that he had been asked by the deceased to draw up a list of assets and subsequently to provide him with a list at monthly intervals because he did not know what they were. Some 2 years before his death Mr A. failed to recognize his second wife (albeit by then they had been separated for 8 years).

On the other side Mrs B. (the Claimant) produced a large number of witnesses who made no reference to any mental deterioration and mostly stated that Mr A. was in full possession of his mental faculties until the date he died. Mr A.'s best friend (who gave evidence for Mrs B.) unwittingly implied that the testator had confused his nephews with his own sons and had imputed the nephews' acts (in forcing him to make the irrevocable trusts) to the sons, but he still went on to say that Mr A. was in full possession of his mental faculties.

In addition to the witness statements there was a huge volume of documentary evidence (which normally would not be available in a case considering testamentary capacity). This could broadly be divided into the following categories:

1. Correspondence with acquaintances, friends, and professional colleagues. It was noticeable that, whilst there was a huge volume of this correspondence, a number of the letters which challenged Mr A. or dealt with difficult subjects requiring his action remained unanswered. Virtually all the other correspondence was answered in a lucid and rational way. In addition, there was a large volume of correspondence with Mr A.'s Spanish Lawyers. Again on the face of it this correspondence was lucid and rational. However, upon deeper consideration it was apparent that Mr A. had forgotten advice that had been given to him previously by his Spanish Lawyer that was central to the issue at hand and was acting in total contradiction to that advice.
2. Mr A. had published a number of articles in his professional area of expertise shortly before his Will was executed and indeed had given lectures on the topic. On the face of it, this strongly suggested that the testator had testamentary capacity.[1] Whilst giving lectures might suggest good mental function, upon deeper consideration and analysis a number of things became evident. Mr A. earlier in his life had a reputation for new and radical thinking in relation to his profession and had contributed toward this subject at an extremely high level for the majority of his life. However, experts for the Defendants stated that the articles and lectures that he was propounding as being new material (which would have been inconsistent with him having impaired mental function) was in fact not new material but had been developed 20 years previously, and that indeed Mr A. had helped in its development at that time.
3. In addition to being an entrepreneur, Mr A. had throughout his life continued his professional work and acquired a reputation in that field. Until he died he continued to act for a number of people including close personal friends. The advice that he gave them appeared at first sight to be extremely technical and inconsistent with impaired mental function. However, an expert in that profession for the Defendants expressed the opinion that the advice he gave in virtually all cases was negligent and that Mr A. had repeatedly fallen back on two inappropriate approaches.

An analysis of this case reveals that there was a lot of evidence both for and against testamentary capacity. There were two expert medical witnesses who provided reports for each side respectively. For the Defendants, the nub of their expert's opinion was that Mr A.:

- had evidence of cerebrovascular dementia consequent upon longstanding insulin-dependent diabetes mellitus, the evidence being mainly memory impairment, personality change, and loss of judgement;
- lacked testamentary capacity because he failed the third *Banks* v. *Goodfellow* test. That is to say, his proper appreciation of the claims on his bounty had been impaired by dementia.

The main opinions of the Claimant's expert were:

- whilst agreeing that the testator had cerebrovascular disease, he thought the grounds for dementia were not conclusive, and that some of the alleged impulsive and capricious behaviour was longstanding, rather than indicative of personality change;

- the episodes of memory impairment and confusion could have been transient hypoglycaemic attacks.

In the event, this case was never contested in Court because the parties reached an out-of-Court settlement, which frequently happens. A number of lessons common to many such cases may be drawn from this one.

1. The medical condition on which a claim for testamentary capacity was disputed was dementia, and the diagnosis of dementia in retrospect can be a contentious matter.
2. A diagnosis of dementia is insufficient to prove lack of testamentary capacity. The *Banks* v. *Goodfellow* test is all-important.
3. The general practitioner certified testamentary capacity, but from the evidence available to the parties he should not have done so. First, the evidence suggested that he had taken little part in the patient's clinical management over the years and did not know him as well as other doctors. Second, he examined the testator's mental state inappropriately, cursorily, and without making proper notes; and third, he clearly did not know what the legal criteria for testamentary capacity were at the time that he certified it as present.
4. Lay witnesses giving opinion as to mental impairment carry little weight. On the other hand, medical evidence backed up by good contemporaneous notes is very compelling.
5. An out-of-Court settlement is often reached which benefits both parties. A full hearing in Court benefits lawyers and expert witnesses, but can drain the disputed estate, or even impoverish one of the parties.
6. Cases, such as this one, can be immensely complex—the medical experts confirmed to each other that they had spent over 20 hours simply reading the documents—but the essential issues always come down to The *Banks* v. *Goodfellow* test.

Notes

1. Of course, the prime test for a sound disposing mind is that of *Banks* v. *Goodfellow*, but evidence of good or impaired mental function clearly does have a bearing on a person's ability to pass that test.

References

Folstein, M. F., Folstein, S. E., and McHugh, P. R. (1975). 'Mini-mental state'. A practical method for grading the mental state of patients for the clinician. *Journal of Psychiatric Research*, **12**, 189–98.

Sherrin, C. H., Barlow, R. F. D., and Wallington, R. A. assisted by Meadway, S. L. (1995). *Williams on Wills*, Vol. 1, *The Law of Wills*. Butterworth, London.

Legal cases

Banks v. *Goodfellow* (1870). 5. LR QB 549.

Beal et al. v. *Henri et al.* (1951). *Dominion Law Reports*, **1**, 260–5.

Broughton and Marston v. *Knight and Others* (1873). LR III Courts of Probate and Divorce 64.

Flynn v *Flynn and others* (1982). *All England Law Reports* 1, 882–92.

O'Neil et al. v. *Royal Trust Co. and McClure et al.* (1946). *Dominion Law Reports*, **4**, 545–68.

Park v. *Park* (1954). All ER 408.

Re Beaney (1978). 2 All ER 595 Ch. D.

Wood and Arthur v. *Smith and Another* (1992). 3 All ER 556.

40 Competence

Seena Fazel

The doctrine of informed consent—that adults have the right to make decisions about their own lives—is a basic ethical and legal principle in medicine and the law. There are three essential components to informed consent—a decision must be made on the basis of adequate information, voluntarily, and competently. The last of these, competence, is particularly important in old age psychiatry as many conditions encountered in this specialty compromise one's competence. Competence is the clinical term for the legal concept of capacity, and the one that I shall use in the remainder of this chapter.

This chapter will examine four major areas: the relevance of competence to old age psychiatry; definitions and concepts of competence; the different competencies; and their assessment. Finally, it will discuss decision-making for incompetent individuals.

The relevance of competence

Competence is particularly important in old age psychiatry for three reasons. First, there are increasing numbers of older people, some of whom may have their competence compromised. Second, the policies of de-institutionalization and community care mean there are more individuals with severe mental illness in the community, for whom issues such as consent to treatment and hospitalization will occasionally arise. Third, decision-making ability may be altered in a number of illnesses that affect patients who are cared for by old age psychiatrists. Delirium, dementia, paraphrenia, affective disorders, and age-related cognitive decline all potentially compromise the decision-making ability of elderly persons. Although many other medical specialties, such as oncology, geriatrics, and neurology, will care for patients with these and other conditions that impair competence, it is psychiatrists who are usually consulted on whether competence has been retained, and to what extent mental illness has influenced a patient's decision-making ability. Governments in some jurisdictions have been moving towards placing competence more centrally in mental health legislation, which will lead to increasing requests for competence assessments.

Definitions and concepts of competence

Basic concepts

Presumption of competence

In England and Wales, and in most other common law jurisdictions, adults are presumed to be competent to give or withhold consent unless proven otherwise. Therefore, health care interventions carried out on individuals who have not given their consent, even if intended for an individual's best interests, may constitute an assault. This does not detract from the doctrine of necessity, which makes it justifiable to intervene medically when competence is unknown, providing the intervention is reasonable and necessary, such as the treatment of serious overdoses in casualty departments. The presumption of competence exists even if the decisions might be detrimental to the health of a person. This was exemplified in England and Wales in the landmark case of *Re C*,[1] a patient suffering from schizophrenia at Broadmoor Hospital, who refused to have his leg amputated although the consensus medical opinion was that he was endangering his life by not undergoing the operation. The courts upheld his right to refuse medical treatment on the basis that he was competent to make that decision.

Approaches to determining competence

Outcome approach

This approach focuses on the decision being made as the criterion for determining competence. With this approach, an individual who makes a decision contrary to conventional medical wisdom or the wishes of those giving treatment may be viewed as incompetent. This approach has been rejected by case law in many jurisdictions, as it contradicts the principle of self-determination and undermines autonomy. The legal position therefore implies that individuals have the right to make decisions about their health even when this is likely to lead to a worse outcome. The ruling in *Re T* states that if a person has capacity, they may refuse any treatment, including lifesaving ones (Kennedy and Grubb 2000).

Status approach

This approach bases an assessment of competence purely on the 'status' of the decision-maker. With this approach, if someone, for example, has a particular psychiatric diagnosis or is above a certain age, the status approach deems them incompetent. The status approach is problematic as it assumes that all those assigned a particular diagnosis or belonging to a certain population are similar to each other. It also does not account for the fact that assessment of competence will depend on the nature of the task. In England and Wales, the status approach has been rejected by case law and by the Mental Health Act Code of Practice. Doctors, however, seem to favour a status approach in some contexts. In a US survey of doctors, 72% said that a diagnosis of dementia automatically rendered someone incompetent; and 66% replied that depression, and 71% that psychosis, established incompetence (Markson *et al.* 1994). In contrast, empirical research has questioned the status approach. For example, 20% of those with dementia in one community sample were capable of completing advance directives (Fazel *et al.* 1999*b*), and 48% of inpatients with an acute schizophrenic episode were competent to make treatment decisions (Grisso and Appelbaum 1995). Some have argued that those with mild depression are more competent than unaffected people as they possess a 'depressive realism' to their decision-making (Sullivan and Youngner 1994). Nevertheless, mental health legislation does incorporate some elements of the status approach; for example, in deeming patients detained under Section 3 of the Mental Health Act 1983 incompetent to give consent to certain treatments, such as electroconvulsive therapy.

Functional approach

This is the favoured approach among US and UK legal jurisdictions, and supported by most researchers in the field. It is based on establishing the extent to which a person has the understanding, knowledge, and skills required to make a particular decision. Competence is therefore decision-specific and time-specific, rather than global or permanent. When asked to perform competence assessments, clinicians should be asking, 'Is the individual competent for this task at this time?' rather than, 'Is this individual competent or not?' An important consequence of the functional approach is that the clinician's focus should be on enhancing competence by improving the relevant functional abilities, rather than on simply administering a test.

Threshold for capacity

One of the difficulties with a functional approach is that there is uncertainty about the threshold for a certain decision. Some have argued for a fixed threshold for certain capacities, such as the ability to pass a sight test for driving, but there will be differences as doctors and cultures hold different views on where the balance exists between upholding the autonomy of individuals and protecting them from harm. The threshold for competence for some decisions will be higher than for others. There is case law in England and Wales that suggests that the more serious the decision, the higher the competence threshold (cf. *Re T*). Some have argued that the threshold for capacity is also dependent on the diagnosis of the individual concerned. This view proposes that those with a psychiatric diagnosis or learning disability should have a higher threshold for competence as they are at greater need of protection (Fazel *et al.* 1999*b*). It is self-evident that there are many individuals in the community who are not competent to perform certain tasks, but society feels a particular responsibility to those who are at risk of harm. Others have contended that the correct threshold for competence may vary from case to case, depending on the clinical consequences of accepting or refusing a treatment, in addition to the risks and benefits of treatment alternatives, in individual cases (Drane 1984).

Abilities relevant to competence

The core abilities relevant to decision-making have been clarified in the research literature in law and medicine (Appelbaum and Grisso 1988). The four main abilities are:

1. *Understanding information relevant to the decision*. This is more than the reception, storage, and retrieval of information. It involves comprehension in 'broad terms' of the nature and purpose of the information presented. One of the ways to test this ability is by asking the individual to paraphrase the information relevant to their decision. In addition, they should be able to identify the choices available to them.
2. *Manipulating information rationally*. This standard refers to the ability to compare the benefits and risks of the various treatment options. It should focus on the process by which the decision is made, rather than the outcome of the decision. The person's decision should be internally coherent, and a 'rational product' of their underlying beliefs, regardless of whether the clinician disagrees with these beliefs. It can be tested by asking individuals the reasons for their choice.
3. *Appreciating the situation and its consequences*. This standard refers to the person's ability to recognize that they have a disorder or problem about which they need to make a decision, on an emotional level as well as an intellectual one, and relate it to their own personal situation. It is tested by ascertaining whether an individual can appreciate the information about the likely consequences of a decision for them and for their family, and can therefore assign values to each benefit and risk.
4. *Communicating choices*. This standard refers to the ability to communicate and maintain choices. It is more than the physical act of communicating choices, and individuals who frequently change their choices without reason should not be deemed competent. This ability can be tested by repeating the question about their decision on a number of occasions.

Types of competence in the elderly

For any given task, the specific requisite abilities must be established, the necessary threshold for each ability determined, and valid and reliable instruments developed to aid in the assessment of these abilities. Some of the instruments validated in the elderly have used clinical vignettes as part of the assessment procedure, and this appears to be a promising approach. Various assessments of competency are now reviewed, focusing on those that can be used in routine clinical practice. Fitness to plead and testamentary capacity are outlined elsewhere in this volume (Chapters 38 and 39). Capacity for other tasks, such as to make a gift, litigate, enter into a contract, vote, and enter into personal relationships are discussed in a joint BMA and Law Society publication (The British Medical Association and The Law Society 1995).

Consent to medical treatment

Competence to consent to medical treatment is probably the most frequently requested competence assessment for clinicians, and consequently the most researched. The criteria for this competence are closely related to the general abilities outlined above. Research has shown that the three standards—understanding, appreciation, and reasoning—are essential components in assessing competence, and that using one standard alone will not identify those who perform badly on the other standards (Grisso and Appelbaum 1995). A study has shown that the other standard, i.e. communicating choices, does not distinguish between those who are competent and those incompetent to make treatment decisions in Alzheimer's disease, and therefore is the least stringent one (Marson *et al.* 1996). Various instruments have been devised to test competence to consent to treatment. For research purposes, the MacArthur tool (the MacArthur Competence Assessment Tool—Treatment; MacCAT-T) is well validated but may be too time-consuming for routine clinical practice (Grisso *et al.* 1997). One instrument that has been developed for use with patients is the Aid to Capacity Evaluation (see Table 40.1) (Etchells *et al.* 1999). The named questions are *suggested* examples rather than rigid prompts.

Some studies have examined the neuropsychological correlates of competence in those with Alzheimer's disease. In general, these investigations have demonstrated that competence to consent to treatment is associated with executive function and frontal lobe function. The criterion of understanding the treatment situation and treatment options is correlated with abstractive capacity, and semantic (but not verbal) memory (Marson *et al.* 1996). The criterion of appreciating the consequences of treatment choices is correlated with verbal fluency and visuomotor

Table 40.1 Competence to consent to treatment: the Aid to Capacity Evaluation[a]

Ability to understand the medical problem
What problem are you having right now?
Why are you in hospital?
Ability to understand the proposed treatment
What is the treatment [for your problem]?
What can we do to help you?
Ability to understand the alternatives to proposed treatment (if any)
Are there any other treatments?
What other options do you have?
Ability to understand the option of refusing the treatment (including withdrawing treatment)
Can you refuse [the treatment]?
Could we stop [the treatment]?
Ability to appreciate the reasonably foreseeable consequences of accepting treatment
What could happen to you if you have [the treatment]?
How could it [the treatment] help you?
Ability to appreciate the reasonably foreseeable consequences of refusing proposed treatment
What could happen to you if you don't have it [the treatment]?
Could you get sicker/die without it [the treatment]?
Ability to make a decision that is not substantially based on hallucinations, delusions, or cognitive signs of depression
Why have you decided to accept/refuse it [the treatment]?
Do you think we are trying to hurt/harm you?
Do you deserve to be treated?
Do you feel that you are being punished?
Do you feel that you are a bad person?

[a]The complete ACE with training materials is on the website: www.utoronto.jcb/

tracking (Marson *et al.* 1996). The criterion of reasoning is correlated with verbal fluency (and not MMSE or verbal memory) (Marson *et al.* 1995). The least stringent standard, of communicating a treatment choice, is correlated with auditory comprehension and dysnomia (Marson *et al.* 1996)

Consent to research

There are no instruments to test ability to consent to research in the elderly. Most researchers have used the general criteria for consent to treatment and applied them to consent to research. For decisions to be made without covert pressure to take part, guidelines published by the Royal College of Psychiatrists in the UK suggest that paying fees or rewards to healthy volunteers or patients should be avoided, beyond expenses incurred in taking part in the research. The guidelines also recommend a period of reflection between explanation of the research study and the final decision to participate, and an assessment of the mental state of the research participant (Royal College of Psychiatrists 1990). Recent work has found that outpatients with major depressive disorder performed quite well on a consent to research assessment, and the extent of their depressive symptoms did not affect the level of their performance on this assessment (Appelbaum *et al.* 1999). Those with schizophrenia did not perform as well as a control group of community-dwelling individuals, but with educational intervention (which lasted over an hour) there were no differences between the two groups in their competence to consent to research (Carpenter *et al.* 2000). Although this study suggested a relationship between cognitive impairment and incompetence, other research has found that elderly patients tend to make the right choices about decisions to participate in research (Stanley *et al.* 1984). The latter study suggested the following three areas as a basis for evaluating this competence:

- reasonable outcome of decision (determined by assessing willingness to participate in higher risk/low-benefit studies);
- quality of reasoning of the decision (determined by showing evidence of appropriate weighing of risks and benefits);
- comprehension of the consent information.

Consent to hospitalization

The American Psychiatric Association appointed a taskforce to draw up some guidelines on the assessment of competence to consent to hospitalization, which suggested in 1993 that two standards should be used. First, the patient must be able to communicate the choice to be voluntarily hospitalized. Second, the patient must understand important information regarding his or her hospitalization, such as awareness of being admitted to a psychiatric hospital, and that release may not be automatic (Appelbaum *et al.* 1998). A useful assessment tool for the elderly has been developed (see Table 40.2) (Levine *et al.* 1994). This study examined the competence to consent to hospitalization in a sample of elderly psychiatric admissions, and found it to be correlated with their Mini-Mental State Examination score and hostility rating on the Brief Psychiatric Rating Scale (BPRS). Interestingly, anxiety and

Table 40.2 An aid to assessing competence to consent to hospitalization

Some people come to hospital of their own free will and others do not; how about yourself?
What type of hospital ward are you on?
What sort of problem are you here for?
Why do you feel that you need to be in hospital for this problem?
What kind of treatment will you receive in the hospital?
If you felt you were ready to leave the hospital and your doctor did not agree, how would you go about leaving?
What if your doctor still feels you are not ready?
Is there someone with whom you could speak about your legal rights as a patient in the hospital?

depression on the BPRS was correlated with higher scores on the competence questionnaire. In studies with younger psychiatric patients, correlates of incompetence to consent to hospitalization were older age and the chronicity of the psychiatric condition (Appelbaum *et al.* 1998).

Financial competence

Competence to take financial decisions comprises a range of cognitive abilities important to the independent functioning of the elderly. Loss of capacity to manage one's financial affairs has important consequences for patients with dementia and their families. There are the economic consequences of not paying bills, and mismanaging one's accounts. The loss of this capacity may also lead to financial exploitation. This can take the form of consumer fraud, and also the undue influence of family and third parties. With the long-term funding of residential and nursing care moving gradually into the private sector, the pressures on older people to protect their assets is increasing. There is one research study examining financial competence in the elderly (Marson *et al.* 2000). The authors identify six domains of financial activity that should be assessed: basic monetary skills; financial conceptual knowledge; cash transactions; chequebook management; bank statement management; and financial judgement (see Table 40.3).

The results of a study using the instrument devised by Marson and colleagues found that only one-quarter of patients with mild Alzheimer's disease (Mini-Mental State Examination score > 19) were able to complete domains 4–6, while those with moderate Alzheimer's (MMSE > 8 and < 20) were unable to complete any of the domains. There were, though, a number of individuals at the lower end of the mild AD range (MMSE 20–23) who were capable of managing their financial affairs.

Advance directives

It is anticipated that the use of advance directives or 'living wills' will increase significantly over the next few decades. A number of commentators,

Table 40.3 An aid to assessing financial competence in the elderly

Domain	Task
Domain 1: Basic monetary skills	
	Identify specific coins and currency
	Indicate relative monetary value of coins and/or currency
	Accurately count groups of coins and/or currency
Domain 2: Financial conceptual knowledge	
	Define a variety of simple financial concepts
	Practical application/computation using financial concepts
Domain 3: Cash transactions	
	Enter into simulated 1-item transaction; verify change
	Enter into simulated 3-item transaction; verify change
	Obtain exact change for vending machine use; verify change
Domain 4: Chequebook management	
	Identify and explain parts of cheque and cheque register
	Enter into simulated transaction and make payment by cheque
Domain 5: Bank statement management	
	Identify and explain parts of a bank statement
	Identify aspects of specific transactions on bank statement
Domain 6: Financial judgement	
	Detect and explain risks in mail fraud solicitation
	Understand investment situation/options; make investment decision

including the British Medical Association, have argued that dementia is one clinical situation for which an advance directive could potentially be useful. An important question is whether individuals with dementia are competent to complete an advance directive. In assessing this competence, it is necessary to test whether an individual is capable of understanding actual possible future situations. An instrument has been developed that tests this competence, which has good psychometric properties and is a patient-centred (see Table 40.4) (Fazel *et al.* 1999*a*). In this approach, patients are not regarded as incompetent solely because of cognitive impairment (such as memory difficulties), which is not critical to competence but can interfere with assessment procedures. It was found that 20% of those with dementia were competent to complete advance directives. In those tested with mild to moderate dementia, those who were competent had significantly higher estimated premorbid IQs than those who were incompetent (Fazel *et al.* 1999*b*).

The assessment of competence

The use of the tools and instruments described above should not undermine the importance of the clinical assessment of competence. The clinical assessment is the 'gold standard', and such tools should be seen as aids to it rather than replacements. This aim should be to enable those

Table 40.4 An aid to assessing competence to complete an advance directive

Case vignettes

Case 1

You are in hospital recovering from a sudden stroke. It has left you half-paralysed from which you are unlikely to improve. You cannot speak but you can understand. You cannot swallow food safely. There is a high risk that food directly enters your windpipe and makes you choke. Your doctor explains that, in order to feed you adequately and safely, he needs to use a feeding tube which passes through your nose into your stomach. This is likely to make you live longer but you need the tube all the time. The other alternative is that you are kept comfortable, but without a feeding tube.

Case 2

You are in a nursing home. Over the past few years you have become forgetful and occasionally confused. You have Alzheimer's dementia. You are able to recognize relatives and nursing-home staff. You are in good physical health. You seem happy and contented. However, your memory problems are going to get worse. One day you pass some blood from your bowel. You can leave it and not have any tests. Or your doctor can organize for you to have some tests to see where the bleeding is coming from, followed by surgery if a cancer is found.

Questions:

Question	Score
1. Can you give a summary of the situation?	Chronic problem (1) Acute problem (1)
2. What treatment would you want if you were in this situation?	Clear answer (not scored)
3. Can you name one other option open to you?	Another treatment option (1)
4. What are the reasons for your choice?	One valid reason (1)
5. What are the problems associated with your choice of treatment?	One problem (1)
6. What will this decision mean for you and your family?	For them (1) For their family (1)
7. What short-term effect will the treatment have?	Short-term effect (1)
8. Can you think of a long-term effect?	Long-term effect (1)
9. Can you repeat what treatment you want?	Repeats answer to question 2 (1)

partially competent to complete the decisions that they face, and the clinical style should reflect this approach.

A systematic assessment should include the following steps. The clinician needs to identify the relevant legal criteria that need to be fulfilled. Background information then needs to be gathered. Medical and psychiatric records prior to the assessment should be read. The examination of the person should aim to establish a diagnosis, if one exists, and to identify any disabilities that may be present. The nature of these disabilities should be clarified—how transient they are, and what impact they may have on the person's ability to undertake the legal test. This may involve the advice of a clinical psychologist (for cognitive impairment) and an occupational therapist (for physical disabilities). An examination of the person's mental state is then required, with particular attention to mood, possible delusions, and any cognitive deficits. An informant history may be useful in the diagnostic process and to identify the underlying values and goals of the person. An understanding of the progression of the person's disease and possible response to treatment will be relevant to the assessment of competence. After the assessment, the clinician needs to make a clear distinction between any diagnosis and disability that exists and how this affects the person's competence (The British Medical Association and The Law Society 1995).

Ways to enable competence

A report of the British Medical Association and The Law Society has identified a number of ways to enhance the competence of those who are being assessed (The British Medical Association and The Law Society 1995):

- Any treatable medical condition that affects competence should be treated before a final assessment is made.
- If a person's condition is likely to improve, such as in delirium, the assessment of capacity should, if possible, be delayed.
- In conditions such as dementia, where competence may fluctuate, the assessment should detail the level of capacity during periods of maximal and minimal disability.
- Some physical conditions that do not directly affect the mental state can interfere with competence, such as problems with communication. There should, therefore, be an assessment of speech, language function, hearing, and sight, and any disabilities discovered must be corrected before any conclusion about competence is reached.
- Care should be taken to provide the best location and timing for a competence assessment. Anxiety may compromise competence, and it may be appropriate to assess the person in their own home. The presence of a third party may also enhance the competence of some persons.
- Education about the nature of the proposed decision may enhance competence. It is important for the clinician to re-explain, and, if necessary, use an information sheet clarifying those aspects of the decision that have not been fully understood. Presenting consent material in small packages may help. Simplifying consent information and using illustrations may also be necessary.

Decision-making for incompetent individuals

When an individual is found not to be competent for a task, there are means to ensure that the appropriate decisions are nevertheless made. Two approaches exist to decision-making in those who are found to be incompetent: advance directives and proxy decision-making. Both are increasingly used in clinical practice but both have important limitations.

Advance directives

An advance directive for medical care or a 'living will' is a statement made by a person when competent about the health care they would want to receive if they become incompetent. They have been widely advocated as a means of extending the autonomy of patients to situations when they are incompetent. However, their impact has been surprisingly small. Despite legislation in the US aimed at encouraging the completion of advance directives, less than 10% of healthy Americans have completed one (Johnston *et al.* 1995). In England and Wales, informed advance refusals of treatment are legally binding, but the legality of other forms of advance health care statements is less clear (Wong *et al.* 1999). The main problems with advance directives are that people, whether competent or not, are not well placed to make decisions concerning their future incompetent selves, and it is often difficult to apply broad principles established in an advance directive to rapidly changing and unanticipated clinical events (Hope 1992). Nevertheless, the informal use of advance directives, including psychiatric ones, as an aid to autonomy is likely to become more common.

Decision-making by proxy

Current legislation within the United Kingdom does not permit those holding power of attorney on behalf of an incompetent person to make proxy treatment or care decisions; although an amendment to the legislation is under consideration by the Government. Proxy decision-making is currently based on 'best interests' or 'substituted judgement'. In England and Wales, the 'best interests' test is favoured. As no person or court can give consent to treatment for an adult who is incompetent, the only legal framework that exists is the common law doctrine of necessity. Here the normative standard is that treatment of an incompetent adult may be carried out if, in accordance with a practice accepted at the time by a responsible body of appropriately skilled medical opinion, it is in the 'best interests' of the person (Wong *et al.* 1999). This approach also permits other action—such as the admission to hospital of a person who lacks competence to make this decision, but is not objecting—without use of the Mental Health Act (1983) (the Bournewood ruling). Commentators have argued for broadening the definition of best interests ('to save their lives or to ensure improvement or prevent deterioration in their physical or mental health') to include the wishes of the individual before their incompetence and the views of significant others, and using the 'least restrictive' treatment option (The Law Commission 1995).

There are two main problems with the 'substituted judgement' approach. The first is that potential proxies, such as family members, have been found to predict poorly the health care preferences of those who later become incompetent. Also, conflicts of interest among family members may lead some proxies to compromise the best interests of the person who has become incompetent. There are no clear ways of resolving the differing opinions of family members that may arise in the course of deciding upon a treatment option for an incompetent person (Wong *et al.* 1999).

Conclusions

This chapter has argued for the relevance of competence to old age psychiatry. The basic concepts of competence—the presumption of competence, the centrality of the functional approach, and the four general abilities of competence—have been outlined. The specific competencies of consent to medical treatment, to participate in research, to consent to hospitalization, to manage one's finances, and to complete advance directives have been discussed and tools described that can aid in the assessment of these competencies. The role of the clinician has been presented, with emphasis on the importance of a comprehensive examination of the mental state of the person being assessed and methods by which the assessing clinician can enhance the competence of the patient. The tools and instruments that are being developed to aid in the assessment of the specific competencies should inform, rather than undermine, the clinical assessment of competence, which remains the 'gold standard'.

Acknowledgements

I am grateful to Drs John McMillan and Séan Whyte for their comments on earlier drafts of this chapter.

Notes

1. All legal cases cited in this chapter are fully referenced in Kennedy and Grubb (1998).

References

Appelbaum, B., Appelbaum, P., and Grisso, T. (1998). Competence to consent to voluntary psychiatric hospitalization: a test of a standard proposed by APA. *Psychiatric Services*, **49**, 1193–6.

Appelbaum, P. and Grisso, T. (1988). Assessing patients' capacities to consent to treatment. *New England Journal of Medicine*, **319**, 1635–8.

Appelbaum, P., Grisso, T., Frank, E., *et al.* (1999). Competence of depressed patients for consent to research. *American Journal of Psychiatry*, **156**, 1380–4.

British Medical Association and the Law Society. (1995). *Assessment of mental capacity: guidance for doctors and lawyers*. British Medical Association, London.

Carpenter, W., Gold, J., Lahti, A., *et al.* (2000). Decisional capacity for informed consent in schizophrenia research. *Archives of General Psychiatry*, **57**, 533–8.

Drane, J. (1984). Competency to give an informed consent: a model for making clinical assessments. *Journal of the American Medical Association*, 252, 925–7.

Etchells, E., Darzins, P., Silberfeld, M., *et al.* (1999). Assessment of patient capacity to consent to treatment. *Journal of General Internal Medicine*, **14**, 27–34.

Fazel, S., Hope, T., and Jacoby, R. (1999*a*). Assessment of competence to complete advance directives: validation of a patient centred approach. *British Medical Journal*, **318**, 493–7.

Fazel, S., Hope, T., and Jacoby, R. (1999*b*). Dementia, intelligence, and the competence to complete advance directives. *Lancet*, **354**, 48.

Grisso, T. and Appelbaum, P. (1995). Comparison of standards for assessing patients' capacities to make treatment decisions. *American Journal of Psychiatry*, **152**, 1033–7.

Grisso, T., Appelbaum, P., and Hill-Fotouhi, C. (1997). The MacCAT-T: A clinical tool to assess patients' capacities to make treatment decisions. *Psychiatric Services*, **48**, 1415–19.

Hope, R. (1992). Advance directives about medical treatment. *British Medical Journal*, **304**, 398.

Johnston, S., Pfeifer, M., and McNutt, R. (1995). The discussion about advance directives. *Archives of Internal Medicine*, **155**, 1025–30.

Kennedy, I. and Grubb, A. (1998). *Principles of Medical Law*. Oxford University Press, Oxford.

Kennedy, I. and Grubb, A. (2000). *Medical Law*. Butterworths Law, London.

Law Commission. (1995). *Mental Incapacity (Report no. 231)*. HMSO, London.

Levine, S., Bryne, K., Wilets, I., *et al.* (1994). Competency of geropsychiatric patients to consent to voluntary hospitalization. *American Journal of Geriatric Psychiatry*, **2**, 300–8.

Markson, L., Kern, D., Annas, G., *et al.* (1994). Physician assessment of patient competence. *Journal of the American Geriatrics Society*, **42**, 1074–80.

Marson, D., Ha, C., Ingram, K., *et al.* (1995). Neuropsychologic predictors of competency in Alzheimer's disease using a rational reasons legal standard. *Archives of Neurology*, **52**, 955–9.

Marson, D., Chatterjee, A., Ingram, K., *et al.* (1996). Toward a neurologic model of competency: Cognitive predictors of capacity to consent in Alzheimer's disease using three different legal standards. *Neurology*, **46**, 666–72.

Marson, D., Sawrie, S., Synder, S., *et al.* (2000). Assessing financial capacity in patients with Alzheimer disease. *Archives of Neurology*, **57**, 877–84.

Royal College of Psychiatrists. (1990). Guidelines for research ethics committees on psychiatric research involving human subjects. *Psychiatric Bulletin*, **14**, 48–61.

Stanley, B., Guido, J., Stanley, M., *et al.* (1984). The elderly patient and informed consent. *Journal of the American Medical Association*, **252**, 1302–6.

Sullivan, M. and Youngner, S. (1994). Depression, competence, and the right to refuse lifesaving medical treatment. *American Journal of Psychiatry*, **15**, 971–8.

Wong, J., Clare, I., Gunn, M., *et al.* (1999). Capacity to make health care decisions: its importance in clinical practice. *Psychological Medicine*, **29**, 437–46.

41 Managing the financial affairs of mentally incapacitated persons in the United Kingdom and Ireland

Denzil Lush

There are three main ways of managing the financial affairs of mentally disordered people. The first is a court-based system whereby a court appoints a manager to look after the property and financial affairs of someone who is mentally incapacitated. The second is a power of attorney that remains in force after the person who made it becomes mentally incapacitated. The third is appointeeship, which applies only to social security benefits and operates on the same basis throughout the entire United Kingdom.

The Court of Protection

The Court of Protection is an office of the Supreme Court of England and Wales. Its function is to protect and manage the property and financial affairs of mentally incapacitated people. The Court's origins date back to the Middle Ages, when the Crown assumed responsibility for the management of the estates of 'lunatics' (the mentally ill) and 'idiots' (the mentally handicapped) in order to protect them from exploitation and abuse. Strictly speaking, the elderly mentally infirm were neither 'lunatics' nor 'idiots', but they were generally accepted within the Court's protective jurisdiction from the beginning of the nineteenth century. This jurisdiction was exercised by the Lord Chancellor, who in 1842 delegated many of his functions to the Master in Lunacy. In 1947 the Office of the Master in Lunacy was renamed the Court of Protection. In 1987 the purely administrative functions of the Court of Protection were transferred the Public Trust Office, which has now been renamed the Public Guardianship Office. The Court of Protection and the Public Guardianship Office are housed in the same building in central London. They have no regional presence, but employ a small number of visitors, known as the Lord Chancellor's Visitors, who operate on a regional basis and make domiciliary visits to patients.

The court's powers are contained in two statutes which operate two fundamentally different schemes: Part VII of the Mental Health Act 1983, and the Enduring Powers of Attorney Act 1985. The Mental Health Act assumes a 'hands on' approach by the Public Guardianship Office to the management of the finances of persons without capacity. The Enduring Powers of Attorney Act assumes that, unless it really needs to intervene, the Court's role in the actual management of someone's affairs will be very much 'hands off'.

The Court of Protection and the Public Guardianship Office look after the affairs of approximately 22 000 patients under the Mental Health Act, who fall into four main client groups:

- the elderly mentally infirm;
- people with mainstream mental illnesses, such as schizophrenia;
- people with learning difficulties; and
- people who have suffered traumatic brain damage as a result of an accident or assault and have been awarded compensation for their personal injuries.

Some 70% of the Court's patients are over the age of 70, and 75% are female. The number of first general orders appointing a receiver under the Mental Health Act has remained constant, at just over 6000 a year, since the Enduring Powers of Attorney Act came into force in 1986. By contrast, the number of applications to register enduring powers of attorney has steadily grown, and is currently around 12 000 a year. The average age of donors of enduring powers when the power is registered is 87.

The Court of Protection has 'power over the purse', but no 'power over the person'. In other words, it can make financial decisions, but cannot make medical or personal decisions, such as where a patient should live, and with whom he or she should have contact. In its report on *Mental incapacity*, published in March 1995, the Law Commission recommended that the present Court should be abolished and that in its place a new Court of Protection should be established. The jurisdiction of the new Court will extend to personal and medical decision-making in addition to financial decision-making, and will be exercised by nominated district judges, circuit judges, and High Court judges sitting throughout England and Wales. The Government has announced that it intends to introduce legislation to implement these proposals as soon as parliamentary time allows.

Competence

Two conditions must be satisfied before the Court of Protection can assume jurisdiction. A person must: (1) have a mental disorder, and (2) be incapable of managing and administering his or her property and affairs. Mental disorder is defined in Section 1(2) of the Mental Health Act 1983 and means 'mental illness, arrested or incomplete development of mind, psychopathic disorder and any other disorder or disability of mind'.

Although the Act defines mental disorder, it does not define the expression 'incapable of managing his property and affairs' and there are no clear criteria as to what this means. The standard textbook on Court of Protection practice, *Heywood & Massey* (Whitehorn 1991), suggests that 'the question of the degree of incapacity of managing and administering a patient's property and affairs must be related to all the circumstances including the state in which the patient lives and the complexity and importance of the property and affairs which he has to manage and administer.' The authority given for this statement is the decision in the case of *Re CAF* in 1962. As a result of several strokes CAF was severely aphasic and incapable not only of communicating instructions but also of initiating thought. She had a life interest in a landed estate and an extensive portfolio in her own right, and it was held that, because of her mental disorder, she was incapable of managing assets of this degree of complexity and importance.

Although this decision was never published in the law reports, there has been a lively debate in the Australian courts as to whether an individual's capacity to manage his or her affairs is specific to that person (following *Re CAF*) or of more universal application. In one case the judge tried to introduce a more objective test and decided that a person must be 'incapable of dealing, in a reasonably competent fashion, with the ordinary routine affairs of man, and by reason of that incompetence there is a real risk that either he or she may be disadvantaged in the conduct of such affairs or that such moneys or property which he or she may possess may be dissipated or lost.' However, in another case a different judge followed *Re CAF* and upheld the subjective test because the Act itself speaks of 'managing *his* affairs', rather than 'the ordinary routine affairs of man.'

Although it is generally held that competence must be specific to individual functions and not a blanket attribute, the capacity to manage one's property and affairs is something of an anomaly. Silberfeld *et al.* (1995) applied some 'generic clinical criteria' to subjects being assessed for different types of competence. These were: (1) the ability to communicate about the subject-matter of the decision; (2) a consistent expression of preferences respecting the subject-matter; (3) the ability to understand and weigh options relating to the subject-matter; and (4) the ability to rationalize choices respecting the subject-matter. To these, Silberfeld and his colleagues added some that were specific to financial competence and which they described as 'suggested by the legal standards'. They did not say what these legal standards were, nor (since they were writing from Canada) to which jurisdiction they were referring. However, the criteria are sensible, straightforward, and commendable as follows:

- knowledge of income;
- knowledge of expenses;
- an ability to handle everyday financial transactions; and
- the ability to delegate financial wishes.

For the clinician assessing an individual patient, it is usually not difficult to determine whether these criteria can be met. For example, as regards the ability to handle everyday transactions, it can be illuminating to show the patient a chequebook and ask her to describe what has to be written on each part of a cheque. The ability to delegate financial wishes raises three further questions, which were suggested by the judge in the case of *White* v. *Fell* (unreported, 12 November 1987, Mr Justice Boreham):

(1) Does she have the insight and understanding of the fact that she has a problem in respect of which she needs advice?
(2) Is she capable of seeking an appropriate adviser and instructing him with sufficient clarity to enable him to understand the problem and to advise her appropriately?
(3) Does she have sufficient mental capacity to understand and make decisions based upon, or otherwise give effect to, such advice as she may receive?

Medical certification

The medical evidence considered by the Court of Protection usually consists of a printed certificate (form CP3), which must be completed by a registered medical practitioner. There is no requirement that the certificate should be completed by a consultant, or by a psychiatrist, neurologist, or geriatrician. In practice, it is usually completed by the patient's general practitioner. Although Whitehead (1987) has argued that the certifying doctor should have 'a good knowledge of psychiatry...and be able to assess an individual's capacity, or otherwise, to handle his or her affairs', it is equally important that the certifying doctor is fully cognizant of the family background and the property and affairs that the patient has to administer.

Occasionally a clinical psychologist completes the form CP3. Although it is acknowledged that some clinical psychologists are experts in assessing cognitive skills, because of the wording of the legislation the Court is unable accept a certificate completed by anyone other than a registered medical practitioner.

Although the Court may be prepared to consider detailed medical reports in another form, the printed form CP3, which was drawn up in consultation with the Royal College of Psychiatrists and the British Medical Association, contains some useful information, sometimes absent from other reports, which assists the Court in making various administrative decisions. For example, the question whether a patient's life expectancy is likely to be under or over 5 years is intended to help the Court decide whether a short-term or long-term investment strategy is required, and the question about Visitors assists the Court in deciding whether or not the patient should be placed on its own Visitors' list.

Form CP3 contains the following statements and questions:

1. I have the following medical qualifications......
2. I am the medical attendant of the above named patient who resides at......and have so acted since......
3. I last examined the patient on the......and in my opinion the patient is incapable by reason of mental disorder of managing and administering his/her property and affairs.
4. My opinion is based on the following diagnosis and the following evidence of incapacity......

5. The present mental disorder has lasted since......
6. Is the patient a danger to himself/herself or others in any way? If yes, give details.
7. Is the patient capable of appreciating his/her surroundings? Please comment.
8. Does the patient need anything to provide additional comfort? If yes, what recommendations do you make?
9. Is there a reasonable prospect of the patient: (a) being moved to a nursing home or residential home; or (b) returning to his/her own home if not living there at present. If yes, when?
10. Is the patient visited by relatives or friends? If yes, (a) how frequently? (b) by whom?
11. What is the patient's age?
12. What is the patient's life expectancy? Under 5 years or over 5 years?
13. Please give a brief summary of the patient's physical condition.
14. What are the patient's prospects of mental recovery?
15. Have you or your family any financial interest in the accommodation in which the patient is living?
16. Additional comments (if any). {exle}

The notes to accompany the medical certificate (form CP3), prepared in conjunction with the Royal College of Psychiatrists and the British Medical Association, state as follows:

- Doctors should be aware that if a person owning real or personal property becomes incapable, by reason of mental disorder, of safeguarding and managing his affairs, an application should be made to the Court of Protection for the appointment of a receiver.
- An application to the Court of Protection for the appointment of a receiver must be supported by a medical certificate stating that, in the doctor's opinion, the patient is incapable of managing and administering his property and affairs by virtue of mental disorder (as defined in Section 1 of the Mental Health Act 1983).
- Criteria for assessing incapacity are not identical with those for assessing the need for compulsory admission to hospital. The fact that a person is suffering from mental disorder within the meaning of the Mental Health Act 1983, whether living in the community or resident in hospital, detained or informal, is not of itself evidence of incapacity to manage his affairs. On the other hand, a person may be so incapable and yet not be liable to compulsory admission to hospital.
- The certifying doctor may be either the person's general practitioner or any other registered medical practitioner who has examined the patient.
- The certificate is given on form CP3 which requires the doctor to state in paragraph 3 the grounds on which he bases his opinion of incapacity. It is this part of the certificate which appears to give the doctor the most difficulty. What is required is not merely a diagnosis (although this may be included) but a simple statement giving clear evidence of incapacity which an intelligent lay person could understand, e.g. reference to defect of short-term memory, of spatial and temporal orientation or of reasoning ability, or to reckless spending (sometimes periodic as in mania) without regard for the future, or evidence of vulnerability to exploitation.
- In many cases of senile dementia, severe brain damage, acute or chronic psychiatric disorder and severe mental impairment the assessment of incapacity should present little difficulty. Cases of functional and personality disorders may give more problems and assessment may depend on the individual doctor's interpretation of mental disorder. The Court tends towards the view that these conditions render a person liable to its jurisdiction where there appears to be a real danger that they will lead to dissipation of considerable assets.
- A person may not be dealt with under the Mental Health Act 1983, and may not be the subject of an application to the Court of Protection, by reason *only* of promiscuity or other immoral conduct, sexual deviancy or dependence on alcohol or drugs.
- The Court attaches considerable importance to receipt by the patient of notice of the proposed proceedings for the appointment of a receiver, since the patient may have an objection, though irrational, to the appointment of a particular person or may, even unwittingly, contribute information of assistance to the Court. The Court is reluctant to exercise its power to dispense with notification, unless it could be injurious to the patient's health, because it is considered that a person has a right to know—or at least be given an opportunity to understand—if the management of his affairs is to be taken out of his hands and thereafter dealt with by someone else on his behalf. If he has no understanding at all, then notification cannot affect him adversely, and a patient who has sufficient insight to appreciate the significance of the Court's

proceedings may need reassurance that they are for his benefit. If the certifying doctor believes that, in a particular case, notification of the proceedings by or under the supervision of the doctor is advisable, he should say so when completing the form CP3.

The British Medical Association makes annual recommendations on the fees medical practitioners may charge for the completion of certificates and other work done in connection with Court of Protection matters. The fees recommended with effect from 1 April 2000 are (a) £84.50 for examining the patient and completing form CP3, and (b) £42.00 for serving on the patient the notice of an application for the appointment of a receiver (form CP7). If travelling is involved a higher fee may be charged.

The Lord Chancellor's Medical Visitors

If there is a problem in establishing whether someone is incapable, by reason of mental disorder, of managing and administering his property and affairs, or if there is conflicting medical evidence, the Court of Protection may ask one of the Lord Chancellor's Medical Visitors to visit the person concerned. The qualifications and functions of the visitors are set out in Sections 102 and 103 of the Mental Health Act 1983. A medical visitor must be a 'registered medical practitioner who appears to the Lord Chancellor to have special knowledge and experience of cases of mental disorder'. There are currently six, all of whom are senior consultant psychiatrists, and each covers a particular circuit of England and Wales.

The visitors have the following rights:

(1) they may interview a patient in private;
(2) they may carry out a medical examination of the patient in private; and
(3) they are entitled to the production of any medical records relating to the patient and may inspect such records.

Receivership

A receiver is a person who is appointed by the Court of Protection to manage a patient's financial affairs on a day-to-day basis. The forms for applying for the appointment of a receiver may be obtained free of charge from the Customer Services Unit at the Public Guardianship Office, Stewart House, 24 Kingsway, London WC2B 6JX. The unit also produces a number of helpful brochures, such as a *Handbook for receivers*, and *The duties of a receiver*.

The following forms should be completed and returned to the Public Guardianship Office:

- two copies of the application (form CP1);
- the Medical Certificate (form CP3);
- the Certificate of Family and Property (form CP5);
- a copy of the patient's Will and other testamentary documents (if any);
- a cheque for the commencement fee of £230 made payable to 'Public Guardianship Office'.

On receiving these documents the Public Guardianship Office will return one copy of form CP1 marked with the date and time when the Court will consider the application. Unless the Court directs otherwise, no attendance on that date will be necessary, and the appointment of a receiver will be purely a paper transaction. An attended hearing will only be necessary if someone objects to the application.

The Public Guardianship Office also sends the applicant a letter addressed to the patient telling him or her the date on which the application will be considered and explaining how representations and observations can be made. Unless the Court directs otherwise, this letter must be personally served on the patient, and the person who serves it must complete a Certificate of Service (form CP7). The letter must be delivered to the patient at least 10 clear days before the date when the application will be considered by the Court.

If the patient's estate is under £10 000 in value, the Court can make a 'short order' authorizing a suitable person to manage the patient's assets, and generally speaking it need no longer be involved in that patient's affairs. In most cases, however, the Court appoints a receiver to deal with the day-to-day management of a patient's affairs, and it has complete discretion as to whom it appoints.

There is no formal order of priority, though traditionally it has preferred to appoint relatives rather than strangers. Some 63% of receivers are members of the patient's family, 13% are solicitors, and 8% are office holders with local authorities, usually the Director of Social Services. In about 10% of cases the Public Trustee is appointed as the 'receiver of last resort', often where the patient is violent, or has been the victim of financial abuse, or comes from a particularly unsuitable family background.

Throughout the world the main characteristics of court-based systems of managing the property of a person without capacity are: (1) an inventory, (2) annual accounting, and (3) security. Receivership in England and Wales is much the same. The inventory is in the certificate of family and property that is submitted with the application for the appointment of the receiver. The receiver is generally required to present an annual account on every anniversary of the order appointing him or her. Where an order is to be made appointing anyone other than the Public Trustee or a professional receiver, the receiver may be required to give security for the due performance of his or her duties. The amount covered by the security bond is usually 1.5 times the patient's annual income. A small premium is payable, and this can be recovered from the patient's estate.

A receiver is entitled to recover his or her reasonable out-of-pocket expenses, such as postage, telephone calls, and travelling expenses, but is granted remuneration only in exceptional circumstances—usually if he or she is a solicitor, accountant, or other professional person.

Receivers have only the powers that are conferred upon them by the first general order or subsequent orders of the Court. Generally speaking, they merely have access to the patient's income, which they are expected to apply for the patient's maintenance. Any dealings with capital and any gifts must be authorized by the Court.

Fees are charged for the services the Court and the Public Trust Office provide. In addition to the commencement fee of £230.00, there are various individual transaction fees, and an annual administration fee of £205.00.

Recovery of the patient

Where a patient's capacity has improved sufficiently to enable him or her to be restored to the management of his or her own affairs, an application can be made to the Court for an order determining proceedings. There is a printed Medical Certificate on the Recovery of a Patient, form CP2, but the quality of certification on recovery is often disappointing, with doctors completing the certificate in a rather laconic and unspecified manner.

Relatively few such orders are made: on average about 100 a year, compared with over 6000 new applications a year for the appointment of a receiver. Among elderly patients recovery is most frequently encountered in stroke cases, and is virtually unknown where patients are suffering from dementia. Cases where there is a temporary remission in a history of chronic mental illness, such as schizophrenia, present particular difficulties and the Court will need to be satisfied that the patient is likely to remain mentally capable of managing his or her affairs for the reasonably foreseeable future. Where the patient has not recovered sufficiently to justify an order determining proceedings, the Court may be willing to consider a less restrictive alternative to receivership and might, for example, authorize a patient who has the capacity to make an enduring power of attorney to create such a power on condition that the attorneys immediately apply to register it with the Court.

Enduring powers of attorney

An enduring power of attorney is a document in which an individual (called 'the donor') appoints one or more other persons to be his or her attorney(s). Unlike an ordinary power of attorney, which is revoked by the donor's subsequent incapacity, an enduring power of attorney endures—or remains in force—after the donor becomes mentally incapacitated, but only if it is registered with the Court of Protection. Once the power has been registered, it cannot be revoked by the donor unless the Court confirms the revocation.

Enduring powers of attorney have been available in England and Wales since March 1986. In contrast to receivership, which is sought *after* mental disorder has been acquired, an enduring power of attorney is *anticipatory* and designed to provide a flexible, less restrictive, and more individual form of agency.

An enduring power of attorney must be in the form prescribed by the Lord Chancellor. The prescribed form consists of three parts. Part A contains some explanatory information. Part B, which is signed by the donor, contains the appointment itself. In Part C the attorneys accept the appointment.

Unless the donor specifically states that it is not to be used until he or she has become mentally incapacitated, the power comes into effect immediately, as soon as it has been signed, and can be operated like an ordinary non-enduring power of attorney. For example, a mentally *un*impaired woman of 70 gives her EPA to her son, who uses it to pay her bills and to write other cheques on her behalf until she dies of a myocardial infarction 8 years later, still mentally unimpaired. Alternatively, an EPA can become effective only later, if and when the donor becomes mentally incapable of managing her affairs.

If the donor wishes to appoint more than one attorney, the appointment must be either joint (where both or all attorneys must act) or joint and several (which allows any one attorney to act independently). Some 60% of donors appoint only one attorney; 34% appoint joint and several attorneys; only 6% appoint joint attorneys.

The prescribed form gives the donor the choice of conferring general authority on the attorney in relation to all his or her property and affairs, or specific authority in respect of a discrete aspect of his or her affairs—98.5% of donors confer general authority on their attorneys.

Attorneys acting under an enduring power, whether registered or unregistered, have limited authority to make gifts of the donor's assets. They may only make seasonal gifts or presents on a birthday, wedding, or wedding anniversary, to people related to or connected with the donor, provided that the value of each such gift is not unreasonable in the circumstances. The donor may, if he or she wishes, include a clause in the power that prohibits the attorneys from making any gifts at all.

An EPA only authorizes an attorney to make decisions regarding the property and financial affairs of the donor. The attorney has no authority to make personal decisions (such as where, or with whom, the donor should live) or decisions relating to medical treatment. It is, of course, good clinical practice to consult with near-relatives on the treatment of mentally impaired patients, and where attorneys are near-relatives, as they most frequently are, their views should certainly be considered. But their rights in their function *as attorney* are limited to the management of the donor's financial affairs. It should also be mentioned here that attorneys acting under a registered EPA do not have the right to make a Will on behalf of the donor. If the donor lacks testamentary capacity, an application must be made to the Court for an order authorizing the execution of a statutory Will (see p. 000).

The Law Commission (1995) has recommended that the Enduring Powers of Attorney Act be repealed and that, instead, it should be possible to make Continuing Powers of Attorney (CPAs) which authorize the attorney to make personal and health care decisions as well as financial decisions on the donor's behalf.

Capacity to create an enduring power of attorney

The Enduring Powers of Attorney Act 1985 does not set out the criteria for the capacity required to create an enduring power. Given the difference between an ordinary power of attorney, which is automatically revoked when the donor becomes mentally incapacitated, it would seem reasonable to assume that a donor may make an enduring power of attorney only when he or she is mentally capable of managing his or her own affairs. However, there is case law to the effect that the donor needs merely to understand the *nature and effect* of the power he or she is donating, and need not necessarily be capable of managing his or her affairs generally. As the judgment in the cases in question, *Re K; Re F* (1988), illustrate not only important legal principles, but also ethical and practical ones related to everyday old age psychiatry, they will be discussed in some detail here.

In *Re K* and *Re F* the then Master of the Court of Protection, Mrs A. B. Macfarlane, dismissed respective applications to register two EPAs because the donors were mentally incapable of managing their affairs when they signed the powers. In the case of *Re K* Master Macfarlane said: 'I accept the strong evidence that on the particular date in question [when she signed the EPA]...Miss K was able to understand that Mr K was to be her attorney under an enduring power of attorney *and that she understood what an enduring power of attorney was* [this author's italics]; but that she was incapable by reason of mental disorder of managing her property and affairs.' In effect, the Master rejected the application to register the EPA because, in her judgment, incapacity to manage one's affairs at the time of donation of the EPA invalidated it.

The attorneys successfully appealed and the judge, Mr Justice Hoffmann, overruled the Master's decision and held that: 'The validity of that act [donation of EPA] depends on whether she understood its nature and effect and not on whether she would hypothetically have been able to perform all the acts which it authorised.' In a later part of the judgment this point was amplified: 'I see no reason why the test for whether it [the EPA] was validly created should be the same as for whether it would have ceased to be exercisable. In principle they are clearly different.' In essence, therefore, this judgment *separated* the capacity to donate an enduring power of attorney from the capacity to manage one's own affairs.

At the end of the judgment, Mr Justice Hoffmann addressed the question of the capacity required to create an enduring power of attorney. He said: 'Plainly one cannot expect that the donor should have been able to pass an examination on the provisions of the 1985 Act. At the other extreme, I do not think that it would be sufficient if he realised only that it gave (the attorney) power to look after his property.' In other words, it is insufficient for the donor merely to express a choice as to who should be the attorney, without knowing what an enduring power of attorney actually is.

The judge then approved a list of the matters which should ordinarily be explained to the donor and which the evidence should show that the donor has understood in order to establish that he or she has understood the nature and effect of creating an enduring power of attorney: in other words for the EPA to be valid. These are:

- the attorney will be able to assume complete authority over the donor's affairs;
- in general, the attorney will be able to do anything with the donor's property which the donor could have done;
- the attorney's authority will continue if the donor should *be or become* incapable, by reason of mental disorder, of managing and administering his or her property and affairs;
- if the donor becomes mentally incapable, he or she cannot revoke the power without confirmation by the Court of Protection.

The judgment in *Re K, Re F* enunciated one further principle relevant to old age psychiatry. It is this. If the donor executes an enduring power of attorney at a time when she is mentally incapable of managing her affairs, it 'means that the obligation to register arises immediately upon execution'. Thus, in certain circumstances, an attorney is obliged to apply to register an EPA as soon as the donor signs the document empowering him to act on his or her behalf. The period between the creation of an EPA and the application to register it is currently less than 1 month in 7% of applications; 1–3 months, 11%; 3–6 months, 9%; 6–12 months, 15%; over 12 months, 58%.

Registration of an enduring power of attorney

When the attorney has reason to believe that the donor *is*, or *is becoming*, mentally incapable of managing her affairs, the attorney must apply for the power to be registered with the Court. The Enduring Powers of Attorney Act 1985 does not specifically require that the donor should be medically examined for this purpose. Carson

(1987), who has highlighted the potential for abuse of an EPA, suggests that as part of its terms donors could require that they be medically examined at regular intervals with the results being submitted to someone who could act upon them if appropriate.

Before making the application to register the power, the attorney must give notice (in the prescribed form EP1) of his or her intention to apply for registration to the donor personally, and to at least three of the donor's closest relatives. There is an order of priority of relatives entitled to receive notice. The list can be found in the excellent explanatory booklet, *Enduring powers of attorney*, published by the Public Guardianship Office and obtainable free of charge from its Customer Services Unit (telephone 020 7664 7300).

Whilst the application to register the power is being made, the attorney's powers are temporarily suspended, except that the attorney still has the power: (1) to maintain the donor and (2) to prevent loss to her estate.

The donor and the relatives have 28 days in which they may object to the registration of the power. There are five grounds on which they may file a valid objection:

1. The instrument is not valid as an enduring power of attorney.
2. The power no longer subsists (in other words, it has been revoked).
3. The application is premature because the donor is not yet becoming mentally incapable.
4. Fraud or undue pressure was used to induce the donor to create the power.
5. Having regard to all the circumstances, the attorney is unsuitable to be the donor's attorney.

If there are no objections, the instrument is registered, with a date stamp and Court seal, and returned to the attorney, whose full authority to act is restored. If there are objections that cannot be resolved otherwise, the Court will impose a solution at an attended hearing. The number of applications that actually result in such a hearing is slightly less than 1%, and the commonest ground of objection is that the attorney is unsuitable. The legal costs involved in a contested application to register an EPA can run into many thousands of pounds and, where there is bitter intersibling rivalry among the donor's children, it may be advisable not to create an EPA in the first place.

When an enduring power of attorney has been registered, the Court generally has no ongoing involvement in the management and administration of the donor's affairs. This is the essential distinction between receivership under the Mental Health Act, on the one hand, and the EPA scheme on the other. Under the former the Court has a continuing responsibility to supervise the receiver. Under the latter, the management of the donor's affairs is firmly vested in the attorney, and the Court only needs to intervene if a problem arises. Nevertheless, the Court does have corrective functions under the Enduring Powers of Attorney Act. For example, it can give directions regarding the management or disposal by the attorney of the property and affairs of the donor, and it can require the attorney to render accounts, furnish information and produce documents. It can also, if necessary, bring the attorneyship to an end.

EPAs and receivership compared

The major advantage of an enduring power of attorney over receivership is that the donor can make her own decision in advance as to who should manage her affairs in the event of incapacity: though with fairness to the Court, it usually takes into account a patient's wishes when deciding whom to appoint as receiver. An EPA can also ensure continuity of agency. For example, an elderly physically frail but mentally fully capable woman gives her daughter an EPA in order to be relieved of the burden of day-to-day affairs. She suffers a stroke and becomes mentally incapable. Apart from the brief statutory period during which the EPA is being registered with the Court of Protection and the power of attorney is temporarily suspended, her daughter continues to act for her.

However, although they are more user-friendly than receivership, EPAs are also more abuser-friendly. Lush (1998) estimated that financial abuse probably occurs in 10–15% of cases, ranging from outright fraud at one end of the spectrum, to the inadvertent mishandling of assets by attorneys who are not fully aware of what they can and cannot do, at the other. There are various reasons why such abuse occurs:

- *The public domain.* An EPA comes into effect immediately, and the attorney may decide not to apply for registration, notwithstanding the subsequent incapacity of the donor, thereby avoiding any scrutiny under the notification procedure. Many powers never enter the public domain.
- *No ongoing supervision by the Court.* The Court has an ongoing responsibility to supervise a receiver, but has no such obligation in respect of an attorney. Although the Court can investigate an attorneyship, it requires a whistleblower to draw any problems to its attention and, although the Court has power to revoke an EPA, this is often as useful as 'closing the stable door after the horse has bolted'. The cost involved in bringing legal proceedings to recover misappropriated funds from fraudulent attorneys is usually prohibitive.
- *Unlimited access to capital and income.* An attorney has unlimited access to the donor's capital and income, and the restrictions contained in the legislation on the extent to which attorneys can make gifts of the donor's property are frequently flouted. Unauthorized gifting is the most widespread form of abuse.
- *No accountability.* Unlike receivers, who have to account annually to the Court, attorneys do not have to account to anyone and some attorneys do not even keep accounts.
- *No security.* A receiver is required to give security for his or her defaults. An attorney is not. In fact, it is impossible for an attorney to obtain security because insurance companies are unwilling to cover such a risk.

If a person suspects that an attorney may be abusing his power, then he or she should contact the Public Guardianship Office (telephone 020 7664 7300). The Public Guardianship Office will require medical evidence that the donor is, or is becoming, mentally incapable, in order to establish that the Court of Protection has jurisdiction to intervene. Lush (1998) suggested various safeguards against abuse: (1) avoiding unprofessional conduct at the time of creating a power, especially where the donor is already mentally incapacitated; (2) greater use of joint powers, and perhaps recommending a professional person to act as joint attorney with a relative; (3) discouraging the use of unregistered powers; and (4) greater discernment when recommending enduring powers of attorney to donors, and ensuring that they are informed not only of the benefits but also of the risks, particularly the risk that the attorney could misuse the power. Although such safeguards are designed to protect the donor, the facility to impose them is an example of the greater flexibility and freedom of choice afforded to both the donor and the attorney under an EPA compared with receivership.

Examples of unprofessional conduct at the time a person is making an enduring power of attorney might include:

- Expressing an opinion on a patient's capacity to make an enduring power without even seeing him or her for that purpose.
- Assessing a patient's capacity to create an enduring power of attorney without applying the tests in *Re K, Re F.*
- Failing to give reasons for deciding why a patient has or does not have the required degree of understanding.
- Mistaking the patient's ability to express a choice as to who should be the attorney, for the ability to understand the actual nature and effect of an enduring power of attorney.
- Making a decision on the basis that it is in the patient's best interests to give a power of attorney rather than that the patient has the capacity to give the power.

Appointeeship

Unlike receivership and attorneyship, which extend to all the property and affairs of a mentally incapacitated person, appointeeship applies solely to their social security benefits. The system is operated by the Secretary of State for Social Security, and the same provisions apply throughout the United Kingdom. There are no statistics on appointeeships, but the number of appointments made each year is probably in the region of 100 000.

If a person who is entitled to social security benefits ('the claimant') is mentally capable, but perhaps physically incapacitated, she can appoint an *agent* to collect her pension or other benefits on her behalf. There are three ways of doing this: (1) If the agency is one-off or short-term, the claimant simply completes the authorization on the back of the order, which says: 'I authorise (*name*) to be my agent and to cash this order for me'. (2) If it is necessary to appoint an agent on a longer term basis, the claimant should complete form BF73, which says: 'Until further notice I authorise (*name*) of (*address*) to cash my order books at (*branch*) Post Office'. The Benefits Agency will issue the agent with a form BF74, or Agency Card. (3) If the claimant is in Part III accommodation, she can complete form BR441 authorizing a local authority official to be his or her signing agent.

Appointeeship, as distinct from agency, is governed by Regulation 33 of the Social Security (Claims and Payments) Regulations 1987. This regulation empowers the Secretary of State to appoint an appointee for a claimant who 'is unable for the time being to act'. The regulation does not actually define this expression, and there are no specific legal criteria for this type of incapacity. Lavery and Lundy (1994) suggested that, in order to have the capacity to claim, receive, and deal with social security benefits, an individual should be able to: (1) understand the basis of possible entitlement; (2) understand and complete the claim form; (3) respond to correspondence from the department; (4) collect or receive the benefits; and (5) manage the benefits in the sense of knowing what the money is for, and be able to choose whether to use it for that purpose and, if so, how.

The Secretary of State will not appoint an appointee if a receiver has already been appointed by the Court of Protection to claim or receive benefits on the claimant's behalf, or if in Scotland the claimant's estate is being administered by a tutor or curator. An enduring power of attorney does not affect appointeeship, though in practice the attorney usually becomes the appointee.

The procedure for appointing an appointee is as follows. The prospective appointee completes form BF56 and returns it to the Benefits Agency. Medical evidence of the claimant's incapacity to act is not usually required. The Benefits Agency visit the claimant to establish whether appointeeship is appropriate and interview the proposed appointee to ensure that he is aware of his responsibilities and is suitable to act. References are sometimes sought. If everything is in order the local benefits supervisor will authorize the appointment on behalf of the Secretary of State. The appointee is notified of the appointment in form BF57, which informs him of his powers and duties.

Whereas an agent only has authority to cash the claimant's order, an appointee can exercise all the rights and duties which the claimant has under the social security legislation: for example, claiming benefits, receiving benefits, notifying the department of any change in the claimant's circumstances, and appealing against the decision of an adjudication officer. Whereas an agent must hand the cash to the claimant straightaway, an appointee is expected to use the cash in the best interests of the claimant and the claimant's dependants, if any.

Appointeeship can also be made for patients in hospital. In such cases it is usual that relatives or close friends will be appointed, but if none can be found a hospital manager may be invited to act. Appointeeship can be revoked at any time if the appointee is thought not to be acting in the claimant's best interests. If the appointee wishes to resign, he must give the Benefits Agency one month's notice.

Managing patients' affairs in Scotland

The legislation in Scotland has recently changed dramatically with the enactment of the Adults with Incapacity (Scotland) Act 2000, which received the Royal Assent on 9 May 2000. Because there are transitional provisions that will apply for some time, the legal provisions prior to the implementation of the Act are summarized below, in addition to the provisions of the Act itself.

Curators

Scotland has no equivalent to the Court of Protection. A *curator bonis* is appointed by the Sheriff Court or Court of Session to manage the property and financial affairs of a person who is incapable of managing his or her own affairs, or incapable of giving instructions for their management. The incapable person for whom the *curator* is appointed is known as a *ward*. Approximately 400 curators are appointed each year.

For the appointment of a curator, a petition or initial writ should be lodged in the Sheriff Court with jurisdiction where the ward resides, or the Court of Session. The petition should give details of the petitioner, the ward, the family, and the ward's estate, and should crave the appointment of the petitioner, or some other named person, or such person as the Court thinks fit, as curator. Traditionally, curators tended to be professional people—such as accountants and solicitors—but in recent years there has been a trend towards the appointment of lay curators, even where the estate has been quite large.

Two medical certificates must be produced showing that the ward is incapable of managing his or her affairs, or is incapable of giving instructions for their management. Unlike the law in England and Wales, the ward need not be incapable by reason of mental disorder. The incapacity may be physical. The medical certificates become out-of-date after 30 days, so they should not be obtained until the law agent is ready to lodge the petition. The Court will order service (unless it dispenses with service) on the ward, his or her relatives, and the Accountant of Court.

Every curator is required to find *caution* (security) prior to entering into his or her duties. The amount is fixed by the Accountant of Court. Caution should be lodged within 1 month of the appointment of the curator. An inventory of the ward's estate as at the date of the curator's appointment—with supporting documentation—should be lodged as soon as possible, and must be lodged within 6 months of the receipt of the bond of caution by the Accountant of Court. The curator must lodge annual accounts with the Accountant of Court for audit within 1 month of the closing date—usually the last day of the month following the anniversary of the curator's appointment. A booklet entitled *Information for families of persons subject to curatory* is issued by the Accountant of Court and may be obtained free of charge from the address below.

Tutors

In addition to curatory, Scots Law also recognizes the concept of tutelage, which until recently had been obsolescent. There are two kinds of tutor, both of whom can only be appointed by the Court of Session after considering evidence of incapacity in two separate medical certificates: a *tutor-dative*, who has only personal decision-making powers, and possibly provides a more personal type of guardianship than that under the Mental Health Act; and a *tutor-at-law*, who has both personal and financial decision-making powers.

In 1992, after a gap of over a century, a tutor-at-law was appointed by the Court of Session. A tutor-at-law has full power over not only the personal welfare of the ward but also his or her financial affairs, and his appointment supersedes that of any existing tutor-dative or curator bonis. Only the nearest male agnate (i.e. male relative on the father's side) may be appointed. A tutor-at-law is subject to the same rules and regulations as apply to curators with regard to caution, lodging an inventory of estate, accounting, and investment. He also comes under the supervision of the Accountant of Court.

Powers of attorney

Scotland has no equivalent statute to the Enduring Powers of Attorney Act 1985. However, by virtue of Section 71 of the Law Reform (Miscellaneous Provisions) (Scotland) Act 1990, all powers of attorney granted since 31 December 1990 continue to be effective after the granter's incapacity, unless the power of attorney itself contains express provisions to the contrary. This section was intended to be a temporary expedient pending the enactment of more comprehensive provisions on continuing and welfare powers of attorney (see below).

Adults with Incapacity (Scotland) Act 2000

Part 2 of the Adults with Incapacity (Scotland) Act 2000 enables people in Scotland to create a continuing power of attorney in respect of their property and finances and/or a welfare power of attorney in respect of personal welfare decisions. There is no prescribed form of continuing power or welfare power, but the document must contain a prescribed form of certificate, completed by a solicitor stating that he or she is satisfied that the granter understood the nature and effect of the power. The attorney has no authority to act under power until it has been registered with the Public Guardian. The Sheriff Court exercises various supervisory functions over attorneys acting under continuing and welfare powers, and can require them to be supervised by the Public Guardian or (in the case of welfare powers) the local authority, and can order them to produce accounts for audit by the Public Guardian. The ultimate sanction is that the Sheriff Court can revoke a continuing or welfare power of attorney.

Part 6 of the Adults with Incapacity (Scotland) Act 2000 replaces the existing system of appointing curators and tutors with a new scheme, whereby the Sheriff Court can make either a 'one-off' intervention order or appoint a guardian to manage the property and finances of an adult with incapacity. Applications for such orders must be accompanied by at least two medical reports, in a prescribed form, completed not more than 30 days before the application is lodged. At least one of the medical reports must be completed by a medical practitioner who is approved for the purposes of Section 20 of the Mental Health (Scotland) Act 1984 as having special expertise in the diagnosis or treatment of mental disorder. Guardianship orders may be limited in time. It is also possible for the Court to appoint interim guardians, joint guardians, and substitute guardians. Intervention orders and guardianship orders must be registered with the Public Guardian. A guardian is required to submit to the Public Guardian an inventory of the estate within 3 months of his appointment, together with a management plan; is expected to account annually, and to provide caution (insurance) against any claims of mishandling funds.

Managing patients' affairs in Northern Ireland

In Northern Ireland the management of mentally incapacitated patients' affairs is controlled by the High Court through the Office of Care and Protection. The relevant legislation, Part VIII of the Mental Health (Northern Ireland) Order 1986 and the Enduring Powers of Attorney (Northern Ireland) Order 1987, is virtually identical to that in England and Wales, except that instead of a receiver a *controller* is appointed to manage a patient's financial affairs. The Office of Care and Protection issues a *Handbook for controllers*, which can be obtained from the address below.

Managing patients' affairs in Ireland

In the Republic of Ireland the management of the property and affairs of mentally incapacitated adults (known as 'wards of court') is overseen by the President of the High Court, who has delegated the day-to-day administration of wardship matters to the Registrar of Wards of Court and his staff. The wardship legislation is contained in the Lunacy Regulation (Ireland) Act 1871. It is possible for a proposed ward to demand a trial by jury to decide the issue of his or her capacity. There have been two such requests in the last 5 years. After the President of the High Court has made an order bringing a person into wardship, he generally appoints a committee (i.e. a person to whom the affairs of the ward are 'committed') to act on the ward's behalf. The committee is authorized to receive the income of the ward; must enter into security with an approved insurance company, and file annual accounts for all sums received and disbursed.

It has been possible to make an enduring power of attorney in the Republic of Ireland since 1 August 1996, when Part II of the Powers of Attorney Act 1996 came into force. The legislation is broadly similar to the Enduring Powers of Attorney Act 1985 in England and Wales. The power must be in a form prescribed by the Minister for Justice. The attorney must apply for the power to be registered with the Office of Wards of Court when he or she has reason to believe that the donor is, or is becoming, mentally incapable. Certain people are entitled to be notified of the attorney's intention to register the power, and there are the same five grounds as in England on which an objection to registration might be sustained.

However, the Irish legislation contains a number of the recommended improvements to the English Act, including a requirement that a registered medical practitioner must state that, in his or her opinion, at the time the document was executed the donor had the mental capacity, with the assistance of such explanations as may have been given, to understand the effect of creating the power. Between 1 August 1996 and 1 August 2000 a total of 100 enduring powers of attorney were registered by the Office of Wards of Court, and there was just one objection to registration. It is possible that the take-up rate for enduring powers of attorney is lower in Ireland than in England and Wales because of the statutory requirement that a medical practitioner must assess the donor's capacity when the power is created.

The main difference between Irish and English enduring powers of attorney is that in Ireland the donor may authorize his or her attorney to make personal welfare decisions, such as:

- where the donor should live;
- with whom the donor should live;
- whom the donor should see and not see;
- what training and rehabilitation the donor should get;
- the donor's diet and dress;
- inspection of the donor's personal papers; and
- housing, social welfare, and other benefits for the donor.

Addresses

For England and Wales:

- Public Guardianship Office, Stewart House, 24 Kingsway, London WC2B 6JX; tel: 020 7664 7300, fax: 020 7664 7168.

For Scotland:

- Supreme Court, Accountant of Court, Parliament Square, Edinburgh EH1 1RQ; tel: 0131 225 2595, fax: 0131 240 6771.
- Office of The Public Guardian, Hadrian House, Callander Business Park, Callander Road, Falkirk FK1 1XR; tel: 01324 678300, fax: 01324 678301.

For Northern Ireland:

- The Office of Care and Protection, Royal Courts of Justice, Chichester Street, PO Box 410, Belfast BT1 3TF; tel: 01232 235 111, fax: 01232 313793.

For the Republic of Ireland:

- The Office of Wards of Court, Aras Ui Dhalaigh, Inns Quay, Dublin 7; tel: 01 888 6000, fax: 01 872 4063.

References

Carson, D. (1987). Being Prepared. In *Making the most of the Court of Protection: a guide to the law relating to the Court of Protection and on making use of the Court's services* (ed. D. Carson), pp. 14–23. King's Fund Centre, London.

Lavery, R. and Lundy, L. (1994). The Social Security Appointee System. *Journal of Social Welfare Law*, No. 3, 313–27.

Law Commission (1995). *Report no 231, Mental Incapacity.* HMSO, London.

Lush, D. (1998). Taking liberties: enduring powers of attorney and financial abuse. *Solicitors Journal*, **142**, 808–9.

Re CAF unpublished.

Re K, Re F (1988). *The Law Reports, Chancery Division*, pp. 310–16; *All England Law Reports*, Vol. 1, p. 358.

Silberfeld, M., Corber, W., Madigan, K. V., and Checkland, D. (1995). Capacity assessments for requests to restore legal competence. *International Journal of Geriatric Psychiatry*, **10**, 191–7.

Whitehead, A. (1987). Medical certification. In *Making the most of the Court of Protection: a guide to the law relating to the Court of Protection and on making use of the Court's services* (ed. D. Carson), pp. 24–31. King's Fund Centre, London.

Whitehorn, N. A. (1991). *Heywood and Massey: Court of Protection Practice*, 12th edition. Sweet and Maxwell, London.

42 Driving and psychiatric illness in later life

Desmond O'Neill

Overview of mobility and health

Mobility and driving evoke a curious response in health care personnel. With most areas of function, we assess and treat people so as to maximize that function. The literature on driving and disease, however, is almost totally biased in favour of the identification of those who should not drive rather than maximizing health and function so that older people can participate and integrate as much as possible in society. This matter assumes great importance in view of the dramatic rise in the proportion of older people in our society. It is further emphasized by the enormous increase in the proportion of older people who wish to continue driving.

Some of this negative attitude stems from a more widespread failure to appreciate the idiosyncratic approach of our society to mobility and safety. At its most striking, a landmark study in the 1960s showed that American motorists felt they were more likely to be involved in a nuclear catastrophe than in a fatal car crash. Despite high-profile campaigns to promote safety on our roads by way of exhortations to reduce speed and avoid alcohol, at virtually every level of transport policy, mobility takes priority over safety. If safety were paramount, the speed limit would be 20 miles per hour and governors would be fitted to car engines to prevent this limit from being exceeded. It is also likely that we would have a more graduated entry to driving in the late teens or early twenties. This is because youth and inexperience breed risky driving behaviours that cause crashes: unfortunately the emphasis of many European governments is to stigmatize older drivers (White and O'Neill 2000). Older drivers are obliged to undergo regular medical checks in most countries of the European Union, despite evidence that this practice is harmful (Hakamies-Blomqvist *et al.* 1996) or ineffective (Rock 1998). This ageist legislation is not based on any factual evidence and reflects the weakness of organized advocacy for older people in Europe. This is despite the fact that older drivers have one of the best safety records of any group of drivers in society (Evans 1988).

It has been suggested that older drivers have a higher crash risk than younger ones, in a 'U'-shaped distribution fashion (Broughton 1988). But comparison of the safety of younger and older drivers is complicated and depends on how the risk is expressed. In the first instance, older people drive fewer miles, which means that the *risk per driver* is closer to that of younger people, despite the latter's *high risk per mile*. It is interesting to note that the very act of driving fewer miles increases the risk of crashes at any age (Hakamies-Blomqvist and Wahlstrom, in press). Also, older people tend to drive on inherently more dangerous roads—rural and suburban highways are more dangerous than motorways. Finally, old people are more fragile and are more likely to suffer death or serious injury for a given severity of crash than young people (Brorsson 1989).

Health and driving

There is a famous illustration in Laurence's pharmacology textbook of the process whereby a new medication is absorbed into medical practice.

This progresses from an initial enthusiastic acceptance, to a sceptical rejection, and finally results in a reasoned assessment of the positive and negative aspects of the drug (Fig. 42.1). This is a similar process to that which occurs when health care professionals encounter the concept of driving and illness for the first time. Initially, working in an environment where a highly selected population are much more likely to have a high burden of disease, it is inevitable that the potential risks should be perceived more readily than the impact on mobility (O'Neill *et al.* 1992). As researchers in the area gain perspective, a totally different concept comes to the fore, that of the major threat posed to the mobility of older people by age-related disease (Metz 2000). Finally, the fusion of both points of view is achieved, whereby an enabling process is developed that encompasses the mechanisms for helping those who can no longer drive to seek alternative methods of transport, secure in the knowledge that a thorough evaluation and rehabilitation were fairly carried out (O'Neill 2000).

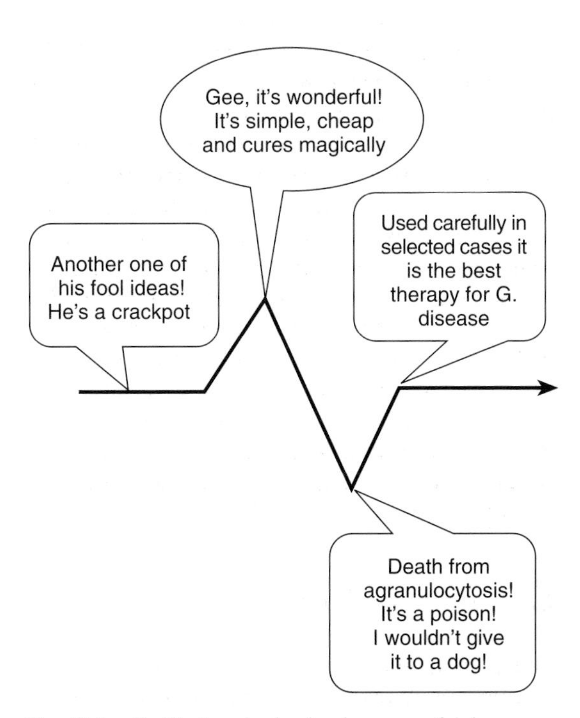

Fig. 42.1 Oscillations in the development of a drug.

Driving is a health-related issue: there is a consistent pattern in many countries whereby cessation of driving relates to illness and loss of function (Campbell *et al.* 1993; Forrest *et al.* 1997; Kostyniuk *et al.* 1998), although driving may persist after other socially useful patterns of mobility have been affected (Hjorthol 2001). This pattern is reflected in several studies of dementia and driving (Foley *et al.* 2000). Older people tend not to discuss concerns about driving with health care providers (Johnson 1998): this is a cause of concern as it is possible that treatable medical causes of driving cessation may be missed.

Although all people with progressive illnesses such as the dementias will eventually decline in cognition, function, and behaviour, it is not clear that this poses a public health risk, despite a somewhat one-sided review of current studies (Dubinsky *et al.* 2000). It is more likely that patients' spontaneous reduction and eventual withdrawal from driving protects the general public from the harmful effects of the illness on driving safety (Trobe *et al.* 1996; Carr *et al.* 2000).

Skills and resources needed for mobility assessment

Many professionals working in the psychiatry of old age feel at a loss when confronted with older people who both drive and have a psychiatric illness. They often do not realize that their many skills used in clinical decision-making also form the basis of making decisions on a patient's driving and mobility. The foundation of these skills was founded on the principles of multidisciplinary assessment, and on the philosophy of advocacy and enabling for older people in the face of nihilism and ageism. In practice, this is seen in the integration of clinical assessment with input from the multidisciplinary team when calculating the risk in other areas of clinical practice, such as deciding on a patient's discharge to home. Elements of this decision-making process include careful multidisciplinary evaluation, discussion with carers, and may involve a trial visit home. Some of the elements of this process are very similar to the assessment of a person's fitness to drive. In driving, as in planning discharge from hospital, relatives may value the patient's security before their independence. In both fields a psychometric model of assessment is unlikely to be helpful. This often surprises clinicians: while psychometric support is important in backing up our diagnostic abilities, it is rarely of help when making decisions about function. For example, the decision that the patient is no longer fit to remain at home and requires placement in a nursing home is much more likely to be taken on the basis of measures of function and behaviour than on psychometry.

The premise that the expertise of those who practise psychiatry with older people already contains some of the elements necessary for mobility assessments is not a charter for dilettantism. Rather, it is a challenge to us to develop the extra resources required to ensure that we have adequate support when making decisions about enhancing the safe mobility of older people. This has many parallels with the task of assessing safety at home or capacity to manage financial affairs: in these cases, it is good practice to liaise with an occupational therapist or a neuropsychologist. There has also been a failure to capitalize on the rich knowledge of psychiatrists: many studies have been more concerned to highlight psychiatrists' lack of knowledge of the driving regulations rather than to draw on their collected wisdom (Elwood 1998). It is likely that their estimates of the parameters of safe mobility in their patient groups would have equal if not greater validity than current driving regulations, which are often arbitrary and sometimes counter-intuitive and unfair.

As a minimum, the assessment of the impact of psychiatric illness on mobility in later life requires a careful medical and psychiatric assessment, a collateral history, and access to occupational therapy and/or neuropsychology as well as access to a specialist driver assessment. There may be a case for developing services at a regional level, particularly for those cases where an unequivocal decision can not be made after the first assessment. A specific concern relates to the funding of such services: although the mobility/risk problem is clearly health-related in origin, Medicare in the United States will not refund specialist driving assessment, and the attendant cost may deter older drivers from seeking help. The psychiatrist will also need to know the local regulations on fitness to drive, the obligations of the patient to disclose relevant illness to the driver licensing authority and insurance company, and an awareness of the local requirements for physician disclosure, if any.

Models of driving behaviour

Driving is an over-learned skill with a significant behavioural input (Ranney 1994). The major advance in this area has been the understanding that a purely cognitive model of driving ability does not adequately reflect the complexity and hierarchical nature of the driving task. We also know that clinicians assessing patients with a range of diseases, including dementia, may not accurately predict their performance on road testing of their driving ability (Heikkila *et al.* 1998). Driver behaviour is complex. One of the simplest and most easily applicable models has been that of Michon's hierarchy (1985) which uses strategic, tactical, and operational factors. The strategic level is the choice of whether or not to travel; the tactical decision is whether or not to overtake; and the operational level is what to do when overtaking and faced with an oncoming car. The strategic and tactical levels are probably more important in terms of driving safety than the operational level. To a certain extent, this has been operationalized for brain damage (head injury and stroke) in Galski's driving model, which in effect adds a behavioural observational element to a battery of cognitive tests and a primitive simulator (Galski *et al.* 1993). It has also been operationalized more closely in a driver screening battery (de Raedt, in press). The most common model for driver assessment is shown in Fig. 42.2.

Not all levels will be required by all patients: a patient with a homonymous hemianopia is barred from driving throughout the European Union, and referral to the social worker to plan alternative transportation is appropriate. Equally, a mild cognitive defect may only require a review

History
- Patient, family/informant
- Driving history

Examination
Functional status
Other illnesses and drugs
Vision
Mental status testing
Diagnostic formulation and prioritization
Disease severity and fluctuations
Remediation
Re-assess
In-depth cognitive/perceptual testing
± On-road Assessment

Overall evaluation of hazard
- Strategic
- Tactical
- Operational

Advice to patient/carer ± DMV
If driving to hazardous, consider alternative mobility strategies

Fig. 42.2 Common Model for Driver Assessments

by the physician and occupational therapist. The overall interdisciplinary assessment should attempt to provide solutions in two areas: maintaining activities, and exploring transport needs. The on-road test can be helpful as it may demonstrate deficits to a patient or carer who is ambivalent about the patient stopping driving. At a therapeutic level, members of the team may be able to help the patient come to terms with the losses associated with stopping driving, where the decision has been objectively taken. The occupational therapist may be able to maximize activities and function and help focus on preserved areas of achievement, while the social worker can advise on alternative methods of transport. This approach should save time and valuable resources for occupational therapy, neuropsychology, and road driver assessors.

In addition to the usual work-up, the medical assessment should include a driving history from patient and carer. Although Hunt has shown a poor correlation between carer assessment and the patient's on-road driving performance (Hunt *et al.* 1993), this single small study is insufficient to discount the collateral history. The Folstein Mini-Mental State Examination would perhaps be the most reasonable choice of a simple screening measure of cognitive impairment: a near-consensus paper in 1996 suggested that those who score 17 or less on a Mini-Mental State Examination require further assessment in a formal way (Lundberg *et al.* 1996). The relatively low cut-off score reflected unease among the participants that reliance on a simple test such as the MMSE would oversimplify the complex task of appropriate assessment of older people with dementia.

The next stage of testing described in the literature has been carried out by occupational therapists and neuropsychologists. None of the studies has been sufficiently large to have a reasonable predictive value or to determine cut-off points on neuropsychological test batteries. This situation parallels that in memory clinics where there is a wide variation in test batteries used. It is likely that the important elements of successful assessment are the choice of key domains, familiarity with a test battery, and the development of an understanding and close liaison between the physician and the occupational therapist and/or neuropsychologist. A wide range of tests has been correlated with driving behaviour, but few have been sufficiently robust to calculate cut-off points for risky driving. All these tests can be criticized for taking an overcognitive view of the driving task.

Specific tests that show a correlation with driving ability in more than one study include the MMSE (above), the Trail-making Test (Maag 1984; Janke and Eberhard 1998; Mazer *et al.* 1998; Stutts *et al.* 1998), and a range of tests of visual attention (Klavora *et al.* 1995; Duchek *et al.* 1998; Marottoli *et al.* 1998; Owsley *et al.* 1998; Trobe 1998), including the Useful Field of View®, a composite measure of preattentive processing, incorporating speed of visual information processing, ability to ignore distractors (selective attention), and ability to divide attention (Owsley *et al.* 1991). A range of other tests have been assessed in single studies (an interesting one is traffic sign recognition (Carr *et al.* 1991); a comprehensive review is available from the US National Highway Transportation Safety Administration (Staplin *et al.* 1999).

In conjunction with the clinical assessment and collateral history, these tests will help to decide which patients require on-road testing, as well as those who are likely to be dangerous to test! The other interesting aspect is that there may be a disparity between scores on a test battery and the clinical assessment of the neuropsychologist. In a small paper by Fox *et al.*, the neuropsychology test scores and the neuropsychology prediction were not found to be significantly associated (Fox *et al.* 1997), suggesting that the clinicians made their decisions on items not formally measured in the neuropsychology test battery.

On-road driver testing is the 'gold standard' and should be offered to all patients who are not clearly dangerous when driving and who are not disqualified from driving for other reasons, such as homonymous hemianopia or convulsions. At least three different road tests have been devised, but the numbers of patients put through these are still relatively small: 27 patients in the Sepulveda Road Test (Fitten *et al.* 1995); 65 in the Washington University Road Test (Hunt *et al.* 1997); and 155 in the Alberta Road Test (Dobbs 1998). The assessor will require a full clinical report, and may choose to use one of the recently developed scoring systems for the on-road testing of patients with dementia. A few countries offer a medical advisory service, for example the Medical Section of the DVLA (Driver and Vehicle Licensing Agency) in the UK.

Functional illness

The role of illness other than dementia has been even less widely studied. Leaving alcohol dependency aside, the overall impression from the literature is that the added risk from schizophrenia and affective disorders is small, although the issue is complicated by the use of psychoactive medications. The emphasis on risk rather than on mobility is similar to the rest of the field, and it is likely that those with psychiatric illness have less mobility than the population as a whole. Buttiglieri and Guenette (1967) found that subjects with psychiatric illness had accident and violation records similar to the general population. Patients with schizophrenia and on depot neuroleptics show a worse performance on a driving test than unmedicated normal controls (Wylie *et al.* 1993), but concrete evidence of an increased crash risk is not available. A Swiss study in 1978 in mostly young and middle-aged people with schizophrenia showed more violations and accidents in those with religious delusions, but was favourable in those with a cautious, anxious character (Sacher 1978). The role of psychiatric intervention has only been assessed in one study. Eelkema *et al.* (1970) found those with alcohol dependency had higher than normal crash rates both before and after hospitalization, whereas those classified as suffering from psychotic and psychoneurotic disorders had higher rates prior to hospitalization and lower ones afterwards. No-one in any of the groups was older than 70, which is a recurring issue in the literature in this area. The one paper dealing with depression and driving in old age is limited to two case reports and is highly conjectural. The use of car crashes as a means of suicide is considered to occur in a very small proportion of cases, despite a suggestion from early studies that this might be a more marked problem. Studies by Tabachnik *et al.* (1966), Schmidt *et al.* (1977), and Isherwood *et al.* (1982) have subsequently shown the risk to be small.

So where does this leave the clinician? Key factors are likely to be the severity and stability of the patient's condition, their insight, impulsiveness, and ability to react appropriately in a strategic and operational fashion. Ideally, medications will be minimized, with due caution given to neuroleptics or long-acting benzodiazepines (see below).

Medications and driving

An area of increasing debate over the last 20 years has been the potential impact of psychoactive medications on driver safety. This interest has paralleled studies showing an impact of these medications on other injuries (Ray 1992), notably falls. Moreover, a number of studies have suggested that physicians should be concerned about diminished driving skills and increased crash risk with these medications (Ray *et al.* 1993; Hemmelgarn *et al.* 1997). In terms of the numbers of prescriptions, the main groups implicated are the benzodiazepines (Hemmelgarn *et al.* 1997) and antidepressants (Ray *et al.* 1992). If a true increased risk can be established and quantified by medication type and dosage, restrictions in prescribing and/or driving may be an achievable component of a crash-prevention strategy.

Demonstrating cause and effect has been problematic. Separating the effects of the disease from those of the medications is not easy: depression, anxiety, and insomnia may have an impact on driving behaviour that might be ameliorated by pharmacological treatment, although current evidence suggests this is likely to be true for depression only. Studies on volunteers do not replicate clinical experience. There is a mini-industry of reaction/braking time tests comparing psychoactive medications. As we have previously seen, operational or reaction factors are less important than strategic or tactical factors, so it is very difficult to give any significant weight to these tests. There is also a danger of trying to extrapolate from them to a real impact on safety.

A parallel here is the theoretical differences between tricyclic antidepressants (TCAs) and selective serotoninergic-reuptake inhibitors (SSRIs) and the risk of falls. Although SSRIs would seem to have theoretical advantages, clinical studies have been unable to show any difference in fall rates between older people on TCAs and SSRIs (Thapa *et al.* 1998). Similarly, there have been difficulties in epidemiological studies in matching controls with cases, in the exclusion of fatalities (more likely to involve alcohol and possibly psychoactive drugs), unreliability in medication recall at interview, lack of diagnostic categorization prior to the crash, and failure to control for the many variables which affect crash risk.

The use of large prescribing databases has helped to reduce uncertainty about prescribed medications among subjects in epidemiological studies. Hemmelgarn and colleagues showed an increased crash risk of 1.5 in the first week of taking a long-acting benzodiazepines among older drivers compared to 1.29 with chronic use, and no increased risk among those on short-acting benzodiazepines (Hemmelgarn *et al.* 1997). A further methodological refinement is reported in a study of a crash population where just over 1% of drivers in a first-ever crash were current users of benzodiazepines (Barbone *et al.* 1998). The authors used a technique whereby subjects acted as their own controls, eliminating the difficulty of finding matching controls and reducing some of the associated confounding effects. The finding of an almost 50% increase in crash risk in users of benzodiazepines should be interpreted cautiously.

While generally consistent with trends in the literature, the risk was concentrated in younger drivers (under 45), and was greatly increased by the presence of alcohol. The absence of an association with increased risk in the elderly, a group who are most sensitive to the effects of benzodiazepines, is noteworthy: if sustained, it suggests that benzodiazepines affect crash-risk by mechanisms other than those which have been traditionally measured by psychometric tests. The lack of an association with tricyclic antidepressants is also a departure from existing data. The restriction of the study to first-time crashes limits the study of those who may demonstrate risky driving behaviour.

Universal advice against driving while taking benzodiazepines is not yet supported by this study, but it should accelerate both epidemiological and policy interest in the subject, as well as clinical caution. An expansion of this style of study should be encouraged, to include all crashes and injury and death from other forms of mobility, such as pedestrians and cyclists. Prospective studies are also needed, perhaps at the time of peri-marketing clinical trials (Ray 1992). In the interim, those who dispense benzodiazepines need to recognize that most adult patients are drivers or potential drivers. Active consideration should be given as to whether the illness is likely to affect driving skills and whether the patient has a past crash history. The patient should be advised not to drive if they cannot abstain from alcohol while taking benzodiazepines. Most importantly, the clinician should ask him/herself whether the patient really needs a benzodiazepine, and if they do, whether it needs to be long-acting.

Practical guidelines

The first priority for the psychiatrist is to ask how the diagnosis affects the patient's mobility: a secondary goal is to assess the potential dangers to safety. The procedures outlined in Fig. 42.2 should be carried out, and, ideally, any permanent decisions on driving should be made when the patient's condition is stabilized and optimized. An interim decision will have to be made until the assessment is completed, which may involve asking the patient to desist from driving temporarily. Some countries have reasonably well-developed guidelines for helping clinicians: however, the evidence-base for the recommendations is unclear, and changes to these regulations may often lag behind advances in clinical practice. For example, the mostly excellent 'At-a-Glance' leaflets from the UK driver licensing authorities (*http://www.dvla.gov.uk/at_a_glance/aag_contents.htm*) seem to assume that hospitalization is still a prerequisite in significant psychiatric illness, whereas ambulatory care is the rule rather than the exception in modern practice. Some of the criteria also seem unnecessarily strict; and as the field of driver assessment matures, it will be important that professional organizations make representations to vehicle licensing authorities to ensure that the regulations are fair. New guidelines from the Association for the Advancement of Automotive Medicine stress the importance of leaving many of the decisions to the specialist, assuming appropriate assessment back-up (Dobbs, in press). In the interim, physicians who feel that the regulations hinder the health, well-being, and mobility of their patient unnecessarily may need to consult their medical defence organization about the clash of ethical responsibilities.

In many cases the decision may be quite clear, either that there are no concerns about driving safety or that the patient is manifestly too unstable or compromised to drive safely. However, in cases where the judgement lies in between, a full assessment including an on-road driving test may be required. Once a decision has been made, the psychiatrist needs to inform the patient of his (the patient's) responsibilities in terms of reporting to the local driver licensing authorities and/or his insurance company: this should be documented in the clinical notes. These responsibilities vary enormously from jurisdiction to jurisdiction. Failure to inform the patient of the relevant requirement may lead to litigation against the doctor. I tend to phrase this by suggesting to the patient that they review their insurance policy documentation. The psychiatrist also needs to be aware of any statutory requirements for physicians to report illnesses such as dementia to departments of motor vehicles (DMVs), as is the case in California and most Canadian provinces. To report a patient without having confidence that a fair and sensitive assessment will be made by the DMV, can pose an ethical dilemma to the physician. It is of some interest that the rate of reporting to the Californian DMV of drivers with dementia by physicians did not increase after the institution of the relevant law.

If the assessment suggests that the patient can drive safely, the decision that driving may continue entails several components. These are:

- duration before review;
- possible restriction;
- driving accompanied;
- licensing authority reporting relationship;
- insurance reporting responsibility.

As dementia is a progressive illness and affective disorders and alcohol dependency are recurrent/relapsing diseases, it is prudent to make any declaration of fitness to drive subject to regular review. For dementia, my own practice is to review again in 6 months, or sooner if any deterioration is reported by the carer. Following evidence that the crash rate is reduced if the driver is accompanied (Bédard *et al.* 1996), it could be sensible to restrict driving to occasions when there is someone else in the car, using the co-pilot paradigm (Shua-Haim and Gross 1996). There is also preliminary evidence from the state of Utah that drivers who have restricted driving licences have lower crash rates (Vernon 1999). Patients should be advised to avoid traffic congestion and not to drive at night or in bad weather. The patient and carers should be advised to acquaint themselves with local driver licensing authority requirements, as well their motor insurance company policy. All the above should be clearly recorded in the medical notes. Except for jurisdictions where there is mandatory reporting of drivers with dementia (e.g. California and some Canadian provinces), there is no obligation on the doctor to break medical confidentiality in these cases.

How do older drivers with dementia deal with driving cessation when driving is no longer possible?

There is strong evidence that drivers with dementia not only limit their own driving and cease driving voluntarily (Foley *et al.* 2000), but also are amenable to pressure from family and physicians. In one of the largest studies 18% of patients stopped driving of their own accord, 23% because of physicians' advice, 42% because of family members, and the rest by a combination of interventions (Trobe *et al.* 1996). There are no data on how patients with dementia compensate for the lack of transport required to fulfil their social, occupational, and health needs. Psychological adaptation to driving cessation may be helped by clarity of diagnosis and psychotherapeutic input, but this has not been subject to a randomized controlled trial. In a single case study, the patient's feelings and fears about giving up driving were explored with him (Bahro *et al.* 1995). The intervention was designed with the patient as collaborator rather than passive recipient of advice, and by dealing with the events at an emotional rather than an intellectual level. The patient was able to grieve about the disease and in particular about the loss of his car. This in turn enabled him to redirect his attention to other meaningful activities that did not involve driving. Although this approach may be hampered by the deficits of dementia, it reflects a more widespread trend towards sharing the diagnosis of dementia with the patient.

What should doctors advise when they assess patients as unfit to drive?

If the assessment supports driving cessation, patients and carers should be advised of this, and a social worker consulted to help maximize transportation options. Giving up driving can have a considerable effect on lifestyle. Normal elderly drivers accept that their physician's advice would be very influential in deciding to give up driving (Rabbitt *et al.* 1996), and many patients with dementia will respond to advice from families or physicians.

The way we deal with driving reflects how we help the patient to deal with the reality of the deficits caused by dementia. If the positive approach described above is not successful, confidentiality may have to be broken for a small minority of cases. Most professional associations for physicians accept that the principle of confidentiality is covered to a degree by a 'common good' principle of protecting third parties when direct advice to the patient is ignored (American Medical Association 1999). Removal of the driving licence alone is unlikely to have much effect on these patients, and the vehicle may need to be disabled (Donnelly and Karlinsky 1990) and all local repair services warned not to respond to calls from the patient!

In the event of a decision to advise cessation of driving, advice from a medical social worker can be helpful in planning strategies for using alternative modes of travel. This may be difficult in a rural setting: one estimate of community transport costs exclusively for older people in the US was $5.14 for a one-way trip in 1983 (Rosenbloom 1993). The political system has not yet woken up to the need for adequate paratransit, i.e. tailored, affordable, and reliable assisted transport which is acceptable to older adults with a physical and/or mental disability (Freund 2000). Tailored transport (paratransit) is expensive, but may have benefits in reducing institutionalization and in improving quality of life.

Screening for dementia among older drivers

Despite the lack of convincing evidence for an older driver 'problem', ageist policies in many jurisdictions have led to screening programmes for older drivers. In the absence of reliable and sensitive assessment tools, this approach is flawed, as illustrated by data from Scandinavia (Hakamies-Blomqvist *et al.* 1996). In Finland there is regular age-related medical certification of a fitness to drive, whereas Sweden has no routine medical involvement in licence renewal. There is no reduction in the number of older people dying in car crashes in Finland compared to Sweden, but there is an increase in the number of those dying as pedestrians and cyclists, possibly in part by unnecessarily removing drivers from their cars. A more minimalist and less medical approach using very simple measures, such as a vision test and a written skill examination may be more helpful (Levy *et al.* 1995): unfortunately this approach is also associated with a reduction in the number of older drivers, a possible negative health impact (Levy 1995). Another approach is opportunistic health screening, perhaps of those older drivers with traffic violations (Johansson *et al.* 1996). It remains to be seen whether these and other screening policies reduce mobility among older people, a practical and civil rights issue of great importance.

References

American Medical Association. (1999). *Ethical and Judicial Affairs Report*. APA, Chicago.

Bahro, M., Silber, E., Box, P., *et al.* (1995). Giving up driving in Alzheimer's disease—an integrative therapeutic approach. *International Journal of Geriatric Psychiatry*, **10**, 871–4.

Barbone, F., McMahon, A., Davey, P., *et al.* (1998). Association of road-traffic accidents with benzodiazepine use. *Lancet*, **352**, 1331–6.

Bédard, M., Molloy, M., and Lever, J. (1996). Should demented patients drive alone? *Journal of the American Geriatrics Society*, **44**, S9.

Brorsson, B. (1989). Age and injury severity. *Scandinavian Journal of Social Medicine*, **17**, 287–90.

Broughton, J. (1988). *The variation of car driver's risk with age* (RR135). Transport and Road Research Laboratory, Crowthorne, Berkshire.

Buttiglieri, M. W. and Guenette, M. (1967). Driving record of neuropsychiatric patients. *Journal of Applied Psychology*, **51**, 96–100.

Campbell, M. K., Bush, T. L., and Hale, W. E. (1993). Medical conditions associated with driving cessation in community-dwelling, ambulatory elders. *Journal of Gerontology*, **48**, S230–4.

Carr, D., Madden, D., Cohen, H. J., *et al.* (1991). The use of traffic identification signs to identify drivers with dementia. *Journal of the American Geriatrics Society*, **39**, A62.

Carr, D. B., Duchek, J., and Morris, J. C. (2000). Characteristics of motor vehicle crashes of drivers with dementia of the Alzheimer type. *Journal of the American Geriatrics Society*, **48**, 18–22. [See comments.]

De Raedt, R. and Ponjaert–Kristoffersen, I. (2000). Can strategic and tactical compensation reduce crash risk in older drivers? *Age and Ageing*, **29**, 517–21.

Dobbs, A. R. *A manual of medical fitness to drive*. Association for the Advancement of Automotive Medicine, Chicago. (In press.)

Dobbs, B., Heller, R. B., and Schopflocher, D. (1998). A comparative approach to identify unsafe older drivers. *Accident Analysis and Prevention*, **30**, 363–70.

Donnelly, R. E. and Karlinsky, H. (1990). The impact of Alzheimer's disease on driving ability: a review. *Journal of Geriatric Psychiatry and Neurology*, **3**, 67–72.

Dubinsky, R. M., Stein, A. C., and Lyons, K. (2000). Practice parameter: risk of driving and Alzheimer's disease (an evidence-based review): report of the quality standards subcommittee of the American Academy of Neurology. *Neurology*, **54**, 2205–11.

Duchek, J. M., Hunt, L., Ball, K., *et al.* (1998). Attention and driving performance in Alzheimer's disease. *Journals of Gerontology. Series B, Psychological Sciences and Social Sciences*, **53**, 130–41.

Eelkema, R., Brosseau, J., Koshnick, R., *et al.* (1970). A statistical study on the relationship between mental illness and traffic accidents. *American Journal of Public Health*, **60**, 459–69.

Elwood, P. (1998). Driving, mental illness and the role of the psychiatrist. *Irish Journal of Psychological Medicine*, **15**, 49–51.

Evans, L. (1988). Older driver involvement in fatal and severe traffic crashes. *Journal of Gerontology*, **43**, S186–93.

Fitten, L. J., Perryman, K. M., Wilkinson, C. J., *et al.* (1995). Alzheimer and vascular dementias and driving. A prospective road and laboratory study [see comments]. *Journal of the American Medical Association*, **273**, 1360–5.

Foley, D. J., Masaki, K. H., Ross, G. W., *et al.* (2000). Driving cessation in older men with incident dementia. *Journal of the American Geriatrics Society*, **48**, 928–30.

Forrest, K. Y., Bunker, C. H., Songer, T. J., *et al.* (1997). Driving patterns and medical conditions in older women. *Journal of the American Geriatrics Society*, **45**, 1214–18.

Fox, G. K., Bowden, S. C., Bashford, G. M., *et al.* (1997). Alzheimer's disease and driving: prediction and assessment of driving performance. *Journal of the American Geriatrics Society*, **45**, 949–53.

Freund, K. (2000). Independent Transportation Network: alternative transportation for the elderly. *TR News*, **206**, 3–12.

Galski, T., Bruno, R. L., and Ehle, H. T. (1993). Prediction of behind-the-wheel driving performance in patients with cerebral brain damage: a discriminant function analysis. *American Journal of Occupational Therapy*, **47**, 391–6.

Hakamies-Blomqvist, L., Johansson, K., and Lundberg, C. (1996). Medical screening of older drivers as a traffic safety measure—a comparative Finnish–Swedish Evaluation study. *Journal of the American Geriatrics Society*, **44**, 650–3.

Hakamies-Blomqvist, L. and Wahlstrom, B. Flattening the U-shaped curve. *Lancet*. (In press.)

Heikkila, V. M., Turkka, J., Korpelainen, J., *et al.* (1998). Decreased driving ability in people with Parkinson's disease. *Journal of Neurology, Neurosurgery and Psychiatry*, **64**, 325–30.

Hemmelgarn, B., Suissa, S., Huang, A., *et al.* (1997). Benzodiazepine use and the risk of motor vehicle crash in the elderly. *Journal of the American Medical Association*, **278**, 27–31.

Hjorthol, R. (2001). *Mobility in an ageing society*. OECD, Paris.

Hunt, L., Morris, J. C., Edwards, D., *et al.* (1993). Driving performance in persons with mild senile dementia of the Alzheimer type. *Journal of the American Geriatrics Society*, **41**, 747–52.

Hunt, L. A., Murphy, C. F., Carr, D., *et al.* (1997). Reliability of the Washington University Road Test. A performance-based assessment for drivers with dementia of the Alzheimer type. *Archives of Neurology*, **54**, 707–12.

Isherwood, J., Adam, K. S., and Hornblow, A. R. (1982). Live event stress, psychosocial factors, suicide attempt and auto-accident proclivity. *Journal of Psychosomatic Research*, **26**, 371–83.

Janke, M. K. and Eberhard, J. W. (1998). Assessing medically impaired older drivers in a licensing agency setting. *Accident Analysis and Prevention*, **30**, 347–61.

Johansson, K., Bronge, L., Lundberg, C., *et al.* (1996). Can a physician recognize an older driver with increased crash risk potential? *Journal of the American Geriatrics Society*, **44**, 1198–204.

Johnson, J. E. (1998). Nursing assessment of older rural drivers. *Journal of Community Health Nursing*, **15**, 217–24.

Klavora, P., Gaskovski, P., Martin, K., *et al.* (1995). The effects of Dynavision rehabilitation on behind-the-wheel driving ability and selected psychomotor abilities of persons after stroke. *American Journal of Occupational Therapy*, **49**, 534–42.

Kostyniuk, L., Shope, J., and Trombley, D. (1998). *The process of reduction and cessation of driving among older drivers: a review of the literature. (HS-042 864, Interim Report)*. University of Michigan Transp Research Institute, Ann Arbor.

Laurence, D. R., Bennett, P. N., and Brown, M. J. (1997). *Clinical Pharmacology* (8th edition). Churchill Livingstone, London.

Levy, D. T. (1995). The relationship of age and state license renewal policies to driving licensure rates. *Accident Analysis and Prevention*, **27**, 461–7.

Levy, D. T., Vernick, J. S., and Howard, K. A. (1995). Relationship between driver's license renewal policies and fatal crashes involving drivers 70 years or older. *Journal of the American Medical Association*, **274**, 1026–30.

Lundberg, C., Johansson, K., Ball, K., *et al.* (1996). Dementia and driving—an attempt at consensus. *Alzheimer's Disease and Associated Disorders*, **11**, 28–37.

Maag, F. (1984). [The effects of mental diseases and behavior problems on the driving of motor vehicles]. *Revue Medicale de la Suisse Romande*, **104**, 879–91.

Marottoli, R. A., Richardson, E. D., Stowe, M. H., *et al.* (1998). Development of a test battery to identify older drivers at risk for self-reported adverse driving events. *Journal of the American Geriatrics Society*, **46**, 562–8.

Mazer, B. L., Korner-Bitensky, N. A., and Sofer, S. (1998). Predicting ability to drive after stroke. *Archives of Physical Medicine and Rehabilitation*, **79**, 743–50.

Metz, D. (2000). Mobility of older people and their quality of life. *Transport Policy*, **7**, 149–52.

Michon, J. A. (1985). A critical review of driver behaviour models: what do we know, what should we do? In *Human behaviour and traffic safety* (ed. L. Evans and R. C. Schwing), pp. 487–525. Plenum, New York.

O'Neill, D. (2000). Safe mobility for older people. *Reviews in Clinical Gerontology*, **10**, 181–92.

O'Neill, D., Neubauer, K., Boyle, M., *et al.* (1992). Dementia and driving. *Journal of the Royal Society of Medicine*, **85** 199–202.

Owsley, C., Ball, K., Sloane, M. E., *et al.* (1991). Visual/cognitive correlates of vehicle accidents in older drivers. *Psychology and Aging*, **6**, 403–15.

Owsley, C., Ball, K., McGwin Jr, G., *et al.* (1998). Visual processing impairment and risk of motor vehicle crash among older adults. *Journal of the American Medical Association*, **279**, 1083–8.

Rabbitt, P., Carmichael, A., Jones, S., *et al.* (1996). *When and why older drivers give up driving*. AA Foundation for Road Safety Research, Basingstoke.

Ranney, T. A. (1994). Models of driving behaviour: a review of their evolution. *Accident Analysis and Prevention*, **26**, 733–50.

Ray, W. A. (1992). Psychotropic drugs and injuries among the elderly: a review. *Journal of Clinical Psychopharmacology*, **12**, 386–96.

Ray, W. A., Fought, R. L., and Decker, M. D. (1992). Psychoactive drugs and the risk of injurious motor vehicle crashes in elderly drivers. *American Journal of Epidemiology*, **136**, 873–83.

Ray, W. A., Thapa, P. B., and Shorr, R. I. (1993). Medications and the older driver. *Clinics in Geriatric Medicine*, **9**, 413–38.

Rock, S. M. (1998). Impact from changes in Illinois drivers license renewal requirements for older drivers. *Accident Analysis and Prevention*, **30**, 69–74.

Rosenbloom, S. (1993). Transportation needs of the elderly population. *Clinics in Geriatric Medicine*, **9**, 297–310.

Sacher, P. (1978). [Schizophrenia and the ability to drive]. *Schweizerische Medizinische Wochenschrift.*, **108**, 373–9.

Schmidt, C. W., Shaffer, J. N., Zlotowitz, H. I., *et al.* (1977). Suicide by vehicular crash. *American Journal of Psychiatry*, **134**, 175–8.

Shua-Haim, J. R. and Gross, J. S. (1996). The 'co-pilot' driver syndrome. *Journal of the American Geriatrics Society*, **44**, 815–17. [See comments.]

Staplin, L. S., Lococo, K. H., Stewart, J., *et al.* (1999). *Safe mobility for older people notebook* (DTNH22-96-C-05140). National Highway Traffic Safety Administration, Washington, DC.

Stutts, J. C., Stewart, J. R., and Martell, C. (1998). Cognitive test performance and crash risk in an older driver population. *Accident Analysis and Prevention*, **30**, 337–46.

Tabachnik, N., Litman, R., Osman, N., *et al.* (1966). Comparative study of accidental and suicidal death. *Archives of General Psychiatry*, **14**, 60–8.

Thapa, P., Gideon, P., Cost, T., *et al.* (1998). Antidepressants and the risk of falls among nursing home residents. *New England Journal of Medicine*, **24**, 875–82.

Trobe, J. D. (1998). Test of divided visual attention predicts automobile crashes among older adults. *Archives of Ophthalmology*, **116**, 665. [Editorial]

Trobe, J. D., Waller, P. F., Cook-Flannagan, C. A., *et al.* (1996). Crashes and violations among drivers with Alzheimer disease. *Archives of Neurology*, **53**, 411–16.

Vernon, D. (1999). *Evaluating drivers licensed with medical conditions in Utah 1992–1996.* Paper presented at the Transportation Research Board, Washington DC.

White, S. and O'Neill, D. (2000). Health and relicencing policies for older drivers in the European Union. *Gerontology*, **46**, 146–52.

Wylie, K. R., Thompson, D. J., and Wildgust, H. J. (1993). Effects of depot neuroleptics on driving performance in chronic schizophrenic patients. *Journal of Neurology, Neurosurgery and Psychiatry*, **56**, 910–13.

Index